ENCYCLOPEDIA OF STEM CELL RESEARCH (2 VOLUME SET)

VOLUME 2

STEM CELLS – LABORATORY AND CLINICAL RESEARCH

Additional books in this series can be found on Nova's website
under the Series tab.

Additional E-books in this series can be found on Nova's website
under the E-books tab.

STEM CELLS AND REGENERATIVE MEDICINE

Additional books in this series can be found on Nova's website
under the Series tab.

Additional E-books in this series can be found on Nova's website
under the E-books tab.

ENCYCLOPEDIA OF STEM CELL RESEARCH (2 VOLUME SET)

VOLUME 2

ALEXANDER L. GREENE
EDITOR

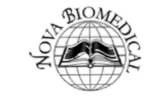

Nova Science Publishers, Inc.
New York

For permission to use material from this book please contact us:
Telephone 631-231-7269; Fax 631-231-8175
Web Site: http://www.novapublishers.com

NOTICE TO THE READER

The Publisher has taken reasonable care in the preparation of this book, but makes no expressed or implied warranty of any kind and assumes no responsibility for any errors or omissions. No liability is assumed for incidental or consequential damages in connection with or arising out of information contained in this book. The Publisher shall not be liable for any special, consequential, or exemplary damages resulting, in whole or in part, from the readers' use of, or reliance upon, this material.

Independent verification should be sought for any data, advice or recommendations contained in this book. In addition, no responsibility is assumed by the publisher for any injury and/or damage to persons or property arising from any methods, products, instructions, ideas or otherwise contained in this publication.

This publication is designed to provide accurate and authoritative information with regard to the subject matter covered herein. It is sold with the clear understanding that the Publisher is not engaged in rendering legal or any other professional services. If legal or any other expert assistance is required, the services of a competent person should be sought. FROM A DECLARATION OF PARTICIPANTS JOINTLY ADOPTED BY A COMMITTEE OF THE AMERICAN BAR ASSOCIATION AND A COMMITTEE OF PUBLISHERS.

Additional color graphics may be available in the e-book version of this book.

LIBRARY OF CONGRESS CATALOGING-IN-PUBLICATION DATA

Encyclopedia of stem cell research / editor, Alexander L. Greene.
     p. ; cm.
  Includes bibliographical references and index.
  ISBN 978-1-51761-835-2 (hardcover)
  1. Stem cells--Encyclopedias. I. Greene, Alexander L.
  [DNLM: 1. Stem Cells. 2. Stem Cell Transplantation. QU 325]
  QH588.S83E532 2010
  616'.02774--dc22
                         2010034298

Published by Nova Science Publishers, Inc. † New York

CONTENTS

In: Encyclopedia of Stem Cell Research (2 Volume Set)   ISBN: 978-1-61761-835-2
Editor: Alexander L. Greene   © 2012 Nova Science Publishers, Inc.

Chapter XXV

STEM CELL TRANSPLANTATION IN LEUKEMIA THE KIDNEY

Terje Forslund

INTRODUCTION

Haematopoietic stem cell transplantation (HSCT) and bone marrow transplantation (BMT) is often used to treat different types of leukaemia (L) like acute myelogenous (AML), chronic myelogenous (CML), acute lymphoblastic (ALL), chronic lymphocytic leukaemia (CLL), and juvenile myelomonocytic leukaemia (JML). In 2002 approximately 17.700 such stem cell transplantations (SCT) were performed in the USA [1]. The total number of HSCTs carried out in Europe in 2004 was 22 216 of which 33 % were allogenic and 67 % autologous [2]. Major differences in transplant rates between the European countries have been reported, however [2]. CLL represents 22-30% of all leukaemia cases worldwide, and the incidence was assumed to be between <1 to 5.5 cases per 100.000 habitants with the highest rates in USA, Ireland and Italy [3]. Further, CML was reported to occur at an incidence of 1-2 cases per 100.000 habitants per year.

During the years 1997 to 2002 Yamamoto and Goodman [4] identified a total of 144,559 leukaemia patients, including 66,067 (46%) acute and 71,860 (50%) chronic leukaemia cases. While the highest rates of AML were observed in Asian-Pacific Islanders (API) the incidence of ALL and promyelocytic leukaemia occurred more often in Hispanics than non-Hispanics, and African-Americans had the highest rates of HTLV-1 positive adult T-cell leukaemia/lymphoma. A sharp increase in the incidence of CML was observed in subjects over 85 years-of-age. Known risk factors could not explain the observed disparities in leukaemia incidence. Lately HSCT treatment has also become available for subjects with advanced age and for patients with co-morbidities.

A new concept for the treatment of CML has emerged with the development of the specific tyrosine kinase inhibitor imatinib mesylate (Gleevec®, USA; Glivec®, Europe), which blocks the BCR/ ABL expression [5,6]. As a result of these new treatment modalities the number of HSCT performed for CML has declined somewhat during the last years [2]. Still, HSCT remains an important treatment option for patients with CML and long-term results with imatinib mesylate are still lacking.

Kidney complications associated to conventional treatment of leukaemia may occur in different ways and was recognized as early as 1943 [7]. Later, after the introduction of BMT treatment, acute renal failure (ARF) and chronic renal failure (CRF), among many other complications, was acknowledged as one of the most frequent and a potentially life-threatening complication. Following BMT, renal failure developed in approximately 40 % of cases, of which 50% required dialysis [8]. With this in mind, pre-existent kidney diseases, previously known or undiscovered, could be present and should be searched for prior to HSCT. Leukaemia may also contribute by producing infiltrations or induce immunological responses within the kidney causing renal failure [9,10]. In some of these cases the leukemic infiltrates may give the impression of or mimic other diseases including Wegener's granulomatosis or sarcoidosis as demonstrated in the kidney biopsy material [11]. Intrarenal granulomas might be found, and together with leukaemia renal failure may develop [12]. Moreover, renal disease may be a direct complication associated to the conditional treatment of leukaemia (see later), occurring shortly after or later in the course after HSCT treatment.

GRADING OF RENAL FUNCTION

Kidney function is graded, scaling from 1 to 5 [13], by nephrologists using the Cockgroft-Gault [14] or the MDRD [15] formula for calculation of creatinine clearance (CrCl) (Table 1). The use of serum (or plasma) creatinine concentration (s-creat) alone is considered not good enough to report kidney function in renal failure (RF) patients. With MDRD calculation renal failure grade 5 is equal to established renal failure or end-stage renal disease (ESRD) with GFR <15 and need for dialysis or kidney transplantation. To evaluate renal complications, nephrotoxicity or renal injury, after HSCT different grading scales of the renal damage have been used as reported [16,17,18].

These three reports [16,17,18] have used a mixed system which combined both CrCl and s-creat with a grading scale from 0 to 3, in which grade 0 was defined as a < 25 % decline in CrCl irrespective of the basis level (table 2).

This grading system might be more easy to use and is very practical in a clinical setting and it is applicable for scientific investigations [15].

Table 1. Stages of CKD

Description and GFR
1.   Kidney damage with normal or increased GFR (> 90 mL/minute/1.73 m^2)
2.   Mild reduction in GFR (60-89 mL/minute/1.73 m^2)
3.   Moderate reduction in GFR (30-59 mL/minute/1.73 m^2)
4.   Severe reduction in GFR (15-29 mL/minute/1.73 m^2)
5.   Kidney failure (GFR < 15 mL/minute/1.73 m^2 or dialysis)

GFR = glomerular filtration rate.

Table 2. Clinical grading of reduction in renal function

Grading of decline in GFR using creatinine clearance (CrCl) and s-creatinine concentration	
Grade 0	Reduction of CrCl < 25 % independent of basis level
Grade 1	Reduction of CrCl > 25 % and less than 2-times increase of s- creat
Grade 2	Reduction of CrCl > 50 % but dialysis treatment not needed
Grade 2 plus	Reduction in CrCl > 50% triple increase in s-creat, no dialysis (ref. 243)
Grade 3	Reduction of CrCl > 50% and need for dialysis treatment

RISK ASSESSMENT AND CO-MORBIDITY

In patients planned for allogenic (allo)-HSCT, several authors have reported methods to assess the risk of complications before performing HSCT, including renal failure and dialysis [19-25]. The most commonly used measure of co-morbidity is the Charlson Index [20,21,22] which initially was developed to predict the one year mortality in patients treated for cancer. The Charlson Index (CI) was later modified to be used to predict co-morbidities and survival in other patients, also for those planned for HSCT [26,27,28]. Even though the CI is very useful, efforts to analyze the impact of co-morbidities on index for many diseases are still not fully developed. In clinical treatment trials, patients with renal failure are most often excluded from such trials, the reason why little is known about the impact of renal disease prior to HSCT. Sorror et al. [28] found that the risk score for moderate to severe renal failure was intermediate, but these findings could not be confirmed in other studies [29].

Algorithms for assessment of cardiac disease [30] and mortality [31] before HSCT in order to identify patients at highest risk, prior to administering any drug, to avoid further worsening of heart involvement and possible organ failure have been proposed [30]. Although these algorithms were suggested for patients treated with HSCT for autoimmune diseases, they may also successfully be applied for patients treated with HSCT for leukemia. Beside a thoroughly questionnaire on the history of previous diseases, a careful physical examination, electrocardiogram (ECG) in order to detect arrhythmias, chest X-ray and echocardiography to assess ventricular function and pressure gradients and leaflets status, and pulmonary circulation should be performed at least in patients with diabetes mellitus, metabolic dysfunction, and hypertension. If necessary, coronary catheterization may be performed prior to HSCT [30]. For later clinical follow-up and cardiac monitoring the measurement of pro-brain natriuretic peptide (pro-BNP) concentration could be of help to evaluate the status of heart failure [30].

DISEASES WITH RENAL INVOLVEMENT

Any disorder, which in general is thought to be a risk for developing kidney dysfunction, should also be considered a risk for developing renal failure after HSCT. Consequently, whatever type of leukaemia suggested for HSCT treatment, it is necessary to identify any pre-existent or co-morbid kidney disease which after HSCT could compromise the renal function further. Disorders, known to constitute a significant risk of morbidity and mortality in the general population, are diabetes mellitus (DM), hypertension (HT), cardiovascular disease (CVD), metabolic syndrome (MBS) and some types of chronic infections [26,32,33,34].

In spite of a report on successful HSCT treatment, performed in a patient with aplastic anemia undergoing hemodialysis (HD) treatment [35], and an observation on remission of IgA nephropathy after HSCT [36], the presence of such diseases (glomerulonephritis (GN) and/or interstitial nephritis (IN)) might have undesirable effects on renal function, morbidity, and mortality in patients selected for HSCT treatment.

HEREDITARY AND INBORN ERRORS

These types of kidney diseases are often known to the family and should easily be recognized using a normal anamnesis questionnaire for renal diseases. Inherited autosomal dominant polycystic kidney disease (ADPKD) and the autosomal recessive polycystic kidney disease (ARPKD) of the young age might be present, as these disorders are being found at increasing frequencies nowadays. At least 4 cases with acute leukemia, developing after renal transplantation due to ADPKD have been reported [37,38,39]. These subjects were given conventional treatment for leukemia and none of them was treated with HSCT. So far, no reports on HSCT in patients with hereditary kidney diseases have come to my knowledge.

Cases mimicking ARPKD, being leukemic were also reported [40,41]. One case had congenital AML presenting as renal masses mimicking ARPKD [40]. A second case, a 5 week-old infant with acute megakaryoblastic leukemia had polycystic aspects of the kidneys at abdominal MRI examination mimicking ARPKD [41].

Alport's syndrome, another inherited disease with glomerular pathology, might be considered a risk for developing renal failure if HSCT should be needed. Patients with Alport's syndrome (not female carriers) will develop progressive renal failure and might be candidates for renal transplantation. However, in any such case if the glomerular filtration rate (GFR) remain within the normal range (GFR > 70 ml/min/1.73m^2) prior to HSCT, these disorders are not expected to have any influence on the course after HSCT.

POSTRENAL AND OBSTRUCTIVE DISEASES

At time being, an increasing amount of leukaemia patients are observed and treated at older age. In men, prostatic disease (hypertrophy and cancer) is more frequently found in this age group. Identification of prostatic disease is made with blood tests i.e. measurement of serum prostatic specific antigen (PSA) concentration and clinical examination (i.e. prostatic palpation). Similarly, women at high age may have urine bladder retraction due to prolapse of the womb and in younger women who have given birth to several children with urine retention might have an increased risk of bladder infection.

Kidney, abdominal, and gynaecological ultrasound examination will identify possible risk factors from urogenital organs. Post-renal obstruction and primary or secondary urinary infection has to be treated properly ahead of HSCT. Presence of any other pathological findings should be properly treated by an urologist or gynaecologist prior to HSCT. Repeat occurrence of urinary infections and retention could point to bladder pathology, or failing of bladder contraction caused by neuropathy or stricture of the urethra, would require cystoscopic examination and urologic intervention.

Identification of pre-transplant cystitis could be important as hemorrhagic cystitis (HC) may develop especially after allo-HSCT [42], for which treatment with hyperbaric oxygen may be indicated. Early HC is a common complication of high-dose of cyclophosphamide caused by its metabolite acrolein. As a routine, mesna that binds to acrolein, enhanced hydration, and forced diuresis with or without urine bladder irrigation may be used to prevent early HC [43]. Late HC after HSCT was associated with recipient anti-adenovirus antibody positivity, total dose of administered busulfan, and chronic GVHD [44].

DIABETES AND HYPERTENSION

The increasing frequency of diabetes mellitus (DM) nephropathy is a general problem in all countries, and some of the patients with DM will develop end-stage renal failure (ESRF). Since a possible genetic relationship between B-cell leukemia and diabetes has been suggested [45], it might be relevant to acknowledge pre-existing DM prior to HSCT. A previous report on positive correlation between ALL and DM type 1 was reported [46], but later reports by these same authors [47] and others [48] were unable to confirm this correlation in well-defined populations. Both pre- and post-transplant treatments may influence DM control, thus survival and prognosis with regard to development of ESRF and later need for dialysis treatment is dependent on close diabetes control after HSCT [49]. The prevalence of new DM type 1 was three times higher in patients treated with HSCT than that of the general population, and the prevalence of DM type 2 was also higher than expected [50].

It is intriguing that treatment of leukaemia with imatinib mesylate (Gleevec®, USA, Glivec®, Europe) also caused a better diabetic control [51].

Although tacrolimus (Prograf®) is evaluated as a possible compound to treat graft-versus host disease (GVHD) in HSCT patients, new DM could develop and pre-existing DM control in diabetic patients may worsen during tacrolimus treatment [52]. Autoimmune polyendocrine failure with DM type 1 and hypothyroidism is a very rare complication after allo-BMT [53] but has not been found after HSCT.

In HSCT subjects, no significant differences between those with or without ARF with regard to pre-existing DM, pre-existing hypertension, or pre-existing cardiomyopathy could be found [16]. According to Parikh et al [16], the only co-morbidity of significance was the pre-existent decrease in GFR prior to HSCT [16]. Hypertension present before and at HSCT has been identified as a risk factor for ARF ($p<0.003$) in HSCT patients [32]. However, survival in patients with hypertension after HSCT did not differ when compared to patients without [32].

Diabetes insipidus (DI) observed in leukemic subjects is of non-renal nature. DI appearing with polyuria and polydipsia may develop as a rare complication of leukemia and is caused by leukemic infiltrations of the pituitary gland [54,55]. Some few cases of DI and leukaemia due to monosomy 7 have been recognised [56,57]. Such cases were not observed after HSCT.

KIDNEY DISEASES ASSOCIATED WITH LEUKAEMIA

Renal diseases observed in patients with leukaemia have been known for more than a half century [7] and may present as acute or chronic renal failure in both acute AML and ALL [58]. Nephrotic syndrome (NS) has been observed associated with CLL and the nephropathy is often discovered simultaneously with the leukaemia [59]. Impaired renal function, present at the time of diagnosis, may in some cases have reached MDRD-grade IV [60]. Renal involvement with leukemic infiltrations in the kidneys, glomerulopathies, with and without NS, was most often reported to occur in CLL [7,9,11,58-70]. Very rarely lymphocytic vasculitis may be present [69]. Leukemic infiltrates was also observed in MML [71]. In most of these cases the infiltrates were unevenly distributed, poorly defined, situated in the renal cortex and medulla, and the histology resembled that of pyelonephritis [71]. CLL may even be found in patients undergoing hemodialysis [71]. While mostly acute and/or chronic renal failure is associated with hyperkalemia, the development of severe hypokalemia by lysozyme-induced renal tubular injury and inappropriate kaliuresis has been reported in a case of AML [72]. NS and ARF was found in some patients with chronic myelomonocytic leukaemia [73,74,75]. Although some authors have suggested a possible relationship between CML and glomerulopathy [74] this remains a matter of debate. Whether immunoglobulin A (IgA) nephropathy may develop in the course of CML is unclear. Biopsy material stained for IgG, IgA, IgM and complement 3 (C_3) and fibrin did reveal strong IgA staining at immunofluorescence in one report suggesting that IgA nephropathy might be observed in patients with CML [74].

The glomerular lesions found simultaneously with or prior to leukaemia treatment, or in association with CLL, have been minimal change GN (MCGN), focal segmental glomerulo-sclerosis (FSGS), membranous GN (MGN), membranoproliferative (also named mesangio-capillary) GN (MPGN), and amyloidosis, all of them often accompanied with NS [76,77,78]. Most often MPGN was described together with CLL [62,63,79,80,81]. Some of these patients, although few at number, presented with manifest NS before the recognition of leukaemia, and some more cases developed NS after debut of leukaemia [76]. As patients with pre-existing GN undergoing hemodialysis treatment with subsequent development of leukaemia was successfully treated with HSCT, they should not be excluded HSCT [82]. Acute renal failure due to MPGN occurring simultaneously with CLL was recently reported [83].

Acute leukemia may develop following kidney transplantation [37,38,39], and in that situation it was assumed that azathioprine and/or cyclophosphamide might have acted as co-factors in the genesis of leukemia [78]. These patients were not given HSCT but in the future such treatment strategies could be possible also after kidney transplantation.

INFECTIONS

Several viruses, among them also cytomegalovirus (CMV) and Epstein Barr virus (EBV) have been identified to constitute a considerable risk for ARF in previous healthy subjects [84] and in immuno-compromised (e.g. patients with HIV and organ transplanted) subjects [85]. About 60 – 80 % of the general population will be serologically positive to CMV and many positive to EBV prior to HSCT. All herpesviruses, including CMV and EBV, share a characteristic ability to remain latent within the body over long periods and a more common problem is the reactivation of the latent virus [86]. Since CMV could have immunosuppressive properties it may contribute to the development of other infections in leukemic HSCT treated patients [87,88], which may contribute to GN and lead to ESRD [89,90,91]. According to Gratwohl et al. [92] infections was the primary cause of death in 10 % of patients (597 deaths) treated with allo-HSCT and out of these 166 patients (28%) a virus-infection was the primary cause. Donor CMV serologic status did not affect outcome after HSCT from a HLA-identical sibling and no effect of donor CMV status on the risk of acute GVHD could be found [88], however. CMV positive donors produced a higher risk for chronic GVHD compared to seronegative donors, 38.5% versus 33.3% (p=0.01), respectively [88]. The situation seemed to change in patients receiving grafts from CMV-seropositive donors as improved survival, event-free survival, and reduced transplantation related mortality was lower in these patients [88].

In non-HSCT, the number of patients with CMV reactivation in lymphoid hematological malignancies was significantly higher (13.6%) than the number of patients (3.9%) with myeloid hematological malignancies [93]. According to this report [93] auto-HSCT did not increase the risk of CMV antigenemia. In contrast to these low values, patients treated with allo-HSCT had a four times higher rate of CMV antigenity (39.1%) in spite of routine prophylaxis [93]. Women with allo-HSCT had significantly higher rate of CMV antigenemia (p<0.006) compared with men with allo-HSCT, and antigenemia increased in a linear fashion with increasing age. Positive antigenemia should be considered a risk for development of disease.

Other viruses, BK polyoma virus infections have been observed in patients with CLL and RF [94,95], and after HSCT adenovirus infection causing hemorrhagic cystitis (HC) and pneumonia could be lethal [96]. Polyoma virus may cause tubulointerstitial nephritis and contribute to RF after HSCT [97]. HC was also reported in a patient with JC virus (John Cunningham virus), a very common virus in the general population [98]. The JC virus, commonly latent in the gastrointestinal tract, may infect epithelial cells of the kidneys [98] where it continues to reproduce with shedding of virus-particles into the urine. During immunosuppression the JC virus may reactivate and give cause to HC and ureteral stenosis [95,99].

The diagnosis of CMV is done by testing for the CMV early antigen, pp65 antigen, in blood and urine. Virus identification and quantitation by means of polymerase chain reaction (PCR) techniques in blood, urine or other samples. Serological tests are considered to be impractical and its usefulness as a diagnostic tool for acute CMV infection is diminishing. The diagnosis may also be made by means of histological examination of kidney biopsy specimen, if a such has been performed.

BK polyoma virus infection may be identified by examination of the urine using a centrifuged sample under a phase-contrast microscope at high-power field (400x). Cells of tubular origin may appear with increased size of the nucleus and contain coarse chromatin inclusion bodies [95]. BK polyoma virus may also be found at electron microscope examination of a kidney biopsy specimen and immunohistochemical analysis.

The recognition of such viruses, which should be searched for, should lead to treatment with anti-viral agents initiated after HSCT and treatments should be continued over long periods of time probably 6 months or more. Side effects of antiviral agents, like neurotoxicity [100] may occur when used in patients with reduced renal function and some of the compounds should eventually be given at smaller doses. The dosage of valganciclovir should be adjusted to the degree of renal impairment [101]. CMV infection reactivation may be observed also when the stem cell donor is CMV negative, and therapy of CMV-reactivation is sometimes difficult to control with single drug treatment [102]. In spite of new diagnostic methods it might be difficult to separate virus-induced from drug-induced RF.

Latent bacterial infections must be excluded and treated prior to HSCT, and routine examination with chest X-ray, orthopantomography of the teeth, urinary and nasal bacterial cultures should be performed to minimize the risk for complications (also renal) after stem cell transplantation. Skin and enteric bacteria infections should be eradicated. Cephalosporins or ciprofloxacin may be given for skin infections and orally metronidazole or vancocin may be used for enteric bacteria.

Patients undergoing HSCT are at high risk of acquiring tuberculosis (Tbc), although the risk of getting Tbc is lower after allo-HSCT than that of solid organ transplantation, and patients with auto-HSCT have the same risk as in the general population [103]. Prophylactic medication, which could compromise renal function, is not needed in patients planned for HSCT. Opportunistic non-tuberculosis mycobacterium infections are more commonly found in Oriental regions [104].

Test for tuberculosis (Mantoux-test) should eventually be performed in all patients prior any pre-treatment and prior to HSCT. Sterile pyuria after HSCT treatment could point to renal tuberculosis and in absence of bacterial urinary infection, staining and cultures for tuberculosis should be performed. Any subject being Mantoux-negative before HSCT who later after HSCT converts to positive, must be considered a candidate for tuberculosis disease. Compounds used to treat tuberculosis are mostly not affecting kidney function much.

RADIATION NEPHROPATHY (RNP)

External beam total body irradiation (TBI) has commonly been used in many preparative regimens for conventional stem cell transplant procedures because of its ability to irreversibly damage DNA, and thus inhibit replication of malignant cells. Potential adverse renal effects of radiation was early recognized and reported in 1906 [105]. Later, in 1926, the first description of experimental nephritis produced by irradiation to dogs was published [106]. The renal pathology in their experiments [106] consisted of interstitial fibrosis, tubular atrophy and glomerular hyalinization. Contrary to the widespread opinion at that time, they found that the kidney was quite susceptible to the exposure of x-rays. A year later, Domagk

[107] observed renal lesions in humans after exposure to irradiation (roentgen rays), the first report with lethal outcome. The importance of the need for a latent period to pass after radiation treatment before the occurrence of renal lesions was recognized [107,108]. The earliest investigators failed to demonstrate renal damage after radiation, probably because the animals died or were killed long before sufficient time had elapsed for the appearance of lesions. Subsequently several investigators have been able to demonstrate significant pathological changes in the kidneys in a variety of animals and in man after radiation treatment [109-112]. The kidney is considered a late-responding tissue when compared to the bone marrow, thus changes within the kidney may be discovered much later after exposition to radiation [113]. This is due to the low mitotic rate in normal kidney tissue, the reason why radiation damage to the kidneys is delayed.

Luxton [109] differentiated four variants of radiation nephropathy (RN). Firstly, the acute radiation nephritis with clinical onset about 6 – 12 months after exposure, secondly, the early chronic radiation nephritis with malignant hypertension developing about 1 to 2 years after radiation. Some patients will develop chronic RN without hypertension, and then again some patients may have chronic RN with benign hypertension [109]. A latent period up to eight years may pass before chronic RF become present after BMT, which is also about the similar time period for developing chronic RN [114]. It is interesting that total body irradiation (TBI) caused an increase in renal blood flow (RBF) and increased glomerular filtration rate (GFR) within a few days after TBI [115]. Similarly, increased GFR is considered the first step in the development of DM-induced nephropathy. Increased GFR was observed in patients with DM and obesity is associated with increased GFR and RBF, glomerulomegaly and in extreme cases also FSGS-disease [116]. Likewise, patients suffering from ADPKD also have hyperfiltration early in the course of the disease [117], before ending up with RF. Some of the vascular mediators of hyperfiltration in DM have been identified [112]. In line with these previous reports [115-117], but in spite of the difficulty to establish a relationship between the increased GFR and RBF after TBI, it is tempting to think that these early hemodynamic changes induced by TBI could be important for the later development of RN and renal failure.

The pathological findings in radiation nephropathy consist of a variable picture including mesangiolysis [113,118], widening of the space between the endothelium and the glomerular basement membrane (GBM). Capillary loop occlusions may be found. Interstitium may be expanded and fibrosis is often observed [113]. The endothelial changes appear to resolve, but the mesangial lesions progress, with hypercellularity and/or hypertrophy, increased mesangial matrix, mesangial sclerosis, and ultimately, glomerulosclerosis. These mesangial changes are similar to those observed in other chronic glomerulopathies [119].

Nephritis caused by TBI is related to the given dose and to the affected volume [120], and according to these authors [120], a minimum of one third of the renal volume needs to be spared from toxic doses. A defined threshold for toxicity based on clinical observations has been suggested [120]. This threshold value needs to be confirmed, however. Renal carcinoma may develop as a very rare complication of radiation-induced damage.

Renal dysfunction after allo-BMT was reported to be strongly related to the delivered TBI dose (and dose per fraction) and to the presence of graft-versus-host disease (GVHD). It was also recommended that renal shielding should be prescribed if a TBI dose greater than 12 Gy (fractionated twice daily over 3 days) was used, and their data suggested that kidney doses higher than 10 Gy should be avoided [121].

In order to reduce the dose of external-beam radiotherapy several attempts using additional radioimmunotherapy (RIT) have been tried. Isotopes In these settings have been a variety of antibodies (anti-CD33, anti-CD45, and anti-CD66) and different isotopes with radio-nucleotide labelling (^{131}I, ^{90}Y, ^{188}Re) have been used. Most reports consisted of Rhenium-188-labelled anti-CD66 monoclonal antibodies (188Re-mAb) or 90-Yttrium antibodies (90Y-mAb) in combination with a lower TBI dose [122]. With the targeted marrow irradiation with radioactively labelled 188Re anti-CD66 antibody the TBI dose was reduced to 6 – 7 Gy [123-125] and in addition renal shielding was used in most cases. Renal toxicity grade 1 was encountered in 9 out of 36 patients, grade 2 in 2 patients, and grade 3 in one patient [124]. Radiation nephropathy was found in one patient requiring dialysis treatment [124]. Along with these results and reports of others [125], the dose limiting organ seemed to be the kidney. Whether (or not) the use of Retin1,1-hydroethylidene-186-diphosphanate (Re-186 HEDP) will be more promising remains to be demonstrated [126]. In the two cases reported so far [126] no nephrotoxicity was found. Similarly, nephrotoxicity and cystitis were absent in four patients treated with high-dose of samarium 153-labeled ethylene-diamine-tetraethylene-phosphonate (^{153}Sm-EDTMP) in high-risk AML [127]. Moreover, although promising reports with the anti-CD33-calicheamin construct, gemtuzumab ozogamicin, in relapsing AML and newly diagnosed AML together with standard chemotherapy, further studies are needed to confirm its efficacy and its renal non-toxicity [128]. A similar approach using RIT and TBI at lower doses in combination has also been reported for patients prior to autologous transplantation [129].

EFFECTS OF CELL PRESERVATION

Cryopreservation is necessary for storage and maintenance of stem cells to be used for autologous and often in allogeneic transplantation [130]. The standard cryoprotectant is dimethyl sulphoxide (DMSO), which prevents freezing damage to living cells [131]. DMSO is a colourless, slightly oily liquid compound that occurs naturally in vegetables, fruits, grains, and animal products. DMSO was first synthesized in 1866 as a by-product of paper manufacturing and was primarily used as an industrial solvent. It was initially introduced for medical use as an anti-inflammatory reagent and is still occasionally used in some autoimmune disorders [132,133] and amyloidosis [134]. DMSO used at concentrations of 10% combined with 0.9% saline and serum albumin, was considered to be safe and non-toxic to stem cells [130]. Other concentrations of DMSO have been tested in vitro [135] and analysed with regard to CD34+ cell viability [136,137], and a 5% DMSO seemed to be just as good as 10% [136,137]. These authors concluded that 5% DMSO may be the optimal dose for cryopreserving PBPC as long as the cells have not been concentrated at much more than 200 x 10 [6] nucleated cells/ml [137].

The most common side effects caused by DMSO consist of nausea, vomiting, and abdominal cramps. In addition, cardiovascular [138], respiratory [139,140], central nervous system [141,142], haemolytic [143] and hepatic toxicity [144] have been reported. Renal side effects attributed to DMSO was reported to occur in 5% of the patients [145]. During cell infusion the patient is exposed to DMSO and also to toxic products of cell lysis. DMSO may cause disruption of red blood cells resulting in the presence of free haemoglobin in the urine in 75 – 100 % of the patients. Due to routinely prophylactic fluid and bicarbonate infusions, ARF is not commonly observed in this setting.

A clear difference was reported with regard to the occurrence of hemoglobinuria after stem cell transplantation between the use of bone marrow (BM) and peripheral blood progenitor cells [146]. As all patients receiving cryopreserved BM had hemoglobinuria, and this symptom was never reported in the auto-PBPC group, they concluded that the high concentration of red cells in BM-HSCT [147] was the leading cause of hemoglobinuria.

Hydroxyethyl starch (HES) has been used as an additive cryopreservating agent and HES have been proven non-toxic to the kidney [147]. HES will not penetrate the cell membrane, and it will form a protective shell around the cell and prevent the cell from dehydration. Trehalose (TRE), a disaccharide that rapidly is hydrolysed to glucose by the enzyme trehalase, has also been used as preservation medium for stem cells [148]. Trehalase is present in humans and most animals at the brush border of the intestinal mucosa, as also in the kidney, liver, and blood plasma [149]. After TRE has entered the kidney it will be cleaved to glucose by trehalase present in the brush border of the kidney proximal tubular cells and almost no amount of intact TRE is excreted in the urine.

Glycerol penetrates the cell slower than DMSO, but it is cryoprotective. Glycerol needs to be removed from the stem cell preparations by washed-out processes prior to re-infusion, making it less suitable for HSCT.

Freezing and thawing of stem cells will contribute to apoptosis and cell debris that may add to the development of RF after HSCT. Among the many mechanisms involved in this setting, activation of caspases during thawing may induce apoptosis [150]. Whether increased caspase-activation also take part in the development of nephrotoxicity is not known, and if so, the addition of caspase inhibitors like the broad-spectrum inhibitor N-benzyloxycarbonyl-Val-Ala-Asp(Ome)-fluoromethylketone (zVAD-fmk) as a cryopreservative could open for future treatment combinations [150]. So far such effects have been tested in animals only and are not available for HSCT patients.

PRE- AND POST- HSCT DRUGS

Drug-related toxicity has a substantial impact on early morbidity and mortality and also contributes to early and late renal dysfunction and failure after both allo-HSCT and auto-HSCT. Compounds that are used prior to HSCT, those used after to effectively prevent acute and late GVHD, and those given to prevent infections or fungi, and are all potentially nephrotoxic.

ANTIBIOTICS

Prevention of bacterial infections is important in patients receiving HSCT, and therefore antibiotics are used to knock out oral and bowel bacterial flora. It is however questionable whether antibiotic pre-treatment will have a positive impact on survival in HSCT patients [151]. Bacterial resistance is another matter of concern. Almost all antibiotics used today, and combination of different antibiotics together with antifungal drugs, used in treatment of patients prior to and after HSCT may have significant impact on kidney function. In addition antivirus compounds that are used in combination (see above) will influence kidney function. Actually, none of the used medicaments will increase kidney function.

Among the various spectrums of side-effects observed with aminoglycosides (Gentamicin, Tobramycin, Amikacin, Netilmicin) nephrotoxicity is recognised especially in patients with DM, dehydration, and high age. Recommended doses and dose adjustments in patients with renal failure are given in table 3. Once daily intravenous dosage is often used today in many hospitals and this way of administration is generally not more toxic to the kidney than dosing three times daily [152]. In elderly patients renal toxicity was observed in about 12 % of the patients [152]. Renal toxicity defined as an increase in s-creat concentration of > 50 % was more often observed in patients given gentamicin (15 %; $p<0.006$) than in those given amikacin [153]. Both compounds produced similar ototoxicity, however. The combination of aminoglycosides with cephalosporins has been considered to produce more renal toxicity than either compound given alone, a matter of dispute, however. In one study, cefotaxime and tobramycin, given either alone or in combination did not confirm increased nephrotoxicity [154]. They concluded that treatment with high doses of cefotaxime did not increase tobramycin nephrotoxicity in patients with normal renal function. The nephrotoxicity of this drug combination is obviously due to the aminoglycoside [154]. Another study comparing ciprofloxacin–piperacillin versus tobramycin–piperacillin in patients with acute leukemia or a bone marrow transplant [155], showed similar responses (17.5% vs. 17.1%, respectively). Abnormal kidney function was observed similarly in both treatment groups and was reported in 21 to 23 % of the patients [155] for which reason treatment had to be discontinued.

Table 3. Recommended dose adjustments for aminoglycosides given by the manufacturer according to kidney function

CrCl. (MDRD) (ml/min/1.73m^2)	S-Creat. (µmol/l)	Dosing interval (hours)			
		Gentamicin 1.5 mg/kg 3.o.d.	Tobramycin 1.5 mg/mg 3.o.d.	Netilmicin 4-6 mg/kg 2.o.d.	Amikacin 7.5 mg/kg/day 2.o.d.
> 70	< 110	8	8	12	12
70 - 35	110 - 176	12	12	15-18	15-18
34 - 25	177 – 255	18	18	24	24
24 – 15	256 – 335	24	24	36	30
14 – 10	336 – 476	36	36	48	36
9 – 5	477 – 636	48 *	48*	72*	>36*

Dosing after each hemodialysis session or according to measured serum through concentration.

These patients had additionally treatment with amphotericin-B and vancomycin, both compounds that may affect kidney function. Interestingly, when they eliminated patients receiving other potential nephrotoxins from their analysis, probable tobramycin-related toxicities were more common than probable ciprofloxacin-related nephrotoxicity [155]. The question whether three times daily should be used or once daily dosing should be used [156,157] remains unanswered, slightly in favour of once daily

Gentamicin

The dose of gentamicin for those with normal kidney function is 3.5 – 5 mg/kg body weight (BW) given i.v., either divided in 3 doses for every 8 hours, or given once daily. The serum level of gentamicin together with serum creatinine concentration should be measured at least 3 times a week in order to achieve the therapeutical concentration without renal toxicity. The dose must be adjusted to the actual renal function Table 2. In hemodialysis patients one dose (4.5 – 5 mg/kg BW) is given after every dialysis session. Prior to start of the next hemodialysis the serum through level should be measured. Depending on the type of hemodialysis and type and size of filter used for HD dose adjustments must be performed [158]. In a small retrospective study, gentamicin, 5 mg/kg BW given once daily, did not produce nephrotoxicity in anyone but one patient [159].

Tobramycin

The recommended daily dose of tobramycin is 3-7 mg/kg BW, and if given divided into three daily doses it should be 3-5 mg/kg BW. Tobramycin may as well be given once daily, and in a prospective study 6 mg/kg BW was found to be as effective as given in 3 daily doses. In that study renal failure with s-creat >110 µmol/l (women) or 120 µmol/l (men) were excluded, and no comments were given with regard to kidney function [160]. In another study [161] although no significant differences in renal function were observed between subjects given tobramycin once daily (increase in max s-creat 32 %) versus every 8 hours (51%; p< 0.054), a clear trend toward better kidney function was observed in those having tobramycin once daily [161]. The doses in this study ranged from 7-9 mg/kg BW in those subjects getting tobramycin once daily and were 2.5 mg when given trice daily.

Amikacin

Amikacin is cleared by glomerular filtration as a non-metabolized molecule. For amikacin the serum through-level should not exceed 10 µg/ml before giving the next dose and peak concentration (measured after 0.5 - 1 hour after last dose) should not be higher than 35 µg/ml. In hematological malignances the dose requirement might be increased without having risk of renal toxicity. Zeitany et al. [162] recommended that in febrile neutropenic patients with an underlying hematologic malignancy, amikacin be initiated at 7.5 to 10 mg/kg per dose every 8 h (2 to 2.5 mg/kg per dose every 8 h for gentamicin) and adjusted within 24 h based on individual pharmacokinetic analysis. Moreover, vancocin did not enhance amikacin-induced tubular nephrotoxicity in leukemic children [163].

Netilmicin

Netilmicin (Netilmicin-sulfate) is a half-synthetic antibiotic soluble in water. Netilmicin peak concentration should be 4-12 µg/ml and not exceed 16 µg/ml when it is given in three times daily dose intervals. Given once daily, the peak concentration may increase to 20-30 µg/ml. Netilmicin could be given as single dose once daily without evidence of nephrotoxicity [164] and monitoring of peak concentrations seamed not necessary unless an increase in serum creatinine concentration was observed. Hemodialysis will remove netilmicin effectively and about 63 % will be removed after an eight-hour dialysis session, less removed at shorter dialysis time. A new dose should be given after every hemodialysis treatment session.

OTHER ANTIBIOTICS

Ciprofloxacin

Ciprofloxacin has been used as part of combination therapy, as modified monotherapy, and as true monotherapy in febrile neutropenic patients [165]. To all regimens with aminoglycosides, the addition of ceftazidime, ciprofloxacin, vancocin, and metronidazole have been given as empiric treatment. In general, the nephrotoxic renal reactions were almost always reversible, some patients will need temporary dialysis, and only some few cases will need dialysis due to chronic renal failure.

Trimethoprim-Sulfamethoxazole

Following HSCT treatment with trimethoprim-sulfamethoxazole (Sulfa-Trimethoprim; ST) is commonly used as prophylaxis against Pneumocystis jiroveci (formerly Pneumocystis carinii) infection and in absence of such prophylaxis about 15-20% of leukemic patients may develop PCI [166]. Infection with Pneumocystis jiroveci pneumonia was also reported to occur after BMT and HSCT [167,168], and may be complicated by other simultaneous virus infections [169]. Treatment with ST may also be protective for toxoplasmosis reactivation after allo-HSCT [170].

Many untoward effects and toxicities due to ST treatment [171,172], among them interstitial nephritis, have been recognised [173,174]. Interstitial nephritis due to ST treatment may also appear without concurrent RF [173]. Interaction between ST and methotrexate, cyclosporine, and many other compounds has also been found. It is recommended to closely follow-up and to make necessary dose adjustments in patients with RF after HSCT. Renal dysfunction changes the pharmacokinetics of both components but disposition are not significantly altered until CrCl is less than 30 ml/min, when its metabolites accumulate and may lead to toxicity. Renal dysfunction, however, does not preclude the use of ST to treat susceptible infections, even when CrCl is less than 15 ml/min [175]. Patients who are intolerant of ST or who have not responded to treatment after 5-7 days of therapy with TMP-

SMZ should be treated with aerosolized pentamidine. In the presence of mild renal failure (stage 2; table 1) kidney function, measured with MDRD calculation for CrCl, may decrease slightly during ST treatment especially in situations where cyclosporine (Cs) is given simultaneously.

ANTIMYCOTICS

Amphotericin-B

The dose of amphotericin-B should be 5 mg/kg BW, and that for liposomal amphotericin-B should be 1.5 or 3.0 mg/kg BW when given of a period of 21 days pr 10 days, respectively. The first dose should be given after a test-dose of 1 mg followed by an observation of 30 minutes for exclusion of anaphylactic reactions. First-aid equipment must be at hand. Impairment of renal function often develops during antifungal treatment with Amphotericin-B (A-B) after HSCT. Acute vasoconstriction of intrarenal arterioles resulting in decreased renal blood flow and reduced glomerular filtration rate, which could be boostered by hyponatremia, is one of the supposed mechanisms of A-B induced nephrotoxicity [176]. Factors contributing to the risk of developing renal failure include the total cumulative dose given, duration of A-B treatment, concomitant use of diuretics, pre-existing renal failure, hypovolemia after HSCT, and the use of other nephrotoxic compounds after HSCT. In a recent report [177], the addition of A-B caused a rapid development of nephrotoxicity in 43 % of patients undergoing BMT or HSCT who concomitantly was treated with other nephrotoxic compounds (e.g. cyclosporine A, antibiotics, and antivirus drugs). However, this report [177] may be different from others as the HSCT treatment was given to patients with multiple myeloma, which distinctly may contribute to development of renal failure.

A significant deterioration in kidney function was observed when A-B-deoxycholate (ABD) was given as a continuous infusion after HSCT [178]. It was assumed that a 24 hours infusion of ABD would improve creatinine clearance and GFR due to less vasoconstriction in the glomerular vascular bed. In the report of Furrer et al. [178] patients treated with ABD had lower concentration of CyA which would actually add to less nephrotoxicity. In spite of the lower CyA levels in ABD treated subjects, s-creat concentration increased and CrCl decreased significantly (p<0.0002) and the grade of renal impairment was still present one year later in ABD treated vs. not ABD treated subjects [178]. The interpretation of their report point to a permanent renal impairment due to ABD treatment, also when given as a 24-hour infusion. Liposomal A-B treatment appeared to be better tolerated in one report [179] which needs to be proven in larger studies.

Fluconazole

Fluconazole (FL) is an antifungal compound often used as prophylaxis in patients given HSCT. FL inhibits cytochrome P450 2C9 in the liver and could provide protection from cyclophosphamide (CY)-related toxicities. Co-administration of FL with CY decreased CY related nephrotoxicity, hepatic toxicity and decreased mortality [180]. The dose should be reduced to half-dose when CrCl decreases by 50 % and a fully dose should be given after every hemodialysis session. No difference in antifungal protection or mortality was found between FL and itraconazole (IC) in allo-HSCT patients [181].

While different doses of systemic antimycotic compounds, amphotericin-B, fluconazole, itraconazole, voriconazole, and caspofungin may be tried with relative efficacy (DR6). However, as stated by these authors, recovery from disseminated fungal infections is unlikely unless the neutropenia of patient resolves [182].

CHEMOTHERAPY

Poor renal function defined as reduced glomerular filtration rate to less than 50 ml/min is considered a relative contraindication for HSCT in patients with CLL. [183], but as mentioned before, HSCT has been successfully performed in a patient undergoing dialysis [35].

Myeloablative (conventional) allo-HSCT consists of high-dose chemotherapy and radiotherapy conditioning regimens to eradicate malignancy, and the allograft serves to rescue the patient from pancytopenia induced by the treatment. A major limitation of this approach is the high degree of acute toxicity that is associated with myeloablative conditioning regimens. Acute renal failure (ARF) occurs frequently after both auto-HSCT and conventional allo-HSCT [185-189].

Cyclophosphamide

Cyclophosphamide (CY) is a highly effective alkylating cytostatic drug used in the conditioning treatment in patients scheduled for HSCT. At doses of greater than 50 mg/kg CY has been associated with impaired water excretion [190-192]. This inability to excrete water, leading to water retention and weight gain during high-dose CY treatment (> 50 mg/kg BW) was reflected by a decreased in urine flow, increased urine osmolality, accompanied by hyponatremia [190]. The nephrotoxic effect of CY, caused mainly by its metabolites is believed to be related to a direct effect on the distal renal tubules and collecting ducts [193]. The mechanisms for the development of water retention, involved anti-diuretic hormone, arginine vasopressin [191,192], and probably vasopressin 2- receptors and aquaporin-2, sited in the collecting duct.

Acrolein, a metabolite of CY (and ifosfamide) is the main molecule responsible for hemorrhagic cystitis (HC) occurring with a frequency of 68% after high dose of CY treatment [194]. Acrolein also accounts for most of the other adverse effects of CY treatment. Acrolein-induced HC is an inflammatory process probably involving several cytokines like tumor necrosis factor (TNF) and interleukins, as also transcription factors such as nuclear factor-kappaB in its pathogenesis [195]. Through these mechanisms a destruction cascade is initiated leading to cell death. Uncontrolled HC may lead to death, and was reported in 4 % of cases [194]. Mesna (2-mercaptoethane sodium sulfonate) is the most common compound used to protect the urine bladder from HC. Mesna is oxidized in the plasma to the dimeric form dimesna of which one third is converted back to mesna by glutathione reductase [196]. About 76% of orally given mesna will be present in the urine where it binds to acrolein preventing acrolein from a direct contact with the uroepithelium [196]. While the use of mesna is most widely used to prevent HC it is not free of adverse reactions and beside hypersensitive reaction also systemic reaction has been described in adults following mesna treatment [197].

Daunorubicin

Daunorubicin (D) is an anthracycline used to treat patients with leukemia. While cardio-toxicity is a well known adverse effect of D treatment, its use is considered relatively safe for the kidney. However, severe drug-related nephropathy has been demonstrated in rat experiments [198]. So far clinical experience in patients with renal dysfunction with a s-creat above 130 μmol/l is still missing. In human, both conventional daunorubicin and liposomal formulations of anthracyclines were comparable with regard to nephrotoxicity and liposomal formulation of daunorubicin showed a toxicity to leukemic cells at least comparable to that of free daunorubicin 199). An increasing dose regimen of daunorubicin in combination with cytarabine and etoposide may be applied with success [200].

Busulfan

Busulfan treatment, often used in the conditioning treatment prior to BMT, brought about microscopic hematuria in 8 out of 50 patients and 5 with macroscopic hematuria, and in addition 5 patients developed severe hemorrhagic cystitis [201]. Clinical symptoms of veno-occlusive disease without any sequelae, was reported in one patient too [201]. These subjects were also treated with cyclophosphamide, which makes the assuming that hemorrhagic complications were more related to cyclophosphamide rather than to busulfan treatment.

Cytocine-Arabinoside

To treat leukaemia cytocine-arabinoside (Ara-C) has been given at different doses, low-dose (100 mg/m^2, daily infusions for 7 days), standard dose (200 mg/m^2, daily infusions during 5 days) and high-dose (3g/m^2 every 12 hours for 2-6 days). The initial half-life of Ara-C is 10 to 15 minutes during which time most of the Ara-C dose is converted by the enzyme cytidine-deaminase to its metabolite uridine-arabinoside. Hepatic dysfunction and renal insufficiency has been considered as risk factors during Ara-C treatment. Hepatorenal syndrome was reported with high-dose regimen [202], and doses as high as 8 g/m^2 over 5 days caused cerebellar toxicity in a patient with renal failure [203]. In the presence of renal failure modifications of high-dose regimen should be applied [204]. High-dose Ara-C treatment may have contributed to acute tumor lysis syndrome in a patient with CML in blast crisis [205]. Whether Ara-C treatment alone or the other treatments given, with high-dose busulfan and cyclophosphamide did contribute to the tumor lysis syndrome, is difficult to decide in their report [205]. However, even low-dose of Ara-C may induce renal dysfunction [206].

Cyclosporine

Renal toxicity caused by cyclosporine (Cs) is a well known entity observed in patients after kidney transplantation. In order to avoid GVHD prophylactic treatment with Cs (alternatively Tacrolimus or Sirolimus) is often administered to patients after HSCT. Initially the dose of Cs (orally 3-5 mg/kg BW) may be adjusted to maintain a blood trough level between 150 and 200 ng/ml and later during the next 2-3 months tapered to values between 80 – 120 ng/ml. Single daily infusion of 3 mg/kg BW of Cs may be used successfully [207] Renal dysfunction was associated with Cs treatment after allo-HSCT but not after auto-HSCT [17]. Cs, tacrolimus, sirolimus and mycophenolate mofetil (MMF) are drugs that together with methyl-prednisolon (MP) often are used to treat nephrotic syndrome and different types of secondary glomerulonephritis if occurring later in the course after HSCT.

Doxorubicin (Adriamycin)

Adriamycin-induced nephropathy (AIN) with heavy proteinuria and NS is a well known entity from animal model experiments [208]. Little is known on the effects of adriamycin (A) in humans, however. It is metabolised in the liver to doxorubicinol and 7-deoxy-doxorubicinol which both have about the similar half-lives. Approximately 5.9 to 6.2 % of the metabolites are excreted by the kidney during the 48 initial hours [209]. It has been assumed that the glomerular injury by A treatment in part might be due to stimulation of free radical production [210]. The hydroxyl radical scavenger dimethylthiourea reduced proteinuria and improved CrCl [211] and curcumin could prevent nephrotoxicity in A treated rats [212]. CyA treatment had no effect on A-induced nephritis in animal experiments [213]. Although no serious renal adverse effects have been reported during treatment with A in patients with normal kidney function a clear deterioration of proximal tubular function could be detected with A and other anthracyclines as expressed by urinary N-acetyl-beta-D-glucosaminidase activity and micro-albuminuria [214]. Apart from small studies on other malignancies than leukaemia [215,216] little is known about the fate of doxorubicin when administered to patients with a CrCl < 30 ml/min.

Fludarabine

Fludarabine phosphate (FP) is well tolerated and its used has produced encouraging results in patients with CLL. Since the kidney eliminates approximately 60% of fludarabine's primary metabolite 2-fluoro-ara-A (2F-ara-A), dose modification is necessary for all patients with impaired renal function including elderly patients. The total body clearance of the 2F-

Ara-A correlates with the CrCl. Intravenous administration was used earlier times, as now an orally compounds has been developed. Beside autohemolytic anemia, tumor lysis syndrome (TLS) during oral FP treatment has been observed [217,218]. In order to avoid toxic effects of FP in ESRD daily dialysis in combination with a reduced dose of FP may be administered [219]. These authors [219] reported that with a 20% FP-dose reduction followed by daily dialysis, a fludarabine exposure that was nearly identical to that of patients with normal renal function was achieved. Fludarabine administration (P = 0.016) had a significant effect on the incidence of CRF [220]. Different degrees of TLS may develop after FP treatment for CLL [221], spanning from life-threatening TLS after a 5-days course [222] and irreversible renal failure [223] with a high mortality rate (20%) in patients with renal failure [224] to reversible ARF after single dose FP treatment [225].

Methotrexate

Methotrexate (M) is an antimetabolite that inhibits the enzyme dihydrofolate reductase in the cytoplasm resulting in depletion or reduction of folates. M and its metabolite 7-hydroxymethotrexate are excreted by the kidney. High doses of M may induce ARF possibly due to precipitation of both M and its metabolite in the renal tubules leading to a decrease in CrCl by 43 - 61% [226]. Accumulation of M due to delayed renal elimination may consequently lead to further M toxicity in other organs [227]. Rescue from this toxicity may be achieved with long-term intravenous leucovorin and thymidine treatment [226,227].

ANTI-VIRAL COMPOUNDS

Acyclovir is usually used for herpes-simplex and herpes zoster virus infections. It is eliminated unchanged by the kidneys by active tubular secretion and competing compounds using the mechanism will cause an accumulation of acyclovir. Concomitant use of acyclovir together with mycophenolate mofetil (MMF) will increase the MMF concentration. In patients with renal failure it is recommended to reduce the dose and patients with a GFR below 10 ml/min the orally given dose should be 200 mg twice daily. Intravenous administration may increase s-creat concentration and development of renal failure has been observed [228]. Dose recommendations and adjustments are shown in table 4.

Valacyclovir, valganciclovir and ganciclovir doses must be reduced in patients with renal failure according to measured CrCl (Table 4). Acute renal failure and have been reported following oral valacyclovir treatment [229] with severe neurotoxicity as a consequence [230]. Similar dose adjustments should be done when famciclovir is administered.

Table 4. Dose adjustments of valacyclovir, valganciclovir and ganciclovir in patients with renal failure according to creatinine clearance

GFR ml/min	Daily dose		
	Valacyclovir	Valganciclovir	Ganciclovir
> 75	2 gr x 4	900 mg x 2	5 mg/kg x 2
50 – 75	1.5 gr x 4	450 mg x 2	2.5 mg/kg x 2
25 – 50	1.5 gr x 3	450 mg x 1	2.5 mg/kg x 1
10 – 25	1.5 gr x 2	450 mg 2:nd d.	1.25 mg/kg x 1
<10 or HD	1.5 gr once	not recommended	1.25 mg/kg/HD

GFR = glomerular filtration rate, HD = hemodialysis.

RENAL COMPLICATIONS AFTER TRANSPLANTATION

Due to the nature of HSCT - myeloablative autologous, myeloablative allogeneic, and non-myeloablative allogeneic transplantation - renal complications are more often recognized after allo-HSCT and less so after auto-HSCT. Some of the renal complications observed after HSCT are common irrespective of whether allo-HSCT or auto-HSCT was performed. However, when describing the complications related to kidney function and pathology, it is important to distinguish between allogenic and auto-HSCT as allo-HSCT carries the burden of graft-versus-host (GVH) reaction which is absent in auto-HSCT.

TUMOR LYSIS SYNDROME (TLS)

Acute tumor lysis syndrome (TLS) may be observed in patients given conventional intensive chemotherapy for leukemia and some other malignancies (non-Hodgkin-lymphoma [231]. TLS may also be a complication to intensive cytostatic treatment of other tumours. TLS is also a complication of conditioning treatment prior to HSCT. It is caused by massive tumor cell destruction that results secondary from chemotherapy and it may be present within a few hours to a few days after initiating the therapy [232]. The risk of developing TLS varies depending on cell proliferation rate and tumor cell mass. TLS may develop also in patients with reduced intensity conditioning [233]. Pre-existent renal failure constitutes a risk factor for TLS after conditioning treatment and after HSCT [234].

The syndrome is characterised by intra-tubular precipitation of intracellular constituents that are released into the tubular lumen consisting of uric acid, phosphate, and xanthine which all have low solubility leading to ARF. Volume depletion constitutes an additional major risk factor for developing TLS. ARF induced by TLS may rapidly progress and temporary hemodialysis treatment may be indicated. In addition, hyperkalemia and hypocalcaemia might lead to cardiac arrhythmia of malignant forms. While the TLS in leukemia patients treated with the i.v. form of fludarabine may appear within 1-2 days, there may be a delay up to 15 to 20 days when fludarabine is given in an oral formulation [235,236].

TLS may be found in 17% of patients with AML [237], and it may be found in patients with ALL and rarely in CLL [218]. Similarly to the TLS found in patients after conventional leukemia treatment, TLS may develop in BMT and HSCT patients causing ARF within a few days (3-5 days) as reported [238,239]. Although TLS is seldom reported in patients with CML treatment with hydroxyurea combined with splenic irradiation or treatment with Ara-C may induce TLS in such patients [205,240].

Treatment of TLS

The treatment should begin immediately if TLS is recognised. Aggressive volume repletion with i.v. fluids (4-5 l/24 hrs) may prevent TLS by increasing GFR, increasing urine production, and decrease precipitation of uric acid, phosphate and xanthine. In general allopurinol, a blocker of uric acid synthesis may be given as prophylaxis, and is initiated prior to HSCT. The daily given dose should be 300 – 600 mg. Recombinant urate oxidase (uricase, rasburicase) which degrades uric acid into allantoin may be used [241] in cases when other treatment failed. Rasburicase treatment was reported to decrease uric acid levels by 85 % significantly better when compared to allopurinol (12%) within 4 hours of i.v. administration [241]. Rasburicase may be given intravenously at doses up to 0.2 mk/kg BW [242]. Allantoin is 5 to 10 times more soluble than uric acid. In addition, alkalinisation of the urine in order to maintain urine pH between 6.5 – 7-5 with intravenous infusion of 5% dextrose containing 100 mmol/L sodium-hydrogen-carbonate (NaHCO3) should be given. The i.v. infusion should be discontinued if serum HCO3 increases to values above 30 mmol/l or if the serum uric acid concentration returns to normal. Haemodialysis treatment should be given early to patients when the above given measures are unsuccessful and renal failure progresses. The prognosis for recovery of ARF due to TLS is generally good.

KIDNEY DISEASES AFTER HSCT

Kidney diseases occurring after allo-HSCT or auto-HSCT may be classified according to the degree of impairment of renal function i.e. acute or chronic renal failure, or divided into those with NS (proteinuria > 3.0 g/day) or those without NS (proteinuria < 3.0 g/day). In addition, the kidney disease may be defined according to pathological changes verified by histological examination of a kidney biopsy specimen. Although a combination of all of these components might be present in many reports on HSCT, some authors describe the occurrence and degree of ARF and NS without any description of histological findings.

ACUTE AND CHRONIC RENAL FAILURE

In allo-HSCT patients ARF may be recognized early within the first days and weeks or much later (CRF) in the course after transplantation (table 5). It must be kept in mind that the incidence of ARF might be different for recipients of BMT compared to those given HSCT.

The difference between BMT and HSCT may in part due to less number of red blood cells and less lysis in HSCT, thereby also less hemoglobinuria [8]. The hypothesis that heme-proteins could play an important part [8] after BMT is probably not similarly valid after HSCT. There are several reasons for ARF and many sequences of events are found and a combination of events is often present (Table 5).

Table 5. Sequences of events causing renal failure after stem cell transplantation

Time after HSCT	Reason for renal failure
Immediately before	Conditioning, cytotoxic and nephrotoxic compounds Obstructive uropathy (cyclophosphamide-induced) Early tumor lysis syndrome
Shortly after (1-7 days)	Toxicity from stored cells (free hemoglobin, cell lysis products) Toxicity from storage medium (DMSO)
10 – 21 days	Marrow aplasia, infections, gastrointestinal complications Acute hepatic toxicity
15 – 25 days	Late tumor lysis syndrome Acute GVHD Hepatorenal syndrome due to veno-occlusive disease
6 mo – 2 years	TBI nephrotoxicity Thrombotic microangiopathy Calcineurin inhibitor toxicity Chronic GVHD *de-novum* kidney disease?

The rate of ARF is different according to type of HSCT with less ARF in patients undergoing auto-HSCT compared to those with allo-HSCT. Most review reports have patient material that includes both BMT and HSCT. Although BMT and HSCT may have similarities in its nature, they are still different with regard to preparative procedures, and it is therefore difficult to make clear conclusions from these reports. Moreover, some reports on HSCT treated patients with renal dysfunction also included patients with solid tumours and multiple myeloma which with regard to ARF may have a different pathophysiology initiated by their primary disease. In the report of Parikh et al. [189] only allo-transplanted with myeloablative treatment was included. This may cause misinterpretation of the mechanisms leading to ARF and CRF. Reports including "clean" leukemia treated HSCT patient material is lacking, and interpretations on renal complications are made from case reports and patient populations with mixed physiopathologies.

As mentioned earlier ARF may be graded from grade 0 (no ARF) to grade 3 (need for dialysis) according to measured plasma creatinine concentration, estimated GFR, and need for dialysis. In a retrospective study including 363 recipients of allo-HSCT after myeloablative treatment the incidence of ARF grades 2 and 3 was 49.6% [32] and the risk of death was highest in patients with ARF grade 3. However, ARF in patients without comorbid conditions have a good prognosis. Oppositely, patients with ARF and comorbid conditions have a much poorer prognosis which led to the conclusion that the prognosis in patients with ARF is rather due to the presence of comorbid conditions than development of ARF by itself [32]. The conditions with highest mortality rate were heart disease requiring observation and treatment in an intensive care unit, thrombotic thrombocytopenic purpura (TTP), sinusoidal occlusion syndrome, and acute GVH-disease [32]. These same investigators [243] also analysed 150 adults receiving non-myeloablative HSCT with regard to development of ARF. In that study they introduced a new grading of ARF in which a tripling of s-creat was called ARF grade 2-plus [243]. Acute GVHD grade III to IV was significantly associated with ARF. Patients with ARF of grade 2-puls had a very high mortality rate (71%), mostly attributed to progression of the primary disease and GVHD [243]. In a smaller study of 26 patients with CML treated with non-myeloablative allo-HSCT, consisting of significantly less doses of radio- and chemotherapy, ARF of some degree was recognised in 38% (10 patients) with the first 100 days after transplantation. One patient required dialysis treatment. The mortality rate was 19% [18] and the mortality rate was significantly higher in those patients who developed ARF [18].

Following myeloablative conditioning moderate to severe ARF was reported in 15 to 20 % [1,8] of patients treated with auto-HSCT. In myeloablative, allo-HSCT treated patients, some degree of renal dysfunction was found in 92 % [189] and ARF in 30 to 60 % [1,8]. While dialysis was needed in 5 to 10 % after auto-HSCT treatment with HD was needed in 20 to 30% after allo-HSCT. Regardless of whether auto- or allo-HSCT treatment had been given, the mortality was equal for all patients requiring dialysis treatment (80%) in those with myeloablative conditioning. According to Parikh et al. [189] the mortality rate was 58 % within the first six months and grade 3 renal dysfunction was associated with a mortality rate of 82.6.%. They analysed 88 patients of which 60 patients had some type of leukemia [189]. The rate of ARF in non-myeloablative HSCT patients was more promising (40%) with less need for dialysis treatment (3-5%), and a mortality rate above 70% if dialysis treatment was required [1,8].

ARF or renal dysfunction was less frequent after auto-BMT treatment in patients with breast cancer [188] as also after myeloablative auto-HSCT treatment [17]. Renal dysfunction was found in 91 % after allo-HSCT and in 52 % after auto-HSCT within the first 100 days after transplantation [17].

Use of vancomycin may contribute to ARF as 28% of patients developed reduced renal function after 11- 20 days of vancocin treatment [244].

Chronic renal failure, defined as occurring later than 6 months after HSCT, is a common complication after BMT [245] and myeloablative allo-HSCT [246] but less often observed after nonmyeloablative HSCT [247].

PATHOLOGY

Nephrotic Syndrome (NS)

Minimal Change GN (MCGN)
The histological picture of MCGN is characterized by normal glomeruli and absence of increased mesangial cellularity or matrix deposition together with negative immuno-

fluorescence stains. The finding of diffuse podocyte foot-process fusions at electron microscopy examination confirms the diagnosis of MCGN. A laser capture micro-dissection combined with Taq-Man quantitative polymerase chain reaction (PCR) technique may be used for differential diagnosis and to exclude leukemia relapse [248]. The above mentioned criteria are not always fulfilled in all reports of MCGN after HSCT. Acute tubular necrosis is not a feature of "pure" MCGN and may point to hypotension, circulatory or a septic-ischemic pathology pattern [249]. Similarly, mononuclear cell infiltrations in the interstitium are not usually observed in patients with MCGN and point to chronic GVHD or reaction to a drug compound (if used) in this population [250]. Hence, in spite of clinical signs of NS with huge proteinuria, most reports on MCGN are combined with other findings in addition to the above mentioned ultrastructural changes [248,249,250]. MCGN may appear both early (median 8 months) after allo-HSCT whereas late NS as a clinical entity may present after 14 months [251] or even as late as 2-3 years after allo-HSCT [251,252].

Similar to people of the general population MCGN may also develop idiopathic or secondary to other causes than, and not necessary always be due to HSCT. As put forward by Humphreys et al., [250] several vaccinations including influenza, pneumococcal, and hepatitis-B vaccines may be linked to MCGN.

Focal Segmental Glomerulosclerosis (FSGS)

It has been suggested that organ specific and autoimmune diseases originate from defects in hematopoietic stem cells [253], and also that FSGS at least in rats could be a stem cell disorder [254]. An immunologic basis involving T cells that are provoked to produce circulatory factors that impair glomerular permeability, in the development of FSGS has been proposed [255]. In this context, the transfer of immature CD34+ cells from patients with either MCGN or FSGS intra-peritoneally to mice resulted in proteinuria and podocyte pathology similar to that observed in humans [256].

Although only case reports exists on biopsy proven FSGS [257,258], the risk of FSGS evolving after discontinuation of immunosuppression given for GVHD exists. Reintroduction of immuno-suppression will eventually lead to remission of the NS [257,259]. The nephrotic syndrome may also present in the absent of GVHD [259]. A single case of kidney biopsy proven FSGS occurring several years after remission of a membranous glomerulonephritis that developed one year after a BMT for ALL has been reported [260]. There are no simple explanations for this phenomenon in whom two different renal diseases with different mechanisms of glomerular injury developing years apart in the same patient. Progressive chronic renal failure due to FSGS may develop late in the course after HSCT, and mesangiolysis may present [257]. In their case [257] the pretransplant irradiation treatment was considered the primary cause of development of FSGS and CRF.

Membranous Nephropathy (MN)

Chronic GVHD is a major complication of allo-HSCT and may occur in 30 - 50% of patients with transplants from HLA-matched siblings and in 60 – 70 % in patients with an unrelated donor [261]. While acute GVHD develops early after allo-HSCT the chronic form of GVHD develops much later (months to years) in the course, and MN was most often related to chronic GVHD in allo-HSCT patients [262]. Membranous nephropathy (MN) or membranous glomerulonephritis is far the most common nephropathy related to chronic GVHD and MN has been reported after both BMT and HSCT [248,251,258,263-268], and may occur as a late complication of chronic GVHD after allo-HSCT [269]. Colombo et al. [270] analysed 279 patients that had been given allo-HSCT whereof 105 of them developed chronic GVHD and six had NS. Four patients had MN. They [270] and others [271] reported that NS was more often seen after peripheral HSCT (24%) than after BMT (3%). It is discussable whether MN also could be a sign of relapse of leukemia [272], but in malignancy associated MN the deposit-class of IgG is different to that of GVHD related [273]. As stated [274], MN is found after both auto-HSCT and allo-HSCT treatment, and MN may respond to anti-B-cell treatment.

Massive proteinuria and microscopic hematuria may be present. Typically granular deposits of IgG and IgM along the glomerular basement membrane and subepithelial electron dense deposits are found in renal biopsies. The deposits of IgG consist almost exclusively of the IgG1 and IgG4 subclass similar to that observed in non-transplanted patients with idiopathic MN [273]. Crescents and antiglomerular basement membrane antibodies are absent. Interstitial infiltrations, tubular atrophy, and vessels are normal. Anti-nuclear antibodies, anti-DNA is typically not found, and tests for different viruses (HBsAg, CMV, EBV, HCV, HIV) are all negative, and BK virus is not found in renal tissues.

Mesangioproliferative GN

Mesangial proliferative glomerulonephritis is a very rare entity in leukemic patients after allo- and auto-HSC. Brukamp et al. [251] reported one case of mesangial proliferative GN after allo-HSCT in a patient with Hodgkin lymphoma and one case with diffuse proliferative GN after BMT for CML was also reported [275]. To my knowledge, only one biopsy-proven case has been reported so far in auto-HSCT for leukemia [276].

IgA Nephropathy

Although some evidence suggesting a role for hematopoietic stem cells in the development of IgA nephropathy exists [36,277], very few cases with IgA nephropathy (one with crescents) have been found after allo-BMT [258,278] and this entity is not found after auto-HSCT.

Membranoproliferative (mesangiocapillary) GN (MPGN)

MPGN is rarely reported after allo-HSCT [279,280] and auto-HSCT [281]. In these reports [279-281] MPGN type I was found. MPGN type-I may occur after infections, often present after HSCT, or may involve defects of the complement system. Speculatively, since MPGN type I may also be familial it in principle possible that it may have been transmitted by stem cells from the donor.

Crescentic GN

Leukemia may develop following the course of CY treatment for Wegener's granulomatosis (WG) [282,283], and it seems that a high CY cumulative dose (>36 g; corresponding to a daily dose of 100 mg) implicates an increased risk for developing AML [284]. Moreover leukemia may develop decades after discontinuation of CY treatment [284].

The serine protease proteinase 3 (PR3) among others [285,286,287] could play a role in the pathogenesis of CY induced AML or CML. Interestingly, patients with high expression of PR3 in CD34+ progenitors before allo-HSCT had a lower incidence of relapse-related deaths and improved over-all survival [287]. These previous observations could make PR3 and other neutrophil granule proteins attractable as target for anti-leukemia vaccines [288].

Among the many manifestations of GVHD in the kidney, serologically and histological proven antineutrophil cytoplasmic antibody (ANCA) associated GN with crescents has been described after allo-HSCT [289] for leukemia, and after auto-HSCT for non-Hodgkin lymphoma [290].

TRANSPLANT-ASSOCIATED MICROANGIOPATHY (TAM)

Thrombotic Thrombocytopenic Purpura (TTP) and Haemolytic Uremic Syndrome (HUS)

Since the first case of TTP was described in 1924 and the clinically similar disease HUS was identified in 1955 [291,292] the presence of an unusually large von Willebrand factor (ULvWF) multimers in plasma and deficiency of von Willebrand factor cleaving protease (vWP-cp) has been discovered and reviewed [293]. This new vWF-cp was designed as ADAMTS-13 (a disintegrin and metalloprotease with thrombospondin type 1 motifs) and the gene was found to be located at chromosome 9q34 [293]. Severely deficiency of ADAMS-13 activity has been recognised in hereditary TTP and decreased activity of and auto-antibodies against ADAMS-13 have been found in some cases of acquired TTP [293], whereas patients with transplant thrombotic microangiopathy (TAM) after HSCT have measurable ADAMS-13 activity [294,295]. The mortality rate is high and the overall mortality rate 61% [296]. Renal failure is a predominant complication of both BMT-HUS and atypical HUS, whereas neurological complications are more prominent in TTP. Almost all cases of TAM are found after allo-BMT [297] and so far only few cases of TTP/HUS were reported after HSCT, among them one was developing TAM three years after auto-HSCT [298].

Although TAM is a well recognized syndrome particularly after allo-HSCT, the pathogenesis is poorly understood. A core set of criteria for diagnosis of TAM has been proposed recently [296]. Different associations to TAM reported and reviewed by Ruutuu et al [296] are: Female sex, unrelated donor, presence of GVHD, fungal or viral infections, and previous treatment with CsA or tacrolimus. Among the ranking criteria for diagnosis of TAM, an sudden and persistent incraese in s-creat and urea is ranked at place 5 out of 27 criteria [296]. Kidneys are almost always affected and seemed to be the primary target, mainly involving glomeruli and arterioles, in TAM after allo-HSCT [299]. In one recent study [300] TAM was found in 22 (17.9%) out of 123 patients given allo-HSCT and multivariate analysis showed that GVHD grade II-IV, treatment with high-dose busulfan and tacrolimus was asociated with a higher risk of develiopng TAM after allo-HSCT. The incidence was not reduced in patients given reduced-intensity conditioing regimens [301].

VENO-OCCLUSIVE DISEASE (VOD)

Hepatic VOD, also called sinusoidal obstruction syndrome, is a well-recognized complication of both allo- and auto-HSCT (for review see ref. 302). VOD is also a significant risk factor for development of acute renal insufficiency and ARF was a predictor for later CRF after BMT [303]. In about 15 % of the patients that developed VOD after HSCT showed a state of moderate hypercoagulability with increased thrombin-antithrombin complex and fibrinogen, and decrease of Factor VII, Protein C, and antithrombin-III [304]. These authors [304] assumed that it was a consequence of marked endothelial damage with increase of von Willebrand Factor and tissue plasminogen activator. It was reported that severe nephrotoxicity (Grade 2 and Grade 3 renal dysfunction) was associated with significantly higher frequencies of sepsis, hepatic toxicity and hepatic VOD, and lung toxicity [189], and similar findings were reported by others too [18]. Parikh et al. [189] found VOD in 9 patients with renal toxicity grade 3 and a significant difference ($p<0.01$) in the frequency of hepatic VOD in grades 0 to 2 (9.8%) versus those with nephrotoxicity grade 3 (31%). Further, the mortality of those 9 patients with nephrotoxicity grade 3 and VOD was 100 % [189]. They also demonstrated a significant different rate of VOD between auto-HSCT (4%) versus 16 % in allo-HSCT recipients [189].

EXAMINATIONS FOR KIDNEY DISEASES AFTER HSCT

Laboratory Tests

Laboratory tests should include routine tests with all hematologic tests and from the point of view of a nephrologist also include plasma- creat, urea (BUN), sodium, potassium, ionized calcium, phosphor, albumin, protein-fraction analysis, and urine bacteriology. Examinations and search for different virus diseases including hepatitis-viruses, EBV, CMV, HIV, and polyoma and BK-virus should be performed if possible before and after HSCT in donor and recipient if allo-HSCT is performed, and also before and after auto-HSCT in order to identify latent recipient or *de-novo* virus infections. It is well known that latent viruses may reappear after transplantations. Before starting conditioning treatment the Mantoux test might give some information about the risk of getting tuberculosis post HSCT. Mantoux testing after HSCT is possibly of no use since strong immunosuppressive medication is used.

Ultrasound Examination (US)

Examination of the kidneys and urinary bladder should be performed by a trained radiologist. The examination will verify kidney size, thickness of parenchyma, and anatomical abnormalities of the kidney, ureters and urine bladder. Combined with doppler-examination some circulatory anomalies might be discovered, although angiography still is the golden standard for evaluation of kidney circulation. The use of radio-contrast medium is also a risk factor that may contribute to the development of acute renal failure (and contrast induced fibrosis) in special risk groups.

Computerised Scan Tomography (CT) and Magnetic Resonance Imaging (MRI)

CT-examination is nowadays often used to diagnose different pathological states and could give additive information with regard to renal pathology and circulation in patients with ARF after HSCT. However, the information gained from CT-examination in this patient population is limited, and the risks of renal complication from contrast media used at CT-examination must be outweighed against the usefulness of the information coming from it.

Similarly, the use of MRI as a diagnostic tool for renal failure after HSCT is very limited to findings of renal infarction, thrombi and circulatory changes that were not found at US-examination. Here too, the necessity of the MRI examination must be evaluated against its usefulness for decision of therapy.

Kidney Biopsy (KB)

It is of no doubt that examination of a kidney biopsy specimen is the most exact way (today) to gain knowledge of histological changes within the kidney after HSCT. A large spectrum of renal diseases was found in patients after treatment with HSCT [305] and in line with their conclusions, the renal biopsy is essential in order to identify the underlying reason, and to be able to give these patients appropriate treatment. In spite of the opinion of some authors KB is the only resort to give the physician some knowledge on the morphology and ideas how to treat a patient with kidney disease.

TREATMENTS

Renal Failure (RF)

Angiotensin converting enzyme inhibitors (ACEi) may eventually be used to treat BMT nephropathy, hypertension and RF [306], but progression of RF to ESRD may still continue in spite of ACEi treatment [251] and intermittent hemodialysis and/or kidney transplantation may be considered in some cases. Although the similar mechanisms are involved when using angiotensin receptor blockade (ARB), no clinical trials exists using this type of medication after HSCT. Recently a report using a combination of the ARB candesartan with the ACEi enalapril which successfully could reduce recurrent proteinuria in a patient with MN after allo-HSCT [307] Thus, probably ARB may be used to treat both hypertension and proteinuria after HSCT.

Nephrotic Syndrome

De novo MCGN with NS may be initially treated successfully with oral prednisone/prednisolon [250] alternatively methyl-prednisolon (MP) at a dose of 1 mg/kg BW (max dose 80 mg) or alternatively prednisolon combined with cyclophosphamide [308] or cyclosporine A (Cs) at an initial daily dose of 5-7 mg/kg BW divided into two or three doses. Later, within the next 2-3 months the Cs dose should be reduced according to through-values. MP may also be combined with tacrolimus (Tacro). Cs or Tacro through levels and plasma/serum creatinine and urea-nitrogen concentration must be controlled for optimal dosing. In cases with decreased glomerular function (GFR< 30 ml/min/1.73 m^2) mycophenolate mofetil (MMF) at doses of 1 g b.i.d. may be tried. The effect of MMF has not been proven in prospective studies, but some reports on improvement exists [249,250]. Treatment of nephrotic syndrome related to chronic GVHD was successfully treated with Cs and steroids with response after 12 weeks of treatment [270].

Most cases with MN and nephrotic syndrome are been treated with a combination of orally given corticosteroids and/or Cs [263,264] and MMF may successfully be added [252]. Similar treatment regimens with steroids and Cs have been used in patients with FSGS following HSCT [257].

GVHD

Patients with chronic GVHD due to relapse or was refractory to previous immunosuppression (Cs and steroids) was given additional sirolimus (S) treatment [309]. In their report [309] 47 patients were given S combined with calcineurin inhibitors (Cs or Tacro), or mycophenolate mofetil or prednisone in whom clinical response was achieved in 38 patients (81%). Complete response was achieved in 18/47 and partial response in 20/47 patients. In the case of development of TAM during that regimen calcineurin inhibitors and S were discontinued, and four patients required plasma exchange treatment. It is to knowledge one case report in which Cs was used for GVHD prophylaxis and withdrawn after one year of treatment then subsequently developing nephrotic syndrome with histology compatible with MCGN [310]. After reintroduction of Cs together with prednisone he recovered [310]. Several others have reported remission of GVHD related NS with steroids and Cs [270], Single case reports on recurrence of NS after Cs withdrawal which was given prophylactic to avoid GVHD related NS has been published [268]. Clinical remission of GVHD related NS has been achieved using short-term methotrexate together with prolonged Cs treatment [271].

Treatment of MPGN type I consists of corticosteroids (prednisone or methyl-prednisolon) which may be given intravenously at alternate day pulses. Treatment may be needed to continue over long periods of time up-to 12 to 66 months [281]. Chlorambucil is a compound seldom used to treat proliferative GN which may be tried in cases with NS due to MPGN type I.

Acute GN with histological findings of crescents in the kidney biopsy specimen should be treated aggressively with cyclophosphamide and steroids and plasma exchange should be considered. Addition of hemodialysis treatment should be started early if RF progress.

Change of immunosuppression should be considered in any case in which current therapy remains ineffective.

Although alpha-interferon has been used to treat nephrotic syndrome in a patient with CLL [311] such therapy has not been tried and is probably not to recommend after allo-HSCT before more experimental data has been presented with alpha-interferon in this setting.

SUPPORTIVE TREATMENTS IN RF

In all cases using the above mentioned treatment combinations for renal disease, and especially if diuretics are added which is almost always the case, there will be a risk of developing thrombotic complications. Therefore addition of low molecule weight heparin, warfarin or low dose acid salicylic acid should be considered. Also gastric ulcer prophylaxis should be given. In the case of low blood haemoglobin concentration subcutaneously administered erythropoiesis stimulating agents should be thought of.

As a last resort, kidney transplantation may be considered in selected patients with chronic renal failure after HSCT.

OTHER TREATMENTS CONNECTED TO RF AFTER HSCT

Thrombotic Microangiopathy (TAM)

The first-line treatment of the idiopathic TTP-HUS syndrome (not associated to BMT or HSCT) is based on plasma-exchange, fresh frozen plasma (FFP) which induces a response and survival rate of approximately 85%, and in addition glucocorticoids, immunoadsorption, vincristine, intravenous immunoglobulin (ivIG) and splenectomy. Cryosupernatant, lacking the larger plasma VWF multimers, has been used as replacement fluid instead of plasma and seemed to be more efficacious if compared with a historical control group in which FFP was used. However, a broad agreement exists that no success is achieved using corticosteroids, immunosuppression, FFP infusion, or plasma-exchange treatment in patients with post-BMT or HSCT induced TAM. Hemodialysis treatment is given if ARF is present. Effective treatment for hematopoietic stem cell transplantation- or neoplasia-associated TAM is unknown, plasma exchange is often used but in severe cases the mortality rate is very high with death occurring either from the underlying neoplasia or the TAM itself. If Cs, Tacro or sirolimus treatment is given, the doses should be reduced and Cs treatment should be discontinued in spite of a better prognosis for sirolimus treated subjects [312]. Recently one report of success using rituximab was published (ref) thus all patients in their study had low levels of ADAMS-13 and the levels of anti-ADAMTS13 antibody did not change significantly with rituximab-induced remission [313]. Blood transfusions are contra-indicated.

As a paradox, one patient with TTP/HUS has been successfully treated with auto-HSCT and CD34+ cell infusion for refractory TTP-HUS syndrome [314].

Veno-Occlusive Disease

Since there are no known effective therapies for VOD prevention is the best strategy for this disease. Heparin is the most used agent in VOD prevention and should eventually be started one week prior to and continued one month after HSCT. This strategy, using a daily dose of 100 U/kg BW may decrease the incidence by about 10 %, alternatively low-molecular-weight heparin (LMWH) may be used [302]. LMWH has the advantage of decreased risk of bleeding and is easier to administer subcutaneously. The use of low-dose prostaglandin E1 (PGE1) is not recommended due to its considerable toxicity. Further, the use of pentoxyphyllin that prevents transcription of tumor necrosis factor-α (TNF-α) thereby stimulating PGI2 and PGE2 did not have beneficial effect either [302].

FUTURE ASPECTS

New discoveries in the field of cell differentiation and regulation have opened for more sophisticated strategies in leukemia therapy. Although several compounds that interact with these new mechanisms of action have been developed, little is known about their effects on kidney function.

Tyrosine kinase inhibitors (TKI) represent a break-through in the treatment of leukemia and imatinib mesylate (IM) was the first TKI to be used to treat CML. Thereafter dasatinib, nilotinib and several other molecules have been developed and shown to be effective in treatment of IM resistant CML [316]. However, both IM and dasatinib may create resistant CML due to mutations in the breakpoint cluster region/Abelson (Bcr-Abl) dependent or independent mechanisms [316]. As a consequence not all patients benefit from this treatment. Since dasatinib is eliminated by the faeces and less than 4% is found in urine renal effects from this compounds is not to be expected. Lately another farnesyl-transferase inhibitor BMS-214662 was found to be effective against CML when tested *in vitro* [317].

Nuclear factor-kB (NF-kB) is a nuclear transcription factor which was first identified by Sen and Baltimore [318]. NF-kB regulates the expression of various gene products or molecules, and several reports have documented that NF- kB activation inhibits apoptosis in cancer cells [319-323]. Bortezomib is an inhibitor of proteasome and NF- kB thereby possessing anti-leukemic activity. Thus, proteasome inhibition (PI) with bortezomib has become one topic of interest as leukemic cells are sensitive to PI whereas normal hematopoietic stem cells are viable after exposure to such compounds. Several clinical studies treating MM or AML with bortezomib in combination with other anti-leukemic agents have been reported [324,325,326] and renal failure was not associated to bortezomib in these reports. On the contrary, renal function was shown to improve during bortezomib treatment for multiple myeloma [327,328] and it may also be used in patients requiring dialysis treatment [329]. However, occurrence of TLS has been reported associated to bortezomib treatment [330].

Inhibition of class I histone deacetylases (HDAC) might offer another mechanism of action to treat hematopoietic malignancies. The depsipeptide romidepsin [331], belinostat and vorinostat are such HDAC inhibitors that have been tested *in vitro* and were also shown to have effect in clinical leukemia [332]. A new oral HDAC inhibitor, R306465, is also a promising compound which has been tested animal experiments [333] and eventually will reach clinical use. Recently, the combination of a protease inhibitor (bortezomib) and romidepsin and belinostat was shown to synergistically cause cell death *in vitro* using cells from patients with CLL [334]. Some concern about cardio-toxicity has been discussed, but so far nothing atypical with regard to kidney function or pathology has been mentioned. None of the HDAC inhibitors has been used in patients conditioned for, or after HSCT.

Some studies have shown that NF-kappaB p65 may play an important role in regulating telomerase by modulating its nuclear translocation [335,336] The enzyme telomerase is a cellular reverse transcriptase that catalyzes the synthesis and extension of telomeric DNA and high telomerase activity are associated with treatment failure of leukemia [337]. Increased telomere loss after allo-HSCT when compared to their donors has been demonstrated [338] which mainly occurs during the first year post-HSCT (339 -341=40-42). Late failure of a successful graft after allo-HSCT is rare, and some individuals in these studies had no demonstrable telomere loss post-transplant. However, the capacity to for self-renewing and/or differentiate seems restricted [342]. Put into a clinical concept, compounds that act on telomeres and telomerase activity in order to prolong life of transplanted hematopoietic cells may, or may not, be retarded by intrinsic mechanisms that limit cell expansion [343].

Although HSC have an enormous capacity to self-renew and/or differentiate, this capacity appears to be finite; for example, murine HSC can only be serially transplanted 5–7 times in mice before hemopoiesis is exhausted [342]. Whether drugs designed to inhibit telomerase expression and/or activity will be effective for the treatment of some forms of leukemia, or will be used as an additive after HSCT, remains to be shown. It is to mention that complete remission has been described in acute ALL patients after receiving prolonged azidothymidine (AZT)/interferon (IFN) treatment [344].

Heat-shock protein 90 (HSP-90) is over-expressed in AML cells [345]. It may play a role in cell survival and resistance to chemotherapy and might signal poor-prognosis. Many years ago several inhibitors of HSP-90, geldanamycin, herbimycin-A, and radicocol, has been isolated and used for different purposes [346]. Geldanamycin has reached a new era as an inhibitor of HSP-90 as it was shown to inhibit malignant cell growth and increase apoptosis in these cells in vitro [345,347], and both cytarabine and rituximab had an additive effect in primary AML cells in vitro [348,349]. Whether these substances will be used clinically during conditional treatment or post-HSCT remains an open question and is to be evaluated within the next years.

CONCLUSION

Treatment schedules used for kidney diseases and renal failure after HSCT are much the same as those in non-HSCT patients. Experiences in this field of nephrology are often achieved from single case reports and only few studies with homologous patient material have been published.

There is no consensus with regard to immunosuppressive treatment schedules for renal failure, nephrotic syndrome, and different types of glomerulonephritis related to GVHD.

Published reports consist of patient materials having a mixture of allo- and auto-HSCT and include patients with both leukemia and other malignancies which per se are known to be complicated with glomerular pathology [315]. Although some of the observations made in patients treated for multiple myeloma with HSCT, the histopathology in multiple myeloma differs widely from that in leukemia. The grading scales previously reported [16,17,18,263] is probably more useful for clinicians to evaluate progression of renal failure (table 2) than that presented in table 1.

In all cases with renal failure, with or without nephrotic syndrome, microscopic or macroscopic hematuria, one should aim for a kidney biopsy to verify the diagnosis. However, contraindications for kidney biopsy, like single kidney and horseshoe kidney, small sized kidneys (length < 10 cm) and kidneys with limited parenchymal thickness (<1.2 cm), untreated hypertension, bleeding diathesis, sepsis or pyuria, must be thoroughly considered. The origin of proteinuria, hematuria and progressive renal failure after hematopoietic stem cell transplantation is caused by many factors that may need different and combined treatment schedules.

REFERENCES

[1]   Humphreys BD. Renal complications of hematopoietic stem cell transplantation. *Nephrology rounds* 2006; 4: 304 - 344 (*www.nephrologyrounds.org*).

[2]   Gratwohl A, Brand R, Apperley J, Crawley C, Ruutu T, Coradini P, Carreras E, Devergie A, Guglielmi C,Kolb H-J, Niederwieser D. Allogenic hematopoietic stem cell transplantation for chronic myeloid leukemia in Europe 2006: transplant activity, long-term data and crrent results. An analysis by the Chronic Leukemia Working Party of the European Group for Blood and Marrow Transplantation (EBMT*). Haematologica* 2006; 91: 513 - 521.

[3]   Redaelli A Laskin BL, Stephens JM, Botteman MF, Pashos CL. The clinical and epidemiological burden of chronic lymphocytic leukaemia. *Eur J Cancer Care* 2004; 13: 279 - 287.

[4]   Yamamoto JF, Goodman MT. Patterns of leukaemia incidence in the United States by subtype and demographic characteristics. 1997 - 2002. *Cancer Causes Control* 2008; 19; 379 - 390.

[5]   Hunter T. Treatment for chronic myelogenous leukemia: the long road to imatinib. *J Clin Invest* 2007; 117: 2036 - 2043.

[6]   Kantarjian HM, Giles F, Quintás-Cardama A, Cortes J. Important therapeutic targets in chronic myelogenous leukemia. *Clin Cancer Res* 2007; 13: 1089 - 1097.

[7]   Merill D, Jackson H. The renal complication of leukemia. *N Engl J Med* 1943; 228: 271 - 275.

[8]   Zager RA. Acute renal failure in the setting of bone marrow transplantation. *Kidney Int* 1994; 46: 1443 - 1458.

[9]   Phillips JK, Bass PS, Majumdar G, Davies DR, Jones NF, Pearson TC. Renal failure caused by leukaemic infiltration in chronic lymphocytic leukaemia. *J Clin Pathol* 1993; 46: 1131 -1133.

[10] Suh WM, Wainberg ZA, deVos S, Cohen AH, Kurtz I, Ngyen MK. Acute lymphoblastic leukaemia presenting as acute renal failure. *Nat Clin Pract Nephrol.* 2007; 3: 106 - 110.

[11] Kamat AV, Goldsmith D, O'Donnel P, van deer Walt J, Carr R. Renal failure with granulomatous interstitial nephritis and diffuse leukemic renal infiltration in chronic lymphocytic leukemia. *Ren Fail* 2007; 29: 763 - 765.

[12] Khan A, Sinks LF, Silhaug M, Champion L. Acute lymphocytic leukemia mimicking renal failure. *CA Cancer J Clin* 1979; 29: 319 - 320.

[13] MacGregor MS, Boag DE, Innes A. Chronic kidney disease: evolving strategies for detection and management of impaired renal function. *Q J Med* 2006; 99: 365 - 375.

[14] Cockroft DW, Gault MH. Prediction of creatinine clearance from serum creatinine. *Nephron* 1976; 16: 31 - 41.

[15] Levey AS, Bosch JP, Lewis JB, Greene T, Rogers N, Roth D. A more accurate method to estimate glomerular filtration rate from serum creatinine: a new prediction equation. Modification of Diet in Renal Disease Study Group. *Ann Intern Med* 1999; 130: 461 - 470.

[16] Parikh CR, Sandmaier BM, Storb RF, Blume KG, Sahebi F, Maloney DG, Maris MB, Nieto Y, Edelstein CL, Schrier RW, McSweeney P. Acute renal failure after nonmyeloablative hematopoietic cell transplantation. *J Am Soc Nephrol* 2004; 15: 1868 - 1876.

[17] Caliskan Y, Besisik, SK, Sargin D, Ecder T. Early renal injury after myeloablative allogenic and autologous hematopoietic cell transplantation. *Bone Marrow Transplant* 2006; 38: 141 - 147.

[18] Liu H, Ding JH, Liu BC, Zhao G, Chen MA. Early renal injury after nonmyeloablative allogenic peripheral blood stem cell transplantation in patients with chronic myelocytic leukemia. *Am J Nephrol* 2007; 27: 336 - 341.

[19] Feinstein AR. The pre-therapeutic classification of co-morbidity in chronic disease. *J Chron Dis.* 1970; 23: 455 – 468.

[20] Charlson ME, Pompei P, Ales KL, et al. A new method of classifying prognostic comorbidity in longitudinal studies: Development and validation. *J Chronic Dis* 1987; 40: 373 - 383.

[21] Charlson M, Szatrowski TP, Peterson J, Gold J. Validation of a combined comorbidity index. *J Clin Epidemiol* 1994; 47: 1245 - 1251.

[22] Extermann M. Measuring comorbidity in older cancer patients (review). *Eur J Cancer* 2000; 36: 453 - 471.

[23] Hemmelgarn BR, Manns BJ, Quan H, Ghali WA. Adapting the Charlson Comorbidity Index for use in patients with ESRD. *Amer J Kidney Dis* 2003; 42: 125 - 132.

[24] Di Iorio B, Cillo N, Cirillo M, De Santo NG. Charlson Comorbidity Index is a predictor of outcomes in incident hemodialysis patients and correlates with phase angle and hospitalization. *Int J Artif Organs* 2004; 27: 330 - 336.

[25] Geraci JM, Escalante CP, Freeman JL, Goodwin JS. Comorbid disease and cancer. The need for more relevant conceptual models in health services research. *J Clin Oncol* 2005; 23: 7399 - 7404.

[26] Alamo J, Shahjahan M, Lazarus HM, de Lima M, Giralt SA. Comorbidity indices in hematopoietic stem cell transplantation: a new report card. *Bone Marrow Transplant* 2005; 36: 475 - 479.

[27] Giles FJ, Borthakur G, Ravandi F, Faderi S, Verstovsek S, Thomas D, Wierda W, Ferrajoli A, Kornblau S, Pierce S, Albitar M, Cortes J, Kantarjian H. The

haematopoietic cell transplantation comorbidity index score is predictive of early death and survival in patients over 60 years of age receiving induction therapy for acute myeloid leukaemia. *Br J Haematol* 2007; 136: 624 - 627.

[28] Sorror ML, Maris MB, Storb R, Baron F, Sandmaier BM, Maloney DG, Storer B. Hematopoietic cell transplantation (HCT)–specific comorbidity index: a new tool for risk assessment before allogeneic HCT. *Blood.* 2005; 106: 2912 - 2919.

[29] Hingorani SR, Guthrie K, Batchelder A, Schoch G, Aboulhosn N, Manchion J, McDonald GB. Acute renal failure after myeloablative hematopoietic cell transplant: incidence and risk factors. *Kidney Int.* 2005; 67: 272 - 277.

[30] Miniati I, Conforti ML, Bernardo P, Tyndall A, Gensini GF, Matucci-Cerinic M. Hematopoietic stem cell transplantation in autoimmune diseases: algorithm for cardiovascular assessment. *Herz* 2007; 32: 43 - 50.

[31] Parimon T, Au DH, Martin PJ, Chien JW. A risk score for mortality after allogenic hematopoietic cell transplantation. *Ann Int Med* 2006; 144: 407 - 414.

[32] Kersting S, Koomans HA, Hené RJ, Verdonck LF. Acute renal failure after allogenic myeloablative stem cell transplantation: retrospective analysis of incidence, risk factors and survival. *Bone Marrow Transplant* 2007; 39: 359 - 365.

[33] Go AS, Chertow GM, Fan D, McCulloch CE, Hsu C. Chronic kidney disease and the risk of death, cardiovascular events, and hospitalization. *New Engl J Med* 2004; 351: 1296 - 1305.

[34] Baker KS, Ness KK, Steinberger J, Carter A, Fransisco L, Burns LJ, Sklar C, Forman S, Weisdorf D, Gurney JG, Bhatia S. Diabetes, hypertension, and cardiovascular events in survivors of hematopoietic cell transplantation: a report from the bone marrow transplantation survivor study. *Blood* 2007; 109: 1765 - 1772.

[35] Hamaki T, Katori H, Kami M, Yamato T, Yamakado H, Itoh T, Ksusmi E, Igarashi M, Ueyama J, Kanda Y, Miyakoshi S, Mineishi S, Morinaga S, Mukai M, Hayashi M, Takaue Y, Hara S, Mutou Y. Successful allogenic blood stem cell transplantation for aplastic anemia in a patient with renal insufficiency requiring dialysis. *Bone Marrow Transplant* 2002; 30: 195 - 198.

[36] Iwata Y, Wada T. Uchiyama A, Miwa A, Nakaya I, Tohyama T, Yamada Y, Kurokawa T, Yoshida T, Ohta S, Yokoyama H, Iida H. Remissionof IgA nephropathy after allogenic peripheral blood stem cell transplantation followed by immunosuppression for acute lymphocytic leukemia. *Internal Med* 2006: 45; 1291 - 1295.

[37] Subar M, Gucalp R, Benstein J, Williams G, Wiernik PH. Acute leukaemia following renal transplantation. *Med Oncol* 1996; 13: 9 - 13.

[38] Burke GW, Cirocco R, Markou M, Temple JD, Allouch M, Roth D, Nery J, Miller J. Early development of acute myelogenous leukemia following kidney transplantation: possible role of multiple serum cytokines. *Leuk Lymphoma* 1995; 19: 173 - 180.

[39] Specchia G, Storlazzi CT, Cunco A, Surace C, Mestice A, Pannunzio A, Rocchi M, Liso V. Acute promyelocytic leukemia with additional chromosome abnormalities in a renal transplant case. *Ann Hematol* 2001; 80: 246 - 250.

[40] Butani L, Paulson TE. Congenital acute myelogenous leukemia presenting as palpable renal masses in a noenate. *J Pediatr Hematol Oncol* 2003; 25: 240 - 242.

[41] Daliphard S, Béhar C, Cornillet-Lefebvre P, Struski S, Sartelet H, Gaillard D. Misleading lead. Acute megakaryoblastic leukemia in an infant mimicking polycystic kidney disease. *Med Pediatr Oncol* 2002; 38: 53 - 54.

[42] Cesaro S, Brugiolo A, Faraci M, Uderzo C, Rondelli R, Favre C, Zecca M, Garetto G, Dini G, Pillon M, Messina C, Znaesco L, Pession A, Locatelli F. Incidence and

treatment of hemorrhagic cystitis in children given hematopoietic stem cell transplantation: a survey from the Italian association of pediatric haematology oncology-bone marrow transplantation group. *Bone marrow transplant* 2003; 32: 925 - 931.

[43]   Haselberger MB, Schwinghammer TL. Efficacy of mesna for prevention of hemorrhagic cystitis after high-dose cyclophosphamide therapy. *Ann Pharmacother* 1995; 29: 918 - 921.

[44]   Yamamoto R, Kusumi E, Kami M, Yuji K, Hamaki T, Saito A, Murasgihe N, Hori A, Kim S-W, Makimoto A, Ueyama J, Tanosaki R, Miyakoshi S, Mori S, Morinaga S, Heike Y, Taniguchi S, Masou S, Takaue Y, Mutou Y. Late hemorrhagic cystitis after reduced-intensity hematopoietic stem cell transplantation (RIST). *Bone Marrow transplant* 2003; 32: 1089 - 1095.

[45]   Ewens KG, George RA, Dharma K, Ziyadeh FN, Spielman RS. Assessment of 115 candidate genes for diabetes nephropathy by transmission/disequilibrium test. *Diabetes* 2005; 54: 3305 - 3318.

[46]   Feltbower RG, McKinney PA, Greaves MF, Parslow RC, Bodansky HJ. International parallels in leukaemia and diabetes epidemiology. *Arch Dis Child* 2004; 89: 54 - 56.

[47]   Feltbower RG, Manda SO, Gilthorpe MS, Greaves MF, Parslow RC, Kinsey SE, Bodansky HJ, McKinney PA. Detecting small-area similarities in the epidemiology of childhood acute lymphoblastic leukemia and diabetes mellitus, type 1. a Bayesian approach. *Am J Epidemiology* 2005; 161; 1168 - 1180.

[48]   Richiardi L, Magnani C, Bruno G, Maule MM, Merletti F, Pastore G. Re:"Detecting small-area similarities in the epidemiology of childhood acute lymphoblastic leukemia and diabetes mellitus, type 1 a Bayesian approach" *Am J Epidemiology* 2005; 162 :1132 - 1133.

[49]   Weiser MA, Cabanillas ME, Konopleva M, Thomas DA, Pierce SA, Escalante CP, Kantarjian HM, O'Brien SM. Relation between the duration of remission and hyperglycemia during induction chemotherapy for acute lymphocytic leukemia with a hyperfractionated cyclophosphamide, vincristine, doxorubicin, and dexamethasone/ methotrexate-cytarabine regimen. *Cancer.* 2004; 100: 79 - 85.

[50]   Hoffmeister PA, Storer BE, Sanders JE. Diabetes mellitus in long-term survivors of pediatric hematopoietic cell transplantation. J Pediatr Hematol Oncol 2004; 26: 81 - 90.

[51]   Lassila M, Allen TJ, Cao Z, Thallas V, Jandeleit-Dahm KA, Candido R, Cooper ME. Imatinib attenuates diabetes-associated atherosclerosis. *Arterioscler Thromb Vasc Biol* 2004; 24: 935 - 42.

[52]   Niwa A, Matsubara H, Adachi S, Fujino H, Higashi Y, Umeda K, Shiota M, Hiramatsu H, Kobayashi M, Watanabe K-I, Yorifuji T, Nakahata T. Diabetes mellitus after stem cell transplantation in a patient with acute lymphoblastic leukemia: Possible association with tacrolimus. *Pediatrics International* 2007; 49: 530 - 532.

[53]   Vialettes B, Maraninchi D, San Marco MP, Birg F, Stoppa AM, Mattei-Zevaco C, Thivolet C, Hermitte L, Vague P, Mercier P. Autoimmune polyendocrine failure--type 1 (insulin dependent) diabetes mellitus and hypothyroidism--after allogenic bone marrow transplantation in a patient with lymphoblastic leukemia. *Diabetologia* 1993; 36: 541 - 546.

[54]   Philippakos D, Kakourus S, Dervenoulas J, Pontidas E. Diabetes insipidus as a complication of acute myelomonocytic leukaemia. *Postgrad Med J* 1983; 59: 93 - 94.

[55] Frangoul HA, Shaw DW, Hawkins D, Park J. Diabetes insipidus as a presenting symptom of acute myelogenous leukemia. *J Pediatr Hematol Oncol* 2000; 22: 457 - 459.

[56] Slater SE, Maccallum PK, Birjandi F, Gibbons B, Lister TA. Acute myelogenous leukemia (ANL) and diabetes insipidus (DI): further association with monosomy 7. *Hematol Oncol* 1992; 10: 221 - 223.

[57] Castagnola C, Morra E, Bernasconi P, Astori C, Santagostino A, Bernasconi C. Acute myeloid leukemia and diabetes insipidus: results in 5 patients. *Acta Haematol* 1995; 93: 1 - 4.

[58] Harris KPG, Hattersley JM, Feehally S, Walls J. Acute renal failure associated with haematological malignances.: a review of 10 years experience. *Eur J Haematol* 1991; 47: 119 - 122.

[59] McLigeyo SO, Notghi A, Thomson D, Anderton JL. Nephrotic syndrome associated with chronic lymphatic leukaemia. *Nephrol Dial Transplant* 1993; 8: 461 - 463.

[60] Moulin B, Ronco PM, Mougenot B, Francois A, Fillastre JP, Mignon F. Glomerulonephritis in chronic lymphocytic leukemia and related B-cell lymphomas. *Kidney Int* 1992; 42: 127 - 135.

[61] Leonard BJ. Chronic lymphatic leukemia and the nephrotic syndrome. *Lancet* 1957; i: 1356 - 1357.

[62] Dathan JRE, Heyworth MF, Maciver AG. Nephrotic syndrome in chronic lymphocytic leukemia. *Br Med J* 1974; 3: 655 - 657.

[63] Seney FD, Federgreen WR, Stein H, Kashgarian M. A review of nephrotic syndrome associated with chronic lymphocytic leukemia. *Arch Intern Med* 1986; 146: 137 - 141.

[64] Martinez-Vea A, Herranz MJ, Llorente A, Carrera M, García C, Razquín S, Oliver JA. Acute renal failure with chronic lymphocytic leukaemia. *Postgrad Med J* 1996; 72: 763 - 755.

[65] Pagniez DC, Fenaux P, Delvallez L, Dequiedt P, Gosselin B, Tacquet A. Reversible renal failure due to specific infiltration in chronic lymphocytic leukaemia. *Am J Med* 1988; 85: 579 - 580.

[66] Saggi S, Calandri C, Muhlfelder T. Choi H, Kahn T, Kaji D. Renal failure due to leukaemic infiltration in chronic lymphocytic leukaemia. *Nephrol Dial Transplant* 1990; 5: 1051 -1052.

[67] Haraldsdottir V, Haanen C, Jordans JG. Chronic lymphocytic leukaemia presenting as renal failure with lymphocytic infiltration of the kidney. *Neth J Med* 1992; 41: 64 - 67.

[68] Comerma-Coma MI, Sans-Boix A, Tuset-Andújar E, Andreu-Navarro J, Pérez-Ruiz A, Naval-Marcos I. Reversible renal failure due to specific infiltration of the kidney in chronic lymphocytic leukaemia. *Nephrol Dial Transplant* 1998; 13: 1550 - 1552.

[69] Quenneville LA, Magil AB. Renal failure due to T-cell mediated lymphocytic vasculitis: an unusual complication of B-cell chronic lymphocytic leukaemia. *Am J Kidney Dis* 2000; 36: E17.

[70] Erten N, Saka B, CaliskanY, Besisik S, Karan MA, Tascioglu C. Acute renal failure due to leukaemic infiltration in chronic lymphocytic leukaemia: a case report. *Int J Clin Pract Suppl* 2005; 147: 53 - 55.

[71] Dodsworth H, Gabriel R. Chronic granulocytic leukaemia in a patient with chronic renal failure on dialysis. *J Clin Pathol* 1981; 34: 58 - 59.

[72] Perazella MA Eisen RN, Frederick WG, Brown E. Renal failure and severe hypokalemia associated with acute myelomonocytic leukemia. *Am J Kidney Dis* 1993; 22: 462 - 467.

[73] Morschhauser T, Wattel E, Pagniez D, Lovi V, Rose C, Bauters F, Fenaux P. Glomerular injury in chronic myelomonocytic leukaemia. *Leuk Lymphoma* 1995; 18: 479 - 483.

[74] Robinson GT Sundaram KR, Dilly SA, Bevan DH, Andrews PA. Renal failure in a patient with chronic myelomonocytic leukaemia. *Nephrol Dial Transplant* 1997; 12: 1500 - 1502.

[75] Schwarze EW. Pathoanatomical features of the kidney in myelomonocytic and chronic lymphocytic leukaemia. *Virchows Arch A Pathol Anat Histol* 1975; 368: 243 - 251.

[76] Eagen JW, Lewis EJ. Glomerulopathies of neoplasia. *Kidney Int* 1977; 11: 297 - 306.

[77] Alpers CE, Cotran RS. Neoplasia and glomerular injury. *Kidney Int* 1986; 30: 465 - 473.

[78] Ziakas PD, Giannouli S, Psimenou E, Nakopoulou L, Voulgarelis M. Membranous glomerulonephitis in chronic lymphocytic leukaemia. *Am J Hematol* 2004; 76: 271 - 274.

[79] Mandelenakis N, Mendoza N, Pirani CL, Pollak VE. Lobular glomerulonephritis and membranoproliferative glomerulonephritis: a clinical and pathologic study based on renal biopsies. *Medicine* 1971; 50: 319 - 355.

[80] Feehally J, Hutchinson RM, MacKay EH, Walls J. Recurrent proteinuria and chronic lymphatic leukaemia. *Clin Nephrol* 1981; 16: 51 - 54.

[81] Touchard G, Preud'homme JL, Aucoutirier P, Giraud C, Gouet, Yver L, Patte D. Nephrotic syndrome associated with chronic lymphocytic leukaemia: an immunological and pathological study. *Clin Nephrol* 1989; 31: 107 - 116.

[82] Bischoff ME, Blau W, Wagner T, Wagenmann W, Dörner O, Basara N, Fauser AA. Total body irradiation and cyclophosphamide is a conditioning regimen for unrelated bone marrow transplantation in a patient with chronic myelogenous leukaemia and renal failure on hemodialysis. *Bone Marrow Transplant* 1998; 22: 591 - 593.

[83] Dwyer JP, Yates KM, Sumner EL, Stone WJ, Wang Y, Koury MJ, Fogo AB, Zent R. Chronic myeloid leukaemia-associated membranoproliferative glomerulonephritis that responded to imatinib mesylate therapy. *Clin Nephrol* 2007; 67: 176 - 81.

[84] Tsai JD, Lee HC, Lin CC, Liang DC, Chen SH, Huang FY. Epstein-Barr virus-associated acute renal failure: diagnosis, treatment, and follow-up. *Pediatr Nephrol* 2003; 18: 667 - 674.

[85] Wade JC. Viral infections in patients with hematological malignancies. *Hematology ASH Education Book* 2006; pp. 368 - 374.

[86] Ryan KJ, Ray CG (editors) (2004). *Sherris Medical Microbiology*, 4th ed., McGraw Hill, pp. 556; 566 - 569.

[87] Deconinck E, Kribs M, Rebibou J-M, Bulabois CE, Ducloux D, Cahn J-Y. Cytomegalovirus infection and chronic graft-versus-host disease are significant predictors of renal failure after allogeneic hematopoietic stem cell transplantation *Haematologia* 2005; 90: 569 - 570.

[88] Ljungman P, Brand R, Einsele H, Frassoni F, Niederwieser D, Cordonnier C. Donor CMV serologic status and outcome of CMV-seropositive recipients after unrelated donor stem cell transplantation: an EBMT megafile analysis. *Blood* 2003; 102: 4255 - 4260.

[89] Weiss MA, Daquioag E, Margolin EG, Pollak VE. Nephrotic syndrome, progressive renal failure and glomerular 'collapse': a new clinicopathologic entity? *Am J Kidney Dis* 1986; 7: 20 - 28.

[90] Detweiler RK, Falk RJ, Hogan SL, Jennette JC. Collapsing glomerulopathy: a clinically and pathologically distinct variant of focal segmental glomerulosclerosis. *Kidney Int* 1994; 45: 1416 - 1424.

[91] Tomlinson L, Boriskin Y, McPhee I, Holwill S, Rice P. Acute cytomegalovirus infection complicated by collapsing glomerulopathy. *Nephrol Dial Transplant* 2003; 18: 187 - 189.

[92] Gratwohl A, Brand R, Frassoni F, Rocha V, Niederwieser D, Reusser P, Einsele H, Cordonnier C. Cause of death after allogeneic haematopoietic stem cell transplantation (HSCT) in early leukaemias: and EBMT analysis of lethal infectious complications and changes over calendar time. *Bone Marrow Transplant* 2005; 36: 757 - 769.

[93] Han XY. Epidemiologic analysis of reactivated cytomegalovirus antigenemia in patients with cancer. *J Clin Microbiol* 2007; 45: 1126 - 1132.

[94] Baudville N, Latham B, Cordingly F, Warr K. Renal failurein a patient with leukemic infiltration of the kidney and polyoma infection. *Nephrol Dial Transplant* 2001; 16: 1059 - 1061.

[95] Fogazzi GB, Furione M, Saglimbeni L, Gatti M, Cantù M, Tarantino A. BK and JC polyomavirus infaction in a patient with chronic lymphocytic leukaemia and renal failure. *Nephrol Dial Transplant* 2002; 17: 1534 - 1535.

[96] Ikegame K, Takimoto T, Takahashi R, Murakami M, Tamaki H, Fujioka T, Kawakami M, Hirabayashi N, Soma T, Sugiyama H, Ogawa H. Lethal adenovirus infection in a patient who had undergone nonmyeloablative stem cell transplantation. *In J Hematol* 2001; 74: 95 - 100.

[97] Stracke S, Helmchen U, von Müller L, Bunjes D, Keller F. Polyoma virus-associated interstitial nephritis in a patient with acute myeloic leukaemia and peripheral blood stem cell transplantation. *Nephrol Dial Transplant* 2003; 18: 2431 - 2433.

[98] Ricciardiello, L., Laghi, L., Ramamirtham, P., Chang, C.L., Chang, D.K., Randolph, A.E. and Boland, C.R. "JC virus DNA sequences are frequently present in the human upper and lower gastrointestinal tract". *Gastroenterology* 2000; 119: 1228 - 1235.

[99] Binet I, Nickeleit V, Hirsch HH. Polyomavirus infections in transplant recipients. Infection in transplantation. *Current Opin Organ Transplant* 2000; 5: 210 - 216.

[100] Peyrière H, Jeziorsky E, Jalabert A, Cociglio M, Benketira A, Blayac JP, Hansel S, Margueritte G, Hillaire-Buys D. Neurotoxicity related to valganciclovir in a child with impaired renal function: usefulness of therapeutic drug monitoring. *Ann Pharmacother* 2006; 40: 143 - 146.

[101] Czock D, Scholle C, Rasche FM, Schaarschmidt D, Keller F. Pharmacokinetics of valganciclovir and ganciclovir in renal impairment. *Clin Pharmacol Ther* 2002; 72: 142 - 150.

[102] Battiwalla M, Paplham P, Almyroudis NG, McCarthy A, Abdelhalim A, Elefante A, Smith P, Becker J, McCarthy PL, Segal BH. Leflunomide failure to control recurrent cytomegalovirus infection in the setting of renal failure after allogenic stem cell transplantation. *Transpl Infect Dis* 2007; 9: 28 - 32.

[103] Akan H, Arslan O, Akan OA. Tuberculosis in stem cell transplant patients. *J Hosp Infect* 2006; 62: 421 - 426.

[104] Au WY, Cheng VCC, Ho PL, Yuen KY, Hung I, Ma SY, Lie AKW, Liang R, Kwong YL. Nontuberculous mycobacterial infections in Chinese hematopopietic stem cell transplantation patients. *Bone Marrow Transplant* 2003; 32: 709 - 714.

[105] Edsall DL. The attitude of the clinician inregard to exposing patients to the x-ray. *JAMA* 1906; 47: 1425 - 1429.

[106] Hartman FW, Bolliger A, Doub HP. Experimental nephritis produced by irradiation. *Am J M Sc* I926; I72: 487 - 500.

[107] Domagk, G. Die R6ntgenstrahlenwirkung auf das Gewebe, im besonderen betrachtet an den Nieren. Morphologische und funktionelle Verinderungen. *Beitr. z. path. Anat. u. z. allg. Path.*, I927; 77: 525 - 575.

[108] Zuelzer WW, Palmer HD, Newton Jr WA. Unusual glomerulonephritis in young children, probably radiation nephritis. Report of three cases. *Am J Pathol* 1950; 26: 1019 - 1039.

[109] Luxton RW. Radiation nephritis. *Q J Med* 1953; 22: 215 - 242.

[110] Baldwin JN, Hagstrom JWC. Acute radiation nephritis. *Calif Me*d 1962; 47: 97 ? 359 – 362

[111] Mogensen CE. Glomerular filtration rate and renal plasma flow in shortterm and long-term juvenile diabetes mellitus. *Scand J Clin Lab Invest* 1971; 28: 91 - 100.

[112] Thomson SC, Vallon V, Blantz RC. Kidney function in early diabetes: the tubular hypothesis of glomerular filtration. *Am J Physiol Renal Physiol* 2004; 286: F8 – F 15.

[113] Cohen EP. Radiation nephropathy after bone marrow transplantation. *Kidney Int.* 2000; 58: 903 - 918.

[114] Oyama Y, Komatsuda A, Imai H, Ohtani H, Hamai K, Wakui H, Miura AB, Nakamoto Y. Late onset bone marrow transplant nephropathy. *Intern Med* 1996; 35: 489 - 493.

[115] Textor SC, Forman SJ, Zipser RD, Carlson JE. Changes in renal blood flow, glomerular filtration, and vasoactive hormones in bone marrow transplant recipients after total body irradiation. In: *Prostaglandin and Lipid Metabolism in Radiation Injury*. Eds: Walden TL & Hughes HN. Plenum Press, New York 1987: pp 305 - 317.

[116] Ritz E. Metabolic syndrome and kidney disease. *Blood Purif* 2008; 26: 59 - 62.

[117] Wong H, Vivian L, Weiler G, Filler G. Patients with autosomal dominant polycystic kidney disease hyperfiltrate early in their disease. *Am J Kidney Dis* 2004; 43: 624 - 628.

[118] Nishi H, Tomida C, Gotoh M, Yamagata K, Akiyama H, Shimokama T. Chronic renal failure with severe mesangiolysis in a hematopoietic stem cell transplant recipient. *Ren Fail* 2006; 28: 519 - 522.

[119] Robbins ME, Bonsib SM. Radiation nephropathy: a review. *Scanning Microsc* 1995; 9: 535 - 560.

[120] Krochak RJ, Baker DG. Radiation nephritis. Clinical manifestations and pathophysiologic mechanisms. *Urology* 1986; 27: 389 - 393.

[121] Miralbell R, Bieri S, Mermillod B, Helg C, Sancho G, Pastoors B, Keller A,. Kurtz JM, Chapuis B. Renal Toxicity after allogenic bone marrow transplantation: the combined effect of total-body irradiation and graft-versus-host disease. *J Cin Oncol* 1996; 14: 579 - 585.

[122] Ringhoffer M, Blumstein N, Neumaier B, Glatting G, von Harsdorf S, Buchmann I, Wiesneth M, Kotzerke J, Zens T, Buck AK, Schauwecker P, Stilgenbauer S, Døhner H, Reske SN, Bunjes D. 188Re or 90Y labelled anti-CD66 antibody as part of a dose-reduced conditioning regimen for patients with acute leukaemia or myelodysplastic

syndrome over the age of 55: results of a phase I-II study. *Br J Haematol* 2005; 130: 604 - 613.

[123] Zens T, Glatting G, Schlenk RF, Buchmann I, Döhner H, Reske SN, Bunjes D. Targeted marrow irradiation with radioactively labelled anti-CD66 monoclonal antibody prior to allogenic stem cell transplantation for patients with leukemia: results of a phase I-II study. *Haematologia* 2006; 91: 285 - 286.

[124] Bunjes D, Buchmann I, Duncker C, Seitz U, Kotzerke J, Wiesneth M, Dohr D, Stefanic M, Buck A, von Harsdorf S, Glatting G, Grimminger W, Karakas T, Munzert G, Döhner H, Bergmann L, Reske SN. Rhenium 188-labeled anti-CD66(a,b,c,e) monoclonal antibody to intensify the conditioning regimen prior to stem cell transplantation for patients with high-risk acute myeloic leukemia or myelodysplastic syndrome: results of a phase I-II study. *Blood* 2001; 98: 565 - 572.

[125] Orchard K, Cooper M. Targeting the bone marrow: applications in stem cell transplantation. *Quart J Nuclear Med*. 2004; 48: 267 - 278.

[126] Döbert N, Martin H, Kranert WT, Klein SA, Mose S, Grünwald F. Re-186 HEDP conditioning therapy in patients with advanced acute lymphoblastic leukemia before allogenic bone marrow transplantation. *Clin Nucl Med*. 2003: 28; 738 - 742.

[127] Rodriguez V, Anderson PM, Litzow MR, Erlandson L, Trotz BA, Arndt CA, Khan SP, Wiseman GA. Marrow irradiation with high-dose 153Samarium-EDTMP followed by chemotherapy and hematopoietic stem cell infusion for acute myelogenous leukemia. *Leuk Lymphoma* 2006; 47: 1583 - 1592.

[128] Jurcic JG. Immunotherapy for acute myeloid leukemia. *Curr Oncology Reports* 2005; 7: 339 - 346.

[129] Sui X, Bensinger W, Press O. Improved conditioning regimens for autologous transplantation using targeted radiotherapy. *Acta Haematol* 2005; 114: 230 - 238.

[130] Berz D, McCormack EM, Winer ES, Colvin GA, Quesenberry PJ. Cryopreservation of hematopoietic cells. *Am J Hematol* 2007; 82: 463 - 472.

[131] Lovelock JE, Bishop MW. Prevention of freezing damage to living cells by dimethyl sulphoxide. *Nature* 1959; 183: 1394 - 1395.

[132] Jimenez RA, Willkens RF. Dimethyl sulfoxide: a perspective of its use in rheumatic diseases. *J Lab Clin Med* 1982; 100: 489 - 500.

[133] Swanson BN. Medical use of dimethyl sulfoxide (DMSO*). Rev Clin Basic Pharmacol* 1985; 5: 1 - 33.

[134] Ravid M, Shapira J, Lang R, Kedar I. Prolonged dimethylsulphoxide treatment in 13 patients with systemic amyloidosis. *Ann Rheum Dis* 1982; 41: 587 - 592.

[135] Bakken AM. Cryopreserving human peripheral blood progenitor cells. *Curr Stem Cell Res Ther* 2006; 1: 47 - 54.

[136] Bakken AM, Bruserud O, Abrahamsen JF. No differences in colony formation of peripheral blood stem cells frozen with 5% or 10% dimethyl sulphoxide. *J Hematother Stem Cell Res* 2003; 12: 351 - 358.

[137] Liseth K, Abrahamsen JF, Bjørsvik S, Grøttebø S, Bruserud Ø. The viability of cryopreserved PBPC depends on the DMSO concentration and the concentration of nucleated cells in the graft. *Cytotherapy* 2005; 7: 328 - 333.

[138] Davis JM, Rowley SD, Braine HG, Piantadosi S, Santos GW. Clinical toxicity of cryopreserved bone marrow graft infusion. *Blood* 1990; 75: 781 - 786.

[139] Benekli M, Anderson B, Wentling D, Bernstein S, Czuczman M, McCarthy P. Severe respiratory depression after dimethylsulphoxide- containing autologous stem cell

infusion in a patient with AL amyloidosis. *Bone Marrow Transplantation* 2000; 25: 299 - 1301.

[140] Miniero R, Vai S, Giacchino M, Giubellino C, Madon E. Severe respiratory depression after autologous bone marrow infusion. *Haematologica* 1992; 77: 98 - 99.

[141] Hoyt R, Szer J, Grigg A. Neurological events associated with the infusion of cryopreserved bone marrow and/or peripheral blood progenitor cells. *Bone Marrow Transplant* 2000; 25: 1285 - 1287.

[142] Hequet O, Dumontet C, El Jaafari-Corbin A, Salles G, Espinouse D, Arnaud P, Thieblemont C, Bouafia F, Coiffier B. Epileptic seizures after autologous peripheral blood progenitor infusion in a patient treated with high-dose chemotherapy for myeloma. *Bone Marrow Transplant* 2002; 29: 544.

[143] Burger J, Gilmore MJ, Jackson B, Prentice HG. Acute haemoglobinaemia associated with the reinfusion of bone marrow buffy coat for autologous bone marrow transplantation. *Bone Marrow Transplant* 1991; 7: 322 - 324.

[144] Zenhausern R, Tobler A, Leoncini L, Hess OM, Ferrari P. Fatal cardiac arrhythmia after infusion of dimethylsulfoxide cryopreserved hematopoietic stem cells in a patient with severe primary cardiac amyloidosis and end-stage renal failure. *Ann Hematol* 2000; 79: 523 - 526.

[145] Windrum P, Morris TC, Drake MB, Niederwieser D, Ruutu T. Variation in dimenthyl sulfoxide use in stem cell transplantation: A survey of EBMT centres. *Bone Marrow Transplant* 2005; 36: 601 - 603.

[146] Alessandrino EP, Bernasconi P, Caldera D, Colombo A, Bonfichi M, Malcovati L, Klersy C, Martinelli G, Maiocchi M, Pagnucco G, Varettoni M, Perotti C, Bernasconi C. Adverse events during bone marrow or peripheral blood progenitor cell infusion: analysis of 126 cases. *Bone Marrow Transplant* 1999; 23: 533 - 537.

[147] Deman A, Peeters P, Sennesael J. Hydroxyethyl starch dosea not impair immediate reanl function in kidney transplant recipients: a retrospective, multicentre analysis. *Nephrol Dial Transplant* 1999; 14: 1517 - 1520.

[148] Buchanan SS, Gross SA, Acker JP, Toner M, Carpenter JF, Pyatt DW. Cryopreservation of stem cells using trehalose: evaluation of the method using a human hematopoietic cell line. *Stem Cells and Development* 2004; 13: 295 - 305.

[149] Richards AB, Krakowka S, Dexter LB, Schmid H, Wolterbeek APM, Waalkens-Berendsen DH, Shigoyuki A, Kurimoto M. Trehalose: a review of properties, history of use and human tolerance, and results of multiple safety studies. *Food and Chem Toxicol* 2002; 40: 871 - 898.

[150] Stroh C, Cassens U, Samraj AK, Sibrowski W, Schulze-Osthoff K, Los M. The role of caspases in cryoinjury: Caspase inhibition strongly improves the recovery of cryopreserved hematopoietic and other cells. *FASEB J* 2002; 16: 1651 - 1653.

[151] Sepkowitz KA. Antibiotic prophylaxis in patients receiving stem cell transplant. *Bone Marrow Transplant* 2002; 29: 367 - 371.

[152] Raveh D, Kopyt M, Hite Y Rudensky B, Sonnenblick M, Yinnon AM. Risk factors for nephrotoxicity in elderly patients receiving once-daily aminoglycosides. *Q J Med* 2002; 95: 291 - 297.

[153] Lerner SA, Schmitt BA, Seligsohn R, Matz GJ. Comparative study of ototoxicity and nephrotoxicity in patients randomly assigned to treatment with amikacin or gentamicin. *Am J Med* 1986; 80: 98 - 104.

[154] Kuhlmann J, Seidel G, Grötsch H. Tobramycin nephrotoxicity: Failure of cefotaxime to potentiate renal toxicity. *Infection* 1982; 10: 233 - 239.

[155] Peacock Jr JE, Herrington DA, Wade JC, Lazarus HM, Reed MD, Sinclair JW, Haverstock DC, Kowalsky SF, Hurd DD, Cushing DA, Harman CP, Donowitz GR, MD. Ciprofloxacin plus Piperacillin Compared with Tobramycin plus Piperacillin as Empirical Therapy in Febrile Neutropenic Patients. A randomized, double-blind trial. *Ann Int Med* 2002; 137: 77 - 86.

[156] Barza M, Ioannidis JP, Cappelleri JC, Lau J. Single or multiple daily doses of aminoglycosides: a meta-analysis. *BMJ* 1996; 312: 38 - 45.

[157] Freeman CD, Strayer AH. Mega-analysis of meta-analysis: an examination of meta-analysis with an emphasis on once-daily aminoglycoside comparative trials. *Pharmacotherapy* 1996; 16: 1093 - 102.

[158] Sowinski KM, Magner SJ, Lucksiri A, Scott MK, Hamburger RJ, Mueller BA. Influence of Hemodialysis on Gentamicin Pharmacokinetics, Removal During Hemodialysis, and Recommended Dosing. *Clin J Am Soc Nephrol* 2008; 3: 355 - 361.

[159] Warkentin D, Ippoliti C, Bruton J, Van Besien K, Champlin R. Toxicity of single daily dose gentamicin in stem cell transplantation. *Bone Marrow Transplant* 1999; 24: 57 - 61.

[160] Torfoss D, Høiby EA, Tangen JM, Holte H, Bø K, Meyer P, Grøttum K, Weyde K, Lauritzsen GF, Sandstad B, Jacobsen A-B, Olsen H, Kvaløy S. Tobramycin once versus three times daily, given with penicillin G, to febrile neutropenic cancer patients in Norway: a prospective, randomized, multicentre trial. *Journal of Antimicrobial Chemotherapy* 2007; 59: 711 - 717.

[161] Sung L, Dupuis LL, Bliss B, Taddio A, Abdolell M, Allen U, Rolland M, Tong A, Taylor T, Doyle J. Randomized controlled trial of once- versus thrice daily tobramycin in febril neutropenic children undergoing stem cell transplantation. *J Natl Cancer Inst* 2003; 95: 1869 - 1877.

[162] Zeitany RG, El Saghir NS, Santhosh-Kumar CR, Sigmon MA. Increased aminoglycoside dosage requirements in hematological malignancy. *Antimicrob Agents Chemother* 1990; 34: 702 - 708.

[163] Goren MP, Baker Jr DK, Shenep JL. Vancomycin does not enhance amikacin-induced tubular nephrotoxicity in children. *Pediatr Infect Dis* 1989; 8: 278 - 282.

[164] Hemsworth S, Nunn AJ, Selwood K, Osborne C, Jones A, Pizer B. Once-daily netilmicin for neutropenic pyrexia in paediatric oncology. *Acta Paediatr* 2005; 94: 268 - 274.

[165] Ghazal HH, Ghazal CD, Tabbara IA. Ceftazidime and ciprofloxacin as empiric therapy in febrile neutropenic patients undergoing hematopoietic stem cell transplantation. *Clin Ther.* 1997; 19: 520 - 526.

[166] Shanker SM, Nania JJ. Management of Pneumocystis jiroveci pneumonia in children receiving chemotherapy. *Paediatr Drugs* 2007; 9: 301 - 309.

[167] Gal AA, Plummer AL, Langston AA, Mansour KA. Granulomatous Pneumocystis carinii pneumonia complicating hematopoietic cell transplantation. *Pathol Res Pract* 2002; 198: 553 - 558.

[168] Saito T, Seo S, Kanda Y, Shoji N, Ogasawara T, Murakami J, Tanosaki R, Tobinai K, Takaue Y, Mineishi S. Early onset Pneumocystis carinii pneumonia after allogeneic peripheral blood stem cell transplantation. *Am J Hematol* 2001; 67: 206 - 209.

[169] Chuu WM, Catlett JP, Perry DJ, Geddes LG, Levit PD, Levy CS, Buick MK, Malkovska V. Concurrent Pneumocystis carinii and cytomegalovirus pneumonia after autologous peripheral blood stem cell transplantation. *Bone Marrow Transplant* 1999; 23: 1087 - 1089.

[170] Bretagne S, Costa JM, Foulet F, Jabot-Lestang L, Baud-Camus F, Cordonnier C. Prospective study of toxoplasma reactivation by polymerase chain reaction in allogeneic stem-cell transplant recipients. *Transpl Infect Dis* 2000; 2: 127 - 132.

[171] Thomas DR, Dover JS, Camp RD. Pancytopenia induced by the interaction between methotrexate and trimethoprim-sulfamethoxazole. *J Am Acad Dermatol*. 1987; 17: 1055 - 1056.

[172] Chandra M, Chandra P, McVicar M, Susin M, Teichberg S. Rapid onset of co-trimoxazole induced interstitial nephritis. *Int J Pediatr Nephrol* 1985; 6: 289 - 292.

[173] Pusey CD, Saltissi D, Bloodworth L, Rainford DJ, Christie JL. Drug associated acute interstitial nephritis: clinical and pathological features and the response to high dose steroid therapy. *Q J Med* 1983; 52: 194 - 211.

[174] Frain JB. Methotrexate toxicity in a patient receiving trimethoprim-sulfamethoxazole. *J Rheumatol* 1987; 14: 194 - 211.

[175] Paap CM, Nahata MC. Clinical use of trimethoprim/sulfamethoxazole during renal dysfunction. *DICP* 1989; 23: 646 - 654.

[176] Heidemann HT, Gerkens JF, Spickard WA, Jackson EK, Branch RA. Amphotericin B nephrotoxicity in humans decreased by salt repletion. *Am J Med* 1983; 75: 476 - 481.

[177] Gubbins PO, Penzak SR, Polston S, McConnell SA, Anaissie E. Characterizing and predicting amphotericin B-associated nephrotoxicity in bone marrow or peripheral blood stem cell transplant recipients. *Pharmacother* 2002; 22: 961 - 971.

[178] Furrer K, Schaffner A, Vavricka SR, Halter J, Imhof A, Schanz U. Nephrotoxicity of cyclosporine A and amphotericin B-deoxycholate as continuos infusion in allogenic stem cell transplantation. *Swiss Med Wkly* 2002; 132: 316 - 320.

[179] Krüger W, Stockschläder M, Sobottka I, Betker R, De Wit M, Kröger N, Grimm J, Arland M, Fiedler W, Erttmann R, Zander AR. Antimycotic therapy with liposomal amphotericin-B for patients undergoing bone marrow or peripheral blood stem cell transplantation. *Leuk Lymphoma* 1997; 24: 491 - 499.

[180] Upton A, McCune JS, Kirby KA, Leisenring W, McDonald G, Batchelder A, Marr KA. Fluconazole coadministration concurrent with cyclophosphamide conditioning may reduce regimen-related toxicity postmyeloablative hematopoietic cell transplantation. *Biol Blood Marrow Transplant* 2007; 13: 760 - 764.

[181] Oren I, Rowe JM, Sprecher H, Tamir A, Benyamin N, Akria L, Gorelik A, Dally N, Zuckerman T, Haddad N, Fineman R, Dann EJ. A prospective randomized trial of itraconazole vs fluconazole for prevention of fungal infections in patients with acute leukemia and hematopoietic stem cell transplant recipients. *Bone Marrow Transplant* 2006; 38: 127 - 134.

[182] Mays SR, Bogle MA, Bodey GP. Cutaneous fungal infections in the oncology patient: recognition and management. *Am J Clin Dermatol* 2006; 7: 31 - 43.

[183] Cigna Health Care Coverage Position 2007: 0418: 1 - 15.

[184] Hamaki T, Katori H, Kami M, Yamato T, Yamakado H, Itoh T, Kusumi E, Igarashi M, Ueyama J, Kanda Y, Miyakoshi S, Mineishi S, Morinaga S, Mukai M, Hayashi M, Takaue Y, Hara S, Mutou Y. Successful allogeneic blood stem cell transplantation for aplastic anemia in a patient with renal insufficiency requiring dialysis. *Bone Marrow Transplant* 2002; 30: 195 - 198.

[185] Zager RA, O'Quigley J, Zager BK, Alpers CE, Shulman HM, Gamelin LM, Steward P, Thomas ED. Acute renal failure following bone marrow transplantation: A retrospective study of 272 patients. *Am J Kidney Dis* 1989; 13: 210 - 216.

[186] Gruss E, Bernis C, Tomas JF, Garcia-Canton C, Figuera A, Motellon JL, Paraiso V, Traver JA, Fernandez-Ranada JM. Acute renal failure in patients following bone marrow transplantation. Prevalence, risk factors and outcome. *Am J Nephrol* 1995; 15: 473 - 479.

[187] Letourneau I, Dorval M, Belanger R, Legare M, Fortier L, Leblanc M. Acute renal failure in bone marrow transplant patients admitted to the intensive care unit. *Nephron* 2002; 90: 408 - 412.

[188] Merouani A, Shpall EJ, Jones RB, Archer PG, Schrier RW. Renal function in high dose chemotherapy and autologous hematopoietic cell support treatment for breast cancer. *Kidney Int* 1996; 50: 1026 - 1031.

[189] Parikh C, McSweeney P, Korulkar D, Ecder T, Merouani A, Taylor J, Sphall E, Jones R, Bearman S, Schrier RW. Renal dysfunction in allogeneic hematopoietic cell transplantation. *Kidney Int* 2002; 62: 566 - 573.

[190] DeFronzo RA, Colvin OM, Braine H, et al. Cyclophosphamide and the kidney. *Cancer* 1974; 33: 483 - 491.

[191] Harlow PJ, DeClerck YA, Shore NA, et al. A fatal case of inappropriate ADH secretion induced by cyclophosphamide therapy. *Cancer* 1979; 44: 896.

[192] Steele TH, Serpick AA, Block JB. Antidiuretic response to cyclophosphamide in man. *J Pharmacol Exp Ther* 1973; 185: 245 - 253.

[193] Schilsky RL. Renal and metabolic toxicities of cancer chemotherapy. *Semin Oncol* 1982; 9: 75 - 83.

[194] Carley ME. The effect of chemotherapy on the function of bladder, ureters and kidneys. *CME Journal of Gynecologic Oncology* 2002; 7:100 - 102.

[195] Korkmaz A, Topal T, Oter S. Pathophysiological aspects of cyclophosphamide and ifosfamide induced hemorrhagic cystitis; implication of reactive oxygen and nitrogen species as well as PARP activation. *Cell Biol Toxicol* 2007; 23: 303 - 312.

[196] Schoenike SE, Dana WJ. Ifosfamide and mesna. *Clin Pharm* 1990; 9: 179 - 191.

[197] Khaw SL, Downie PA, Waters KD, Ashley DM, Heath JA. Adverse hypersensitivity reactions to mesna as adjunctive therapy for cyclophosphamide. *Pediatr Blood Cancer* 2007: 49; 341 - 343.

[198] Deprez-DeCampeneere D, Jaenke R, Trouet A. Comparative cardiac and renal toxicity in the rat and the rabbit. *Cancer Treat Rep* 1982; 66: 395 - 397.

[199] Pea F, Russo D, Mchieli M, Baraldo M, Ermacora A, Damiani D, Baccarani M, Furlanut M. Liposomal daunorubicin plasmatic and renal disposition in patients with acute leukemia. *Cancer Chemother Pharmacol* 2000; 46: 279 - 286.

[200] Novitzky N, Thomas V, Abrahams L, du Toit C, McDonald A. Increasing dose intensity of anthracycline antibiotics improves outcome in patients with acute myelogenous leukemia. *Am J Hematol* 2004; 76: 319 - 329.

[201] Tutschka PJ, Copelan EA, Klein JP. Bone marrow transplantation for leukemia following a new busulfan and cyclophosphamide regimen. *Blood* 1987; 70: 1382 - 1388.

[202] Kirtley DW, Votaw ML, Thomas E. Jaundice and hepatorenal syndrome associated with cytosine arabinoside. *J Natl Med Assoc* 1990; 82: 217 - 218.

[203] Hasle H. Cerebellar toxicity during cytarabine therapy associated with renal insufficiency. *Cancer Chemother Pharmacol* 1990; 27: 76 - 78.

[204] Smith GA, Damon LE, Rugo HS, Ries CA, Linker CA. High-dose cytarabine dose modification reduces the incidence of neurotoxicity in patients with renal insufficiency. *J Clin Oncol* 1997; 15: 833 - 839.

[205] Przepiorka D, Gonzales-Chambers R. Acute tumor lysis syndrome in a patient with chronic myelogenous leukemia in blast crisis: role of high-dose Ara-C. *Bone Marrow Transplant* 1990; 6: 281 - 282.

[206] Tanaka M, Kanamori H, Yamaji S, Mishima A, Fujita H, Fujisawa S, Murata T, Koharazawa H, Matsuzaki M, Mohri H. Low-dose cytarabine-induced hepatic and renal dysfunction in a patient with myelodysplastic syndrome. *Anticancer Drugs* 1999; 10: 289 - 91.

[207] Nawa Y, Hara M, Tanimoto K, Nakase K, Kozuka T, Maeda Y. Single-dose daily infusion of cyclosporine for prevention of Graft-versus-host disease after allogeneic bone marrow transplantation from HLA allele-matched, unrelated donors. *Int J Hematol* 2006; 83: 159 - 163.

[208] Bertani T, Poggi A, Pozzoni R, Delaini F, Sacchi G, Thoua Y, Mecca G, Remuzzi G, Donati MB. Adriamycin-induced nephrotic syndrome in rats: sequence of pathologic events. *Lab Invest* 1982; 46: 16 - 23.

[209] Mross K, Maessen P, vande Vijgh WJ, Gall H, Boven E, Pinedo HM. Pharmacokinetics and metabolism of epidoxorubicin and doxorubicin in humans. *J Clin Oncol* 1988; 6: 517 - 526.

[210] Mimnaugh EG, Trush MA, Gram TE. A possible role for membrane lipid peroxidation in anthracyclines nephrotoxicity. *Biochem Pharmacol* 1986; 35: 4327 - 4335.

[211] Milner LS, Wei SH, Houser MT. Amelioration of glomerular injury in doxorubicin hydrochloride nephrosis by dimethylthiourea. *J Lab Clin Med* 1991; 118: 427 - 434.

[212] Venkatesan N, Punithavathi D, Venkatesan A. Curcumin prevents adriamycin nephrotoxicity in rats. *Br J Pharmacol* 2000; 129: 231 - 234.

[213] Japaulo EG, Soares V. Effect of cyclosporine on adriamycin induced nephritis. *Ren Fail* 2002; 24: 577 - 584.

[214] Bárdi E, Bobok I, v-Oláh A, Kappelmayer J, Kiss C. Anthracycline antibiotics induce acute renal tubular toxicity in children with cancer. *Pathol Oncol Res* 2007; 13: 249 - 253.

[215] Králicková P, Melichar B, Malir F, Roubal T. Renal tubular dysfunction and urinary zinc excretion in breast cancer patients treated with anthracycline-based combination chemotherapy. *J Exp Clin Cancer Res* 2004; 23: 579 - 584.

[216] Li Y, Finkel KW, Hu W, Liu J, Coleman R, Kavanagh JJ. Pegylated liposomal doxorubicin treatment in recurrent gynaecologic cancer patients with renal dysfunction. *Gynecol Oncol* 2007; 106: 375 - 380.

[217] List AF, Kummett TD, Adams JD, Chun HG. Tumour lysis syndrome complicating treatment of chronic lymphocytic leukaemia with fludarabine phosphate. *Am J Med* 1990; 89: 388 - 390.

[218] Calvo-Villas JM, Urcuyo BM, Umpierrez AM, Sicilia F. Acute tumor lysis syndrome during oral fludarabine treatment for chronic lymphocytic leukemia. Role of treatment with rasburicase. *Onkologie* 2008; 31: 197 - 199.

[219] Horwitz ME, Spasojevic I, Morris A, Telen M, Essell J, Gasparetto C, Sullivan K, Long G, Chute J, Chao N, Rizzieri D. Fludarabine-based nonmyeloablative stem cell transplantation for sickle cell disease with and without renal failure: clinical outcome and pharmacokinetics. *Biol Blood Marrow Transplant* 2007; 13: 1422 - 1426.

[220] Delgado J, Cooper N, Thomson K, Duarte R, Jarmulowicz M, Cassoni A, Kottaridis P, Peggs K, Mackinnon S. The importance of age, fludarabine, and total body irridiation in the incidence and severity of chronic renal failure after allogeneic hematopoietic cell transplantation. *Biol Blood Marrow Transplant*. 2006; 12: 75 - 83.

[221] Frame JN, Dahut WL, Crowley S. Fludarabine and acute tumor lysis in chronic lymphocytic leukemia. *N Engl J Med* 1992; 327: 1396 - 1397.

[222] Hussain K, Mazza JJ, Clouse LH. Tumor lysis syndrome (TLS) following fludarabine therapy for chronic lymphocytic leukemia (CLL): case report and review of the literature. *Am J Hematol* 2003; 72: 212 - 215.

[223] Timuragaoglu A, Karadogan I, Undar L. Irreversible renal failure in a patient with chronic lymphocytic leukemia treated with fludarabine. *Ann Hematol* 1999; 78: 109 - 110.

[224] Cheson BD, Frame JN, Vena D, Quashu N, Sorensen JM. Tumor lysis syndrome: an uncommon complication of fludarabine therapy of chronic lymphocytic leukemia. *J Clin Oncol* 1998; 16: 2313 - 2320.

[225] Nunes R, Passos-Coelho JL, Miranda N, Nave M, Leal da Costa F, Abecasis M. Reversible acute renal failure following single administration of fludarabine. *Bone Marrow Transplantation* 2004; 33: 671.

[226] Abelson HT, Fosburg MT, Beardsley GP, Goorin AM, Gorka C, Link M, Link D. Methotrexate-induced renal impairment: clinical studies and rescue from systemic toxicity with high-dose leucovorin and thymidine. *J Clin Oncol* 1983; 1: 208 - 216.

[227] van den Bongard HJGD, Mathôt RAA, Boogerd W, Schornagel JH, Soesan M, Schellens JHM, Beijnen JH. Successful rescue with leucovorin and thymidine in a patient with high-dose Methotrexate induced acute renal failure. *Cancer Chemother Pharmacol* 2001; 47: 537 - 540.

[228] Mihara A, Mori T, Nakazato T. Ikeda Y, Okamoto S. Acute renal failure caused by intravenous acyclovir for disseminated varicella zoster virus. *Scand J Infect Dis* 2007; 39: 94 - 95.

[229] Sugimoto T, Yasuda M, Sakaguchi M, Koyama T, Uzu T, Kashiwagi A, Isshiki K, Kanasaki M. Oliguric acute renal failure following oral valacyclovir therapy. *QJM* 2008; 101: 164 - 166.

[230] Carlon R, Possamai C, Corbanese. Acute renal failure and severe neurotoxicity following valacyclovir. *Intensive Care Med* 2005; 31: 1953.

[231] Cairo MS, Bishop M. Tumour lysis syndrome: new therapeutic strategies and classification. *Br J Haematol* 2004; 127: 3 - 11.

[232] Chasty RC, Liu-Yin JA. Acute tumour lysis syndrome. *Br J Hosp Med* 1993; 49: 488 - 492.

[233] Linck D, Basara N, Tran V, Vucinic V, Hermann S, Hoelzer D, Fauser AA. Peracute onset of severe lysis syndrome immediately after 4Gy fractionated TBI as part of reduced intensity preparative regimen in a patient with T-ALL with high tumor burden. *Bone Marrow Transplant* 2003; 31: 935 - 937.

[234] Sallan S. Management of acute TLS. *Semin Oncol* 2001; 28 (Suppl. 5): 9 - 12.

[235] Michallet AS, Tartas S, Coiffier B: Optimizing management of tumor lysis syndrome in adults with hematologic malignancies. *Support Cancer Ther* 2005; 2: 159 - 66.

[236] Rioufol C, Coiffier B. Acute tumor lysis syndrome during oral fludarabine treatment for CLL – a rare event that might be observed more frequently in the future. *Onkologie* 2008; 31: 157 - 158.

[237] Montesinos P, Lorenzo I, Martín G, Sanz J, Pérez-Sirvent ML, Martínez D, Ortí G, Algarra L, Martínez J, Moscardó F, de la Rubia J, Jarque I, Sanz G, Sanz MA. Tumor lysis syndrome in patients with acute myeloid leukemia: identification of risk factors and development of a predictive model. *Haematologica* 2008; 93: 67 - 74.

[238] Nomdedeu J, Martino R, Sureda A, Huidobro G, Lopéz R, Brunet S, Domingo-Albós A. Acute tumor lysis syndrome complicating therapy for bone marrow transplantation in a patient with chronic lymphocytic leukemia. *Bone Marrow Transplant* 1994; 13: 659 - 660.

[239] Fleming DR, Henslee-Downey PJ, Coffey CW. Radiation-induced acute tumor lysis syndrome in the bone marrow transplant setting. *Bone Marrow Transplant* 1991; 8: 235 - 236.

[240] Chen SW, Hwang WS, Tsau CJ, Liu HS, Huang GC. Hydroxyurea and splenic irradiation-induced tumour lysis syndrome: a case report and review of the literature. *J Clin Pharm Ther*. 2005; 30: 623 - 625.

[241] Hochberg J, Cairo MS. Tumor lysis syndrome: current perspective. *Haematologica* 2008; 93: 9 - 13.

[242] Pui CH, Jeha S, Irwin D, Camitta B. Recombinant urate oxidase (rasburicase) in the prevention and treatment of malignancy-associated hyperuricemia in pediatric and adult patients: results of a compassionate-use trial. *Leukemia* 2001; 15: 1505 - 1509.

[243] Kersting S, Dorp SV, Theobald M, Verdonck LF. Acute renal failure after nonmyeloablative stem cell transplantation in adults. *Biol Blood Marrow Transplant*. 2008; 14: 125 - 131.

[244] Mae H, Ooi J, Takahashi S, Tomonari A, Tsukada N, Konuma T, Hongo E, Kato S, Kasahara S, Oiwa-Monna M, Kurokawa Y, Tojo A, Asano S. Early renal injury after myeloablative cord blood transplantation in adults. *Leukemia and Lymphoma* 2008; 49: 538 - 542.

[245] Cohen EP. Renal failure after bone-marrow transplantation. *Lancet* 2001; 357: 6 - 7.

[246] Kersting S, Hen\e RJ, Koomans HA, Verdonck LF. Chronic kidney disease after myelo-ablative allogeneic hematopoietic stem cell transplantation. *Biol Blood Marrow Transplant* 2007; 13: 1169 - 1175.

[247] Kersting S, Verdonck LF. Chronic kidney disease after nonmyeloablative stem cell transplantation in adults. *Biol Blood Marrow Transplant* 2008; 14: 403 - 408.

[248] Romagnani P, Lazzeri E, Mazzinghi B, Lasagni L, Guidi S, Bosi A, Cirami C, Salvadori M. Nephrotic syndrome and renal failure after allogeneic stem cell transplantation: Novel molecular diagnostic tools for a challenging differential diagnosis. *Am J Kidney Dis* 2005; 46: 550 - 556.

[249] Silva S, Maximino J, Henrque R, Paiva A, Baldaia, Campilho F, Pimentel P, Loureiro A. Minimal change nephrotic syndrome after stem cell transplantation: a case report and literature review. *J Med Case Reports* 2007; 1: 121 - 127.

[250] Humphreys BD, Vanguri V, HendersonJ, Antin JH. Minimal-change nephrotic syndrome in a hematopoietic stem-cell transplant recipient. *Nature Clin Pract Nephrol* 2006; 2: 535 - 539.

[251] Brukamp K, Doyle AM, Bloom RD, Bunin N, Tomaszewski JE, Čižman B. Nephrotic syndrome after hematopoietic cell transplantation: Do glomerular lesions represent renal Graft-versus-host disease? *Clin Am J Soc Nephrol* 2006; 1: 685 - 694.

[252] Sato Y, Hara S, Fujimoto S, Yamada K, Sakamaki H, Eto T. Minimal change nephrotic syndrome after allogenic hematopoietic stem cell transplantation. *Int Medicine* 2004; 43: 512 - 515.

[253] Ikehara S, Kawamura M, Takao F, Inaba M, Yasumizu R, Than S, Hisha H, Sugiura K, Koide Y, Yoshida T, Ida T, Imura H, Good RA. Organ-specific and systemic autoimmune diseases originate from defects in hematopoietic stem cells. *Proc Natl Acad Sci* 1990; 87: 8341 - 8344.

[254] Nishimura M, Toki J, Sugiura K, Hashimoto F, Tomita T, Fujishima H, Hiramatsu Y, Nishioka N, Nagata N, Takahashi Y, Ikehara S. Focal segmental glomerulosclerosis, a type of intractable chronic glomerulonephritis, is a stem cell disorder. *J Exp Med* 1994; 179: 1053 - 1058.

[255] Ritz E. Pathogenesis of "idiopathic" nephrotic syndrome. *N Engl J Med* 1994; 330: 61 - 62.

[256] Sellier-Leclerc A-L, Duval A, Riveron S, Macher M-A, Deschenes G, Loirat C, Verpont M-C, Peuchmaur M, Ronco P, Monteiro RC, Haddad E. A humanized mouse model of idiopathic nephrotic syndrome suggests a pathogenic role for immature cells. *J Am Soc Nephrol* 2007; 18: 2732 - 2739.

[257] Heras M, Saiz A, Sánchez R, Fernandez-Reyes MJ, Mampaso F, Queizán JA, Molina A, Vázquez L, Alvarez-Ude F. Nephrotic syndrome resulting from focal segmental glomerulosclerosis in a peripheral blood stem cell transplant patient. *J Nephrol* 2007; 20: 495 - 498.

[258] Chan GS, Lam MF, Au WY, Chim S, Tse KC, Lo SH, Fung SH, Lai KN, Chan KW. Clinicopathologic analysis of renal biopsies after haematopoietic stem cell transplantation. *Nephrology (Carlton)* 2008; 23: (Epub ahead of print).

[259] Chien YH, Lin KH, Lee TY, Lu MY, Tsau YK. Nephrotic syndrome in a bone marrow transplant recipient without chronic graft-versus-host disease. *J Formos Med Assoc* 2000; 99: 503 - 506.

[260] Chan GS, Chim S, Fan YS, Chan KW. Focal segmental glomerulosclerosis after membranous glomerulonephritis in remission: temporal diversity of glomerulopathy after bone marrow transplantation. *Hum Pathol* 2006; 37: 1607 - 1610.

[261] Perotta S, Conte ML, LaManna A, Indolfi P, Rossi F, Locatelli F, Nobili B. Membranous glomerulopathy in children given allogeneic hematopoietic stem cell transplantation. *Haematologica* 2005; 90: 89 - 91.

[262] Srinivasan R. Balow JE, Sabnis S, Lundqvist A, Igarashi T, Takahashi Y, Austin H, Tisdale AH, Barrett J, Geller N, Childs R. Nephrotic syndrome: an under-recognised immune-mediated complication of non-myeloablative allogenic haematopoietic cell transplantation. *Br J Haematol* 2005; 131: 74 - 79.

[263] Tsusumi C, Miyazaki Y, Fukushima T, Yoshida S, Taguchi J, Miyake C, Miyazaki M, Kohno S, Jinnai I, Tomonaga M. Membranous nephropathy after allogeneic stem cell transplantation: report of 2 cases. *Int J Hematol* 2004; 79: 193 - 197.

[264] Lin J, Markowitz GS, Nocolaides M, Hesdorffer CS, Appel GB, D'Agati VD, Savage DG. Membranous glomerulopathy associated with graft-versus-host dsease following allogeneic stem cell transplantation. Report of 2 cases and review of the literature. *Am J Nephrol* 2001; 21: 351 - 356.

[265] Sato N, Kishi K, Yagisawa K, Kasama J, Karasawa R, Shimada H, Nishi S, Ueno M, Ito K, Koike T, Takahashi H, Moriyama Y, Arakawa M, Shibata A. Nephrotic syndrome in a bone marrow transplant recipient with chronic-graft-versus-host disease. *Bone Marrow Transplant* 1995; 16: 303 - 305.

[266] Barbara JA, Thomas AC, Smith PS, Gillis D, Ho JO, Woodrofe AJ. Membranous nephropathy with graft-versus host disease in a bone marrow transplant recipient. *Clin Nephrol* 1992; 37: 115 - 8.

[267] Yorioka N, Taniguchi Y, Shimote K, Komo T, Yamakido M, Hyodo H, Kimura A, Taguchi T. Membranous nephropathy with chronic graft-versus host disease in a bone marrow transplant recipient. *Nephron* 1998; 80: 371 - 2.

[268] Hiesse C, Goldschmidt E, Santelli G, Charpentier B, Machover D, Fries D. Membranous nephropathy in a bone marrow transplant recipient. *Am J Kidney Dis* 1988; 11: 188 - 91.

[269] Cupelli L, Niscola P, Tendas A, Dentamoro T, Scaramucci L, Piccioni D, Perotti A, Palumbo R, deFabritiis P. Long term follow-up of a membranous glomerulopathy as late complication of chronic graft-versus-host disease folloeing allogeneic stem cell transplantation. *Int J Hematol* 2008; 87: 449 - 450.

[270] Colombo AA, Rusconi C, Esposito C, Bernasconi C, Caldera D, Lazzarino M, Alessandrino EP. Nephrotic syndrome after allogeneis hematopoietic stem cell transplantation as a late complication of chronic graft-versus-host disease. *Transplantation* 2006; 81: 1087 - 1092.

[271] Arat, Arslan O, Beksac M, Keven K, Nergizoglu G, Erturk S. Hematopoietic cell transplantation-related nephropathy. *Am J Kidney Dis* 2001; 38: 218 - 219.

[272] Stevenson WS, Nankivell BJ, Hertzberg MS. Nephrotic syndrome after stem cell transplantation. *Clinical Transplant* 2005; 19: 141 - 144.

[273] Terrier B, Delmas Y, Hummel A, Presne C, Glowacki F, Knebelmann B, Combe C, Lesavre P, Maillard N, Noël LH, Patey-Mariaud de Serre N, Nusbaum S, Radford I, Buzyn A, Fakhouri F. Post-allogeneic haematopoietic stem cell transplantation membranous nephropathy: clinical presentation, outcome and pathogenic aspects. *Nephrol Dial Transplant.* 2007; 22: 1369 - 1376.

[274] Troxell ML, Pilapil M, Miklos DB, Higgins JP, Kambham N. Renal pathology in hematopoietic cell transplantation recipients. *Modern Pathol* 2008; 21: 396 - 406.

[275] Suehiro T, Masutani K, Yokoyama M, Tokumoto M, Tsuruya K, Fukuda K, Kanai H, Katafuchi R, Nagatoshi Y, Hirakata H. Diffuse proliferative glomerulonephritis after bone marrow transplantation. *Clin Nephrol* 2002; 58: 231 - 237.

[276] Forslund T, Anttinen J, Hallman H, Heinonen K, Pitkänen R. Mesangial proliferative glomerulonephritis after autologous stem cell transplantation. *Am J Kidney Dis* 2006; 48: 314 - 320.

[277] Imasawa T, Utsunomiya Y. Stem cells in renal biology: bone marrow transplantation for the treatment of IgA nephropathy. *Exp. Nephrol* 2002; 10: 51 - 58.

[278] Kimura S, Horie A, Hiki Y, Yamamoto C, Suzuki S, Kuroda J, Deguchi M, Kato G-i, Karasuno T, Hiraoka A, Yoshikawa T, Maekawa T. Nephrotic syndrome with crescent formation and massive IgA deposition following allogeneic bone marrow transplantation for natural killer cell leukemia/lymphoma. *Blood* 2003; 101: 4219 - 4221.

[279] D'Amico G, Ferrario F. Mesangiocapillary glomerulonephritis. *Am Soc Nephrol* 1992;2:(Suppl 10): 159 - 66.

[280] Kemper MJ, Güngör T, Halter J, Schanz U, Neuhaus TJ. Favorable long-term outcome of nephrotic syndrome after allogeneic hematopoietic stem cell transplantation. *Clin Nephrol* 2007; 67: 5 - 11.

[281] Sakarcan A, Neuberg RW, McRedmond KP, Islek I. Membranoproliferative glomerulonephritis develops in a child with autologous stem cell transplant. *Am J Kidney Dis* 2002; 40: E19.

[282] Wheeler GE. Cyclophosphamide-associated leukemia in Wegener's granulomatosis. *Ann Intern Med* 1981; 94: 361 - 362.

[283] Kunitomi A, Ishikawa T, Tajima K, Konaka Y, Yagita M. Bone marrow transplantation with a reduced-intensity conditioning regimen in a patient with Wegener

granulomatosis and therapy-related leukemia. *In J Hematol* 2006; 83: 262 - 265.

[284] Faurschou M, Sørensen IJ, Mellemkjaer L, Loft AG, Thomsen BS, Tvede N, Baslund B. Malignancies in Wegener's granulomatosis: incidence and relation to cyclophosphamide therapy in a cohort of 293 patients. *J Rheumatol* 2008; 35: 100 - 105.

[285] Musette P, Labbaye C, Dorner M, Cayre YE, Casanova J-L, Kourilsky P. Wegener's autoantigen and leukemia. *Blood* 1991; 77: 1398 - 1399.

[286] van der Geld YM, Limburg PC, Kallenberg CG. Proteinase 3, Wegener's autoantigen: from gene to antigen. *J Leukoc Biol* 2001; 69: 177 - 190.

[287] Yong AS, Rezvani K, Savani BN, Eniafe R, Mielke S, Goldman JM, Barrett AJ. High PR3 or ELA2 expression by CD34+ cells in advanced-phase chronic myeloid leukemia is associated with improved outcome following allogeneic stem cell transplantation and may improve PR1 peptide-driven graft-versus leukemia effects. *Blood* 2007; 110: 770 - 775.

[288] Barrett J, Rezvani K. Neutrophil granule proteins as targets of leukemia-specific immune responses. *Curr Opin Hematol* 2006; 13: 15 - 20.

[289] Nouri-Majelan N, Sandgol H, Ghafari A, Rahimian M, Najafi F, Mortazavizadeh M, Moghaddasi S. Antineutrophil cytoplasmic antibody-associated glomerulonephritis in chronic graft-versus-host disease after allogenic hematopoietic stem cell transplantation. *Transplant Proc* 2005; 37: 3213 - 3215.

[290] Kingdon EJ, Johnston RE, Pawson R, Prentice HG, Potter MN, Burns A, Powis SH: ANCA+ vasculitis after autologous PBSC transplantation *Nephrol Dial Transplant* 2002;17: 285 - 287.

[291] Moschcowitz E. Hyaline thrombosis of the terminal arterioles and capillaries: a hitherto undescribed disease. *Proc N Y Pathol Soc* 1924; 24: 21 - 24.

[292] Gasser C, Gautier E, Steck A, Siebenmann RE, Oechslin R. Hämolytisch-urämische Syndrome: bilaterale Nierenrindennekrosen bei akuten erworbenen hämolytischen Anämien. *Schweiz Med Wochenschr* 1955; 85: 905 - 909.

[293] Lämmle B, Kremer Hovinga JA, Alberio L. Thrombotic thrombocytopenic purpura. *J Thromb Haemost* 2005; 3: 1663 - 1675.

[294] van der Plas RM, Schiphorst ME, Huizinga EG, Hene RJ, Verdonck LF, Sixma JJ, Fijnheer R. von Willebrand factor proteolysis is deficient in classic, but not in bone marrow transplantation-associated, thrombotic thrombocytopenic purpura. *Blood* 1999; 93: 3798 -802.

[295] Vesely SK, George JN, La¨ mmle B, Studt JD, Alberio L, El-Harake MA, Raskob GE. ADAMTS-13 activity in thrombotic thrombocytopenic purpura-hemolytic uremic syndrome: relation to presenting features and clinical outcomes in a prospective cohort of 142 patients. *Blood* 2003; 102: 60 - 68.

[296] Ruutu T, Barosi G, Benjamin RJ, Clark RE, George JN, Gratwohl A, Holler E, Iacobelli M, Kentouche K, Lämmle B, Moake JL, Richardson P, Socié G, Zeigler Z, Niederwieser D, Barbui T; European Group for Blood and Marrow Transplantation; European Leukemia Net. Diagnostic criteria for hematopoietic stem cell transplant-associated microangiopathy: results of a consensus process by an International Working Group. *Haematologica.* 2007; 92: 95 - 100.

[297] George JN, Li X, McMinn JR, Terrell DR, Vesely SK, Selby GB. Thrombotic thrombocytopenic purpura - hemolytic uremic syndrome following allogeneic HPC transplantation: a diagnostic dilemma. *Transfusion* 2004; 44: 294 - 304.

[298] González-Vicent M, Díaz MA, Madero L. An uncommon case of late thrombotic thrombocytopenic purpura (42 months) after autologous peripheral blood stem cell (PBSC) transplantation in a child. *Bone marrow transplant* 1999; 23: 735 - 736.

[299] Siami K, Kojouri K, Swisher KK, Selby GB, George JN, Laszik ZG. Thrombotic microangiopathy after allogeneic hematopoietic stem cell transplantation: an autopsy study. *Transplantation* 2008; 85: 22 - 28.

[300] Nakamae H, Yamane T, Hasegawa T, Nakamae M, Terada Y, Hagihara K, Ohta K, Hino M. Risk factor analysis for thrombotic microangiopathy after reduced-intensity or myeloablative allogeneic hematopoietic stem cell transplantation. *Am J Hematol* 2006; 81: 525 - 531.

[301] Shimoni A, Yeshurun M, Hardan I, Avigdor A, Ben-Bassat I, Nagler A. Thrombotic microangiopathy after allogeneic stem cell transplantation in the era of reduced-intensity conditioning: the incidence is not reduced. *Biol Blood Marrow Transplant* 2004; 10: 484 - 493.

[302] Kumar S, deLeve LD, Kamath PS, Tefferi A. Hepatic veno-occlusive disease (sinusoidal obstruction syndrome) after hematopoietic stem cell transplantation. *Mayo Clin Proc* 2003; 78: 589 - 598.

[303] Kist-van Holthe JE, Goedvolk CA, Brand R, van Weel MH, Bredius RG, van Oostayen JA, Vossen JM, van der Heijden BJ. Prospective study of renal insufficiency after bone marrow transplantation. *Pediatr Nephrol* 2002; 17: 1032 - 1037.

[304] Villalón L, Avello AG, César J, Odriozola J, López J, Oteyza JP, Laraña JG, Cantalapiedra A, Navarro JL. Is veno-occlusive disease a specific syndrome or the exacerbation of physiopathologic hemostatic changes in hematopoietic stem cell transplantation (HSCT)? *Thromb Res* 2000; 99: 439 - 446.

[305] Chang A, Hingorani S, Kowalewska J, Flowers ME, Aneja T, Smith KD, Meehan SM, Nicosia RF, Alpers CE. Spectrum of renal pathology in hematopoietic cell transplantation: a series of 20 patients and review of the literature. *Clin J Am Soc Nephrol* 2007; 2: 1014 - 1023.

[306] Ichida S, Okada K, Itoh M, Okada R, Katoh N, Kasai M, Yuzawa Y. Bone marrow transplant nephropathy successfully treated with angiotensin-converting enzyme inhibitor. *Clin Exp Nephrol* 2006; 10: 78 - 81.

[307] Osugi Y, Yamada H, Hosoi G, Noma H, Ikemiya M, Ishii T, Sako M. Treatment with candesartan combined with angiotensin-converting enzyme inhibitor for immunosuppressive treatment-resistant nephrotic syndrome after allogeneic stem cell transplantation. *Int J Hematol* 2006; 83: 454 - 458.

[308] Akar H, Keven K, Celebi H, Orhan D, Nergizoğlu G, Erbay B, Tulunay O, Ozcan M, Ertürk S. Nephrotic syndrome after allogeneic peripheral blood stem cell transplantation. *J Nephrol* 2002; 15; 79 - 82.

[309] Jurado M, Vallejo C, Pérez-Simón JA, Brunet S, Ferra C, Balsalobre P, Pérez-oteyza J, Espigado I, Romero A, Caballero D, Sierra J, Ribera JM, Díez JL. Sirolimus as part of immunosuppressive therapy for refractory chronic graft-versus-host disease. *Biol Blood Marrow Transplant* 2007; 13: 701 - 706.

[310] Oliveira JSR, Bahia D, Franco M, Balda C, Stella, Kerbauy J. Nephrotic syndrome as a clinical manifestation of graft-versus-host disease (GVHD) in a marrow transplant recipient after cyclosporine withdrawal. *Bone Marrow Transplant* 1999; 23: 99 - 101.

[311] Nakayama S, Yabe H, Nagai K. Nephrotic syndrome associated with chronic lymphocytic leukaemia successfully treated with interferon-alpha. *Jpn J Clin Haematol* 1990; 31: 1924 -8.

[312] Cutler C, Henry NL, Magee C, Li S, Kim HT, Alyea E, Ho V, Lee SJ, Soiffer R, Antin JH. Sirolimus and thrombotic microangiopathy after allogeneic hematopoietic stem cell transplantation. *Biol Blood Marrow Transplant* 2005; 11: 551 - 557.

[313] Au WY, Ma ES, Lee TL, Ha SY, Fung AT, Lie AK, Kwong YL. Successful treatment of thrombotic microangiopathy after haematopoietic stem cell transplantation with rituximab. *Br J Haematol* 2007; 137: 475 - 478.

[314] Musso M, Porretto F, Crescimanno A, Bondi F, Polizzi V, Scalone R, Iannitto E, Mariani G. Successful treatment of resistant thromotic thrombocytopenic purpura/hemolytic uremic syndrome with autologous peripheral blood stem cell and progenitor (CD34+) cell transplantation. *Bone Marrow Transplant* 1999; 24: 207 - 209.

[315] Humphreys BD, Soiffer RJ, Magee CC. Renal failure associated with cancer and its treatment: an update. *Am J Soc Nephrol* 2005; 16: 151 - 161.

[316] Ramirez P, DiPersio JF. Therapy options in imatinib failures. *The Oncologist* 2008; 13: 424 – 434.

[317] Copland M, Pellicano F, Richmond L, Allan EK, Hamilton A, Lee FY, Weinmann R, Holyoake TL. BMS-214662 potently induces apoptosis of chronic myeloid leukemia stem and progenitor cells and synergizes with tyrosine kinase inhibitors. *Blood* 2008; 111: 2843 - 2853.

[318] Sen R, Baltimore D. Inducibility of kappa immunoglobulin enhancer-binding protein Nf-kappa B by a posttranslational mechanism. *Cell* 1986; 47: 921 - 928.

[319] Brach MA, Kharbanda SM, Herrmann F, Kufe DW. Activation of the transcription factor kappa B in human KG-1 myeloid leukemia cells treated with 1-beta-D-arabinofuranosyl-cytosine. *Mol Pharmacol* 1992; 41: 60 - 63.

[320] Sreenivasan Y, Sarkar A, Manna SK. Mechanism of cytosine arabinoside-mediated apoptosis: role of REL A (p65) dephosphorylation. *Oncogene* 2003; 22: 4356 - 4369.

[321] Wang C-I, Mayo MW, Baldwin AS Jr. TNF and cancer therapy induced apoptosis: potentiation by inhibition of NF-kB. *Science* 1996; 274: 784 - 787.

[322] Boland MP, Foster SJ, O'Neill LA. Daunorubicin activates NFkappaB and induces kappaB-dependent gene expression in HL-60 promyelocytic and Jurkat T lymphoma cells. *J Biol Chem* 1997; 272: 12952 - 12960.

[323] Beg AA, Baltimore D. An essential role for NF-kB in preventing TNF-a induced cell death. *Science* 1996; 274: 782 - 784.

[324] Pineda-Roman M, Zangari M, van Rhee F, Anaissie E, Szymonifka J, Hoering A, Petty N, Crowley J, Shaughnessy J, Epstein J, Barlogie B. VTD combination therapy with bortezomib-thalidomide-dexamethasone is highly effective in advanced and refrectory multiple myeloma. *Leukemia* 2008; Apr 24 (Epub ahead of print).

[325] Attar EC, DeAngelo DJ, Supko JG, D'Amato F, Zarieh D, Sirulnik A, Wadleigh M, Ballen KK, McAfee S, Miller KB, Levine J, Galinsky I, Trehu EG, Schenkein D, Neuberg D, Stone RM, Amrein PC: Phase I and pharmacokinetic study of bortezomib in combination with idarubicin and cytarabine in patients with acute myelogenous leukemia. *Clin Cancer Res* 2008; 14: 1446 - 1454.

[326] Gil L, Styczynski J, Dytfeld D, Debski R, Kazmierczak M, Kolodziej B, Rafinska B, Kubicka M, Nowicki A, Komarnicki M, Wysocki M. Activity of bortezomib in adult de novo and relapsed acute myeloid leukemia. *Anticancer Res* 2007; 27: 4021 - 4025.

[327] Forslund T, Sikiö A, Anttinen J. IgA nephropathy in a patient with IgG lambda light-chain plasmacytoma: a rare coincidence. *Nephrol Dial Transplant* 2007; 22: 2705 - 2708.

[328] Malani AK, Gupta V, Rangineni R. Bortezomib and dexamethasone in previously untreated multiple myeloma associated with renal failure and reversal of renal failure. *Acta Haematol* 2006; 116: 255 - 258.

[329] Chanan-Khan AA, Kaufman JL, Mehta J, Richardson PG, Miller KC, Lonial S, Munshi NC, Schlossman R, Tariman J, Shinghal S. Activity and safety of bortezomib in multiple myeloma patients with advanced renal failure: a multicenter retrospective study. *Blood* 2007; 109: 2604 - 2606.

[330] Terpos E, Politou M, Rahemtulla A. Tumor lysis syndrome in multiple myeloma after bortezomib (VELCADE) administration. *J Cancer Res Clin Oncol* 2004; 130: 623 - 625.

[331] Byrd JC, Shinn C, Ravi R, Willis CR, Waselenko JK, Flinn IW, Dawson NA, Grever MR. Depsipeptide (FR901228): a novel therapeutic agent with selective, in vitro activity against human B-cell chronic lymphocytic leukemia cells. *Blood* 1999; 94: 1401 - 1408.

[332] Glaser KB. HDAC inhibitors: clinical update and mechanism-based potential. *Biochem Pharmacol* 2007; 74: 659 - 671.

[333] Arts J, Angibaud P, Mariën A, Floren W, Janssens B, King P, van Dun J, Janssen L, Geerts T, Tuman RW, Johnson DL, Andries L, Jung M, Janicot M, van Emelen K. R306465 is a novel potent inhibitor of class I histone deacetylases with broad-spectrum antitumoral activity against solid and haematological malignancies. *Br J Cancer* 2007; 97: 1344 - 1353.

[334] Dai Y, Chen S, Kramer LB, Funk VL, Dent P, Grant S. Interactions between bortezomib and romidepsin and belinostat in chronic lymphocytic leukemia cells. *Cli Cancer Res* 2008; 14; 549 - 558.

[335] Akiyama M, Hideshima T, Hayashi T, Tai YT, Mitsiades CS, Mitsiades N, Chauhan D, Richardson P, Munshi NC, Anderson KC. Nuclear factor-κB p65 mediates tumor necrosis factor α-induced nuclear translocation of telomerase reverse transcriptase protein. *Cancer Res* 2003; 63: 18 - 21.

[336] Sinha-Datta U, Horikawa I, Michishita E, Datta A, Sigler-Nicot JC, Brown M, Kazanji M, Barrett JC, Nicot C. Transcriptional activation of hTERT through the NFκB pathway in HTLV-1- transpformed cells. *Blood* 2004; 104: 2523 - 2531.

[337] Devemy E, Li B, Tao M, Horvath E, Chopra H, Fisher L, Nayini J, Creech S, Venugopal P, Yang J, Kaspar C, Hsu W, Preisler HD. Poor prognosis acute myelogenous leukemia:3-biological and molecular biological changes during remission induction therapy. *Leuk Res* 2001; 25: 783 - 791.

[338] Notaro R, Cimmino A, Tabarini D, Rotoli B, Luzatto L. In vivo telomere dynamics of human hematopoietic stem cells. *Proc Natl Acad Sci USA* 1997; 94: 13782 - 13785.

[339] Mathioudakis G, Storb R, McSweeney PA, Torok-Storb B, Lansdorp PM, Brümmendorf TH, Gass MJ, Bryant EM, Storek J, Flowers MED, Gooley T, Nash RA. Polyclonal hematopoiesis with variable telomere shortening in human long-term allogeneic marrow graft recipients. *Blood* 2000; 96: 3991 - 3994.

[340] Rufer N, Brümmendorf TH, Chapuis B, Helg C, Lansdorp PM, Roosnek E. Accelerated telomere shortening in hematological lineages is limited to the first year following stem cell transplantation. *Blood* 2001; 97: 575 - 577.

[341] Brummendorf TH, Rufer N, Baerlocher GM Roosnek E, Lansdorp PM. Limited telomere shortening in hematopoietic stem cells after transplantation. *Ann N Y Acad Sci* 2001; 938: 1 - 7; discussion 7 - 8.

[342] Harrison DE, Astle CM, Delaittre JA. Loss of proliferative capacity in immunohemopoietic stem cells caused by serial transplantation rather than aging. *J Exp Med* 1978; 147: 1526 -1531.

[343] Drummond MW, Balabanov S, Holyoake TL, Brümmendorf TH. Concise review: Telomere biology in normal and leukemic hematopoietic stem cells. *Stem Cells* 2007; 25: 1853 - 1861.

[344] Hermine O, Allard I, Levy V, Arnulf B, Gessain A, Bazarbachi A; French ATL therapy group. A prospective phase II clinical trial with the use of zidovudine and interferon-alpha in the acute and lymphoma forms of adult T-cell leukemia/lymphoma. *Hematol J.* 2002; 3: 276 - 282.

[345] Flandrin P, Guyotat D, Duval A, Cornillon J, Tavernier E, Nadal N, Campos L. Significance of heat-shock protein (HSP:) 90 expression in acute myeloid leukemia cells. *Cell Stress Chapreones* 2008; Apr.3. (E-pub ahead of print).

[346] Uehara Y. Natural product origins of HSP90 inhibitors. *Curr Cancer Drug Targets* 2003; 3: 325 - 330.

[347] Jeon YK, Park CH, Kim KY, Li YC, Kim J, Kim YA, Paik JH, Park BK, Kim CW, Kim YN. The heat-shock protein 90 inhibitor, geldanamycin, induces apoptotic cell death in Epstein-Barr virus-positive `MK/T-cell lymphoma by Akt down-regulation. *J Pathol* 2007; 213: 170 - 179.

[348] Al Shaer L, Walsby E, Gilkes A, Tonks A, Walsh V, Mills K, Burnett A, Rowntree C. Heat shock protein 90 inhibition is cytotoxic to primary AML cells expressing mutant FLT3 and results in altered downstream signalling. *Br J Haematol* 2008; 141: 483 - 493.

[349] Johnson AJ, Wagner AJ, Cheney CM, Smith LL, Lucas DM, Guster SK, Grever MR, Lin TS, Byrd JC. Rituximab and 17-allylamino-17-demethoxygeldanamycin induce synergistic apoptosis in B-cell chronic lymphocytic leukaemia. *Br J Haematol* 2007; 139: 837 - 844.

In: Encyclopedia of Stem Cell Research (2 Volume Set)   ISBN: 978-1-61761-835-2
Editor: Alexander L. Greene

ChapterXXVI

NEW INSIGHTS IN THE DEVELOPMENT OF BIOLOGICAL CHIMERAS: GENOMIC INSTABILITY AND EPITHELIAL CHIMERISM AFTER HEMATOPOIETIC STEM CELL TRANSPLANTATION

Alexandros Spyridonidis[1], Yannis Metaxas[2], Maria Themeli[1],
Hartmut Bertz[2], Nicholas Zoumbos[1] and Juergen Finke[2]*

[1]Division of Hematology, University of Patras Medical Center, Patras, Greece
[2]Department of Hematology and Oncology, Albert-Ludwigs University Medical Center,
Freiburg, Germany

ABSTRACT

Allogeneic hematopoietic stem cell transplantation (allo-HSCT) in humans results in true biological chimeras. While circulating hematopoietic and immune cells and their tissue derivatives (e.g., Kupffer cells, Langerhans cells) become donor genotype after transplantation, other cells remain recipient in origin. This unphysiological formation of biological chimeras is not free of consequences. The first sequel which has been recognized in the development of chimerical organisms after allo-HSCT is the graft versus host reaction, in which the new developed immune cells from the graft recognize the host's epithelial cells as foreign and kill them. There is now accumulating evidence that there are also other consequences in the co-existence of two genetically distinct populations in the transplant recipient. First, epithelial cells with donor-derived genotype emerge. Second, epithelial tissues of the host acquire genomic alterations. The current

---

* Correspondence concerning this article should be addressed to: A. Spyridonidis, M.D. Division of Hematology, University of Patras Medical Center, 26500 Rio/Patras, Greece. Tel: +30-2610-999247. Fax: +30-2610-993950; E-mail: spyridonidis@med.upatras.gr; Supported by Landesstiftung Baden Württemberg.

chapter discusses existing data on these recently discovered phenomena and focuses on their pathogenesis, clinical significance and therapeutic implications.

INTRODUCTION

Bone marrow (BM) consists one of the largest organs of our body. BM in adults has a weight of about 2.6 kg as compared to the 1.6 kg of the liver. The function of BM as the hematopoietic organ was first recognized in 1868 by Neumann in Germany and Bizzazero in Italy [1,2]. Nearly 70 years later, Lorenz and colleagues showed that the hematopoietic activity of BM is transplantable by demonstrating that mice receiving an intravenous infusion of BM could be protected from the lethal effects of ionizing irradiation on hematopoiesis [3]. The first attempts to translate this exciting discovery into the clinic were disappointing [4]. Further research in bigger animals led to the first successful clinical BM transplantations (BMT) in the late ´60s, especially from the group of E. Donall Thomas who was therefore acknowledged with the Nobel Prize in 1990 [4]. The last 30 years BMT has become a standard treatment for many hematological malignancies and is now increasingly used also as immunotherapy for the treatment of solid tumours [4,5]. Continuous experimental and clinical research led to further characterization and identification of the hematopoietic stem cells (HSC) within the BM leading to the refinement of this procedure which is now called Hematopoietic Stem Cell Transplantation (HSCT) or Hematopoietic Cell Transplantation (HCT).

As it is known, during allogeneic HCT (allo-HCT) the patient-recipient receives a preparative conditioning regimen (e.g., chemotherapy, radiotherapy) to destroy his hematopoiesis and immune system. This practice is followed by the administration of HSC harvested from the donor. The donor's HSC engraft, proliferate and finally reconstitute hematopoiesis in the recipient. The result is the creation of a biological chimera, a term used to describe the presence of tissues of different genetic origin in the same organism. The hematopoietic cells derive from the donor whilst the other tissues (e.g. epithelium) are genetically derived from the patient-recipient. This unphysiological formation of biological chimeras is not free of consequences. The first sequel which has been recognized in the development of chimeric organisms after allo-HCT is the graft versus host reaction (GvHR) in which the new developed immune cells from the graft recognize the host's epithelial cells as foreign and kill them [6]. There is now accumulating evidence that there are also other consequences in the co-existence of two genetically distinct populations in the transplant recipient. First, epithelial cells with donor-derived genotype emerge, a phenomenon which was initially misinterpreted and falsely described as "stem cell plasticity". Second, epithelial tissues of the host acquire genomic alterations. In the following we discuss existing data on these recently discovered phenomena occurring after allogeneic HCT and focus on their pathogenesis, clinical significance and their clinical and therapeutic implications.

A. EPITHELIAL CHIMERISM AFTER ALLOGENIC HCT

Since the first experiments in mice performed by Lorenz et al., [3] researchers continued to perform murine and other animal bone marrow transplantations in order to understand this procedure in detail. The research was mainly focused on the hematopoiesis and immune-reconstitution in the transplanted animals and little attention has been paid to the effects of the Hematopoietic Cell Transplantation (HCT) on the non-hematopoietic tissues such as epithelium. A surprising result in 1998 revolutionized the bone marrow transplantation field and stem cell research. Ferrari et al., [7] presumed that fibroblasts, cells which normally make connective tissue, could also transdifferentiate to muscle cells. Therefore, the researchers injected purified fibroblasts in chemically-damaged muscles of mice and as controls they injected BM cells devoid of fibroblasts. To their surprise, new muscle cells were generated only in the mice that got the BM without the fibroblasts. This finding led to the speculation that BM is the source of tissue-specific stem cells. Indeed, a series of experimental hematopoietic cell transplantations performed in animals soon after the report by Ferrari et al. showed that the infusion of unfractionated bone marrow cells or bone-marrow cell subsets with high hematopoietic activity into irradiated mice, gave rise to hepatocytes, skin cells, pneumocytes, intestinal epithelium, pancreas cells, skeletal muscle, myocardium, neurons, and endothelium of donor origin[8-12]. Typically, in those experiments donor cells expressed either green fluorescent protein (GFP) or β-galactosidase (β-gal) and tissue-specific donor-derived cells after the transplantation were detected by expression of these markers in the tissue(s) of interest. These experimental animal results led to the exploration of similar events in humans. In humans, scientists mostly studied sex-mismatched allogeneic transplanted women and searched for Y+/tissue-specific cells. Indeed, many studies suggested the generation of donor-derived hepatocytes, cholangiocytes and colonic cells, among other epithelial cells [13-15]. Moreover, some of them claimed that up to 17% of the epithelial cells found were of donor origin. These initial reports proposing the robust generation of epithelial cells after murine or human HCT were published in reputable journals, and revealed probable new aspects of ontogenesis while also engendered expectations for novel therapies both in the scientific and the popular press. However, at the same time a significant number of studies failed to detect donor-derived epithelial cells after allo-HCT in similar experimental systems [16-18]. The debate on the developmental potential of adult hematopoietic stem cells became even more confusing since terms implicating mechanisms, such as "plasticity" and "transdifferentiation", were used in order to describe the above mentioned observations. To minimize confusion scientists started to use more precise terms in order to describe their findings. Epithelial chimerism or tissue-specific chimerism, like "myocardial chimerism", is used when cells obtained from hematopoietic tissues of a donor are transplanted into a host, and then marked donor cells are identified as epithelial cells in the host. On the other hand, the term "plasticity" is a functional characterization and is used only if stringent criteria are fulfilled, such as robust detection of epithelial chimerism, documentation of functionality of the chimerical epithelial cells and clonal analysis of the chimerical cells to verify their origin from a hematopoietic stem cell [19].

These new findings in HCT opened a new and very exciting era for intensive research for both stem cell biologists and clinicians. Moreover, it raised a significant number of questions to be answered. Does epithelial chimerism after HSC represent a real phenomenon? If epithelial chimerism really exists, is it an incidental by-product of transplantation without ancillary biological significance or does it have any clinical consequences? How does epithelial chimerism after HCT occur and which patterns does it follow? Are the chimerical epithelial cells functional and may HCT contribute to non-hematopoietic tissue repair? Adult hematopoietic stem cells do really transdifferentiate into non-hematopoietic lineages?

Epithelial Chimerism after Allogeneic HCT is Real

Initial studies claiming to detect epithelial chimerism (or even more plasticity) after HCT were treated with doubt, because of methodological limitations. Alternative explanations were given for some of the suspected chimeric events found within histological sections. In animal models, the unanticipated endogenous β-gal signal might lead to false positive results when ROSA mice are used as donors for HCT [20,21]. Lymphocytes entering epithelial tissues via the circulation, might act as "contaminants" and be easily mistaken as donor-derived epithelial cells, if the expression of hematopoietic markers is not examined. Tissue macrophages can down-regulate the expression of hematopoietic specific markers (CD45+) and therefore escape their detection as hematopoietic cells, if appropriate macrophage specific markers are not used [22]. Furthermore, in recent years it became clear that microscopic examinations of tissues may be tricky. Tissue is a compact, three-dimensional structure and this has to be taken in mind when interpretating the results of microscopic examinations. Indeed, overlapping cells in histological sections may produce artefacts showing marker co-localisation apparently within the same cell, although the markers are actually expressed in different cells [23]. Furthermore, the detection of tissue chimerism in female patients by the Y-chromosome is complicated by the fact that Y-chromosome material has been also found in maternal tissues from women which had a male fetus or had received blood transfusions from male donors [24]. These studies clearly show that detection of epithelial chimerism after HCT is not straightforward and requires unequivocal detection systems, like the use of combined stains within a single section and the use of laser scanning confocal and deconvolution microscopic methods for three dimensional analysis.

Despite the above methodological limitations, several carefully designed studies in recent years demonstrated that epithelial chimerism after HCT may in fact occurs. In an elegant study Spyridonidis et al [23] applied a three-dimensional analysis on single colon sections from transplanted women after triple stain with donor specific, epithelial-specific and hematopoietic-specific markers, and could clearly show that epithelial chimerism after human HCT is a real phenomenon. This study was in accordance to other studies which strongly implied similar events in a human setting [15,23,25-27]. Because, as mentioned before, cells can wrap one another making tissue analysis very difficult, scientists further analysed isolated single epithelial cells for their origin after transplantation. Tran et al [28] and Metaxas et al [29] found that isolated buccal epithelial cells obtained by oral scraping from allo-transplanted women, contained the Y-chromosome within their nucleus, as detected by FISH, suggesting that HCT results in generation of individual epithelial cells with donor-derived genotype.

Are the Chimeric Epithelial Cells Functional?

The finding that transplanted cells derived from adult hematopoietic tissues are directly involved in the generation of epithelial cells raises the question of whether the generated cells are functional and whether HCT could functionally contribute to tissue repair by replacing damaged epithelia. In some animal HCT models, liver cells, pneumocytes and kidney tubular epithelial cells bearing donor specific DNA were found to express mRNA-albumin, mRNA-surfactant B and a specific cytochrome P450 enzyme (CYP1A2) respectively, indicating an appropriate cellular function [14]. However, since these cells appeared as isolated single cells it seems unlikely that they play an important role in the homeostasis, regeneration and function of epithelial tissue, at least in the setting of clinical HCT. In 2000, Lagasse et al., [30] went a step further by demonstrating a robust and functional epithelial chimerism in a mice model of fatal hereditary tyrosinemia type I. The researchers performed transplantations of purified hematopoietic stem cells from ROSA wild-type mice to transgenic mice homozygous deficient for fumarylacetoacetate hydrolase (FAH–/–). These mice show progressive liver failure and renal tubular damage unless treated with 2-(2-nitro-4-trifluoro-methylbenzyol)-1,3-cyclohexanedione (NTBC). Three weeks after transplantation, they discontinued NTBC to allow selection of liver repopulating cells. They found that in contrast to control mice the transplanted mice survived the NTBC withdrawal and seemed clinically healthy. The liver of the survived mice revealed a high amount of donor-derived cells, presented as ß-gal+ nodes within damaged liver and making about 30–50% of the liver mass. Taken together, the results indicated that the donor-derived chimeric cells were responsible for the survival of the mice. The restoration of liver function through HCT in mice suffering from a lethal liver disease is a ground-breaking experiment, which has been reproduced in several laboratories [31,32], and proves that murine HC-derived cells are directly involved in the generation of functional hepatocytes. In a similar experimental model, Hess et al., [33] could restore damaged pancreatic function of streptozocin treated mice by transplantation of *c-kit+* BM stem cells. Many studies since then were performed in order to find out the mechanism by which HCT may restore liver and pancreas function and rescue the mice. In the FAH-/- model hematopoietic cells were involved in the generation of functional hepatocyte-like cells through fusion. In the streptozocin treated mice the authors suggested that the HCT initiated the proliferation of endogenous pancreatic cells. A "paracrine effect" of BM-derived cells through release of cytokines within the damaged organ, or induction of neovascularization from BM-derived endothelial cells [34] are two possible mechanisms which may explain how the transplantation induced the endogenous tissue repair processes.

Aiming to find out whether besides murine HSC also human HSC has the potential to restore damaged organ function, Wang et al., [35] examined liver repopulation by human HSC in xenograft models. The authors treated NOD/SCID and NOD/SCID/β_2 microglobulin-null mice with carbon tetrachloride (CCl$_4$) in order to induce liver damage and then transplanted them with highly purified human hematopoietic stem cells. One month after transplantation the researchers detected human albumin in the serum of the mice, indicating that human derived albumin-secreting cells emerged. When they analyzed tissue sections of the liver, they detected human albumin along with human DNA sequences on hepatocyte-like liver cells. Almeida et al., [36] performed similar studies in a mammalian non-injury model as they analyzed liver sections of sheep having undergone *in utero* HCT from human cells. As in the study of Wang, the researchers detected human hepatocyte-like cells and human albumin in the transplanted sheep.

Such reports suggesting that HCT may functionally contribute to non-hematopoietic tissue regeneration and restoration of damaged organ, stimulated investigators to seek rapid clinical translation. Human clinical trials investigating regenerative properties of HC-derived adult cells have already been started, especially in patients with heart diseases [37,38]. However, for the clinical application of hematopoietic cells for regenerative purposes much remains to be determined. Whether observations made in selected experimental models also happen in humans is unclear. More importantly, the exact mechanism into how transplanted cells may actually improve organ function has not been elucidated. On the other side, such procedures may in fact cause opposite effects than tissue regeneration. In a very elegant study in mice, Houghton et al., [39] showed that transplanted bone marrow cells may transform into cancer cells under conditions of chronic inflammatory signals. The researchers used a Helicobacter felis (H. felis) C57BL/6 mouse strain which develops severe chronic gastritis and intestinal metaplasia after infection with H. felis [40]. These mice underwent bone marrow transplantation from ROSA26 transgenic mice expressing a non-mammalian β-galactosidase enzyme, so that bone marrow cells could be tracked by X-galactosidase (Xgal) staining. After hematopoietic reconstitution, the C57BL/6 mice were infected with H. felis, resulting in chronic inflammation of their gastric mucosa. The researchers observed that over time the dysplasia of the epithelium increased in severity, finally ending in the development of gastric cancer. When they examined sections of the gastric carcinoma they noticed that the majority of the glands stained blue with X-gal indicating their donor origin. A very recent study by Cogle et al., [41] supported these results, even in a human setting, although the mechanisms suggested for the occurrence of the phenomenon differed between the two studies. Houghton et al based on their observations of the numerous donor-derived cancer cells proposed the bone marrow as a source for epithelial cancer, whereas Cogle et al., for the exact opposite reason thought that bone-marrow cells rather adopt a cancerous phenotype via developmental mimicry.

Factors Contributing to the Development of Epithelial Chimerism after Allogeneic HCT

Epithelial chimerism after HCT is a rare and focal event with less than 1%, and probably less than 0.1%, of the overall tissue epithelial cells to contain donor genetic material. The reported higher incidence of epithelial chimerism found in some human studies (up to 17%) is most likely a methodological artefact resulting from counting the intraepithelial lymphocytes within the tissue as donor-derived epithelial cells. Although epithelial chimerism has been found in most of the epithelial tissues tested irrespective of the presence or absence of tissue damage, it seems that injury and high cell turnover play a role both in the occurrence and extent of chimeric events [8,30,42]. Most studies suggest that the more the degree of the tissue damage the greater the percentage of the detected chimeric cells [29,42-44]. For example the percentage of the buccal chimeric cells in the allo-transplanted patients has been found to significantly correlate with the degree of oral mucositis in the early post transplantation period [29]. A recent study aimed to determine the degree of tissue damage required to produce chimeric events [45]. They used a mouse model having undergone allogeneic HCT and estimated the chimeric lung epithelial cells after various doses of irradiation. They concluded that only doses causing apparent tissue damage led to emergence of chimeric lung cells. A possible scenario explaining these results is that bone-marrow derived cells support tissue homeostasis when the extent of damage overwhelms the endogenous capacity of tissue regeneration.

Another critical factor for the development of chimerism in non-hematopoietic tissues is the type of tissue itself. It is suggested that the presence as well as the extent of this phenomenon is taking place in a tissue-dependent manner [46], with some tissues favouring the development of chimerical cells and others not. To further support this notion, a recent study addressed the presence of donor-derived epithelial cells in multiple organs after HCT in murine embryos. They concluded that the different types of analyzed tissues showed variable degrees of chimerical events, although hematopoietic engraftment was always the same [47]. This could be attributed to micro-environmental cues provided by the tissue, which could induce a cell fate change in bone-marrow derived cells [48,49]. Finally, there could be other factors affecting the emergence of epithelial chimerism, such as time elapsed after HCT. Herzog et al. [45] in mice and Metaxas et al. [29] in humans showed that time after HCT correlated positively with the degree of chimeric epithelial cells detected. Whatever the factors contributing to epithelial chimerism might be, they shed no light on the exact mechanisms responsible for this phenomenon.

Plasticity of Bone-Marrow Derived Cells?

Krause et al., [50] demonstrated that a single cell capable of long-term reconstitution of hematopoiesis in lethally irradiated mice was also capable of differentiating into epithelial cells of the liver, lung, gastrointestinal tract and skin. The researchers used a membrane bound dye (PKH26) along with the stem cell markers CD34 and SCA-1 to track hematopoietic stem cells in sex-mismatched serial transplantations. After transplanting a first series of female mice with such cells isolated from male donors and establishing long-term hematopoiesis in them, they subsequently transplanted single hematopoietic stem cells from their bone marrow to a second series of female mice. They sacrificed those secondary recipients after having established long-term repopulation of the hematopoietic system and evaluated different epithelial tissues for the presence of donor-derived non-hematopoietic cells. They detected such cells in different percentages, with the higher numbers being present in the alveoli of the lungs. These results suggested that in the adult bone marrow resides a cell(s) capable of both reconstituting the hematopoietic lineage and differentiating to non-hematopoietic cells, making the study of Krause et al. the best example of possible plasticity potential of hematopoietic stem cells. However, even this elegant study had some limitations and could not fulfil the previously mentioned criteria for demonstration of plasticity. First, there was no 3D analysis of the examined tissues and there was no analysis of single chimeric cells; therefore overlapping events and hematopoietic "contaminants" residing within the examined tissue could not be unequivocally excluded. Second, there was no detection of robust epithelial chimerism. Third, although the researchers searched for tissue-specific genes, there was no clear evidence regarding the function of the chimeric cells. Fourth, there was no clonal analysis of the chimeric cells. And finally, the conclusion that "transdifferentiation" occurred, which was based on the detection of donor-derived epithelial cells after transplantation of a single hematopoietic cell, is not beyond question, since contaminants in the purified cell population cannot be entirely excluded. Taken together, the study of Krause et al lies very close, but the unambiguous proof of epithelial chimerism after HCT due to developmental plasticity and transdifferentiation of hematopoietic cells has not been clearly given. Transdifferentiation is observed in lower vertebrates [51] and in some in vitro experiments with adult mammalian cells, but has been never clearly and unequivocally demonstrated that such an event could also occur naturally *in vivo*. Recently, Takahashi et al [52] went a step further to this direction by demonstrating that differentiated fibroblasts can re-differentiate *in vitro* to embryonic-like stem cells, which are subsequent able to give rise *in vivo* to whole mice when injected to blastocysts. Now other studies emerge in accordance to this new concept [53,54], and it remains to be seen, if this phenomenon could take place in a large scale setting in *in vivo* experiments.

Possible Mechanisms Underlying Epithelial Chimerism

Other mechanisms have been suggested in order to explain how epithelial chimerism after HCT occurs. Avital et al., [55] and Ratajczak et al., [56] found cells in the BM and peripheral blood that express various early markers for hepatocytes (albumin, HNF-4, C/Eba, CYP3A2, CK19, fetoprotein) myocytes (Myf-5, MyoD), and neurons (GFAP, nestin), suggesting that tissue specific progenitors may exist in the BM and may also circulate in the blood. Others speculated that a universal type of stem cell, akin to an embryonic stem cell, exists in adult BM. Verfaillie et al. isolated "multipotent adult progenitor cells" (MAPCs) in the murine and human bone marrow capable to differentiate both in vitro and in vivo to various cell types such as muscle, cartilage, bone, liver, and different types of neurons and brain cells [57]. However, this work has not been replicated from other groups in its entirety [58] and Verfaillie et al. recently published some corrections of their initial work regarding mainly the detectable surface proteins of the presumed differentiated progenies of MAPCs [59]. Recently, the group of Ratajczak described another rare population of pluripotent stem cells in adult mice bone marrow [60] and in human cord blood [61] naming them Very Small Embryonic Like cells (VSELs) and having the phenotype CD45-/Lin-/CXCR4+/Oct-4+/Nanog+/SSEA- 1+. [62]. The authors showed that these cells have morphology and a phenotype similar to embryonic stem cells and possess the capacity to differentiate into all three germ lines in cultures *in vitro*. There is evidence that MAPCs and VSELs may be the same cell, as sharing many of their markers [63]. However, it is not unambiguously shown whether this capacity exist in a significant percentage *in vivo* or is induced mainly through *in vitro* manipulation [64].

Another proposed mechanism aiming to explain epithelial chimerism after allogeneic HCT is the fusion of bone-marrow derived stem cells with tissue-specific differentiated cells.

However, different studies exploring this probability have yielded contradictory results. Vassilopoulos et al., [65] showed that in FAH–/– mice fusion was the principal mechanism for the generation of chimeric liver cells, and Wang et al., [66] agreed. However, in uninjured tissues fusion events are shown in a far smaller percentage [11]. Perhaps the liver regeneration in the FAH–/– liver favours the formation of heterokaryons through fusion, which could not be the case in other tissues. Furthermore, other studies in animal models using Cre/lox technology implied that fusion events may generally not occur during the generation of epithelial chimerism [12]. The results of our own group, where we detected only one X-chromosome in chimeric Y-chromosome positive buccal cells after male to female transplantation, were consisted with non-fusion mechanism for the generation of epithelial chimerism in humans [67] However, both studies have serious limitations since the Cre-recombinase enzyme is not expressed in all cells and X-chromosomes could be lost after cell fusion [35,68].

Table 1. Studies showing either epithelial chimerism or functionality of chimeric cells or plasticity potential of hematopoietic stem cells in animal and human setting

Epithelial Chimerism		Functional Epithelial Chimerism		Plasticity potential	
animal	human	animal	human	animal	human
Jang et al. Ianus et al. Mezey et al. Harris et al.	Alison et al. Theise et al. Körbling et al. Tran et al. Metaxas et al. Spyridonidis et al.	Lagasse et al. Wang et al. Houghton et al.	never shown	Krause et al.	never shown

Recent findings suggest a novel mechanism explaining epithelial chimerism after allogeneic HCT. Jang et al., [8] found that when murine hematopoietic stem cells, enriched through phenotypical and functional assays (Fr25lin- PKH+ 2-d homed HSC), were co-cultured with injured liver separated by a barrier they may convert into liver-like cells. In a similar experimental system, Quesenberry et al., [69] found that injured lung tissue induced *in vitro* bone marrow cells to express lung proteins. When these *in vitro* converted bone marrow cells were transplanted into lethally irradiated mice they were found again as type II pneumocytes. The group of Quesenberry went a step further and tried to find out which factors from the injured lung tissue induce the ectopic expression of lung proteins on bone marrow derived cells. Ultracentrifugation of the lung-conditioned medium revealed that the fraction able to induce lung-protein expression was the one which contained microvesicles carrying lung-specific mRNA. These microvesicles showed the ability to enter into subpopulations of the marrow cells thus mediating the marrow cell phenotype conversion. The authors suggest that the cell cycle status of the stem cells might relate to the ease of microvesicle cell entry into them. Thus, a possible scenario after HCT is that hematopoietic stem cells engraft in the tissues, incorporate microvesicles containing tissue-specific mRNA released from the tissue in case of injury and alter this way their phenotype leading to the observed epithelial chimerism.

Another mechanism explaining epithelial chimerism after allogeneic HCT which needs further exploration is horizontal gene transfer [70]. In this case, genetic material released from the hematopoietic-derived donor cells will be transferred, incorporated into the nucleus and eventually expressed by the recipient epithelial cell, ultimately leading to the emergence of epithelial cells with donor-derived genome. Horizontal gene transfer is well described in prokaryotic organisms as a mechanism for functional and phenotypic change in order to adapt to different enviromental conditions [71]. Horizontal gene transfer has also been shown in eukaryotic organisms both *in vitro* and *in vivo* [70,72]. Large fragments of plasmid DNA fed to mice passed into the bloodstream and integrated into the nucleus of white blood cells, spleen and liver cells [73].

Table 2. Proposed mechanisms for the development of epithelial chimerism

Possible Mechanism	Reference
tissue-specific progenitors in the bone marrow	Avital et al.
multipotent adult progenitor cells, very small embryonic like cells	Verfaillie et al., Ratajczak et al.
fusion	Vassilopoulos et al., Wang et al.
transdifferentiation of terminally differentiated cells	Brockes et al, Takahashi et al.
Horizontal transfer of tissue-specific microvesicles	Quesenberry et al.

B. GENOMIC INSTABILITY IN EPITHELIUM AFTER ALLOGENIC HCT

DNA is a reactive molecule and constantly attacked and modified by external and internal agents. A mammalian DNA molecule can undergo about 100.000 modifications per day and replicates with an error rate of one error per 10^{10} nucleotides [76]. Genome integrity is a basic element of the cellular homeostasis. To maintain genome integrity and ensure its stable inheritance during their replication, cells are equipped with several mechanisms, including DNA repair mechanisms, cell-cycle checkpoints and programmed cell death [77]. The term genomic instability (GI) describes the failure to transmit an accurate copy of the entire genome from one cell to its two daughter cells. The existence of genomic instability is a sign of the above mechanisms' failure, and has been correlated with cancer and cancerous transformation [78].

Microsatellites (MS) are short tandem repeat sequences (repeat units range from 1-6 bp in length) dispersed throughout the genome. There are more than 1 million MS loci in the human genome which comprises approximately 3% of the genome. MS are among the most variable types of DNA sequence in the genome. Their polymorphism derives mainly from variability in length rather than in primary sequence. Though highly polymorphic, as their length varies in a population, they are inherited stably and are unique to each individual, which means that the length of a MS is the same in all the cells of the same person [79]. For this reason the detection of different MS polymorphisms with PCR-based assays can be used for linkage mapping, paternity test, forensic purposes as well as for chimerism quantification after allo-HCT [79,80]. The term MS instability (MSI) describes alterations in the length of a MS locus detected by PCR amplification of an individual's DNA [77]. The detection of MSI is considered to be indicative of a general genomic instability -which means the accumulation of mutations in the cells- and has been related to carcinogenesis [79,81]. MSI was first detected and described in individuals with a type of hereditary colon cancer (HNPCC, hereditary non-polyposis colorectal carcinoma) which is caused by mutation of DNA-mismatch-repair gene MSH2 [81]. Besides HNPCC, MSI has also been reported in several sporadic cancers (colorectal, bladder, skin, lung, ovarian) [81-84]. Recently, MSI has also been observed in chronic inflammatory diseases such as ulcerative colitis and rheumatoid arthritis [85,86]. The exact mechanisms through which chronic inflammation may lead to these genomic alterations are the subject of continuing debate. The biologic significance of genomic instability in chronic inflammation settings is yet unknown. Whilst in ulcerative colitis MSI has been associated with increased cancer risk [87], there is no such indication in rheumatoid arthritis [86].

After allogeneic HCT, epithelial tissues become injured through the preparative regimen and are then potentially attacked by alloreactive T cells. Graft-versus-host (GvH) reactions are complex processes developing after allo-HCT involving recruitment of alloreactive T-lymphocytes, release of cytokines (TNF-α, IL-1), production of free radicals and cellular cytotoxicity, among others [6,88]. The net effect of these alloantigeneic reactions is tissue stress and apoptosis which we recognize clinically as GvH-disease (GvHD). Transplant survivors, especially those who suffer from chronic GvHD, are at risk for the development of secondary epithelial cancers [89]. The pathogenesis of solid tumours post-transplant is unknown.

Faber et al. [90] hypothesized that chronic tissue stress due to interaction of donor-derived lymphocytes with host epithelium in the biological chimeras developed after HCT may cause genomic alterations and therefore analysed epithelial tissues from allo-transplanted patients at molecular level. The authors found frequent genomic alterations measured as MSI in non-neoplastic epithelial tissues of patients who underwent allogeneic HCT. These genomic alterations were found only in allo-transplanted patients but not after autologous HCT or intensive chemotherapy, and therefore they suggested that allogeneic reactions after allo-HCT, e.g., GvH reactions, are substantially involved in the mutation process. In subsequent analyses performed in additional 70 patients who underwent allo-HCT, the authors confirmed their previous results by demonstrating GI in non-neoplastic tissues of nearly 50% of the allo-transplanted patients, especially in old recipients and those who suffered from chronic GvHD (unpublished results). The observation that biological chimeras after allo-HCT acquire genomic alterations initiates scientific questions and opens a new investigation field.

What does the GI found in non-neoplastic tissues after transplantation point out? Replication errors during DNA synthesis occur with a certain probability in all cells and may result in a change of the length of MS loci, which are sequences particularly prone to DNA polymerase slippage because of their repetitive nature [79,91,92]. The mismatch repair (MMR) system recognizes and corrects these genomic alterations [76]. Whenever the DNA error cannot be repaired, apoptosis pathways are activated [77]. Thus, cells with MS alterations which escaped repair will not replicate and therefore in molecular studies should not become apparent among the large excess of the surrounding normal cells [93]. However, if deficient DNA repair is coupled with a failure to elicit an apoptotic response, this association may result in a growth advantage sufficient to generate a detectable clonal population of cells that share genetic alterations. Therefore, the detection of MSI in clinical samples indicates the presence of a cell population which i) was exposed to a factor which caused MSI, ii) failed to repair the genetic damage through their DNA repair mechanisms, iii) did not go to apoptosis through activation of DNA-damage checkpoints and finally iv) multiplied and perhaps acquired a growth advantage so as to create a detectable clonal population (Figure 1).

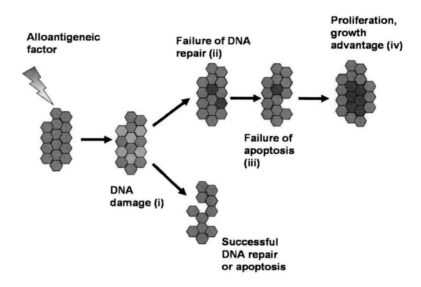

Figure 1. Emergence of genomic instable clones after allogeneic HCT. (i) A cell population is constantly exposed to an allogeneic factor which causes DNA damage (ii) Some cells fail to repair DNA damage through DNA repair mechanisms. (iii) Failure of apoptosis of damaged cells through DNA-damage checkpoints activation. (iv) Proliferation of damaged cells and perhaps acquisition of growth advantage so as to create a detectable clonal population.

i) Factors Inducing GI in the Allotransplanted Recipients

As mentioned before, MSI in non-neoplastic epithelial tissues has been found only in patients treated with myeloablative or reduced-intensity chemotherapy and allogeneic HCT but not in patients after myelosuppressive chemotherapy or myeloablative chemotherapy combined with autologous HCT. In addition, MSI was found also many years after HCT [90]. It is very likely that the alloantigeneic GvH reactions and the following tissue stress could be the the driving force in producing detectable MSI in the allografted patients. Several hypotheses could be made on which of the elements of this inflamed environment could be responsible for causing MSI and by which mechanism. During GvHD, donor activated lymphocytes and macrophages are recruited in the patient's tissues [6,88]. These activated cells produce mediator molecules such as cytokines (IFN-γ, TNF-α, IL-1 etc) and reactive oxygen species (ROS) such as H_2O_2, $OH^{\cdot}$, $O_2^{\cdot}$. These factors have been shown to cause DNA damage in various experimental systems [94].

ROS can cause base pair mutations, deletions and insertions among other DNA structural alterations through different mechanisms [94]. Oxidants have been shown to induce mutations directly by chemical modification of DNA bases or conformational change of DNA that diminishes the accuracy of DNA polymerases [94]. *In vitro* experiments demonstrated that H_2O_2 can cause induction of MSI not only in MMR-deficient but also at higher concentrations in MMR-proficient human colorectal cancer cell lines [95]. Thus, even with an intact MMR system free radicals produced in inflamed tissues could cause such direct DNA damage which overwhelms the capacity of repair pathways. Oxidants may also facilitate the accumulation of mutations and the creation of MSI indirectly by oxidative damage of DNA repair proteins [96] or through DNA methylation and silencing of DNA repair genes [97]. Besides the effect of oxidants in the DNA repair machinery, ROS may also alter the DNA-damage checkpoints such as p53, facilitating this way the survival of cells with genomic alterations [98].

Inflammatory cytokines may also induce DNA damage in epithelial cells [99,100]. A nitric oxide (NO) pathway is mainly involved in the cytokine-induced DNA damage. Cytokines such as TNF-α and IFN-γ, which are released in increased amounts in GvHD areas, may cause activation of nuclear factor κB (NFκB) which induces the expression of iNOS (inducible NO synthase) in the epithelial cells. NO produced by cytokine activated cells can be auto-oxidized leading to the formation of reactive radicals called reactive nitrogen species (RNS) which, like ROS, are mutagenic agents with the potential to chemically modify DNA bases by deamination, nitration or oxidation. In addition, NO may affect DNA repair processes by inhibiting DNA repair enzymes through sulfhydryl-nitrosylation of cystein residues of their DNA binding sites [94,99]. Therefore, NO might be another key player in the induction of MSI after allo-HCT. NO may indeed be the link between chronic alloantigeneic stimulation, relaxation of DNA repair mechanisms and GvHD induced genomic instability. NO has been shown to be an important mediator in GvHD pathology [88]. Increased levels of circulating NO characterize GvHD and iNOS inhibition leads to decreased GvHD severity in animal models [101,102]. In addition, plasma levels of NO have been associated with GvHD severity in humans [103].

Taken together, oxidative stress like the one produced in the biological chimera due to the interaction between donor T cells and host epithelium may lead to accumulation of genomic alterations in the recipient cells either by overwhelming the capacity for DNA repair or by directly inactivating DNA repair pathways.

ii) Failure of DNA Repair

The presence of MSI in non-neoplastic tissues after allo-HCT means that a replication error occurred and escaped from the DNA repair mechanisms. As mentioned before, oxidative stress may influence the function of the DNA repair machinery. The normal function of the MMR system has been identified as crucial to MS stability [76,91]. It consists of several proteins (MSH2, MSH3, MSH6, MLH1, PMS2) with different functions who recognize base-base mismatches or insertion-deletion loops and correct them [104]. It has been shown that mutation rates of MS are increased in MMR deficient cell lines compared to MMR proficient ones [105]. MMR deficiency could be attributed to mutations, epigenetic changes or post-translational modifications, as mentioned previously. MSI in HNPCC has been correlated to mutations within MMR genes [81] and suppressed expression of MMR proteins has been found in several types of characterized as MSI-high cancers and cancer cell lines [106-108]. Suppressed expression of MMR could also be due to epigenetic changes as many MSI-high sporadic cancers have been found to lack hMLH1 expression because of methylation of hMLH1 gene promoter [109,110]. Although mutations and silencing of MMR genes are usually responsible for high levels of MSI, low levels of MSI have been observed in some cancers with no known MMR mutations or promoter hypermethylation [81]. MMR deficiency can be attained also without mutation or epigenetic change, through a deregulation of expression of one of its subunits. MSH2 forms two different complexes with MSH3 and MSH6 with different activity. MSH3 and MSH6 compete each other for binding with MSH2. Thus, overexpression of either of MSH3 or MSH6 can lead to decreased activity of the other's complex with MSH2 [76]. In the subset of chronic tissue stress, ROS (reactive oxygen species) or RNS (reactive nitrogen species) may impair MMR function by post-translational modifications of MMR proteins [94].

Although the MMR system is responsible for correcting DNA strand loops typical for MSI, recent studies suggest that the different DNA repair systems do not act independently and that MSI may be attributable to alterations in DNA repair pathways distinct from MMR [111,112]. In addition, since all the types of DNA repair mechanisms use the same types of polymerases for final DNA synthesis [104], excess activity of one repair mechanism may result in reduction of the activity of the other. Hofseth et al. demonstrated in an elegant study that the chronic inflammation in ulcerative colitis leads to MSI through excessive activity of BER enzymes and therefore insufficient MMR activity [111]. It has been also shown that imbalanced expression of Polβ can be associated with MSI and chromosome instability [112,113]. The exact DNA repair defect behind the observed genomic instability found in allotransplanted patients needs to be elucidated.

iii) Failure of DNA Damage Checkpoints

Besides the DNA repair proteins, cells are equipped with additional DNA protective mechanisms (ATM, p53 etc.) which detect unrepaired DNA and lead the cell to cycle arrest or apoptosis [77]. So, even in the case of repair mechanisms failure to correct DNA damage, cells which exhibit genomic instability (GI) will not further proliferate and thus they shouldn't be detected among the rest of the normal cells which proliferate normally. Inactivation of p53 and the failure of cellular demise has been suggested as playing a mechanistic role in the occurrence of MSI in sporadic tumors and in chronically inflamed tissue [81,86,114-116]. Furthermore, it is interesting that solid tumours post-transplant exhibit p53 mutations [89,117]. The pattern of p53 expression in GvHD-affected and genome instable epithelium in allotransplanted patients needs further evaluation.

iv) Growth Advantage of GI Clones in the Allotransplanted Recipients

Another interesting hypothesis is whether cells with instable MS gain an immunologic survival advantage in contrast to normal cells and thus, they can be detected after allo-HCT. In vitro experiments have shown that cells which display MSI can escape T-cell mediated destruction through inhibition of HLA antigen expression and abnormal presentation of peptide fragments [118,119]. The inhibition of HLA expression can be caused by mutations in HLA transcriptional areas or by instability of MS located near the HLA gene complex. After allogeneic HCT the recipient's epithelial cells stimulate through HLA system the new immune system which derives from the donor. This could lead to immune mediated epithelial cell destruction, which we recognize clinically as GvHD. Therefore, if genomic instable cells reduce expression of HLA genes then they will acquire an immunologic survival advantage. Whilst the normal cells will undergo destruction by the donor derived immune system, the MSI displaying cells will not be recognized by the donor's T-cells. This hypothesis is surely challenging and should be further investigated.

Clinical Significance of GI in Allotransplanted Patients

MSI has been shown to be an indicator of genomic instability [79]. It is very likely that mutations occur not only in non-transcribed MS but also in coding regions of the genome [120]. Mutations in coding genes might be responsible for the protean post-transplant GvHD-related clinical syndromes and phenotypes such as scleroderma, Sjögren syndrome, musculoskeletal or pulmonary disease and many others. In addition to serving as an indicator for genomic instability, mutations of MS may directly contribute to evolution of post-transplant diseases. Although MS were thought to consist "junk" DNA dispersed in non-coding regions throughout the genome, there is evidence that MS distribution is not random and that there are MS within genes which play a regulatory role in gene expression [91]. TGFRII, IGFIIR and BAX genes are paradigms of transcribed genes which contain MS within their coding regions [81,120]. Changes in the lengths of these repetitive sequences when found within coding regions of specific genes have been shown to result in gene inactivation or modification of function of the gene and cause disease in humans like Huntington's disease and myotonic dystrophy [120].

MSI has been mainly associated with cancer [81] or cancer risk in chronic inflammatory diseases [87]. In hereditary nonpolyposis colorectal carcinoma the MMR deficiency plays an aetiological role in the development of MSI and carcinogenesis [81]. MS alterations are also common in various sporadic cancers such squamous cancers [81]. It is interesting that squamous cell carcinomas are the most common secondary tumours after allogeneic HCT [121] and are associated with chronic alloantigeneic stimulation through GvHD. Therefore, the hypothesis that MSI may characterize a precancerous state of the epithelial cell seems logical. Our preliminary results in the analysis of nearly 70 allogeneic recipients suggest such an association (unpublished data). Genome analyses in allografted recipients may indeed identify specific genomic alterations which might be responsible for, or used as molecular biomarkers of post-transplant diseases, including secondary cancer.

Taken together, it seems that in the GvHD tissue environment cytokines, ROS and NO induce genomic alterations in epithelium by acting through several different but communicating pathways. The oxidative stress damages the DNA causing mutations such as MS length alterations. The induction of mutations is facilitated by a relaxation of DNA repair system mediated by NO or ROS. The cells may survive due to a possible inactivation of the DNA-checkpoint apoptotic mechanisms. Furthermore, the donor-derived immune system in an allogeneic setting may attack the recipient-derived, normal epithelial cells, yet spare cells with an MSI phenotype, providing in this way a selective growth advantage for the cells with novel repeat lengths. Elucidating the ultimate mechanisms underlying the genomic instability following alloantigeneic reactions in the chimeric organism is a major challenge. Findings may provide more information about GvHD pathology and pathogenesis of post transplantation clinical outcomes such as secondary malignancies and GvHD related syndromes. Focusing on the pathways through which the alloantigeneic reaction causes genomic instability may bring up novel therapeutic targets for the protection of the epithelium during GvHD and the prevention of malignant transformation.

CONCLUSION

Although allogeneic HCT has been a part of clinical practice for more than 30 years, the consequences of the unphysiological creation of these biological chimeras are still not fully explored. Development of epithelial cells with donor-derived genotype and accumulation of genomic alterations in the epithelial tissues are only two newly recognized phenomena caused by the co-existence of two genetically distinct populations in the transplant recipient. The ultimate mechanisms and the clinical consequences of these are still under investigation. It is unclear whether these two phenomena, which are both presented in the host epithelium, occur independently or are indeed aetiologically linked. A possible scenario which needs further experimental proof is the following. The transplanted and engrafted bone marrow produces continuously hematopoietic cells, like leukocytes and lymphocytes, in the recipient. Since these cells have a limited life span, they undergo apoptosis and charge constantly the host environment with donor DNA. The donor-derived apoptotic DNA fragments are than taken up and cleared by the recipient's mesenchymal and epithelial cells. It is possible that part of the donor-derived DNA is incorporated into recipient nucleus through horizontal gene transfer leading to occurrence of epithelial cells with donor-derived genome. Induction of genomic DNA damage through the conditioning for the allogeneic HCT leads to an increased frequency of illegitimate DNA integration [122-124]. On the other side, the incorporation of the foreign DNA in the host genome may result extensive physical rearrangements at the site of integration including deletions, duplications and translocations [125-128] leading this way to the detected genomic instability of the chimeric epithelium. Lymphocyte-epithelial interactions between the two genetically distinct cell populations in the transplant recipient should be investigated more precisely not only in cellular but also in molecular level.

ACKNOWLEDGMENTS

We would like to thank all our colleagues from the Department of Hematology in Patras University Medical Center, Patras, Greece and the Department of Hematology-Oncology in Albert-Ludwigs University Medical Center, Freiburg, Germany. We especially thank Miguel Waterhouse (Freiburg) and Eleni Lagadinou (Patras) for critical discussions and helping by preparing the manuscript. This work was supported by Landesstiftung Baden Württemberg.

REFERENCES

[1]   Bizzazero, Sulla functione hemapoetica del midollo delle ossa. *Gaz Med Ital Lomb*, 1868. 28: p. 381.

[2]   Neumann, áber die Bedeutung des Knochenmarks fór die Blutbildung. *Zbl Med Wiss*, 1868. 6: p. 689-672.

[3]   Lorenz E, C.D., Uphoff D, Modification of acute irradiation injury in mice and guinea pigs by bone marrow injection. *Radiology*, 1951. 58: p. 863-877.

[4]   Little, M.T. and R. Storb, History of haematopoietic stem-cell transplantation. *Nat Rev Cancer,* 2002. 2(3): p. 231-8.

[5]   Bolan, C.D., et al., Prospective evaluation of cell kinetics, yields and donor experiences during a single large-volume apheresis versus two smaller volume consecutive day collections of allogeneic peripheral blood stem cells. *Br J Haematol*, 2003. 120(5): p. 801-7.

[6]   Zeiser, R., et al., Immunopathogenesis of acute graft-versus-host disease: implications for novel preventive and therapeutic strategies. *Ann Hematol*, 2004. 83(9): p. 551-65.

[7]   Ferrari G, C.-D.A.G., Coletta M, Paolucci E, Stornaiuolo A, Cossu G, Mavilio F., Muscle regeneration by bone marrow-derived myogenic progenitors. *Science*, 1998. 279: p. 1528-30.

[8]   Jang, Y.Y., et al., Hematopoietic stem cells convert into liver cells within days without fusion. *Nat Cell Biol*, 2004. 6(6): p. 532-9.

[9]   Ianus A, H.G., Theise ND, Hussain MA, In vivo derivation of glucose- competent pancreatic endocrine cells from bone marrow without evidence of cell fusion. *J Clin Invest*, 2003. 111: p. 843- 850.

[10]   Mezey, E., et al., Turning blood into brain: cells bearing neuronal antigens generated in vivo from bone marrow. *Science*, 2000. 290(5497): p. 1779-82.

[11]   Camargo FD, G.R., Capetenaki Y, Jackson KA, Goodell MA, Single hematopoietic stem cells generate skeletal muscle through myeloid intermediates. *Nat Med*, 2003. 91: p. 1520- 1527.

[12]   Korbling, M., et al., Recombinant human granulocyte-colony-stimulating factor-mobilized and apheresis-collected endothelial progenitor cells: a novel blood cell component for therapeutic vasculogenesis. *Transfusion*, 2006. 46(10): p. 1795-802.

[13]   Alison MR, P.R., Jeffrey R, Dhillon AP, Quaglia A, Jacob J, Novelli M, Prentice G, Williamson J, Wright NA, Hepatocytes from nonhepatic adult stem cells. *Nature*, 2000. 406: p. 257.

[14]   Theise, N.D., et al., Derivation of hepatocytes from bone marrow cells in mice after radiation-induced myeloablation. *Hepatology*, 2000. 31(1): p. 235-40.

[15] Anderlini, P., et al., Long-term follow-up of normal peripheral blood progenitor cell donors treated with filgrastim: no evidence of increased risk of leukemia development. *Bone Marrow Transplant*, 2002. 30(10): p. 661-3.

[16] Castro RF, J.K., Goodell MA, Robertson CS, Liu H, Shine HD., Failure of bone marrow cells to transdifferentiate into neural cells in vivo. *Science*, 2002. 297: p. 1299.

[17] Wagers, A.J., et al., Little evidence for developmental plasticity of adult hematopoietic stem cells. *Science*, 2002. 297(5590): p. 2256-9.

[18] Ono, K., et al., Preservation of hematopoietic properties in transplanted bone marrow cells in the brain. *J Neurosci Res*, 2003. 72(4): p. 503-7.

[19] Holden C, V.G., Stem cells. Plasticity: time for a reappraisal? *Science*, 2002. 296: p. 2126-9.

[20] Wagers, A.J., Sherwood R.I., Christensen J.L., Weissman I.L., Response to comment on "Little evidence for developmental plasticity of adult hematopoietic stem cells". *Science*, 2003. 299: p. 1317.

[21] Theise, N.D., D.S. Krause, and S. Sharkis, Comment on "Little evidence for developmental plasticity of adult hematopoietic stem cells". *Science*, 2003. 299(5611): p. 1317; author reply 1317.

[22] Spyridonidis, A., R. Mertelsmann, and J. Finke, Hematopoietic stem cell transplantation: more than just hematopoietic? *J Cancer Res Clin Oncol*, 2004.

[23] Spyridonidis, A., et al., Epithelial tissue chimerism after human hematopoietic cell transplantation is a real phenomenon. *Am J Pathol*, 2004. 164(4): p. 1147-55.

[24] Bianchi DW, Z.G., Weil GJ, Sylvester S, DeMaria MA, Male fetal progenitor cells persist in maternal blood for as long as 27 years postpartum. *Proc Natl Acad Sci USA*, 1996. 93: p. 705- 708.

[25] Cogle, C.R., et al., Bone marrow transdifferentiation in brain after transplantation: a retrospective study. *Lancet*, 2004. 363(9419): p. 1432-7.

[26] Okamoto, R., et al., Damaged epithelia regenerated by bone marrow-derived cells in the human gastrointestinal tract. *Nat Med*, 2002. 8(9): p. 1011-7.

[27] Mattsson, J., et al., Lung epithelial cells and type II pneumocytes of donor origin after allogeneic hematopoietic stem cell transplantation. *Transplantation*, 2004. 78(1): p. 154-7.

[28] Tran SD, P.S., Dutra A, Barrett AJ, Brownstein MJ, Key S, Pak E, Leakan RA, Kingman A, Yamada KM, Baum BJ, Mezey E, Differentiation of human bone marrow-derived cells into buccal epithelial cells in vivo: a molecular analytical study. *Lancet*, 2003. 361: p. 1084- 1088.

[29] Metaxas Y, Z.R., Schmitt-Graeff A, Waterhouse M, Faber P, Follo M, Bertz H, Finke J, Spyridonidis A, Human hematopoietic cell transplantation results in generation of donr-derived epithelial cells. *Leukemia*, 2005. 19: p. 1287-1289.

[30] Lagasse E, C.H., Al-Dhalimy M, Reitsma M, Dohse M, Osborne L, Wang X, Finegold M, Weissman IL, Grompe M., Purified hematopoietic stem cells can differentiate into hepatocytes in vivo. *Nat Med*, 2000. 6: p. 1229-34.

[31] Willenbring, H., et al., Myelomonocytic cells are sufficient for therapeutic cell fusion in liver. *Nat Med*, 2004. 10(7): p. 744-8.

[32] Camargo FD, F.M., Goodell MA, Hematopoietic myelomonocytic cells are the major source of hepatocyte fusion partners. *J Clin Invest*, 2004. 113: p. 1266-1270.

[33] Hess, D., et al., Bone marrow-derived stem cells initiate pancreatic regeneration. *Nat Biotechnol*, 2003. 21(7): p. 763-70.

[34] Rafii, S. and D. Lyden, Therapeutic stem and progenitor cell transplantation for organ vascularization and regeneration. *Nat Med*, 2003. 9(6): p. 702-12.

[35] Wang Xiuli, S.G., McNamara G, Hao QL, Crooks GM, Nolta JA, Albumin- expressing hepatocyte- like cells develop in the livers of immune- deficient mice that received transplants of highly purified human hematopoietic stem cells. *Blood*, 2003. 101: p. 4201- 4208.

[36] Almeida-Porada, G., et al., Formation of human hepatocytes by human hematopoietic stem cells in sheep. *Blood*, 2004. 104(8): p. 2582-90.

[37] Stamm, C., Westphal B, Kleine HD, et al., Autologous bone-marrow stem-cell transplantation for myocardial regeneration. *Lancet*, 2003. 361: p. 45-46.

[38] Bolli R, J.H., Dawn B, Bone marrow cell-mediated cardiac regeneration: A veritable revolution. *J Am Coll Cardiol*, 2005. 46: p. 1659-1661.

[39] Grigg, A.P., et al., Optimizing dose and scheduling of filgrastim (granulocyte colony-stimulating factor) for mobilization and collection of peripheral blood progenitor cells in normal volunteers. *Blood*, 1995. 86(12): p. 4437-45.

[40] Roth K, K.S., Martin S, Lorenz R, Cellular immune responses are essential for the development of Helicobacter felis-associated gastric pathology. *J Immunol*, 1999. 163: p. 1490-1497.

[41] Cogle CR, T.N., DongTao F, Ucar D et al, Bone marrow contributes to epithelial cancers in mice and humans as developmental mimicry. *Stem Cells*, 2007. online ahead publish.

[42] Abedi, M., et al., Tissue injury in marrow transdifferentiation. *Blood Cells Mol Dis*, 2004. 32(1): p. 42-6.

[43] Spyridonidis A, T.T., Zeiser R et al, Stem cell plasticity: The debate begins to clarify. *Stem Cell Reviews*, 2005. 1(1): p. 37-43.

[44] Idilman R, K.I., Erden E, et al, Evaluation of the effect of transplant-related factors and tissue-injury on donor-derived hepatocyte and gastrointestinal epithelial cell repopulation following hematopoietic cell transplantation. *Bone Marrow Transplant*, 2006. 37: p. 199-206.

[45] Herzog, E.L., Van Arnam J, Hu BuQu, Krause DS, Threshold of lung injury required for the appearance of marrow-derived lung epithelia. *Stem Cells*, 2006. 24: p. 1986-1992.

[46] Vieyra DS, J.K., Goodell MA, Plasticity snd tissue regenerative potential of bone marrow-derived cells. *Stem Cell Reviews*, 2005. 1(1): p. 65-69.

[47] Bruscia, E., Ziegler EC, Price JE et al., Engraftment of donor-derived epithelial cells in multiple organs following bone marrow transplantation into newborn mice. *Stem Cells*, 2006. 24: p. 2299-2308.

[48] Muller-Borer, B.J., et al., Adult-derived liver stem cells acquire a cardiomyocyte structural and functional phenotype ex vivo. *Am J Pathol*, 2004. 165(1): p. 135-45.

[49] Jang, Y.Y., Sharkis SJ, Stem cell plasticity: A rare cell, not a rare event. *Stem Cell Reviews*, 2005. 1(1): p. 45-51.

[50] Krause DS, T.N., Collector MI, Henegariu O, Hwang S, Gardner R, Neutzel S, Sharkis SJ., Multi-organ, multi-lineage engraftment by a single bone marrow-derived stem cell. *Cell*, 2001. 105: p. 369-77.

[51] Brockes JP, K.A., Plasticity and reprogramming of differentiated cells in amphibian regeneration. *Nat Rev Mol Cell Biol*, 2002. 3: p. 566- 574.

[52] Takahashi K, Y.S., Induction of pluripotent stem cells from mouse embryonic and adult fibroblast cultures by defined factors. *Cell*, 2006. 126: p. 663-676.

[53] Okita, K., Ichisaka T, Yamanaka S, Generation of germline-competent induced pluripotent stem cells. *Nature*, 2007. 448: p. 313-317.

[54] Wernig M, M.A., Foreman R et al, In vitro reprogramming of fibroblasts into a pluripotent ES-cell-like state. *Nature*, 2007. 448: p. 318-324.

[55] Avital I, I.D., Aoki T, Tyan DB, Cohen AH, Ferraresso C, Rozga J, Arnaout WS, Demetriou A, Isolation, characterization, and transplantation of bone marrow- derived hepatocyte stem cells. *Biochem Biophys Res Commun*, 2001. 288: p. 156- 164.

[56] Ratajczak, M.Z., et al., Stem cell plasticity revisited: CXCR4-positive cells expressing mRNA for early muscle, liver and neural cells 'hide out' in the bone marrow. *Leukemia*, 2004. 18(1): p. 29-40.

[57] Jiang Y, J.B., Reinhardt RL, Schwartz RE, Keene CD, Ortiz- Gonzalez XR, Reyes M, Lenvik T, Lund T, Blackstad M, Du J, Aldrich S, Lisberg A, Low WC, Largaespada DA, Verfaillie CM, Pluripotency of mesenchymal stem cells derived from adult marrow. *Nature*, 2002. 418: p. 41- 49.

[58] Check, Stem-cell paper corrected. *Nature*, 2007. 447: p. 763.

[59] Jiang Y, J.B., Reinhardt RL, Schwartz RE, Keene CD, Ortiz- Gonzalez XR, Reyes M, Lenvik T, Lund T, Blackstad M, Du J, Aldrich S, Lisberg A, Low WC, Largaespada DA, Verfaillie CM, Pluripotency of mesenchymal stem cells derived from adult marrow. *Nature,* 2007. 447: p. 880-881.

[60] Kucia M, R.R., Campbell FR, Zuba-Surma E, Majka M, Ratajczak J, Ratajczak Z, A population of very small embryonic-like (VSEL) CXCR4+SSEA-1+Oct-4+ stem cells identified in adult bone marrow. *Leukemia*, 2006. 20: p. 857-869.

[61] Kucia M, H.M., Wysoczynski M, et al, Morphological and molecular characterization of novel population of CXCR4+ SSEA-4+ Oct-4+ very small embryonic-like cells purified from human cord blood- preliminary report. *Leukemia*, 2007. 21: p. 297-303.

[62] Anjos-Afonso F, B.D., Nonhematopoietic/endothelial SSEA-1+ cells define the most primitive progenitors in the adult murine bone marrow mesenchymal compartment. *Blood*, 2007. 109: p. 1298-1306.

[63] Ratajczak MZ, M.B., Wojakowski W, Ratajczak J, Kucia M, A hypothesis for an embryonic origin of pluripotent Oct-4+ stem cells in adult bone marrow and other tissues. *Leukemia*, 2007. 21: p. 860-867.

[64] Gurtner GC, C.M., Longaker MT, Progress and potential for regenerative medicine. *Annu Rev Med*, 2007. 58: p. 299-312.

[65] Vassilopoulos, G., P.R. Wang, and D.W. Russell, Transplanted bone marrow regenerates liver by cell fusion. *Nature*, 2003. 422(6934): p. 901-4.

[66] Wang, X., et al., Cell fusion is the principal source of bone-marrow-derived hepatocytes. *Nature*, 2003. 422(6934): p. 897-901.

[67] Metaxas, Z., Schmitt-Graeff, Waterhouse, Faber, Follo, Bertz, Finke, Spyridonidis, Human hematopoietic cell transplantation results in generation of donor-derived epithelial cells. *Leukemia*, 2005. 19: p. 1287-1289.

[68] Vogel G, Developmental biology. More data but no answers on powers of adult stem cells. *Science*, 2004. 305: p. 27.

[69] Quesenberry, P.J., Colvin G, Dooner G, Dooner M, Aliotta JM, Johnson K, The stem cell continuum: Cell cycle, injury, and phenotype lability. *Ann NY Acad Sci*, 2007. online pre-publication.

[70] Bergsmedh, A., et al., Horizontal transfer of oncogenes by uptake of apoptotic bodies. *Proc Natl Acad Sci U S A*, 2001. 98(11): p. 6407-11.

[71] Jain, R., M.C. Rivera, and J.A. Lake, Horizontal gene transfer among genomes: the complexity hypothesis. *Proc Natl Acad Sci U S A*, 1999. 96(7): p. 3801-6.

[72] Holmgren, L., et al., Horizontal transfer of DNA by the uptake of apoptotic bodies. *Blood*, 1999. 93(11): p. 3956-63.

[73] Schubbert, R., et al., Foreign (M13) DNA ingested by mice reaches peripheral leukocytes, spleen, and liver via the intestinal wall mucosa and can be covalently linked to mouse DNA. *Proc Natl Acad Sci U S A*, 1997. 94(3): p. 961-6.

[74] Mezey E, K.S., Vogelsang G, Szalayova I, Lange GD, Crain B, Transplanted bone marrow generates new neurons in human brains. *Proc Natl Acad Sci USA*, 2003. 100: p. 1364- 1369.

[75] Verfaillie, C.M., M.F. Pera, and P.M. Lansdorp, Stem cells: hype and reality. *Hematology (Am Soc Hematol Educ Program)*, 2002: p. 369-91.

[76] Jiricny, J., Replication errors: cha(lle)nging the genome. *Embo J*, 1998. 17(22): p. 6427-36.

[77] Zhivotovsky, B. and G. Kroemer, Apoptosis and genomic instability. *Nat Rev Mol Cell Biol*, 2004. 5(9): p. 752-62.

[78] Sieber, O.M., K. Heinimann, and I.P. Tomlinson, Genomic instability--the engine of tumorigenesis? *Nat Rev Cancer*, 2003. 3(9): p. 701-8.

[79] Ellegren, H., Microsatellites: simple sequences with complex evolution. *Nat Rev Genet*, 2004. 5(6): p. 435-45.

[80] Spyridonidis, A., et al., Capillary electrophoresis for chimerism monitoring by PCR amplification of microsatellite markers after allogeneic hematopoietic cell transplantation. *Clin Transplant*, 2005. 19(3): p. 350-6.

[81] Boland, C.R., et al., A National Cancer Institute Workshop on Microsatellite Instability for cancer detection and familial predisposition: development of international criteria for the determination of microsatellite instability in colorectal cancer. *Cancer Res*, 1998. 58(22): p. 5248-57.

[82] Sood, A.K., et al., Application of the National Cancer Institute international criteria for determination of microsatellite instability in ovarian cancer. *Cancer Res*, 2001. 61(11): p. 4371-4.

[83] Xu, L., et al., Microsatellite instability at AAAG repeat sequences in respiratory tract cancers. *Int J Cancer*, 2001. 91(2): p. 200-4.

[84] Danaee, H., et al., Microsatellite instability at tetranucleotide repeats in skin and bladder cancer. *Oncogene*, 2002. 21(32): p. 4894-9.

[85] Chen, S.H., X. Li, and X.J. Huang, Effect of recombinant human granulocyte colony-stimulating factor on T-lymphocyte function and the mechanism of this effect. *Int J Hematol*, 2004. 79(2): p. 178-84.

[86] Sohn, S.K., et al., Harvesting peripheral blood stem cells from healthy donors on 4th day of cytokine mobilization. *J Clin Apher*, 2003. 18(4): p. 186-9.

[87] Willenbucher, R.F., et al., Genomic instability is an early event during the progression pathway of ulcerative-colitis-related neoplasia. *Am J Pathol*, 1999. 154(6): p. 1825-30.

[88] Teshima, T. and J.L. Ferrara, Understanding the alloresponse: new approaches to graft-versus-host disease prevention. *Semin Hematol*, 2002. 39(1): p. 15-22.

[89] Deeg, H.J. and G. Socie, Malignancies after hematopoietic stem cell transplantation: many questions, some answers. *Blood*, 1998. 91(6): p. 1833-44.

[90] Faber, P., et al., Frequent genomic alterations in epithelium measured by microsatellite instability following allogeneic hematopoietic cell transplantation in humans. *Blood*, 2006. 107(8): p. 3389-96.

[91]   Li, Y.C., et al., Microsatellites: genomic distribution, putative functions and mutational mechanisms: a review. *Mol Ecol*, 2002. 11(12): p. 2453-65.

[92]   Mirkin, S.M., Expandable DNA repeats and human disease. *Nature,* 2007. 447(7147): p. 932-40.

[93]   Mao, L., et al., Microsatellite alterations as clonal markers for the detection of human cancer. *Proc Natl Acad Sci U S A*, 1994. 91(21): p. 9871-5.

[94]   Wiseman, H. and B. Halliwell, Damage to DNA by reactive oxygen and nitrogen species: role in inflammatory disease and progression to cancer. *Biochem J*, 1996. 313 (Pt 1): p. 17-29.

[95]   Gasche, C., et al., Oxidative stress increases frameshift mutations in human colorectal cancer cells. *Cancer Res*, 2001. 61(20): p. 7444-8.

[96]   Chang, C.L., et al., Oxidative stress inactivates the human DNA mismatch repair system. *Am J Physiol Cell Physiol*, 2002. 283(1): p. C148-54.

[97]   Seril, D.N., et al., Oxidative stress and ulcerative colitis-associated carcinogenesis: studies in humans and animal models. *Carcinogenesis*, 2003. 24(3): p. 353-62.

[98]   Cerutti, P.A., Oxy-radicals and cancer. *Lancet*, 1994. 344(8926): p. 862-3.

[99]   Jaiswal, M., et al., Inflammatory cytokines induce DNA damage and inhibit DNA repair in cholangiocarcinoma cells by a nitric oxide-dependent mechanism. *Cancer Res*, 2000. 60(1): p. 184-90.

[100] Seidelin, J.B. and O.H. Nielsen, Continuous cytokine exposure of colonic epithelial cells induces DNA damage. *Eur J Gastroenterol Hepatol*, 2005. 17(3): p. 363-9.

[101] Drobyski, W.R., et al., Inhibition of nitric oxide production is associated with enhanced weight loss, decreased survival, and impaired alloengraftment in mice undergoing graft-versus-host disease after bone marrow transplantation. *Blood*, 1994. 84(7): p. 2363-73.

[102] Flanagan, D.M., et al., Nitric oxide participates in the intestinal pathology associated with murine syngeneic graft-versus-host disease. *J Leukoc Biol*, 2002. 72(4): p. 762-8.

[103] Choi, I.C., et al., Plasma nitric oxide is associated with the occurrence of moderate to severe acute graft-versus-host disease in haemopoietic stem cell transplant recipients. *Haematologica*, 2001. 86(9): p. 972-6.

[104] Christmann, M., et al., Mechanisms of human DNA repair: an update. *Toxicology*, 2003. 193(1-2): p. 3-34.

[105] Boyer, J.C., et al., Sequence dependent instability of mononucleotide microsatellites in cultured mismatch repair proficient and deficient mammalian cells. *Hum Mol Genet*, 2002. 11(6): p. 707-13.

[106] Boyer, J.C., et al., Microsatellite instability, mismatch repair deficiency and genetic defects in human cancer cell lines. *Cancer Res*, 1995. 55(24): p. 6063-70.

[107] Liu, J., et al., Microsatellite instability and expression of hMLH1 and hMSH2 proteins in ovarian endometrioid cancer. *Mod Pathol*, 2004. 17(1): p. 75-80.

[108] Yao, Y., et al., Alterations of DNA mismatch repair proteins and microsatellite instability levels in gastric cancer cell lines. *Lab Invest*, 2004. 84(7): p. 915-22.

[109] Kane, M.F., et al., Methylation of the hMLH1 promoter correlates with lack of expression of hMLH1 in sporadic colon tumors and mismatch repair-defective human tumor cell lines. *Cancer Res*, 1997. 57(5): p. 808-11.

[110] Fleisher, A.S., et al., Hypermethylation of the hMLH1 gene promoter in human gastric cancers with microsatellite instability. *Cancer Res*, 1999. 59(5): p. 1090-5.

[111] Hofseth, L.J., et al., The adaptive imbalance in base excision-repair enzymes generates microsatellite instability in chronic inflammation. *J Clin Invest*, 2003. 112(12): p. 1887-94.

[112] Yamada, N.A. and R.A. Farber, Induction of a low level of microsatellite instability by overexpression of DNA polymerase Beta. *Cancer Res*, 2002. 62(21): p. 6061-4.

[113] Bergoglio, V., et al., Deregulated DNA polymerase beta induces chromosome instability and tumorigenesis. *Cancer Res*, 2002. 62(12): p. 3511-4.

[114] Ahrendt, S.A., et al., Microsatellite instability at selected tetranucleotide repeats is associated with p53 mutations in non-small cell lung cancer. *Cancer Res*, 2000. 60(9): p. 2488-91.

[115] Hussain, S.P., et al., Increased p53 mutation load in noncancerous colon tissue from ulcerative colitis: a cancer-prone chronic inflammatory disease. *Cancer Res*, 2000. 60(13): p. 3333-7.

[116] Inazuka, M., et al., Analysis of p53 tumour suppressor gene somatic mutations in rheumatoid arthritis synovium. *Rheumatology (Oxford)*, 2000. 39(3): p. 262-6.

[117] Zouvelou C, B.H., Faber P, Spyridonidis A, p53 mutations in secondary malignancies after allogeneic hematopoietic cell transplantation. *Biology of Blood and Marrow Transplantation*, 2007. 13(2): p. 53.

[118] Hirata, T., et al., Characterization of the immune escape phenotype of human gastric cancers with and without high-frequency microsatellite instability. *J Pathol*, 2007. 211(5): p. 516-23.

[119] Kloor, M., et al., Immunoselective pressure and human leukocyte antigen class I antigen machinery defects in microsatellite unstable colorectal cancers. *Cancer Res*, 2005. 65(14): p. 6418-24.

[120] Li, Y.C., et al., Microsatellites within genes: structure, function, and evolution. *Mol Biol Evol*, 2004. 21(6): p. 991-1007.

[121] Curtis, R.E., et al., Impact of chronic GVHD therapy on the development of squamous-cell cancers after hematopoietic stem-cell transplantation: an international case-control study. *Blood*, 2005. 105(10): p. 3802-11.

[122] Bode, J., et al., Fatal connections: when DNA ends meet on the nuclear matrix. *J Cell Biochem Suppl*, 2000. Suppl 35: p. 3-22.

[123] Shcherbakova, O.G. and M.V. Filatov, Camptothecin enhances random integration of transfected DNA into the genome of mammalian cells. *Biochim Biophys Acta*, 2000. 1495(1): p. 1-3.

[124] Bennett, C.L., et al., Haematological malignancies developing in previously healthy individuals who received haematopoietic growth factors: report from the Research on Adverse Drug Events and Reports (RADAR) project. *Br J Haematol*, 2006. 135(5): p. 642-50.

[125] Covarrubias, L., Y. Nishida, and B. Mintz, Early postimplantation embryo lethality due to DNA rearrangements in a transgenic mouse strain. *Proc Natl Acad Sci U S A*, 1986. 83(16): p. 6020-4.

[126] Covarrubias, L., et al., Cellular DNA rearrangements and early developmental arrest caused by DNA insertion in transgenic mouse embryos. *Mol Cell Biol*, 1987. 7(6): p. 2243-7.

[127] Kato, S., R.A. Anderson, and R.D. Camerini-Otero, Foreign DNA introduced by calcium phosphate is integrated into repetitive DNA elements of the mouse L cell genome. *Mol Cell Biol*, 1986. 6(5): p. 1787-95.

[128] Robins D, R.S., Henderson A, Axel R, Transforming DNA integrates into the host chromosome. *Cell*, 1981. 23: p. 29-39.

In: Encyclopedia of Stem Cell Research (2 Volume Set)   ISBN: 978-1-61761-835-2
Editor: Alexander L. Greene   © 2012 Nova Science Publishers, Inc.

Chapter XXVII

THE EVOLVING ROLE OF HEMATOPOIETIC STEM CELL TRANSPLANTATION IN NON-HODGKIN LYMPHOMA

Koji Kato[*], *Smitha Mellacheruvu and Shin Mineishi*

Blood and Marrow Transplantation Program,
University of Michigan; Comprehensive Cancer Center, MI, US

ABSTRACT

Autologous hematopoietic stem cell transplantation (auto-HSCT) is widely accepted as an effective therapy for patients with relapsed diffuse large B-cell lymphoma (DLBL). Although some of these patients can expect to be cured, many patients will relapse. In addition, follicular lymphoma (FL) and mantle cell lymphoma (MCL) are rarely cured with auto-HSCT. To reduce the incidence of relapse after auto-HSCT, more and more attempts have been made to combine the transplantation with so-called "targeted therapy" such as rituximab before, during, and after HSCT. The other approach to reduce relapse is allogeneic HSCT (allo-HSCT) through graft-versus-lymphoma (GVL) effect. The GVL effect may be prominent in FL and MCL, while it is much less in DLBL. Allo-HSCT has been increasingly used in patients with non-Hodgkin lymphoma (NHL), although it is associated with high non-relapse mortality (NRM). Recently, reduced-intensity stem cell transplantation (RIST) has opened a new era for allo-HSCT. It was developed based on the knowledge that GVL effect is the main anti-tumor effect in allo-HSCT. Because RIST is associated with less morbidity and mortality, it can be applied to many patients with NHL who could not undergo myeloablative allogeneic stem cell transplantation (MAST).

Although HSCT has been developing in NHL with the introduction of new treatment and improvements of supportive care, there are still many unsolved questions, especially regarding optimal timing and optimal types for each disease categories in NHL. In this

[*] Corresponding Author: Koji Kato, MD, PhD; Blood and Marrow Transplantation Program, University of Michigan Comprehensive Cancer Center; Address: 5303 CCGC 1500E. Medical Center Drive, Ann Arbor, MI 48109-0914, USA; Phone: 1-734-936-8456 ; FAX: 1-734-936-8788 ; E-mail: kojikato@umich.edu

review, we would like to attempt to evaluate the efficacy of HSCT for NHL and also to provide future perspectives.

Keywords: Non-Hodgkin lymphoma; Hematopoietic stem cell transplantation; Reduced-intensity stem cell transplantation; Graft-versus-lymphoma effect; Immunotherapy;

1. INTRODUCTION

Non-Hodgkin lymphoma (NHL) is a heterogeneous group of lymphoid malignancies. The incidence of NHL has increased by 50% over the past two decades. A subset of patients with NHL will be cured with standard chemotherapies and/or an irradiation therapy, but significant numbers will either fail to achieve remission or relapse after remission.[1-4] Salvage chemotherapy can be used to re-induce remission, however, it is rarely curable.[5] High dose chemotherapy (HDC) followed by autologous hematopoietic stem cell transplantation (auto-HSCT) can overcome the resistance of tumor cells to standard treatments by intensified dose of chemotherapy and/or irradiation therapy and improve the survival.[6]

It is important to recognize that the incidence of both indolent and aggressive lymphomas increases with ages, making these the most common diagnosed in patients over 60 years. Along with improved supportive care and reduced non-relapse mortality (NRM), elderly NHL patients with older more than 60 years are now considered eligible for auto-HSCT.[7-9] Allogeneic HSCT (allo-HSCT) has been generally considered for NHL patients with chemo-refractory disease despite salvage chemotherapies[10] and relapse after auto-HSCT.[11] Although allo-HSCT has provided the possibility of cure for many patients with NHL through through graft-versus-lymphoma (GVL) effect,[11-13] many of them can not tolerate for intensive conditioning regimens because of their old age or medical co-morbidities.[13] Reduced-intensity stem cell transplantation (RIST) has recently been developed and allowed allo-HSCT to be explored in those patients.[14-16]

Some of the most significant advances in the therapy of NHL have occurred in the past two decades. Targeted therapies, such as rituximab and radioimmunotherapeutic agents, also play a very important role in the progress of HSCT for NHL.[17-22] Investigators are trying to combine these new therapeutic modalities with HSCT.

2. CLASSIFICATION OF NON-HODGKIN LYMPHOMA

Changes in the understanding of NHL have resulted in the evolution of numerous clinical and pathologic classification schemes over the last 50 years.[23, 24] Lymphomas were categorized predominantly by morphology in Rappaport classification,[25] by morphology and clinical prognosis in the Working Formulation,[26] or by cell lineage and differentiation in the Lukes and Collins[27] or Kiel classification.[28] These lymphoma classification schemes were largely replaced in 1994 by the revised European-American Lymphoma (REAL) classification, which incorporated morphologic, immunophenotypic, genotypic, and clinical features into disease subtype definition.[29] In 2001, the World Health Organization (WHO) introduced a new classification of hematological malignancies based on the REAL classification.[30] The WHO classification stratifies according to the lineage. Lymphomas are categorized into 3 groups: B-cell neoplasms, T/NK-cell neoplasms, and Hodgkin lymphoma (HL). Similar to the REAL classification, each disease entity is defined according to a combination of morphology, immunophenotype, genetic feature, and clinical features. In addition, for each neoplasm, a cell origin is postulated. The WHO classification has been adopted worldwide as the consensus classification for clinical and pathologic use. However, more than 30 different subtypes are recognized within the classification and, in addition, marked heterogeneity exists within subtypes. Recently several studies attempted to further classify these lymphomas using gene expression profile. These analyses, focusing on the importance of the site of origin of these tumors, provided further information on some of the variants of each lymphoma listed in the WHO classification.[31]

Thus, lymphoma classification has undergone major revisions over the last decade. These revisions made it possible to make accurate histological diagnoses and to allow the optimal selection of treatment options, while made it difficult to compare recent results to previous data and to establish long-term follow up after transplantation.[32]

3. PROGNOSTIC FACTORS

The management of patients with NHL is complicated because of the diversity of classification and the heterogeneity within each subtype. Despite these complexities, we need to provide as accurate predictions of prognosis as possible for each patient and offer an appropriate treatment. Through the evaluation of prognostic factors for each patient, we may be moving towards individual risk-stratified therapy.

The International Prognostic Index (IPI) predicts the likelihood for cure with chemotherapy for patients with diffuse large B-cell lymphoma (DLBL).[33] The Follicular Lymphoma International Prognostic Index (FLIPI)[34] and the Prognostic Index of T cell lymphoma (PIT)[35] are also used for patients with follicular lymphoma (FL) and peripheral T-cell lymphoma, unspecified (PTCL-U), respectively (table 1). The introduction of fluorodeoxyglucose-positron emission tomography (FDG-PET) in the assessment of response for patients with NHL allows physicians to make a decision more precisely.[36-38] In addition, many molecular markers have been examined recently and some of them have been shown to be predictive of outcome.[39, 40]

Diffuse Large Cell Lymphoma

For patients with diffuse large B-cell lymphoma (DLBL), the IPI predicts the likelihood for cure with chemotherapy. The IPI is based on the sum total of scores in 5 adverse risk factors: age ($\leq$ 60 years versus > 60 years), Ann Arbor stage (I-II versus III-IV), performance status (0-1 versus $\geq$ 2), number of extranodal sites (0-1 versus $\geq$ 2), and serum LDH level (normal or below versus above normal). Low (0-1 of risk factors), low/intermediate (2 of risk factors), high/intermediate (3 of risk factors), and high risk (4-5 of risk factors) were identified with overall survival (OS) at 5-year of 73%, 51%, 43%, and 26%, respectively. The age-adjusted IPI (aaIPI), applied for patients 60 years or older, is consisted of 3 factors of the IPI with the exception of age and the number of extranodal sites. Low (0 of risk factors), low/intermediate (1 of risk factors), high/intermediate (2 of risk factors), and high risk (3 of risk factors) were identified with OS at 5-year of 83%, 69%, 46%, and 32%, respectively.[33] However, the IPI was examined before the era of rituximab. Shen LH et al reported revised IPI is a better predictor of outcome than the IPI for patients with DLBL treated with rituximab and CHOP.[41]

FDG-PET is a more sensitive and specific imaging modality than CT for DLBL. Several investigators addressed the role of FDG-PET in early response assessment during induction chemotherapy and post-treatment remission assessment. Early restaging FDG-PET scan (early FDG-PET) performed after 1 to 4 cycles of induction chemotherapy have been shown to be predictive of outcome.[37]

Based on a gene expression profile, 2 major subtypes have been identified; one is germinal center B-cells (GCB) type and the other activated peripheral blood B-cells (ABC).[31] The GCB type has been described as IPI-independent prognostic factors compared to ABC type with CHOP-like regimen with 60% versus 35% of 5-year OS. Evaluating prognostic factors by genomics/proteomics may become more popular in the near future.

Table 1. Clinical prognostic models

1. International Prognostic Index (IPI)			
Risk group	IPI scores	5-yr OS	
Low	0,1	73%	
Low/intermediate	2	51%	
High/intermediate	3	43%	
High	4,5	26%	
1. Age: greater than 60			
2. Ann Arbor stage: stage III/IV			
3. More than one extranodal site			
4. LDH: >normal			
5. ECOG performance status: ≥ 2			
2. Age Adjusted IPI (aaIPI)			
Risk group	IPI scores	5-yr OS	
Low	0	83%	
Low/intermediate	1	69%	
High/intermediate	2	46%	
High	3	32%	
1. Ann Arbor stage: stage III/IV			
2. LDH: >normal			
3. ECOG performance status: ≥ 2			
3. Follicular Lymphoma International Prognostic Index (FLIPI)			

Risk group	FLIPI scores	5-yr OS	10-yr OS
Low	0,1	90.6%	70.7%
Intermediate	2	77.6%	50.9%
High	≥3	52.5%	35.5%
1. Age: greater than 60			
2. Ann Arbor stage: stage III/IV			
3. Hb <12g/dl			
4. LDH: >normal			
5. Number of nodal area: >4			
4. Prognostic Index for Peripheral T-cell Lymphoma, Unspecified (PIT)			
Risk group	PIT scores	5-yr OS	10-yr OS
Group 1	0	62.3%	54.9%
Group 2	1	52.9%	38.8%
Group 3	2	32.9%	18.0%
Group 4	3,4	18.3%	12.6%
1. Age: greater than 60			
2. LDH: >normal			
3. ECOG performance status: ≥2			
4. Bone marrow involvement			

Follicular Lymphoma

The FLIPI has become widely used for the clinical risk assessment of FL, which was based on the sum total scores of 5 adverse prognostic factors: age ($\leq$ 60 years versus > 60 years), Ann Arbor stage (I-II versus III-IV), hemoglobin level (< 120 g/L versus $\geq$ 120 g/L), number of nodal areas ($\leq$ 4 versus > 4), and serum LDH level (normal or below versus above normal). Low (0-1 of adverse factors), intermediate (2 adverse factors), and high risk group ($\geq$ 3adverse factors) were identified with OS at 10-year of 71%, 51%, and 36%, respectively.[34] As the FLIPI was validated by the data of patients diagnosed before 1992, however, it must be revalidated using rituximab.

Three pathological grades are recognized by the WHO classification based on the proportion of centroblasts seen in neoplastic follicles. Grade 1 and 2 of FL are likely to behave indolently, whereas grade 3 of FL appears to behave more aggressively and has often been treated similarly to DLBL. However, the correlation of pathological grade to clinical outcome has been still controversial.

Transformation of FL (t-FL) to high- or intermediate-grade histology is well recognized, occurring in the range of 30-70% of patients during course of their disease.[42, 43] In general, the prognosis of patients with t-FL is very poor despite combination chemotherapy, with 1 year of a median survival after transformation.[42, 44] Based on the results in patients with chemo-sensitive relapsed DLBL, auto-HSCT has also been applied to patients with t-FL. Transformation is usually defined as a loss of follicular architecture and evolution toward diffuse mixed or diffuse large cell lymphoma. The WHO criteria define any area of DLBL within a FL indicates transformation. It means that the cases which lack clear indolent period are included in t-FL. In addition, grade 1 or 2 FL that progress to grade 3 FL is occasionally included in t-FL.[45] The lack of the uniform definition of "transformation" makes the interpretation of outcome results of t-FL difficult.

Compared to DLBL, the utility of FDG-PET for FL has been unclear. FDG uptake in NHL has been described to correlate well with lymphoma grading, and false negative FDG-PET studies has been reported in FL.[46]

The detection of Bcl-2/IgH rearrangement by PCR is being used as a molecular residual disease (MRD).[47] Some studies showed that molecular remission after standard chemotherapy or auto-HSCT may be associated with a prolonged survival.

Peripheral T-Cell Lymphoma/NK-Cell Lymphoma

Peripheral T-cell lymphomas (PTCL) are a rare (fewer than 10% of all NHL) and heterogeneous subset of lymphomas with a poorer prognosis compared with B-cell lymphomas. T-cell and NK-cell phenotype have been demonstrated to be an independent adverse risk factor in all group except for anaplastic lymphoma kinase (ALK)-positive lymphoma, with about 30% of OS at 5-year.[48-51] Hepatosplenic $\gamma\delta$ T-cell lymphoma, Adult T-cell leukemia/lymphoma (ATLL), enteropathy-associated T-cell lymphoma, and extranodular NK/T cell lymphoma, which are rare, have aggressive behavior and are incurable diseases with conventional chemotherapy.

Similar to DLBL and FL, several studies have addressed the utility of IPI in PTCL.[52] Recently, the PIT has been applied to PTCL-U according to the WHO classification.[35] The PIT incorporates age, performance status, LDH, and bone marrow involvement. Compared to patients with low PIT score (0 factor), patients with high PIT scores (3 or 4 factors) have a poorer outcome in conventional chemotherapy (62% in low risk group versus 18% in high risk group at 5-year OS).

Preliminary data suggest that chemokine receptor expression may distinguish subsets of T helper cells and correlates with histology and prognosis. CXC chemokine receptor (CXCR) 3 expression was observed in angioimmunoblastic T-cell lymphoma (AILT), while CC chemokine receptor (CCR) 5 was observed with poor prognosis histologies including ALCL and ATLL. Moreover, CCR4 expression in PTCL-U was an independent poor prognostic factor.[53, 54] A gene expression study in T-cell lymphomas separated PTCL-U into 3 groups according to the overexpression of cyclin D2, NF-κB1 and Bcl-2, and interferon (IFN)-γ/JAK/STAT pathway.[55] However, further study is needed whether these groups correlate with clinical outcome.

Future prognostic models in NHL are likely to incorporate FDG-PET, immunophenotype and gene expression profiling as well as clinical data. Based on these prognostic models, patients with NHL who have poor prognostic factors at diagnosis or relapse may benefit from HSCT than standard chemotherapy.

4. CONDITIONING REGIMENS

Autologous Transplantation

HDC is used to overcome resistance that may occur in malignant cells. The cyclophosphamide (Cy) and total body irradiation (TBI) combination has been widely used in NHL.[6, 56, 57] Also various conditioning regimens such as CVB (cyclophosphamide, etoposide, carmustine)[58-60] and BEAM (carmustine, etoposide, cytarabine, melphalan)[61] have been used recently. TBI-containing regimen improved the outcome in FL,[56] on the other hand, chemotherapy-based conditioning regimens without TBI have shown better outcomes in DLBL.[62] These different outcomes may be due to the difference in sensitivity to radiation therapy between indolent and aggressive lymphomas. More importantly, a significant proportion of the patients treated with auto-HSCT subsequently has developed secondary myelodysplasia (MDS) or acute myeloid leukemia (AML), and retrospective analyses demonstrated that chemotherapy-based conditioning regimens were associated with a lower incidence of MDS/AML than TBI-conditioning regimens.[63, 64]

TBI should be avoided in patients who have received prior radiotherapy or for whom radiotherapy after auto-HSCT is planned, to avoid pulmonary complications.[65] Idiopathic pneumonia syndrome (IPS) in non-TBI regimens may have lower incidence after auto-HSCT than TBI-containing regimens. The lung toxicity by carmustine, which is a part of CVB or BEAM regimens, has been observed at relatively high incidence.[66]

Relapse remains the main cause of death after auto-HSCT. Residual lymphoma cells in the graft may account for some relapses after auto-HSCT.[67, 68] Rituximab has been used together with stem cell mobilization chemotherapy (in-vivo purging) and shown to be effective.[47, 69-72] The use of immunotherapy, such as rituximab, ^{131}I-tositumomab or ^{90}Y-ibritumomab, as a part of the conditioning regimen for auto-HSCT has produced promising results with improved disease control without a significant increase in toxicity.[73] Rituximab, an anti-CD20 chimeric antibody that works via complement-mediated cytotoxicity as well as by antibody-dependent cell-mediated cytotoxicity, effectively eliminates circulating B cells for an extended period of time after its administration. The use of rituximab has become a standard therapy as an adjunct to initial or salvage chemotherapy.[2, 3] A few studies were reported about the use of rituximab in the peri-transplant period. The MD Anderson Cancer Center (MDACC) used pre-mobilization rituximab followed by BEAM in combination with high-dose rituximab (1000 mg/m^2) after auto-HSCT.[18] Sixty-seven patients with aggressive NHL were treated with this approach. Although follow-up is short at 20 months, 2-year OS and DFS were 87% and 67%, respectively, and these results were significantly better than historical controls. Rituximab has been shown to be active in patients with less disease burden, and it is appealing to give maintenance in patients with MRD following HSCT.[74] Several studies of rituximab maintenance therapy after auto-HSCT are ongoing. Despite the lack of randomized trials, some investigators tended to incorporate rituximab into the peri-transplant period. Press et al reported promising results of a high dose ^{131}I-tositumomab in combination with HDC followed by auto-HSCT.[19-21] More recently, Vose et al demonstrated a very good long-term survival using a standard dose ^{131}I-tositumomab-BEAM treatment.[75] Currently, phase 3 is ongoing through Bone Marrow

Transplant Clinical Trials Network (BMT-CTN) to compare ^{131}I-tositumomab-BEAM to rituximab-BEAM.

One of serious adverse effects of anti-CD20 antibody in the peri-transplant period is an increase in the incidence of opportunistic infections due to organisms such as bacteria or cytomegalovirus due to B-cell depletion and resulting hypogammaglobulinemia after HSCT.[76, 77] Transient neutropenia is another cause of infections[78, 79] and occurred in 6 of 23 patients treated with rituximab after HSCT.[17] Some reports have demonstrated impairment of harvest of stem cells and subsequent delayed recovery of the platelets after transplantation. It is still controversial whether the use of rituximab or radioimmunotherapy affects the efficiency of mobilization, purging of malignant cells in the graft, or immune recovery after HSCT.[80-82] The effect of rituximab and radioimmunotherapy in the peri-transplant period should be carefully evaluated in a future study.

Allogeneic Transplantation

Allo-HSCT has several advantages over auto-HSCT such as avoiding the re-infusion of malignant cells and the reduction of the risk of relapse through GVL effect. The GVL effect is considered to be prominent in mantle cell lymphoma (MCL) and FL, while it is much less in DLBL.[83] Allo-HSCT may be recommended for NHL patients with refractory disease at transplantation or relapse after auto-HSCT. Similar to auto-HSCT, TBI/Cy has often been used for patients with NHL,[84] as well as chemotherapy-based conditioning such as CVB[85] and busulfan/cyclophosphamide (Bu/Cy).[86] On the other hand, many of them can not tolerate for intensive conditioning regimens because of their old age or medical co-morbidities.[87, 88]

Since the mid-1990s, investigators started to realize that, it is not absolutely necessary to destroy the bone marrow of the host to create a space for donor cells to engraft. However, it is still necessary to provide enough immune suppression to the host to ensure the engraftment of donor stem cells. Based on these findings, reduced-intensity stem cell transplantation (RIST) has been developed. RIST regimens are generally less intensive in terms of chemotherapy dose, but provide enough immunosuppression. In this type of regimens, anti-tumor effect is mainly mediated by GVL effect, rather than the direct cytotoxic effect of conditioning regimens. Likewise, in RIST, it is not the effect of conditioning regimen itself, but graft-versus host (GVH) effect, to eradicate the host hemopoiesis. Since a few groups have reported successful RIST in the late 1990s,[14-16] it has been used worldwide as one of the treatment options for hematological malignancies including NHL. More than a few different nomenclatures have been proposed to classify RIST regimens, and it is now quite confusing. We have previously proposed a classification of RIST regimens (figure 1).[89, 90]

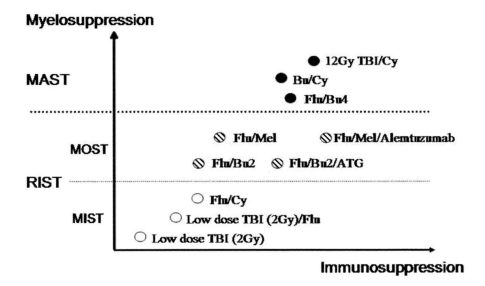

Figure 1. Classification of conditioning regimens in allogeneic hematopoietic stem cell transplantation. TBI indicates total body irradiation; Flu, fludarabine; Cy, cyclophosphamide; Bu, busulfan; ATG, anti-thymocyte globulin; Mel, melphalan; MAST, myeloablative stem cell transplantation; RIST, reduced-intensity stem cell transplantation; MOST, moderate-intensity stem cell transplantation; MIST, minimal-intensity stem cell transplantation.

In our classification, RIST is divided into minimal-intensity stem cell transplantation (MIST) and moderate-intensity stem cell transplantation (MOST). MIST conditioning was originally developed at Fred Hutchinson Cancer Research Center (FHCRC) involving low-dose TBI (2Gy), either alone or in combination with fludarabine (Flu). With this type of minimal-intensity regimen, if donor stem cells are not infused after conditioning, host's own hemopoiesis recovers within 30 days, and patient may have very short or no period of cytopenia. In MOST, the conditioning regimen partly destroys the host hemopoiesis. Host's own hemopoiesis may recover in cases of graft rejection or loss of graft, but it may take much longer than in MIST. With myeloablative stem cell transplantation (MAST), on the other hand, host's hemopoiesis may not recover at all, or it takes more than 3-6 months to recover if graft is lost. The patients can not survive if no rescue stem cells are given in case of engraftment failure in MAST.

Flu is most popular agent to be used in RIST regimens in combination with Bu, melphalan (Mel), low-dose TBI, Cy, or others.[15] Other nucleoside analogues such as cladribine or pentostatin are also being used.[91, 92] Antibodies against T-cells, such as anti-thymocyte globulin (ATG)[15] or alemtuzumab[93], have also been used to both facilitate engraftment and prevent GVHD. The importance of serotherapy in anti-tumor responses (ATG in T-cell lymphoma or alemtuzumab in CD52 expressing low-grade lymphoma) remains unclear. Similar to auto-HSCT, several groups has tested rituximab or radioimmunotherapy combined with RIST for anti-tumor effect. Whether the use of these agents in peri-transplant period in RIST changes the survival, the incidence of GVHD or infections is to be determined.

RIST has been used for over a decade, and many issues have been clarified. The importance of dose intensity may be different in different NHL. Also, the efficacy of GVL may be different disease by disease. Thus, all RIST regimens should not be considered equivalent in NHL. Accordingly, the likelihood of success after RIST is highly dependent on the type of NHL. Recent studies showed that despite lower NRM with RIST, relapse rate was higher and there was no significant difference in survival compared to MAST.[94] As it has become more apparent that intensity of conditioning regimens is important to prevent relapse, myeloablative regimens with attenuated toxicity have been developed for older or medically unfit patients. One of these regimens, Flu with myeloablative dose of intravenous Bu (Flu/Bu4) achieved 100 day NRM below 10% and comparable survival with conventional regimens in to AML and MDS.[95] Another approach is auto-HSCT followed by RIST in refractory NHL to reduce tumor burden by auto-HSCT followed by RIST as immunotherapy.[96] This approach has been the most popular in multiple myeloma.[96-98]

Although RIST has opened a many new possibilities for allo-HSCT, GVHD still remains the major obstacle. Prophylaxis and treatment of GVHD have been investigated in many studies including ones using etanercept,[99] sirolimus,[100] pentostatin,[101] alemtuzumab[102] or extracorporeal photopheresis.[101, 103] Lowsky et al reported a unique regimen using 8Gy of total lymphoid irradiation in 10 fractions with ATG.[104] They claimed that this regimen induces NKT cells, and they showed that incidence of GVHD was very low while GVL effect seemed to be preserved.

5. STEM CELL SOURCE AND MANIPULATION

Autologous Transplantation

Randomized clinical trials show that auto-HSCT using growth factor-mobilized peripheral blood stem cell (PBSC) result in earlier engraftment and lower cost than using cells from bone marrow (BM).[105] At present, mobilized PBSC has been used in most cases of auto-HSCT except for the cases of poor mobilization. Recently AMD3100, a reversible inhibitor of stromal cell-derived factor (SDF)-1α and CXCR4 which play key regulatory roles in stem cell trafficking and retention by the marrow[106] has been explored in patients with poor mobilization using chemotherapy and/or granulocyte colony stimulating factor (G-CSF) or granulocyte monocyte colony stimulating factor (GM-CSF) in clinical trials, and the results were encouraging.[107]

Allogeneic Transplantation

Up to 60% of allo-HSCT is being done with PBSC, in contrast to 90% in auto-HSCT. Many prospective studies comparing allogeneic peripheral blood stem cell transplantation (allo-PBSCT) with allogeneic bone marrow transplantation (allo-BMT) has been conducted mainly in leukemias. The meta-analysis using data from these 9 randomized trials demonstrated that allo-PBSCT is associated with a significant risk of extensive chronic

GVHD, a decreased relapse rate, and improvement in OS and DFS in patients with late-stage diseases.[108] However, these most patients in these studies were leukemias and only few cases of NHL were included.

There are few published data regarding allo-HSCT for NHL from unrelated donor including umbilical cord blood.[109-111] Some investigators suggested that the use of unrelated donor may be associated with more potent GVL effect, less relapse and improved survival.[112] Considering that many patients do not have an HLA-identical sibling donor, the alternative donor source should be actively sought.

6. HSCT FOR ELDERLY PATIENTS WITH NHL

Increasing age is associated with poorer survival in patients treated with conventional therapy.[113, 114] In fact, age is one of the important prognostic factors in the IPI, the FLIPI, and the PIT. Poorer prognosis may be due to either different biology in the elderly patients or due to intolerance to therapy. To overcome the poor prognosis, HSCT has been increasingly applied to elderly patients especially after the introduction of RIST. It should be mentioned that HSCT is clearly more toxic than conventional therapies and that recovery from HSCT may take much longer than expected in younger patients.

Autologous Transplantation

Along with developments in supportive care, morbidity and mortality associated with auto-HSCT have decreased. NRM has been in the range of 5-10%.[8, 9] This is higher than NRM (2-3%) in younger patients. TBI has not been used much in this age group. Instead, CBV or BEAM have been used.[8, 9] No large studies have been conducted in this age group. Based on small single center studies, efficacy of auto-HSCT in elderly patients with NHL may be comparable to that observed in younger population. Mobilization of progenitor cells is unsuccessful in about 10% of patients with NHL.[115] Age does not seem to affect the success of progenitor cell mobilization in NHL patients mobilized with intermediate-dose Cy and G-CSF.[116] Further studies are needed to decrease toxicity of HDC in the elderly patients where co-morbid conditions may exist. Careful evaluation of patients based on clear eligibility criteria is very important in elderly patients.

Allogeneic Transplantation

RIST was originally developed to reduce NRM, so that older patients can tolerate. Many studies have confirmed that the early post-transplant (<100 days) NRM following RIST are much less than that after MAST,[117] and investigators use higher age limit for RIST. However, mortality from acute GVHD may occur even after day 100 in patients who received RIST and GVHD mortality seems to be the same as that of MAST. Some investigators also reported that the incidence of acute GVHD was higher in elderly patients and/or donors than in younger patients and/or donors.[118, 119] Therefore, in most literatures, NRM at 2-year after RIST is about 20%, which is still lower than that after MAST (30%), but may not be as impressive as the difference in day 100 mortality.[87, 88, 120] Quality of life (QOL) after allo-HSCT has also become an important issue. According to previous studies, patient's age and chronic GVHD may adversely affect QOL after allo-HSCT.[121, 122]

In a retrospective study, the FHCRC group compared RIST with MAST from unrelated donors. Although patients who underwent RIST had significantly more pre-transplant co-morbidities, were older, and had more often failed preceding myeloablative allo- or auto-HSCT, they experienced fewer toxicities than patients who underwent MAST.[88] It has been shown that medical co-morbidity, not necessarily physiological age, is more related with the outcome of HSCT. The Charlson comorbidity index was applied to RIST recipients and a direct relationship between comorbidity scores and outcome was found.[123]

7. Transplant Indications and Outcomes

This section highlights the use of both auto-HSCT and allo-HSCT according to each disease categories. These results are summarized in table 2.

7.1. Diffuse Large Cell Lymphoma

Autologous Transplantation as Consolidation in First Remission
Several randomized studies reported conflicting results on the impact of auto-HSCT in the first-line treatment for aggressive NHL (table 2).[58, 124-133] There was no evidence that auto-HSCT improved OS and event-free survival (EFS) in patients with good risk. The role of it in patients with poor risk is still unclear. Auto-HSCT should not be further investigated in patients with good risk, but highly quality studies in patients with poor risk are warranted.[134, 135]

Autologous Transplantation as a Salvage Therapy
The randomized PARMA study established auto-HSCT as a standard therapy for relapsed aggressive lymphoma that is still sensitive to conventional dose salvage chemotherapy (table 2).[6] Of the initial 215 patients younger than 60 years of age who were in first or second relapse, only 109 were randomized, with most of the remaining patients excluded because of failure to respond to salvage therapy with DHAP (dexamethazone, cytrabine, cisplatin). The 5-year EFS was 46% for the auto-HSCT group compared to 12% for salvage chemotherapy group (p=0.001). OS was also higher in the auto-HSCT group (53% versus 32%, p=0.038). Even patients with primary induction failure may have a benefit from auto-HSCT if these patients remain chemo-sensitive to disease after salvage chemotherapy.[136, 137]

Thus, auto-HSCT has been shown to produce superior OS compared with conventional salvage chemotherapy in patients with chemo-sensitive relapsed disease. However, only 30-40% of patients are cured by auto-HSCT. Several prognostic factors that predict for outcome of auto-HSCT in patients with relapsed or refractory NHL have been reported. Further analysis of the PARMA study showed that the IPI at the time of relapse was highly correlated with OS in the conventional salvage therapy group but not in the auto-HSCT group.[138] In contrast, time to relapse (<12 months versus >12 months from diagnosis to relapse) was found to be an independent prognostic factor for both EFS and OS regardless of the treatment group. The Memorial Sloan-Kettering Cancer Center also evaluated the aaIPI at the initiation of second-chemotherapy in 150 patients with relapsed or refractory DLBL followed by auto-HSCT.[139] They confirmed the predictive value of the aaIPI, showing that patients with a score of 2 or 3 at the time of relapse had 4-year progression-free survival (PFS) and OS of only 16% and 18%. Several groups have reported high predictive value of FDG-PET for lymphoma in the setting of auto-HSCT, showing that the positivity of pre-transplant FDG-PET may predict clinical outcome in NHL after auto-SCT.[36, 46] Spaepen et al retrospectively analyzed the impact of FDG-PET before auto-HSCT in 60 patients (19 HL, and 41 NHL) who had failed induction therapy or had chemo-sensitive relapses.[36] Thirty patients had negative FDG-PET before auto-HSCT, and 25 of these remained in remission at the median follow-up of 4 years. Two patients died from NRM without relapse and only 3 patients had relapsed. Of the 30 patients with positive FDG-PET before auto-HSCT, 26 patients relapsed at a median of 402 days and 16 died of progressed disease. Only 4 patients remained in remission.

Other novel approaches may be required for those patients with poor prognostic factors such as chemo-refractory disease, positive FDG-PET before auto-HSCT, and high aaIPI at the time of relapse. [62, 140]

Allogeneic Transplantation

Certainly several studies have shown long-term disease control following allo-HSCT in NHL,[12, 70, 141-143] however, the role of allo-HSCT in DLBL remains undefined yet. The European Group for Blood and Marrow Transplantation (EBMT) analyzed the data of aggressive lymphoma retrospectively,[144] which showed about equal the 4-year PFS of 35% in allo-HSCT and 39% in auto-HSCT. Allo-HSCT tends to be reserved for younger NHL patients with bone marrow involvement, chemo-resistance, or patients who relapsed after auto-HSCT.[11, 145-147]

Only small studies have been done for RIST in DLBL. Available reports showed that RIST for chemo-refractory DLBL was associated with poor outcome.[102] Because of rapid disease progression, RIST may not be able to control the tumor burden until the time GVL effects start to work. To overcome this problem, auto-HSCT followed by RIST has been tried in DLBL with moderate success.[96]

Table 2. Prospective randomized studies of auto-HSCT for NHL

Study	Disease	Status at transplant	Therapy	No	OS	p	PFS/EFS	p
Italy, Milan[124]	DLBL	Up-front, 1st remission	MACOP-B	50	55%	—	49%	—
			Auto-HSCT	48	81% (7yr)	0.09	76% (7yr)	0.004
Italy, NHLCSG[125]	Aggressive NHL	Up-front	VACOP-B	61	65%		48%	
			Auto-HSCT	63	65% (6yr)	0.5	60% (6yr)	0.4
GELA LNH 87-2[58]	Aggressive NHL	Up-front CR1	A/NCVB	111	49%		39%	
		aalPI;HI/H	Auto-HSCT	125	64% (8yr)	0.04	55% (8yr)	0.02
EORTC[126]	Aggressive NHL	Up-front IPI;L/LI(70%)	CHVmP/BV	96	77%		56%	
			Auto-HSCT	98	68% (5yr)	0.34	61% (5yr)	0.71
GELA LNH 93-3[127]	Aggressive NHL	Up-front aalPI; HI/H	ACVBP	181	60%		51%	
			Auto-HSCT	189	46% (5yr)	0.007	39% (5yr)	0.01
Germany, HGLSG[128]	Aggressive NHL	Up-front	CHOEP	154	63%		49%	
			Auto-HSCT	158	62% (3yr)	0.68	59% (3yr)	0.22
Italy, multi-center[129]	Aggressive NHL	Up-front aalPI; HI/H	MACOP-B	75	65%		49%	
			Auto-HSCT	75	64% (5yr)	0.95	61% (5yr)	0.21
GOELAMS[130]	Aggressive NHL	Up-front aalPI; L/LI/HI	CHOP	99	56%		37%	
			Auto-HSCT	98	71% (5yr)	0.076	55% (5yr)	0.037
IIL[131]	Aggressive NHL	Up-front IPI; HI/H	MegaCEOP	66	63%		48%	

Study	Disease	Status at transplant	Therapy	No	OS	p	PFS/EFS	p
HOVON[132]	Aggressive NHL	Up-front PR1	Auto-HSCT	60	49% (5yr)	0.060	43% (6yr)	0.56
			CHOP	35	85%		53%	
Study	Disease	Status at transplant	Therapy	No	OS	p	PFS/EFS	p
Italy, multi-center[133]	Aggressive NHL	Up-front PR1	Auto-HSCT	34	56% (4yr)	>0.1	41% (4yr)	>0.1
			DHAP	27	59%		52%	
PARMA[6]	Aggressive NHL	Salvage for relpase	Auto-HSCT	22	73% (55mo)	0.4	73% (55mo)	0.3
			DHAP	54	32%		12%	
		Chemo-sensitive	Auto-HSCT	55	53% (5yr)	0.038	46% (5yr)	0.001
GLSG[158]	FL	Up-front	CHOP like +IFN-α	154	NA	NA	33%	<0.0001
			Auto-HSCT	153	NA		64.7% (5yr)	
GOELAMS[159]	FL	Up-front	CHVP +IFN-α	80	84%	0.493	48%	0.05
			Purged auto-HSCT	86	78% (5yr)		60% (5yr)	
GELA[160]	FL	Up-front	CHVP +IFN-α	209	71%		28%	
			Auto-HSCT	192	76% (7yr)	0.53	38% (7yr)	0.11
EBMT CUP[71]	FL	Salvage for relpase	CHOP like	24	46%		26%	
		Chemo-sensitive	Unpurged auto-HSCT	33	71%	0.079	58%	
			Purged auto-HSCT	32	77% (4yr)		55% (2yr)	0.0037

Table 2. (Continued)

European MCL Network[7]	MCL	Up-front CR/PR	IFN-α maintenance	60	83%		17mo	
			Auto-HSCT	62	77% (3yr)	0.018	39mo (median)	0.01

Auto-HSCT, autologous hematopoietic stem cell transplantation; NHL, non-Hodgkin's lymphoma; OS, overall survival; PFS, progression-free survival; EFS, event-free survival; DLBL, diffuse large B-cell lymphoma; FL, follicular lymphoma; MCL mantle cell lymphoma; CR, complete remission; PR, partial remission; IPI, international prognostic index; aaIPI, Age adjusted IPI; MACOP-B, methotrexate, doxorubicin, cyclophosphamide, vincristine, prednisone, and bleomycin; VACOP-B, etoposide, doxorubicin, cyclophosphamide, vincristine, prednisone, and bleomycin; ACVB, doxorubicin, cyclophosphamide, vindesine, and bleomycin; CHVmP/BV, cyclophosphamide, doxorubicin, teniposide, prednisone, bleomycin, and vincristine; ACVBP, doxorubicin, cyclophosphamide, vindesine, bleomycin, and prednisone; CHOEP, cyclophosphamide, doxorubicin, vincristine, etoposide, and prednisone; CHOP, cyclophosphamide, doxorubicin, vincristine, and prednisone; CEOP, cyclophosphamide, epirubicin, vincristine, and prednisone; DHAP, cisplatin, cytarabine, and dexamethasone; CHVP, cyclophosphamide, doxorubicin, teniposide, and prednisone; IFN, interferon; NA, not available.

7.2. Follicular Lymphoma

Although the introduction of anti-CD20 antibody has altered the landscape of treatment in FL, FL is considered an incurable disease. [148-154] Auto-HSCT is shown in several studies to induce remissions and may change the natural history. However, there was little evidence that auto-HSCT conferred any survival advantage compared with conventional treatment for FL.

Autologous Transplantation as Consolidation in First Remission

Auto-HSCT has been used for advanced-stage FL patients in first complete or partial remission as a consolidation therapy.[155-157] The role of auto-HSCT in patients with FL under the age of 60 during first remission was explored in 3 phase 3 randomized trials (table 2). The GLSG (German Low-Grade Lymphoma Study Group) study recruited 307 previously untreated patients, and patients who responded after induction chemotherapy were randomly assigned to auto-HSCT or IFN-α maintenance.[158] Among 240 evaluable patients, the 5-year PFS was 64.7% in the auto-HSCT arm and 33.3% in the IFN-α arm ($p<$ 0.001). There was no difference between 2 arms in OS. Similar results were reported by the GOELAM (Groupe Ouest Est des Leucemies Aigues et des Maladies du Sang).[159] In this study, 172 patients with newly diagnosed advanced FL were randomly assigned either to chemotherapy and IFN-α or to HDC followed by purged auto-HSCT. Patients who received auto-HSCT had a higher response rate than patients who received chemotherapy and IFN-α (81% versus 69%, p = 0.045) and a longer median PFS (not reached versus 45 months), but there was no difference in OS between the 2 groups because of an excess of secondary malignancies in the auto-HSCT arm. The advantage of auto-HSCT was restricted to patients with high risk according to the FLIPI. The Group d'Etude des Lymphome d'Adulte (GELA) study enrolled 401 patients with previously untreated advanced stage FL who were randomly assigned to receive CHVP (cyclophosphamide, doxorubicin, teniposide, prednisone) plus IFN-α compared with 4 courses of CHOP followed by HDC with auto-HSCT.[160] Similar to 2 previous studies, this study also did not show a significant survival benefit for those randomized to auto-HSCT. These results show that auto-HSCT should be reserved for relapsed patients.

Autologous Transplantation as a Salvage Therapy

Several phase 2 studies demonstrated that auto-HSCT as a salvage treatment prolongs OS and disease-free survival (DFS) for patients with chemo-sensitive relapsed FL.[56, 57, 161-163] The GELA study compared results in patients who underwent auto-HSCT or received standard chemotherapy after relapse.[162] Patients in the auto-HSCT group had a superior in OS and DFS to chemotherapy (58% versus 38% in OS and 42% versus 16% in DFS, respectively). The EBMT sponsored CUP (conventional chemotherapy, unpurged and purged autograft) study is the only prospective randomized trial to address the role of auto-HSCT in patients with relapsed FL (table 2).[71] After 3 initial cycles of chemotherapy (usually a CHOP-like regimen), patients with chemo-sensitive diseases were randomized to one of the 3 treatment arms: further conventional chemotherapy, auto-HSCT using ex-vivo purged graft or auto-HSCT using unpurged graft. The study was closed early because of slow accrual with

140 of the planned 250 patients accrued and only 89 patients randomly assigned to treatment. A median follow-up was 69 months. The results of the study suggested a PFS and OS advantage in auto-HSCT over conventional chemotherapy, with 4-year OS of 46% for the chemotherapy arm versus 71% for the unpurged and 77% for the purged auto-HSCT arms, respectively. In this study, there was no clear evidence of benefit in purging. Thus, auto-HSCT provides a survival benefit in patients with chemo-sensitive relapsed FL.

Allogeneic Transplantation

Allo-HSCT used to be used in FL patients who were not candidates for auto-HSCT due to chemo-refractory disease or massive bone marrow involvement. Several retrospective studies have demonstrated a lower risk of relapse in comparison with auto-HSCT, but the higher incidence of NRM has offset any significant difference in survival.[164, 165] The International Bone Marrow Transplant Registry (IBMTR)/Autologous Blood and Marrow Transplant Registry (ABMTR) compared the outcomes of 904 patients with FL who received allo-HSCT between 1990 and 1999 to those who received auto-HSCT.[13] A total of 176 patients received allo-HSCT from HLA matched sibling and 728 received auto-HSCT (131 purged and 597 unpurged). The 5-year probabilities of survival of 51% were comparable to that of auto-HSCT. The NRM rates were higher and the relapse rates at 5-year were significantly lower in the allo-HSCT group compared to the purged and unpurged auto-HSCT groups. There were few late relapses beyond 1 year in the allo-HSCT group.

Because of the high NRM rates in allo-HSCT for FL, several groups have utilized RIST. The first report of RIST for FL was from the MDACC.[166] They reported the results of 20 patients with relapsed low-grade lymphoma (including 18 patients with FL), who underwent RIST. In 9 cases, rituximab was added to the preparative regimen. All 20 achieved a complete remission (CR) after transplantation, including 6 molecular remissions (by polymerase chain reaction for bcl-2 gene rearrangement). Two-year OS and DFS were both 84%; none of the patients have relapsed, with a median follow-up period of 21 months. Data from the EBMT on 52 patients with low-grade NHL underwent RIST are also encouraging although limited in the length of follow-up.[167] Most cases (85%) were chemo-sensitive at the time of RIST. OS and PFS at 2-year were 65 and 54%, respectively. Longer follow-up is needed to confirm the possible plateau in survival.

7.3. Transformed Follicular Lymphoma

The prognosis of patients with t-FL is generally very poor, and conventional chemotherapy is of limited benefit. The median OS historically ranges from 2.5 to 22 months.[42, 168]

Autologous Transplantation

Except for the patients with limited disease who have not been previously treated for FL, most patients with t-FL will relapse quickly following conventional treatment.[42, 168-172] In a series from the Dana-Farber Cancer Institute in which 21 patients have undergone anti-B-cell purged auto-HSCT for FL transformed into DLBL,[173] DFS at 5-year was 46% with follow-up from 12 to 120 months. A series from the Stanford University reported 17 patients with t-FL including 13 patients transplanted at first relapse, and only 6 patients in CR at transplant.[163] The 4-year DFS and OS were 49% and 50%, respectively. Berglund et al reported 11 patients with chemo-sensitive disease who underwent auto-HSCT.[174] The follow-up time was the longest of all reports series, with OS and DFS 81% and 72% at 74 months. Similar results with larger numbers of patients in t-FL were reported by the EBMT.[175] Fifty patients with chemo-sensitive t-FL who underwent auto-HSCT were compared with 200 case-matched patients with low-grade FL and 200 case-matched patients with de novo high- or intermediate-grade lymphoma who underwent auto-HSCT. OS and DFS with t-FL were 51 and 30% at 5 years, respectively. There were no significant differences in OS and DFS between the t-FL group and the low-grade FL or de novo high- or intermediate-grade lymphoma groups. An increased LDH level at auto-HSCT was identified as an adverse risk factor. A subgroup of patients with residual chemo-sensitive disease who attained CR after auto-HSCT had an OS at 5 years of 69%. All 3 patients with chemo-resistant disease at the time of auto-HSCT died of relapsed or progressive disease. A series from Chen et al included 35 patients with t-FL. At median follow-up of 52 months, OS and PFS at 5-year was 37% and 36%, respectively.[176]

Results of these studies suggest that aggressive therapy with auto-HSCT is a reasonable treatment option for selected patients less than age 60 and with chemo-sensitive disease. However, the number of reported patients was very small, and it is still unclear whether survival curve in auto-HSCT becomes plateau after 5 years. In addition, alternative therapies may be required for patients with chemo-refractory t-FL. The development of secondary AML/MDS as well as relapse after auto-HSCT further hampers the treatment outcome.[63, 174, 177]

Allogeneic Transplantation

There is an increased incidence of late relapse following auto-HSCT, which has led to further investigations utilizing allo-HSCT for t-FL. However, there are no conclusive data yet in allo-HSCT for t-FL. MAST for younger patients with t-FL may result in a significantly decreased relapse rate, providing both GVL and anti-tumor effect through conditioning high-dose chemotherapy. To decrease NRM, RIST in t-FL is worth of further investigation.[166]

7.4. Mantle Cell Lymphoma

MCL is an aggressive and generally incurable disease with standard-dose chemotherapy.[32, 178-180] HSCT plays an important role in the treatment of MCL. However, the exact role of HSCT in MCL has not been clearly established due to the absence of large prospective studies.

Autologous Transplantation

A retrospective analysis was performed using the pooled data from the EBMT and ABMTR registries on the outcome of 195 MCL patients who had been treated with auto-HSCT.[181] After a median follow-up of 3.9 years, OS at 2- and 5-year were 76% and 50%, and PFS at 2- and 5-year were as 55% and 33%, respectively. Patients who were transplanted in first CR were less likely to die from MCL than beyond first CR. Results were similar in a retrospective analysis of 69 patients at Stanford University and City of Hope who underwent auto-HSCT.[182] Patients who were in first CR at the time of transplant had 3- and 5-year OS/DFS rates of 93%/74% and 77%/50%, respectively. In comparison, the OS/DFS at 3 and 5 years for patients who were not in first remission at the time of transplantation were 64%/51% and 39%/21%, respectively. The median time to relapse in the group transplanted in first CR was 32 months compared to 10.5 months if not in CR. Taken together, auto-HSCT may improve prognosis when performed at first CR. However, the results vary among studies because of differences in patient selection, induction and conditioning regimens, the number of prior therapies, and remission status at the time of transplantation. Therefore, it is difficult to draw definite conclusions regarding the role of auto-HSCT for MCL.

Recently, the European MCL Network reported the results of the first prospective randomized trial comparing upfront auto-HSCT versus IFN-α after CHOP-like induction regimen with or without rituximab in 122 patients that achieved at least partial remission (PR) (table 2).[7] PFS was significantly longer in the auto-HSCT group (median 39 months versus 17 months, $p=0.0108$). Longer follow-up is needed to assess impact on OS, which was not significantly different (83% versus 77%, $p=0.18$) at 3 years. In a subset analysis, patients who underwent auto-HSCT in CR had the greatest benefit. However, most patients continue to relapse even though they were in CR at transplant, showing that auto-HSCT may not be curative for MCL.

Various strategies have been employed to improve the outcome of auto-HSCT for MCL. Dose intensification of chemotherapy has been attempted. The use of hyper-CVAD (fractionated cyclophosphamide, doxorubicin, vincristine, dexamethasone) alternating with high-dose methotrexate and cytarabine as initial therapy for MCL may result in better transplant outcome for eligible patients.[183] Rituximab has been incorporated into conditioning regimens and maintenance therapy for MCL.[184, 185] Pott et al reported that an MRD kinetics study of bone marrow or peripheral blood during the first year following auto-HSCT.[186] They concluded that MRD elimination after transplantation is highly predictive of a favorable prognosis with a median PFS of 92 months in the MRD negative group compared with 21 months in the MRD-positive group ($p <0.001$), making molecular remission a desirable goal in the treatment of MCL. However, the longer-term impact of pre-transplant or post-transplant rituximab for MCL is not yet clear. Incorporation of radioimmunotherapy into conditioning regimens has been also attempted. Gopal et al evaluated the efficacy of ^{131}I -tositumomab in combination with etoposide and cyclophosphamide followed by auto-HSCT in 16 relapsed MCL patients. OS and PFS at 3-year were 93% and 61%, respectively.[187] This approach is thought to be feasible, and further study is warranted.

Allogeneic Transplantation

MCL has been associated with a high risk of relapse after conventional chemotherapy or auto-HSCT. Due to the advanced age of the majority of patients with MCL, the opportunity to perform MAST in MCL has been limited. In most series, PFS at 3-year in MAST has been reported to be about 50%, and most patients underwent allo-HSCT as a salvage therapy.[188-

190] A series of 16 patients with MCL demonstrated that OS and EFS at 3-year following MAST from a sibling donor were both 55%, although a high NRM of 38% was reported.[191]

Recently, some investigators reported the outcomes with RIST in MCL. The MDACC analyzed 18 patients conditioned predominantly with Flu/Cy and high-dose rituximab.[192] All 16 patients had chemo-sensitive MCL. DFS at 2-year was 82% with only 3 relapses reported. Two patients received donor lymphocyte infusion (DLI) resulting in one sustained CR and one PR lasting for 1 year. The FHCRC reported 33 refractory or relapsed MCL patients (16 related donors and 17 unrelated donors) undergoing MIST using Flu/2Gy TBI.[112] DFS and OS at 2-year were 60% and 64%, respectively. Morris et al assessed 10 patients underwent MOST using alemtuzumab-based regimens. Nine of 10 patients had chemo-sensitive MCL and four had a prior auto-HSCT. NRM was 20% and 3-year PFS and OS were 50 and 60%, respectively. These results suggest that RIST is effective in MCL, and may be able to salvage some patients who had chemo-refractory disease or relapsed after auto-HSCT.

Further studies comparing auto- and allo-HSCT are needed, stratified by disease status. New agents, such as Bortezomib,[193] Thalidomide,[194] and Temsirolimus,[171, 195] have been studied in relapsed/refractory MCL as a single agent or in combination with other drugs. In future, some of these agents may be used in the HSCT settings.

7.5. Peripheral T-Cell Lymphoma and NK-Cell Neoplasms

PTCL and NK neoplasms are a heterogenous group of NHL. These diseases have a geographic variation, with more nodal disease in North America and Europe, including PTCL-U, anaplastic large cell lymphoma (ALCL) and AILT; and more extranodal disease in Asia due to Epstein-Barr virus-related NK/T lymphoma and ATLL. The progress in treatments has been slow due to the rarity of the diseases, inadequate pathological classification, relative chemo-resistance, and lack of well-designed clinical trials.

Autologous Transplantation

Some retrospective studies using auto-HSCT in relapsed or refractory patients with T-cell lymphoma showed that this approach was an effective salvage treatment, resulting in approximately DFS of 30% and OS of 40% at 3-4 years.[196-198] Several prognostic factors at the time of transplantation have been identified and they are almost similar to those described in DLBL, such as chemo-sensitive disease and low IPI.[52] In addition, results were more favorable in ALK-positive ALCL compared to the other PTCL subtypes. Patients with ALK-positive ALCL in first CR have the best outcome among this subtype of NHL with OS at 5-year of more than 80%, thus auto-HSCT should not be recommended to patients with ALK-positive ALCL in first CR. Patients with AILT[199] or enteropathy-associated T-cell lymphoma[200] have so poor prognosis after chemotherapy that the use of auto-HSCT is favored in first remission by some investigators.

Similar to DLBL, PTCL patients with chemo-sensitive relapsed disease should be offered auto-HSCT and also patients with poor prognostic factors may be indicated for auto-HSCT in first CR.[201] However, no randomized studies have been performed to compare auto-HSCT versus standard chemotherapy in this group.

Allogeneic Transplantation

Very few studies have addressed the role of allo-HSCT in T/NK-cell lymphomas.[202] Similar to the outcome of B-cell lymphomas, the rate of NRM after MAST was quite significant. It is noteworthy, however, that OS at 5-year was 41% and especially 76% for patients in CR, suggesting a curative potential of allo-HSCT.[142] Corradini et al recently reported the outcome of RIST for 17 patients with relapsed or refractory PTCL (9 patients with PTCL-U, 4 with AILT, and 4 with ALK-negative ALCL).[203] Eight patients had a disease relapse after auto-HSCT. The estimated 3-year OS and PFS were 81% and 64%, respectively. The NRM at 2-year was 6%. DLI induced a response in 2 patients who had progression after RIST. They suggested that RIST for PTCL is a feasible treatment but cytoreduction of tumor prior to allo-HSCT is necessary.

Table 3. Proposed indication of transplantation for non-Hodgkin lymphoma

Disease	Disease status at transplantation	Auto-HSCT	Allo-HSCT
DLBL	CR1; low risk	NR	NR
	CR1; high risk	D	NR
	≥CR2, Chemo-sensitive disease; low risk	R	NR
	≥CR2, Chemo-sensitive disease; high risk	D	D
	Chemo-refractory disease	NR	D
FL	CR1; low risk	NR	NR
	CR1; high risk	D	NR
	≥CR2, Chemo-sensitive disease	D	D
	Chemo-refractory disease	NR	D
MCL	CR1	D	D
	≥CR2, Chemo-sensitive disease	D	D
	Chemo-refractory disease	NR	D
PTCL	CR1	D	D
	CR1, ALK-positive ALCL	NR	NR
	≥CR2, Chemo-sensitive disease	D	D
	Chemo-refractory disease	NR	D
	ATLL	NR	D
	Hepatosplenic γδ T-cell lymphoma	NR	D

Auto-HSCT, autologous hematopoietic stem cell transplantation; Allo-HSCT, allogeneic hematopoietic stem cell transplantation; DLBL, diffuse large B-cell lymphoma; FL, follicular lymphoma; MCL, mantle cell lymphoma; PTCL, peripheral T-cell lymphoma; CR, complete remission; ALK, anaplastic lymphoma kinase ; ATLL, adult T-cell leukemia/lymphoma; R, recommended; D, developmental; NR, not recommended.

ATLL is caused by human T-cell leukemia virus type I (HTLV-I) and has an extremely poor prognosis with projected 2- and 4-year survival rates of 16.7% and 5.0% for the acute type and 21.3% and 5.7% for the lymphoma type, respectively.[204] Neither intensified chemotherapy nor auto-HSCT has improved the prognosis.[205, 206] Encouraging results in allo-HSCT for ATLL have been reported by several groups with approximately 40% OS at 3-year.[207-209] Okamura et al reported the utility of RIST for ATLL through possible GVL effect.[210, 211] Allo-HSCT from unrelated HTLV-I-negative donors is feasible treatment for ATLL to avoid possible transmission of HTLV-I from sibling HLA-matched donors with positive HTLV-I.[110, 212, 213]

Hepatosplenic γδ T-cell lymphoma is a rare disease with a poor prognosis and some case reports suggest the cure potential of allo-HSCT.[214]

A Japanese group evaluated the utility of HSCT for NK-cell lineage tumors.[215] OS at 4-year was 39% with a median follow-up of 50 months; this was significantly better than that of patients who did not undergo HSCT (21%, $p=0.0003$). The probability after relapse in allo-HSCT was as low as 17%, even though most of them (60%) were in non-remission at transplantation.

Many targeted therapies, such as anti-IL-2 receptor antibodies,[216] alemtuzumab,[217] and anti-CCR4 antibody,[53] have been introduced in the treatment of PTCL recently. However, there are few data regarding these agents in the HSCT setting for PTCL, and the role of these remains unclear.

CONCLUSION

HSCT has become increasingly important in the treatment scheme of NHL. The use of RIST has extended the benefits of HSCT to a wider range of patients. In addition, the introduction of novel agents, including rituximab, radioimmunotherapy, and other target therapies, open the new possibilities. Emerging data from molecular markers and gene expression profiling may also help us to understand the pathophysiology of NHL and to identify new targets for therapy.

As advances in HSCT have led to an increasing number of patients to be cured, late effects after HSCT have become of major clinical importance. Secondary malignancies are one of the late effects, which have increasingly been recognized. It is still unclear whether the incidence of secondary AML/MDS is lower in radioimmunotherapy compared to TBI-containing regimen.[218] More effective surveillance and early diagnosis may lead patients to have a better chance of cure with increased awareness and evolving understanding of risk factors.

Most recent studies in HSCT, particularly using new agents such as targeted therapies, have still short follow-up. To define the role of HSCT in the era of "targeted therapy", well organized clinical trials and careful follow-up are needed.

REFERENCES

[1]   Fisher RI, Gaynor ER, Dahlberg S, et al. Comparison of a standard regimen (CHOP) with three intensive chemotherapy regimens for advanced non-Hodgkin's lymphoma. *N. Engl. J. Med.* 1993; 328:1002-6.

[2]   Coiffier B, Lepage E, Briere J, et al. CHOP chemotherapy plus rituximab compared with CHOP alone in elderly patients with diffuse large-B-cell lymphoma. *N. Engl. J. Med.* 2002; 346:235-42.

[3]   Feugier P, Van Hoof A, Sebban C, et al. Long-term results of the R-CHOP study in the treatment of elderly patients with diffuse large B-cell lymphoma: a study by the Groupe d'Etude des Lymphomes de l'Adulte. *J. Clin. Oncol.* 2005; 23:4117-26.

[4]   Pfreundschuh M, Trumper L, Osterborg A, et al. CHOP-like chemotherapy plus rituximab versus CHOP-like chemotherapy alone in young patients with good-prognosis diffuse large-B-cell lymphoma: a randomised controlled trial by the MabThera International Trial (MInT) Group. *Lancet Oncol.* 2006; 7:379-91.

[5]   Rodriguez-Monge EJ, Cabanillas F. Long-term follow-up of platinum-based lymphoma salvage regimens. The M.D. Anderson Cancer Center experience. *Hematol. Oncol. Clin. North Am.* 1997; 11:937-47.

[6]   Philip T, Guglielmi C, Hagenbeek A, et al. Autologous bone marrow transplantation as compared with salvage chemotherapy in relapses of chemotherapy-sensitive non-Hodgkin's lymphoma. *N. Engl. J. Med.* 1995; 333:1540-5.

[7]   Dreyling M, Lenz G, Hoster E, et al. Early consolidation by myeloablative radiochemotherapy followed by autologous stem cell transplantation in first remission significantly prolongs progression-free survival in mantle-cell lymphoma: results of a prospective randomized trial of the European MCL Network. *Blood.* 2005; 105:2677-84.

[8]   Buadi FK, Micallef IN, Ansell SM, et al. Autologous hematopoietic stem cell transplantation for older patients with relapsed non-Hodgkin's lymphoma. *Bone Marrow Transplant.* 2006; 37:1017-22.

[9]   Jantunen E, Itala M, Juvonen E, et al. Autologous stem cell transplantation in elderly (>60 years) patients with non-Hodgkin's lymphoma: a nation-wide analysis. *Bone Marrow Transplant.* 2006; 37:367-72.

[10]   Philip T, Armitage JO, Spitzer G, et al. High-dose therapy and autologous bone marrow transplantation after failure of conventional chemotherapy in adults with intermediate-grade or high-grade non-Hodgkin's lymphoma. *N. Engl. J. Med.* 1987; 316:1493-8.

[11]   Baron F, Storb R, Storer BE, et al. Factors associated with outcomes in allogeneic hematopoietic cell transplantation with nonmyeloablative conditioning after failed myeloablative hematopoietic cell transplantation. *J. Clin. Oncol.* 2006; 24:4150-7.

[12]   Ratanatharathorn V, Uberti J, Karanes C, et al. Prospective comparative trial of autologous versus allogeneic bone marrow transplantation in patients with non-Hodgkin's lymphoma. *Blood.* 1994; 84:1050-5.

[13]   van Besien K, Loberiza FR, Jr., Bajorunaite R, et al. Comparison of autologous and allogeneic hematopoietic stem cell transplantation for follicular lymphoma. *Blood.* 2003; 102:3521-9.

[14]   Giralt S, Estey E, Albitar M, et al. Engraftment of allogeneic hematopoietic progenitor cells with purine analog-containing chemotherapy: harnessing graft-versus-leukemia without myeloablative therapy. *Blood.* 1997; 89:4531-6.

[15]   Slavin S, Nagler A, Naparstek E, et al. Nonmyeloablative stem cell transplantation and cell therapy as an alternative to conventional bone marrow transplantation with lethal cytoreduction for the treatment of malignant and nonmalignant hematologic diseases. *Blood.* 1998; 91:756-63.

[16]   Khouri IF, Keating M, Korbling M, et al. Transplant-lite: induction of graft-versus-malignancy using fludarabine-based nonablative chemotherapy and allogeneic blood

progenitor-cell transplantation as treatment for lymphoid malignancies. *J. Clin. Oncol.* 1998; 16:2817-24.

[17] Flinn IW, O'Donnell PV, Goodrich A, et al. Immunotherapy with rituximab during peripheral blood stem cell transplantation for non-Hodgkin's lymphoma. *Biol. Blood Marrow Transplant.* 2000; 6:628-32.

[18] Khouri IF, Saliba RM, Hosing C, et al. Concurrent administration of high-dose rituximab before and after autologous stem-cell transplantation for relapsed aggressive B-cell non-Hodgkin's lymphomas. *J. Clin. Oncol.* 2005; 23:2240-7.

[19] Press OW, Eary JF, Appelbaum FR, et al. Radiolabeled-antibody therapy of B-cell lymphoma with autologous bone marrow support. *N. Engl. J. Med.* 1993; 329:1219-24.

[20] Press OW, Eary JF, Appelbaum FR, et al. Phase II trial of 131I-B1 (anti-CD20) antibody therapy with autologous stem cell transplantation for relapsed B cell lymphomas. *Lancet.* 1995; 346:336-40.

[21] Press OW, Eary JF, Gooley T, et al. A phase I/II trial of iodine-131-tositumomab (anti-CD20), etoposide, cyclophosphamide, and autologous stem cell transplantation for relapsed B-cell lymphomas. *Blood.* 2000; 96:2934-42.

[22] Nademanee A, Forman S, Molina A, et al. A phase 1/2 trial of high-dose yttrium-90-ibritumomab tiuxetan in combination with high-dose etoposide and cyclophosphamide followed by autologous stem cell transplantation in patients with poor-risk or relapsed non-Hodgkin lymphoma. *Blood.* 2005; 106:2896-902.

[23] Aisenberg AC. Historical review of lymphomas. *Br. J. Haematol.* 2000; 109:466-76.

[24] Harris NL, Jaffe ES, Diebold J, Flandrin G, Muller-Hermelink HK, Vardiman J. Lymphoma classification--from controversy to consensus: the R.E.A.L. and WHO Classification of lymphoid neoplasms. *Ann. Oncol.* 2000; 11 Suppl 1:3-10.

[25] Rappaport H. Tumors of the hematopoietic system. In: Atlas of Tumor Pathology. Washington, DC: *Armed Forces Institute of Pathology,* 1966:47-61.

[26] National Cancer Institute sponsored study of classifications of non-Hodgkin's lymphomas: summary and description of a working formulation for clinical usage. The Non-Hodgkin's Lymphoma Pathologic Classification Project. *Cancer.* 1982; 49:2112-35.

[27] Lukes RJ, Collins RD. Immunologic characterization of human malignant lymphomas. *Cancer.* 1974; 34:suppl:1488-503.

[28] Stansfeld AG, Diebold J, Noel H, et al. Updated Kiel classification for lymphomas. *Lancet.* 1988; 1:292-3.

[29] Harris NL, Jaffe ES, Stein H, et al. A revised European-American classification of lymphoid neoplasms: a proposal from the International Lymphoma Study Group. *Blood.* 1994; 84:1361-92.

[30] Jaffe E, Harris N, Stein H, Vardiman J, eds. World Health Organization Classification of Tumours. *Pathology and Genetics of Tumours of Haematopoietic and Lymphoid Tissues.* Lyon,France: IARC Press, 2001.

[31] Alizadeh AA, Eisen MB, Davis RE, et al. Distinct types of diffuse large B-cell lymphoma identified by gene expression profiling. *Nature.* 2000; 403:503-11.

[32] Armitage JO, Weisenburger DD. New approach to classifying non-Hodgkin's lymphomas: clinical features of the major histologic subtypes. Non-Hodgkin's Lymphoma Classification Project. *J. Clin. Oncol.* 1998; 16:2780-95.

[33] A predictive model for aggressive non-Hodgkin's lymphoma. The International Non-Hodgkin's Lymphoma Prognostic Factors Project. *N. Engl. J. Med.* 1993; 329:987-94.

[34] Solal-Celigny P, Roy P, Colombat P, et al. Follicular lymphoma international prognostic index. *Blood*. 2004; 104:1258-65.

[35] Gallamini A, Stelitano C, Calvi R, et al. Peripheral T-cell lymphoma unspecified (PTCL-U): a new prognostic model from a retrospective multicentric clinical study. *Blood*. 2004; 103:2474-9.

[36] Spaepen K, Stroobants S, Dupont P, et al. Prognostic value of pretransplantation positron emission tomography using fluorine 18-fluorodeoxyglucose in patients with aggressive lymphoma treated with high-dose chemotherapy and stem cell transplantation. *Blood*. 2003; 102:53-9.

[37] Spaepen K, Stroobants S, Dupont P, et al. Early restaging positron emission tomography with (18)F-fluorodeoxyglucose predicts outcome in patients with aggressive non-Hodgkin's lymphoma. *Ann. Oncol.* 2002; 13:1356-63.

[38] Haioun C, Itti E, Rahmouni A, et al. [18F]fluoro-2-deoxy-D-glucose positron emission tomography (FDG-PET) in aggressive lymphoma: an early prognostic tool for predicting patient outcome. *Blood*. 2005; 106:1376-81.

[39] Rosenwald A, Wright G, Chan WC, et al. The use of molecular profiling to predict survival after chemotherapy for diffuse large-B-cell lymphoma. *N. Engl. J. Med.* 2002; 346:1937-47.

[40] Shipp MA, Ross KN, Tamayo P, et al. Diffuse large B-cell lymphoma outcome prediction by gene-expression profiling and supervised machine learning. *Nat. Med.* 2002; 8:68-74.

[41] Sehn LH, Berry B, Chhanabhai M, et al. The revised International Prognostic Index (R-IPI) is a better predictor of outcome than the standard IPI for patients with diffuse large B-cell lymphoma treated with R-CHOP. *Blood*. 2007; 109:1857-61.

[42] Bastion Y, Sebban C, Berger F, et al. Incidence, predictive factors, and outcome of lymphoma transformation in follicular lymphoma patients. *J. Clin. Oncol.* 1997; 15:1587-94.

[43] Montoto S, Davies AJ, Matthews J, et al. Risk and clinical implications of transformation of follicular lymphoma to diffuse large B-cell lymphoma. *J. Clin. Oncol.* 2007; 25:2426-33.

[44] Hubbard SM, Chabner BA, DeVita VT, Jr., et al. Histologic progression in non-Hodgkin's lymphoma. *Blood*. 1982; 59:258-64.

[45] Lerner RE, Burns LJ. Transformed lymphoma: an Achilles' heel of non-Hodgkin's lymphoma. *Bone Marrow Transplant*. 2003; 31:531-7.

[46] Cremerius U, Fabry U, Wildberger JE, et al. Pre-transplant positron emission tomography (PET) using fluorine-18-fluoro-deoxyglucose (FDG) predicts outcome in patients treated with high-dose chemotherapy and autologous stem cell transplantation for non-Hodgkin's lymphoma. *Bone Marrow Transplant*. 2002; 30:103-11.

[47] Gribben JG, Freedman AS, Neuberg D, et al. Immunologic purging of marrow assessed by PCR before autologous bone marrow transplantation for B-cell lymphoma. *N. Engl. J. Med.* 1991; 325:1525-33.

[48] Melnyk A, Rodriguez A, Pugh WC, Cabannillas F. Evaluation of the Revised European-American Lymphoma classification confirms the clinical relevance of immunophenotype in 560 cases of aggressive non-Hodgkin's lymphoma. *Blood*. 1997; 89:4514-20.

[49] Gisselbrecht C, Gaulard P, Lepage E, et al. Prognostic significance of T-cell phenotype in aggressive non-Hodgkin's lymphomas. Groupe d'Etudes des Lymphomes de l'Adulte (GELA). *Blood*. 1998; 92:76-82.

[50] Morabito F, Gallamini A, Stelitano C, et al. Clinical relevance of immunophenotype in a retrospective comparative study of 297 peripheral T-cell lymphomas, unspecified, and 496 diffuse large B-cell lymphomas: experience of the Intergruppo Italiano Linformi. *Cancer.* 2004; 101:1601-8.

[51] Armitage JO, Vose JM, Weisenburger DD. Towards understanding the peripheral T-cell lymphomas. *Ann. Oncol.* 2004; 15:1447-9.

[52] Majhail NS, Burns LJ. Hematopoietic stem cell transplantation in the treatment of peripheral T-cell lymphomas. *Curr. Hematol. Rep.* 2005; 4:252-9.

[53] Ishida T, Iida S, Akatsuka Y, et al. The CC chemokine receptor 4 as a novel specific molecular target for immunotherapy in adult T-Cell leukemia/lymphoma. *Clin. Cancer Res.* 2004; 10:7529-39.

[54] Tsuchiya T, Ohshima K, Karube K, et al. Th1, Th2, and activated T-cell marker and clinical prognosis in peripheral T-cell lymphoma, unspecified: comparison with AILD, ALCL, lymphoblastic lymphoma, and ATLL. *Blood.* 2004; 103:236-41.

[55] Ballester B, Ramuz O, Gisselbrecht C, et al. Gene expression profiling identifies molecular subgroups among nodal peripheral T-cell lymphomas. *Oncogene.* 2006; 25:1560-70.

[56] Freedman AS, Neuberg D, Mauch P, et al. Long-term follow-up of autologous bone marrow transplantation in patients with relapsed follicular lymphoma. *Blood.* 1999; 94:3325-33.

[57] Apostolidis J, Gupta RK, Grenzelias D, et al. High-dose therapy with autologous bone marrow support as consolidation of remission in follicular lymphoma: long-term clinical and molecular follow-up. *J. Clin. Oncol.* 2000; 18:527-36.

[58] Haioun C, Lepage E, Gisselbrecht C, et al. Survival benefit of high-dose therapy in poor-risk aggressive non-Hodgkin's lymphoma: final analysis of the prospective LNH87-2 protocol--a groupe d'Etude des lymphomes de l'Adulte study. *J. Clin. Oncol.* 2000; 18:3025-30.

[59] Stiff PJ, Dahlberg S, Forman SJ, et al. Autologous bone marrow transplantation for patients with relapsed or refractory diffuse aggressive non-Hodgkin's lymphoma: value of augmented preparative regimens--a Southwest Oncology Group trial. *J. Clin. Oncol.* 1998; 16:48-55.

[60] Stein RS, Greer JP, Goodman S, et al. Intensified preparative regimens and autologous transplantation in refractory or relapsed intermediate grade non-Hodgkin's lymphoma. *Bone Marrow Transplant.* 2000; 25:257-62.

[61] Caballero MD, Rubio V, Rifon J, et al. BEAM chemotherapy followed by autologous stem cell support in lymphoma patients: analysis of efficacy, toxicity and prognostic factors. *Bone Marrow Transplant.* 1997; 20:451-8.

[62] Caballero MD, Perez-Simon JA, Iriondo A, et al. High-dose therapy in diffuse large cell lymphoma: results and prognostic factors in 452 patients from the GEL-TAMO Spanish Cooperative Group. *Ann. Oncol.* 2003; 14:140-51.

[63] Friedberg JW, Neuberg D, Stone RM, et al. Outcome in patients with myelodysplastic syndrome after autologous bone marrow transplantation for non-Hodgkin's lymphoma. *J. Clin. Oncol.* 1999; 17:3128-35.

[64] Milligan DW, Ruiz De Elvira MC, Kolb HJ, et al. Secondary leukaemia and myelodysplasia after autografting for lymphoma: results from the EBMT. EBMT Lymphoma and Late Effects Working Parties. European Group for Blood and Marrow Transplantation. *Br. J. Haematol.* 1999; 106:1020-6.

[65] Gulati S, Yahalom J, Acaba L, et al. Treatment of patients with relapsed and resistant non-Hodgkin's lymphoma using total body irradiation, etoposide, and cyclophosphamide and autologous bone marrow transplantation. *J. Clin. Oncol.* 1992; 10:936-41.

[66] Schmitz N, Diehl V. Carmustine and the lungs. *Lancet.* 1997; 349:1712-3.

[67] Leonard BM, Hetu F, Busque L, et al. Lymphoma cell burden in progenitor cell grafts measured by competitive polymerase chain reaction: less than one log difference between bone marrow and peripheral blood sources. *Blood.* 1998; 91:331-9.

[68] Brenner MK, Rill DR, Moen RC, et al. Gene-marking to trace origin of relapse after autologous bone-marrow transplantation. *Lancet.* 1993; 341:85-6.

[69] Galimberti S, Marasca R, Caracciolo F, et al. The role of molecular monitoring in autotransplantation for non-Hodgkin's lymphoma. *Bone Marrow Transplant.* 2002; 29:581-7.

[70] Bierman PJ, Sweetenham JW, Loberiza FR, Jr., et al. Syngeneic hematopoietic stem-cell transplantation for non-Hodgkin's lymphoma: a comparison with allogeneic and autologous transplantation--The Lymphoma Working Committee of the International Bone Marrow Transplant Registry and the European Group for Blood and Marrow Transplantation. *J. Clin. Oncol.* 2003; 21:3744-53.

[71] Schouten HC, Qian W, Kvaloy S, et al. High-dose therapy improves progression-free survival and survival in relapsed follicular non-Hodgkin's lymphoma: results from the randomized European CUP trial. *J. Clin. Oncol.* 2003; 21:3918-27.

[72] van Heeckeren WJ, Vollweiler J, Fu P, et al. Randomised comparison of two B-cell purging protocols for patients with B-cell non-Hodgkin lymphoma: in vivo purging with rituximab versus ex vivo purging with CliniMACS CD34 cell enrichment device. *Br. J. Haematol.* 2006; 132:42-55.

[73] Magni M, Di Nicola M, Devizzi L, et al. Successful in vivo purging of CD34-containing peripheral blood harvests in mantle cell and indolent lymphoma: evidence for a role of both chemotherapy and rituximab infusion. *Blood.* 2000; 96:864-9.

[74] Brugger W, Hirsch J, Grunebach F, et al. Rituximab consolidation after high-dose chemotherapy and autologous blood stem cell transplantation in follicular and mantle cell lymphoma: a prospective, multicenter phase II study. *Ann. Oncol.* 2004; 15:1691-8.

[75] Vose JM, Bierman PJ, Enke C, et al. Phase I trial of iodine-131 tositumomab with high-dose chemotherapy and autologous stem-cell transplantation for relapsed non-Hodgkin's lymphoma. *J. Clin. Oncol.* 2005; 23:461-7.

[76] Hoerr AL, Gao F, Hidalgo J, et al. Effects of pretransplantation treatment with rituximab on outcomes of autologous stem-cell transplantation for non-Hodgkin's lymphoma. *J. Clin. Oncol.* 2004; 22:4561-6.

[77] Shortt J, Spencer A. Adjuvant rituximab causes prolonged hypogammaglobulinaemia following autologous stem cell transplant for non-Hodgkin's lymphoma. *Bone Marrow Transplant.* 2006; 38:433-6.

[78] Lemieux B, Tartas S, Traulle C, et al. Rituximab-related late-onset neutropenia after autologous stem cell transplantation for aggressive non-Hodgkin's lymphoma. *Bone Marrow Transplant.* 2004; 33:921-3.

[79] Cairoli R, Grillo G, Tedeschi A, D'Avanzo G, Marenco P, Morra E. High incidence of neutropenia in patients treated with rituximab after autologous stem cell transplantation. *Haematologica.* 2004; 89:361-3.

[80]   Buckstein R, Imrie K, Spaner D, et al. Stem cell function and engraftment is not affected by "in vivo purging" with rituximab for autologous stem cell treatment for patients with low-grade non-Hodgkin's lymphoma. *Semin. Oncol.* 1999; 26:115-22.

[81]   Benekli M, Hahn T, Shafi F, et al. Effect of rituximab on peripheral blood stem cell mobilization and engraftment kinetics in non-Hodgkin's lymphoma patients. *Bone Marrow Transplant.* 2003; 32:139-43.

[82]   Kamezaki K, Kikushige Y, Numata A, et al. Rituximab does not compromise the mobilization and engraftment of autologous peripheral blood stem cells in diffuse-large B-cell lymphoma. *Bone Marrow Transplant.* 2007; 39:523-7.

[83]   Peggs KS, Mackinnon S, Linch DC. The role of allogeneic transplantation in non-Hodgkin's lymphoma. *Br. J. Haematol.* 2005; 128:153-68.

[84]   Long GD, Amylon MD, Stockerl-Goldstein KE, et al. Fractionated total-body irradiation, etoposide, and cyclophosphamide followed by allogeneic bone marrow transplantation for patients with high-risk or advanced-stage hematological malignancies. *Biol. Blood Marrow Transplant.* 1997; 3:324-30.

[85]   Law LY, Horning SJ, Wong RM, et al. High-dose carmustine, etoposide, and cyclophosphamide followed by allogeneic hematopoietic cell transplantation for non-Hodgkin lymphoma. *Biol. Blood Marrow Transplant.* 2006; 12:703-11.

[86]   Fernandez HF, Tran HT, Albrecht F, Lennon S, Caldera H, Goodman MS. Evaluation of safety and pharmacokinetics of administering intravenous busulfan in a twice-daily or daily schedule to patients with advanced hematologic malignant disease undergoing stem cell transplantation. *Biol. Blood Marrow Transplant.* 2002; 8:486-92.

[87]   Diaconescu R, Flowers CR, Storer B, et al. Morbidity and mortality with nonmyeloablative compared with myeloablative conditioning before hematopoietic cell transplantation from HLA-matched related donors. *Blood.* 2004; 104:1550-8.

[88]   Sorror ML, Maris MB, Storer B, et al. Comparing morbidity and mortality of HLA-matched unrelated donor hematopoietic cell transplantation after nonmyeloablative and myeloablative conditioning: influence of pretransplantation comorbidities. *Blood.* 2004; 104:961-8.

[89]   Kassim AA, Chinratanalab W, Ferrara JL, Mineishi S. Reduced-intensity allogeneic hematopoietic stem cell transplantation for acute leukemias: 'what is the best recipe?' *Bone Marrow Transplant.* 2005; 36:565-74.

[90]   Kato K, Khaled Y, Mineishi S. Reduced-intensity stem cell transplantation for hematological malignancies: Current status and the future. *Current Stem Cell Research and Therapy.* 2007; 2:149-62.

[91]   Saito T, Kanda Y, Kami M, et al. Therapeutic potential of a reduced-intensity preparative regimen for allogeneic transplantation with cladribine, busulfan, and antithymocyte globulin against advanced/refractory acute leukemia/lymphoma. *Clin. Cancer Res.* 2002; 8:1014-20.

[92]   Giralt S, Thall PF, Khouri I, et al. Melphalan and purine analog-containing preparative regimens: reduced-intensity conditioning for patients with hematologic malignancies undergoing allogeneic progenitor cell transplantation. *Blood.* 2001; 97:631-7.

[93]   Chakraverty R, Peggs K, Chopra R, et al. Limiting transplantation-related mortality following unrelated donor stem cell transplantation by using a nonmyeloablative conditioning regimen. *Blood.* 2002; 99:1071-8.

[94]   Alyea EP, Kim HT, Ho V, et al. Comparative outcome of nonmyeloablative and myeloablative allogeneic hematopoietic cell transplantation for patients older than 50 years of age. *Blood.* 2005; 105:1810-4.

[95] de Lima M, Couriel D, Thall PF, et al. Once-daily intravenous busulfan and fludarabine: clinical and pharmacokinetic results of a myeloablative, reduced-toxicity conditioning regimen for allogeneic stem cell transplantation in AML and MDS. *Blood.* 2004; 104:857-64.

[96] Carella AM, Cavaliere M, Lerma E, et al. Autografting followed by nonmyeloablative immunosuppressive chemotherapy and allogeneic peripheral-blood hematopoietic stem-cell transplantation as treatment of resistant Hodgkin's disease and non-Hodgkin's lymphoma. *J. Clin. Oncol.* 2000; 18:3918-24.

[97] Garban F, Attal M, Michallet M, et al. Prospective comparison of autologous stem cell transplantation followed by dose-reduced allograft (IFM99-03 trial) with tandem autologous stem cell transplantation (IFM99-04 trial) in high-risk de novo multiple myeloma. *Blood.* 2006; 107:3474-80.

[98] Bruno B, Rotta M, Patriarca F, et al. A comparison of allografting with autografting for newly diagnosed myeloma. *N. Engl. J. Med.* 2007; 356:1110-20.

[99] Uberti JP, Ayash L, Ratanatharathorn V, et al. Pilot trial on the use of etanercept and methylprednisolone as primary treatment for acute graft-versus-host disease. *Biol. Blood Marrow Transplant.* 2005; 11:680-7.

[100] Cutler C, Kim HT, Hochberg E, et al. Sirolimus and tacrolimus without methotrexate as graft-versus-host disease prophylaxis after matched related donor peripheral blood stem cell transplantation. *Biol. Blood Marrow Transplant.* 2004; 10:328-36.

[101] Chan GW, Foss FM, Klein AK, Sprague K, Miller KB. Reduced-intensity transplantation for patients with myelodysplastic syndrome achieves durable remission with less graft-versus-host disease. *Biol. Blood Marrow Transplant.* 2003; 9:753-9.

[102] Morris E, Thomson K, Craddock C, et al. Outcomes after alemtuzumab-containing reduced-intensity allogeneic transplantation regimen for relapsed and refractory non-Hodgkin lymphoma. *Blood.* 2004; 104:3865-71.

[103] Couriel DR, Hosing C, Saliba R, et al. Extracorporeal photochemotherapy for the treatment of steroid-resistant chronic GVHD. *Blood.* 2006; 107:3074-80.

[104] Lowsky R, Takahashi T, Liu YP, et al. Protective conditioning for acute graft-versus-host disease. *N. Engl. J. Med.* 2005; 353:1321-31.

[105] Vose JM, Sharp G, Chan WC, et al. Autologous transplantation for aggressive non-Hodgkin's lymphoma: results of a randomized trial evaluating graft source and minimal residual disease. *J. Clin. Oncol.* 2002; 20:2344-52.

[106] Liles WC, Broxmeyer HE, Rodger E, et al. Mobilization of hematopoietic progenitor cells in healthy volunteers by AMD3100, a CXCR4 antagonist. *Blood.* 2003; 102:2728-30.

[107] Devine SM, Flomenberg N, Vesole DH, et al. Rapid mobilization of CD34+ cells following administration of the CXCR4 antagonist AMD3100 to patients with multiple myeloma and non-Hodgkin's lymphoma. *J. Clin. Oncol.* 2004; 22:1095-102.

[108] Allogeneic peripheral blood stem-cell compared with bone marrow transplantation in the management of hematologic malignancies: an individual patient data meta-analysis of nine randomized trials. *J. Clin. Oncol.* 2005; 23:5074-87.

[109] Izutsu K, Kanda Y, Ohno H, et al. Unrelated bone marrow transplantation for non-Hodgkin lymphoma: a study from the Japan Marrow Donor Program. *Blood.* 2004; 103:1955-60.

[110] Kato K, Kanda Y, Eto T, et al. Allogeneic bone marrow transplantation from unrelated human T-cell leukemia virus-I-negative donors for adult T-cell leukemia/lymphoma:

retrospective analysis of data from the Japan Marrow Donor Program. *Biol. Blood Marrow Transplant.* 2007; 13:90-9.

[111] Yuji K, Miyakoshi S, Kato D, et al. Reduced-intensity unrelated cord blood transplantation for patients with advanced malignant lymphoma. *Biol. Blood Marrow Transplant.* 2005; 11:314-8.

[112] Maris MB, Sandmaier BM, Storer BE, et al. Allogeneic hematopoietic cell transplantation after fludarabine and 2 Gy total body irradiation for relapsed and refractory mantle cell lymphoma. *Blood.* 2004; 104:3535-42.

[113] Vose JM, Armitage JO, Weisenburger DD, et al. The importance of age in survival of patients treated with chemotherapy for aggressive non-Hodgkin's lymphoma. *J. Clin. Oncol.* 1988; 6:1838-44.

[114] Bertini M, Boccomini C, Calvi R. The Influence of advanced age on the treatment and prognosis of diffuse large-cell lymphoma (DLCL). *Clin. Lymphoma.* 2001; 1:278-84.

[115] Kuittinen T, Nousiainen T, Halonen P, Mahlamaki E, Jantunen E. Prediction of mobilisation failure in patients with non-Hodgkin's lymphoma. *Bone Marrow Transplant.* 2004; 33:907-12.

[116] Jantunen E, Mahlamaki E, Nousiainen T. Feasibility and toxicity of high-dose chemotherapy supported by peripheral blood stem cell transplantation in elderly patients (>/=60 years) with non-Hodgkin's lymphoma: comparison with patients <60 years treated within the same protocol. *Bone Marrow Transplant.* 2000; 26:737-41.

[117] Scott BL, Sandmaier BM, Storer B, et al. Myeloablative vs nonmyeloablative allogeneic transplantation for patients with myelodysplastic syndrome or acute myelogenous leukemia with multilineage dysplasia: a retrospective analysis. *Leukemia.* 2006; 20:128-35.

[118] Hagglund H, Bostrom L, Remberger M, Ljungman P, Nilsson B, Ringden O. Risk factors for acute graft-versus-host disease in 291 consecutive HLA-identical bone marrow transplant recipients. *Bone Marrow Transplant.* 1995; 16:747-53.

[119] Gaziev D, Polchi P, Galimberti M, et al. Graft-versus-host disease after bone marrow transplantation for thalassemia: an analysis of incidence and risk factors. *Transplantation.* 1997; 63:854-60.

[120] Valcarcel D, Martino R, Sureda A, et al. Conventional versus reduced-intensity conditioning regimen for allogeneic stem cell transplantation in patients with hematological malignancies. *Eur. J. Haematol.* 2005; 74:144-51.

[121] Chiodi S, Spinelli S, Ravera G, et al. Quality of life in 244 recipients of allogeneic bone marrow transplantation. *Br. J. Haematol.* 2000; 110:614-9.

[122] Diez-Campelo M, Perez-Simon JA, Gonzalez-Porras JR, et al. Quality of life assessment in patients undergoing reduced intensity conditioning allogeneic as compared to autologous transplantation: results of a prospective study. *Bone Marrow Transplant.* 2004; 34:729-38.

[123] Sorror ML, Maris MB, Storb R, et al. Hematopoietic cell transplantation (HCT)-specific comorbidity index: a new tool for risk assessment before allogeneic HCT. *Blood.* 2005; 106:2912-9.

[124] Gianni AM, Bregni M, Siena S, et al. High-dose chemotherapy and autologous bone marrow transplantation compared with MACOP-B in aggressive B-cell lymphoma. *N. Engl. J. Med.* 1997; 336:1290-7.

[125] Santini G, Salvagno L, Leoni P, et al. VACOP-B versus VACOP-B plus autologous bone marrow transplantation for advanced diffuse non-Hodgkin's lymphoma: results of

a prospective randomized trial by the non-Hodgkin's Lymphoma Cooperative Study Group. *J. Clin. Oncol.* 1998; 16:2796-802.

[126] Kluin-Nelemans HC, Zagonel V, Anastasopoulou A, et al. Standard chemotherapy with or without high-dose chemotherapy for aggressive non-Hodgkin's lymphoma: randomized phase III EORTC study. *J. Natl. Cancer Inst.* 2001; 93:22-30.

[127] Gisselbrecht C, Lepage E, Molina T, et al. Shortened first-line high-dose chemotherapy for patients with poor-prognosis aggressive lymphoma. *J. Clin. Oncol.* 2002; 20:2472-9.

[128] Kaiser U, Uebelacker I, Abel U, et al. Randomized study to evaluate the use of high-dose therapy as part of primary treatment for "aggressive" lymphoma. *J. Clin. Oncol.* 2002; 20:4413-9.

[129] Martelli M, Gherlinzoni F, De Renzo A, et al. Early autologous stem-cell transplantation versus conventional chemotherapy as front-line therapy in high-risk, aggressive non-Hodgkin's lymphoma: an Italian multicenter randomized trial. *J. Clin. Oncol.* 2003; 21:1255-62.

[130] Milpied N, Deconinck E, Gaillard F, et al. Initial treatment of aggressive lymphoma with high-dose chemotherapy and autologous stem-cell support. *N. Engl. J. Med.* 2004; 350:1287-95.

[131] Vitolo U, Liberati AM, Cabras MG, et al. High dose sequential chemotherapy with autologous transplantation versus dose-dense chemotherapy MegaCEOP as first line treatment in poor-prognosis diffuse large cell lymphoma: an "Intergruppo Italiano Linfomi" randomized trial. *Haematologica.* 2005; 90:793-801.

[132] Verdonck LF, van Putten WL, Hagenbeek A, et al. Comparison of CHOP chemotherapy with autologous bone marrow transplantation for slowly responding patients with aggressive non-Hodgkin's lymphoma. *N. Engl. J. Med.* 1995; 332:1045-51.

[133] Martelli M, Vignetti M, Zinzani PL, et al. High-dose chemotherapy followed by autologous bone marrow transplantation versus dexamethasone, cisplatin, and cytarabine in aggressive non-Hodgkin's lymphoma with partial response to front-line chemotherapy: a prospective randomized Italian multicenter study. *J. Clin. Oncol.* 1996; 14:534-42.

[134] Strehl J, Mey U, Glasmacher A, et al. High-dose chemotherapy followed by autologous stem cell transplantation as first-line therapy in aggressive non-Hodgkin's lymphoma: a meta-analysis. *Haematologica.* 2003; 88:1304-15.

[135] Greb A, Bohlius J, Trelle S, et al. High-dose chemotherapy with autologous stem cell support in first-line treatment of aggressive non-Hodgkin lymphoma - results of a comprehensive meta-analysis. *Cancer Treat. Rev.* 2007; 33:338-46.

[136] Kewalramani T, Zelenetz AD, Hedrick EE, et al. High-dose chemoradiotherapy and autologous stem cell transplantation for patients with primary refractory aggressive non-Hodgkin lymphoma: an intention-to-treat analysis. *Blood.* 2000; 96:2399-404.

[137] Vose JM, Zhang MJ, Rowlings PA, et al. Autologous transplantation for diffuse aggressive non-Hodgkin's lymphoma in patients never achieving remission: a report from the Autologous Blood and Marrow Transplant Registry. *J. Clin. Oncol.* 2001; 19:406-13.

[138] Guglielmi C, Gomez F, Philip T, et al. Time to relapse has prognostic value in patients with aggressive lymphoma enrolled onto the Parma trial. *J. Clin. Oncol.* 1998; 16:3264-9.

[139] Hamlin PA, Zelenetz AD, Kewalramani T, et al. Age-adjusted International Prognostic Index predicts autologous stem cell transplantation outcome for patients with relapsed or primary refractory diffuse large B-cell lymphoma. *Blood.* 2003; 102:1989-96.

[140] Moskowitz CH, Nimer SD, Glassman JR, et al. The International Prognostic Index predicts for outcome following autologous stem cell transplantation in patients with relapsed and primary refractory intermediate-grade lymphoma. *Bone Marrow Transplant.* 1999; 23:561-7.

[141] Chopra R, Goldstone AH, Pearce R, et al. Autologous versus allogeneic bone marrow transplantation for non-Hodgkin's lymphoma: a case-controlled analysis of the European Bone Marrow Transplant Group Registry data. *J. Clin. Oncol.* 1992; 10:1690-5.

[142] Dhedin N, Giraudier S, Gaulard P, et al. Allogeneic bone marrow transplantation in aggressive non-Hodgkin's lymphoma (excluding Burkitt and lymphoblastic lymphoma): a series of 73 patients from the SFGM database. Societ Francaise de Greffe de Moelle. *Br. J. Haematol.* 1999; 107:154-61.

[143] Schimmer AD, Jamal S, Messner H, et al. Allogeneic or autologous bone marrow transplantation (BMT) for non-Hodgkin's lymphoma (NHL): results of a provincial strategy. Ontario BMT Network, Canada. *Bone Marrow Transplant.* 2000; 26:859-64.

[144] Peniket AJ, Ruiz de Elvira MC, Taghipour G, et al. An EBMT registry matched study of allogeneic stem cell transplants for lymphoma: allogeneic transplantation is associated with a lower relapse rate but a higher procedure-related mortality rate than autologous transplantation. *Bone Marrow Transplant.* 2003; 31:667-78.

[145] Radich JP, Gooley T, Sanders JE, Anasetti C, Chauncey T, Appelbaum FR. Second allogeneic transplantation after failure of first autologous transplantation. *Biol. Blood Marrow Transplant.* 2000; 6:272-9.

[146] Freytes CO, Loberiza FR, Rizzo JD, et al. Myeloablative allogeneic hematopoietic stem cell transplantation in patients who experience relapse after autologous stem cell transplantation for lymphoma: a report of the International Bone Marrow Transplant Registry. *Blood.* 2004; 104:3797-803.

[147] Feinstein LC, Sandmaier BM, Maloney DG, et al. Allografting after nonmyeloablative conditioning as a treatment after a failed conventional hematopoietic cell transplant. *Biol. Blood Marrow Transplant.* 2003; 9:266-72.

[148] Dana BW, Dahlberg S, Nathwani BN, et al. Long-term follow-up of patients with low-grade malignant lymphomas treated with doxorubicin-based chemotherapy or chemoimmunotherapy. *J. Clin. Oncol.* 1993; 11:644-51.

[149] Marcus R, Imrie K, Belch A, et al. CVP chemotherapy plus rituximab compared with CVP as first-line treatment for advanced follicular lymphoma. *Blood.* 2005; 105:1417-23.

[150] Liu Q, Fayad L, Cabanillas F, et al. Improvement of overall and failure-free survival in stage IV follicular lymphoma: 25 years of treatment experience at The University of Texas M.D. Anderson Cancer Center. *J. Clin. Oncol.* 2006; 24:1582-9.

[151] Hiddemann W, Kneba M, Dreyling M, et al. Frontline therapy with rituximab added to the combination of cyclophosphamide, doxorubicin, vincristine, and prednisone (CHOP) significantly improves the outcome for patients with advanced-stage follicular lymphoma compared with therapy with CHOP alone: results of a prospective randomized study of the German Low-Grade Lymphoma Study Group. *Blood.* 2005; 106:3725-32.

[152] Press OW, Unger JM, Braziel RM, et al. A phase 2 trial of CHOP chemotherapy followed by tositumomab/iodine I 131 tositumomab for previously untreated follicular non-Hodgkin lymphoma: Southwest Oncology Group Protocol S9911. *Blood.* 2003; 102:1606-12.

[153] Kaminski MS, Tuck M, Estes J, et al. 131I-tositumomab therapy as initial treatment for follicular lymphoma. *N. Engl. J. Med.* 2005; 352:441-9.

[154] Horning SJ, Rosenberg SA. The natural history of initially untreated low-grade non-Hodgkin's lymphomas. *N. Engl. J. Med.* 1984; 311:1471-5.

[155] Freedman AS, Gribben JG, Neuberg D, et al. High-dose therapy and autologous bone marrow transplantation in patients with follicular lymphoma during first remission. *Blood.* 1996; 88:2780-6.

[156] Horning SJ, Negrin RS, Hoppe RT, et al. High-dose therapy and autologous bone marrow transplantation for follicular lymphoma in first complete or partial remission: results of a phase II clinical trial. *Blood.* 2001; 97:404-9.

[157] Ladetto M, Corradini P, Vallet S, et al. High rate of clinical and molecular remissions in follicular lymphoma patients receiving high-dose sequential chemotherapy and autografting at diagnosis: a multicenter, prospective study by the Gruppo Italiano Trapianto Midollo Osseo (GITMO). *Blood.* 2002; 100:1559-65.

[158] Lenz G, Dreyling M, Schiegnitz E, et al. Myeloablative radiochemotherapy followed by autologous stem cell transplantation in first remission prolongs progression-free survival in follicular lymphoma: results of a prospective, randomized trial of the German Low-Grade Lymphoma Study Group. *Blood.* 2004; 104:2667-74.

[159] Deconinck E, Foussard C, Milpied N, et al. High-dose therapy followed by autologous purged stem-cell transplantation and doxorubicin-based chemotherapy in patients with advanced follicular lymphoma: a randomized multicenter study by GOELAMS. *Blood.* 2005; 105:3817-23.

[160] Sebban C, Mounier N, Brousse N, et al. Standard chemotherapy with interferon compared with CHOP followed by high-dose therapy with autologous stem cell transplantation in untreated patients with advanced follicular lymphoma: the GELF-94 randomized study from the Groupe d'Etude des Lymphomes de l'Adulte (GELA). *Blood.* 2006; 108:2540-4.

[161] Bierman PJ, Vose JM, Anderson JR, Bishop MR, Kessinger A, Armitage JO. High-dose therapy with autologous hematopoietic rescue for follicular low-grade non-Hodgkin's lymphoma. *J. Clin. Oncol.* 1997; 15:445-50.

[162] Brice P, Simon D, Bouabdallah R, et al. High-dose therapy with autologous stem-cell transplantation (ASCT) after first progression prolonged survival of follicular lymphoma patients included in the prospective GELF 86 protocol. *Ann. Oncol.* 2000; 11:1585-90.

[163] Cao TM, Horning S, Negrin RS, et al. High-dose therapy and autologous hematopoietic-cell transplantation for follicular lymphoma beyond first remission: the Stanford University experience. *Biol. Blood Marrow Transplant.* 2001; 7:294-301.

[164] van Besien K, Sobocinski KA, Rowlings PA, et al. Allogeneic bone marrow transplantation for low-grade lymphoma. *Blood.* 1998; 92:1832-6.

[165] Hosing C, Saliba RM, McLaughlin P, et al. Long-term results favor allogeneic over autologous hematopoietic stem cell transplantation in patients with refractory or recurrent indolent non-Hodgkin's lymphoma. *Ann. Oncol.* 2003; 14:737-44.

[166] Khouri IF, Saliba RM, Giralt SA, et al. Nonablative allogeneic hematopoietic transplantation as adoptive immunotherapy for indolent lymphoma: low incidence of

toxicity, acute graft-versus-host disease, and treatment-related mortality. *Blood.* 2001; 98:3595-9.

[167] Robinson SP, Goldstone AH, Mackinnon S, et al. Chemoresistant or aggressive lymphoma predicts for a poor outcome following reduced-intensity allogeneic progenitor cell transplantation: an analysis from the Lymphoma Working Party of the European Group for Blood and Bone Marrow Transplantation. *Blood.* 2002; 100:4310-6.

[168] Oviatt DL, Cousar JB, Collins RD, Flexner JM, Stein RS. Malignant lymphomas of follicular center cell origin in humans. V. Incidence, clinical features, and prognostic implications of transformation of small cleaved cell nodular lymphoma. *Cancer.* 1984; 53:1109-14.

[169] Vose JM, Wahl RL, Saleh M, et al. Multicenter phase II study of iodine-131 tositumomab for chemotherapy-relapsed/refractory low-grade and transformed low-grade B-cell non-Hodgkin's lymphomas. *J. Clin. Oncol.* 2000; 18:1316-23.

[170] Kaminski MS, Estes J, Zasadny KR, et al. Radioimmunotherapy with iodine (131)I tositumomab for relapsed or refractory B-cell non-Hodgkin lymphoma: updated results and long-term follow-up of the University of Michigan experience. *Blood.* 2000; 96:1259-66.

[171] Witzig TE, Gordon LI, Cabanillas F, et al. Randomized controlled trial of yttrium-90-labeled ibritumomab tiuxetan radioimmunotherapy versus rituximab immunotherapy for patients with relapsed or refractory low-grade, follicular, or transformed B-cell non-Hodgkin's lymphoma. *J. Clin. Oncol.* 2002; 20:2453-63.

[172] Horning SJ. Treatment approaches to the low-grade lymphomas. *Blood.* 1994; 83:881-4.

[173] Friedberg JW, Neuberg D, Gribben JG, et al. Autologous bone marrow transplantation after histologic transformation of indolent B cell malignancies. *Biol. Blood Marrow Transplant.* 1999; 5:262-8.

[174] Berglund A, Enblad G, Carlson K, Glimelius B, Hagberg H. Long-term follow-up of autologous stem-cell transplantation for follicular and transformed follicular lymphoma. *Eur. J. Haematol.* 2000; 65:17-22.

[175] Williams CD, Harrison CN, Lister TA, et al. High-dose therapy and autologous stem-cell support for chemosensitive transformed low-grade follicular non-Hodgkin's lymphoma: a case-matched study from the European Bone Marrow Transplant Registry. *J. Clin. Oncol.* 2001; 19:727-35.

[176] Chen CI, Crump M, Tsang R, Stewart AK, Keating A. Autotransplants for histologically transformed follicular non-Hodgkin's lymphoma. *Br. J. Haematol.* 2001; 113:202-8.

[177] Miller JS, Arthur DC, Litz CE, Neglia JP, Miller WJ, Weisdorf DJ. Myelodysplastic syndrome after autologous bone marrow transplantation: an additional late complication of curative cancer therapy. *Blood.* 1994; 83:3780-6.

[178] Bosch F, Lopez-Guillermo A, Campo E, et al. Mantle cell lymphoma: presenting features, response to therapy, and prognostic factors. *Cancer.* 1998; 82:567-75.

[179] Lenz G, Dreyling M, Hoster E, et al. Immunochemotherapy with rituximab and cyclophosphamide, doxorubicin, vincristine, and prednisone significantly improves response and time to treatment failure, but not long-term outcome in patients with previously untreated mantle cell lymphoma: results of a prospective randomized trial of the German Low Grade Lymphoma Study Group (GLSG). *J. Clin. Oncol.* 2005; 23:1984-92.

[180] Romaguera JE, Fayad L, Rodriguez MA, et al. High rate of durable remissions after treatment of newly diagnosed aggressive mantle-cell lymphoma with rituximab plus hyper-CVAD alternating with rituximab plus high-dose methotrexate and cytarabine. *J. Clin. Oncol.* 2005; 23:7013-23.

[181] Vandenberghe E, Ruiz de Elvira C, Loberiza FR, et al. Outcome of autologous transplantation for mantle cell lymphoma: a study by the European Blood and Bone Marrow Transplant and Autologous Blood and Marrow Transplant Registries. *Br. J. Haematol.* 2003; 120:793-800.

[182] Molina A, Popplewell L, Kashyap A, Nademanee A. Hematopoietic stem cell transplantation in the new millennium: report from City of Hope National Medical Center. *Clin. Transpl.* 2000:317-42.

[183] Ritchie DS, Seymour JF, Grigg AP, et al. The hyper-CVAD-rituximab chemotherapy programme followed by high-dose busulfan, melphalan and autologous stem cell transplantation produces excellent event-free survival in patients with previously untreated mantle cell lymphoma. *Ann. Hematol.* 2007; 86:101-105.

[184] Mangel J, Leitch HA, Connors JM, et al. Intensive chemotherapy and autologous stem-cell transplantation plus rituximab is superior to conventional chemotherapy for newly diagnosed advanced stage mantle-cell lymphoma: a matched pair analysis. *Ann. Oncol.* 2004; 15:283-90.

[185] Gianni AM, Magni M, Martelli M, et al. Long-term remission in mantle cell lymphoma following high-dose sequential chemotherapy and in vivo rituximab-purged stem cell autografting (R-HDS regimen). *Blood.* 2003; 102:749-55.

[186] Pott C, Schrader C, Gesk S, et al. Quantitative assessment of molecular remission after high-dose therapy with autologous stem cell transplantation predicts long-term remission in mantle cell lymphoma. *Blood.* 2006; 107:2271-8.

[187] Gopal AK, Rajendran JG, Petersdorf SH, et al. High-dose chemo-radioimmunotherapy with autologous stem cell support for relapsed mantle cell lymphoma. *Blood.* 2002; 99:3158-62.

[188] Ganti AK, Bierman PJ, Lynch JC, Bociek RG, Vose JM, Armitage JO. Hematopoietic stem cell transplantation in mantle cell lymphoma. *Ann. Oncol.* 2005; 16:618-24.

[189] Kasamon YL, Jones RJ, Diehl LF, et al. Outcomes of autologous and allogeneic blood or marrow transplantation for mantle cell lymphoma. *Biol. Blood Marrow Transplant.* 2005; 11:39-46.

[190] Laudi N, Arora M, Burns L, et al. Efficacy of high-dose therapy and hematopoietic stem cell transplantation for mantle cell lymphoma. *Am. J. Hematol.* 2006; 81:519-24.

[191] Khouri IF, Lee MS, Romaguera J, et al. Allogeneic hematopoietic transplantation for mantle-cell lymphoma: molecular remissions and evidence of graft-versus-malignancy. *Ann. Oncol.* 1999; 10:1293-9.

[192] Khouri IF, Lee MS, Saliba RM, et al. Nonablative allogeneic stem-cell transplantation for advanced/recurrent mantle-cell lymphoma. *J. Clin. Oncol.* 2003; 21:4407-12.

[193] Goy A, Bernstein S, Kahl B, et al. Bortezomib in patients with relapsed or refractory mantle cell lymphoma (MCL): preliminary results of the PINNACLE study. *J. Clin. Oncol.* 2005; 23:6563 [meeting abstracts].

[194] Kaufmann H, Raderer M, Wohrer S, et al. Antitumor activity of rituximab plus thalidomide in patients with relapsed/refractory mantle cell lymphoma. *Blood.* 2004; 104:2269-71.

[195] Witzig TE, Geyer SM, Ghobrial I, et al. Phase II trial of single-agent temsirolimus (CCI-779) for relapsed mantle cell lymphoma. *J. Clin. Oncol.* 2005; 23:5347-56.

[196] Rodriguez J, Caballero MD, Gutierrez A, et al. High-dose chemotherapy and autologous stem cell transplantation in peripheral T-cell lymphoma: the GEL-TAMO experience. *Ann. Oncol.* 2003; 14:1768-75.

[197] Blystad AK, Enblad G, Kvaloy S, et al. High-dose therapy with autologous stem cell transplantation in patients with peripheral T cell lymphomas. *Bone Marrow Transplant.* 2001; 27:711-6.

[198] Song KW, Mollee P, Keating A, Crump M. Autologous stem cell transplant for relapsed and refractory peripheral T-cell lymphoma: variable outcome according to pathological subtype. *Br. J. Haematol.* 2003; 120:978-85.

[199] Schetelig J, Fetscher S, Reichle A, et al. Long-term disease-free survival in patients with angioimmunoblastic T-cell lymphoma after high-dose chemotherapy and autologous stem cell transplantation. *Haematologica.* 2003; 88:1272-8.

[200] Jantunen E, Juvonen E, Wiklund T, Putkonen M, Nousiainen T. High-dose therapy supported by autologous stem cell transplantation in patients with enteropathy-associated T-cell lymphoma. *Leuk. Lymphoma.* 2003; 44:2163-4.

[201] Rodriguez J, Conde E, Gutierrez A, et al. The results of consolidation with autologous stem-cell transplantation in patients with peripheral T-cell lymphoma (PTCL) in first complete remission: the Spanish Lymphoma and Autologous Transplantation Group experience. *Ann. Oncol.* 2007; 18:652-7.

[202] Rodriguez J, Munsell M, Yazji S, et al. Impact of high-dose chemotherapy on peripheral T-cell lymphomas. *J. Clin. Oncol.* 2001; 19:3766-70.

[203] Corradini P, Dodero A, Zallio F, et al. Graft-versus-lymphoma effect in relapsed peripheral T-cell non-Hodgkin's lymphomas after reduced-intensity conditioning followed by allogeneic transplantation of hematopoietic cells. *J. Clin. Oncol.* 2004; 22:2172-6.

[204] Shimoyama M. Diagnostic criteria and classification of clinical subtypes of adult T-cell leukaemia-lymphoma. A report from the Lymphoma Study Group (1984-87). *Br. J. Haematol.* 1991; 79:428-37.

[205] Yamada Y, Tomonaga M, Fukuda H, et al. A new G-CSF-supported combination chemotherapy, LSG15, for adult T-cell leukaemia-lymphoma: Japan Clinical Oncology Group Study 9303. *Br. J. Haematol.* 2001; 113:375-82.

[206] Tsukasaki K, Maeda T, Arimura K, et al. Poor outcome of autologous stem cell transplantation for adult T cell leukemia/lymphoma: a case report and review of the literature. *Bone Marrow Transplant.* 1999; 23:87-9.

[207] Utsunomiya A, Miyazaki Y, Takatsuka Y, et al. Improved outcome of adult T cell leukemia/lymphoma with allogeneic hematopoietic stem cell transplantation. *Bone Marrow Transplant.* 2001; 27:15-20.

[208] Kami M, Hamaki T, Miyakoshi S, et al. Allogeneic haematopoietic stem cell transplantation for the treatment of adult T-cell leukaemia/lymphoma. *Br. J. Haematol.* 2003; 120:304-9.

[209] Fukushima T, Miyazaki Y, Honda S, et al. Allogeneic hematopoietic stem cell transplantation provides sustained long-term survival for patients with adult T-cell leukemia/lymphoma. *Leukemia.* 2005; 19:829-34.

[210] Okamura J, Utsunomiya A, Tanosaki R, et al. Allogeneic stem-cell transplantation with reduced conditioning intensity as a novel immunotherapy and antiviral therapy for adult T-cell leukemia/lymphoma. *Blood.* 2005; 105:4143-5.

[211] Harashima N, Kurihara K, Utsunomiya A, et al. Graft-versus-Tax response in adult T-cell leukemia patients after hematopoietic stem cell transplantation. *Cancer Res.* 2004; 64:391-9.

[212] Nakase K, Hara M, Kozuka T, Tanimoto K, Nawa Y. Bone marrow transplantation from unrelated donors for patients with adult T-cell leukaemia/lymphoma. *Bone Marrow Transplant.* 2006; 37:41-4.

[213] Tamaki H, Matsuoka M. Donor-derived T-cell leukemia after bone marrow transplantation. *N. Engl. J. Med.* 2006; 354:1758-9.

[214] Sallah S, Smith SV, Lony LC, Woodard P, Schmitz JL, Folds JD. Gamma/delta T-cell hepatosplenic lymphoma: review of the literature, diagnosis by flow cytometry and concomitant autoimmune hemolytic anemia. *Ann. Hematol.* 1997; 74:139-42.

[215] Suzuki R, Suzumiya J, Nakamura S, et al. Hematopoietic stem cell transplantation for natural killer-cell lineage neoplasms. *Bone Marrow Transplant.* 2006; 37:425-31.

[216] Waldmann TA, White JD, Carrasquillo JA, et al. Radioimmunotherapy of interleukin-2R alpha-expressing adult T-cell leukemia with Yttrium-90-labeled anti-Tac. *Blood.* 1995; 86:4063-75.

[217] Enblad G, Hagberg H, Erlanson M, et al. A pilot study of alemtuzumab (anti-CD52 monoclonal antibody) therapy for patients with relapsed or chemotherapy-refractory peripheral T-cell lymphomas. *Blood.* 2004; 103:2920-4.

[218] Bennett JM, Kaminski MS, Leonard JP, et al. Assessment of treatment-related myelodysplastic syndromes and acute myeloid leukemia in patients with non-Hodgkin lymphoma treated with tositumomab and iodine I131 tositumomab. *Blood.* 2005; 105:4576-82.

In: Encyclopedia of Stem Cell Research (2 Volume Set)   ISBN: 978-1-61761-835-2
Editor: Alexander L. Greene   © 2012 Nova Science Publishers, Inc.

Chapter XXVIII

EFFICIENT IN VIVO GENE TRANSFER INTO RAT BONE MARROW PROGENITOR CELLS USING SV40-DERIVED VIRAL VECTORS: MIGRATION AND DIFFERENTIATION OF TRANSDUCED BONE MARROW-RESIDENT CELLS TO OTHER ORGANS

Jean-Pierre Louboutin*, Alena A. Chekmasova,
Bianling Liu and David S. Strayer
Department of Pathology, Anatomy, and Cell Biology, Thomas Jefferson University,
Philadelphia, PA, US

ABSTRACT

Gene transfer to hematopoietic stem cells (HSCs) has been mainly attempted *ex vivo* and has been limited by transplantation-related problems in homing and engraftment, as well as by cytokine-induced loss of self-renewal capacity. The goal is usually to provide long-term gene expression in the differentiated progeny of HSCs. We attempted to circumvent such limitations by transducing HSCs directly in their native environment, the bone marrow (BM). To do this, an efficient method of gene transfer to resting HSCs is needed. Tag-deleted SV40-derived vectors (rSV40s) fit this description. Rats received direct injection of SV(Nef-FLAG) into the femoral BM cavities. The vector is a rSV40 carrying a marker gene (FLAG epitope). Control rats received an unrelated rSV40 or saline. Peripheral blood cells (5%) and femoral marrow cells (25%) expressed FLAG for the entire study (16 months). Flow cytometry analysis demonstrated transgene expression

* Correspondence concerning this article should be addressed to: JP Louboutin, MD, PhD, Department of Pathology, Anatomy, and Cell Biology, Thomas Jefferson University, 1020 Locust street, 251 JAH, Philadelphia, PA 19107, USA. Email address: jplouboutin@hotmail.com.

in multiple hematopoietic cell lineages, including granulocytes, CD3+ T lymphocytes and CD45R+ B lymphocytes, indicating successful gene transfer to long-lived progenitor cells with multilineage capacity. FLAG expression was also assessed in different organs at 1, 4 and 16 months. FLAG+ macrophages were detected throughout the body, and were very prominent in the spleen. FLAG+ cells were also common in pulmonary alveoli. The latter included immunologically identifiable alveolar macrophages and type II pneumocytes. FLAG+ pneumocytes were not detected at 1 month, infrequent at 4 months and common at 16 months after intramarrow injection. Rare liver cells were positive for both FLAG and ferritin, indicating that some hepatocytes also expressed this BM-delivered transgene. In the CNS, FLAG-expressing cells were mainly detected in the dentate gyrus (DG) of the hippocampus and in the periventricular subependymal zone (PSZ). These areas are involved in spontaneous adult neurogenesis. DG and PSZ FLAG+ cells were virtually nonexistant before 1 month and were rare at 4 months, but they were abundant 16 months after BM injection. Approximately 5% of DG cells were FLAG+. Of these, 48.6% were neurons, 49.7% were microglial cells and 1.6% were astrocytes, as determined by double immunostaining for FLAG and CNS lineage markers. DG and PSZ studies of control animals were negative. Thus: (a) direct intramarrow administration of rSV40 vectors provides efficient gene transfer to rat BM progenitor cells; (b) fixed tissue phagocytes may be accessible to gene delivery by intramarrow transduction of their progenitors; (c) transduced BM-resident cells or their derivatives may migrate to other organs (lungs, brain) and may differentiate into cells specific of these organs and (d) intramarrow injection of rSV40s does not detectably transduce parenchymal cells of other organs.

A. INTRODUCTION

Hematopoietic stem cells (HSCs) are among the most promising targets for gene tranfer because of their unique lifelong ability to proliferate and to differentiate into all of the cell lineages in the peripheral blood (PB). It has been suggested that gene delivery to HSCs could potentially be used to treat selected genetic diseases, and be applicable to the therapy of such acquired diseases as AIDS, cancer, as well as neurodegenerative and autoimmune disorders. Moreover, reports of HSC plasticity (i.e., the ability to develop into cells of nonhematopoietic lineages) may open new fields for HSC gene delivery.

Human HSC gene therapy clinical trials have generally yielded disappointing results, the main exception being successful treatment of severe combined immune deficiency (SCID-X1 and adenosine deaminase [ADA]-SCID) [Cavazzana-Calvo et al., 2000; Aiuti et al., 2002]. However, successful gene transfer has been hampered by low transduction efficiency of human HSCs because oncoretroviruses, the viral vector used for this purpose clinically, require cell division in order to integrate into host genome [Roe et al., 1993]. By contrast, primitive HSCs are naturally quiescent [Mahmud et al., 2001].

Different strategies have been developed to overcome this obstacle, using different cytokines in various combinations to elicit cell division. Unfortunately, cytokine treatments often lead to HSC differentiation, limiting plutipotency and compromising the capacity to replenish the stem cell pool. Moreover, such *ex vivo* treatment necessitates transplantation of the gene-modified HSC, which involves complications related to bone marrow (BM) cell homing and engraftment [Tavassoli and Hardy, 1990; Peters et al., 1995; Liu et al., 2003].

The challenge of HSC gene delivery might be approached using different paradigms, for example, applying both novel vector systems and direct *in situ* gene delivery to HSCs. Recombinant simian virus 40-derived viral vectors (rSV40s) transduce nondividing cells, including neurons and HSCs, efficiently and can achieve long term transgene expression *in vitro* and *in vivo*, although levels of protein production tend to be lower than with other vector systems [Strayer et al., 1997; Strayer et al., 2000; Strayer et al., 2002a; Cordelier et al., 2003]. Efficient transduction of hematopoietic progenitor cells using SV40 viral vectors *ex vivo* has been demonstrated [Rund et al., 1998; Strayer et al., 2000].

In a recent study [Liu et al., 2005], an *in vivo* gene transfer approach using percutaneous intrafemoral BM injection to deliver rSV40s directly into the BM cavity is described.

B. In vivo Gene Transfer into Rat Bone Marrow Progenitor Cells using rSV40 Viral Vectors

SV40 Viral Vectors Transduce Unstimulated Rat BM Cells *in vitro* Efficiently

Before attempting intramarrow administration using rSV40 vectors, gene delivery was first tested in rat BMMNCs (bone marrow mononuclear cells) selected from rat femurs and tibias using Ficoll-Hypaque. Freshly isolated rat BMMNCs were transduced with SV(Nef-FLAG), a rSV40 carrying a marker gene (FLAG epitope) appended to HIV-1 Nef protein, for 2 hours without cytokine stimulation. Cells were cultured for 3 weeks after transduction, in the presence of IL-3, IL-6, and stem cell factor. Control cells were mock-transduced and cultured under the same conditions. Seven and 21 days after transduction, the cultured cells were analyzed for FLAG expression using immunostaining. FLAG expression was detected in almost all SV(Nef-FLAG) exposed BMMNCs either 7 or 21 days after transduction. Percentages of FLAG-expressing cells were identical in transduced cells at both time points, indicating a persistent transgene expression delivered by the rSV40 viral vector. Control cells were negative (Figure 1). These results demonstrate that SV40 viral vectors transduce rat BMMNCs with very high efficiency and that they deliver sustained transgene expression.

In vivo Transduction of BM Cells by Direct Intramarrow Injection of SV(Nef-FLAG)

To test the transduction efficiency of BM cells *in vivo*, six rats were injected with SV(Nef-FLAG), at a dose of 10^{11} IU/femur. Four rats received the control vector SV(BUGT); four were given saline.

The specificity of immunostaining to detect FLAG expression was assessed in BM smears 7 days after intramarrow injection of SV(Nef-FLAG) (Figure 2A). FLAG expression was only seen in BM cells from SV(Nef-FLAG)-treated animals immunostained with anti-FLAG antibody. Cells from control (SV(BUGT)- or saline-injected) animals were negative, as were all BM specimens when the primary antibody was omitted or replaced by a non-immune isotype-matched immunoglobulin.

Two rats were killed each on day 7 and day 42 after injection. BM cells were assayed for FLAG expression by flow cytometry after intracellular immunostaining. Percentages of BM cells expressing FLAG ranged from 20 to 30%. Data from 1 and 6 weeks were almost identical (Figure 2B).

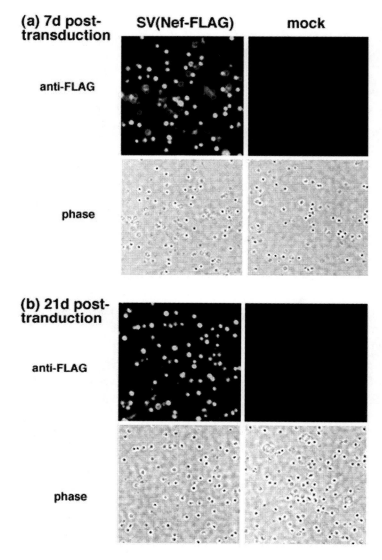

Figure 1. FLAG expression in rat BMMNCs transduced with SV(Nef-FLAG) in vitro. After selection by centrifugation over Ficoll-Hypaque and transduction with SV(Nef-FLAG) or (negative control) SV(BUGT), FLAG expression in transduced rat BMMNCs was analyzed by immunostaining. (A) Seven days after transduction. (B) 21 days after transduction. (This research was originally published in Blood. Liu B, Daviau J, Nichols CN, Strayer DS. In vivo gene transfer into rat bone marrow progenitor cells using rSV40 viral vectors. *Blood*. 2005; 106: 2655-2662. Copyright The American Society of Hematology).

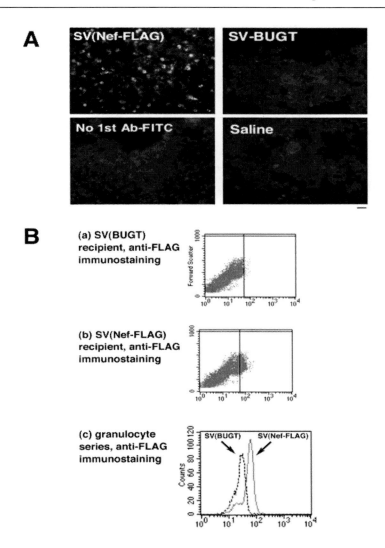

Figure 2. Detection of FLAG in BM cells of rats injected with SV(FLAG). A. Immunostaining for FLAG in bone marrow of SV(Nef-FLAG) recipients or control (SV(BUGT) or saline) recipients, 7 days after injection into the femoral bone marrow cavities. Bone marrow from SV(Nef-FLAG) recipients was also immunostained with a non-immune isotype-matched antibody. Bar: 60μm. B. One week after being injected with SV(Nef-FLAG) or SV(BUGT), BM cavities of the femurs with PBS were flushed and BM cells were lysed with ammonium chloride, permeabilized, immunostained for FLAG, and analyzed by FACS. (a) FACS scattergram for FLAG expression in BM cells of a representative control rat (SV(BUGT) recipient) one week after injection; (b) of a representative SV(Nef-FLAG) recipient rat one week after transduction. (c) Double immunostaining of BM cells from these rats for granulocyte lineage marker (CD11b)+ FLAG, comparing SV(BUGT) recipient (dashed line) and SV(Nef-FLAG) recipent (solid gray line). (This research was originally published in: Blood. Liu B, Daviau J, Nichols CN, Strayer DS. In vivo gene transfer into rat bone marrow progenitor cells using rSV40 viral vectors. *Blood*. 2005; 106: 2655-2662. Copyright The American Society of Hematology and in: Journal of Gene Medicine. Louboutin JP, Liu B, Chekmasova AA, Reyes, BAS, van Bockstaele EJ, Strayer DS. Delivering genes to the organ-localized immune system: long term results of direct intramarrow transduction. *J Gene Med* 2007; 9: 843-851).

In vivo rSV40 Gene Delivery by Intramarrow Injection Results in high Levels of Transgene Expression in Rat PB Cells

SV(Nef-FLAG) vectors were injected at 2×10^{11} IU/animal into the BM cavity of both femurs of rats. Control rats received a control vector, SV(BUGT). Gene expression of FLAG was then followed in PB cells by PB sampling and FACS analysis every 2 weeks up to 56 weeks. Within the first 2 weeks of injection, FLAG was expressed in between 7 and 10% of PB leukocytes (average 9%), then decreased to between 0.5 and 1% at week 8 after injection, rising thereafter to stabilize at week 12 between 3.5 and 10% (average: 6%) for the remainder of the 13-month follow-up period. Comparing test animals to the ones given SV(BUGT), the percentages of FLAG-positive cells in the PB were significantly (p at least < 0.05) above background levels for each biweekly time point. These results show that BM injection with rSV40 vectors provides efficient *in vivo* gene transfer to primitive BM progenitor cells with long-term hematopoietic capacity.

BM Injection of rSV40 Vectors Transduces Progenitor Cells that Differentiate into Multiple Lineages

FLAG expression was followed over time by flow cytometry in granulocytes, and T and B lymphocytes in PB of rats whose BM was injected with SV(Nef-FLAG). Sustained FLAG expression was demonstrated in different hematopoietic lineages. FLAG expression in granulocytes was between 1.2 and 8.8% of total nucleated cells, and between 7.5 and 55.4% of PB granulocytes. Lower percentages of CD3- and CD45R-positive cells (B lymphocytes) expressed the transgene (0.13 to 1.9%, and 0.2 and 3.5% respectively), perhaps reflecting persistence of circulating cells of their long-lived lineages that exited the BM before gene delivery (Figure 3). Similar data were obtained for T cell subsets and other circulating blood cell lineages. These findings show that *in vivo* injection of rSV40 vectors into the BM transduced a BM progenitor cell population(s) with long term multilineage potential very efficiently.

Long Term Transgene Expression in Rat BM Cells after rSV40 Gene Delivery by Percutaneous Intramarrow Injection

Femoral BM cells were analyzed for FLAG expression by flow cytometry, 13 to 16.5 months after intramarrow injection. Percentages of FLAG-positive cells ranged from 2 to 40% of all nucleated cells (average: 15.9%). Percentages of FLAG expressing femoral BM leukocytes averaged about 15% of all nucleated cells, but an average of 49% of all granulocyte marker-positive cells in the BM expressed FLAG, while lower percentages were seen in BM T-lymphocytes or B lymphocytes (Figure 4).

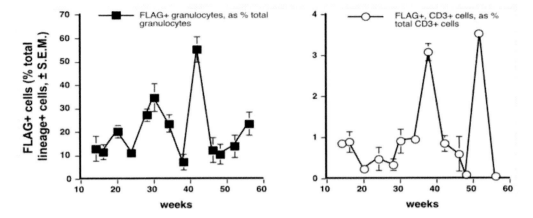

Figure 3. Detection of FLAG expression by FACS in both PB granulocytes and lymphocytes of rats whose BM has been in jected with SV(Nef-FLAG). Blood from the rats injected with SV(Nef-FLAG) was double-immunostained for FLAG and mature leukocyte lineage markers. Lineage marker expression and FLAG among the several hematopoietic subpopulations was tested by FACS 14 weeks after the injection into the BM. Time course of FLAG expression in PB granulocytes and CD3+ lymphocytes of rats injected with SV(Nef-FLAG). (This research was originally published in Blood. Liu B, Daviau J, Nichols CN, Strayer DS. In vivo gene transfer into rat bone marrow progenitor cells using rSV40 viral vectors. *Blood*. 2005; 106: 2655-2662. Copyright The American Society of Hematology).

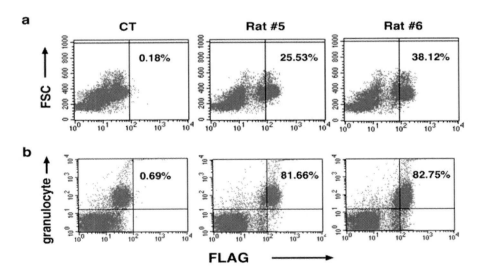

Figure 4. Long term FLAG expression seen in BM cells of rats injected with SV(Nef-FLAG). FACS analysis of FLAG expression in BM cells of rats that received SV(Nef-FLAG) or negative control SV(BUGT) into the BM 16 months earlier. A. Representative dot plots for FLAG expression in BM cells in rats injected with SV(Nef-FLAG) and in control rat. FSC: Forward scatter. The proportion of FLAG-positive cells as a percentage of total nucleated cells are shown. B. Representative FACS dot plots for FLAG expression in BM granulocytes in the same rats. Percentages of FLAG-positive granulocytes shown are relative to total granulocyte-positive cells. (This research was originally published in Blood. Liu B, Daviau J, Nichols CN, Strayer DS. In vivo gene transfer into rat bone marrow progenitor cells using rSV40 viral vectors. *Blood*. 2005; 106: 2655-2662. Copyright The American Society of Hematology).

At 16 months after the injection, there was no difference in the percentages of FLAG-positive cells in the BM from the femur and the tibia, suggesting that BM progenitor cells may not be stationary within the hematopoietic system but may migrate and redistribute among the various blood-forming areas of the BM over time.

The effectiveness of HSC transduction using oncoretroviral vectors has significantly improved in recent years [Halene et al., 1999; Cavazzano-Calvo et al., 2000; Abonour et al., 2000]. However, extensive *ex vivo* cytokine stimulation to induce cell division is still obligatory for oncoretroviral gene delivery to HSCs which are mostly in G0 phase in the BM. Lentiviral vectors have elicited interest because they can transduce nondividing cells, including HSCs [Naldini et al., 1996]. However, fully quiescent G0 cells are not well transduced by lentiviral vectors [Korin and Zack., 1998; Sutton et al., 1999], and effective lentiviral gene transfer to HSCs still requires *ex vivo* cytokine stimulation [Zielske and Gerson, 2003]. Moreover, HIV-based lentiviral vector gene transfer to primitive HSCs in nonhuman primates has yielded disappointing results [Horn et al., 2002; An et al., 2000, 2001]. For these and other reasons, clinical trials of lentiviral HSC gene therapy have been long in coming [Josephson et al., 2002].

Because the consequences of combined cytokine stimulation and reimplantation are problematic, we and others have begun to test *in vivo* gene transfer to HSCs as a potential alternative to conventional *ex vivo* gene delivery. Consequently, viral vectors that transduce nondividing cells permanently should be considered potential vehicles for HSC-directed gene transfer. Long-term transduction in rabbits was achieved using retrovirus-mediated gene transfer to HSC by direct *in vivo* administration [Nelson et al., 1997]. Effective *in vivo* gene transfer into short-term reconstituting HSCs with multiple lineage potential was seen in mice given retroviral vectors by direct intrafemoral BM injection to correct a defect in Jak3 [McCauslin et al., 2003]. *In vivo* retroviral gene transfer to HSCs of neonatal sheep using BM injection achieved long-term transgene expression (0.9% of PB cells were transgene-expressing lymphocytes, and 1.8% were transgene-expressing granulocytes/monocytes) [Porada et al., 2000].

We have pursued a similar strategy, except that we used rSV40 viruses to deliver a marker gene. rSV40s were employed in the current study because they transduce cells in G0 with high efficiency and provide permanent transgene expression. We observed efficient, sustained gene transfer to rat BM progenitor cells: direct injection of a BM compartment with 10% to 15% of the total BM pool resulted in an average of 6% of nucleated blood cells expressing the transgene. This may be attributed to the efficiency of rSV40 vectors in transducing the targeted BM progenitor cells. Transgene expression continued undiminished for the 16 month duration of these studies. This is consistent with other studies in which rSV40 transduction of several organs has proven long-lived [Strayer and Milano, 1996; Strayer et al., 2002a, b; Duan et al., 2004]. Thus, direct *in vivo* BM injection may be an alternative to *ex vivo* transduction.

Intramarrow injection avoids the extensive *ex vivo* cytokine treatment that is used to induce HSC mitosis, which is needed for *ex vivo* oncoretroviral or lentiviral transduction of HSC. The use of rSV40s in our studies circumvents the requirement that HSCs be in mitosis at the time of transduction, as these vectors integrate into genomes of nondividing HSCs and other cells.

rSV40 vectors injected into the femoral BM cavity *in vivo* transduced cells capable of differentiating into granulocytes and lymphocytes. It is not clear if these cells were true "stem" cells. HSCs are a very low percentage of the BM cell pool and rodents lack an agreed-upon HSC cell membrane marker. Although rSV40 vectors are very effective in transducing mature lymphocytes [Strayer et al., 1997; Goldstein et al., 2002; Cordelier et al., 2002], the percentages of total cells in the blood and BM that expressed both FLAG and lymphocyte markers were lower than for granulocytes. Unlike neutrophils that turn over very rapidly, lymphocytes are long-lived and the transduced progenitors in the BM might not necessirily proliferate and differentiate into mature lymphocytes in the absence of a systemic stress that would increase demand for more lymphocytes.

Percentages of transgene-expressing cells in the BM of injected rats were much higher than in the PB. Although femoral BM is only about 10% of the total marrow pool in the rat, it is of interest to note that the tibia contained similar percentages of FLAG-positive cells 16 months after transduction. These findings suggest that intrafemoral BM injection may reach more progenitor cells than simply those present at the time of injection. As well, resident marrow progenitors may circulate among the marrow-containing bones.

One of the transgene markers used, the FLAG epitope, was appended to a carrier protein, in this case, HIV-1 Nef. This approach, using an antibody-recognized intracellular antigen, differs from techniques used in other studies. "Traditional" marker genes, such as the fluorescent proteins, or β-galactosidase, are not expressed well when delivered by rSV40 vectors. The reasons for this are not entirely clear, but the COS-7 cells that package these vectors appear to recognize and inactivate invertebrate or prokaryote DNAs (MS Strayer, et al., in preparation). Other mammalian DNAs, and genes from mammalian viruses, are largely expressed effectively by these vectors. Nonetheless, levels of protein expression, though durable and not prone to silencing post-transduction, tend to be lower than are seen with, e.g., adenoviral vectors– perhaps for the same reasons.

It may be possible to increase percentages of transgene-positive cells further using multiple inoculations, preferably into different BM sites. We attempted to inject other bones in the rat, but more distal accessible long bones (i.e., tibia) contain much less marrow than the femur, and other bones like the sternum and the iliac crest proved too fragile for our injection technique.

Repeated vector dosing may also be tried, since the majority of BM cells, even in the femur, were not transduced with a single injection. This approach increases numbers of rSV40-transduced cells in studies *in vivo* targeting other organs [Strayer and Milano, 1996; Strayer et al., 2002a, b; Sauter et al., 2000; Duan et al., 2004]. In this respect, rSV40 vectors have a unique advantage: repeated studies have shown that they do not elicit detectable neutralizing immune responses, and that consecutive administrations may be given in rapid sequence or with lengthy time intervals in between. Thus multiple dosing is possible without loss of gene delivery efficiency [McKee and Strayer, 2002]. The transparency of the virus to the immune system, which accounts for this unique capability, probably reflects the virus' unusual route of entry, which avoids antigen processing even in transduction of professional antigen presenting cells [Yamada and Kasamatsu 1993; Anderson et al., 1996; Chen and Norkin, 1999; Pelkmans et al., 2001, 2002]. The absence of detectable neutralizing antibodies, by whatever the mechanism, allows for multiple administrations of rSV40s without loss of gene transfer efficacy due to vector-specific immune responses [Anderson et al., 1996; Chen and Norkin; Pelkmans et al., 2001, 2002].

We have demonstrated that rSV40s are effective gene delivery vehicles for use in the BM. Their lack of antigenicity and ability to transduce nondividing cells make rSV40 vectors attractive vehicles for direct *in vivo* BM gene transfer in settings where efficient and sustained gene transfer is desired. We will now examine some of the possibilities suggested by these results.

C. DELIVERING GENES TO THE ORGAN-LOCALIZED IMMUNE SYSTEM AFTER DIRECT INTRAMARROW TRANSDUCTION

Reports of unexpected transdifferentiation of stem cells into mature derivative cell types raised expectations of possible novel cellular therapies in regenerative medicine [Masson et al., 2004; Kashofer and Bonnet, 2005]. It is well known that embryonic stem (ES) cells are totipotent and can generate all or most tissues [Wilmut et al., 2002]. Over the past several years, many studies have suggested that some tissue specific or adult stem cells may possess the potential to differentiate into cells of other tissues [Krause et al., 2001; Lagasse et al., 2002; Jiang et al., 2002]. Several possible mechanisms might be invoked to explain these phenomena, and recent experiments have raised controversy about the mechanism(s) involved. One possibility is transdifferentiation of a committed cell directly into another cell type as a response to environmental cues [Labarge and Blau, 2002; Lapidos et al., 2004; Camargo et al., 2003]. Practically, the clinical utility of direct transdifferentiation would be limited by the number of cells that can be introduced into an organ without removing resident cells. On the other hand, if BM cells can give rise to other tissues, they could in theory repopulate organs from a small number of progenitors. Recent data from animal studies support such a model [Jang et al., 2004; Brittan et al., 2005; Harris et al., 2004; Schwarz et al., 2002; Jiang et al., 2003]. However, it has been suggested that if there are BM resident cells with extensive capacity to differentiate into nonhematopoietic cell types, they may not be HSCs. Rather this activity may reflect the presence in the BM of distinct, tissue-specific stem cells, or BM-resident pluripotent stem cells [Wagers et al., 2002]. It has been also demonstrated that fusion of host and donor cells can give rise to mature tissue cells without transdifferentiation or dedifferentiation [Weimann et al., 2003a; Alvarez-Dolado et al., 2003; Vassilopoulos et al., 2003; Wang et al., 2003; Camargo et al., 2004; Willenbring et al., 2004; Kashofer et al., 2005; Stadtfel and Graf, 2005].

Several of the results concerning transdifferentiation are based on experimental conditions including transplantation of HSCs into irradiated recipients [Krause et al., 2001; Lagasse et al., 2002]. However, *ex-vivo* manipulation of HSCs with multiple cytokines, as is necessary for transduction with retroviral or lentiviral vectors, often leads to differentiation and loss of pluripotency, and so compromises replenishment of the stem cell pool. *Ex vivo* treatment also requires reimplantation (transplantation), subsequent homing to the BM *in vivo* and successful engrafment. These processes lead to significant loss of transplanted cells. Finally, besides HSCs, the BM compartment contains committed progenitor cells, noncirculating stromal cells that have the ability to develop into mesenchymal lineages.

Although some other investigators have claimed intramarrow gene delivery [Halene et al., 1999; Abonour et al., 2000; Nelson et al., 1997], the lineages and distribution of transgene–expressing cells in the body after intramarrow gene delivery have not been reported. Thus, to study the consequences of intramarrow injection as well as the differentiated progeny of transduced BM progenitor cells, we examined the population of transgene-expressing cells in the major organs after direct injection of rSV40 viral vectors into the BM of rats [Louboutin et al., 2007a] as previously described [Liu et al., 2005].

Transgene Expression of FLAG in the Spleen

Numerous FLAG-expressing cells were seen in the spleen, both 4 and 16 months after intramarrow injection of SV(Nef-FLAG) (Figure 5A). No FLAG expression was detectable in animals injected with either saline or SV(BUGT), or when the primary antibody was omitted or replaced by a non-immune isotype-matched antibody. Very few FLAG-positive cells were detected when spleens were assayed 1 month after BM injection (not shown). Most FLAG+ cells were in the marginal zone (MZ). Very few were in germinal centers (GC) (Figure 5B). By double immunostaining, FLAG-positive cells in the MZ mostly co-expressed macrophage markers, CD68 or CD11b. Some transgene-expressing cells also coimmunostained for CD68 outside the GC and the MZ, probably in the red pulp where macrophages are known to express CD68. Some FLAG-expressing cells coimmunostained for CD3, but very few were CD45R-positive (Figure 5C). Studies done 4 and 16 months after transduction gave similar results.

Transgene Expressing Alveolar Macrophages and Alveolar Pneumocytes in the Lung

FLAG-positive cells were detected in pulmonary alveoli (Figure 6A), but not in conducting airways (bronchi or trachea, not shown). Alveolar FLAG+ cells were mainly detectable 4 and 16 months after BM injection, the numbers increasing from 2.5% of all alveolar cells at 4 months to 4.6% at 16 months. Controls were negative (Figure 6A). Many FLAG-positive cells coimmunostained for the macrophage marker, ED1 (Figure 6B). However, a significant number of ED1-negative, FLAG+ cells, coexpressed TTF1, a marker of alveolar type II cells (Figure 6C), suggesting that BM progenitors may have given rise to alveolar epithelial progeny. Four months after BM injection with SV(Nef-FLAG), 65.8 +/- 7.5% of FLAG-positive alveolar cells were ED1-positive, 32.4 +/- 2.8% of FLAG-positive cells were TTF-1-positive, and 1.8 +/- 0.2% of FLAG-positive were neither ED1-, or TTF-1- positive. Sixteen months after BM injection, the percentages of FLAG-positive /ED1-positive cells, FLAG-positive/TTF-1-positive, FLAG-positive/TTF-1- and ED1-negative were 63.6 +/- 7.2%, 35.2 +/- 3.7 %, and 1.1 +/- 0.2 %, respectively.

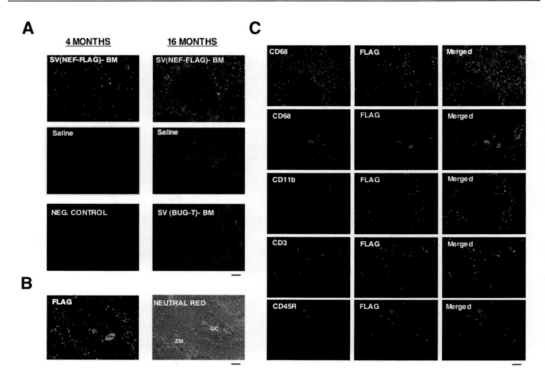

Figure 5. Transgene expression in spleen cells 4 and 16 months after injection of SV(Nef-FLAG) into the BM. A. FLAG-expressing spleen cells 4 and 16 months after injection of SV(Nef-FLAG) into the BM. Spleens from saline and SV(BUGT) recipients are also shown, as is the immunostaining of SV(Nef-FLAG) recipient spleen sections when the primary antibody was replaced by a non-immune isotype-matched antibody (neg. control). Bar: 100µm. B. Localization of FLAG+ cells mostly at the periphery of germinal centers (GC). Left, immunofluorescence with anti-FLAG antibody. Right, neutral red staining of the same section. The marginal zone (ZM) and germinal center are indicated. Bar: 100µm. C. Lineages of FLAG-positive cells in the spleen. Spleen sections from recipients of intramarrow SV(Nef-FLAG) 16 months earlier were immunostained for FLAG and for markers of macrophages CD68 (ED1) and CD11b, mainly in the ZM. The second row of CD68 coimmunostaining is a higher magnification of a field from the first row. Coimmunostaining for CD3 and CD45R is shown below. Bar: 100 µm, except in the second row: 50 µm. (This research was originally published in Journal of Gene Medicine. Louboutin JP, Liu B, Chekmasova AA, Reyes, BAS, van Bockstaele EJ, Strayer DS. Delivering genes to the organ-localized immune system: long term results of direct intramarrow transduction. *J Gene Med* 2007; 9: 843-851).

Rare Transgene-Expressing Cells in Liver, Kidney and Muscle

Less than 1% of cells in the liver were FLAG-positive. Such cells were, if not abundant, more numerous at 16 months after intramarrow injection than after 4 months (Figure 7A, B, C). No transgene expression was detected in livers of control animals, injected with saline or with SV(BUGT), or when the primary antibody was replaced by a non-immune isotype-matched antibody or omitted (Figure 7A). FLAG-positive cells generally coimmunostained with CD68, a marker of liver Kuppfer cells, (Figure 7B). However, coimmunostaining for FLAG and ferritin, the latter a marker of hepatocytes, was also seen in occasional cells

(Figure 7C). At 4 and 16 months after injection of SV(Nef-FLAG) into the BM, fewer than 1% of the cells in the kidney were positive for FLAG (Figure 7D). These cells were interstitial cells, that coimmunostained for CD68 (Figure 7E); no FLAG immunostaining was seen in the glomeruli. Control animals were totally negative.

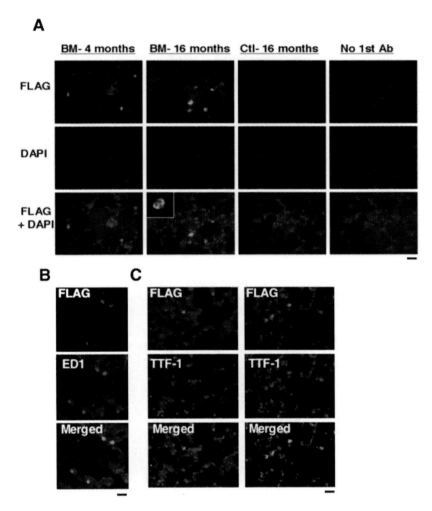

Figure 6. Transgene expression in the lung. A. Cryostat sections of lung from rats whose BM has been injected by SV(Nef-FLAG) 4 and 16 months previously, with DAPI staining and overlays. Controls shown include lung sections from animals injected with SV(BUGT) and immunostaining performed when the primary antibody was replaced by a non-immune isotype-matched antibody (right column). Bar: 50 µm. B. FLAG-positive cells coimmunostained with ED1, a marker of macrophages. Note that FLAG-positive cells were not all CD68-positive. Bar: 50 µm. C. FLAG-positive cells coimmunostained with TTF-1, a marker of type II alveolar cells (right column). Note that FLAG-positive cells are not all TTF-1-positive (left column). Bar: 50 µm. (This research was originally published in Journal of Gene Medicine. Louboutin JP, Liu B, Chekmasova AA, Reyes, BAS, van Bockstaele EJ, Strayer DS. Delivering genes to the organ-localized immune system: long term results of direct intramarrow transduction. *J Gene Med* 2007; 9: 843-851).

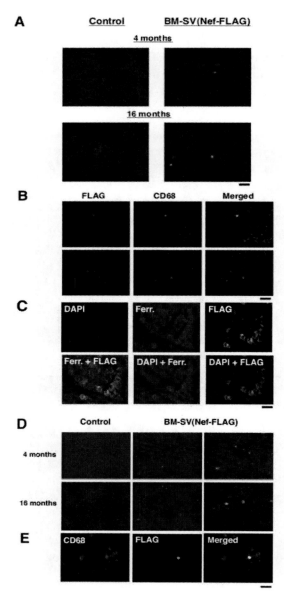

Figure 7. Expression of FLAG in liver and kidneys from rats whose BM had been injected 4 and 16 months previously by SV(Nef-FLAG). A. Immunostaining of the liver at 4 and 16 months after intramarrow transduction. No expression was seen in animals injected with SV(BUGT) (control, not shown). Bar: 100 μm. B. Demonstration that some, but not all, FLAG-positive cells coimmunostained with CD68, a marker of Kuppfer cells in the liver, 16 months after injection of the BM by SV(Nef-FLAG). Bar: 100 μm. C. Demonstration that rare FLAG+, centronucleated, cells in the liver coimmunostained for ferritin, a hepatocyte marker 16 months after injection of the BM by SV(Nef-FLAG). Bar: 50 μm. D. Immunostaining of cryostat sections of kidney 4 and 16 months after injection of SV(Nef-FLAG) in the BM. Control sections were from animals injected with SV(BUGT). E. Coimmunostaining of FLAG and CD68 in the kidney. Bar: 100 μm in D, 50 μm in E. (This research was originally published in Journal of Gene Medicine. Louboutin JP, Liu B, Chekmasova AA, Reyes, BAS, van Bockstaele EJ, Strayer DS. Delivering genes to the organ-localized immune system: long term results of direct intramarrow transduction. *J Gene Med* 2007; 9: 843-851).

Different muscles (Extensor Digitorum Longus-EDL-, Soleus,-SOL-, Tibialis Anterior-TA) were studied and showed the same pattern. Scattered FLAG-positive cells were seen in the interstitium peripheral to muscle fibers (Figure 8A). FLAG-positive cells were also positive for ED1 (Figure 8B), but not for N-CAM, marker of satellite cells, or MyoD, marker of regenerating muscle fibers, on the samples examined (Figure 8C). No FLAG expression was detected in cardiac myocytes (Figure 8D). Again, controls were negative.

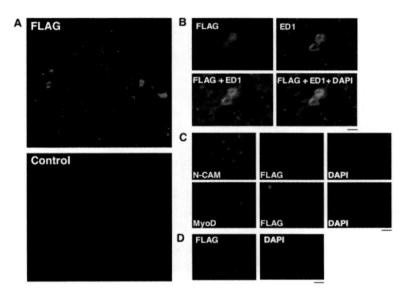

Figure 8. Expression of FLAG in skeletal and heart muscle from rats 16 months after intramarrow injection of SV(Nef-FLAG). A. Rare FLAG-positive cells are seen are at the periphery of the muscle fibers. No expression is seen when the primary antibody was replaced by a non-immune isotype-matched antibody (control). Bar: 15 μm. B. FLAG-positive cells coimmunostained with ED1, a marker of macrophages. Bar: 20 μm. C. FLAG-positive cells did not coimmunostain with MyoD, a marker of regenerating muscle fiber, neither a coimmunostaining between N-CAM, a marker of satellite cells and FLAG was seen. Bar: 100 μm. D. No FLAG-expression was detected in the heart. Bar: 100 μm. (This research was originally published in Journal of Gene Medicine. Louboutin JP, Liu B, Chekmasova AA, Reyes, BAS, van Bockstaele EJ, Strayer DS. Delivering genes to the organ-localized immune system: long term results of direct intramarrow transduction. *J Gene Med* 2007; 9: 843-851).

We sought here to address three main issues: (a) the extent to which intramarrow delivery of recombinant SV40-derived vectors led to detectable gene transfer outside of the BM; (b) the potential of such intramarrow transduction to achieve long-term genetic modification of cell populations, such as tissue macrophages, that are relatively inaccessible to transduction and (c) whether cells not usually considered to be of BM origin expressed transgene delivered to the BM, to suggest that they might derive in part from BM-resident cell populations.

We found no evidence that intramarrow injection of rSV40 vectors led to transduction beyond the BM. For example, in the kidneys, which are highly susceptible to rSV40 transduction [Strayer and Milano, 1996], we detected no transgene expression in those epithelial cells at any time. Transgene expression in phagocytes in those tissues therefore probably reflects transduction of their hematopoietic progenitors.

Noncirculating lymphocytes and tissue phagocytes have long been problematic targets for gene delivery. These long-lived populations are thought to be key reservoirs where HIV-1 persists, even in patients who are currently on antiretroviral therapy and have no detectable circulating HIV-1 [Cavert et al., 1997; Lafeuillade et al., 2001; Finzi et al., 1997; Natajaran et al., 1999; Chun et al., 1998; Finzi et al., 1999; Zhang et al., 1998]. The ability to modify these cell populations genetically is of substantial potential importance in approaching AIDS-related gene therapy. Our studies document that intramarrow transduction with rSV40s (and, possibly, other vectors as well) can provide stable, long-term transgene expression to these cells. After 16 months, transgene-expressing cells were found in hematopoietic organs like the spleen, and also in tissue phagocytes in the lungs, kidneys, liver, muscle and brain [see following paragraph and Louboutin et al., 2006]. These findings have potential application for gene transfer in other settings, including inherited defects of macrophages and T lymphocytes, or to enhance or regulate immune responses.

We also assessed the extent to which nonhematopoietic cell populations outside the marrow could be accessible to transduction by intramarrow gene delivery. Krause reported that BM cells can migrate to the conducting airways and differentiate into epithelial cells [Krause et al., 2001]. Bronchiolar progenitor cells are thought to be Clara cells [Hong et al., 2004]. We did not observe FLAG-expressing cells in either the larger airways or bronchioles. Type II cells are thought to be the alveolar progenitor cells: they can replenish themselves and give rise to the terminally differentiated type I alveolar lining cells [Wu and Wei, 2004]. In this study, over 4.5% of alveolar cells expressed the transgene, suggesting that BM-derived cells could migrate to the alveoli. Since these FLAG+ cells were mainly seen at the 16 month time point, our data suggest that at least some type II cells in adults may derive from precursors in the BM.

Some studies suggest that BM-derived cells may be progenitors for hepatocytes [Krause et al., 2001; Petersen et al., 1999; Theise et al., 2000], especially following moderate to severe liver injury [Wilmut et al., 2002]. However, it seems that HSCs may rarely acquire hepatocyte phenotype (frequency <10-4) [Thorgeirsson and Grisham., 2006], most likely via differentiation through the macrophage-monocyte lineage [Vassilopoulos et al., 2003]. Cells of the myeloid lineage, rather than HSCs themselves, may also fuse with hepatocytes and so impact to their expression of genes delivered to the BM [Camargo et al., 2003].

In the present study, very few transgene-expressing cells were detected in the liver. Almost all of these cells expressed the ED1 macrophage marker. Nonetheless, a very small population of hepatocytes, identified as such by immunopositivity for ferritin, did express the transgene that had been delivered into the BM. Because organ injury was not part of our studies, our findings reflect normal physiology of cell turnover in rats and suggest that BM-resident progenitors or their derivatives may *trans*-differentiate into, or fuse with, hepatocytes very infrequently at most. Currently, we are testing whether liver injury can trigger the development of transgene-positive hepatocytes in animals transduced with intramarrow rSV40s.

Other tissues examined showed only occasional stromal cells that expressed FLAG detectably. These were largely immunopositive for macrophage markers. Thus FLAG-expressing myocytes were not detected in skeletal muscle or the heart. BM-derived cells may be precursors for regenerating skeletal myocytes following injury or in Duchenne muscular dystrophy [Ferrari et al., 1998; Fukada et al., 2002; Gussoni et al, 1999; Gussoni et al., 2002]. Camargo *et al.,* [2003] showed that a cell of the macrophage lineage contributed to myotubes in a model of muscle injury, confirming previous reports of a role for blood borne macrophages in muscle regeneration [Lescaudron et al., 1999]. Injury was not involved in our studies and FLAG+ skeletal or cardiac myocytes were not detected.

Our results confirm that derivatives of BM-resident progenitor cells can be transduced by SV(Nef-FLAG), migrate to different organs and that they either differentiate into, or fuse with, other cell types. As well, *in vivo* BM injection of SV40-derived vectors may be a safe alternative to current gene delivery approaches to BM transduction, and may allow access to long-lived resident tissue phagocyte and lymphocyte populations that have been difficult to reach by other means. It should be noted that the femoral marrow is responsible for about 10% of total hematopoiesis in the adult rat. Considering the manner in which transduction was performed, any cell population in the BM at the time of vector injection might have been transduced. Our studies thus do not establish the identity of the BM cell population(s) that lead to transgene expression in the different organs studied: they may be of hematopoietic, stromal or other origin.

D. Rat BM Progenitor Cells Transduced in situ by rSV40 Vectors Differentiate into Multiple Central Nervous System Cell Lineages

Gene delivery to the brain has focused mainly on transducing neurons directly. However, an alternative approach may be to consider those areas of the brain where neurogenesis continues well into adult life: the dentate gyrus (DG) of the hippocampus, and the periventricular subependymal zone. These cells produce new neurons throughout life, and also participate in repair of brain lesions. One might then genetically engineer brain stem cells *in situ* so that their proliferation after injury of the brain would lead to functional brain cells expressing the transgene. However, the number of progenitor cells is very limited in the adult brain and adult stem cells may have a shorter life span and different properties than pluripotent stem cells. We therefore tested whether some BM progenitor cells, transduced *in vivo* by direct injection of a rSV40 vector into the BM, were able to migrate in the brain and to differentiate into central nervous system cell lineages [Louboutin et al., 2006].

Transgene Expression in Cells with Neuronal Phenotype in the Dentate Gyrus

We focused the study on the DG, part of the hippocampus, composed of the granule cell layer (GCL), formed by an inner (upper) and outer (lower) blades, surrounding the hilus area. Sixteen months after injection of SV(Nef-FLAG) directly into the BM, FLAG expression was observed in some cells with neuronal morphology in the DG. No FLAG expression was seen in the DG in control animals either injected with saline or injected with a control vector, or when the primary antibody was replaced by a non-immune isotype-matched immunoglobulin (Figure 9A). The appearance of transgene-expressing cells in the DG progressed overtime: no FLAG-expressing cells were observed in the DG one month after injection of SV(Nef-FLAG) into the BM and very few were seen 4 months after injection of the vector into the BM. Some of the FLAG-expressing cells coimmunostained for NeuN, a neuronal marker, in the GCL as well as in the hilus area (Figure 9A). The morphology of NeuN-positive FLAG-expressing cells was strongly suggestive of neurons from the DG, with some characteristics of basket and pyramidal cells (Figure 9A). FLAG-expressing cells that were not NeuN positive were also observed in the same areas, suggesting that neurons were not the only cell type expressing the transgene (Figure 9A).

The percentage of NeuN-positive cells expressing FLAG was measured on several serial cryostat sections (at least 5 sections) for each sample examined. The inner and outer blades of the GCL were examined as well as the hilus area. Sixteen months after *in situ* injection of SV(Nef-FLAG) into the bone marrow, the percentage of NeuN-positive cells expressing FLAG was about 2.4% in the different areas examined. Such cells were too few to enumerate at earlier time points.

Transgene Expression in non Neuronal Cells in the Dentate Gyrus

FLAG expression was observed in cells with the morphology of microglial cells (Figure 9B). Some of the FLAG-expressing cells coimmunostained with antibodies against CD11b-C3bi, and CD68, markers of microglial cells (Figure 9B). Very rare GFAP-positive cells were expressing FLAG (not shown). Morphometric studies showed that 48.6% of the FLAG-expressing cells were NeuN-positive and that 49.7% of the FLAG-positive cells were expressing markers of microglial cells; only 1.6% of FLAG-positive cells were GFAP positive.

FLAG Expression in the Periventricular Subependymal Zone

Transgene expression in the periventricular subependymal zone (PSZ) followed similar kinetics. At 1 and 4 months post-BM injection, there were respectively no or few cells positive for the transgene, while at 16 months, numerous FLAG-positive cells were found in the PSZ. As in the DG, about 50% of FLAG-positive cells were stained by NT (Figure 9C). Thus, FLAG-expressing cells can be found in other areas of the brain besides the DG.

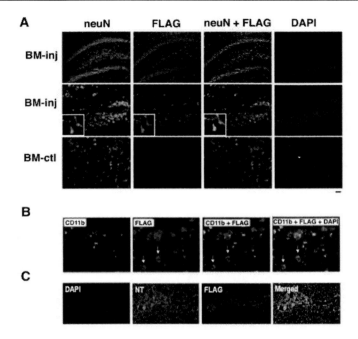

Figure 9. Transgene expression in CNS cells following bone marrow-directed gene delivery. A. Cryostat sections of the dentate gyrus (DG) from rats whose bone marrow (BM) had been injected by SV(Nef-FLAG) 16 months previously were simultaneously immunostained for NeuN and FLAG. Nuclei were stained by DAPI. The overlay composite highlights the many FLAG-positive cells that also labeled for NeuN (first row-low magnification- and second row- high magnification). Inserts show higher magnifications of cells positive for FLAG and NeuN. Control groups are shown in the third row (rats whose BM has been injected with a control SV40 vector). Bar: first row: 120 micrometers; second and third rows: 30 micrometers. B. Transduction of bone marrow leads to expression of the transgene in microglial cells. Sections of DG from the animals described in A, above, coimmunostained for CD11b (microglial cell marker) and FLAG. Note that not all FLAG-expressing cells are CD11b-positive. Note neuron-like cells positive for FLAG (arrow). C. Expression of FLAG in the periventricular subependymal zone after injection of SV(Nef-FLAG) in the BM. Brain cryostat sections immunostained for FLAG and stained for Neurotrace (NT) 16 months after injection of SV(Nef-FLAG) into the bone marrow. No expression of FLAG was seen when the primary antibody was replaced by a non-immune isotype-matched immunoglobulin (not shown), or when the BM was injected with a control SV vector (not shown). (This research was originally published in Stem Cells. Louboutin JP, Liu B, Reyes BAS, van Bockstaele EJ, Strayer DS. Rat bone marrow progenitor cells transduced in situ by rSV40 vectors differentiate into multiple CNS cell lineages. *Stem Cells* 2006; 24: 2801-2809).

It is unlikely that the transgene expression observed reflects direct transduction of the DG and PSZ, even though rSV40 vectors transduce CNS cells effectively when given by direct intracerebral injection [Cordelier et al., 2003; Agrawal et al., 2006; Agrawal et al., 2007; Louboutin et al., 2007b,c]. Virtually no FLAG-expressing cells were detected within the first few weeks after transduction and very few were seen at 4 months. Only at the 16 month time point were substantial numbers of FLAG-positive cells detected, while direct transduction is readily detected within 4 to 7 days.

As mentioned above, cell-cell fusion has been implicated in the detection of marked BM stem cells in other organs [Alvarez-Dolado et al., 2003; Weimann et al, 2003a,b]. Our data do not rule out this possible explanation for our results with CNS or elsewhere. However, BM stromal cells in culture can express neuronal and glial antigens when exposed to epidermal growth factor and brain-derived neurotrophic factor, or when grown together with fetal mesencephalic or striatal cells [Sanchez-Ramos et al., 2000]. As well, BM stromal cells injected into neonatal brain ventricles can differentiate to express neuronal and astrocytic marker proteins [Kopen et al., 1999]. Therefore, reported data suggest that BM-derived cells can *trans*-differentiate into CNS cells [Mezey et al., 2000], even if alternative explanations for these observations have not been completely ruled out.

Thus, transdifferentiation seems the most likely, if not the only explanation for our observations. Neural stem cells reside in the PSZ and hippocampus, and can give rise to all three major types of CNS cells [Scheffler et al., 1999]. These progenitors may provide the cells for the constant remodeling that goes on in the olfactory bulbs and hippocampus [Thomas et al., 1996; van Praag et al., 2002]. In the absence of stress or injury to the brain, the apparent differentiation of BM progenitors is most likely a physiologic phenomenon.

There is evidence that the adult rodent brain may undergo neurogenesis, especially in the DG and PSZ, after various types of injury [Magavi et al., 2000; Scharfman et al., 2000; Jin et al., 2001]. However, our rats sustained no injury to the CNS. Along these lines, both experimental and human data in which male HSC of BM were transplanted into female recipients showed CNS neurons bearing Y chromosome [Mezey et al., 2000; Mezey et al., 2003a; Cogle et al., 2004]. This process took a long time, which is consistent with our present observations [Tamaki et al., 2002; Weimann et al., 2003a,b; Cogle et al., 2004].

The mechanism(s) by which such *trans*-differentiation would occur are not clear, but would have to involve both homing to the CNS and maturation into CNS cells. Several molecular species have been suggested as being involved in homing, including vascular and extracellular matrix molecules [Prockop, 1997; Doetsch et al., 1999; Mezey et al., 2000; Palmer et al., 2000; Shors et al., 2001]. Several cell membrane proteins have been implicated, including CXCR4 and its ligand, SDF-1 [Ma et al., 1998; Klein et al., 2001; Hatch et al. 2002]. How transdifferentiation would occur is, similarly, unclear [Steindler and Pincus, 2002]. Diverse molecular signals have been reported to be involved, including neural cell adhesion molecules [Lois et al., 1996], proteins regulating cell cycle transit [Zindy et al., 1999] and transcription factors [Yang et al., 1996]. The potential involvement of extracellular matrix has attracted considerable attention [Palmer et al., 2000; Shors et al., 2001].

Our finding that multiple lineages of CNS cells expressed a transgene delivered by rSV40 vectors to the BM long after the initial injection suggests that these cells were likely to have originated from progenitors in the BM. About 5% of DG cells were FLAG-positive, which is similar to the percentage of transgene-expressing peripheral blood cells and alveolar cells, and reflects approximately half of the contribution made by femoral BM to hematopoiesis in the rat.

Transgene expression delivered by rSV40 vectors tend to endure for long periods of time [Sauter et al., 2000; Duan et al., 2004]. In contrast, that delivered by other integrating vectors tends to wane. Thus, expression of proteins is less reliable as a marker of transduced BM cells if transgene expression declines over time [Castro et al., 2002; Wagers et al., 2002; Yagi et al., 2004] than other assays based on DNA analysis [Mezey et al., 2003b]. Most studies suggesting BM to CNS transdifferentiation utilized FISH assays. Furthermore, since the detection of BM-derived markers in neurons requires considerable time [Weimann et al.,

2003a,b; Tamaki et al., 2002], it is possible that negative results reported in some studies [Castro et al., 2002] might in part reflect short time intervals between treating the animals and harvesting the brains.

The results in the present study suggest that transdifferentiation of BM resident cells into neurons occurs. However the ultimate proof that such BM cells can migrate to the brain and differentiate into CNS-specific cells may require that the putative cells that undergo transdifferentiation be isolated from the CNS and that functional studies show CNS-specific cell functions. The present observations suggest that gene delivery to the BM may be a way to provide long-term transgene expression in the neurons, microglia and astrocytes in the brain, particularly the dentate gyrus. The therapeutic implications of these findings remain to be explored.

REFERENCES

Abonour, R; Williams, DA; Einhorn, L; et al. Efficient retrovirus mediated transfer of the multidrug resistance 1 gene into autologous human long term repopulating hematopoietic stem cells. *Nat Med* 2000; 6:652-658.

Agrawal, L; Louboutin, JP; Reyes, BAS; et al. Antioxidant enzyme gene delivery to protect from HIV-1 gp120-induced neuronal apoptosis. *Gene Ther* 2006; 13: 1645-1656.

Agrawal, L; Louboutin, JP; Strayer, DS. Preventing HIV-1 Tat-induced neuronal apoptosis using antioxidant enzymes: mechanistic and therapeutic implications. *Virology* 2007; 363: 462-472.

Aiuti, A; Slavin, S; Aker, M; *et al.* Correction of ADA-SCID by stem cell therapy combined with nonmyeloabrasive conditioning. *Science* 2002; 296: 2410-2413.

Alvarez-Dolado, M; Pardal, R; Garcia-Verdugo, JM; et al. Fusion of bone-marrow-derived cells with Purkinje neurons, cardiomyocytes and hepatocytes. *Nature* 2003; 425: 968-973.

An, DS; Wersto, RP; Agricola, BA; *et al.* Marking and gene expression by a lentivirus vector in transplanted human and nonhuman primate CD34(+) cells. J Virol 2000; 74: 1286-1295.

An, DS; Kung, SK; Bonifacino, A; et al. Lentivirus vector-mediated hematopoietic stem cell gene transfer of common gamma-chain cytokine receptor in rhesus macaque. *J Virol* 2001; 75: 3547-3555.

Anderson, HA; Chen, Y; Norkin, LC. Bound simian virus 40 translocates to caveolin-enriched membrane domains, and its entry is inhibited by drugs that selectively disrupt caveolae. *Mol Biol Cell* 1996; 7: 1825-1834.

Brittan, M; Braun, KM; Reynolds, LE; et al. Bone marrow cells engraft within the epidermis and proliferate in vivo with no evidence of cell fusion. *J Pathol* 2005; 205: 1-13.

Camargo, FD; Green, R; Capetanaki, Y; et al. Single hematopoietic stem cells generate skeletal muscle through myeloid intermediates. *Nat Med* 2003; 9: 1520-1527.

Camargo, FD; Finegold, M; Goodell, MA. Hematopoietic myelomonocytic cells are the major source of hepatocyte fusion partners. *J Clin Invest* 2004; 113: 1266-1270.

Castro, RF; Jackson, KA; Goodell, MA; et al. Failure of bone marrow cells to transdifferentiate into neural cells in vivo. *Science* 2002; 297: 1299.

Cavazanna-Calvo, M; Hacein-Bey, S; de Saint-Basile, G; et al. Gene therapy of human severe combined immunodeficiency (SCID)-X1 disease. *Science* 2000; 288: 669-672.

Cavert, W; Notermans, DW; Staskus, K; et al. Kinetics of response in lymphoid tissues to antiretroviral therapy of HIV-1 infection. *Science* 1997; 276: 960-964.

Chen, Y; Norkin, LC. Extracellular simian virus 40 transmits a signal that promotes virus enclosure within caveolae. *Exp Cell Res* 1999; 10: 83-90.

Chun, TW; Engel, D; Berrey, MM; et al. Early establishment of a pool of latently infected, resting CD4(+) T cells during primary HIV-1 infection. *Proc Natl Acad Sci USA* 1998; 95: 8869-8873.

Cogle, CR; Yachnis, AT; Laywell, ED; et al. Bone marrow transdifferentiation in brain after transplantation: a retrospective study. *Lancet* 2004; 363: 1432-1437.

Cordelier, P; Calarota, S; Strayer, DS. Trans-activated IFNa2 delivered to T cells by SV40 inhibits early stages in the HIV-1 replicative cycle. *J Hematother Stem Cell Res* 2002; 11: 817-828.

Cordelier, P; van Bockstaele, E; Calarota, SA; et al. Inhibiting AIDS in the central nervous system: gene delivery to protect neurons from HIV. *Mol Ther* 2003; 7: 801-810.

Doetsch, F; Caille, I; Lim, DA; et al. Subventricular zone astrocytes are neural stem cells in the adult mammalian brain. *Cell* 1999; 97: 703-716.

Duan, YY; Wu, J; Zhu, JL; et al. Gene therapy for human alpha1-antitrypsin deficiency in an animal model using SV40-derived vectors. *Gastroenterology* 2004; 127: 1222-1232.

Ferrari, G; Cusella-de Angelis, G; Coletta, M; et al. Muscle regeneration by bone marrow-derived myogenic progenitors. *Science* 1998; 279: 1526-1530.

Finzi, D; Hermankova, M; Pierson, T; et al. Identification of a reservoir for HIV-1 in patients on highly active antiretroviral therapy. *Science* 1997; 278: 1295-1300.

Finzi, D; Blankson, J; Siliciano, JD; et al. Latent infection of CD4+ T cells provides a mechanism for lifelong persistence of HIV-1, even in patients on effective combination therapy. *Nat Med* 1999; 5: 512-517.

Fukada, S; Miyagoe-Suzuki, Y; Tsukihara, H; et al. Muscle regeneration by reconstitution with bone marrow or fetal liver cells from green fluorescent protein-gene transgenic mice. *J Cell Sci* 2002; 115: 1285-1293.

Goldstein, H; Pettoello-Mantovani, M; Anderson, CM; et al. Gene therapy delivered in vivo using an SV40-derived vector inhibits the development of in vivo HIV-1 infection of Thy/liv-SCID/hu mice. *J Infect Dis* 2002; 185: 1425-1430.

Gussoni, E; Soneoka, Y; Strickland, CD, et al. Dystrophin expression in the mdx mouse restored by stem cell transplantation. *Nature* 1999; 401: 390-394.

Gussoni, E; Bennett, RR; Muskiewicz, KR; et al. Long-term persistence of donor nuclei in a Duchenne muscular dystrophy patient receiving bone marrow transplantation. *J Clin Invest* 2002; 110: 807-814.

Halene, S; Wang, L; Cooper, RM; et al. Improved expression in hematopoietic and lymphoid cells in mice after transplantation of bone marrow transduced with a modified retroviral vector. *Blood* 1999; 94: 3349-3357.

Harris, RG; Herzog, EL; Bruscia, EM; et al. Lack of a fusion requirement for development of bone marrow-derived epithelia. *Science* 2004; 305: 90-93.

Hatch, HM; Zheng, D; Jorgensen, ML; et al. SDF-1alpha/CXCR4: a mechanism for hepatic oval cell activation and bone marrow stem cell recruitment to the injured liver of rats. *Cloning Stem Cells* 2002; 4: 339-351.

Hong, KU; Reynolds, SD; Watkins, S; et al. Basal cells are a multipotent progenitor capable of renewing the bronchial epithelium. *Am J Pathol* 2004; 164: 577-588.

Horn, PA; Morris, JC; Bukovsky, AA; et al. Lentivirus-mediated gene transfer into hematopoietic repopulating cells in baboons. *Gene Ther* 2002; 9: 1464-1471.

Jang, Y; Collector, MI; Baylin, SB; et al. Hematopoietic stem cells convert into liver cells within days without fusion. *Nat Cell Biol* 2004; 6: 532-539.

Jiang, Y; Jahagirdar, BN; Reinhardt, RL; et al. Pluripotency of mesenchymal stem cells derived from adult marrow. *Nature* 2002; 418: 41-49.

Jiang, Y; Henderson, D; Blackstad, M; et al. Neuroectodermal differentiation from mouse multipotent adult progenitor cells. *Proc Natl Acad Sci USA* 2003; 100 (Suppl 1): 11854-11860.

Jin, K; Minami, M; Lan, JQ; et al. Neurogenesis in dentate subgranular zone and rostral subventricular zone after focal cerebral ischemia in the rat. *Proc Natl Acad Sci U S A* 2001; 98: 4710-4715.

Josephson, NC; Vassilopoulos, G; Trobridge, GD; et al. Transduction of human NOD/SCID-repopulating cells with both lymphoid and myeloid potential foamy virus vectors. *Proc Natl Acad Sci USA* 2002; 99: 8295-8300.

Kashofer, K; Bonnet, D. Gene therapy progress and prospects: stem cell plasticity. *Gene Ther* 2005; 12: 1229-1234.

Klein, RS; Rubin, JB; Gibson, HD; et al. SDF-1 alpha induces chemotaxis and enhances sonic hedgehog-induced proliferation of cerebellar granule cells. *Development* 2001; 128: 1971-1981.

Kopen, GC; Prockop, DJ; Phinney, DG. Marrow stromal cells migrate throughout forebrain and cerebellum, and they differentiate into astrocytes after injection into neonatal mouse brains. *Proc Natl Acad Sci U S A* 1999 96: 10711-10716.

Korin, YD; Zack, JA. Progression to the G1b phase of the cell cycle is required for completion of human immunodeficiency virus type 1 reverse transcription in T cells. *J Virol* 1998; 72: 3161-3168.

Krause, DS; Theise, ND; Collector, MI; et al. Multiorgan, multi-lineage engraftment by a single bone marrow-derived stem cell. *Cell* 2001; 105: 369-377.

Labarge, MA; Blau, HM. Biological progression from adult bone marrow to mononucleate muscle stem cell to multinucleate muscle fiber in response to injury. *Cell* 2002; 111: 589-601.

Lafeuillade, A; Khiri, H; Chadapaud, S; et al. Persistence of HIV-1 resistance in lymph node mononuclear cell RNA despite effective HAART. *AIDS* 2001; 15: 1965-1999.

Lagasse, E; Connors, H; Al Dhalimy, M; et al. Purified hematopoietic stem cells can differentiate into hepatocytes in vivo. *Nat Med* 2002; 6: 1229-1234.

Lapidos, KA; Chen, YE; Earley, JU; et al. Transplanted hematopoietic stem cells demonstrate impaired sarcoglycan expression after engraftment into cardiac and skeletal muscle. *J Clin Invest* 2004; 114: 1577-1585.

Lescaudron, L; Peltekian, E; Fontaine-Perus, J; et al. Blood borne macrophages are essential for the triggering of muscle regeneration following muscle transplant. *Neuromuscul Disord* 1999; 9: 72-80.

Liu, B; Buckley, SM; Lewis, ID; et al. Homing defect of cultured hematopoietic cells in the NOD/SCID mouse is mediated by FAS/CD95. *Exp Hematol* 2003; 31: 824-832.

Liu, B; Daviau, J; Nichols, CN; et al. In vivo gene transfer into rat bone marrow progenitor cells using rSV40 viral vectors. *Blood* 2005; 106: 2655-2662.

Lois, C; Garcia-Verdugo, JM; Alvarez-Buylla, A. Chain migration of neuronal precursors. *Science* 1996; 271: 978-981.

Louboutin, JP; Liu, B; Reyes, BAS; et al. Rat bone marrow progenitor cells transduced in situ by rSV40 vectors differentiate into multiple CNS cell lineages. *Stem Cells* 2006; 24: 2801-2809.

Louboutin, JP; Liu, B; Chekmasova, AA; et al. Delivering genes to the organ-localized immune system: long term results of direct intramarrow transduction. *J Gene Med* 2007a; 9: 843-851.

Louboutin, JP; Reyes, BAS; Agrawal, L; et al. Strategies for CNS-directed gene delivery: in vivo gene transfer to the brain using SV40-derived vectors. *Gene Ther* 2007b; 14: 939-949.

Louboutin, JP; Agrawal, L; Reyes, BAS; et al. Protecting neurons from HIV-1 gp120-induced oxidant stress using both localized intracerebral and generalized intraventricular administration of antioxidant enzymes delivered by SV40-derived vectors. *Gene Ther* 2007c; 14: 1650-1661.

Ma, Q; Jones, D; Borghesani, PR; et al. Impaired B-lymphopoiesis, myelopoiesis, and derailed cerebellar neuron migration in CXCR4- and SDF-1-deficient mice. *Proc Natl Acad Sci USA* 1998; 95: 9448-9453.

McCauslin, CS; Wine, J; Cheng, L; et al. In vivo retroviral gene transfer by direct intrafemoral injection results in correction of the SCID phenotype in Jak3 knock-out animals. *Blood* 2003; 102: 843-848.

McKee, HJ; Strayer, DS. Immune responses against SIV envelope glycoprotein, using recombinant SV40 as a vaccine delivery vector. *Vaccine* 2002; 20: 3613-3625.

Magavi, SS; Leavitt, BR; Macklis, JD. Induction of neurogenesis in the neocortex of adult mice. *Nature* 2000; 405: 951-955.

Mahmud, N; Devine, SM; Weller, KP; et al. The relative quiescence of hematopoietic stem cells in nonhuman primates. *Blood* 2001; 97: 3061-3068.

Masson, S; Harrison, DJ; Plevris, JN, et al. Potential of hematopoietic stem cell therapy in hepatology: a critical review. *Stem Cells* 2004; 22: 897-907.

Mezey, E; Chandross, K; Harta, G; et al. Turning blood into brain: cells bearing neuronal antigens generated in vivo from bone marrow. *Science* 2000; 290:1779-1782.

Mezey, E; Key, S; Vogelsang, G; et al. Transplanted bone marrow generates new neurons in human brains. *Proc Natl Acad Sci U S A* 2003a; 100: 1364-1369.

Mezey, E; Nagy, A; Szalayova, I; et al. Comments on: "Failure of bone marrow cells to transdifferentiate into neural cells in vivo". *Science* 2003b; 299: 1184.

Naldini, L; Blomer, U; Gallay, P; et al. In vivo gene delivery and stable transduction of nondividing cells by a lentiviral vector. *Science* 1996; 272: 263-267.

Natarajan, V; Bosche, M; Metcalf, JA; et al. HIV-1 replication in patients with undetectable plasma virus receiving HAART. Highly active antiretroviral therapy. *Lancet* 1999; 353: 119-120.

Nelson, DM; Metzgar, ME; Dohanue, RE; et al. *In vivo* retrovirus-mediated gene transfer into multiple hematopoietic lineages in rabbits without preconditioning. *Hum Gene Ther* 1997; 8: 747-754.

Palmer, TD; Willhoite, AR; Gage, FH. Vascular niche for adult hippocampal neurogenesis. *J Comp Neurol* 2000; 425: 479-494.

Pelkmans, L; Kartenbeck, J; Helenius, A. Caveolar endocytosis of simian virus 40 reveals a new two-step vesicular-transport pathway to the E.R. *Nature Cell Biol* 2001; 3: 473-483.

Pelkmans, L; Puntener, D; Helenius, A. Local actin polymerization and dynamin recruitment in SV40-induced internalization of caveolae. *Science* 2002; 296: 535-539.

Peters, SO; Kittler, ELW; Ramshaw, HS; et al. Murine marrow cells expanded in culture with IL-3, IL-6, and SCF acquire an engraftment defect in normal hosts. *Exp Hematol* 1995; 23: 461-469.

Petersen, BE; Bowen, WC; Patrene, KD; et al. Bone marrow as a potential source of hepatic oval cells. *Science* 1999; 284: 1168-1170.

Porada, CD; Tran, ND; Zhao, Y; et al. Neonatal gene therapy: transfer and expression of exogenous genes in neonatal sheep following direct injection of retroviral vectors into the bone marrow space. *Exp Hematol* 2000; 28: 642-650.

Prockop, DJ. Marrow stromal cells as stem cells for nonhematopoietic tissues. *Science* 1997; 276: 71-74.

Roe, T; Reynolds, TC; Yu, G; et al. Integration of murine leukemia virus DNA depends on mitosis. *EMBO J* 1993; 12: 2099-2108.

Rund, D; Dagan, M; Dalyot-Herman, N; et al. Efficient transduction of human hematopoietic cells with the human multidrug resistance gene 1 via SV40pseudovirions. *Hum Gene Ther* 1998; 9: 649-657.

Sanchez-Ramos, J; Song, S; Cardozo-Pelaez, F; et al. Adult bone marrow stromal cells differentiate into neural cells in vitro. *Exp Neurol* 2000; 164: 247-256.

Sauter, BV; Parashar, B; Chowdhury, NR; et al. A replication-deficient rSV40 mediates liver-directed gene transfer and a long-term amelioration of jaundice in gunn rats. *Gastroenterology* 2000; 119: 1348-1357.

Scharfman, HE; Goodman, JH; Sollas, AL. Granule-like neurons at the hilar/CA3 border after status epilepticus and their synchrony with area CA3 pyramidal cells: functional implications of seizure-induced neurogenesis. *J Neurosci* 2000; 20: 6144-6158.

Scheffler, B; Horn, M; Blumcke, I; et al. Marrow-mindedness: a perspective on neuropoiesis. *Trends Neurosci* 1999; 22: 348-357.

Schwartz, RE; Reyes, M; Koodie, L; et al. Multipotent adult progenitor cells from bone marrow differentiate into functional hepatocyte-like cells. *J Clin Invest* 2002; 109: 1291-1302.

Shors, TJ; Miesegaes, G; Beylin, A; et al. Neurogenesis in the adult is involved in the formation of trace memories. *Nature* 2001; 410: 372-376.

Stadtfel, M; Graf, T. Assessing the role of hematopoietic plasticity for endothelial and hepatocyte development by non-invasive lineage tracing. *Development* 2005; 132: 203-213.

Steindler, DA; Pincus, DW. Stem cells and neuropoiesis in the adult human brain. *Lancet* 2002; 359: 1047-1054.

Strayer, DS; Milano, J. SV40 mediates stable gene transfer in vivo. *Gene Ther 1996*; 3: 581-587.

Strayer, DS; Kondo, R; Milano, J; et al. Use of SV40-based vectors to transduce foreign genes to normal human peripheral blood mononuclear cells. *Gene Ther* 1997; 4: 219-225.

Strayer, DS; Pomerantz, RJ; Yu, M; et al. Efficient gene transfer to hematopoietic progenitor cells using SV40-derived vectors. *Gene Ther* 2000; 7: 886-895.

Strayer, DS; Branco, F; Zern, MA; et al. Durability of transgene expression and vector integration: recombinant SV40-derived gene therapy vectors. *Mol Ther* 2002a; 6: 227-237.

Strayer, DS; Zern, MA; Chowdhury, JR. What can SV40-derived vectors do for gene therapy? *Curr Opin Mol Ther* 2002b; 4: 313-323.

Sutton, RE; Reitsma, MA; Uchida, N; et al. Transduction of human progenitor hematopoietic stem cell by human immunodeficiency virus type 1 based vectors is cell cycle dependent. *J Virol* 1999; 73: 3649-3660.

Tamaki, S; Eckert, K; He D; et al. Engrafment of sorted/expended human nervous system stem cells from fetal brain. *J Neurosci Res* 2002; 69: 976-986.

Tavassoli, M; Hardy, CL. Molecular basis of homing of intravenously transplanted stem cells to the marrow. *Blood* 1990; 76: 1059-1070.

Theise, ND; Badve, S; Saxena, R; et al. Derivation of hepatocytes from bone marrow cells in mice after radiation-induced myeloablation. *Hepatology* 2000; 31:235-240.

Thomas, LB; Gates, MA; Steindler, DA. Young neurons from the adult subependymal zone proliferate and migrate along an astrocyte, extracellular matrix-rich pathway. *Glia* 1996; 17: 1-14.

Thorgeirsson, SS; Grisham, JW. Hematopoietic cells as hepatocyte stem cells: a critical review of the evidence. *Hepatology* 2006; 43: 2-8.

van Praag, H; Schinder, AF; Christie, BR; et al. Functional neurogenesis in the adult hippocampus. *Nature* 2002; 415: 1030-1034.

Vassilopoulos, G; Wang, PR; Russell, DW. Transplanted bone marrow regenerates liver by cell fusion. *Nature* 2003; 422: 901-904.

Wagers, AJ; Sherwood, RI; Christensen, JL; et al. Little evidence for developmental plasticity of adult hematopoietic stem cells. *Science* 2002; 297: 2256-2259.

Wang, X; Willenbring, H; Akkari, Y; et al. Cell fusion is the principal source of bone-marrow-derived hepatocytes. *Nature* 2003; 422: 897-901.

Weimann, JM; Johannson, CB; Trejo, A; et al. Stable reprogrammed heterokaryons form spontaneously in Purkinje neurons after bone marrow transplant. *Nat Cell Biol* 2003a; 5: 959-966.

Weimann, JM; Charlton, CA; Brazelton, TR; et al. Contribution of transplanted bone marrow cells to Purkinje neurons in human adult brains. *Proc Natl Acad Sci U S A* 2003b; 100: 2088-2093.

Willenbring, H; Bailey, AS; Foster, M; et al. Myelomonocytic cells are sufficient for therapeutic cell fusion in liver. *Nat Med* 2004; 10: 744-748.

Wilmut, I; Beaujean, N; de Sousa, PA; et al. Somatic cell nuclear transfer. *Nature* 2002; 419: 583-586.

Wu, M; Wei, YQ. Development of respiratory stem cells and progenitor cells. *Stem Cell Dev* 2004; 13: 607-613.

Yagi, T; McMahon, EJ; Takikita, S; et al. Fate of hematopoietic cells in demyelinating mutant mouse, twitcher, following transplantation of GFP+ bone marrow cells. *Neurobiol Dis* 2004; 16: 98-109.

Yamada, M; Kasamatsu, H. Role of nuclear pore complex in simian virus 40 nuclear targeting. *J Virol* 1993; 67: 119-130.

Yang, XW; Zhong, R; Heintz, N. Granule cell specification in the developing mouse brain as defined by expression of the zinc finger transcription factor RU49. *Development* 1996; 122: 555-566.

Zhang, H; Dornadula, G; Beumont, M; et al. Human immunodeficiency virus type 1 in the semen of men receiving highly active antiretroviral therapy. *N Engl J Med* 1998; 339: 1803-1809.

Zielske, SP; Gerson, SL. Cytokines, including stem cell factor alone, enhance lentiviral transduction in nondividing human LTCIC and NOD/SCID repopulating cells. *Mol Ther* 2003; 7: 325-333.

Zindy, F; Cunningham, JJ; Sherr, CJ; et al. Postnatal neuronal proliferation in mice lacking Ink4d and Kip1 inhibitors of cyclin-dependent kinases. *Proc Natl Acad Sci U S A* 1999; 96: 13462-13467.

In: Encyclopedia of Stem Cell Research (2 Volume Set)   ISBN: 978-1-61761-835-2
Editor: Alexander L. Greene   © 2012 Nova Science Publishers, Inc.

Chapter XXIX

STEM CELLS AND THEIR USE IN REGENERATIVE THERAPY OF THE RETINA

Abed Namavari

INTRODUCTION

Sight is one of the most crucial senses for patient quality of life. Indeed, many patients consider their quality of vision to be more important than many other essential physical functions. As such, the role of ophthalmic pathology in a growing geriatric population and the limitations of current vision therapies have gained profound significance. In particular, diseases of the retina have a notable impact on elderly patients and progress in therapies for retinal impairments have become increasingly important over the past decade.

In this context, it is understandable why the novel possibility of stem cell tissue engineering for retinal repair has garnered much excitement in the scientific community. Tissue engineered therapies and stem cell technologies are rapidly becoming more clinically applicable, and accordingly, the use of such treatments for the retina has gained prominence.

In this chapter, we discuss the current state of progress in the retinal application of stem cell therapies and tissue engineering technologies. We begin with a brief review of clinical pathologies that are applicable for regeneration therapies, discuss the regeneration of the various cell types that compose the retina, delineate the issues affecting current transplantation modalities, and conclude with a brief discussion of necessary future progress.

CLINICAL SIGNIFICANCE OF RETINAL REGENERATION

As illustrated in Figure 1, the retina is a highly organized, complex structure that is comprised of:

1) the retinal pigment epithelium (RPE)

2) the photoreceptors, including rods, and cones
3) several types of neurons, including ganglion cells and neurons that interconnect
    the photoreceptors to the ganglion cells

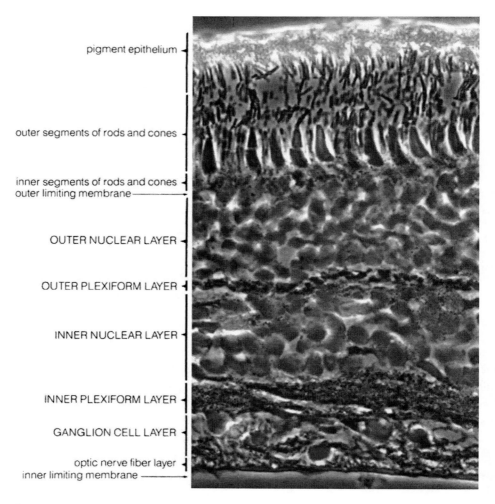

pigment epithelium

outer segments of rods and cones

inner segments of rods and cones
outer limiting membrane

OUTER NUCLEAR LAYER

OUTER PLEXIFORM LAYER

INNER NUCLEAR LAYER

INNER PLEXIFORM LAYER

GANGLION CELL LAYER

optic nerve fiber layer
inner limiting membrane

Figure 1.

In addition, the retina is vascularized, with blood vessels of the choroids and branches of the central retinal artery providing nutrients to the tissue.

When studying the retina, it is important to consider the photoreceptors and the adjacent retinal pigment epithelium as one functional unit. The destabilization of any one component can affect the viability of the photoreceptors, and this has consequent effects on the function of the tissue. Pathologically, dying photoreceptors cause progressive degeneration of functional retinal tissue, and clinically, this results in gradual blindness [1]. Several diseases fit this description; two prominent ones are Retinitis Pigmentosa (RP) and Age-related Macular Degeneration (AMD). RP and AMD, combined, are the leading cause of blindness in the western world.

Retinitis Pigmentosa

RP is an inherited, progressively debilitating disease that affects 1 in 3500 people [2-4]. Most of identified mutations that cause RP target photoreceptors, but some affect retinal pigment epithelial (RPE) cells as well. Clinically, the patient experiences a gradual loss in rod function, beginning at the periphery and progressing towards the retinal center; in later stages, only the fovea is spared.

Age-Related Macular Degeneration

AMD affects 30% of people over age 75. It appears to be due to RPE dysfunction as well as histological changes in Bruch's membrane [5,6]. These changes include lipid deposition, protein-crosslinking, and reduced permeability to nutrients. AMD appears to be multi-factorial; dietary and environmental factors as well as heritable traits appear to be associated with the disease. In AMD, neovascularization is on the major causes of the visual impairment. The pathological neovascularization has been attributed to angiogenesis, whereby new vessels grow from existing ones.

Pathological Angiogenesis

It appears that hematopoietic stem cells play an important role in this pathological angiogenesis process. However, the physiology of postnatal angiogenesis is not particularly clear. Recently, it has been demonstrated that circulating endothelial progenitor cells may be recruited to the diseased areas and may be the source of the new vessels [7]. These hematopoietic stem cells (HSCs) are multipotent cells capable of self-renewal and give rise to committed progenitors (lymphoid and myeloid). The role of HSCs is to replenish the cells of the blood and lymph for the life of the individual. HSCs differentiate into two classes of endothelial progenitors, identified by cell-surface markers: CD34+ and CD133+. Of these two, a specific subset of the CD34+ leukocytes has been shown to home to ischemic sites of the retina and express endothelial antigens [7-10].

In situations where neovascularization is required for therapy, these principles have been used to enhance blood flow [11]. In fact, these HSCs have already been adapted for cardiac function improvement in human clinical trials.

There is some information advocating an important role for these endothelial progenitor cells in proliferative diabetic retinopathy and subretinal neovascularization associated with AMD. Grant et al. demonstrated that adult HSCs provide functional hemangioblast activity during retinal neovascularization. Adult mice engrafted with HSCs expressing green fluorescent protein (GFP) were subjected to retinal ischemia using a laser ablation technique. The resulting new vessels demonstrated significant repopulation with GFP+ endothelial cells [12].

Similarly, Otani et al. demonstrated that endothelial progenitor cell-enriched HSCs stably incorporated into forming retinal vasculature [13]. However, multiple factors that remain unclear, including the regulatory process involved in such incorporation, the factors that control differentiation, the process of recruitment to angiogenesis sites, the competition between localized endothelial cells and blood-borne progenitors, and the role of extracellular matrix components.

One of the key chemical cues identified in the overall process is VEGF. VEGF contributes to postnatal neovascularization by mobilizing bone-marrow-derived endothelial progenitor cells [14]; these progenitors are responsive to VEGF and show high levels of VEGFR2 expression.

The potential therapeutic role of HSCs remains unclear. However, understanding the molecular mechanisms governing their behavior will likely prove crucial in designing therapies for pathologic neovascularization.

Regenerative Therapy

RP and AMD currently have very few applicable therapies. Only recently have the advent of growth-factor inhibitors and other cell-specific therapies delayed the progression of these diseases. Despite these recent advances, no currently approved treatment aims to regenerate functional retinal tissue, and thus, regenerative tissue engineering presents itself as a possible solution. However, regenerative therapies currently face a multitude of challenges before they can become clinically applicable. To understand the regenerative potential of the retina, we begin with a discussion of the properties of retinal progenitor cells. These cells are a recent discovery and have changed our perception of retinal development altogether.

RETINAL STEM AND PROGENITOR CELLS

Identification of Retinal Progenitor Cells

The vertebrate retina has seven major classes of cells. The development of the adult mammalian retina is a coordinated process that involves the proliferation, migration, and maturation of all these cell classes.

Lower Vertebrates

The retinal development process, as well as the characteristics of retinal progenitor cells, began with the study of fish and amphibian eyes. In these species, the retina continually regenerates by adding new cells of all types. These new cells arise from the ciliary marginal zone (CMZ), a region at the peripheral edge of the retina. The CMZ cells progressively differentiate toward the central retina. In other words, the youngest and least differentiated stem cells are closer to the periphery (most anterior), the progenitors (retinoblasts – slightly more differentiated) are in the middle, and the postmitotic cells are at the center (most posterior).

Interestingly, the least differentiated cells exist where the RPE folds and adjoins the retina. Lineage trace studies show that these cells generate clones both for the RPE as well as the interior retinal layers. In contrast, the most central and posterior cells of the CMZ, although undifferentiated in appearance, do not exhibit mitotic potential [15].

Rodents

Retinal progenitor cells have also been identified in rodents, initiated by the lower vertebrate findings above. These retinal progenitors display 2 key properties of stem cells:

1. They proliferate and express the neurofilament *nestin*, a marker for neuroectodermal stem cells [16].
2. They prove to be multi potential and give rise to cells that can differentiate into retinal cells.

The third key characteristic of stem cells is their potential to self-renew, and it is unclear whether the rodent retinal progenitors display this property. A study by Ahmad et al. did not show this self-renewal capability; however, the cells were isolated a late neurogenic stage, which limits their self-renewal capability altogether. Some authors conclude that this represents a lack of true stem cell capability. However, others contend that the cells may indeed have self-renewal capability at an earlier embryological stage [17].

When these rodent progenitor cells were injected into the subretinal space of rats, they did not integrate into the retina, but did survive and express the photoreceptor-specific markers opsin and RET-P1 [18].

Other investigators have also studied pigmented cells from the ciliary margin (PCM). These cells also express nestin and are capable of self renewal. Tropepe et al. studied the ability of PCM in rodents to proliferate clonally in vitro using a neural stem-cell colony-forming assay [19]. When cultured in sphere colonies known to promote differentiation, PCM cells show a formation where a small number of nestin-positive cells remain confined to the centers of the colonies and peripherally localized cells express different mature retinal markers. These studies suggest that the mammalian PCM is an evolutionarily conserved region, akin to the CMZ of the lower vertebrates.

This discovery has greatly advanced transplantation research capabilities. Studies have been initiated which have investigated the potential of brain-derived neural progenitor cells, embryonic retinal progenitor cells, bone marrow-derived stem cells, and embryonic stem cells from the inner mass of the mouse blastocyst to incorporate and differentiate into functional layers of the retina.

Human Retinal Progenitor Cells

Such retinal progenitors in human eyes were first isolated from retinoblastoma tumors by Lee et al., [15] These tumors, a form of malignant early-childhood ocular tumors, contain clusters of nonneoplastic progenitor cells that express nestin, alpha-tubulin III [20], and neural retinal leucinezipper protein (NRL) [21]. NRL is a protein that is activated in cells of retinal origin.

These cells were labeled with a fluorescent dye and transplanted into the vitreous space of neonatal rat eyes. After 2 to 3 weeks, the cells showed an ability to migrate into the retina and to localize in each nuclear layer of the retina. This suggests an ability of these cells to recognize and respond to retinal-specific developmental signals, an indication of progenitor or stem cell status.

There are two theories as to why these progenitor cells are present in the retinoblastoma tumor. One possibility, as previous studies have proposed, is that retinoblastoma may originate from Human Retinal Progenitor Cells (HRPCs) [22,23]. Another possibility is that the HRPC migration is a response to tissue damage induced by tumor growth. Similar responses have been noted in the spinal cord [24]. The HRPCs may retard tumor growth through secretion of various factors to induce tumor cell maturation [22]. However, it has not been proven that these cells serve in a tumor-inhibition manner; they may promote tumor progression or retard tumor cell apoptosis instead. Nonetheless, it is clear that retinal progenitor cells are present in the ciliary margin of human eyes from these studies.

Characteristics of Retinal Stem Cells

The population of such cells, however, is quite small. In adult human eyes, only 0.2% of pigmented cells in ciliary margin are thought to have the stem cell properties of:

1) Controlled proliferation
2) Multipotential differentiation
3) Self-renewal

In vitro, these cells clonally proliferate and form sphere colonies. These colonies can differentiate into:

1) Photoreceptors
2) Intermediate neurons
3) Muller glia [19,25]. These retinal glia may not simply be a retinal phenotype with limited functionality. Fisher et al. showed evidence in the chick that Muller glia may have the potential to become RPCs themselves [26]. These glia also seem to play an important role in the generation of precursor cells from embryonic components [25].
4) Other yet-unidentified intraretinal cells. Wang et al. proposed that intraretinal collagen fiber synthesis, which is critical in the structure of the adult vitreous, may in fact be the function of a retinal phenotype derived from the HRPCs [27].

Regulation of RSCs

The regulation of this process of phenotypical differentiation and proliferation is currently unclear. It is evident that a multitude of transcription factors, including Pax6, Six3, Rx1, Chx10, and Hes1 play a role. The cyclin-dependent kinase inhibitor protein, p27Kip1 is also implicated (Levine et al. 2000). Several growth factors have also been associated, including FGF2, EGF, and IGF-1 [19,26,28]. As mentioned previously, certain cellular components, including Muller glia, may play a role themselves.

RSC Markers

The identification of cells with progenitor capability is a task unto itself, primarily because the receptors often used for such identification are regulatory markers, and the regulatory markers are unknown. Nonetheless, current researchers utilize a variety of surface and nuclear markers to isolate cells with progenitor capability.

The classic marker for neural stem cells is nestin [16]. This intermediate filament is a component of the cytoskeleton of immature neuroepithelial cells. This marker is not specific for stem cells, but *in vitro*, it can be used to confirm the presence of highly plastic neural cells [29]. How this filament confers progenitor capability is currently not well understood.

Additional markers of interest include Notch, Numb, Musashi-1, and Presenilin. Nuclear markers such as FGFR4, Fz9, Sox2, and Nucleostemin have also been cited as possible neural stem cell markers [30,31].

Of these various possibilities, surface markers are of notable interest, since they present a method of obtaining an enriched yield of stem cells, and since they can be potential drug targets. In addition to Notch, CD133, CD15, and glycolipid GD2 ganglioside are other such markers [32,33]. Other surface molecules can be used indirectly to enhance the yield of a cell cluster. For example, ABCG2 transport is known to extrude Hoechst 33342 dye; this property can be used to isolate a cellular subpopulation [34,35].

Other less specific markers of CNS stem cells include vimentin, Ki-67, Cyclin D1, NCAM, CD9, CD81, CD34, CD95 (Fas), and MHC Class 1. While no marker thus far has proved to be a single identifier of retinal progenitor status, the use of a combination of markers will likely be effective. A comprehensive understanding of transcriptional activity will also clarify the utility of markers, especially for the prospective isolation of neural cells with retinal progenitor capability.

Future Utility of Human RPCs

Despite the limited knowledge of RPCs currently, it is clear that further investigation of HRPCs will delineate two important concepts in the understanding of the retina. First, these cells are likely to be the key in elucidating the mechanisms that regulate retinal development. Second, these cells may lead to therapeutic applications to restore retinal cell loss or to deliver drugs and genes. Ultimately, these will likely prove to be extraordinarily beneficial in medical therapies.

REGENERATION OF RETINAL CELLS

Strategies for Therapy

In general, retinal diseases affect neurons (including the photoreceptors), the RPE, and/or the vasculature. This allows for 3 main targets for future cell therapy:

1. Endothelium
2. RPE cells
3. Photoreceptors

The regeneration of each cellular component of the retina will be discussed separately. Then, the current transplantation techniques used to target these 3 areas and applicable challenges will be explored.

Endothelial Cell Regeneration

Clinical Utility

The regeneration, or the prevention of improper regeneration, of retinal vasculature is critical in several retinal diseases.

In Age-related Macular Degeneration (AMD), Bruch's membrane is disrupted and choroidal vessels invade the retina. This leads to subsequent retinal detachment and photoreceptor death. In this situation, the endothelial neovascularization needs to be blocked and photoreceptor regeneration promoted.

Diabetic retinopathy shares a similar vascularization course. Neovascularization induces retinal detachment in this case as well. Again, this endothelial regeneration needs to be prevented for preservation of visual function.

On the other hand, the pathology of Retinitis Pigmentosa (RP) is caused by the degeneration of retinal vessels. This is linked to the subsequent degeneration of photoreceptors. In this case, endothelial regeneration needs to be promoted and the photoreceptors and the retinal vessels need to be replaced.

Characteristics

One of the fundamental roles of endothelial cells in the retina is trophic support for retinal cell survival. Otani et al. [13,36] showed that in photoreceptor loss in *rd1* and *rd10* mice, blood vessels also degenerate. A lineage-negative population of bone marrow cells was transplanted into the mouse vitreous. These cells stabilized blood vessels and protected cones against degeneration. However, the cones did not retain full activity. The transplanted cell population included endothelial progenitor cells and hemangioblasts able to generate endothelial progenitor cells and blood cells. It is unclear whether cones are preferentially preserved in this transplantation model.

It appears that endothelial cells interact with glial cells for direction and alignment. Indeed, in diseases with neovascularization as a leading pathological process, glial hyperplasia and increased specific gene expression are clearly evident. These activated glia favor neovascularization and accept bone-marrow-derived endothelial progenitors. This suggests that the activated glia could serve as therapy targets in diseases such as AMD and diabetic retinopathy, where unnecessary vascularization needs to be blocked.

Preliminary experiments in this regard have shown some promise. Murine bone marrow cells were genetically engineered with the T2 fragment of the tryptophanyl-tRNA synthetase, which is an anti-angiogenic factor. These cells, when injected into the vitreous, prevented the formation of mouse retinal vessels during development [13]. This suggests that the manipulation of progenitor cells with anti-angiogenic genes may help prevent vascularization in pathologic processes.

Retinal Pigment Epithelium Regeneration

The RPE is a cell monolayer. The degeneration of this layer in AMD is well established from several clinical trials [37-39]. Thus, the regeneration of this layer is of critical clinical importance.

As such, researchers have begun studying RPE transplantation in animal models and limited clinical trials. The most common animal model used is the RCS (Royal College Surgeon) rat. The RCS rat contains a mutation in the Mertk gene, which leads to a loss of phagocytic ability in the rat RPE cells. This leads to the accumulation of photoreceptor outersegment debris and eventual photoreceptor death. Thus, it is considered an appropriate model for AMD. In this model, transplanted RPE cells showed the ability to eliminate the debris accumulation and maintain visual function in the transplanted area [1].

This subsequently led to the generation of human RPE cell lines immortalized by the SV40 Large T antigen [40], and the use of a spontaneous immortazlied adult human RPE cell line (ARPE 19) [41] with ability to retain CNS connections. None of these lines, or those used in the RCS rat, have thus far shown evidence of tumor formation, suggesting that refinement of this technique may indeed lead to clinical progress in AMD therapy.

Clinical studies with RPE transplantation have had some positive results as well. In one study, RPE tissue translocation into the fovea of AMD patients and ablation of choroidal neo-vascularization led to the maintenance of foveal fixation in several patients, suggesting the possible benefit of RPE regeneration in AMD pathologies. However, in this study, the vision rescue was transient. In similar studies where autologous RPE was used, another limitation was noted – current methods of harvesting a sufficient number of autologous healthy RPE cells are limited. Thus, the understanding of the mechanisms that govern proper survival and integration of new RPE cells, as well as improvements in the yield methods of autologous RPE cells, will be important in the continued development of regenerative therapies.

Neuronal Regeneration

The portion of the retina interior to the retinal pigment epithelium is an intricate organization of several phenotypes of neural derivates (Figure 1). Consequently, the regeneration of this component of the retina presents many difficulties. However, some studies have shown preliminary evidence of natural differentiation and organization.

In one study, adult rat stem-cell derived hippocampal progenitors were injected into the vitreous of newborn rats [42]. In the developing eye, these cells showed morphological change into neuroglial, amacrine, bipolar, horizontal, and photoreceptor cell types in retinal layer locations appropriate for each phenotype. However, these cells did not acquire the specialized markers of the retina. Some researchers attribute this to a possible lack of exogenous cues in the newborn rat that ordinarily would have been present in the adult one. This study suggests that exogenous cues and the retinal environment may be sufficient to provide structure and induce differentiation, if the source progenitors can survive in the transplant area. When understood, the mechanisms that control this retinal neuron organization process will, nonetheless, improve the efficacy of progenitor transplantation.

RETINA CELL TRANSPLANTATION

The clinical applicability of stem and progenitor transplantation is the driving factor in its continued research. In this regard, there are 2 main sources of retinal stem cells (RSCs) for use in transplantation:

1) Cells located in the retina – Generates all retinal cells during development
2) Cells of the pigmented ciliary margin – Generates all retina phenotypes in vitro

The adult RSCs of the ciliary region have been shown to have greater renewal capacity than fetal HRPCs [43].

As mentioned previously, studies in small animals have revealed that the adult RSCs can generate different retinal phenotypes in the correct locations, at least transiently. This capability is further limited to diseased or injured areas, lending further credence to various transplantation therapy theories.

Genetic Modification of Stem Cells

One such transplantation theory is that of genetically modified retinal stem cells. The premise of retinal stem cell gene modification stems from experiments using neural stem cells. Initial studies showed that adult rat neural stem cells (NSCs) migrate and differentiate into neurons in an injured [44,45] or degenerating [46] retina, but not a healthy one. These studies suggested that extrinsic factors drive the expression of certain genes in the stem cells, which in turn causes necessary differentiation. Such a concept opens the door for manipulation of stem cells and subsequent transplantation to injured retinal regions.

Some researchers have pursued this strategy already. When transfected with genes coding for transcription factors known to control photoreceptor differentiation and survival, adult mouse RSCs generate cells committed to the photoreceptor pathway. These genes include Crx [47], Otx2 [48], and Crx plus NeuroD [49]. Such induction of differentiation was not achieved with mesencephalic neural stem cells, showing that certain intrinsic factors in the adult RSCs are necessary for the action of the transfected genes. Interestingly, those photoreceptors induced with Crx showed hyperpolarization responses to light stimuli, indicating that there is some functionality present. It is not been studied whether Otx2 would have a similar effect in the long tem.

One of the difficulties in this gene modification technique has been the achievement of appropriate opsin levels. Photoreceptors have the potential to die if the opsin expression in the cell varies less than 50% or more than 125% of normal levels [50]. In addition to influencing differentiation, Crx is known to affect opsin expression. Thus, Crx expression needs to be controlled during and after transplantation to ensure photoreceptor survival.

An alternative gene proposed for this technique is the melanopsin gene, which induces photosensitivity in non-neural cells. Melanopsin is situated in the retinal ganglia and is involved in circadian rhythm and pupil reflex actions [51]. This gene may have a role in induction of light-responsive neurons. However, it has not been tested in transplantation settings thus far.

Challenges of Transplantation

There are numerous challenges in the transplantation of stem and progenitor cells for retinal regeneration. We can categorize these into 4: Delivery, Survival, Differentiation, and Integration. Each of these challenges will be reviewed briefly before discussing some of the current target solutions to overcome them.

Delivery

Cell delivery is a formidable challenge that must be solved before transplantation modalities can become clinically applicable. This is especially true of transplants to the subretinal space of the eye, which is the preferred location of grafts in retinal disease.

Modern surgical techniques allow delivery of a sheet of cells to the subretinal space. The less preferable alternative would be the injection of cell suspensions or crude tissue aggregates. The sheet delivery is beneficial for most cell types, particularly RPE grafts and neuroretinal cells. One benefit of such a delivery is easy *in vivo* monitoring, utilizing GFP expression in grafted cells.

Survival

The survival of transplanted cells is another major hurdle. Many researchers suggest that the survival of grafted stem or progenitor cells is often less than 1% after 2-4 weeks [30]. With the limited knowledge of factors affecting the survival of retinal progenitors, and neural progenitors altogether, the solution to this problem may be quite complex. As discussed above, certain genes and environmental factors may indeed affect several aspects of a graft, such as the importance of Crx for differentiation and survival.

Differentiation

One of the primary challenges in this process is a targeted differentiation of transplanted stem and progenitor cells. The genetic modification theory was discussed above as one presumable method. Some studies have identified particular factors that affect cell differentiation into various retinal phenotypes. For example, RSCs derived from newborn radial glial cells have been shown to commit to the retinal ganglion fate with just one single factor [52].

However, such specific targets have not been identified for the photoreceptor fate, and this differentiation remains one of the toughest, and yet one of the most important, hurdles.

One study showed that with sequential stimulation with FGF-2 and B27 of RSCs from radial glia, approximately 30% of cells became committed to the photoreceptor fate, including the expression of several photoreceptor specific markers [53]. However, this commitment was transient and the cells did not survive long-term. A similar, more recent study revealed that fetal RPCs cultivated in the presence of several growth factors markedly favor differentiation into photoreceptors *in vivo*.

However, in other studies [54,55], the results have been quite different. In one, mouse RSCs transplanted into damaged retinas showed poor differentiation altogether, suggesting that some other prior differentiation in vitro may be needed. Similar studies support this observation that retinal stem cells can regenerate retinal cells in vivo, but a previous commitment needs to be achieved to generate photoreceptors after transplantation.

These conflicting results make it difficult to identify exactly what intrinsic and extrinsic factors favor the appearance of photoreceptors. This ability will be important to delineate for successful transplantation of progenitors in injured retina.

Integration

Mouse and rat cell transplantation studies have shown robust integration into rodent models of retinal degeneration. In these studies, the primary cells were prepared as aggregates [56] or in full-thickness sheets containing the RPE layer [57].

Interesting results were shown by MacLaren et al. who studied the behavior of immature primary photoreceptors after efficient transplantation. They showed efficient integration of the normal or the degenerating retina, including restoration of some vision. Specifically, they showed effectiveness with postmitotic cells committed to the photoreceptor fate isolated from the retina between PN1 and PN7; younger and older cells did not show this ability. The results also showed the formation of correct synapses, response of the transplanted cells to glutamate stimulation, and improved pupil light reflex in rhodopsin knockout mice [58]. The data suggest that if immature photoreceptors are transplanted at a particular stage in the development process, they can be compatible with various cell replacement strategies.

However, given the limited source of fetal retinal cells, the difficulty comes in translating these strategies to stem cells. These cells, with a capacity to generate an unlimited number of progeny, are excellent sources for regenerative tissue. Thus far, their integration capabilities have been limited. In porcine models where neuroepithelial stem cell neurospheres have shown a sustained capacity to differentiate in vivo, the cells do not integrate the retina [59]. As the molecular mechanisms governing these cells are better understood, the integration properties will hopefully improve as well.

TISSUE ENGINEERING STRATEGIES

Current research has begun to explore various strategies to address the multiple difficulties associated with retinal and stem cell transplantation. These strategies include various tissue engineering techniques, including the use of artificial scaffolds.

It is clear that direct subretinal or intravitreal injection of dissociated cells or tissue aggregates give rise to disorganized or incorrectly localized grafts [29]. In this context, cell polarity and continuity are integral to positive graft outcome. To meet this challenge, investigators have started using biodegradable polymers as a substrate to obtain organized sheets of cells for transplantation. In tissues such as bone, cartilage, and blood vessels, the benefits of biodegradable polymer/stem cell composites are well known.

The idea behind these designs arose from a lack of tissue availability and the observation that cells alone were often not capable of recreating complex tissues. This is likely true for the retina as well, where that complex organization is of prime importance in function. In the other tissues, cells grown under the appropriate conditions on a three-dimensional biodegradable scaffold have often recreated complex tissue structures [60-63].

Biodegradable scaffolds allow for temporary support as the tissue forms, avoiding long-term foreign body reactions. Numrous hydrogels, polymers such as polycaprolactone, polylactic-co-glycolic acid (PLGA), polylactic acid (PLA), polyglycolic acid (PGA), and various copolymers have all been shown to have the biodegradable properties useful in transplantation. They have been shown to be biocompatible in the CNS [64] and can undergo surface modification to improve attachment or initiate differentiation [65,66]. These polymer structures can be seeded with stem cells and grafted easily.

One of the most important benefits of these substrates includes much improved differentiation potential. These constructs can also be readily monitored in vivo if the transplanted cells bear GFP, which allows for non-invasive quantification of survival over time.

These various benefits of tissue engineered scaffolds can serve as excellent complements to the other processes necessary in retinal transplantation. The combination of stem cells, tissue engineering, and transplantation will permit the repair and replacement of diseased retina. Further study in larger animals will improve our understanding of how to incorporate tissue engineering strategies with cell biology and transplantation techniques.

ALTERNATIVE CELL SOURCES

Another method of overcoming the limitations of retinal progenitor transplantation is to use stem cells not derived from the retina. These cells are often easier to acquire, and with growing knowledge of differentiation properties, they may be transformed into retinal phenotypes. Examples include: brain-derived neural progenitor cells, bone marrow derived stem cells, embryonic stem cells, and progenitor cells of other tissues. We specifically address two types of these cells:

1) Limbal Stem Cells
2) Embryonic Stem Cells

Limbal Stem Cells

Limbal stem cells have shown transplantable capacity to reconstitute corneal epithelium. They can be easily expanded and differentiated. Interestingly, they also show some capability to transform into neuronal cells, and a possibility for retinal transformation seems to exist.

Zhao et al. showed that rat limbal stem cells can be committed to a neural progenitor fate with EGF and FGF-2, and then differentiated into neuron-like cells by adding serum [67]. These cells did not show complete differentiation and lacked appropriate electrophysiological function.

In rat transplantation studies, when placed in a mechanically injured retina, the limbal stem cells migrated to different retinal layers. In addition, they expressed markers that were specific to the lamina into which they incorporated [56]. Although this does not represent transformation into functionally repaired tissue, further investigation will reveal whether limbal stem cells can be utilized in autologous retinal cell transplantation.

Embryonic Stem Cells

Embryonic Stem (ES) cells, although perhaps controversial, have shown capability to transform into retinal phenotypes through multiple methods. The co-incubation of ES cells with developing retinal cells has shown to generate cells expressing retinal markers, suggesting a profound environmental impact on ES behavior. Similarly, the co-incubation of ES cells with PA6 stromal cells and FGF-2 generates an eye-like structure with a lens and 4 retinal neuron types, partially surrounded by an RPE layer [68]. Wnt2b stimulation of this eye-like structure yields colonies of RPE cells [69].

Transplanted ES cells stimulated by retinoic acid show a capacity to integrate a diseased retina and to differentiate into three or more retinal cell types. The transplanted cells also seem to delay degeneration in the integrated area, suggesting potential clinical utility.

To definitively attain specific retinal phenotypes, various researchers have designed several different methods of ES cell selective differentiation. To attain photoreceptors, mouse ES cells were first studied. Ikeda et al. transformed these mouse ES cells into rostral brain progenitors and then used Wnt, Nodal antagonist, and activin to transform these into retinal progenitors. Finally, these RPCs were co-cultured with embryonic retinal cells to attain a photoreceptor fate. In their study, approximately 36% of the cells acquired the photoreceptor phenotype [70].

To generate human photoreceptors from ES cells, several methods have been developed:

1) Sequential stimulation with Noggin and then with EGF and FGF-2 generates cells that express several retinal genes. Subretinal injection of these differentiated cells showed the potency to adopt a retinal fate [71].
2) In another sequential stimulation method, Dickkopf-1 was used to inhibit Wnt signaling in addition to Noggin use. This generated differentiated ES cells of a forebrain phenotype. To these, FGF-2 was added for 3 weeks. This also leads to the expression of several retinal progenitor markers and allows the generation of retinal cells in vitro [72].

Some investigators have also explored the generation of retinal ganglion cells from ES cells. In mice models, gene transfer methods have been successful in this regard. Specifically, the genes for various transcription factors such as Rx/rax and Chx10, can induce the differential of retinal neurons with electrophysiological characteristics of retinal ganglion cells [73].

The generation of RPE cells has also been explored. Some success has been attained by culturing human ES cells in a complex medium containing substitutes of serum. This method was shown to be efficient in 18 different hES cell lines [74]. These RPE cells cannot be greatly expanded, but the protocol appears to be sufficiently reproducible to compensate for this limited passage ability. These differentiated cells were transplanted into the subretinal space of RCS rats and showed improved retinal function and visual behavior.

These impressive studies show the potential of ES cells in retinal therapy. However, multiple steps remain. One of the key elements in using ES cells is that cell sorting is required to isolate the properly differentiated cells from potential tumorigenic ones. Additionally, the functional benefits of the successfully differentiated and transplanted ES cells remain unclear.

CONCLUSION

The *in vitro* and animal studies have improved our understanding of retinal pathogenesis and regenerative therapy immensely. However, one of the most important steps needed is to translate these therapeutic ideas into larger mammals that better represent the human retina. In particular, larger animals have a more representative vitreal space and a higher cone/rod ratio in comparison to rodents.

Of larger animals, the pig appears to have several advantages over other animal models. The size, structure, and shape of the pig eye closely resemble that of humans and allow the application of standard human surgical techniques. In addition, GFP-expressing transgenic animals [75,76] and disease models of human retinal dystrophies [77,78] are also readily available in the pig. Several investigators have begun adapting transplantation studies into this setting already.

In addition to animal model changes, a better molecular understanding of all the factors involved in retinal development and progenitor differentiation and integration will likely be critical in improving the therapeutic effectiveness of regenerative transplantation. Advances in cell biology, transplantation techniques, and tissue engineering will truly be the future of ophthalmology and will greatly advance the care of the multitude of patients afflicted by debilitating retinal diseases.

REFERENCES

[1]   Lund RD, Kwan AS, Keegan DJ, Sauvé Y, Coffey PJ, Lawrence JM. Cell Transplantation as a Treatment for Retinal Disease. *Prog Retin Eye Res*. 2001 Jul;20(4):415-49.

[2]   Bunker CH, Berson EL, Bromley WC, Hayes RP, Roderick TH. Prevalence of retinitis pigmentosa in Maine *Am J Ophthalmol*. 1984 Mar;97(3):357-65.

[3]   Bundey S, Crews SJ. A study of retinitis pigmentosa in the City of Birmingham. I Prevalence. *J Med Genet.* 1984 Dec;21(6):417-20.

[4]   Kaplan J, Bonneau D, Frézal J, Munnich A, Dufier JL. Clinical and genetic heterogeneity in retinitis pigmentosa. *Hum Genet.* 1990 Oct;85(6):635-42.

[5]   Green WR, Enger C. Age-related macular degeneration histopathologic studies. *Ophthalmology.* 1993 Oct;100(10):1519-35.

[6]   Zarbin MA. Age-related macular degeneration: review of pathogenesis. *Eur J Ophthalmol.* 1998 Oct-Dec;8(4):199-206.

[7]   Asahara T, Murohara T, Sullivan A, Silver M, van der Zee R, Li T, Witzenbichler B, Schatteman G, Isner JM. Isolation of putative progenitor endothelial cells for angiogenesis. *Science.* 1997 Feb 14;275(5302):964-7.

[8]   Crosby JR, Kaminski WE, Schatteman G, Martin PJ, Raines EW, Seifert RA, Bowen-Pope DF. Endothelial cells of hematopoietic origin make a significant contribution to adult blood vessel formation. *Circ Res.* 2000 Oct 27;87(9):728-30.

[9]   Grant MB, Caballero S, Brown GA, Guthrie SM, Mames RN, Vaught T, Scott EW. The contribution of adult hematopoietic stem cells to retinal neovascularisation. *Adv Exp Med Biol.* 2003;522:37-45.

[10]   Rafii S, Lyden D. Therapeutic stem and progenitor cell transplantation for organ vascularisation and regeneration. *Nat Med.* 2003 Jun;9(6):702-12.

[11]   Schatteman GC, Hanlon HD, Jiao C, Dodds SG, Christy BA. Blood-derived angioblasts accelerate blood flow restoration in diabetic mice. *J Clin Invest.* 2000 Aug;106(4):571-8.

[12]   Grant MB, May WS, Caballero S, Brown GA, Guthrie SM, Mames RN, Byrne BJ, Vaught T, Spoerri PE, Peck AB, Scott EW. Adult hematopoietic stem cells provide functional hemangioblast activity during retinal neovascularisation. *Nat Med.* 2002 Jun;8(6):607-12.

[13]   Otani A, Kinder K, Ewalt K, Otero FJ, Schimmel P, Friedlander M. Bone-marrow derived stem cells target retinal astrocytes and promote or inhibit retinal angiogenesis. *Nat Med.* 2002 Sep;8(9):1004-10. Epub 2002 Jul 29.

[14]   Asahara T, Takahashi T, Masuda H, Kalka C, Chen D, Iwaguro H, Inai Y, Silver M, Isner JM. VEGF contributes to postnatal neovascularization by mobilizing bone marrow-derived endothelial progenitor cells. *EMBO J.* 1999 Jul 15;18(14):3964-72.

[15]   Pantcheva MB, Mukai S. Stem cells in ophthalmology. *Int Ophthalmol Clin.* 2001 Fall;41(4):241-54.

[16]   Lendahl U, Zimmerman LB, McKay RD. CNS stem cells express a new class of intermediate filament protein. *Cell.* 1990 Feb 23;60(4):585-95.

[17]   Ahmad I, Dooley CM, Thoreson WB, Rogers JA, Afiat S. In vitro analysis of a mammalian retinal progenitor that gives rise to neurons and glia. *Brain Res.* 1999 Jun 12;831(1-2):1-10.

[18]   Chacko DM, Rogers JA, Turner JE, Ahmad I. Survival and differentiation of cultured retinal progenitors transplanted in the subretinal space of the rat. *Biochem Biophys Res Commun.* 2000 Feb 24;268(3):842-6.

[19]   Tropepe V, Coles BL, Chiasson BJ, Horsford DJ, Elia AJ, McInnes RR, van der Kooy D. Retinal stem cells in the adult mammalian eye. *Science*. 2000 Mar 17;287(5460):2032-6.

[20]   Sullivan KF. Structure and utilization of tubulin isotypes. *Annu Rev Cell Biol*. 1988;4:687-716.

[21]   Swaroop A, Xu JZ, Pawar H, Jackson A, Skolnick C, Agarwal N. A conserved retina-specific gene encodes a basic motif/leucine zipper domain. *Proc Natl Acad Sci U S A*. 1992 Jan 1;89(1):266-70.

[22]   Kyritsis AP, Tsokos M, Triche TJ, Chader GJ. Retinoblastoma--origin from a primitive neuroectodermal cell? *Nature*. 1984 Feb 2-8;307(5950):471-3.

[23]   Verhoeff FH, Jackson E. Minutes of the proceedings of the sixty-second annual meeting. *Trans Am Ophthalmol Soc* 1926; 24: 38-43.

[24]   Johansson CB, Momma S, Clarke DL, Risling M, Lendahl U, Frisén J. Identification of a neural stem cell in the adult mammalian central nervous system. *Cell*. 1999 Jan 8;96(1):25-34.

[25]   Layer PG, Rothermel A, Willbold E. From stem cells towards neural layers: A lesson from re-aggregated embryonic retinal cells. *Neuroreport*. 2001 May 25;12(7):A39-46.

[26]   Fischer AJ, Reh TA. Potential of Müller glia to become neurogenic retinal progenitor cells. *Glia*. 2003 Jul;43(1):70-6.

[27]   Wang J, McLeod D, Henson DB, Bishop PN. Age-dependent changes in the basal retinovitreous region. *Invest Ophthalmol Vis Sci*. 2003 May;44(5):1793-800.

[28]   Akagi T, Haruta M, Akita J, Nishida A, Honda Y, Takahashi M. Different characteristics of rat retinal progenitor cells from different culture periods. *Neurosci Lett*. 2003 May 8;341(3):213-6.

[29]   Young MJ. Stem cells in the mammalian eye: a tool for retinal repair. *APMIS*. 2005 Nov-Dec;113(11-12):845-57.

[30]   Cai J, Wu Y, Mirua T, Pierce JL, Lucero MT, Albertine KH, Spangrude GJ, Rao MS. Properties of a fetal multipotent neural stem cell (NEP cell). *Dev Biol*. 2002 Nov 15;251(2):221-40.

[31]   Tsai RY, McKay RD. A nucleolar mechanism controlling cell proliferation in stem cells and cancer cells. *Genes Dev*. 2002 Dec 1;16(23):2991-3003.

[32]   Uchida N, Buck DW, He D, Reitsma MJ, Masek M, Phan TV, Tsukamoto AS, Gage FH, Weissman IL. Direct isolation of human central nervous system stem cells. *Proc Natl Acad Sci U S A*. 2000 Dec 19;97(26):14720-5.

[33]   Klassen H, Schwartz MR, Bailey AH, Young MJ. Surface markers expressed by multipotent human and mouse neural progenitor cells include tetraspanins and non-protein epitopes. *Neurosci Lett*. 2001 Oct 26;312(3):180-2.

[34]   Bhattacharya S, Jackson JD, Das AV, Thoreson WB, Kuszynski C, James J, Joshi S, Ahmad I. Direct identification and enrichment of retinal stem cells/progenitors by Hoechst dye efflux assay. *Invest Ophthalmol Vis Sci*. 2003 Jun;44(6):2764-73.

[35]   Scharenberg CW, Harkey MA, Torok-Storb B. The ABCG2 transporter is an efficient Hoechst 33342 efflux pump and is preferentially expressed by immature human hematopoietic progenitors. *Blood*. 2002 Jan 15;99(2):507-12.

[36] Otani A, Dorrell MI, Kinder K, Moreno SK, Nusinowitz S, Banin E, Heckenlively J, Friedlander M. Rescue of retinal degeneration by intravitreally injected adult bone marrow-derived lineage-negative hematopoietic stem cells. *J Clin Invest.* 2004 Sep;114(6):765-74.

[37] Algvere PV, Gouras P, Dafgård Kopp E. Long-term outcome of RPE allografts in non-immunosuppressed patients with AMD. *Eur J Ophthalmol.* 1999 Jul-Sep;9(3):217-30.

[38] Peyman GA, Blinder KJ, Paris CL, Alturki W, Nelson NC Jr, Desai U. A technique for retinal pigment epithelium transplantation for age-related macular degeneration secondary to extensive subfoveal scarring. *Ophthalmic Surg.* 1991 Feb;22(2):102-8.

[39] Weisz JM, Humayun MS, De Juan E Jr, Del Cerro M, Sunness JS, Dagnelie G, Soylu M, Rizzo L, Nussenblatt RB. Allogenic fetal retinal pigment epithelial cell transplant in a patient with geographic atrophy. *Retina.* 1999;19(6):540-5.

[40] Kanuga N, Winton HL, Beauchéne L, Koman A, Zerbib A, Halford S, Couraud PO, Keegan D, Coffey P, Lund RD, Adamson P, Greenwood J. Characterization of genetically modified human retinal pigment epithelial cells developed for in vitro and transplantation studies. *Invest Ophthalmol Vis Sci.* 2002 Feb;43(2):546-55.

[41] Coffey PJ, Girman S, Wang SM, Hetherington L, Keegan DJ, Adamson P, Greenwood J, Lund RD. Long-term preservation of cortically dependent visual function in RCS rats by transplantation. *Nat Neurosci.* 2002 Jan;5(1):53-6.

[42] Takahashi M, Palmer TD, Takahashi J, Gage FH. Widespread integration and survival of adult-derived neural progenitor cells in the developing optic retina. *Mol Cell Neurosci.* 1998 Dec;12(6):340-8.

[43] Kelley MW, Turner JK, Reh TA. Regulation of proliferation and photoreceptor differentiation in fetal human retinal cell cultures. *Invest Ophthalmol Vis Sci.* 1995 Jun;36(7):1280-9.

[44] Guo Y, Saloupis P, Shaw SJ, Rickman DW. Engraftment of adult neural progenitor cells transplanted to rat retina injured by transient ischemia. *Invest Ophthalmol Vis Sci.* 2003 Jul;44(7):3194-201.

[45] Nishida A, Takahashi M, Tanihara H, Nakano I, Takahashi JB, Mizoguchi A, Ide C, Honda Y. Incorporation and differentiation of hippocampus-derived neural stem cells transplanted in injured adult rat retina. *Invest Ophthalmol Vis Sci.* 2000 Dec;41(13):4268-74.

[46] Young MJ, Ray J, Whiteley SJ, Klassen H, Gage FH. Neuronal differentiation and morphological integration of hippocampal progenitor cells transplanted to the retina of immature and mature dystrophic rats. *Mol Cell Neurosci.* 2000 Sep;16(3):197-205.

[47] Furukawa T, Morrow EM, Cepko CL. Crx, a novel otx-like homeobox gene, shows photoreceptor-specific expression and regulates photoreceptor differentiation. *Cell.* 1997 Nov 14;91(4):531-41.

[48] Nishida A, Furukawa A, Koike C, Tano Y, Aizawa S, Matsuo I, Furukawa T. Otx2 homeobox gene controls retinal photoreceptor cell fate and pineal gland development. *Nat Neurosci.* 2003 Dec;6(12):1255-63. Epub 2003 Nov 16.

[49] Akagi T, Akita J, Haruta M, Suzuki T, Honda Y, Inoue T, Yoshiura S, Kageyama R, Yatsu T, Yamada M, Takahashi M. Inoue et al., Iris-derived cells from adult rodents

and primates adopt photoreceptor-specific phenotypes. *Invest Ophthalmol Vis Sci.* 2005 Sep;46(9):3411-9.

[50] Tan E, Wang Q, Quiambao AB, Xu X, Qtaishat NM, Peachey NS, Lem J, Fliesler SJ, Pepperberg DR, Naash MI, Al-Ubaidi MR. The relationship between opsin overexpression and photoreceptor degeneration. *Invest Ophthalmol Vis Sci.* 2001 Mar;42(3):589-600.

[51] Berson DM. Strange vision: ganglion cells as circadian photoreceptors. *Trends Neurosci.* 2003 Jun;26(6):314-20.

[52] Angénieux B, Schorderet DF, Arsenijevic Y. Epidermal growth factor is a neuronal differentiation factor for retinal stem cells in vitro. *Stem Cells.* 2006 Mar;24(3):696-706. Epub 2005 Sep 22.

[53] Merhi-Soussi F, Angénieux B, Canola K, Kostic C, Tekaya M, Hornfeld D, Arsenijevic Y. High yield of cells committed to the photoreceptor fate from expanded mouse retinal stem cells. *Stem Cells.* 2006 Sep;24(9):2060-70. Epub 2006 Apr 27.

[54] Klassen HJ, Ng TF, Kurimoto Y, Kirov I, Shatos M, Coffey P, Young MJ. Multipotent retinal progenitors express developmental markers, differentiate into retinal neurons, and preserve light-mediated behavior. *Invest Ophthalmol Vis Sci.* 2004 Nov;45(11):4167-73.

[55] Chacko DM, Das AV, Zhao X, James J, Bhattacharya S, Ahmad I. Transplantation of ocular stem cells: the role of injury in incorporation and differentiation of grafted cells in the retina. *Vision Res.* 2003 Apr;43(8):937-46.

[56] Kwan AS, Wang S, Lund RD. Photoreceptor layer reconstruction in a rodent model of retinal degeneration. *Exp Neurol.* 1999 Sep;159(1):21-33.

[57] Aramant RB, Seiler MJ. Progress in retinal sheet transplantation. *Prog Retin Eye Res.* 2004 Sep;23(5):475-94.

[58] MacLaren RE, Pearson RA, MacNeil A, Douglas RH, Salt TE, Akimoto M, Swaroop A, Sowden JC, Ali RR. Retinal repair by transplantation of photoreceptor precursors. *Nature.* 2006 Nov 9;444(7116):203-7.

[59] Klassen H, Kiilgaard JF, Zahir T, Ziaeian B, Kirov I, Scherfig E, Warfvinge K, Young MJ. Progenitor cells from the porcine neural retina express photoreceptor markers after transplantation to the subretinal space of allorecipients. *Stem Cells.* 2007 May;25(5):1222-30. Epub 2007 Jan 11.

[60] Freed LE, Vunjak-Novakovic G, Biron RJ, Eagles DB, Lesnoy DC, Barlow SK, Langer R. Biodegradable polymer scaffolds for tissue engineering. *Biotechnology (N Y).* 1994 Jul;12(7):689-93.

[61] Pomahac B, Svensjö T, Yao F, Brown H, Eriksson E. Tissue engineering of skin. *Crit Rev Oral Biol Med.* 1998;9(3):333-44.

[62] Temenoff JS, Mikos AG. Review: tissue engineering for regeneration of articular cartilage. *Biomaterials.* 2000 Mar;21(5):431-40.

[63] Atala A. Tissue engineering for bladder substitution. *World J Urol.* 2000 Oct;18(5):364-70.

[64] Langer R. Biomaterials in drug delivery and tissue engineering: one laboratory's experience. *Acc Chem Res.* 2000 Feb;33(2):94-101.

[65]   Lavik EB, Hrkach JS, Lotan N, Nazarov R, Langer R. A simple synthetic route to the formation of a block copolymer of poly(lactic-co-glycolic acid) and polylysine for the fabrication of functionalized, degradable structures for biomedical applications. *J Biomed Mater Res*. 2001 May 1;58(3):291-4.

[66]   Cook AD, Hrkach JS, Gao NN, Johnson IM, Pajvani UB, Cannizzaro SM, Langer R. Characterization and development of RGD-peptide-modified poly(lactic acid-co-lysine) as an interactive, resorbable biomaterial. *J Biomed Mater Res*. 1997 Jun 15;35(4):513-23.

[67]   Zhao X, Das AV, Thoreson WB, James J, Wattnem TE, Rodriguez-Sierra J, Ahmad I. Adult corneal limbal epithelium: a model for studying neural potential of non-neural stem cells/progenitors. *Dev Biol*. 2002 Oct 15;250(2):317-31.

[68]   Hirano M, Yamamoto A, Yoshimura N, Tokunaga T, Motohashi T, Ishizaki K, Yoshida H, Okazaki K, Yamazaki H, Hayashi S, Kunisada T. Generation of structures formed by lens and retinal cells differentiating from embryonic stem cells. *Dev Dyn*. 2003 Dec;228(4):664-71.

[69]   Aoki H, Hara A, Nakagawa S, Motohashi T, Hirano M, Takahashi Y, Kunisada T. Embryonic stem cells that differentiate into RPE cell precursors in vitro develop into RPE cell monolayers in vivo. *Exp Eye Res*. 2006 Feb;82(2):265-74. Epub 2005 Sep 16.

[70]   Ikeda H, Osakada F, Watanabe K, Mizuseki K, Haraguchi T, Miyoshi H, Kamiya D, Honda Y, Sasai N, Yoshimura N, Takahashi M, Sasai Y. Generation of Rx+/Pax6+ neural retinal precursors from embryonic stem cells. *Proc Natl Acad Sci U S A*. 2005 Aug 9;102(32):11331-6. Epub 2005 Aug 2.

[71]   Banin E, Obolensky A, Idelson M, Hemo I, Reinhardtz E, Pikarsky E, Ben-Hur T, Reubinoff B. Retinal incorporation and differentiation of neural precursors derived from human embryonic stem cells., *Stem Cells*. 2006 Feb;24(2):246-57. Epub 2005 Aug 25.

[72]   Lamba DA, Karl MO, Ware CB, Reh TA. Efficient generation of retinal progenitor cells from human embryonic stem cells. *Proc Natl Acad Sci U S A*. 2006 Aug 22;103(34):12769-74. Epub 2006 Aug 14.

[73]   Tabata Y, Ouchi Y, Kamiya H, Manabe T, Arai K, Watanabe S. Specification of the retinal fate of mouse embryonic stem cells by ectopic expression of Rx/rax, a homeobox gene. *Mol Cell Biol*. 2004 May;24(10):4513-21.

[74]   Lund RD, Wang S, Klimanskaya I, Holmes T, Ramos-Kelsey R, Lu B, Girman S, Bischoff N, Sauvé Y, Lanza R. Human embryonic stem cell-derived cells rescue visual function in dystrophic RCS rats. *Cloning Stem Cells*. 2006 Fall;8(3):189-99.

[75]   Park KW, Cheong HT, Lai L, Im GS, Kühholzer B, Bonk A, Samuel M, Rieke A, Day BN, Murphy CN, Carter DB, Prather RS. Production of nuclear transfer-derived swine that express the enhanced green fluorescent protein. *Anim Biotechnol*. 2001 Nov;12(2):173-81.

[76]   Lai L, Park KW, Cheong HT, Kühholzer B, Samuel M, Bonk A, Im GS, Rieke A, Day BN, Murphy CN, Carter DB, Prather RS. Transgenic pig expressing the enhanced green fluorescent protein produced by nuclear transfer using colchicine-treated fibroblasts as donor cells. *Mol Reprod Dev*. 2002 Jul;62(3):300-6.

[77]   Petters RM, Alexander CA, Wells KD, Collins EB, Sommer JR, Blanton MR, Rojas G, Hao Y, Flowers WL, Banin E, Cideciyan AV, Jacobson SG, Wong F. Genetically engineered large animal model for studying cone photoreceptor survival and degeneration in retinitis pigmentosa. *Nat Biotechnol.* 1997 Oct;15(10):965-70.

[78]   Li ZY, Wong F, Chang JH, Possin DE, Hao Y, Petters RM, Milam AH. Rhodopsin transgenic pigs as a model for human retinitis pigmentosa. *Invest Ophthalmol Vis Sci.* 1998 Apr;39(5):808-19.

In: Encyclopedia of Stem Cell Research (2 Volume Set)   ISBN: 978-1-61761-835-2
Editor: Alexander L. Greene   © 2012 Nova Science Publishers, Inc.

Chapter XXX

VASCULAR TISSUE ENGINEERING: CURRENT APPROACHES AND STRATEGIES

Shannon L. M. Dahl[*]
Humacyte, Inc., Durham, NC, US

ABSTRACT

A myriad of approaches have been used to create tissue engineered blood vessels over the past 20 years. In this chapter, current approaches and strategies for culturing blood vessels are reviewed. First, scaffold choices are discussed with respect to their impact on vessel strength; persistence or degradation; and ability to facilitate cellular attachment, growth, and extracellular matrix production. Cell sourcing strategies are reviewed with respect to their impact on vessel strength, ability to adhere to scaffolds, and feasibility for translation to clinical use. Culture strategies also are discussed, and where possible, compositional characteristics of tissue engineered blood vessels cultured are highlighted. Implantation of tissue engineered blood vessels into large animal models is reviewed with an emphasis on graft functionality, cellular retention or infiltration, remodeling of extracellular matrix, and remaining challenges. Two human clinical trials focused on tissue engineered blood vessels are described. Future directions are proposed based on the advantages and roadblocks of different strategies. The topics reviewed within this chapter are applicable not only to the development of tissue engineered blood vessels, but also to other engineered tissues.

INTRODUCTION

Cardiovascular diseases lead to more deaths in the United States than any other disease. More than 15 million patients suffer from coronary heart disease, with more than 400,000

---

[*] Correspondence concerning this article should be addressed to: Shannon L. M. Dahl, E-mail: dahl@humacyte.com; T.: 919-475-9911.

coronary artery bypass procedures performed per year [1]. Further, peripheral artery disease affects approximately 8 million Americans [1]. Conduits are needed for coronary and peripheral artery disease patients, as well as for patients who suffer from other vascular diseases. Synthetic grafts, such as expanded polytetrafluoroethylene (ePTFE), often are used for large-diameter (> 6 mm) vascular grafting applications, but synthetic grafts have poor patency rates in small diameter, low-flow settings [2-4]. Tissue engineered blood vessels (TEBVs) currently are being evaluated as an alternate source for vascular grafting conduit in two clinical applications. Pending the outcomes of current and future clinical trials, TEBVs have the potential to serve as conduits for many vascular grafting procedures.

TEBVs often are created using the traditional paradigm for tissue engineering, in which cells are seeded within a scaffold and cultured in vitro for a period of time ranging from hours [5,6] to months [7,8]. The approach of seeding cells on a scaffold for a short time period, such as hours, requires the scaffold to provide mechanical integrity. In contrast, long term cell culture may generate an extracellular matrix that provides mechanical integrity. TEBVs require mechanical properties that are sufficient for surgical handling and long term cyclic straining in vivo, an endothelium for small diameter applications, and immunocompatibility with the host. In this chapter, we present an overview of the literature on scaffolds and cell sources for TEBVs. Strategies behind choosing combinations of scaffolds and cells are discussed. Finally, preclinical and clinical studies with TEBVs are reviewed.

SCAFFOLD CHOICES

Many scaffolds have been used for cellular seeding, including biologically derived materials, synthetic polymers, combinations of synthetic and biologic materials, and decellularized tissues. In addition, some groups use no scaffolds. Mimicking a native vessel in terms of composition, structure, and function, remains the gold standard for vascular tissue engineering. Thus, scaffold choices generally aim to provide compositional similarity to native vessels, to provide mechanical similarity to native vessels, or to facilitate cellular production of extracellular matrix with compositional and mechanical similarity to native vessels.

Biopolymer Scaffolds

Formation of TEBVs was first reported by Weinberg and Bell in 1986 [9]. Cells were suspended in a solution of type I collagen monomers, and collagen fibrillogenesis occurred with an increase in temperature [9]. Smooth muscle cells (SMCs) were mixed with collagen to create a medial layer, and fibroblasts and collagen were mixed to form an outer adventitial layer. Endothelial cells (ECs) adhered to the lumen and displayed antithrombogenic activity. These layered gel based constructs were very weak, with burst pressures of less than 10 mmHg [9]. In order to withstand physiologic pressures (typically 70–120 mmHg in humans), constructs were wrapped with multiple layers of Dacron to impart strength.

In the past decade, gel-based constructs have been further evaluated [10-13]. Biopolymer scaffolds, such as collagen and fibrin hydrogels are attractive from the standpoint that they do not contain synthetic materials. Collagen gel materials, however, typically are derived from bovine type I collagen, which may stimulate an immune response upon implantation into other species, including humans. The same concern exists for fibrin-based constructs, which are formed by mixing SMCs with fibrinogen and bovine thrombin to promote fibrin fibril formation. SMCs embedded in collagen hydrogels failed to generate significant amounts of new extracellular matrix proteins during culture [14], which explains their weak burst pressures. Mechanical strengths of collagen gel constructs have been improved by nonenzymatic crosslinking (glycation) [15] or exposure to cyclic strains during culture [12,16]. Even with these improvements, collagen gel-based constructs have not achieved strengths suitable for clinical use without additional structural supports. Fibrin gel based TEBVs, however, were stronger and stiffer than collagen-based constructs [13]. Strengths of fibrin based constructs were likely related to the ability of SMCs embedded within fibrin gels to synthesize extracellular matrix proteins, including collagen and elastin during a 4 – 6 week in vitro culture period [13,17-19]. Synthesis of elastin is rarely achieved in vitro, and thus elastin in fibrin-based constructs is an impressive accomplishment. Although short (1–2 mm in length) fibrin-based constructs have impressive mechanical properties, generating longer tubes leads to highly variable mechanical properties [20]. If generation of long grafts with consistently robust mechanical properties is achieved, fibrin-based constructs will show greater promise for clinical use.

Another biological material that has been evaluated for use as a TEBV scaffold is esterified hyaluronic acid (HYAFF) [21]. HYAFF degrades within 40 days [22], and its biocompatibility has been established in a subcutaneous rat model [23]. ECs formed a subendothelial matrix composed of collagen IV, collagen VIII, fibronectin, and laminin within 7 days of seeding on HYAFF felts [24], which suggests that HYAFF may be a good material to promote a mature intact endothelial ultrastructure. HYAFF also has supported vascular SMC attachment and growth, which reached a maximum at 7 days [21]. After 2 weeks of culture with SMCs, mechanical testing revealed that HYAFF constructs had higher stiffnesses and lower ultimate tensile strengths than native porcine arteries [21].

Degradable Synthetic Polymer Scaffolds

Multiple approaches use synthetic materials to create TEBVs. Polyglycolic acid (PGA) and poly-l-lactic acid (PLLA) are degradable polymers commonly used for tissue engineering applications. Both materials have been approved by the U.S. Food and Drug Administration for several medical uses. PGA degrades more rapidly than PLLA. PGA and PLLA may be used independently or in combination (e.g., polylactic-co-glycolic acid, or PLGA) to tailor polymer degradation rates. See Gunatillake and Adhikari [25] for a review of common biodegradable synthetic polymers for tissue engineering applications. Degradation data for common synthetic polymer scaffolds are shown in Table 1. PGA or PLLA often have been formed into nonwoven felts with high porosities, which allows cells to migrate easily into the scaffold [26]. Prior to seeding with cells, PGA or PLLA felts often undergo surface treatment to improve cell attachment. This may include surface hydrolysis with sodium hydroxide [27,28], plasma treatment [29], or coating with extracellular matrix components [30]. In one approach, Niklason et al., seeded SMCs onto tubular PGA scaffolds and cultured constructs with pulsatile cyclic strains [8]. PGA scaffolds supported cellular synthesis of collagen. During 8 weeks in culture, more than 80% of the PGA scaffold degraded, and the PGA scaffold stopped providing mechanical support after 3 weeks in culture [31]. TEBVs cultured using PGA scaffolds were strong enough to withstand surgical handling, and the mechanical properties were derived primarily from collagen [8,32].

Table 1. Reported Degradation Profiles of Common Synthetic Polymer Scaffolds

Polymer	Evaluation Day	Percent Polymer Remaining	References
HYAFF	40	0	[22]
PGA	60	0-20	[6, 31]
P(CL/LA)	168	0	[5]
PLLA	161	~30	[33]
PLLA	730	0	[5]
PCL-PU	30	>98	[34]
PCL-PU	56	~84	[35]
P4-HB	169	P4-HB visible, but not quantified	[36]

Polyurethane (PU) scaffolds also have been used to generate TEBVs. Degradable forms of PU are commonly formed by including soft segments of polyester, such as polycaprolactone (PCL) [34,37]. The degradation rate of PU may be tailored [35,38], but PU typically degrades more slowly than PGA or PLLA [31,35]. PU has high compliance, which has made it popular as a scaffold for vascular graft applications [39,40]. New processing solvents have reduced the concern of cytotoxicity, which historically has been associated with PU scaffolds [40]. PU may be tailored such that it supports EC adhesion, proliferation, and release of von Willebrand factor (vWF), nitric oxide and ICAM-1 under physiological stimuli [35,37].

Poly-4-hydroxybutyrate (P4-HB) is a scaffold that degrades slowly. P4-HB coated with collagen type I has been seeded with vascular ECs, SMCs, and fibroblasts over a 4-day period prior to implantation as a pulmonary artery patch in an ovine model [36]. P4-HB scaffolds withstood surgical handling and supported collagen, elastin, and glycosaminoglycan deposition in vivo [36,41]. Tubular P4-HB-based TEBVs have been wrapped with small intestine submucosa (SIS) for additional mechanical support, but even with the extra support, P4-HB-based TEBVs dilated after 24 weeks in vivo [42]. The authors hypothesized that increased elastin synthesis was necessary to prevent dilatation in future studies [42].

Multilayer structures also have been used as scaffolds. For example, Watanabe et al. used a structure consisting of a PGA scaffold coated with a copolymer of L-lactide and ε-caprolactone, or P(CL/LA) [43]. After seeding these scaffolds with autologous femoral vein cells and culturing for one week in vitro, constructs were implanted into the inferior vena cava in an autologous canine model. Strength provided by the synthetic scaffold was sufficient for surgical handling. Further, the polymer provided mechanical support in vivo as extracellular matrix was formed in the graft. The details of mechanical graft integrity during polymer degradation and extracellular matrix deposition were not evaluated within the first 3 months in vivo. However, given that no remnant polymer was seen after 3 months and that all grafts were intact at 3 months, a functional balance of polymer degradation and matrix deposition was achieved to maintain mechanical integrity in vivo. Further, the absence of inflammatory cells in grafts suggested that PGA with P(CL/LA) was well tolerated in a canine model.

Electrospinning has generated synthetic polymers with fiber diameters that mimic diameters of native extracellular matrix proteins [44,45]. Further, electrospinning has created scaffolds containing a mixture of synthetic polymers and native proteins [46-48]. For example, Lee et al. recently have electrospun nanofiber scaffolds comprised of 45% collagen, 15% elastin, and 40% biodegradable polymer by weight [48]. Collagen and elastin concentrations in these electrospun scaffolds mimic protein concentrations found in native arteries. Telemeco et al. have shown that cells infiltrated electrospun collagen scaffolds in vivo within 7 days, but cells failed to readily infiltrate electrospun gelatin, PGA, or PLA scaffolds [49]. This study suggests that in vivo cellular infiltration may be regulated in part by fiber material. Electrospun materials, however, generally are less porous than nonwoven felts, which also reduces cellular infiltration [49].

Decellularized Tissues as Scaffolds

Autologous culture of TEBVs requires long culture periods of up to 24 weeks [50]. For the many patients who require near-term vascular replacements, a faster graft development strategy is needed. Decellularized scaffolds of native or tissue-engineered origin may serve as constructs onto which autologous cells may be seeded for short time periods prior to implantation. Decellularized scaffolds also may be implanted without cells in large-diameter vascular grafting applications.

Many tissue engineers work towards the goal of designing TEBVs that match native arterial tissue in terms of composition, organization, and function [51]. Given that native vascular tissues already posses the ideal composition and organization of extracellular matrix proteins, decellularized native tissues are attractive as scaffolds for TEBVs. Several groups have used decellularized native porcine tissues as acellular scaffolds [52-56].

The successful widespread clinical use of porcine-derived SIS has popularized the approach of using decellularized native tissues. An acellular vascular graft was created by Huynh et al. by rolling sheets of acellular porcine SIS around a mandrel and cross-linking the construct with 1-ethyl-3(3-dimethylaminopropyl) carbodiimide hydrochloride [54]. The construct was lined with dense fibrillar bovine type I collagen and a heparin-benzalkonium chloride complex. No cells were seeded onto SIS-based TEBVs. Prior to implant, constructs had high burst pressures of 931 ± 284 mmHg. During a 90 day implant period in rabbits, SIS-based scaffolds supported SMC infiltration, became endothelialized, and remained patent. Thus, decellularized native tissues show potential as vascular grafts.

TEBVs also have been created by decellularizing vascular porcine tissues. Teebken et al. enzymatically decellularized porcine thoracic aortas with trypsin, DNAse, and RNAse [55]. Scanning electron microscopy and histology showed that collagen and elastin fibers were well conserved following decellularization treatments. Human saphenous vein ECs or myofibroblasts were seeded onto acellular constructs and cultured for 4 days in vitro. Although cells adhered to porcine constructs, neither cell type infiltrated the acellular construct. The inability of seeded cells to penetrate decellularized native arteries has been observed by other investigators as well [57].

Porcine native arteries also have been decellularized using detergents. For example, decellularization has been accomplished with Triton X-100 and ammonium hydroxide, or with sodium dodecyl sulfate (SDS) and CHAPS [58]. Decellularized porcine arteries supported attachment of human saphenous vein ECs [52], porcine cells [59], and sheep peripheral blood endothelial precursor cells [56]. Decellularized native arteries were consistently less elastic than their cellular counterparts, but retained collagen and elastin architectures as seen by histology [52,59].

Decellularization of native vessels largely preserves the architecture of the native extracellular matrix. Organized collagen and elastin are desirable for graft strength and compliance, respectively. Decellularization of human cadaver tissues has advantages over that of xenogenic tissues, as allogeneic extracellular matrix proteins are non-immunogenic [60,61]. However, cadaver tissues often are harvested from the elderly, who may have diseased arteries with plaque or calcification. Thus, availability of healthy tissues from cadavers is a concern. In contrast, animal-derived tissues rarely contain plaque or calcification due to the significantly shorter lifespan of animals and the early time points at which animals are sacrificed to procure healthy tissues. Both human and animal donors, however, are prone to a variety of viruses and diseases, and thus the approach of decellularizing native tissues likely will require significant routine testing for donor health as well as graft performance.

Culturing TEBVs from human cells, and then decellularizing engineered constructs, may alleviate concerns associated with decellularized xenogenic or cadaveric tissues. For example, one human donor cell population that is known to be free of viruses and disease may be used to create many TEBVs. In contrast, xenogenic and cadaveric tissues vary between donors with respect to viral load, disease state, and other properties. The approach of using decellularized TEBVs as scaffolds has been investigated by our group [59]. Porcine SMCs were cultured on biodegradable PGA scaffolds for 8 weeks to create collagenous TEBVs. TEBVs were then decellularized with SDS and CHAPS. Decellularized constructs supported adhesion of allogeneic cells [59].

No Scaffolds

TEBVs also have been produced without the use of any biologic or synthetic scaffolds. In the self assembly method, SMCs and fibroblasts were cultured in separate flasks and stimulated with ascorbic acid to produce an extracellular matrix [7]. Sheets of tissue were then rolled around a mandrel, with an acellular inner layer, an SMC medial layer, and a fibroblast outer layer. Constructs were cultured for at least 9 weeks in bioreactors after tube formation [7]. Constructs cultured from umbilical vein SMCs and young adult skin fibroblasts had burst pressures higher than those of human saphenous veins [7], which is an impressive achievement for engineered tissue. Recently, this approach has been used to culture grafts from adult human skin fibroblasts and saphenous vein ECs (without SMCs), and has been called "sheet-based tissue engineering" [62]. This approach focuses on culturing completely autologous TEBVs, which minimizes risk of immunogenic complications. Sheet-based TEBVs have begun testing in human clinical trials [50].

A completely in vivo approach also has been employed to culture TEBVs. Campbell and colleagues implanted a silastic mandrel into the peritoneal cavity of rats or rabbits for 2 weeks, which resulted in the formation of a collagenous construct (~0.18 mm in thickness) around the implanted mandrel [63]. TEBVs cultured in vivo contained myofibroblasts, macrophages, and a mesothelial cell layer. When implanted as autologous vascular grafts, elastic lamellae began to form 1 month after implant. Growth of TEBVs in vivo has also been performed using mandrels covered by synthetic scaffolds to support cell infiltration, proliferation, and matrix deposition within synthetic scaffolds. Scaffolds used in this approach have included PGA (degradable) [64], polypropylene (non-degradable) [64], and Dacron (non-degradable) [65].

CELL SEEDING STRATEGIES

One approach is to implant acellular constructs with the thought that grafts will remodel *in vivo*. Remodeling may involve infiltration of native cells that provide contractile function and may lead the extracellular matrix to behave mechanically more like native arterial tissue [54]. Biological conduits are more compliant than ePTFE and thus may lessen the burden of significant compliance mismatch associated with ePTFE. Given that compliance mismatch leads to an increased risk of thrombosis [66,67], compliant biological grafts may have lower rates of thrombosis than ePTFE grafts. Like ePTFE, decellularized biological constructs may function without cells at diameters of 6 mm and above. Two significant advantages of implanting completely acellular TEBVs are that acellular TEBVs (1) are available immediately at the time of a specified patient need and (2) obviate the need for a biopsy procedure to harvest autologous cells.

It is commonly thought that small diameter vascular graft (< 6mm) applications require an endothelial layer to prevent thrombosis [68]. This is based largely on the findings that endothelialization has reduced platelet aggregation on ePTFE grafts [69] and has improved long-term patency of ePTFE grafts in clinical studies [70]. ECs frequently are seeded onto TEBVs just days prior to implant. Grafts seeded with ECs typically are preconditioned to shear stresses in vitro, which theoretically improves EC retention on TEBVs following exposure to high shear stresses in vivo. Without preconditioning in vitro, up to 80% of ECs seeded onto ePTFE grafts detach upon exposure to blood flow [71]. Several techniques have attempted to accelerate EC attachment to vascular grafts, including pressure sodding of ePTFE grafts [72] and magnetic seeding [73,74], thought these techniques have yet to be used routinely in tissue engineering applications.

Although some approaches only incorporate endothelial cells to simplify graft preparation, inclusion of SMCs or fibroblasts within the wall of the graft may also provide useful benefits. SMCs and fibroblasts produce collagen in vitro, and therefore have been used to generate the extracellular matrix of TEBVs during long-term autologous culture [7,8].

Other approaches use only short-term cell seeding of SMCs, which are contractile cells, to reduce the probability of graft dilatation upon implantation. Given that biological constructs typically are weaker than ePTFE, there is a concern about dilatation of biologic grafts. However, SMC phenotype in culture differs greatly from that in vivo. Specifically, cultured SMCs are significantly less contractile than native SMCs [75], and thus may require a differentiation period to regain a contractile phenotype following implantation and thereafter may actively resist graft dilatation. SMC phenotype also may impact the phenotype of ECs seeded onto a tissue engineered construct [76].

Autologous Cell Sources

Ideally, minimally invasive procedures would be used to harvest cells or to harvest tissues from which cells may be isolated. Once a biopsy has been acquired, ECs and SMCs, stem cells, or precursor cells may be isolated. Isolated cells may be seeded onto TEBVs immediately. Cells may also be propagated in vitro for expansion, differentiation, or assistance in graft formation.

Although saphenous vein harvest is invasive, both ECs and SMCs have been isolated successfully from human saphenous veins [55,62,77-81]. Some reports indicate that autologous vein harvest fails to consistently yield a sufficient number of cells for seeding a graft [6], and that in vitro expansion of human vein ECs leads to poor attachment and growth on vascular graft surfaces [82]. However, others indicate successful long-term culture (>10 passages) of ECs with consistent phenotype after isolation from saphenous veins and subsequent purification by immunoisolation with Ulex europeaus I lectin [52]. Saphenous vein ECs seeded onto decellularized porcine aortas displayed functional characteristics, including prostaglandin I_2 production and release of vasoactive agents [52]. Although saphenous vein harvest is a routine procedure for many coronary artery bypass procedures and therefore may be accepted clinically as an option for cell procurement, less invasive procedures surely would be preferred.

Several approaches for creating TEBVs require isolated cells to proliferate repeatedly during long-term in vitro culture. For example, autologous SMCs may be isolated from saphenous vein [79] or fibroblasts may be isolated from skin biopsies [62]. Cells isolated from elderly patients, however, tolerate fewer population doublings than cells from younger donors [83], and synthesize less collagen than cells from younger donors [80]. Infection of human saphenous vein SMCs with the telomerase reverse transcriptase subunit (hTERT) to extend cell lifespan has been investigated for tissue engineering applications [80,84,85]. TEBVs cultured with hTERT-infected SMCs had higher burst pressures and higher cell densities than TEBVs without hTERT [80]. In safety studies, human SMCs infected with hTERT were not found to be cancerous in comparison with non-infected cells [85]. Thus, hTERT has the potential to improve the lifespan of human adult cells used for TEBV production.

Autologous stem and progenitor cells are desirable cell sources for TEBVs, as they may be isolated using less invasive procedures than saphenous vein biopsies and guided towards differentiation into vascular cell phenotypes. Stem cells also have the potential to undergo more population doublings than isolated adult differentiated cells. Popular cell sources that include stem or progenitor cells are bone marrow, peripheral blood, and adipose tissue.

Bone marrow cells (BMCs) may be aspirated from bone marrow, centrifuged, and seeded onto scaffolds as multipotent cells [5]. This approach minimizes graft preparation time, eliminates exposure to serum, and minimizes risk of contamination due to culture [5]. The approach of seeding the mononuclear fraction of BMCs onto grafts has been used clinically with success [6]. Canine implant studies have shown that bone marrow-derived cells will differentiate into vascular cells in vivo [5].

TEBVs have been constructed not only using bone marrow-derived cells seeded onto scaffolds and implanted the same day of isolation [5,6,86], but also using BMCs cultured for a period of days to achieve differentiation, expansion, or labeling prior to implant [19,86]. For example, bone marrow-derived mesenchymal stem cells (MSCs) may be used to seed TEBVs. In vitro studies showed that MSCs and control ECs resisted platelet adhesion at similar levels [87]. In vivo studies showed that MSC-seeded constructs displayed less luminal thrombus formation than unseeded grafts, indicating that MSCs may provide antithrombogenic properties for TEBVs.

Bone marrow also contains endothelial progenitor cells (EPCs) and SMC progenitor cells [88]. EPCs have been derived from bone marrow using positive selection with anti-CD34 [89], but poor yield is a problem [90]. SMC progenitors from bone marrow may be guided towards differentiation into SMCs by 2-mercaptoethanol and ascorbic acid [91] or by exposing the cells to cyclic strain in culture [92]. Expression of SMC markers following exposure to cyclic strain reveals an exciting potential for use of SMC progenitors from bone marrow during long-term in vitro TEBV culture. Further, it is possible that SMC progenitors from bone marrow may be guided towards SMCs in vivo in response to physiologic cyclic strains.

EPCs also have been derived from peripheral blood, using positive selection with anti-CD34 and anti-Flk-1 [93] or and anti-AC133 [94]. Expression of EC markers, including CD34, CD31, Flk-1, Tie-2, and E selectin, in cells isolated from peripheral blood and plated on fibronectin-coated flasks for 7 days, closely resembled expression in human umbilical vein ECs [93]. EPCs derived from sheep produced NO when seeded on porcine decellularized arteries in vitro, and implanted EPC-seeded grafts remained patent for up to 130 days, likely also as a result of NO production [56]. Isolating EPCs from peripheral blood or bone marrow often results in selection of very few positive cells, and culture of the cells is not always successful [90]. Thus, autologous EPCs (either from peripheral blood or bone marrow) may not be appropriate as a clinical cell source for adults with cardiovascular risk factors given the lack of consistency in isolation and culture outcomes [95]. Interestingly, umbilical cord blood contains high concentrations of EPCs, and therefore may serve as a clinically useful EPC source for repair of congenital cardiac defects [96]. If successful routine isolation is achieved from adult donors, EPCs may serve as a potential cell source to line the lumens of TEBVs.

Adipose-derived stem cells (ASCs) have been isolated via liposuction from adult patients undergoing vascular procedures, and thus may serve as a cell source for TEBVs with greater cell yields than EPCs in bone marrow [97]. ASCs have been isolated by enzymatically digesting subcutaneous fat, adhering cells to tissue culture plates for one week, and then negatively selecting for CD31 and CD45 [97]. The resulting cell population was positive for

CD13, CD29, and CD90 [97], which are common ASC surface antigens [98]. ASCs cultured with vascular endothelial growth factor (VEGF) expressed CD31, endothelial nitric oxide synthase (eNOS), and vWF, which are features of ECs [97]. Thus, ASCs derived from adult adipose tissue in patients with vascular disease may provide cells with an EC phenotype for tissue engineering applications with greater consistency and yield than EPCs derived from bone marrow [95,97].

Adipose tissue also contains differentiated ECs within capillaries. These microvascular ECs may be isolated quickly and thereby provide an immediate cell source in the operating room for tissue engineering applications. High yields of microvascular ECs were isolated from liposuction aspirates in a 1.5 hour procedure [72] and immediately formed an endothelial layer on synthetic grafts using a pressure sodding technique [99]. Together, these early reports showed great promise for clinical utility of microvascular ECs, yet clinical trials with microvascular EC-seeded grafts yielded mixed results with evidence of intimal thickening in microvascular EC-seeded grafts [100]. Further purification of the microvascular cell population to achieve an EC purity of greater than 90% has reduced thrombogenicity [101]. Thus, eliminating contaminating cells in microvascular EC isolates may improve the clinical potential of microvascular ECs for tissue engineering applications.

Allogeneic Cells

The possibility of utilizing allogeneic cells in TEBVs has the appeal of (1) eliminating invasive procedures for cell isolation and (2) expediting the time between a patient's identified need for a vascular graft and the availability of a vascular graft for that patient. For example, a graft with allogeneic cells may be available quickly if it is cryopreserved or otherwise stored to maintain cell viability. In contrast, use of autologous cells requires time for cell harvest and a cell culture period and/or a cell seeding procedure. TEBVs containing allogeneic cells rarely are implanted, however, because there is a risk of rejection associated with mismatches between donor and recipient major histocompatibility complex (MHC) antigens.

One potential use of allogeneic cells is to create a universal EC cell source, which may be used to line the lumen of any vascular graft. To reduce the risk of MHC mismatch, allogeneic ECs have been modified genetically to downregulate MHC class I expression via an intracellularly expressed antibody directed against MHC class I molecules [102].

Another possibility is to culture TEBVs from allogeneic cells and then decellularize grafts prior to implant. The benefits of this approach include having allogeneic cell banks that improve consistency in quality across large numbers of manufactured TEBVs, as well as provided biologic acellular grafts that may be available off the shelf for immediate implant or for seeding with cells prior to implant. Allogeneic cells used to culture TEBVs may be stem cells or cells from young donors. Another possible approach would be to transfect allogeneic adult cells with telomerase to extend cell lifespan [80]. Using allogeneic cell sources that tolerate many population doublings would minimize donor testing requirements and ensure consistency in quality across large batches of cultured TEBVs. Using allogeneic cells with normally expressed MHCs, however, likely would require removal of allogeneic cells prior to implant to reduce the risk of rejection.

Interestingly, allogeneic human embryonic stem cells may be tolerated in tissue engineered constructs. A recent study compared lymphocyte infiltration at one month in implanted human adult skin, undifferentiated human embryonic stem cells, and differentiated tissue fragments derived from human embryonic stem cell-induced teratomas [103]. Leukocyte infiltration was significant in human adult skin samples, absent in undifferentiated human embryonic stem cell samples, and minor in transplanted teratomas [103]. This study suggests that the immunostimulatory capacity of human embryonic stem cells is lower than that of adult human cells [103]. Several studies have focused on differentiation of human embryonic stem cells towards an EC phenotype, and have shown the potential of these cells to form blood vessels [104-106]. Human embryonic stem cells adhere to PLLA/PLGA (50%/50%) scaffolds, suggesting that they may be used for tissue engineering applications [104]. Further scientific study is required to understand human embryonic stem cells and their derivatives, such as differentiated ECs, must be performed prior to clinical use [107]. In addition, ethical controversies regarding the use of human embryonic stem cells must be addressed [108,109]. Yet, human embryonic stem cells and their differentiated derivatives show promise as potential allogeneic cell sources for tissue engineered constructs.

LARGE ANIMAL MODELS

Discussion of animal models in this chapter is limited to large animals, which contain large vessels that that allow implantation of vascular grafts with diameters of ≥ 3 mm. Dogs, pigs, and sheep are the common large animal models used for cardiac and vascular surgery [110], with dogs and pigs used more frequently for vascular applications and sheep used more frequently for heart valve studies [111]. Pigs grow rapidly, and heavy adult pigs are hard to handle [112]. Dogs, on the other hand, maintain adult weights that are easy to handle. Sheep have long necks, which makes it easy to work with their carotid arteries. Sheep also have large arteries, which allow testing of large diameter grafts. Pigs and sheep are comparable in price, and both are cheaper than dogs [113]. Dogs have been used for circulatory research for centuries [114], but given their status as a companion animal, their use in research is not popular in Western countries [112]. Nonetheless, the Society for Vascular Surgery and the International Society for Cardiovascular Surgery recommend dogs as the preferred preclinical animal model for many vascular studies [115].

Each animal has physiologic differences that affect graft outcomes. Pigs are less susceptible to hematogenous infection than dogs [116]. In addition, pigs endothelialize grafts quickly, whereas sheep and dogs endothelialize grafts more slowly [117]. It has been proposed that the rate of endothelial outgrowth may depend more on animal senescence than on interspecies variability [118]. Studies with sheep and pigs often use juvenile animals that are quick to endothelialize, whereas studies with dogs are often performed in adult animals, which leads to slower endothelialization [118]. Sheep have a higher incidence of clotting than dogs [119], but are slower to form neointimal hyperplasia than pigs [117]. Dogs can be hypercoagulable, which presents a stringent test of graft thrombogenicity [115]. Almost all animal models endothelialize vascular grafts more rapidly than humans, and therefore, absence of thrombus in animal models does not always translate into absence of thrombus in humans [111]. Animal models, however, provide a physiologic indicator of vascular graft function that cannot be predicted fully by in vitro studies.

Nonhuman primates have been used in rare cases to evaluate vascular grafts. Primates are phylogenetically closer to humans than pigs, dogs, or sheep, and therefore serve as a better model for human-based tissues. In addition, the clotting and fibrinolytic systems of primates are more closely related to humans [120]. Primates, however, are significantly more expensive than any other animal [113], and difficult to handle and maintain [112]. In addition, a limited number of primates are available, and therefore, it is more difficult to procure primates than pigs or dogs.

Comparisons of animal models for TEBV evaluation are difficult to perform. Isolation of cells from bone marrow, peripheral blood, or adipose tissue may rely on antibodies, which may not be available or equivalent in effectiveness for all species. Further, cellular growth and cellular protein synthesis may vary between species and with animal age. Thus, an attempt to create similar TEBVs for multiple species may not be possible based on the fact that cells from each species behave differently. Challenges based on differences between species in cellular behavior also are present during the translation of technology from animal testing to human clinical use.

Dogs

With a long history of use for vascular graft testing, the canine model remains popular. Dogs have been used to evaluate the approach of seeding bone marrow cells onto scaffolds. In one study, PLLA/P(CL/LA) scaffolds (8 mm in diameter) were incubated with autologous mononuclear bone marrow cells for 1.5–2 hours prior to implantation into the inferior vena cava of adult beagles [5]. No obstruction or thrombus was noted in grafts followed for 2–8 weeks or for 2 years, and almost complete endothelialization was seen at 4 weeks [5]. Further, seeded bone marrow cells differentiated in vivo into ECs and possibly also into SMCs [5]. One graft was evaluated 2 years after implant, and showed collagen and elastin deposition in addition to ECs and SMCs. A similar study was performed using a PGA/P(CL/LA) scaffold [121]. These studies support the feasibility of generating functional grafts using the approach of isolating cells, seeding them onto scaffolds, and implanting the constructs within hours of cell seeding.

Bone marrow cells also have been differentiated in vitro into cells with vascular phenotypes prior to scaffold seeding and canine implantation. Decellularized allogeneic canine carotid arteries (3 mm in diameter) were seeded with autologous bone marrow-derived cells with vascular phenotypes, cultured in vitro for 1 week, and implanted as end-to-end carotid interposition grafts in mongrel dogs [57]. Grafts seeded with cells remained patent up to 8 weeks. In contrast, all non-seeded grafts developed occlusive thrombus by 2 weeks. After 8 weeks in vivo, seeded grafts contained cells that stained positive for alpha-smooth muscle actin and smooth muscle myosin heavy-chain in the medial layer of the graft, and for vWF in the lumen of the graft, suggesting the presence of SMCs and ECs, respectively. Further, grafts explanted at 8 weeks contained collagen and elastin in an organizational pattern that resembled native vascular tissue.

The dog model has been used to study TEBVs with EPCs from peripheral blood. A type I collagen gel tube was wrapped with segmented PU to provide mechanical reinforcement [122]. Scaffolds (4.5 mm in diameter) were lined with autologous EPCs and implanted as end-to-end carotid artery interposition grafts in mongrel dogs for 1 or 3 months [122]. Of 12 implanted grafts, 11 were patent and 1 was partially occluded and dilated at one month. Three months after implantation, staining showed that cells in the lumens of the grafts were positive for vWF, cells in the middle of the collagen gel were positive for alpha-smooth muscle actin, and cells permeating the PU were positive for vimentin (likely fibroblasts) [122]. Further, collagen and proteoglycans were seen in histological sections 3 months after implantation, suggesting that the grafts were remodeling in vivo. The authors concluded that EPC-seeded grafts were promising for clinical use, but given the difficulties associated with consistent isolation and proliferation of EPCs from peripheral blood (harvest success rate of 15%), they suggested focusing future studies on EPCs derived from bone marrow [122].

TEBVs containing human cells also have been tested in dogs. The sheet-based tissue engineering approach was used to create TEBVs (4.2 mm in diameter) from human skin fibroblasts and saphenous vein ECs [62]. TEBVs were implanted as end-to-end interposition grafts in a canine femoral artery model with immunosuppression and anticoagulation therapy [62]. Even with immunosuppression, a massive immune response was seen at 14 days, indicating that the dog model is not appropriate for long-term testing of TEBVs that contain human cells [62].

Pigs

Swine have been used to evaluate the function of autologous and xenogenic tissue engineered constructs. Small caliber TEBVs were formed by culturing bovine or autologous porcine SMCs on PGA scaffolds. Two days after seeding with autologous ECs, TEBVs were implanted into the saphenous arteries of Yucatan miniature swine for up to 4 weeks with anticoagulation therapy, and with immunosuppression in the case of the xenograft [8]. TEBVs cultured with pulsatile strains in vitro remained patent at 4 weeks, whereas TEBVs cultured in static conditions in vitro formed thrombi at 3 weeks post implantation [8]. An inflammatory response was visible in the xenograft at 4 weeks post implantation, yet the graft remained patent [8]. Thus, a porcine model with immunosuppression was suitable for testing grafts of xenogenic origin for short implant periods.

Sheep

Sheep, which have large vessels, primarily have been used to test TEBVs with large diameters. TEBVs (15 mm in diameter) were formed on a P4-HB scaffold with autologous SMCs and ECs, and were implanted as descending aorta interposition grafts in a juvenile sheep model [41,42]. Tubular grafts were wrapped with SIS to provide mechanical support and to stimulate angiogenesis [42]. Grafts resisted thrombus and dilatation up to 6 weeks in vivo. Non-occluding thrombus was seen in grafts implanted for 12 and 24 weeks, and dilatation was seen at 24 weeks. Most of the graft remodeling occurred within 3 weeks of implantation, with increases in cellularity and collagen deposition, and minimal deposition of elastin [42]. The absence of leukocyte or giant cell infiltration, the absence of calcification, matrix deposition, and good long-term patency were positive outcomes for this technology. Evidence of dilatation at 6 months was worrisome, and the authors suggested that future studies should focus on elastic fiber formation [42].

TEBVs also have been tested in a large diameter venous ovine model. PGA/P(CL/LA) scaffolds (1.3 cm in diameter) were seeded with bone marrow-derived vascular cells, cultured for 7 days in vitro, and then implanted as interposition grafts in the inferior vena cava in a juvenile lamb model [86]. After 4 weeks in vivo, no thrombus or calcification was seen, about half of the polymer remained in the grafts, ECs and SMCs were present in the graft, and small amounts of extracellular matrix had been deposited [86].

Sheep carotid artery models have been used to evaluate small diameter grafts. Porcine iliac arteries (4 mm in diameter) were decellularized and seeded with autologous ovine EPCs isolated from peripheral blood of 1–2-week-old sheep [56]. EPC-seeded grafts implanted in an ovine carotid artery interposition model in juvenile sheep (~ 30 kg) remained patent with no signs of thrombus, obstruction, or aneurismal dilation at 15 (n = 3) or 130 days (n = 4). In contrast, non-EPC seeded grafts developed significant thrombus that occluded flow by day 5 in 3 of 4 grafts. The original anatomic features of implanted conduits, especially elastin, were retained at 130 days. A confluent monolayer of ECs was seen on EPC-seeded grafts explanted at both 15 and 130 days, and some of ECs also expressed the label used to identify EPCs at implant, indicating that EPCs were retained on the constructs in vivo. After 130 days, contractile SMCs had infiltrated the intimal layer. EPC-seeded grafts implanted for 130 days relaxed in response to acetylcholine, which was likely an NO-mediated response. The authors suggest that the NO activity of EPCs on implanted grafts contributed to high patency rates.

Sheep also have been used to evaluate TEBVs in a small diameter vein model. Ovine bone marrow-derived smooth muscle progenitor cells were embedded in fibrin gels, cultured for 2 weeks in vitro, seeded with bone marrow-derived endothelial cells, cultured for an additional 10 days, and implanted as jugular vein interposition grafts in a juvenile ovine model for 5 weeks [19]. Grafts were 4 mm in diameter. Explanted grafts contained ECs, SMCs, collagen, and elastin. The authors propose that bone marrow-derived smooth muscle progenitor cells may have a higher elastogenic potential than mature vascular smooth muscle cells [18,19].

Juvenile sheep are attractive as a model to study adaptation of TEBVs during biological growth, which is complete by 2 years of age in sheep [123]. PGA/P4-HB scaffolds (18 mm in diameter) cultured with myofibroblasts and seeded with ECs were implanted to replace an excised segment of pulmonary artery in juvenile sheep (~ 28 kg) [123]. No thrombus, calcification, stenosis, or aneurysm was seen in any graft at up to 100 weeks. TEBVs increased in length and diameter as the animals progressed through their biological growth cycle. Cellularity and glycosaminoglycan content of TEBVs at all explanted time points (20–100 weeks) were similar to those of native pulmonary arteries. Collagen content in the TEBVs increased during the 100-week implant period, and all explanted grafts had higher collagen densities than native pulmonary arteries. Explanted TEBVs were stronger and stiffer, but less compliant, than native pulmonary arteries. The authors suggest that TEBVs continue remodel up to 100 weeks in vivo, and that their findings support the possibility of using TEBVs to repair congenital defects.

Primates

Human-derived TEBVs were implanted in immunosuppressed cynomolgus primates [62]. Three grafts with diameters of 4.2 mm were implanted as iliac or aortic interposition grafts for 6–8 weeks. Grafts remained patent, resisted dilatation, were endothelialized, and showed evidence of remodeling [62]. A moderate immune response to the human TEBVs was seen in these immunosuppressed primates [62].

HUMAN CLINICAL TRIALS

Two clinical trials are underway for TEBVs. One clinical study evaluated the use of TEBVs as conduits for extracardiac total cavopulmonary connection (n = 23) in patients 1–24 years of age [6,124]. Grafts were constructed by seeding scaffolds made of P(CL/LA) and PGA or PLLA (12–24 mm in diameter) with mononuclear bone marrow cells. Cells were incubated on scaffolds for 2 to 4 hours to support cell attachment prior to implantation. Anticoagulation therapy included continuous injections of heparin in the early postoperative period, and after discharge from the hospital, 3 to 6 months of warfarin sodium and aspirin. One patient died 3 months postoperatively, but the death was not associated with the TEBV. Within the first week after operation, maximum values of C-reactive protein and maximum white blood cell counts were similar to those in a control group of patients. No thrombosis, stenosis, or obstruction of the TEBVs was seen at up to 32 months follow-up. Further, no calcification was seen, which is impressive given that young patients have high calcium turnover [6]. In addition, no aneurysm formation was seen, although graft diameters were increased by approximately 10% at follow-up. This study showed that TEBVs were functional up to at least 32 months in a high-diameter, low-pressure setting. Proving in vivo clinical utility is a promising step for the entire field of tissue engineering. Additional monitoring of graft function and remodeling during growth will be informative for understanding the future applicability of TEBVs to pediatric patients.

A second clinical trial evaluated TEBVs as arteriovenous grafts in an adult population (29–89 years of age) [125]. Ten patients were enrolled in a study with autologous TEBVs that were cultured with the sheet-based approach using biopsies of skin and superficial vein as cell sources [50,125]. After 3 months *in vivo*, grafts were punctured for hemodialysis access [125]. Of six grafts implanted to date, 2 have developed complications, including aneurysm, thrombosis, and dilatation [125]. One of the grafts became aneurismal near a site used for repeated puncturing. Following repair at 11.5 months, the aneurismal graft continued to function until the patient received a kidney transplant at 13 months. The TEBV withstood more than 200 punctures. One patient died with a functioning graft. A third graft was lost to thrombosis and dilatation at 12 weeks. The remaining three patients had no complications at up to 5 months post implantation. Given that primary patency rates for ePTFE used for upper extremity arteriovenous hemodialysis accesses are less than 50% at one year [126], the outcomes of this TEBV clinical study to date show promise for clinical use.

CONCLUSION

Many technologies show potential for advancing the field of vascular tissue engineering. Scaffolds with variable degradation properties may be chosen to provide support either for *in vitro* culture or for *in vivo* use. Alternatively, scaffolds may be made from decellularized tissues or may not be used at all. Advances in cell sourcing, particularly in stem and progenitor cell isolation, will likely play an important role in providing an autologous cell choice for TEBVs. Continued research in scaffold generation and cell sourcing may provide improvements for second and third generation TEBV products.

Preclinical evaluation of TEBVs in large animal models provides useful information that cannot be acquired in vitro. Although large animal studies are the best possible predictors of graft success prior to clinical trials, challenges exist with using outcomes of animal studies to predict success in humans. Thus, clinical trials must be performed. Technologies with successful outcomes in preclinical animal studies warrant testing in human clinical trials [5,6,124]. Technologies that are human-based and experience complications in xenogenic animal models also may warrant testing in human clinical trials [62,125].

The first two uses of TEBVs in the clinic yielded encouraging outcomes for the entire field of vascular tissue engineering, and particularly for approaches using PLLA, PGA, P(CL/LA) and sheet-based tissue engineering. These studies also show that isolation of sufficient numbers of autologous cells is feasible using bone marrow in a pediatric population, or using skin and veins in an adult population. Longer term clinical follow-ups will be important to determine the durability and long-term patency of TEBVs. Comparison studies relating the efficacy of TEBVs to that of grafts currently in clinical use, such as ePTFE, will be necessary to determine when TEBVs should be used instead of ePTFE or other grafts. It will be exciting to monitor the outcomes of ongoing and future clinical trials for TEBVs as the field of vascular tissue engineering transitions from research to the possibility of routine clinical use.

REFERENCES

[1]   Rosamond, W; Flegal, K; Friday, G; Furie, K; Go, A; Greenlund, K, et al. Heart disease and stroke statistics—2007 update: A report from the American Heart Association statistics committee and stroke statistics subcommittee. *Circulation* 2007;115:e69-e171.

[2]   Hehrlein, F; Schlepper, M; Loskot, F; Scheld, H; Walter, P; Mulch, J. The use of expanded polytetrafluoroethylene (PTFE) grafts for myocardial revascularization. *J Cardiovasc Surg* 1984;25:549-553.

[3]   Sayers, RD, Raptis, S., Berce, M., Miller, J.H. Long-term results of femorotibial bypass with vein or polytetrafluoroethylene. *British Journal of Surgery* 1998;85:934-938.

[4]   O'Donnell, TF, Jr.; Mackey, W; McCullough, JL, Jr.; Maxwell, SL, Jr.; Farber, SP; Deterling, RA, et al. Correlation of operative findings with angiographic and noninvasive hemodynamic factors associated with failure of polytetrafluoroethylene grafts. *J Vasc Surg* 1984;1:136-48.

[5]   Matsumura, G; Miyagawa-Tomita, S; Shin'oka, T; Ikada, Y; Kurosawa, H. First evidence that bone marrow cells contribute to the construction of tissue-engineered vascular autografts in vivo. *Circulation* 2003;108:1729-34.

[6]   Shin'oka, T; Matsumura, G; Hibino, N; Naito, Y; Watanabe, M; Konuma, T, et al. Midterm clinical result of tissue-engineered vascular autografts seeded with autologous bone marrow cells. *J Thorac Cardiovasc Surg* 2005;129:1330-8.

[7]   L'Heureux, N; Paquet, S; Labbe, R; Germain, L; Auger, FA. A completely biological tissue-engineered human blood vessel. *FASEB Journal* 1998;12:47-56.

[8]   Niklason, LE; Gao, J; Abbott, WM; Hirschi, K; Houser, S; Marini, R, et al. Functional arteries grown in vitro. *Science* 1999;284:489-493.

[9]   Weinberg, CB; Bell, E. A blood vessel model constructed from collagen and cultured vascular cells. *Science* 1986;231:397-400.

[10]   Hirai, J; Matsuda, T. Venous reconstruction using hybrid vascular tissue composed of vascular cells and collagen: Tissue regeneration process. *Cell Transplantation* 1996;5:93-105.

[11]   Tranquillo, RT; Girton, TS; Bromberek, BA; Triebes, TG; Mooradian, DL. Magnetically orientated tissue-equivalent tubes: Application to a circumferentially orientated media-equivalent. *Biomaterials* 1996;17:349-357.

[12]   Seliktar, D; Black, RA; Vito, RP; Nerem, RM. Dynamic mechanical conditioning of collagen-gel blood vessel constructs induces remodeling in vitro. *Annals of Biomedical Engineering* 2000;28:351-362.

[13]   Grassl, ED; Oegema, TR; Tranquillo, RT. A fibrin-based arterial media equivalent. *J Biomed Mater Res* 2003;66A:550-561.

[14]   Thie, M; Schlumberger, W; Semich, R; Rauterberg, J; Robenek, H. Aortic smooth muscle cells in collagen lattice culture: Effects on ultrastructure, proliferation and collagen synthesis. *Eur J Cell Biol* 1991;55:295-304.

[15]   Girton, TS; Oegema, TR; Tranquillo, RT. Exploiting glycation to stiffen and strengthen tissue equivalents for tissue engineering. *Journal of Biomedical Materials Research* 1999;46:87-92.

[16]   Isenberg, BC; Tranquillo, RT. Long-term cyclic distention enhances the mechanical properties of collagen-based media-equivalents. *Ann Biomed Eng* 2003;31:937-49.

[17]   Long, JL; Tranquillo, RT. Elastic fiber production in cardiovascular tissue-equivalents. *Matrix Biology* 2003;22:339-350.

[18]   Swartz, DD; Russell, JA; Andreadis, ST. Engineering of fibrin-based functional and implantable small-diameter blood vessels. *Am J Physiol Heart Circ Physiol* 2005;288:H1451-60.

[19]   Liu, JY; Swartz, DD; Peng, HF; Gugino, SF; Russell, JA; Andreadis, ST. Functional tissue-engineered blood vessels from bone marrow progenitor cells. *Cardiovasc Res* 2007;75:618-28.

[20]   Isenberg, BC; Williams, C; Tranquillo, RT. Endothelialization and flow conditioning of fibrin-based media-equivalents. *Ann Biomed Eng* 2006;34:971-85.

[21]   Remuzzi, A; Mantero, S; Colombo, M; Morigi, M; Binda, E; Camozzi, D, et al. Vascular smooth muscle cells on hyaluronic acid: Culture and mechanical characterization of an engineered vascular construct. *Tissue Eng* 2004;10:699-710.

[22]   Campoccia, D; Doherty, P; Radice, M; Brun, P; Abatangelo, G; Williams, DF. Semisynthetic resorbable materials from hyaluronan esterification. *Biomaterials* 1998;19:2101-27.

[23]   Benedetti, L; Cortivo, R; Berti, T; Berti, A; Pea, F; Mazzo, M, et al. Biocompatibility and biodegradation of different hyaluronan derivatives (hyaff) implanted in rats. *Biomaterials* 1993;14:1154-60.

[24]   Turner, NJ; Kielty, CM; Walker, MG; Canfield, AE. A novel hyaluronan-based biomaterial (hyaff-11) as a scaffold for endothelial cells in tissue engineered vascular grafts. *Biomaterials* 2004;25:5955-64.

[25]   Gunatillake, PA; Adhikari, R. Biodegradable synthetic polymers for tissue engineering. *Eur Cell Mater* 2003;5:1-16.

[26]   Freed, LE; Vunjak-Novakovic, G; Biron, RJ; Eagles, DB; Lesnoy, DC; Barlow, SK, et al. Biodegradable polymer scaffolds for tissue engineering. *Bio/Technology* 1994;12:689-693.

[27]   Gao, J; Niklason, LE; Langer, RS. Surface hydrolysis of poly(glycolic acid) meshes increases the seeding density of vascular smooth muscle cells. *Journal of Biomedical Materials Research* 1998;42:417-424.

[28]   Atthoff, B; Hilborn, J. Protein adsorption onto polyester surfaces: Is there a need for surface activation? *J Biomed Mater Res B Appl Biomater* 2007;80:121-30.

[29]   Chu, CF; Lu, A; Liszkowski, M; Sipehia, R. Enhanced growth of animal and human endothelial cells on biodegradable polymers. *Biochim Biophys Acta* 1999;1472:479-85.

[30]   Ye, Q; Zund, G; Jockenhoevel, S; Schoeberlein, A; Hoerstrup, SP; Grunenfelder, J, et al. Scaffold precoating with human autologous extracellular matrix for improved cell attachment in cardiovascular tissue engineering. *Asaio J* 2000;46:730-3.

[31]   Prabhakar, V; Grinstaff, MW; Alarcon, J; Knors, C; Solan, AK; Niklason, LE. Engineering porcine arteries: Effects of scaffold modification. *J Biomed Mater Res* 2003;67A:303-311.

[32]   Niklason, LE; Abbott, WA; Gao, J; Klagges, B; Hirschi, KK; Ulubayram, K, et al. Morphologic and mechanical characteristics of engineered bovine arteries. *Journal of Vascular Surgery* 2001;33:628-638.

[33]   Jonnalagadda, S; Robinson, DH. Effect of thickness and PEG addition on the hydrolytic degradation of PLLA. *J Biomater Sci Polym Ed* 2004;15:1317-26.

[34]   Skarja, GA; Woodhouse, KA. In vitro degradation and erosion of degradable, segmented polyurethanes containing an amino acid-based chain extender. *J Biomater Sci Polym Ed* 2001;12:851-73.

[35]   Guan, J; Wagner, WR. Synthesis, characterization and cytocompatibility of polyurethaneurea elastomers with designed elastase sensitivity. *Biomacromolecules* 2005;6:2833-42.

[36]   Stock, UA; Sakamoto, T; Hatsuoka, S; Martin, DP; Nagashima, M; Moran, AM, et al. Patch augmentation of the pulmonary artery with bioabsorbable polymers and autologous cell seeding. *J Thorac Cardiovasc Surg* 2000;120:1158-67.

[37]   Williamson, MR; Black, R; Kielty, C. Pcl-pu composite vascular scaffold production for vascular tissue engineering: Attachment, proliferation and bioactivity of human vascular endothelial cells. *Biomaterials* 2006;27:3608-16.

[38]   Santerre, JP; Woodhouse, K; Laroche, G; Labow, RS. Understanding the biodegradation of polyurethanes: From classical implants to tissue engineering materials. *Biomaterials* 2005;26:7457-70.

[39]   Tiwari, A; Salacinski, H; Seifalian, AM; Hamilton, G. New prostheses for use in bypass grafts with special emphasis on polyurethanes. *Cardiovasc Surg* 2002;10:191-7.

[40]   Guan, J; Fujimoto, KL; Sacks, MS; Wagner, WR. Preparation and characterization of highly porous, biodegradable polyurethane scaffolds for soft tissue applications. *Biomaterials* 2005;26:3961-71.

[41]   Opitz, F; Schenke-Layland, K; Richter, W; Martin, DP; Degenkolbe, I; Wahlers, T, et al. Tissue engineering of ovine aortic blood vessel substitutes using applied shear stress and enzymatically derived vascular smooth muscle cells. *Ann Biomed Eng* 2004;32:212-22.

[42]   Opitz, F; Schenke-Layland, K; Cohnert, TU; Starcher, B; Halbhuber, KJ; Martin, DP, et al. Tissue engineering of aortic tissue: Dire consequence of suboptimal elastic fiber synthesis in vivo. *Cardiovasc Res* 2004;63:719-30.

[43]   Watanabe, M; Shin'oka, T; Tohyama, S; Hibino, N; Konuma, T; Matsumura, G, et al. Tissue-engineered vascular autograft: Inferior vena cava replacement in a dog model. *Tissue Eng* 2001;7:429-39.

[44]   Li, WJ; Cooper, JA, Jr.; Mauck, RL; Tuan, RS. Fabrication and characterization of six electrospun poly(alpha-hydroxy ester)-based fibrous scaffolds for tissue engineering applications. *Acta Biomater* 2006;2:377-85.

[45]   Li, WJ; Laurencin, CT; Caterson, EJ; Tuan, RS; Ko, FK. Electrospun nanofibrous structure: A novel scaffold for tissue engineering. *J Biomed Mater Res* 2002;60:613-21.

[46]   He, W; Yong, T; Teo, WE; Ma, Z; Ramakrishna, S. Fabrication and endothelialization of collagen-blended biodegradable polymer nanofibers: Potential vascular graft for blood vessel tissue engineering. *Tissue Eng* 2005;11:1574-88.

[47]   Stitzel, J; Liu, J; Lee, SJ; Komura, M; Berry, J; Soker, S, et al. Controlled fabrication of a biological vascular substitute. *Biomaterials* 2006;27:1088-94.

[48]   Lee, SJ; Yoo, JJ; Lim, GJ; Atala, A; Stitzel, J. In vitro evaluation of electrospun nanofiber scaffolds for vascular graft application. *J Biomed Mater Res A* 2007.

[49]   Telemeco, TA; Ayres, C; Bowlin, GL; Wnek, GE; Boland, ED; Cohen, N, et al. Regulation of cellular infiltration into tissue engineering scaffolds composed of submicron diameter fibrils produced by electrospinning. *Acta Biomater* 2005;1:377-85.

[50]   L'Heureux, N; Dusserre, N; Marini, A; Garrido, S; de la Fuente, L; McAllister, T. Technology insight: The evolution of tissue-engineered vascular grafts--from research to clinical practice. *Nat Clin Pract Cardiovasc Med* 2007;4:389-95.

[51]   Mitchell, SL; Niklason, LE. Requirements for growing tissue engineered vascular grafts. *Cardiovascular Pathology* 2003;12:59-64.

[52]   Amiel, GE; Komura, M; Shapira, O; Yoo, JJ; Yazdani, S; Berry, J, et al. Engineering of blood vessels from acellular collagen matrices coated with human endothelial cells. *Tissue Eng* 2006;12:2355-65.

[53]   Badylak, SF; Lantz, GC; Coffey, A; Geddes, LA. Small intestinal submucosa as a large diameter vascular graft in the dog. *J Surg Res* 1989;47:74-80.

[54]   Huynh, T; Abraham, G; Murray, J; Brockbank, K; Hagen, P-O; Sullivan, S. Remodeling of an acellular collagen graft into a physiologically responsive neovessel. *Nature Biotechnology* 1999;17:1083-1086.

[55]   Teebken, OE; Bader, A; Steinhoff, G; Haverich, A. Tissue engineering of vascular grafts: Human cell seeding of decellularised porcine matrix. *Eur J Vasc Endovasc Surg* 2000;19:381-6.

[56]   Kaushal, S; Amiel, GE; Guleserian, KJ; Shapira, OM; Perry, T; Sutherland, FW, et al. Functional small-diameter neovessels created using endothelial progenitor cells expanded ex vivo. *Nat Med* 2001;7:1035-40.

[57]   Cho, SW; Lim, SH; Kim, IK; Hong, YS; Kim, SS; Yoo, KJ, et al. Small-diameter blood vessels engineered with bone marrow-derived cells. *Ann Surg* 2005;241:506-15.

[58]   Livesy, SA; del Campo, AA; Nag, A; Nichols, KB; Coleman, C, Livesy, SA; del Campo, AA; Nag, A; Nichols, KB; Coleman, CLivesy, SA; del Campo, AA; Nag, A; Nichols, KB; Coleman, Cs; LifeCell Corporation, assignee. Method for processing and preserving collagen-based tissues for transplantation. United States. 1994 Aug 9.

[59]   Dahl, SLM; Koh, J; Prabhakar, V; Niklason, LE. Decellularized native and engineered arterial scaffolds for transplantation. *Cell Transplantation* 2003;12:659-666.

[60]   Allaire, E; Bruneval, P; Mandet, C; Becquemin, JP; Michel, JB. The immunogenicity of the extracellular matrix in arterial xenografts. *Surgery* 1997;122:73-81.

[61]   Sclafani, AP; Romo, T, 3rd; Jacono, AA; McCormick, S; Cocker, R; Parker, A. Evaluation of acellular dermal graft in sheet (AlloDerm) and injectable (micronized alloderm) forms for soft tissue augmentation. Clinical observations and histological analysis. *Arch Facial Plast Surg* 2000;2:130-6.

[62]   L'Heureux, N; Dusserre, N; Konig, G; Victor, B; Keire, P; Wight, TN, et al. Human tissue-engineered blood vessels for adult arterial revascularization. *Nat Med* 2006;12:361-365.

[63]   Campbell, JH, Efendy, J.L., Campbell, G.R. Novel vascular graft grown within recipient's own peritoneal cavity. *Circulation Research* 1999;85:1173-1178.

[64]   Chue, WL; Campbell, GR; Caplice, N; Muhammed, A; Berry, CL; Thomas, AC, et al. Dog peritoneal and pleural cavities as bioreactors to grow autologous vascular grafts. *J Vasc Surg* 2004;39:859-67.

[65]   Sparks, CH. Silicone mandril method for growing reinforced autogenous femoro-popliteal artery grafts in situ. *Ann Surg* 1973;177:293-300.

[66]   Davies, AH; Magee, TR; Baird, RN; Sheffield, E; Horrocks, M. Vein compliance: A preoperative indicator of vein morphology and of veins at risk of vascular graft stenosis. *British Journal of Surgery* 1992;79:1019-1021.

[67]   Abbott, WM; Megerman, J; Hasson, JE; L'Italien, GJ; Warnock, DJ. Effect of compliance mismatch on vascular graft patency. *Journal of Vascular Surgery* 1987;5:376-382.

[68]   Seifalian, AM; Tiwari, A; Hamilton, G; Salacinski, HJ. Improving the clinical patency of prosthetic vascular and coronary bypass grafts: The role of seeding and tissue engineering. *Artif Organs* 2002;26:307-20.

[69]   Ortenwall, P; Wadenvik, H; Kutti, J; Risberg, B. Endothelial cell seeding reduces thrombogenicity of Dacron grafts in humans. *J Vasc Surg* 1990;11:403-10.

[70]   Deutsch, M; Meinhart, J; Fischlein, T; Preiss, P; Zilla, P. Clinical autologous in vitro endothelialization of infrainguinal ePTFE grafts in 100 patients: A 9-year experience. *Surgery* 1999;126:847-855.

[71]   Rosenman, JE; Kempczinski, RF; Pearce, WH; Silberstein, EB. Kinetics of endothelial cell seeding. *J Vasc Surg* 1985;2:778-84.

[72]   Williams, SK; Jarrell, BE; Rose, DG; Pontell, J; Kapelan, BA; Park, PK, et al. Human microvessel endothelial cell isolation and vascular graft sodding in the operating room. *Ann Vasc Surg* 1989;3:146-52.

[73]   Perea, H; Aigner, J; Hopfner, U; Wintermantel, E. Direct magnetic tubular cell seeding: A novel approach for vascular tissue engineering. *Cells Tissues Organs* 2006;183:156-65.

[74]   Shimizu, K; Ito, A; Arinobe, M; Murase, Y; Iwata, Y; Narita, Y, et al. Effective cell-seeding technique using magnetite nanoparticles and magnetic force onto decellularized blood vessels for vascular tissue engineering. *J Biosci Bioeng* 2007;103:472-8.

[75]   Thyberg, J. Differentiated properties and proliferation of arterial smooth muscle cells in culture. *Int Rev Cytol* 1996;169:183-265.

[76]   Leung, BM; Sefton, MV. A modular tissue engineering construct containing smooth muscle cells and endothelial cells. *Ann Biomed Eng* 2007.

[77]   Kadletz, M, Moser, R., Preiss, P., Deutsch, M., Zilla, P., Fasol, R. In vitro lining of fibronectin coated PTFE grafts with cryopreserved saphenous vein endothelial cells. *Thoracic & Cardiovascular Surgeon* 1987;35:143-147.

[78]   Bader, A; Steinhoff, G; Strobl, K; Schilling, T; Brandes, G; Mertsching, H, et al. Engineering of human vascular aortic tissue based on a xenogeneic starter matrix. *Transplantation* 2000;70:7-14.

[79]   Grenier, G; Remy-Zolghadri, M; Guignard, R; Bergeron, F; Labbe, R; Auger, FA, et al. Isolation and culture of the three vascular cell types from a small vein biopsy sample. *In Vitro Cell Dev Biol Anim* 2003;39:131-9.

[80]   Poh, M; Boyer, M; Solan, A; Dahl, SL; Pedrotty, D; Banik, SS, et al. Blood vessels engineered from human cells. *The Lancet* 2005;365:2122-2124.

[81]   Tiwari, A; Salacinski, HJ; Hamilton, G; Seifalian, AM. Tissue engineering of vascular bypass grafts: Role of endothelial cell extraction. *Eur J Vasc Endovasc Surg* 2001;21:193-201.

[82]   Radomski, JS; Jarrell, BE; Pratt, KJ; Williams, SK. Effects of in vitro aging on human endothelial cell adherence to dacron vascular graft material. *J Surg Res* 1989;47:173-7.

[83]   Bierman, EL. The effect of donor age on the in vitro life span of cultured human areterial smooth-muscle cells. *In Vitro* 1978;14:951-955.

[84]   McKee, JA; Banik, SS; Boyer, MJ; Hamad, NM; Lawson, JH; Niklason, LE, et al. Human arteries engineered in vitro. *EMBO Rep* 2003;4:633-638.

[85]   Klinger, RY; Blum, JL; Hearn, B; Lebow, B; Niklason, LE. Relevance and safety of telomerase for human tissue engineering. *Proc Natl Acad Sci U S A* 2006;103:2500-5.

[86]   Roh, JD; Brennan, MP; Lopez-Soler, RI; Fong, PM; Goyal, A; Dardik, A, et al. Construction of an autologous tissue-engineered venous conduit from bone marrow-derived vascular cells: Optimization of cell harvest and seeding techniques. *J Pediatr Surg* 2007;42:198-202.

[87]   Hashi, CK; Zhu, Y; Yang, GY; Young, WL; Hsiao, BS; Wang, K, et al. Antithrombogenic property of bone marrow mesenchymal stem cells in nanofibrous vascular grafts. *Proc Natl Acad Sci U S A* 2007;104:11915-20.

[88]   Charbord, P; Lerat, H; Newton, I; Tamayo, E; Gown, AM; Singer, JW, et al. The cytoskeleton of stromal cells from human bone marrow cultures resembles that of cultured smooth muscle cells. *Exp Hematol* 1990;18:276-82.

[89]   Shi, Q, Raffi, S., Wu, M.H., Wijelath, E.S., Yu, C., Ishida, A., Fujita, Y., Kothari, S., Mohle, R., Sauvage, L.R., Moore, M.A., Storb, R.F., Hammond, W.P. Evidence for circulating bone marrow-derived endothelial cells. *Blood* 1998;92:362-367.

[90]   Ishikawa, M; Asahara, T. Endothelial progenitor cell culture for vascular regeneration. *Stem Cells Dev* 2004;13:344-9.

[91]   Arakawa, E; Hasegawa, K; Yanai, N; Obinata, M; Matsuda, Y. A mouse bone marrow stromal cell line, TBR-B, shows inducible expression of smooth muscle-specific genes. *FEBS Lett* 2000;481:193-6.

[92]   Hamilton, DW; Maul, TM; Vorp, DA. Characterization of the response of bone marrow-derived progenitor cells to cyclic strain: Implications for vascular tissue-engineering applications. *Tissue Eng* 2004;10:361-9.

[93]   Asahara, T, Murohara, T., Sullivan, A., Silver, M., van der Zee, R., Li, T., Witzenbichler, B., Schatteman, G., Isner, J.M. Isolation of putative progenitor endothelial cells for angiogenesis. *Science* 1997;275:964-967.

[94]   Peichev, M; Naiyer, AJ; Pereira, D; Zhu, Z; Lane, WJ; Williams, M, et al. Expression of VEGFR-2 and AC133 by circulating human CD34(+) cells identifies a population of functional endothelial precursors. *Blood* 2000;95:952-8.

[95]   Dzau, VJ; Gnecchi, M; Pachori, AS; Morello, F; Melo, LG. Therapeutic potential of endothelial progenitor cells in cardiovascular diseases. *Hypertension* 2005;46:7-18.

[96]   Schmidt, D; Breymann, C; Weber, A; Guenter, CI; Neuenschwander, S; Zund, G, et al. Umbilical cord blood derived endothelial progenitor cells for tissue engineering of vascular grafts. *Ann Thorac Surg* 2004;78:2094-8.

[97]   DiMuzio, P; Tulenko, T. Tissue engineering applications to vascular bypass graft development: The use of adipose-derived stem cells. *J Vasc Surg* 2007;45 Suppl A:A99-103.

[98]   Katz, AJ; Tholpady, A; Tholpady, SS; Shang, H; Ogle, RC. Cell surface and transcriptional characterization of human adipose-derived adherent stromal (hADAS) cells. *Stem Cells* 2005;23:412-23.

[99]   Rupnick, MA; Hubbard, FA; Pratt, K; Jarrell, BE; Williams, SK. Endothelialization of vascular prosthetic surfaces after seeding or sodding with human microvascular endothelial cells. *J Vasc Surg* 1989;9:788-95.

[100]   Schmidt, SP; Meerbaum, SO; Anderson, JM; Clarke, RE; Zellers, RA; Sharp, WV. Evaluation of expanded polytetrafluoroethylene arteriovenous access grafts onto which microvessel-derived cells were transplanted to "improve" graft performance: Preliminary results. *Ann Vasc Surg* 1998;12:405-11.

[101]   Arts, CH; Blankensteijn, JD; Heijnen-Snyder, GJ; Verhagen, HJ; Hedeman Joosten, PP; Sixma, JJ, et al. Reduction of non-endothelial cell contamination of microvascular endothelial cell seeded grafts decreases thrombogenicity and intimal hyperplasia. *Eur J Vasc Endovasc Surg* 2002;23:404-12.

[102]   Doebis, C; Schu, S; Ladhoff, J; Busch, A; Beyer, F; Reiser, J, et al. An anti-major histocompatibility complex class I intrabody protects endothelial cells from an attack by immune mediators. *Cardiovasc Res* 2006;72:331-8.

[103]   Drukker, M; Katchman, H; Katz, G; Even-Tov Friedman, S; Shezen, E; Hornstein, E, et al. Human embryonic stem cells and their differentiated derivatives are less susceptible to immune rejection than adult cells. *Stem Cells* 2006;24:221-9.

[104]   Levenberg, S; Huang, NF; Lavik, E; Rogers, AB; Itskovitz-Eldor, J; Langer, R. Differentiation of human embryonic stem cells on three-dimensional polymer scaffolds. *Proc Natl Acad Sci U S A* 2003;100:12741-6.

[105]   Levenberg, S; Golub, JS; Amit, M; Itskovitz-Eldor, J; Langer, R. Endothelial cells derived from human embryonic stem cells. *Proc Natl Acad Sci U S A* 2002;99:4391-6.

[106]   Gerecht-Nir, S; Ziskind, A; Cohen, S; Itskovitz-Eldor, J. Human embryonic stem cells as an in vitro model for human vascular development and the induction of vascular differentiation. *Lab Invest* 2003;83:1811-20.

[107]   Levenberg, S; Zoldan, J; Basevitch, Y; Langer, R. Endothelial potential of human embryonic stem cells. *Blood* 2007;110:806-14.

[108]   Brock, DW. Is a consensus possible on stem cell research? Moral and political obstacles. *J Med Ethics* 2006;32:36-42.

[109]   Parker, C. Ethics for embryos. *J Med Ethics* 2007;33:614-616.

[110]   Bianco, RW; Grehan, JF; Grubbs, BC; Mrachek, JP; Schroeder, EL; Schumacher, CW, et al. Large animal models in cardiac and vascular biomaterials research and testing. In: Ratner, BD, Schoen, FJ, Hoffman, AS, Lemons, JE, editors. *Biomaterials science: An introduction to materials in medicine.* Second ed. Elsevier Science & Technology Books; 2004.

[111]   Northup, SJ. In vitro assessment of tissue compatibility. In: Ratner, BD, Schoen, FJ, Hoffman, AS, Lemons, JE, editors. *Biomaterials science: An introduction to materials in medicine.* Second ed. Elsevier Science & Technology Books; 2004.

[112]   Narayanaswamy, M; Wright, KC; Kandarpa, K. Animal models for atherosclerosis, restenosis, and endovascular graft research. *Journal of Vascular and Interventional Radiology* 2000;11:5-17.

[113]   Rashid, ST; Salacinski, HJ; Hamilton, G; Seifalian, AM. The use of animal models in developing the discipline of cardiovascular tissue engineering: A review. *Biomaterials* 2004;25:1627-37.

[114]   Svedsen, P; Hau, J. *Handbook of laboratory animal science, animal models.* Vol. II. Boca Raton, FL: CRC Press Inc.; 1994.

[115]   Abbott, WM; Callow, A; Moore, W; Rutherford, R; Veith, F; Weinberg, S. Evaluation and performance standards for arterial prostheses. *J Vasc Surg* 1993;17:746-56.

[116]   Ricci, MA; Mehran, RJ; Petsikas, D; Mohamed, F; Guidoin, R; Marois, Y, et al. Species differences in the infectability of vascular grafts. *J Invest Surg* 1991;4:45-52.

[117]   Ueberrueck, T; Tautenhahn, J; Meyer, L; Kaufmann, O; Lippert, H; Gastinger, I, et al. Comparison of the ovine and porcine animal models for biocompatibility testing of vascular prostheses. *J Surg Res* 2005;124:305-11.

[118]   Zilla, P; Bezuidenhout, D; Human, P. Prosthetic vascular grafts: Wrong models, wrong questions and no healing. *Biomaterials* 2007;28:5009-27.

[119]   Ortenwall, P; Bylock, A; Kjellstrom, BT; Risberg, B. Seeding of ePTFE carotid interposition grafts in sheep and dogs: Species-dependent results. *Surgery* 1988;103:199-205.

[120]   Mason, RG; Read, MS. Some species differences in fibrinolysis and blood coagulation. *J Biomed Mater Res* 1971;5:121–128.

[121]   Matsumura, G; Ishihara, Y; Miyagawa-Tomita, S; Ikada, Y; Matsuda, S; Kurosawa, H, et al. Evaluation of tissue-engineered vascular autografts. *Tissue Eng* 2006;12:3075-83.

[122]   He, H, Shirota, T., Yasui, H., Matsuda, T. Canine endotehlial progenitor cell-lined hybrid vascular graft with nonthrombogenic potential. *Journal of Thoracic and Cadiovascular Surgery* 2003;126:455-464.

[123]   Hoerstrup, SP; Cummings Mrcs, I; Lachat, M; Schoen, FJ; Jenni, R; Leschka, S, et al. Functional growth in tissue-engineered living, vascular grafts: Follow-up at 100 weeks in a large animal model. *Circulation* 2006;114:I159-66.

[124]   Shin'oka, T; Imai, Y; Ikada, Y. Transplantation of a tissue-engineered pulmonary artery. *N Engl J Med* 2001;344:532-3.

[125]   L'Heureux, N; McAllister, TN; de la Fuente, LM. Tissue-engineered blood vessel for adult arterial revascularization. *N Engl J Med* 2007;357:1451-3.

[126]   Huber, TS; Carter, JW; Carter, RL; Seeger, JM. Patency of autogenous and polytetrafluoroethylene upper extremity arteriovenous hemodialysis accesses: A systematic review. *J Vasc Surg* 2003;38:1005-11.

In: Encyclopedia of Stem Cell Research (2 Volume Set)   ISBN: 978-1-61761-835-2
Editor: Alexander L. Greene   © 2012 Nova Science Publishers, Inc.

Chapter XXXI

SKELETAL MUSCLE TISSUE ENGINEERING USING ADIPOSE TISSUE DERIVED STEM CELLS

MiJung Kim [*] *and Yu Suk Choi*

Department of Laboratory Medicine,
University of Ulsan College of Medicine/Cell and Molecular Biology Laboratory,
Asan Institute for Life Sciences, Asan Medical Center, University of Ulsan, Seoul, Korea

ABSTRACT

The use of adult stem cells for cell-based tissue engineering and regeneration represents a promising approach for repairing damaged tissue. This emerging field of regenerative medicine will require a reliable source of stem cells in addition to biomaterial scaffolds and growth factors. Recent studies have shown that stem cells can be isolated from a wide variety of tissues including bone marrow, muscle, and adipose tissue. The cellular component of this regenerative approach will play a key role in bringing tissue-engineered constructs from the laboratory bench to the clinical bedside. An ideal source of stem cells still remains undefined, however, and may differ depending upon the required application.

Muscle tissue engineering approaches could revolutionize current therapies for irreversible skeletal muscle damage and muscular dystrophies, and may significantly improve the quality of life of millions of patients. Skeletal muscle tissue engineering approaches rely mainly on myoblasts and biomaterials; however, myoblasts lack expansion capability. Cells from other sources, including adult stem cells, are being investigated to overcome this problem. Several cell sources have been proposed for creation of engineered skeletal tissue, but the literature to date unfortunately does not assist in the identification of an ideal cell source. We describe here the advantages and limitations of candidate cell sources for skeletal muscle tissue engineering.

[*] Correspondence concerning this article should be addressed to: Associate Professor of Dept. of Laboratory Medicine, University of Ulsan College of Medicine / Cell & Molecular Biology Lab., AILS, Seoul, Korea. e-mail: mjkimhsc@korea.com, Fax: 82-2-3010-4182.

As with bone marrow, adipose tissue is a mesoderm-derived organ that contains a stromal population including microvascular endothelial cells, smooth muscle cells, and stem cells. This population shares many characteristics with its bone marrow counterpart including extensive proliferative potential and an ability to undergo multilinear differentiation. Adipose tissue also has the ability to dynamically expand and shrink throughout the life of an adult. This capacity is mediated by the presence of vascular and non-vascular cells that provide a pool of stem and progenitor cells with unique regenerative capacities. Human adipose tissue-derived adult stem cells (ASCs) therefore meet many of the requirements of "ideal" cells for stem cell therapy and tissue engineering. ASCs have been used in cell-based tissue engineering of hard tissues such as bone and cartilage, but their capacity to assist in regeneration of damaged muscle has not yet been investigated in detail.

Here we review recent progress in the muscle tissue engineering field and describe one of our experiments as an example of successful skeletal muscle tissue engineering. We engineered skeletal muscle tissue using a combination of ASCs and injectable PLGA spheres. These findings suggest that mixtures of ASCs and injectable scaffolds may provide excellent tools for muscle tissue engineering and that such combinations may find applications in clinical settings requiring muscle tissue regeneration therapy.

1. INTRODUCTION

Loss of voluntary power of skeletal muscle may result from interruption of innervation or may occur because of deficiency in or loss of muscle mass. Muscle loss or deficiency may be primary in congenital anomalies such as Prune-belly syndrome and advanced forms of anal atresia, or may be secondary after radical resection of malignant tumors, trauma, or surgical interventions. Intrinsic diseases such as muscular dystrophies (Duchenne type or Steinert's disease), periodic diseases (Myasthenia gravis), developmental defects (hypoplasia or aplasia), and endocrine or metabolic disturbances, are also responsible for functional losses of skeletal muscle [1].

Skeletal muscles are composed of bundles of highly oriented and dense muscle fibers, each being a multinucleated cell derived from a myoblast. The muscle fibers in native skeletal muscle are closely packed together in an extracellular three-dimensional matrix to form an organized tissue with high cell density and an advanced degree of cellular orientation, to generate longitudinal contraction. After muscle injuries, myofibers become necrotic and are removed by macrophages [2]. A specialized myoblast subpopulation termed satellite cells, scattered below the basal lamina of myofibers, is capable of muscle regeneration [3]. The incidence of satellite cells in skeletal muscle is very low (1–5%) and depends on age and muscle fiber composition [4]. These cells usually remain in a quiescent and undifferentiated state but can enter the mitotic cycle in response to specific local factors [5]. Such factors include proliferation and fusion of myoblasts to form multinucleated and elongated myotubes, which self-assemble to form a more organized structure, namely the muscle fiber [3]. Satellite cells migrate to and proliferate in injured areas and can also form a connective tissue network ("muscle fibrosis"). This process is termed "scar tissue formation" and leads to loss of muscle functionality [5,6].

Tissue engineering is a fast-developing field that aims to create or regenerate tissues and organs by using combinations of cells, scaffolds, and/or biomolecules. Tissue engineering strategies promise to revolutionize current therapies for irreversible skeletal muscle damage, such as are caused by the muscular dystrophies, and to significantly improve the quality of life of millions of patients. Skeletal muscle tissue engineering approaches rely mainly on the use of combinations of myoblasts and biomaterials, which can deliver cells safely to defective sites and then provide appropriate environments for tissue assembly and neovascularization. Because myoblasts lack expansion capacity, cells from other sources, including adult stem cells, are being investigated for use in muscle tissue engineering [7].

In addition to cells, the second element necessary in cell-based tissue engineering is the scaffold, which must be biocompatible, biodegradable, and possess considerable stability, thus allowing for successful integration between newly formed tissue and host tissue. Unlike hard tissue such as bone and cartilage, muscle tissue engineering may require rather soft and flexible biomaterial scaffolds in therapeutic applications. Injectable biodegradable scaffolds such as PLGA spheres may fulfill these requirements.

2. CELLS FOR SKELETAL MUSCLE TISSUE ENGINEERING

The optimal cell source for engineered skeletal tissue must meet several requirements. Cells should be easy to harvest, capable of proliferating to fill a void, nonimmunogenic, and either show myoblast functions or have the capacity to differentiate into functional muscle cells. Unfortunately, a cell source with all these desirable features remains undescribed in the literature. Several cell sources have been proposed for skeletal tissue engineering, as shown in table 1, which describes the advantages and limitations of seven cell sources [8–15].

Table 1. Advantages and disadvantages of various sources of stem cells

Cells	Easy Accessibility	High Expandability	Myogenic Capacity	Autologous Origin
Skeletal Myoblast	Yes	Depends on age	Yes	Yes
MDSCs	Yes	No	Yes	Yes
ESCs	No	Yes	Yes	No
BMSCs	Yes	Depends on age	Yes	Yes
UCBCs	Yes	Yes	Yes	No
HSCs	Yes	Yes	Debated	Yes
ASCs	Yes	Yes	Yes	Yes

* MDSC; muscle-derived stem cell, ESC; embryonic stem cell, BMSC; bone marrow-derived stem cell, UCBC; umbilical cord blood stem cell, HSC; hematopoietic stem cell, ASC; adipose tissue-derived stem cell.

2.1. Muscle-Derived Cells (MDCs)

Different populations of muscle-derived progenitor cells appear to exhibit varying degrees of pluripotency. The best-characterized muscle progenitor cells are satellite cells [16]. In addition to participating in the formation of myofibers, muscle satellite cells can also differentiate into other lineages, such as osteogenic, chondrogenic, and adipogenic cells [17,18]. Other populations of muscle-derived cells are mostly distinct from satellite cells [19] and can be divided into many different subpopulations by examining surface marker profiles and the abilities of the cells to undergo myogenic differentiation. Muscle-derived stem cells (MDSCs) can be separated into two main subpopulations: CD45+ cells and CD45- cells, based on their relationships to hematopoietic cells. CD45+ cells isolated from normal muscle have a very limited myogenic potential *in vitro* and *in vivo*, but they possess a high degree of hematopoietic potential [20]. In contrast, CD45- cells readily differentiate into myogenic lineages both *in vitro* and *in vivo* [20,21] and can also differentiate into other lineages, such as blood cells [22].

The different populations of muscle-derived cells are closely related. For example, CD45+ cells, which normally possess low myogenic potential, can undergo active myogenesis during muscle injury by responding to the combined signaling of Wnt 5a, Wnt 5b, and Wnt 7a [23]. Thus, the differentiation potential of muscle-derived cells may be modified by environmental cues. This published study also demonstrated that CD 45+ muscle-derived cells are the resident muscle stem cells responsible for regeneration of injured muscle when the pool of satellite cells has been depleted because of cardiotoxin insult [23]. More research is, however, necessary to determine the relative contributions of different populations of muscle progenitor cells, including CD45+ cells, CD45- cells, and satellite cells, to muscle regeneration after common injuries that do not lead to the depletion of a particular group of cells. Nevertheless, it has been shown that under the influence of environmental factors (such as Wnt signaling), CD45+ muscle-derived cells can contribute to muscle regeneration [8].

2.2. Embryonic Stem Cells

Embryonic stem (ES) cells, which are multipotent cells derived from the inner cell mass of the pre-implantation blastocyst, have the potential to be useful as a new approach for cell transplantation therapy [24,25]. When transferred to suspension cultures, mouse ES cells begin to differentiate into multicellular aggregates of differentiated and undifferentiated cells, termed embryoid bodies (EBs) which resemble early post-implantation embryos. Cell differentiation in EBs is disorganized and frequently varies from one EB to another, even in the same culture [24]. Although EBs develop skeletal muscle cells and other cells *in vitro*, transplantation of EBs, without any induction to direct development along a specific pathway, leads to a failure of integration into recipient tissues and often results in teratoma formation in transplanted tissues [26]. Growth factors which selectively promote myogenic differentiation have not yet been identified.

ES cells may have a developmental advantage over myogenic precursor cells derived from muscle or bone marrow in their capacity to form differentiated skeletal muscle tissue *in vivo*. Compared to other forms of cell transplantation [27–31], in which occasional dystrophin-positive myonuclei were seen within multinucleate myotubes, ES cell transplantation results in the development of normally organized and vascularized skeletal muscle tissue *in vivo* [10].

Many results indicate that ES cells can contribute to the formation of new viable muscle tissue [24–26]. There are, however, disadvantages to the use of human ES cells. 1) ES cells are mainly derived from IVF surplus embryos, which are of allogenic origin, and this may result in rejection by the recipient's immune system; 2) the isolation and use of ES cells are still topics of intense ethical debate, and; 3) ES cells are by definition tumorigenic when undifferentiated. This emphasizes the need for a thorough understanding of the pathways of differentiation of ES cells into myoblasts. Only then can ES cells be used for regenerating damaged muscle tissue. The alternative adult stem cells may have fewer restrictions on use.

2.3. Bone Marrow-Derived Stem Cells (BMSCs)

Ferrari et al., first described transdifferentiation of BMSCs into skeletal muscle [30]. Unfractionated BMSCs from C57/M*lacZ* transgenic mice were injected into the chemically injured tibialis anterior muscle of immunodeficient mice. Two to five weeks later, four of six mice that received unfractionated BMSCs exhibited β-gal$^+$ nuclei within the damaged muscle [30]. After bone marrow transplantation, intravenously injected BMSCs also homed to damaged muscle and differentiated to show a skeletal muscle phenotype [30]. Subsequent studies with mouse models of Duchenne muscular dystrophy demonstrated that *mdx* transgenic mice transplanted with wild-type bone marrow contained donor-derived cells that were positive for muscle-specific markers (myogenin and Myf-5), and expressed dystrophin [31]. Similarly, when irradiated mice were transplanted with EGFP+ BMSCs, BMSC-derived satellite cells and multinucleated muscle fibers could be identified in recipient mice. Although these studies indicate that BMSCs can differentiate into a skeletal muscle phenotype, the specific type of BMSC that exhibits this plastic behavior remains to be identified.

2.4. Adipose Tissue-Derived Stem Cells (ASCs)

Adipose tissue has recently been identified as an alternative, uniquely abundant, and accessible source of pluripotent cells. In adult mammals, adipose tissue and an association of adipocytes are held together in a framework of collagen fibers [11]. In addition to mature adipocytes, adipose tissue contains the stromal vascular fraction (SVF), which is composed of a heterogeneous cell population including adipose precursor cells of varying degrees of differentiation, vascular cells, and a supportive stroma. As with BMSCs, adipose tissue-derived stem cells (ASCs) can differentiate *in vitro* into adipogenic, chondrogenic, osteogenic and myogenic cells [32], as well as into other non-mesenchymal lineages such as neurons and hepatocytes [33,34] in the presence of lineage-specific inductive media. Also, heterogeneous population of ASCs has been shown to include progenitors of endothelial cells. Recently, short-term cultures of ASCs have been shown to develop into regenerating muscle fibers with low efficiency after transplantation into damaged muscles. The full myogenic potential of freshly isolated ASCs and their ability to respond to myogenic cues producing terminally differentiated myotubes are largely unknown, however.

2.5. Summary

Stem cell-based skeletal muscle tissue engineering is potentially a powerful application for skeletal muscle diseases. As seen above, we have considered four stem cell candidates for skeletal muscle tissue engineering. ES cells and MDCs have been studied in much more detail than have ASCs, however, but the use of ES cells is associated with ethical and immunogenic rejection problems. MDSCs and MSCs do not replicate to any great extent *in vitro*, and are restricted in donor expandability. ASCs, which can be obtained by minimally invasive procedures from subcutaneous fat, are highly expandable in culture and can be readily induced to differentiate into muscle tissue-forming cells by exposure to well-established myogenic media. Adipose tissue is routinely available in liter quantities from patients undergoing liposuction.

3. SCAFFOLDS FOR SKELETAL MUSCLE TISSUE ENGINEERING

In addition to cells, the second element necessary for cell-based tissue engineering is the scaffold, which must be biocompatible, biodegradable, and possess considerable stability, thus allowing for successful integration between the newly formed tissue and the host tissue. Biomaterials provide mechanical stability to the construct in the short term and serve as templates for the three-dimensional organization of the developing tissue. The effective repair and regeneration of injured tissues and organs depend on early re-establishment of the blood flow needed for metabolic support. An implantable biomaterial should be three-dimensional and highly porous to enable cell growth and flow transport of nutrients and metabolic waste. The scaffold should be biodegradable and should have a surface chemistry suitable for cell attachment and proliferation. Furthermore, the scaffold should be capable of easy laboratory processing to form a variety of shapes and sizes [35].

Many attempts have been made to reconstruct skeletal muscle tissue *in vitro* [36–40]; the results of these studies taken together suggest it is indeed feasible to engineer bioartificial muscles. With current technology, however, tissue-engineered skeletal muscle analogs are far from clinical reality. Morphologically, these materials fall short of actual skeletal muscle in many respects, including small diameters of myofibers, low myofiber organization, and excessive extracellular matrix content. Because myofibers need to be packed parallel to each other to generate sufficient force for muscle contraction [39,41], the lack of structural organization in engineered constructs results in too little active force capacity for utility in clinical applications.

Injectable biodegradable scaffolds, such as poly(lactic-co-glycolic acid) (PLGA) spheres, provide appropriate rigidity, self-aggregate, and function similarly to porous scaffolds *in vivo*. In addition, we have shown that adipose tissue can be generated from PLGA spheres combined with BMSCs or ASCs. PLGA is a highly biocompatible material approved by the United States Food and Drug Administration (FDA) for certain human clinical applications, including bioresorbable surgical sutures and screws. Moreover, these scaffolds have not been observed to result in any post-operation scars [42–45].

4. ENGINEERING SKELETAL MUSCLE TISSUE

Much work has been done using the cells and scaffolds mentioned above, but skeletal muscle tissue engineering still remains challenging. We will introduce one of our previous experiments as an example of successful skeletal muscle tissue engineering using PLGA [44].

4.1. Isolation and Culture of Adipose Tissue-Derived Stem Cells

A variety of terms have been used to describe the plastic-adherent cell population isolated from collagenase digests of adipose tissue, such as adipose-derived stem cells (ADCs), adipose-derived adult stem (ADAS) cells, and processed lipoaspirate (PLA) cells. Fortunately, the International Fat Applied Technology Society has recently clarified the situation and adopted the standard terminology "adipose tissue-derived stem cells (ASCs)". ASCs are one of several populations in the stromal vascular fraction, which is a heterogeneous population of stem cells, microvascular endothelial cells, fibroblasts, and smooth muscle cells. ASCs can be isolated by liposuction using a very simple and minimally invasive method. Figure 1 is a graphical representation of our study. Our concept was to cure skeletal muscle failure in patients using a combination of tissue engineering techniques with autologous adult stem cells. Briefly, we collected lipoaspirate samples from young, healthy plastic surgery patients by liposuction, digested the samples with collagenase for 1 h, lysed red blood cells, washed the remaining cells, and plated them on dishes. Each raw lipoaspirate (~ 300ml) was washed extensively with an equal volume of phosphate buffered saline (PBS) and the extracellular matrix was digested at 37°C for 30 min with 0.075% (w/v) collagenase (Sigma; St. Louis, MO). Enzyme activity was neutralized with Dulbecco's modified Eagle's medium (DMEM; Gibco; Grand Island, NY) containing 10% (v/v) fetal bovine serum (FBS), and the suspension was then centrifuged at 800G for 10 min (Sorvall RT 7 Plus). The pellet, containing the high density stromal vascular fraction (SVF) was resuspended in 0.16 M NH_4Cl and incubated at room temperature for 5 min to lyse any remaining red blood cells. The SVF was collected by centrifugation at 800G for 5 min, filtered through a 100 μm nylon mesh to remove cellular debris, and incubated overnight at 37°C in a humidified atmosphere containing 5% (v/v) CO_2 in control medium (DMEM, 10% [v/v] FBS, 1% [w/v] antibiotic/antimycotic solution). Each plate was washed extensively with PBS to remove residual nonadherent red blood cells. The resulting cell population, the ASCs, was maintained at 37°C in a humidified atmosphere containing 5% (v/v) CO_2 in control medium.

Sub-passaging yielded spindle-shaped cells which readily expanded in simple growth media. We used these stem cells in previous studies for adipose tissue and muscle tissue engineering (figure 2) [43,44]. Figure 3 shows the cells, and describes expression of cell surface markers. ASCs are positive for CD 73, CD 90, and CD 105, but are negative for CD 34 and CD 45. These results are similar to those obtained using bone marrow stromal cells [43].

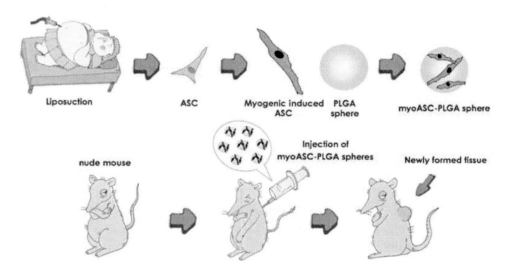

Figure 1. Schematic diagram of skeletal muscle tissue engineering using ASCs.

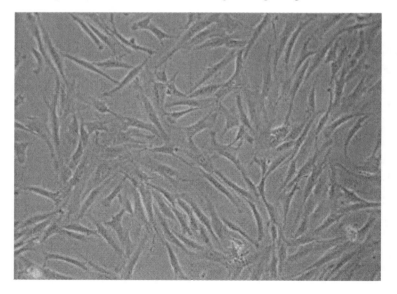

Figure 2. Morphology of adipose tissue-derived adult stem cells (ASCs). Human primary ASCs were cultured for 7 days in complete medium (DMEM, 10% [w/v] FBS, 1% [w/v] antibiotics). After the second passage, the ASCs appeared to assume a more uniform fibroblast-like shape (magnification x100).

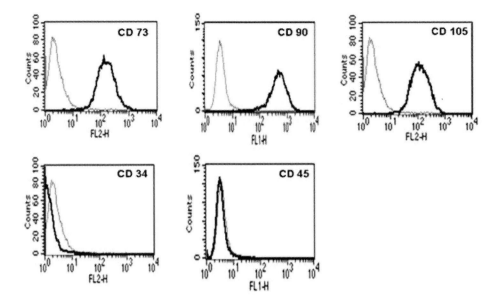

Figure 3. Characterization of ASCs using flow cytometry.

4.2. Preparation of Scaffolds and *In Vitro* Cultivation of ASC-Scaffold Mixtures

PLGA [85:15] (MW = 90,000; Purac; Park Road Blair, Nebraska) was dissolved 12:100 (w/v) in dichloromethane, added dropwise to a stirred solution of 0.27% (w/v) polyvinyl alcohol (PVA; MW = 30,000–70,000, Sigma), and stirred for 72 h, allowing for complete evaporation of the solvent. The spheres were isolated by filtration, washed with deionized water, air-dried for 2 h, and vacuum-dried for an additional 24 h. The spheres were separated into size ranges of 100–150 μm using commercially available sieves and stored desiccated until further use.

4.3. Myogenic Potency of Adipose Tissue-Derived Stem Cells

For muscle regeneration, we first verified that *in vitro* cultures of ASCs could differentiate into muscle cells. We found that the myogenic induction of ASCs was time-dependent; the length of culture time in myogenic medium was an important factor. During very early stages of myogenic differentiation in myogenic conditioned medium, ASCs started to differentiate into a myogenic lineage expressing Myo D at day 7 (figure 4).

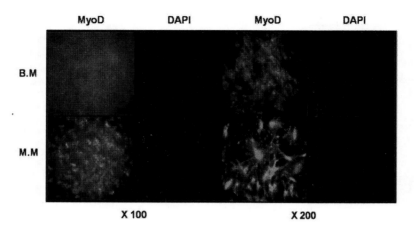

Figure 4. Myogenic differentiation of ASCs *in vitro* culture in myogenic conditioned medium at day 7. Myo D and DAPI staining were done for differentiation and cellularity, respectively. (B.M.;basal media, M.M.;myogenic media, X100, X200;each magnification designated).

ASCs can transdifferentiate into cells of other lineages, but, at terminal differentiation, they have the properties of mature muscle cells. We therefore myogenically induced ASCs for 3 weeks, at which stage they expressed both Myo D1 and MYS, confirming that they had differentiated into muscle cells of early to intermediate stages (figures 5 and 6). Because ASCs can differentiate into various cell types, it was possible for injected ASCs attached to PLGA spheres to differentiate into undesirable cell lineages. To ascertain whether any ASCs had differentiated into osteocytes, chondrocytes, or adipocytes, we cultured cells in myogenic medium for 42 days, and stained these cells with alizarin red S, safranin O, or oil red O. Cells did not stain with these chemicals and we found no significant differences between cells grown thereafter in myogenic media and cells grown in nondifferentiating control media. Once induced in myogenic medium, the ASCs were committed to the myogenic lineage and differentiated into muscle cells, suggesting that injected ASCs would not differentiate *in vivo* into cells of other lineages.

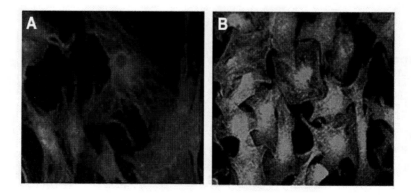

Figure 5. MyoD1 expression by ASCs cultured in myogenic media. ASCs were stained with Myo D1-FITC and visualized using a confocal microscope on day 0 (A) or day 42 (B).

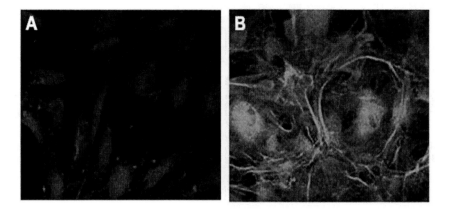

Figure 6. Myosin heavy-chain (MYS) expression by ASCs cultured in myogenic media. ASCs were stained with MYS-FITC and visualized using a confocal microscope on day 0 (A) or day 42 (B).

4.4. *In Vivo* Study

PLGA spheres, either alone or attached to ASCs, were cultured in myogenic media for 21 days and injected subcutaneously into the necks of six athymic nude mice for each group; six untreated mice served as controls. After 30 and 60 days, the mice were sacrificed and newly formed tissues were harvested (figure 7). We observed newly formed tissues under the skins of mice injected with ASCs attached to PLGA, but not in control groups. A gross view of incised dorsal skin showed that the largest volume of newly formed tissue was regenerated 60 days after mice were injected with ASCs attached to PLGA.

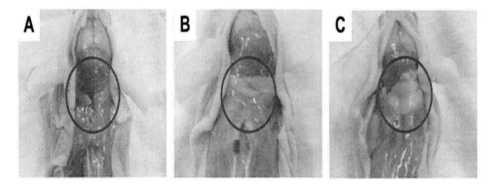

Figure 7. Gross images of newly formed tissue in untreated nude mice (A), and in nude mice injected with ASCs attached to PLGA, after 30 days (B) and 60 days (C).

H and E staining showed that muscle tissues were regenerated in mice injected with ASCs attached to PLGA at 60 day post-injection, and the regenerated muscle tissue was morphologically similar to native muscle (figure 8). When we stained regenerated tissues with FITC-Myo D1, we found morphologies similar to that of native muscle, and myogenic markers were expressed at both 30 and 60 day post-injection (figure 9). This finding was confirmed by MYS staining and by RT-PCR, in that messages encoding Myo D1 and MYS were observed at both 30 and 60 day post-injection; at 60 days, the band intensities were similar to those observed in native muscle tissue (data not shown).

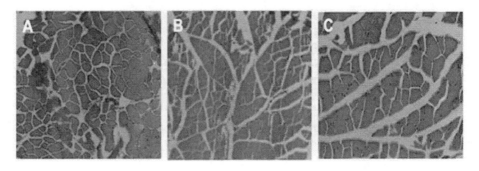

Figure 8. H&E staining of engineered skeletal muscle of nude mice injected with ASCs attached to PLGA after 30 days (A) or 60 days (B), and of native skeletal muscle (C).

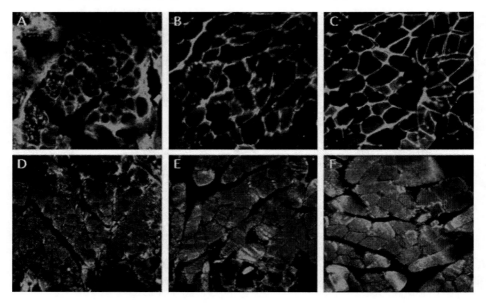

Figure 9. Myo D1 and Mys expression in engineered skeletal muscle of nude mice injected with ASCs attached to PLGA after 30 (A,D) or 60 days (B,E), and in native skeletal muscle (C,F), stained with FITC-antibodies to MyoD1(A-C) and MYS(D-F).

4.5. Summary

We have shown that ASCs attached to PLGA spheres generated skeletal muscle tissue when injected subcutaneously into nude mice. These findings suggest that ASCs and injectable spheres are useful materials for skeletal muscle tissue engineering, and indicate that this combination can be used in a clinical setting for such engineering.

5. DISCUSSION

Our ASCs have several important advantages compared to previously reported stem cell systems. ASCs can easily be isolated from patients by liposuction and can be efficiently expanded *in vitro*. Furthermore, injection of ASCs should encounter few ethical problems, because the employment of these cells avoids controversies surrounding the use of ES cells. In addition, PLGA, the scaffolding material, has been clinically approved by the U.S. FDA [45]. Autologous transplantation of ASCs should minimize the risks of immune rejection. Although our results indicate that the combination of ASCs and injectable PLGA spheres can participate in the process of skeletal muscle tissue engineering and give rise to fully differentiated muscle tissue, there are still problems that must be solved prior to clinical use.

First, questions that remain to be answered by researchers studying ASCs are similar to those encountered by others working in the stem cell field, and involve such issues as 1) the efficiency of myogenic differentiation, 2) the mechanisms underlying development from stem cells to mature muscle cells, 3) the cell viability and proliferation capacity of differentiated cells, and, 4) contractile functions of differentiated cells.

Second, the major obstacle in the engineering of thick complex tissues such as skeletal muscle is that of vascularization, which is necessary to maintain cell viability during tissue growth and for the induction of structural organization. Most approaches to engineering new tissue have relied on the host for vascularization. Although this approach has been useful in many tissues, it has not been very successful in thick highly vascularized tissue such as muscle, which must have an abundant blood vessel supply. Also, researchers need to evaluate the contractile function of their engineered tissue.

ACKNOWLEDGMENTS

This research was supported by a grant to Dr. MiJung Kim (#SC3280) from the Stem Cell Research Center of the 21st Century Frontier Research Program, funded by the Ministry of Science and Technology, Republic of Korea and from Asan Foundation (#2000-133), Seoul, Korea.

REFERENCES

[1]   Saxena, AK; Marler, J; Benvenuto, M; Willital, GH; Vacanti, JP. Skeletal muscle tissue engineering using isolated myoblasts on synthetic biodegradable polymers: preliminary studies. *Tissue Eng*, 1999, 5, 525-532.

[2]   Hurme, T; Kalimo, H; Lehto, M; Jarvinen, M. Healing of skeletal muscle injury: and ultrastructural and immunohistochemical study. *Med. Sci. Sports Exerc*, 1991, 23, 801-810.

[3]   Campion, DR. The muscle satellite cell: a review. *Int. Rev. Cytol*, 1984, 87, 25-251.

[4]   Allen, RE; Temm-Grove, CJ; Sheehan, SM; Rice, G. Skeletal muscle satellite cell culture. *Methods Cell Biol*, 1997, 52, 155-176.

[5]   Hill, M; Wernig. A; Goldspink, G. Muscle satellite (stem) cell activation during local tissue injury and repair. *J. Anat*, 2003, 203, 89-99.

[6]   Li, Y; Huard, J. Differentiation of muscle-derived cells into myofibroblasts in injured skeletal muscle. *Am. J. Pathol*, 2002, 161, 895-907.

[7]   Bach, AD; Beier, JP; Stern-Staeter, J; Horch, RE. Skeletal muscle tissue engineering. *J. Cell Mol. Med*, 2004, 8, 413-422.

[8]   Peng, H; Huard, J. Muscle-derived stem cells for musculoskeletal tissue regeneration and repair. *Transpl. Immunol*, 2004, 12, 311-319.

[9]   Dawn, B; Bolli, R. Adult bone marrow-derived cells: Regenerative potential, plasticity, and tissue commitment. *Basic Res. Cardiol*, 2005, 100, 494-503.

[10] Bhagavati, S; Xu, W. Generation of skeletal muscle from transplanted embryonic stem cells in dystrophic mice. *Biochem. Biophys. Res. Commun*, 2005, 333, 644-649.

[11] Di Rocco, G; Iachininoto, MG; Tritarelli, A; Straino, S; Zacheo, A; Germani, A; Crea, F; Capogrossi, MC. Myogenic potential of adipose-tissue-derived cells. *J. Cell Sci*, 2006, 119, 2945-2952.

[12] Sinanan, AC; Buxton, PG; Lewis, MP. Muscling in on stem cells. *Biol. Cell*, 2006, 98, 203-214.

[13] Dellavalle, A; Sampaolesi, M; Tonlorenzi, R; Tagliafico, E; Sacchetti, B; Perani, L; Innocenzi, A; Galvez, BG; Messina, G; Morosetti, R; Li, S; Belicchi, M; Peretti, G; Chamberlain, JS; Wright, WE; Torrente, Y; Ferrari, S; Bianco, P; Cossu, G. Pericytes of human skeletal muscle are myogenic precursors distinct from satellite cells. *Nat. Cell Biol*, 2007, 9, 255-267.

[14] Levenberg, S; Rouwkema, J; Macdonald, M; Garfein, ES; Kohane, DS; Darland, DC; Marini, R; van Blitterswijk, CA; Mulligan, RC; D'Amore, PA; Langer, R. Engineering vascularized skeletal muscle tissue. *Nat. Biotechnol*, 2005, 23, 879-884.

[15] Dezawa, M; Ishikawa, H; Itokazu, Y; Yoshihara, T; Hoshino, M; Takeda, S; Ide, C; Nabeshima, Y. Bone marrow stromal cells generate muscle cells and repair muscle degeneration. *Science*, 2005, 309, 314-317.

[16] Partridge, TA. Cells that participate in regeneration of skeletal muscle. *Gene Ther*, 2002, 9, 752-753.

[17] Asakura, A; Komaki, M; Rudnicki, M. Muscle satellite cells are multipotential stem cells that exhibit myogenic, osteogenic, and adipogenic differentiation. *Differentiation*, 2001, 68, 245-253.

[18] Wada, MR; Inagawa-Ogashiwa, M; Shimizu, S; Yasumoto, S; Hashimoto, N. Generation of different fates from multipotent muscle stem cells. *Development*, 2002, 129, 2987-2995.

[19] Asakura, A; Seale, P; Girgis-Gabardo, A; Rudnicki, MA. Myogenic specification of side population cells in skeletal muscle. *J. Cell Biol*, 2002, 159, 123-134.

[20] McKirmey-Freeman,SL; Jackson, KA; Camargo, FD; Ferrari, G; Mavilio, F; Goodell, MA. Muscle-derived hematopoietic stem cells are hematopoietic in origin. *Proc. Natl. Acad. Sci. USA*, 2002, 99, 1341-1346.

[21] Qu-Petersen, Z; Deasy, B; Jankowski, R; Ikezawa, M; Cummins, J; Pruchnic, R; Mytinger, J; Cao, B; Gates, C; Wernig, A; Huard, J. Identification of a novel population of muscle stem cells in mice: potential for muscle regeneration. *J. Cell Biol*, 2002, 157, 851-864.

[22] Cao B, Zheng B, Jankowski RJ, Kimura S, Ikezawa M, Deasy B, Cummins J, Epperly M, Qu-Petersen Z, Huard J. Muscle stem cells differentiate into haematopoietic lineages but remain myogenic potential. *Nat. Cell Biol*, 2003, 5, 640-646.

[23] Polesskaya, A; Seale, P; Rudnicki, MA. Wnt signalling induces the myogenic specification of resident CD45+ adult stem cells during muscle regeneration. *Cell*, 2003, 113, 841-852.

[24] Odorico JS, Kaufman DS, Thomson JA. Multilineage differentiation from human embryonic stem cell lines. *Stem cells*, 2001, 19, 193-204.

[25] Thomson JA, Itskovitz-Eldor J, Shapiro SS, Waknitz MA, Swiergiel JJ, Marshall VS, Jones JM. Embryonic stem cells lines derived from human blastocysts. *Science*, 1998, 282, 1145-1147.

[26] Smith, AG. Embryo-derived stem cells: of mice and men. *Annu. Rev. Cell Dev. Biol*, 2001, 17, 435-462.

[27] Chamberlain, JS. Gene therapy of muscular dystrophy. *Hum. Mol. Genet*, 2002, 11, 2355-2362.

[28] Smythe, GM; Hodgetts, SI; Grounds, MD. Problems and solutions in myoblast transfer therapy. *J. Cell. Mol. Med*, 2001, 5, 33-47.

[29] Gibson, AJ; Karasinski, J; Relvas, J; Moss, J; Sheratt, TG; Strong, PN; Watt, DJ. Dermal fibroblasts convert to a myogenic lineage in mdx mouse muscle. *J. Cell Sci*, 1995, 108, 207-214.

[30] Ferrari, G; Cusella-De Angelis, G; Coletta, M; Paolucci, E; Stornaiulo, A; Cossu, G; Mavilio, F. Muscle regeneration by bone marrow derived progenitors. *Science*, 1998, 279, 1528-1530.

[31] Gussoni, E; Soneoka, Y; Strickland, CD; Buzney, EA; Khan, MA; Flint, AF; Kunkel, LM; Mulligan, RC. Dystrophin expression in the mdx mouse restored by stem cell transplantation. *Nature*, 1999, 401, 390-391.

[32] Zuk, PA; Zhu, M; Mizuno, H; Huang, J; Futrell, JW; Katz, AJ; Benhaim, P; Lorenz, HP; Hedrick, MH. Multilineage cells from human adipose tissue: implications for cell-based therapies. *Tissue Eng*, 2001, 7, 211-228.

[33] Safford, KM; Hicok, KC; Safford, SD; Halvorsen, YD; Wilkison, WO; Gimble, JM; Rice, HE. Neurogenic differentiation of murine and human adipose-derived stromal cells. *Biochem. Biophys. Res. Commun*, 2002, 294, 371-379.

[34] Seo, M; Suh, SY; Bae, YC; Jung, JS. Differentiation of human adipose stromal cells into hepatic lineage in vitro and in vivo. *Biochem. Biophys. Res. Commun*, 2005, 328, 258-264.

[35] Hutmacher, DW. Scaffold design and fabrication technologies for engineering tissues-stat of the art and future perspectives. *J. Miomater. Sci. Polym. Ed*, 2001, 12, 107-124.

[36] Powell, CA; Smiley, BL; Mills, J; Vandenburgh, HH. Mechanical stimulation improves tissue-engineered human skeletal muscle. *Am. J. Physiol. Cell Physiol*, 2002, 283, C1557-C1565

[37] Kosnik Jr, P; Dennis. RG; Faulkner, JA. Functional development of engineered skeletal muscle from adult and neonatal rats. *Tissue eng*, 2001, 7, 573-584.

[38] Okano, T; Satoh, S; Oka, T; Matsuda, T. Tissue engineering of skeletal muscle: highly dense, highly oriented hybrid muscular tissue biomimicking native tissues. *ASAIO J*, 1997, 43, M749-M753.

[39] Saxena, AK; Willital, GH; Vacanti, JP. Vascularized three-dimensional skeletal muscle tissue-engineering. *Biomed. Mater Eng*, 2001, 11, 275-281.

[40] Mulder, MM; Hitchcock, RW; Tresco, PA. Skeletal myogenesis on elastomeric substrates: implications for tissue engineering. *J. Miomater Sci. Polym. Ed*, 1998, 44, 355-370.

[41] Vandenburgh, HH. Functional assessment and tissue design of skeletal muscle. *Ann. N Y Acad. Sci*, 2002, 961, 201-202.

[42] Choi, YS; Park, SN; Suh, H. Adipose tissue engineering using mesenchymal stem cells attached to injectable PLGA spheres. *Biomaterials*. 2005, 26, 5855-5863.

[43] Choi, YS; Cha, SM; Lee, YY; Kwon, SW; Park, CJ; Kim, M. Adipogenic differentiation of adipose tissue derived adult stem cells in nude mouse. *Biochem. Biophys. Res. Commun*, 2006, 345, 631-637.

[44] Kim, M; Choi, YS; Yang, SH; Hong, HN; Cho, SW; Cha, SM; Pak, JH; Kim, CW; Kwon, SW; Park, CJ. Muscle regeneration by adipose tissue-derived adult stem cells attached to injectable PLGA spheres. *Biochem. Biophys. Res. Commun*, 2006, 348, 386-392.

[45] Food and Drug Administration. Web site: <*www.fda.gov*>

In: Encyclopedia of Stem Cell Research (2 Volume Set) ISBN: 978-1-61761-835-2
Editor: Alexander L. Greene © 2012 Nova Science Publishers, Inc.

Chapter XXXII

OLFACTORY NEUROBLASTOMA

Zhichun Lu and Honggang Liu [*]

Department of Pathology, Beijing Tongren Hospital, Capital Medical University,
P.R. China

ABSTRACT

Olfactory neuroblastoma (ONB), also known as esthesioneuroblastoma, is a rare malignant neoplasm arising from the olfactory neuroepithelium in the upper nasal cavity. It accounts for 3% of all intranasal tumors [1]. The ONB incidence is reported at 4 cases per ten million inhabitants [2]. There are more than 1000 cases being reported in the literature since it was first described in 1924 [3].

This paper provides an overview of the disease and highlights the updates in physiology, anatomy, histopathology, molecular biology, clinical feature, treatment, prognosis and predictive factors based on the literature reviews.

1. PHYSIOLOGY

The function of olfaction mainly depends on the olfactory cells in the mucosa of the olfactory region. The olfactory cells play important roles in recognition, alert, enhancement of appetite, or emotion. The ONB patients may experience a series of nasal symptom and abnormity of olfaction, such as nasal obstruction, rhinorrhea, epistaxis, rhinogenic headache, olfactory dysfunction, hyposmia, and anosmia.

[*] Correspondence concerning this article should be addressed to: Hong-gang Liu, Prof. MD, Ph.D Department of Pathology, Beijing Tongren hospital, Capital Medical University, P.R.China. E-mail: liuhg1125@163.com.

2. ANATOMY AND HISTOLOGY

Olfactory region lies in the middle of the top nasal cavity, including the region of olfactory cleft such as the upper nasal septum and the outboard of the nasal cavity. Olfactory region is covered with the pseudostratified, non-ciliated columnar epithelium which is composed of the basal cells located against the basement membrane, the olfactory neurosensory cells, and the sustentacular supporting cells, the processes of which extend on the luminal surface. The basal cells constitute a stem cell compartment that regenerates not only physiologically for self-maitenance but also for tissue repair after trauma or environmental insults. Those stem cells can differentiate into olfactory neurosensory cells and/or sustentacular supporting cells. The olfactory neurosensory cell is a bipolar neuronal cell with olfactory hair. The terminal of the olfactory cell swells to form olfactory vesicle, which emits 10-30 cilia to sense smell. The base of the olfactory cell emits axon to form Remak's nerve fiber, which enters the encephalic cavity though the pores of the cribriform plate and terminates at the olfactory bulb.

3. PATHOLOGICAL CHARACTERISTICS

3.1. Histogenesis

ONB is possibly originated from the neuroepithelium in the olfactory mucosa or the neuroectodermal structure in the olfactory placode [4]. However the exact origin of the neoplasm cells remains unclear due to their multidirectional differentiation. In the World Health Organization Classification of Head and Neck Tumors [5], ONB was originated from the basal cells of the olfactory neuroepithelium.

The olfactory neuroepithelium is a unique neurosensory organ, because olfactory neurons are continuously renewed every 40 days throughout adult life [6,7]. Three types of cells are classically recognized in the olfactory mucosa: the basal cells, the olfactory neurosensory cells, and the sustentacular supporting cells. The spherical basal cells constitute a stem-cell compartment, which confers to this tissue its peculiar ability to regenerate and differentiate into the olfactory neurosensory cells and the sustentacular supporting cells [8,9]. The basal cells express [10] neural cell adhesion molecule (NCAM) [11] and the mammalian homologue of Drosophila achaete-scute (MASH) gene [12]. Immature olfactory cells express [8,9] GAP43, a 24 kDa membrane-associated protein kinase C involved in turnover of polyphosphoinositide [13], and HASH, the human homologue of the MASH gene. With maturation, the olfactory cells migrate towards the luminal surface and express olfactory marker protein (OMP) [14] and NCAM, but not GAP43 [8,9,15]. ONB tumors were found to express HASH, the human homologue of the MASH gene, but stained negative for OMP [16]. Other indirect evidence that ONB originates from olfactory stem cells comes from transgenic mice, in which the SV40T oncogene was inserted under control of the olfactory marker protein gene promoter region [17]; these mice did not develop ONB but adrenal and sympathetic ganglia neuroblastoma. Therefore, the currently available evidence connects ONB with the basal progenitor cells of the olfactory epithelium. Some authors have proposed

[18] that ONB belonged to the Ewing's sarcoma family [19] or the primitive neuroectodermal tumours (PNET) [20], because of the identification in some cases of translocation t(1 1:22), which is regarded as specific for Ewing's sarcoma [21]. Studies with fluorescence in situ hybridization [22,23] (FISH) and Real-time PCR (RT-PCR) [23,24] have not proved this translocation in ONB. Therefore, ONB should be seen as a distinct entity from Ewing's /PNET.

3.2. Etiology

No clear etiological agent has been documented in human beings. The injections of diethyinitrosamine into Syrian hamsters [25] and N-nitrosopiperidine into rats [26] have produced tumors histologically identical to the human olfactory neuroblastoma. In 1990, Koike *et al* [27] reported three cases of olfactory neuroblastoma in cats in which the feline and murine leukemia virus, a type C retrovirus, was observed in the neoplasm cell cytoplasm. However the role of the virus in human ONB needs further exploration.

3.3. Morphological Characteristics

The gross appearance of the tumor tissue is pink to red brown, vascular nasal mass, polypoid, soft, friable, and hemorrhagic. Microscopically, neoplasm cells of ONB are arranged in nests or lobules with intervening fibrovascular septa and marked microvascularity. Common features of the neoplasm cells are small round or fusiform with almost nonexistent cytoplast, indistinct karyotheca. Nuclei are hyperchromatic with punctuate or fine chromatin distribution and small nucleoli. The neoplasms take on distinct fibrillar and reticulate intracellular background which resembles other neural tumors. The Homer-Wright pseudorosette pattern or the Flexner-Wintersteiner rosette pattern may be present. Rosettes consist of a central space ringed by columnar cells with radially oriented nuclei.

The ONB cells at different differential stages vary morphologically. Some tumor cells are large, with abundant cytoplast, and line in solid nests, which is of neuroepithelial character. Other tumor cells are anaplastic hyperchromatic small cells that show many mitotic figures and scant cytoplasm, which is of neuroblastoma character. Another tumor cells have the characters of both neuroepithelioma and neuroblastomawhich not only coexist sometimes but also interchange in certain cases [4].

Base on the cell characters described above, Liu *et a.,l* [28] ummarized the histomorphologic characters of the ONB as follows: (1the neoplastic cells are arranged in round or elliptical epithelioid nest or lobules structure (figures 1a) ; (2) the neoplastic epithelioid lobular structure was retiformly rounding up by the hyperplastic vasculature (figure 1a) which will transform into hemagioma-like structure when the vasculature proliferation is prominent (figure 1b) (3) the neoplastic cells are round with fusiform or round nuclei and sparse, pink or clear cytoplasm (figure 1c) (4) The Homer-Wright pseudorosettes (figure 1d) or Flexner-Wintersteiner rosettes are present in most cases but vary with numbers and patterns; (5) band like neurofilament could be seen in ONB with well differentiation (figure 1e) (6) some neoplastic cells show squamous differentiation (figure 1f) or/and glandular differentiation without identifiable basilar membrane (figure 1g) (7) in poorly differentiated tumor, the anaplastic tumor cell nests will be separated with dense stroma (figure 1h). As described as above, the poorly differentiated ONB usually contains the features in (1), (3), (7) and necrosis as well; and the well differentiated ONB always includes (4) and (6). Vasculature proliferation and band like neurofilament represent in all the tumors with variable differentiation.

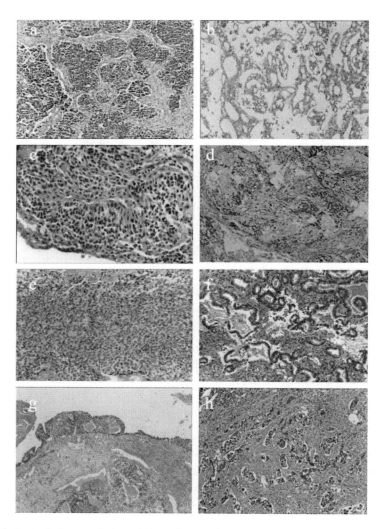

Figure 1. Morphological characteristics of ONB. (a) neoplasm cells of ONB are arranged in nests or lobules with interwoven fibrovascular septa HE33; (b) sparse tumor cells in a background with microvasculature proliferation and focal hemangioma-like structures HE25; (c) the neoplastic cells with small round nuclei and scant, eosinophilic cytoplasm HE40; (d) the neoplastic cells in neurofibrillar background which resembles cerebral tumors HE 20; (e) Homer-Wright pseudorosettes is consisted of cells arranged radially towards the core HE66; (f) glandular differentiation without identifiable basement membrane HE 20; (g) the neoplastic cell transformation from adjacent normal olfactory mucosal epithelium HE25; (h) tumor cell islands with dense anaplastic stroma HE33.

However, other histopathologic features can also be seen in some atypical ONB, such as calcification (figures 2a, 2b) and rhabdomyoblast differentiation (figures 2c, 2d). The morphologic features of metastatic lesion sometimes differ from those of primary tumors. (figures 2e, 2f).

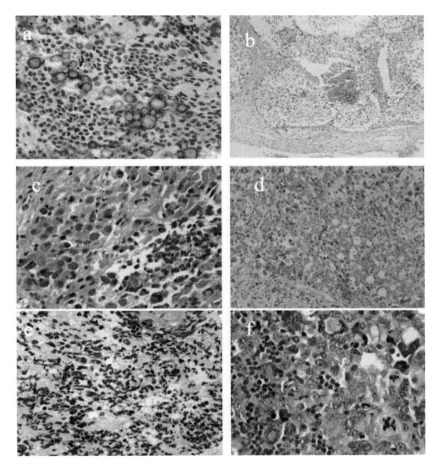

Figure 2. The atypical ONB. (a) stromal calcification HE40; (b) stromal calcification HE 10; (c) rhabdomyoblast differentiation. Oval rhabdomyoblast cells was frequently observed to have abundant eosinophilia cytoplasm and a nucleus sometimes displaced towards the periphery of the cell body HE40; (d) positive stain for desmin in cytoplasm of rhabdomyoblast cells Desmin20; (e) the small and round neoplastic cells in loose arrangement in primary tumor HE40; (f) metastatic tumor in the cervical lymph node from the same patient of (e): metastatic tumor cells are large and som e ha ve multiple nuclei, significantly different from the primary ones HE40.

3.4. Pathological Grading

In 1924, ONB was first histologically classified by Berger [3] into three subsgrades: olfactory neuroepitheliuma with true rosettes (Flexner-Wintersteiner rosettes), olfactory neuroblastoma with pseudorosettes (Homer-Wright rosettes), and esthesioneurocytoma without true rosettes and pseudorosettes.

In 1988, Hyams [29] proposed a pathological grading system (table 1), which classified ONB into four grades based on neoplasm biological features and histological features. This grading scheme could reportedly provide prognostic information and is more useful to clinic. Grade I is well differentiated, the characters of which are of distinct lobular architecture, plentiful vascularized fibrous stroma and neurofibrillary matrix. The neoplastic cells are well-differentiated, with uniform, small round nuclei, and scant cytoplasm. Homer-Wright rosettes are frequently seen. Mitotic activity and necrosis are absent. Grade II also has lobular architecture, vascularized fibrous stroma, and neurofibrillary matrix. However, the neoplastic nuclei show increased pleomorphism and mitotic activity. Homer-Wright rosettes and local necrosis may be observed. Grade III is more anaplastic and hyperchromatic and has increased mitotic activity as compared to grade I or grade II tumor. Flexner-Wintersteiner rosettes and necrosis can be seen. It is hard to see lobular architecture and vascularized fibrous stroma. Grade IV is poorly differentiated, without lobular architecture and rosettes. Neoplasm cells have high mitotic activity and karyon anaplasia. Necrosis is frequently seen. The lower grade ONB is well differentiated, and it could be easily recognized and diagnosed successfully by light microscopy. However, the higher histological grade tumors are hard to differentiate from other small-cell nasal neoplasms by light microscopy due to the anaplastic hyperchromatic small cells characters. In these cases, immunohistochemical staining and electron microscopy become important in establishing the diagnosis.

Table 1. Hyams histopathological grading system

Grade	LA preservation	Mitotic index	Nuclear polymorphism	Fibrillary matrix	Rosettes	Necrosis
I	+	Zero	None	Promonent	HW	None
II	+	Low	Low	Present	HW	None
III	+/-	Moderate	Moderate	Low	FW	Rare
IV	+/-	High	High	Absent	None	Frequent

LA lobular architecture; HWHomer-Wright; FW Flexner- Wintersteiner.

3.5. Immunohistochemistry and Differential Diagnosis

Neurospecific enolase (NSE) is the most consistently expressed marker, whose positive rate could reach 100%. Although the specificity of NSE is not strong, most of the pathologists also believe that NSE is an unsubstituted marker for establishing the diagnosis of ONB figure 3a. The immunoreactivity of neurofilament (NF) is usually low and its positive rates in ONB vary in different reports figure 3b. S-100 protein staining is typically limited to the sustentacular cells located along the periphery of the neoplastic lobules (figures 3c, 3d). Chromogranin and synaptophysin are specific and broad-spectrum markers of neural and neuroendocrine tumor. The express of chromogranin is related to the neuroendocrine particle. The poor differentiation of tumor always expresses the low immunoreactivity of chromogranin (figure 3e). Synaptophysin is unrelated to the tumor differentiation, but it has higher sensitivity than NF and chromogranin (figure 3f). So, in neural and neuroendocrine markers, NES, chromogranin and synaptophysin play an important role in diagnosis of ONB, and NF, S-100 protein could be adjuvant markers of diagnosis. Cytokeratin and AE1/AE3 are usually negative, but they can show some positive cells in some cases (figures 3g, 3h).

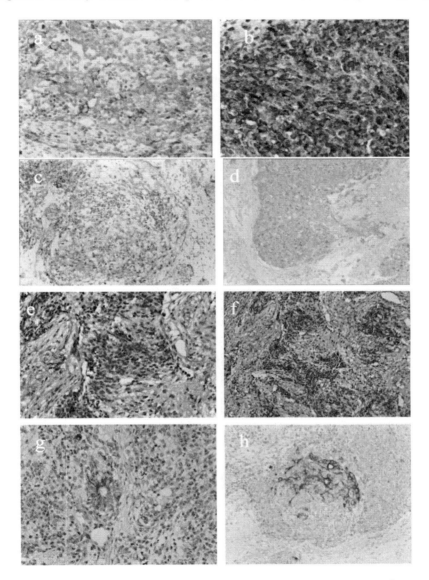

Figure 3. Immunohistochemical studies in ONB. (a) micrograph reveals positive stain for NSE in cytoplasm of most tumor cells NSE20; (b) positive reaction to NF antibody NF40; (c) S-100 protein is typically limited to the sustentacular cells located along the periphery of the neoplastic lobules S-100 20; (d) the same as (c) S-100 10; (e)immunoreactivity to Chromogranin appeared in well differentiated tumor cells Chromogranin20; (f) immunostain for synaptophysin 10; (g)immunostain for Cytokeratin can be occasionally positive in some cases. Cytokeratin 20; (h) positive reaction for AE1/AE3 can be occasionally appeared in some cases. AE1/AE310.

Epithelial membrane antigen (EMA), leukocyte common antigen (LCA), HMB-45, desmin, and CD99 are absent [19,30,31,32]. The proliferation markers including Ki-67 and MIB-1 have shown a high proliferative index of 10-50% and the flow cytometric analysis has shown frequent polyploidy or aneuploid [33,34]. P53 tumour suppressor gene stained variably, and there are conflicting data on the prognostic role of the P53 tumour suppressor gene mutations [35,36].

The differential diagnosis of ONB includes a group of small round cell malignant neoplasms occurred in the sinonasal tract, i.e., malignant lymphoma, embryonal rhabdomyosarcoma, mucosal malignant melanoma, Ewing's/PNET, sinonasal undifferentiated carcinoma and sinonasal neuroendocrine carcinoma.

The key point of distinguishing ONB from mucosal malignant melanoma is based on the lack of expression of HMB45 antibody and the pattern of S-100 protein staining. In the malignant melanoma, S-100 protein expresses a diffuse and strong immunopositivity in most cells, whereas in ONB the stain is scattered and peripheral. Distinguishing ONB from embryonal rhabdomyosarcoma is based on the lack of desmin, vimentin, myoglobin, MyoD 1, myosin, and sarcomeric actin. However, when ONB is accompanied by rhabdomyoblasts differentiation, the group of markers above must combine morphological characters of neoplasm cells in order to be used to establish diagnosis. ONB can be distinguished from lymphoma based on the lack of common leucocyte antigen immunostaining. Most sinonasal lymphoma is non-Hodgkin diffuse large cell tumors and has a mass of necrosis. It seems difficult to distinguish Ewing's/PNET from the poorly differentiated ONB, which had been regarded as a member of the Ewing's/PNET family before. With the use of CD99 protein and detection of the EWS-FLI1 hybrid transcripts, ONB could also be differentiated from Ewing's/PNET [37]. Recent research shows that CD99 isn't a specific and sensitive marker of Ewing's/PNET, and it could also express in rhabdomyoma [38] thusCD99 should not be used by itself to distinguish between esthesioneuroblastoma and Ewing's/PNET. The immunohistochemical differentiation of sinonasal undifferentiated carcinoma from ONB is based on a positive stain with cytokeratin antibodies, such as low molecular weight and epithelial membrane antigen (EMA) [39]. Another neoplasm, which is distinguished from ONB, is sinonasal neuroendocrine carcinoma. Cytokeratins immunopositivity, especially in a punctuate paranuclear distribution, is the main diagnostic maker for the differentiation from ONB [40].

3.6. Electron Microscopy

The tumor was mainly composed of round to oval cells, with scant cytoplasm, with a high nuclear/cytoplasmic ratio. In cytoplasm, there are numerous membrane-bound dense core neurosecretory granules measuring 50-250 nm in diameter. Cytoplasmic processes containing microtubules, mirofilaments, and membrane-bound granules were present [41,42] (figure 4).

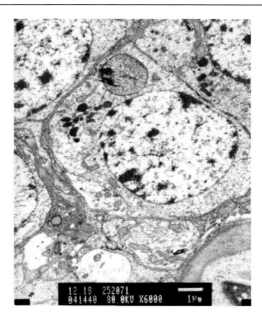

Figure 4. Electron microscopy shows membrane-bound dense core neurosecretory granules. Bar,1 m.

4. GENETIC AND MOLECULAR ANALYSIS

In 1995 [16], immature olfactory neurons was found to express hASH- 1, but OMP, which is expressed in mature olfactory neurons only, was not. Based on the results of this study, the authors suggested that ONB might develop from immature olfactory neurons rather than mature ones. Recently, Paulette et al., [43] used real-time polymerase chain reaction (RT-PCR) to determine the value of hASH 1 messenger RNA (mRNA) levels in differentiating ONB from other poorly differentiated tumors in sinonasal cavity. All of the ONB cases were positive, and other poorly differentiated tumors were negative. Therefore, they concluded that the hASH 1 mRNA level might be a useful tool for distinguishing ONB from the poorly differentiated tumors of the sinonasal cavity.

In former research, ONB was included within the Ewing sarcoma family of tumor [44] or the primitive neuroectodernal tumors (PNET) [19] because the translocation t (11:22) (q24; q12) and trisomy 8, which is regarded as specific molecular abnormality for Ewing's sarcoma, had been identified in certain ONB cases [21]. By using immunocytochemistry, cytogenetic analysis, fluorescent in situ hybridization, and reverse transcriptase PCR, recent studies showed that neither EWS/FLI- 1, EWS/ERG and EWS/FEV fusion nor MIC2 expression were found in any ONB tumor [22,23,45]. Therefore, ONB should be considered as an entity distinct from Ewing's/PNET family.

By using comparative genomic hybridization (CGH), Riazimand et al., [46] analyzed three ONB cases and revealed multiple recurrent aberrations including DNA overrepresentations on chromosomes 1 9p/q, partial gains on chromosomes 8q, 15q, and 22q, and deletions on chromosome 4q. Beside these common aberrations, several single gains and losses occurred, that is, gains on chromosomes 6p, 10q, 1p, 9q, and 13q. These findings also gave evidence that ONB was not included in the pPNET family. You et al., [47] analyzed 22 cases of ONB and revealed that consensus deletion regions were most frequently observed on chromosomes 1p , 2q , 3p/ q , 4p/ q , 5p/ q , 6q , 8p/ q , 9p , 10p/ q , 11p , 1 2q , 1 3q , 1 8q , and 21 q. DNA overrepresentations were identified on chromosomes 1p, 7q, 9q, 11q, 14q, 16p/ q, 17p/ q, 19p/ q, 20p/ q and 22p/ q. Thus, the genetic pattern of ONB was distinct from that of other small round cell tumor types and neuroblastomas. The deletion on chromosome band 1p21-p31 was associated with poor prognosis.

5. CLINICAL FEATURES AND STAGING

5.1. Clinical Features

The early study showed that the age of the patients with ONB fell in the range of 3~79 and there were two disease peaks, 10-20 and 50-60, indicating the bimodal age distribution in the second and sixth decade of life [2,4]. However, recent study only revealed a single peak of age distribution from 50~60 [48,49]. There is no gender and racial difference [50]. The most common site of the occurrence of ONB is in the olfactory mucosa region, including the top of nasal cavity, the upper nasal septum and the supersurface of concha nasalis superior. The neoplasm cells usually infiltrate focally adjacent sinus maxillaries, ethmoid sinus, sphenoid sinus and frontal sinus. Furthermore it may also involve base of skull and orbit [4]. The main symptoms are unilateral nasal obstruction and epistaxis. The less common symptoms include rhinorrhea, headache, anosmia, excessive lacrimation, and diplopia-visual disturbances [51,52,53]. Generally, the mean time delay between the appearance of the first symptom and the diagnosis is from six months to about one year [50]. The neoplasm could metastasize by lymphatic and hematogenous routes. The most common site of the metastasis is the cervical lymph node [54]. And metastasis could also occur in distant organs, i.e. lungs, pleura, brain, trachea, and bone [55].

5.2. Clinical Staging

In 1976, Kadish [56] staging was proposed, which is a comprehensively accepted clinical staging based on the clinical spread of neoplasm. It includes three stages: stage AB and C (table 2). In 1993, Morita et al., [57] modified Kadish staging by adding stage D based on the clinical need table 3. Nowadays, in predicting recurrence of ONB or biological behavior, there are no more valuable prognostic indicators than the Kadish staging system [58]. Eduardo et al., [49] found the Kadish staging system to be prognostically significant for 2-year and 5-year survival, despite there were no significant differences between groups with regard to 10-year survival. And all recurrence occurred in patients whose disease was initially Kadish stage C. These findings indicate that early-stage disease (stages A and B) has improved survival and a lower incidence of recurrence compared with stage C disease. However, because the range of the stage C of Kadish staging is too broad, taking the advantage of the radiologic advances, Biller tumor staging (table 4) [59] and a modified TNM staging system (table 5) [50] were proposed based on the tumor-node-metastasis system. This allows patients, treated either by surgery or by radiotherapy, to be staged reliably.

Table 2. Kadish tumor staging

Type	Extension
A	tumor limited to the nasal cavity
B	tumor involving the nasal and paranasal cavities
C	tumor extending beyond the nasal and paranasal cavities, including involvement of the cribriform plate, base of the skull, orbit or intracranial cavity

Data from Kadish *et al.*

Table 3. Modified Kadish tumor staging

Type	Extension
A	tumor limited to the nasal cavity
B	tumor involving the nasal and paranasal cavities
C	tumor extending beyond the nasal and paranasal cavities, including involvement of the cribriform plate, base of the skull, orbit or intracranial cavity
D	tumor with metastasis to cervical nodes or distant sites

Data from Kadish et al and Morita *et al.*

Table 4. Biller tumor staging

Stage	Description
T1	tumor in the nasal cavity sinuses(except sphenoid) with or without erosion of anterior cranial fossa bone
T2	periorbital or anterior cranial fossa extension
T3	brain involvement w/re spectable margins
T4	unresectable tumor

Data from Biller *et al.*

Table 5. Modified TNM staging system

Stage	Characteristics
T1	Tumor involving the nasal cavity or paranasal sinuses(excluding the sphenoid sinus) sparing the most superior ethmoidal cells
T2	Tumor involving the nasal cavity or paranasal sinuses(including the sphenoid sinus) with extension to or erosion of cribriform plate ,
T3	Tumor extending into the orbit or protruding into the anterior cranial fossa without dural invasion
T4	Tumor involving the brain
N0	No cervical lymph node metastases
N1	Any form of cervical lymph node metastases
M0	No metastases
M1	Any distant metastases

Data from Dulguerov *et al.*

6. IMAGING

CT and MRI could provide the most valuable information about the exact margins of the tumor extension, especially the relationship between the tumor and the important surrounding apparatus, such as orbital cavity, optic nerve, intracranial cavity and encephalon. It is crucial for the preoperation staging and helpful for the surgeons to make management plans.

Since MRI could display tumor multiplanarly without spurious shadow of the bone, it is better than CT in displaying the tumor in the nasal cavity, the nasal sinus or the tumor invading into intracranial cavity. However, CT is more sensitive than MRI in displaying the bone invasion, calcification, ossification, because calcification isn't a characteristic representation in the MRI image. The contrast-enhanced CT scanning can display the blood supply which could also be revealed by angiographic studies [60].

7. TREATMENT

Treatment modalities used for ONB include surgery, radiation, and chemotherapy. Unfortunately, there is no consensus regarding the treatment of ONB. The combination of surgery and radiotherapy is the most frequently used approach which could achieve the highest cure rates.

7.1. Surgery

Intracranial extension and the close relationship to the ethmoid roof and cribriform plate of ONB require the craniofacial resection, which permits *en bloc* resection of the tumor with better assessment of any intracranial extension and protection of the brain and optic nerves. According to literatures, the advent of craniofacial resection has clearly improved local control and reduced the recurrence rate. Based on the report from the University of Virginia, the recurrence rate was 60% before the adoption of craniofacial resection compared with 40% afterwards [50,61].

Some authors recommended surgery alone in early-stage disease. Biller et al., [59] advocated craniofacial resection alone with negative margins as treatment for patients with Kadish stage A/B disease. Similarly, Morita et al., [57] reported that surgical resection alone was effective for low-grade tumors if tumor-free margins could be achieved. But with the using of combined treatment, surgical resection alone isn't the ideal treatment in local control and reducing the recurrence rate. Dulgherov and Calcaterra [50] reported 86% local control with combined treatment compared with 17% with surgery alone. O'Connor et al [62] observed none recurrence after the combined approach compared with 75% rate after surgery alone. Foote et al., [63] reported that, when postoperative radiation was added, local control improved from 72.7% to 85.9% and strongly advocated the use of postoperative radiation to improve local control. From 20 of 24 ONB cases treated with a combination of surgery and radiation, Eduardo et al got the similar result. Thus, the addition of radiation to surgery with a combined craniofacial approach seems to be the ideal treatment and to significantly improve local control and reduce recurrence of ONB.

7.2. Radiotherapy

Currently, it is believed that radiotherapy should play a role in the management of ONB, particularly in patients who have had incomplete surgical resection or who present with residual disease [64,65].

Standard radiotherapeutic techniques include external megavoltage beam and a three-field technique. An anterior port is combined with wedge lateral fields to provide a homogeneous dose distribution. The doses range from 55 Gy to 65 Gy, and in the most doses above 60 Gy. Stereotactic irradiation as an overall minimally invasive treatment modality can also be successful in some patients if combined with intranasal access, although long-term data with these procedures are lacking here [66]. Stereotactic irradiation could improve target coverage and sparing of organs at risk [67] and associate with a lower complication rate compared to conventional radiotherapy [68].

At present, radiation combined with craniofacial approach is considered to be the best treatment. The optimum point in time for RT has been discussed in multiple studies. Preoperative RT can achieve reduction of tumor size and improve the prospects for radical resection [61,69,70], but may on the other hand obscure the actually required extent of resection after tumor shrinkage [59,71]. Postoperative RT is preferred in most cases. The dose required to achieve local tumor control is on the order of 50 to 70 Gy depending on the radicality of the operation [48,50,57,63,72].

7.3. Chemotherapy

Despite ONB is regarded as a chemosensitive tumor based on multiple responses to treatment [73], chemotherapy as a single modality therapy does not appear to be curative. Klepin et al., [74] reported that chemotherapy should not be used as a single-modality therapy for initial treatment but may provide additional benefit when used in combination with radiation and surgery, particularly in advanced-stage disease. Combination chemotherapy should be considered as initial therapy for unresectable tumors and metastasis disease and salvage therapy in disease recurrence.

Neoadjuvant chemotherapy has been used to decrease the tumor burden before resection. The study from University of Virginia over a 20-year period [70] showed two thirds of 34 cases had a significant reduction of tumor burden with adjuvant therapy. The patients who responded to neoadjuvant therapy had lower rate of disease-free related mortality. Multiple agents of chemotherapy have been used, including DTIC, actinomycin, MTX, BCNU, procarbazine, platinum regimens, etoposide, cyclophosphamide, vincristine, and doxorubicin. Some large referral centers advocate routine use of systemic preoperative chemotherapy in stage C disease. For example, routine use of cyclophosphamide (650 mg/m2) and vincristine (1.5 mg/m2; maximal dose, 2 mg) was administered every 3 weeks for six cycles.

Combination of chemotherapy with radiation and surgery has been demonstrated to improve survival in the published University of Virginia experience [73]. High-dose chemotherapy with stem cell rescue has been reported as primary and salvage therapy. Mishima *et al* [75] published a study of 12 patients who were treated with combination chemotherapy and radiation therapy with or without autologous stem cell transplant. Response to primary chemotherapy was high (75%). All four patients treated with autologous transplantation obtained a complete remission.

7.4. Recommended Treatment

Therefore, the treatment recommended as following [76]:

- Kadesh A: Surgery combined with radiotherapy in selected cases.
- Kadesh B: Radiotherapy before or after surgery to the primary tumor site and subclinical lymph nodes. Adjunctive chemotherapy may be added to this treatment.
- Kadesh C or D: Preoperative chemotherapy, radiotherapy, or both followed by surgery. The value of adjuvant chemotherapy has yet to be elucidated further, along with the timing of the surgery and the radiotherapy.

8. PROGNOSIS AND PREDICTIVE FACTORS

8.1. Metastasis

The most common metastasis is cervical lymph node metastasis. In 2002, Rinaldo *et al* [77] reported a cumulative incidence of 23.4% of synchronous and metachronous lymph node metastasis from 15 institutions worldwide. In 2003, Alfio et al., [78] have calculated a cumulative metastatic rate of 23.5% of cervical lymph nodes in 494 cases of ENB from 26 institutions worldwide. In the some year, Monroe et al., [54] reported that the incidence of cervical metastases in nine publications ranged from 17% to 33%, and pointed out that elective neck radiotherapy is effective in preventing cervical recurrence and should be considered in all patients with Kadish stage B and C disease. And, Koka et al., [72] concluded that neck lymphadenopathy may increase the risk for the development of distant metastases and has been correlated with poor prognosis.

Distant metastasis usually happens, and all histologic grades have the capacity to metastasize. Approximately 10%~60% patients will experience distant metastasis [55]. The prognosis of patients with distant metastases is uniformly fatal. When metastases occur in central nervous system (CNS), the prognosis is poor. The following implications has been proposed [79]: (1) most patients in whom CNS metastases developed had Kadish stage C disease at diagnosis; (2) there was a highly variable time to onset of CNS metastases, ranging from 1 to 228 months after initial diagnosis of ONB; (3) survival after CNS metastases was generally less than 2 years; and (4) the treatment regimen that appeared to result in the longest survival after CNS metastases included surgical resection of the metastatic lesion followed by radiation, chemotherapy, or both.

8.2. Recurrences

Recurrences are noted in 37% to 62% of cases, 70% to 80% of these occurring within the first 2 years [61,69,80,81]. However, these tumors can appear even after more than 10 years [56,58]. Median survival after recurrences was only 12 months [33,31].

The most frequent recurrence is local, with rates around 30%. Craniofacial resection followed by radiotherapy is associated with fewer recurrences, approximately 10% [50,63]. Importantly, different from results with most other skull base tumors, salvage after local recurrence is possible in 33 to 50% of cases. Morita [57] and Eriksen [71] proposed that the degree of histopathologic differentiation was the most important and the only significant risk factor for development of a recurrence.

8.3. Survival Rates

From the University of Virginia's experience [70], the overall 5- and 10-year survival rates have been reported to be 81% and 54% respectively. Disease-free survival at 5 years was 86% for stage A and B and 60% for stage C. In 2003 Argiris et al [51] retrospectively analyzed 227 cases from nine institutions in the world to reveal 57% of Kadish C disease. They observed that the average rate of 5-year survival was 67% (51 %-92%) and of 5-year disease-free survival was 54% (33%-75%).

8.4. Prognosis Factors

The study of prognosis factors has been being a field. An important factor for patient survival and prognosis is the degree of histopathologic differentiation of the tumor, such as histologic grading (Hyams system), proliferation rate, and ploidy. The Hyams system was correlated with clinical outcome and a significantly higher 5-year survival for low-grade tumors (80%) than for high-grade tumors (40%) [57]. Eriksen et al [71] also demonstrated that patients with high-grade tumors survived for a shorter period of time on average. In addition, other authors proposed that Hyams system was not only indicative of survival, but also predictive for the utility of chemotherapy [82,83].

In the case of immunohistochemistry, Hirose and colleagues [35] found that a high degree of S-100 immunopositivity and a low (<10%) Ki-67 labelling index were associated with better survival. And there are conflicting data on the prognostic role of the P53 tumor suppressor gene mutations [35,36].

Furthermore, previous reports identified age greater than 50 years, female gender, tumor recurrence, and metastasis as negative prognostic factors [50]. The meta-analysis data from the Johns Hopkins [48] and the university of Texas M.D. Anderson Cancer Center [49], confirmed the conclusion of Koka et al., [72] the only negative prognostic factor was the presence of cervical nodal metastasis at the time of diagnosis of primary cases. Gender, age, recurrence, race, side of presentation, history of tobacco, alcohol use, and family history of cancer had no significant prognostic effect.

8.5. Recommended Follow-Up

ONB, as a neoplastic disease with a long natural history characterized by frequent local and regional recurrences after conventional treatment [80], should be warranted a long-term follow-up of patients.

The follow-up protocol has been suggested as followings [84]: Continued clinical follow-up is indicated annually thereafter, investigated on the basis of symptoms. MRI with gadolinium should be performed 2 to 4 months after completion of all therapy, and should be repeated every 4 to 6 months for 5 years, and then annually for the patient's lifetime [80,85]. An annual chest radiograph should be performed to exclude the presence of metastases.

REFERENCES

[1]   Broich G, Pagliari A, Ottaviani F, et al. Esthesioneuroblastoma: a general review of the case published since the discovery of the tumor in 1924. *Anticancer Res*, 1997, 17:2683-2706.
[2]   Theilgaard S.A, Buchwald C, Ingeholm P, et al. Esthesioneuroblastoma: A Danish demographic study of 40 patients registered between 1978 and 2000. *Acta Otolaryngologica*, 2003, 123: 433-439.
[3]   Berger L, Luc R, Richard D. L'esthesioneuroepitheliome olfactif. *Bull. Assoc. Fr. Etude Cancer*, 1924, 13:410-421.
[4]   Rosai J, Rosai and Ackeman's *Surgical Pathology*, ninth edition 2004.1.316-317
[5]   Barnes L.W. Eveson J.W., Reichart P, et al. World Health Organization Classification of Tumour. *Pathology and Genetics of Head and Neck Tumours*. IARC Press: Lyon, 2005,66-70.
[6]   Graziadej PP. Cell dynamics in the olfactory mucosa. *Tissue Cell*. 1973; 5: 1131.
[7]   Graziadei PP, Levine RR, Monti Graziadei GA. Plasticity of connections of the olfactory sensory neuron: regeneration into the forebrain following bulbectomy in the neonatal mouse. *Neuroscience*. 1979; 4: 713 27.
[8]   Verhaagen J, Oestreicher AB, Gispen WH, Margolis FL. The expression of the growth associated protein B50/GAP43 in the olfactory system of neonatal and adult rats. *J. Neurosci*. 1989; 9: 68391.
[9]   Margolis FL, Verhaagen J, Biffoe t Sa,l . Regulation of gene expression in the olfactory neuroepithelium: a neurogenetic matrix. *Prog. Brain Res*. 1991; 89: 97 122.
[10]   Miragall F, Kadmon G, Husmann M, Schachner M. Expression of cell adhesion molecules in the olfactory system of the adult mouse: presence of the embryonic form of N-CAM. *Dev. Biol*. 1988; 129: 51631.

[11] Cunningham BA, Hemperly JJ, Murray BA, et al. Neural cell adhesion molecule: structure, immunoglobulin-like domains, cell surface modulation, and alternative RNA splicing. *Science.* 1987; 236: 799806.

[12] Guillemot F, Lo LC, Johnson JE, et al. Mammalian achaete-scute homolog 1 is required for the early development of olfactory and autonomic neurons. *Cell* 1993; 75: 46376.

[13] Benowitz LI, Routtenberg A. A membrane phosphoprotein associated with neural development, axonal regeneration, phospholipid metabolism and synaptic plasticity. *Trends Neurosci.* 1987; 10: 52732.

[14] Margolis FL. A brain protein unique to the olfactory bulb. *Proc. Natl. Acad. Sci. USA.* 1972; 69: 1221 24.

[15] Nibu K, Li G, Zhang X, et al. Olfactory neuron-specific expression of NeuroD in mouse and human nasal mucosa. *Cell Tissue Res.* 1999; 298: 40514.

[16] Carney ME, O Reilly RC, Sholevar B, et al. Expression of the human Achaetescute 1 gene in olfactory neuroblastoma (esthesioneuroblastoma). *J. Neurooncol.* 1995; 26: 3543.

[17] Servenius B, Vernachio J, Price J, et al. Metastasizing neuroblastomas in mice transgenic for simian virus 40 large T (SV40T) under the olfactory marker protein gene promoter. *Cancer Res.* 1994; 54: 5198205.

[18] Delattre O, Zucman J, Melote t Ta,l . The Ewing family of tumors: a subgroup of small-round-cell tumors defined by specific chimeric transcripts. *N. Engl. J. Med.* 1994; 331: 29499.

[19] Sorensen PH, Wu JK, Berean KW, et al. Olfactory neuroblastoma is a peripheral primitive neuroectodermal tumor related to Ewing sarcoma. *Proc. Natl. Acad. Sci. USA.* 1996; 93: 103843.

[20] Nelson RS, Perlman EJ, Askin FB. Is esthesioneuroblastoma a peripheral neuroectodermal tumor? *Hum. Pathol.* 1995; 26: 63941.

[21] Delattre O, Zucman J, Melote t Ta,l . The Ewing family of tumors: a subgroup of small-round-cell tumors defined by specific chimeric transcripts. *N. Engl. J. Med.* 1994; 331: 29499.

[22] Kumar S, Perlman E, Packe t Sa,l . Absence of EWS/FL1 1 fusion in olfactory neuroblastomas indicates these tumors do not belong to the Ewings sarcoma family. *Hum. Pathol.* 1999; 30: 1356 60.

[23] Mezzelani A, Tornielli S, Minoletti F, et al. Esthesioneuroblastoma is not a member of the primitive peripheral neuroectodermal tumour-Ewings group. *Br. J. Cancer.* 1999; 81: 58691.

[24] Pellin A, Boix J, Blesa JR, Noguera R, Carda C, Llombart-Bosch A. EWS/FLI-1 rearrangement in small round cell sarcomas of bone and soft tissue detected by reverse transcriptase polymerase chain reaction amplification. *Eur. J. Cancer.* 1994; 30A: 82731.

[25] Herrold KM. Induction of olfactory neuroepithelial tumors in Syrian hamsters by diethylnitrosamine. *Cancer.* 1964; 30: 101424.

[26] Vollrath M, Altmannsberger M. Chemically induced esthesioneuroepithelioma: ultrastructural findings. *Ann. Otol. Rhinol. Laryngol.* 1989; 98: 25666.

[27] Koike K, Jay G, Hartley JW, et al. Activation of retrovirus in transgenic mice: association with development of olfactory neuroblastoma. *J. Virol.* 1990; 64: 3988-91.

[28] Liu HG, Zhang SZ, He CY. Study on pathological features and diagnosis, differential diagnosis of olfactory neuroblastoma. *Zhonghua Bing Li Xue Za Zhi*, 2003 Oct, 32(5):432-436.

[29] Hyams VJ, Batsakis JG, Michaels L. *Olfactory neuroblastoma. In: Tumors of the upper respiratory tract and ear, Fascicle 25*, Second Series. Washington DC: Armed Forces Institute of Pathology, 1988, 240-248.

[30] Axe S, Kuhajda FP. Esthesioneuroblastoma: intermediate filaments, neuroendocrine, and tissue-specific antigens. *Am. J. Clin. Pathol.* 1987; 88: 13945.

[31] Frierson HF Jr, Ross GW, Mills SE, Frankfurter A. Olfactory neuroblastoma: additional immunohistochemical characterization. *Am. J. Clin. Pathol.* 1990; 94: 547 53.

[32] Lund VJ, Milroy C. Olfactory neuroblastoma: clinical and pathological aspects. *Rhinology.* 1993; 31: 1 6.

[33] Tatagiba MSamii MDankoweit-Timpe EAguiar PHOs terwald L, Babu R, Ostertag H(1995). Esthesioneuroblastomas with intracranial extension. Proliferative potential and management. *Arq. Neuropsiquiatr.* 53:577-586.

[34] Varvares RK (1996). Olfactory neuroblastoma: an immunohistochemical, ultrastructual, and flow cytometric study. *Cancer.* 77: 1957-1959.

[35] Hirose T, Scheithauer BW, Lopes MB, et al. Olfactory neuroblastoma: an immunohistochernical, ultrastructural, and flow cytometric study. *Cancer.* 1995; 76: 419.

[36] Papadaki H, Kounelis S, Kapadia SB, et al. Relationship of p53 gene alterations with tumor progression and recurrence in olfactory neuroblastoma. *Am. J. Surg. Pathol.* 1996; 20: 71521.

[37] Perlman EJ, Dickman PS, Askin FB, et al. Ewings sarcomaroutine diagnostic utilization of MIC2 analysis: a Pediatric Oncology Group/Childrens Cancer Group Intergroup Study. *Hum. Pathol.* 1994; 25: 30407.

[38] Folpe AL, Hill CE, Parham DM, O'Shea PA, Weiss SW.Immunohistochemical detection of FLI-1 protein expression: a study of 132 round cell tumors with emphasis on CD9 9-positive mimics of Ewing's sarcoma/primitive neuroectodermal tumor. *Am. J. Surg. Pathol.* 2000 Dec; 24(12):1657-62.

[39] Smith SRSom PFahmy ALawson WSacks S Brandwein M. A. clinicopathological study of sinonasal neuroendocrine carcinoma and sinonasal undifferentiated carcinoma. *Laryngoscope.* 2000 Oct;1 10(10 Pt 1):1617-22

[40] Perez-Ordonez B, Caruana SM, Huvos AG, Shah JP. Small cell neuroendocrine carcinoma of the nasal cavity and paranasal sinuses. *Hum Pathol* 1998; 29: 82632.

[41] Vartanian RK. Olfactory neuroblastoma: an immunohistochemical, ultrastructural and flow cytometric study. *Cancer.* 1996 May 1, 77(9):1957-1959.

[42] Choi HS, Anderson PJ. Olfactory neuroblastoma: an immuno-electron microscopic study of S-100 protein-positive cells. *J. Neuropathol. Exp. Neurol.* 1986 Sep; 45(5): 576-87.

[43] Paulette M, Margaret B, Mounia A, et al. Human achaete-scute Homologue (hASH1)mRNA level as adiagnostic marker to distinguish esthesioneuroblastoma from poorly differentiated tumors arising in the sinonasal tract. *Am. J. Clin. Pathol,* 2004, 122:100-105.

[44] Sorensen PHB, Wu JK, Berean KW, Lim JF, Donn W, Frierson HF, Reynolds LP, Lopez-Terrada D and Trichet J (1996) Olfactory neuroblastoma is a peripheral primitive neuroectodermal tumor related to Ewing sarcoma. *Proc. Natl. Acad. Sci. USA.* 93: 1038–1043

[45] Argani P, Perez-Ordonez B, Xiao H, Caruana SM, Huvos AG and Ladanyi M (1998) Olfactory neuroblastoma is not related to the Ewing family of tumors absence at EWS/FLI1 gene fusion and MIC2 expression. *Am. J. Surg. Pathol.* 22: 39 1–398

[46] Szymas J, Wolf G, Kowalczyk D, Nowak S, Petersen I(1997) Olfactory neuroblastoma: detection of genomic imbalances by comparative genomic hybridization. *Acta Neurochir. (Wien)* 139:839-844

[47] You XJ, Petersen I, Arps H, et al. Cytogenetic aberrations of esthesioneuroblastoma studied by comparative genomic hybridization. *Zhonghua Zhong Liu Za Zhi*, 2005 Jan, 27(1):16-21.

[48] Resto VA, Eisele DW, Forastiere A, et al. Esthesioneuroblastoma: the Johns Hopkins experience. *Head Neck.* 2000;22:550–558.

[49] Eduardo M. Richard H. Adel K. James L. Franco D. Olfactory neuroblastoma: The 22-Year Experience at one Comprehensive Cancer Center. *Head Neck.* 2005 Feb;27(2): 138-149

[50] Dulguerov P, Calcaterra T. Esthesioneuroblastoma: the UCLA experience 1970–1990. *Laryngoscope.* 1992;102: 843–850.

[51] Argiris A, Dutra J, Tseke P, Haines K. Esthesioneuroblastoma: the Northwestern University experience. *Laryngoscope.* 2003, 113:155–160.

[52] Constantinidis J, Steinhart H, Koch M, Buchfelder M, Schaenzer A, Weidenbecher M, Iro H.Olfactory neuroblastoma: the University of Erlangen-Nuremberg experience 1975-2000. *Otolaryngol. Head Neck Surg.* 2004 May; 130(5):567-74.

[53] Lund VJ, Howard D, Wei W, Spittle M. Olfactory neuroblastoma: past, present, and future? *Laryngoscope.* 2003 Mar; 1 13(3):502-7.

[54] Monroe AT, Hinerman RW, Amdur RJ, et al. Radiation therapy for esthesioneuroblastoma: rationale for elective neck irradiation. *Head Neck.* 2003;25:529–534.

[55] Barnes L, Brandwein M, Som PM. Diseases of the nasal cavity, paranasal sinuses, and nasopharynx. In: Barnes L, ed. *Barnes Surgical Pathology of the Head and Neck.* 2nd ed. New York: Marcel Dekker, Inc; 2000.

[56] Kadish S, Goodman M, Wang CC. Olfaeiory neuroblastoma. A clinical analysis of 17 cases. *Cancer.* 1976;37:1571-1576

[57] Morita A, Ebersold MJ, Olsen KD, et al. Esthesioneuroblastoma: prognosis and management. *Neurosurgery.* 1993;32 :706-715.

[58] Levine PA, Gallagher R, Cantrell RW: Esthesioneuroblastoma: reflections of a 21-year experience. *Laryngoscope.* 109: 1539–1543, 1999

[59] Biller HF, Lawson W, Sachdev VP, et al: Esthesioneuroblastoma: surgical treatment without radiation. *Laryngoscope.* 100: 1199–1201, 1990

[60] Woodhead P, Lioyd GA (1988). Olfactory neuriblastoma: imaging by magnetic resonance, CT and conventional techniques. *Clin. Otolaryngol.* 13:387-394.

[61] Spaulding CA, Kranyak MS, Constable WC, Stewart FM. Esthesioneuroblastoma: a comparison of two treatment eras. *Int. J. Radiat. Oncol. Biol. Phys.* 1988; 15: 58190

[62] O'Connor TA, McLean P, Juillard GJF, Parker RG. Olfactory neuroblastoma. *Cancer.* 1989;63:2426–2428.

[63] Foote RL, Morita A, Ebersold MJ, et al. Esthesioneuroblastoma: the role of adjuvant radiation therapy. *Int. J. Radiat. Oncol. Biol. Phys.* 1993;27:835–842.

[64] Slevin NJ, Irwin CJR, Banerjee SS, et al.: Olfactory neural tumors—the role of external beam radiotherapy. *J. Laryngol. Otol.* 1996, 110:1012–1016.

[65] Eich HT, Staar S, Micke O, et al.: Radiotherapy of esthesioneuroblastoma. *Int. J. Radiat. Oncol. Biol. Phys.* 2001, 49:155–160.

[66] Walch C, Stammberger H, Anderhuber W, et al. The minimally invasive approach to olfactory neuroblastoma: combined endoscopic and stereotactic treatment. *Laryngoscope.* 2000;1 10:635-40.

[67] Zabel A, Thilmann C, Milker-Zabel S, et al.: The role of stereotactically guided conformal radiotherapy for local tumour control of esthesioneuroblastoma. *Strahlenther. Onkol.* 2002, 178:187–191.

[68] Battacharyya N, Thornton AF, Joseph MP, et al. Successful treatment of esthesioneuroblastoma and neuroendocrine carcinoma with combined chemotherapy and proton radiation. *Arch. Otolaryngol. Head Neck Surg.* 1997;123:34-40.

[69] Eden BV, Debo RF, Larner JM, et al. Esthesioneuroblastoma— long term outcome and patterns of failure-the University of Virginia experience. *Cancer.* 1994;73:2556- 62.

[70] Polin RS, Sheehan JP, Chenelle AG, et al. The role of preoperative adjuvant treatment in the management of esthesioneuroblastoma: the University of Virginia experience. *Neurosurgery.* 1998;42: 1029-37.

[71] Eriksen JG, Basthold L, Krogdahl AS, et al. Esthesioneuroblastoma. What is the optimal treatment? *Acta Oncol.* 2000;39:231-5.

[72] Koka VN, Julieron M, Bourhis J, et al. Aesthesioneuroblastoma. *J. Laryngol. Otol.* 1998;112:628-33.

[73] Sheehan JM, Sheehan JP, Jane JA, et al.: Chemotherapy for esthesioneuroblastoma. *Neurosurg. Clin. North Am.* 2000, 11:693–701.

[74] Klepin HD, McMullen KP, Lesser GJ. Esthesioneuroblastoma. *Curr. Treat Options Oncol.* 2005 Nov;6(6):509-1 8.

[75] Mishima Y, Nagasaki E, Terui Y, et al.: Combination chemotherapy (cyclophosphamide, doxorubicin, and vincristine with continuous-infusion cisplatin and etoposide) and radiotherapy with stem cell support can be beneficial for adolescents and adults with esthesioneuroblastoma. *Cancer.* 2004, 101:1437–1444.

[76] Bradley PJ, Jones NS, Robertson I. Diagnosis and management of esthesioneuroblastoma. Curr Opin Otolaryngol. *Head Neck. Surg.* 2003 Apr;11(2):112-8.

[77] Rinaldo A. Ferlito A, Shaha AR, et al. Esthesioneuroblastoma and cervical lymph node metastases: Clinical and iherapeiilic implications. *Acta Otoiaryngol.* 2002Mar: 1 22(2):2 15-21

[78] Ferlito A, Rinaldo A, Rhys-Evans PH. Contemporary clinical commentary: esthesioneuroblastoma: an update on management of the neck. *Laryngoscope.* 2003 Nov; 1 13(11):1935-8.

[79] Shaari CM, Catalano PJ, Sen C, Post K. Central nervous system metastases from esthesioneuroblastoma. *Otolaryngol. Head Neck Surg.* 1996; 114:808–812.)

[80] Olsen KD, DeSanto LW. Olfactory neuroblastoma: biologic and clinical behavior. *Arch. Otolaryngol.* 1983;109:797-802.

[81] Elkon D, Hightower SI, Lim ML, et al. Esthesioneuroblastoma. *Cancer.* 1 979;44: 1087-94.

[82] McElroy EA, Buckner JC, Lewis JE. Chemotherapy for advanced esthesioneuroblastoma: the Mayo Clinic experience. *Neurosurgery.* 1998;42: 1023–1 028.

[83] Sakata K, Aoki Y, Karasawa K, et al. Esthesioneuroblastoma: a report of seven cases. *Acta Oncol.* 1993; 32:399–402.

[84] Girod D, Hanna E, Lawrence L: Esthesioneuroblastoma. *Head Neck.* 2001, 23:500–505.

[85] Simon JH, Zhen W, Mc Culloch TM, et al.: Esthesioneuroblastoma: the University of
      Iowa experience 1978–1998. *Laryngoscope*. 2001, 111:488–493.

In: Encyclopedia of Stem Cell Research (2 Volume Set)   ISBN: 978-1-61761-835-2
Editor: Alexander L. Greene   © 2012 Nova Science Publishers, Inc.

Chapter XXXIII

DOES NEURAL PHENOTYPIC PLASTICITY FROM NON-NEURAL CELLS REALLY EXIST?

S. Wislet-Gendebien[1,2,*], F. Wautier[1], E. Laudet[1] and B. Rogister[1,3]

[1]Center for Cellular and Molecular Neuroscience, University of Liège,
Liège, Belgium
[2]Centre for Research in Neurodegenerative Diseases, University of Toronto, Canada
[3]Department of Neurologie, CHU, Université de Liège, Belgium

ABSTRACT

Cellular therapies are promising approaches in the treatment of several neurological diseases such as Parkinson's disease [Isacson et al., 2001] or Huntington's disease [Dunnett et al., 2000], but also for spinal cord injury [Hall et al., 2001]. One main problem concerns the origin and nature of the cells to be used for such procedures. In this context, recent studies suggest that somatic stem cells (stem cells from foetal or adult tissues) might be able to exhibit more plasticity than previously thought as they seem able to differentiate into many cell types, including cell types which are not encountered in their tissue origin. This last property, named phenotypic plasticity of somatic stem cells, is thus the capacity for a stem cell to develop in several phenotypes depending on their environment. Several recent reports suggest that bone marrow mesenchymal stem cells (MSC) could be a source of somatic stem cells suitable for cell replacement strategies in the treatment of central nervous system (CNS) disorders. MSC can differentiate into many types of mesenchymal cells, i.e. osteocytes, chondrocytes and adipocytes, but can also differentiate into non-mesenchymal cell, i.e. neural cells in appropriate *in vivo* and *in vitro* experimental conditions [Kopen et al., 1999; Brazelton et al, 2000; Mezey et al, 2000; Wislet-Gendebien et al., 2003, 2005]. Some works have attributed the neural phenotypic plasticity to "transdifferentiation" [Krause et al., 2001; Orlic et al., 2001; Priller et al., 2001; Wislet-Gendebien et al., 2005], while some other works suggested that this neural plasticity could be explained by cell fusion [Terada et al., 2002; Ying et al.,

---

* Correspondence concerning this article should be addressed to: S. Wislet-Gendebien, Telephone: +1416 978 0773; Fax: +1416 978 1878; e-mail: sabine.wislet@utoronto.ca.

2002; Vassilopoulos et al., 2003; Alvarez-Dolado et al., 2003]. These observations could suggest that mesenchymal cells are heterogeneous and there are two cell populations able to adopt a neural phenotype: one which is able to fuse with already-present neurons and a second one which is really able to differentiate in neurons. In the first part of this chapter, we will review the studies realized on the potential neural phenotypic plasticity of the mesenchymal stem cells. The second part of this chapter will focus on recent studies demonstrating that stem cells isolated from adipose, skin and umbilical cord cells have the ability to differentiate into neural cells [Nagase et al., 2007; McKenzie et al., 2006; Fallahi-Sichani et al., 2006]. This ability could be attributed to the presence of neural crest stem cells in those tissues [Fernandes et al., 2007; Crane and Trainor, 2006]. Consequently, we will address the question of the potential presence of neural crest stem cells in bone marrow.

INTRODUCTION

Embryologists and developmental biologists have introduced the stem cell concept several years ago. A stem cell, by definition, is an undifferentiated cell that can produce daughter cells that can either remain a stem cell (a process called self-renewal) or commit to a pathway leading to differentiation. The first stem cell (and probably the more symbolic) is the fertilized egg which results from the fusion of two haploid germinal stem cells. Once fertilized, the egg undergoes a series of divisions, yielding two, then four, then eight identical cells. These cells are *totipotent* (Figure 1), meaning that each one, if isolated and allowed to develop, can form a new viable embryo. This is how identical (homozygous) twins result from a single fertilized egg. Beside this particular type of stem cells, two other types of stem cells can be distinguished according to their origin and their potential of differentiation: embryonic stem cells (ES) and somatic stem cells (SSC) [Stanford et al., 1998]. After the eight-cell stage (in human, two or three days after fertilization), the cells continue to divide, but lose the ability to form a new embryo because trophoblastic differentiation is no more observed at this stage of development. The embryo takes the form of a hollow sphere, known as a blastocyst, containing an inner cell mass. ES are isolated for the inner mass of the blastocyte and are able to differentiate into the three germ layer cell types [Amit et al., 2000, Itskovitz-Eldor et al., 2000, Schuldiner et al., 2000]. This property is also call *pluripotentiality*. ES are not considered to be totipotent because they cannot produce all of the extra-embryonic tissues required for a full organism development. SSC are isolated from fetal (after gastrulation stage) or adult tissues and have a more restricted potential of differentiation also defined as *multipotentiality*. Currently, SSC have been isolated from various organs or tissues: brain [Davis and Temple, 1994], blood [Domen and Weissman, 1999], epidermis [Gandarillas and Watt, 1997], intestine [Potten et al., 2003], bone marrow [Bianco and Robey, 1999], pancreas [Lechner and Habener, 2003], liver [Sell, 1990], cornea [Wu et al., 2001] and skeletal muscles [Seale and Rudnicki, 2000]. It was classically admitted that SSC support tissue homeostasis by replacing lost cells. This function relies on the self-renewing capacity which, together with asymmetrical division, prevents the drying up of stem cell stocks and on the differentiation into mature cells to replace the lost cells.

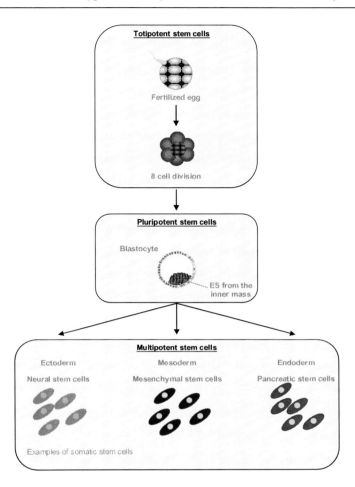

Figure 1. Stem cell types, origin and potential of differentiation. Totipotent stem cells results from the fusion of two haploid germinal stem cells and the first divisions of the zygote. Pluripotent stem cells are issued from the inner mass of the blastocyte, also named embryonic stem cells (ES). Multipotent stem cells also defined as somatic stem cells, have a more restricted potential of differentiation than the ES although this potential is not already well defined and seems to vary between somatic stem cells of various organs and tissues.

However, while a great number of organs or tissues contain somatic stem cells, it appears that, most of the time, those cells are quiescent or weakly active and, at least in some organs, are unable to efficiently repair the damaged tissue. This is especially true for neural stem cells which are found in the subependymal layer of the subventricular zone (SVZ) and the *dentate gyrus* (DG) of the hippocampus in adult mammals [Gage, 2002]. Those cells, while still able to proliferate and differentiate *in vitro* into neurons, astrocytes and oligodendrocytes [McKay, 1997], seem unable to sufficiently do so *in vivo* to ensure brain homeostasis as we define it above [Li et al., 2003]. These two neurogenic zones are only able to form a small microneurons population for olfactory bulb (SVZ) or CA1 (DG) [Hagg, 2005]. By contrast, mesenchymal stem cells (MSC) remain able to proliferate and differentiate into adipocytes, osteocytes, fibroblasts and chondrocytes during the whole life and thus guarantee such homeostasis for these cell types and tissues [Bianco and Robey, 1999].

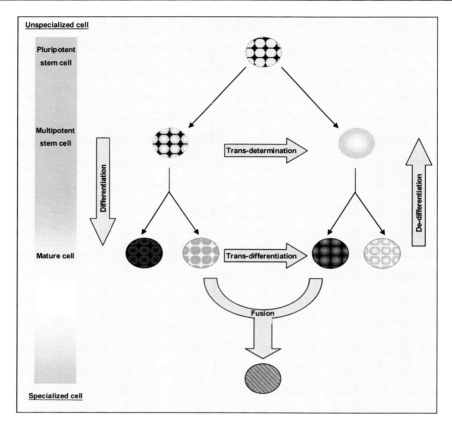

Figure 2. Phenotypic plasticity of somatic stem cells. The six different modes of phenotype acquisition can explain the unusual differentiation properties of the somatic stem cells: differentiation, trans-determination, trans-differentiation, fusion, real pluripotent behaviour and trophic factor influences.

Over the last decade, researchers have challenged the concept of tissue restriction of SSC and demonstrated that those stem cells have more differentiation abilities than previously thought. This ability, also refereed as stem cell *phenotypic plasticity*, can be defined as a cell property where a same genotype can express different phenotype in function of the environmental conditions. Such kind of plasticity can be adaptative or non-adaptative. Six different mechanisms of differentiation, described by the embryologists during the development could explain the phenotypic plasticity of SSC: de-differentiation, trans-differentiation, the fusion, the trans-determination, true pluripotent stem cell behaviour and the influence of trophic factors (Figure 2):

- *De-differentiation.* De-differentiation refers to the gain in differentiation potential that would occur if mature cells were pushed back up the hierarchical model of lineage restriction. After injury, some amphibians regenerate limbs, tail, and even brain and spinal cord by de-differentiation at the injury site [Tsonis, 2000; Stocum, 2003]. Normally, primordial germ cells transplanted into blastocysts are fate-restricted to germ cells. However, environmental manipulation allows these cells to contribute to all somatic tissues. For instance, oligodendrocyte precursor cells can be induced to generate neurospheres and subsequently neurons *in vitro* [Kondo and Raff, 2000, 2004]. Whether de-differentiation of mammalian cells occurs under normal circumstances or in repair remains unclear.

- *Fusion.* Investigators recognized in the 1960s that differentiated cell fate could be altered in the rather extreme experimental conditions used when a somatic cell nucleus was injected into an enucleated egg, and the cloning of mammals provides proof of principle [Hochedlinger and Jaenisch, 2006]. Nonetheless, much of our knowledge about cell fusion has been derived from studies involving heterokaryons-cells fused *in vitro*. Typically, specialized functions are lost in these cells, although they may be regained after chromosome loss. Silent genes may be activated; for example, synthesis of human muscle proteins occurs in human amniotic fibroblasts after fusion with mouse muscle cells [Clegg et Hauschka, 1987]. It has been postulated that gene dosage (the relative genetic contribution of the two fused cell types) is important both to novel gene activation in heterokaryons and to the suppression of malignancy in hybrids. The formation of (non-dividing) heterokaryons indicates that differentiated cell phenotype can be altered without DNA replication and cell division.

- *Transdifferentiation.* In transdifferentiation, a mature cell assumes the phenotype and function of another fully differentiated cell. This mechanism occurs during normal oesophageal development, when smooth muscle cells switch to skeletal muscle [Reddy and Kablar, 2004]. Moreover, the transdifferentiation is encountered in various organs which are the target of a chronic inflammation leading to metaplasia [Slack, 2007]. Some reports of transdifferentiation without chronic inflammation have been based on morphological characteristics and lineage-specific markers alone. However, to fulfil the criteria for transdifferentiation, multilineage engraftment and functional activity must also be demonstrated.

- *Transdetermination.* Transdetermination is the redirection of lineage-committed stem cells or precursors to an alternative lineage [Johnston, 2005]. This happens during development in drosophila, but it is extremely difficult to establish definitively that cells are irreversibly committed to a lineage before transdetermination, either at single cell or population level.

- *True pluripotent cells.* True pluripotent cells may persist beyond embryogenesis and, if provided with the appropriate signals, differentiate into cells of multiple lineages. Presently, our knowledge of cell markers is inadequate to define cell populations accurately, so it is possible that cells with true pluripotency issued from adult organisms will have contaminated experiments previously reported as examples of transdifferentiation. However, if the presence of an adult reserve of stem cells is confirmed, the question of why such cells fail to effectively contribute to repair in disease states must be addressed. Stem cells of various origins, including bone marrow, do have tropism for inflammation suggesting that signals may be released from areas of tissue damage into the circulation.

- *Trophic factors.* Stem cells could also play a part in promoting functional recovery by means other than cell replacement. The production of trophic factors might confer resistance to disease, or promote the survival, migration, and differentiation of endogenous precursors. Certainly, bone-marrow cells are known to produce a wide variety of cytokines and exert paracrine effects [Wislet-Gendebien et al., 2004]. Moreover, these trophic factors could be concentrated in discrete functional localisations, the so-called "niche", where trophic factors should also include paracrine and extracellular influences [Scadden, 2006].

The finding of stem cell plasticity carries significant implications for potential cell therapy. For example, if differentiation can be redirected, stem cells of abundant source and easy access, such as bone marrow or umbilical cord blood, could be used to substitute stem cells in tissues that are difficult to isolate, such as heart and nervous system tissue. In this therapeutical objective, numerous studies have been performed on the plasticity of the mesenchymal stem cells. In this chapter, we will discuss the different studies of neural phenotypic plasticity of mesenchymal stem cells and the pathway used by those cells to express some neural characteristics.

NEURAL PHENOTYPIC PLASTICITY OF MESENCHYMAL STEM CELLS: MECHANISM(S) OF DIFFERENTIATION

Mesenchymal stem cells (MSC) are isolated from various tissues i.e. bone marrow, adipose tissue and muscles. Those cells are characterized by the expression of numerous surface antigens, but none of them appears to be exclusively expressed on MSC. It is classically admitted that those cells need to be positive for STRO-1, CD13, CD49a, CD29, CD44, CD90 (Thy1.1), VCAM-1 and p75-NGFr markers, but negative for CD11b, CD34 and CD45 [reviewed by Herzog, 2003]. As a high proliferate and accessible source of cells, MSC have been intensively studied for their potential use in restorative approaches for degenerative diseases and traumatic injuries. In the central nervous system (CNS), stem cell-based strategies have been proposed to replace lost neurons in degenerative diseases such as Parkinson's disease, Huntington's disease, and amyotrophic lateral sclerosis [Lou Gehrig's disease), or to replace lost oligodendrocytes in demyelinating diseases such as multiple sclerosis. However, even if some studies, which we will be described later in this chapter, demonstrated that MSC derived from adult tissues could be good candidates for cell replacement therapy, a better knowledge of the mechanisms underlying the phenotypic plasticity of somatic stem cells is a prerequisite before considering their use in the treatment of neurological diseases.

During the last decade, different studies have shown that MSC are able to adopt neural phenotypes. Those studies can be classified in 3 groups: A) *In vivo* studies; B) neural phenotypic plasticity induce *in vitro* using chemical agents and C) neural phenotypic plasticity *in vitro* using co-culture. Those studies have been summarized in the Table 1 and will be briefly described in the following paragraphs.

Table 1. Summary of the *in vivo* / *in vitro* neural phenotypic plasticity of the MSC

Group	Experimental conditions	in vivo	in vitro	type of cell-like obtained	Immunological characteristics after experiment	References
A	Injection of MSC into the lateral ventricle of neonatal mice	+		Astrocytes	GFAP	Kopen et al., 1999
	Intravascular delivery of MSC into lethally irradiated mice	+		Neurons Astrocytes	NeuN, NF-H, βIII-tubulin GFAP	Brazelton et al., 2000
	Injection of MSC into injured spinal cord	+		Neurons Astrocytes	NSE, NF GFAP	Deng et al., 2006
B	Retinoic acid and BDNF treatment		+	Neurons Astrocytes	NeuN, Nestin, βIII-tubulin GFAP	Sanchez-Ramos et al., 2000
	Retinoic acid and BDNF treatment		+	Neurons Astrocytes	NeuN, Nestin, βIII-tubulin GFAP	Sanchez-Ramos et al., 2002
	Beta-mercaptoethanol treatment		+	Neurons	NeuN, NF-H, βIII-tubulin	Woodbury at al., 2000
	Beta-mercaptoethanol treatment		+	Neurons	NeuN, NF-H, βIII-tubulin	Woodbury at al., 2002
	Isobutylmethylxanthine and dibutyryl cAMP treatment		+	Neurons	NSE vimentin	Deng et al., 2001
	Neurotrophin NT3 treatment		+	Neurons	NeuN	Podovan et al., 2003
	Culture with bFGF and EGF		+	Neurons	Tuj1, NF, MAP2 and NeuN	Locatelli et al., 2003
	Induction with RA and Shh GDNF, dibutyryl AMPc and PACAP		+	Neurons	NF-L and synapsin	Tzeng et al., 2004
	bFGF and ganglioside GM1 treatment		+	Neurons Astrocytes	NSE GFAP	Zhang et al., 2004
	BDNF transfection and retinoic acide treatment		+	Neurons Astrocytes	NeuN GFAP	Zhao et al., 2004
	GDNF, IL-1beta, mesencephalic glial-cell-conditioned medium and flash-frozen mesencephalic membrane fragments.		+	Dopaminergic neurons	NSE, MAP2ab and TH	Guo et al., 2005
	Culture with RA, IBMX, dAMPc and ascorbic acid		+	neurons	NSE and NeuN	Hellmann et al., 2006
	Conditionned medium from hippocampus and cerebellum		+	Neurons	GAP-43 and NF	Rivera et al., 2006
C	Co-culture of MSC with neural stem cells		+	astrocytes	GFAP	Wislet-gendebien et al., 2003
	Co-culture of MSC with atrocytes		+	Neurons astrocytes	NF-200 GFAP	Jiang et al., 2002 and 2003
	Co-culture with fetal midbrain cells		+	Neurons astrocytes	NeuN GFAP	Sanchez-Ramos et al., 2000
	Co-culture of MSC with cerebellar granule neurons		+	Neurons astrocytes	Tuj1, NF-M and NeuN GFAP	Wisletgendebien-et al., 2005

1. *In Vivo* Studies

One of the first studies was realised by Kopen et al. [1999] who injected mouse MSC into the lateral ventricle of neonatal mice. By 12 days post-injection, grafted MSC migrated throughout the forebrain and cerebellum without disrupting the host brain architecture and some MSC labelled by BrdU incorporation before grafting were characterized within the striatum and the hippocampus by their expression of glial fibrillary acidic protein (GFAP) and, therefore, recognized as mature astrocytes. Brazelton et al. [2000] demonstrated that after intravascular delivery of genetically-marked adult mouse bone marrow into lethally irradiated normal adult hosts, donor-derived cells in the brain expressed neuronal and astroglial proteins. Lee et al. [2003] transplanted MSC stereotaxically into the brains of mice subjected to focal cerebral infarct. A large number of grafted cells survived after injection in the normal side of the brain 4 weeks after transplantation. MSC can then migrate into CNS lesions and differentiate there into neurons or astrocytes. After inducing the neuronal differentiation of MSC using cryptotanshinone, an AMP-kinase inhibitor extracted from the roots of *Salvia miltiorrhiza* [Kim et al, 2006], Deng et al. [2006] demonstrated that MSC-derived neuron-like cells are able to restore spinal cord function when grafted into injured monkey spinal cord.

2. *In Vitro* Studies

Several studies were also performed *in vitro* and demonstrated in different ways the MSC ability to express neural markers. Sanchez-Ramos et al. [2000 and 2002] treated a subset of both human and murine bone marrow cells with retinoic acid and BDNF. This treatment allows MSC to express markers of immature neurons. Likewise, Woodbury et al. [2000 and 2002] found that β-mercaptoethanol (BME) added to cultivated adult rat MSC rapidly induced a transition into neuron-like cells, but not into glial cells. Deng et al. [2001] reported that compounds that increase intracellular cAMP levels such as isobutylmethylxanthine (IBMX) and dibutyryl cAMP (db-cAMP), stimulated cultured human MSC to exhibit neural cell morphology. Padovan et al. [2003] demonstrated that human MSC express an immature neuronal marker (β-III-tubulin) when they are stimulated with neurotrophins such as neurotrophin3 (NT3) or brain-derived neurotrophic factor (BDNF). Zhang et al. [2004] demonstrated that a combination of basic fibroblast growth factor (bFGF) with ganglioside GM1 may synergistically promote the transformation of adult rat MSC into neurons and astrocyte-like cells. More recently, Guo et al. [2005] demonstrated that MSC treated with IBMX for 2 days and replace in a differentiating medium containing GDNF, IL-1β, mesencephalic glial-cell-conditioned medium and flash-frozen mesencephalic membrane fragments are able to differentiate into dopaminergic neuron-like cells. Likewise, Rivera et al. [2006] demonstrated that soluble factors derived from adult hippocampus, cortex or cerebellum are sufficient to induce the expression of several neuronal markers like GAP-43 and neurofilament by MSC.

Most of those *in vitro* and *in vivo* studies have only characterized the morphological and immunological characteristic of the MSC-derived neural-like cells. Few studies, however, have demonstrated that beside their immunological similarities, MSC-derived neuron-like cells can also exhibit some neuron specific functionalities. Zhao et al., [2004] demonstrated that, after being transfected with the BDNF gene via a recombinant retroviral vector, human MSC become able to differentiate into neural cells when they are treated with all-trans-retinoic acid (RA). Those MSC-derived neural cells express neural-specific proteins such as NeuN, O4 and glial fibrillary acidic protein (GFAP). Electrophysiological analyses using the whole-cell patch-clamp technique recorded voltage-dependent K^+/Ca^{2+} currents with a resting membrane potential of -65.4±6.07mV. Similarly, we recently demonstrated that adult rats MSC are able to differentiate into excitable neuron-like cells when they are co-cultivated with mouse cerebellar granule neurons [Wislet-Gendebien et al., 2005]. First we demonstrated that those cells express several neuronal markers (NeuN and β-III-tubulin), an axonal marker (neurofilament protein recognized by the monoclonal antibody, SMI31) and a dendritic marker (MAP2ab). Electrophysiological recordings of these nestin-positive MSC-derived neuron-like cells (MDN) were performed and three maturation stages were observed. At 4–6 days of co-culture, MDN showed some neurotransmitter responsiveness (GABA, glycine, serotonin and glutamate) and voltage-gated K^+ currents inhibited by TEA (tetraethylammonium). At that stage, MDN do not express functional sodium voltage-gated channels and have a low membrane potential (V_{rest}) (-37.6±3mV, $n = 61$). During the second week of co-culture, MDN started to display Na^+ currents reversely inhibited by TTX (tetrodotoxin) and were able to fire single action potential spikes. In those older co-cultures, the V_{rest} reaches a more negative value which is closer to the value usually measured in neurons (7–9 days, -50.3±2mV, $n = 76$ and 10–15 days, -56.7±2.3mV, $n = 97$).

Altogether those studies suggest that MSC have some real potential to mimic immunological and functional characteristic of neural cells. Different ways of differentiation have been proposed to explain the unusual abilities of MSC: fusion, real pluripotency and trophic factors.

- *Fusion:* Alvarez-Dolado et al. used an elegant approach based on Cre/lox recombination methodology to detect cell fusion events and demonstrated that after being intravenously injected in X-irradiated animals, bone marrow-derived cells fuse spontaneously *in vivo* with hepatocytes in liver, Purkinje neurons in the cerebellum and cardiac muscle in the heart, resulting in the formation of bi-nucleated cells. For this study, they used as donor mice expressing ubiquitously the Cre-recombinase gene under the control of a hybrid cytomegalovirus enhancer/β-actin (ACTB) promoter and the conditional Cre reporter mouse line R26R12 as a host animal. In these mice, the LacZ reporter gene is exclusively expressed after the excision of a lox P-flanked (floxed) stop cassette by Cre-mediated recombination. When Cre-expressing cells fuse with R26R12 cells, Cre recombinase excises the floxed stop cassette of the reporter gene in the R26R12 nuclei, resulting in expression of LacZ in the fused cells. Consequently, fused cells can be detected easily by 5-bromo-4-chloro-3-indolyl-beta-d-galactoside (X-gal) staining. To study cell fusion *in vivo*, R26R12 reporter mice were lethally irradiated, and two days later were grafted with bone marrow from mice constitutively expressing Cre recombinase and green fluorescent protein (GFP) under the control of the β-actin promoter. In all animals, cells labelled with X-gal were only found in brain, heart and liver (animals examined 10 months after grafting: in brain 5 cells/1.5×10^6 Purkinje neurons; in liver 59 cells/5.5×10^5 hepatocytes; in heart 71 cells/7500 cardiomyocytes). In the same study, they co-cultured bone marrow stromal cells from R26R12 reporter mice with Cre-positive multipotent progenitor cells isolated from postnatal brain and grown as neurospheres. After 4 days *in vitro*, a small proportion of LacZ-positive cells (1–2 cells per 80,000 cells) were found in these co-cultures. Weimann et al. injected intravenously GFP-expressing MSC in X-irradiated mice and observed after at least 6 weeks, that some Purkinje cells in the host animal were GFP-positive [2003]. However, these GFP-positive Purkinje neurons are characterized by the presence of two nuclei and when only male GFP-MSC donor cells are injected into female receiver animals, one nucleus is recognized by a Y-chromosome probe by in situ hybridisation. The frequency of cell fusion events in these experiments seems to be roughly the same as described above.

- *True pluripotent cells:* We recently analysed the mechanism underlying the neural phenotypic plasticity of nestin-positive MSC when these cells are co-cultivated with cerebellar granule neurons (CG) [Wislet-Gendebien et al., 2005]. Three sets of experiments were performed. The first group involved the analysis of the DNA content of nestin-positive MSC and CG before and after co-culture. In all cases, we never observed a significant difference in ploidy which could explain how 60% of the MSC show some neural differentiation (40% as astrocytes and 20% as neuron-like cells). Although the sensitivity of this technique does not allow us to rule out that some fusion events can take place, we performed two other experiments. Rats MSC were co-cultivated with granule cerebellar neurons cultivated from green-mice expressing the Green Fluorescent Protein (GFP) under the control of the actin promoter [Okabe et al., 1997]. Thereafter, double labellings with GFAP and M2 antibodies on one hand, and Tuj1 (anti-β-III-tubulin) and M6 antibodies on the other hand were performed. M2 and M6 recognize respectively and specifically mouse astrocytes and mouse neurons [Lagenaur et al., 1981]. We could observe that: (1) all GFAPpositive/ GFP-negative and Tuj1-positive/GFP-negative cells are also negative for M2 and M6, respectively, allowing us to conclude that those cells are of rat origin and thus likely derive from the MSC population, (2) all the cells which were recognized either by the M2 or by the M6 antibodies were also GFP-positive, ruling out a down-regulation of GFP expression during the co-culture period. Finally, nestin-positive MSC were cultivated for 5 days on paraformaldehyde-fixed GFP-positive granule cerebellar neurons in the presence of CG-conditioned medium (which has been centrifuged and filtered). In such conditions, we observed that $16.1 \pm 2.6\%$ ($n = 8$) nestin-positive MSC-derived cells were NeuN-positive and $23.1 \pm 2.1\%$ ($n = 7$) nestin-positive MSC-derived cells were GFAP-positive. Note that the level of GFP fluorescence in the fixed cells maintained for 5 days in culture remains stable. Although some rare fusion events cannot be excluded in these three sets of experiments using a co-culture paradigm, we can conclude that most MSC-derived neuron-like cells appear as a consequence of a differentiation process of nestin-positive MSC.

- *Trophic factors:* As described above, Podovan et al. [2003], Zhao et al. [2004], Zhang et al. [2004] and Rivera et al. [2006] demonstrated that several factors like GDNF, bFGF, NT3 or unknown factors contain in neural cell conditioned medium are able to orientate the MSC toward a neural fate, although most of these studies are only based on an immunological approaches except for Zhao et al. which infect cells with retroviruses (see above).

All of these results suggest that the mechanisms underlying the neural phenotypic plasticity of MSC could vary as a function of the environment and/or the cell status. We have also to consider that bone marrow mesenchymal stem cells are an heterogeneous population suggesting that some cells would be more subjected for cell fusion while the other would respond to environmental factors (like trophic factors) and/or adopt a true pluripotent stem cell behaviour. Cell fusion could be a hallmark of precursors or progenitors of monocytes and/or osteoclasts, two well-known cell types which usually fused with other cells or with themselves.

COULD NEURAL CREST STEM CELLS BE PRESENT IN THE BONE MARROW?

Beside MSC, other cell types form different tissues were studied for their potential ability to differentiate into neural cells, i.e., adipose tissue, umbilical cord cells, and skin cells. Adipose tissue, like bone marrow, is derived from the embryonic mesoderm. While available literature conflicts about the presence of certain cell receptor antigens, there is general agreement that adipose-derived stem cells and bone marrow stromal cells share adhesion and receptor molecules but are distinct for several adhesion markers with known function in hematopoietic stem cell homing and mobilization that is unique to the bone marrow function [Gronthos et al., 2001; De Ugarte et al., 2003]. Other similarities of adipose-derived stem cells to bone marrow stromal cells is that both stem cell types are capable of differentiating into chondrocytes, osteoblasts, and myocytes [Sanchez-Ramos et al., 2000; Zuk et al., 2001; Safford et al., 2004]. To date, there have been several publications that demonstrate neural cell differentiation of adipose-derived stem cells both *in vivo* and *in vitro* [reviewed by Kokai et al. 2005]. According to those studies, it appears that adipose-derived stem cells can express, under specific conditions, neural markers like nestin, NF-M, NeuN, NSE, Map2, S100 and GFAP.

The mononuclear fraction of umbilical cord blood cells (UCBmf) is rich in stem/progenitor cells. Like bone marrow stem cells, UCBmf cells are capable of self-renewal [Kim et al., 2005], proliferation, subsequent lineage commitment for multiple differentiated cell types [Goodwin et al., 2001]. Moreover those cells can be used to reconstitute the blood and immune systems [reviewed by Broxmeyer, 2005] in various haematological diseases. Some of these pluripotent mesodermal cells have recently been shown to differentiate into cells derived from other germ layers both *in vitro* and *in vivo* [Kong et al., 2004]. It has been show that UCBmf are able to express numerous markers of either stemness or neural fate *in vitro* such as nestin, Musashi1, Oct-4, TuJ1, NCAM, vimentin, GFAP, S100, GalC and

MAP2 [McGuckin et al., 2005; Chen et al., 2005]. Further, these cells express neurotrophic receptors trkB, trkC and p75NTR and cytokine receptor CXCR4 [Sanchez-Ramos et al., 2006; Chen et al., 2005].

Similarly, recent evidence indicates that multipotent stem cell populations are present in the mammalian dermis. These cells, defined skin-derived stem cells (SKS), were isolated from the embryo and adult mouse dermis, expanded, and differentiated into cells of various lineages when cultured in optimized media [Toma et al., 2001 and Jahoda et al., 2003]. Like bone marrow and UCBmf cells, the SKS are able to express some neural markers, i.e., nestin, NF-H, NF-M, beta-III-tubulin, Map2, GAP43 and GFAP [Toma et al., 2001, Gorio et al., 2004, Kawase et al., 2004 and Collo et al., 2006].

Beside the ability to express some neural marker that adipose, umbilical cord and skin cells share, recent studies reported that neural crest stem cells can be isolated from those tissue [Reviewed by Crane and Trainor, 2006; Fernandes et al., 2007]. Therefore, in the second part of this chapter, we will analyse the possibility that neural crest stem cells can be isolated from adult bone marrow.

Origin of the Neural Crest Cells

In early vertebrate development, the neural crest is specified in the embryonic ectoderm at the boundary of the neural plate and the ectoderm. Once specified, the neural crest cells (NCCs) undergo a process of epithelium to mesenchyme transition (EMT) that will confer them the ability to migrate. The EMT involves different molecular and cellular machineries and implies deep changes in cell morphology and in the type of cell surface adhesion and recognition molecules. When the EMT is complete, they delaminate from the neural folds/neural tube and migrate along characteristic pathways to differentiate into a wide variety of derivates (Figure 3) [reviewed by Kalcheim, 2000]. Classically, the neural crest can be divided in four main domains, each with characteristic derivatives and functions: the *cranial* (*cephalic*), the *trunk*, the *vagal* and *sacral*, and the *cardiac* neural crest cells [Le Lièvre et Le Douarin, 1975].

- The *cranial neural crest* arises in the anterior and populates the face and the pharyngeal arches giving rise to cartilage, bone, cranial neurons of the peripheral nervous system, glial and connective tissue of the face. Cells that migrated into the pharyngeal arches play an inductive role in the thymus and thyroid gland development.
- The *trunk neural crest* is a transient structure which disappears soon after the neural tube closes, lies between the vagal and sacral neural crest and gives rise to two groups of cells. One group migrates dorso-lateral and populates the skin, forming pigment cells and the other migrates ventro-lateral through the anterior sclerotome to become the epinephrine-producing cells of the adrenal gland and the neurons of the sympathetic nervous system. Some cells remain in the sclerotome to form the dorsal root ganglia.

- The *vagal* and *sacral neural crest* arises in the neck and tail and populates the gut, forming the parasympathetic neurons that regulate peristalsis and control blood vessel dilation.
- *Cardiac neural crest* cells as the cranial neural crest cells can differentiate into melanocytes, neurons, cartilage and connective tissue, but can also more specifically produce the entire muscular-connective tissue wall of the large arteries as they arise from the heart as well as contributing to the septum that separate pulmonary circulation from the aorta.

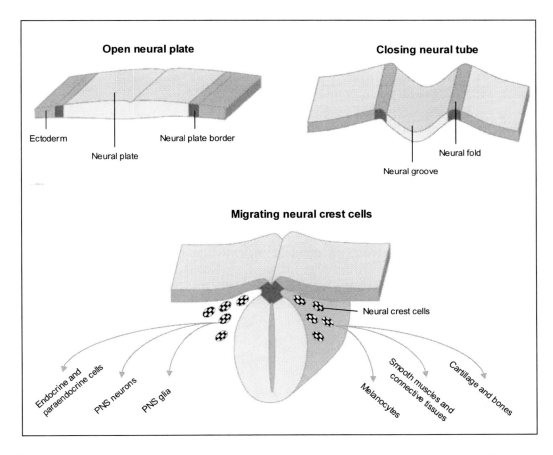

Figure 3. Neurulation and neural crest migration. As neurulation proceeds, the neural plate rolls up and the neural plate border becomes the neural folds. Near the time of neural tube closure (depending on the species), the neural crest cells go through an epithelial to mesenchymal transition (EMT) and delaminate from the neural folds or dorsal neural tube and migrate along defined pathways.

Molecular Pathways Underlying the Formation of the Neural Crest Stem Cells

A large body of *in vitro* studies as well as analyses of gene mutations in mice has led to the identification of several growth factor/receptor signalling pathways implicated in the development of specific neural crest derivative subtypes [reviewed by Anderson, 1997; Le Kalcheim, 2000; Sieber-Blum, 1997]. In mice, neural crest stem cells are defined by expression of two markers: p75NGFR (low-affinity nerve growth factor receptor) and the transcription factor Sox10 [Stemple et Anderson, 1992; Rao et Anderson, 1997; Paratore et al., 2001; Kim et al., 2003].

A number of signals have been implicated in the formation of the neural crest, including members of the *Wnt*, *FGF* and *BMP* families. These secreted proteins (extrinsic factors) regulate early expression of transcription factors, cell adhesion molecules, extracellular glycoproteins, etc. while intrinsic factors act to stabilize the competence of the epithelium to form neural crest [Knecht and Bronner-Fraser, 2002] and, moreover, some also regulate subsequent developmental events, such as delamination and initiation of migration [Kalcheim, 2005, LaBonne and Bronner- Fraser, 2000].

1) Extrinsic Factors Regulation the Neural Crest Formation

The formation of neural crest has traditionally been considered as a classic example of induction, in which signals from one tissue elicit differentiation in a responding competent tissue [Liem et al., 1995; Selleck and Bronner-Fraser, 1995; Mancilla and Mayor, 1996]. As described in the Figure 4, signals inducing the formation of the neural crest formation are sent by the mesoderm as well as the epidermis. *A) Signals from the mesoderm*: a graded signal from the mesoderm is responsible for neural crest induction. Members of the *Wnt* (wingless/INT) family of secreted glycoproteins may mediate the neural crest inducing ability of paraxial mesoderm [Bang et al., 1999]. Likewise, a member of the fibroblast growth factor (FGF) family, *FGF-8*, mediates the inductive effects of paraxial mesoderm. Several studies suggested that FGF's ability to induce neural crest is dependent on Wnt signaling [LaBonne and Bronner-Fraser, 1998]. *B) Signals from ectoderm*: a gradient of *BMP* signalling acts initially to specify epidermal, neural, and border (prospective neural crest) fates in the ectoderm. Both Wnt and FGF signals have been proposed to play a role in this process [Mayor et al., 2000; LaBonne and Bronner-Fraser, 1998; Marchant et al., 1998; Bastidas et al., 2004]. Wnt proteins play significant roles in neural crest cell development at different developmental times [reviewed in Wu *et al.*, 2003]. *Wnt6* is synthesized in the epidermal ectoderm and might mediate crest specification [Garcia-Castro *et al.*, 2002]. Slightly later, *Wnt1* and *Wnt3a* are present in the dorsal neural tube following initial specification of crest cells [Dickinson *et al.*, 1995]. Wnt3a is intense already opposite the segmental plate while Wnt1 becomes apparent slightly later, opposite epithelial somites and concomitant with BMP relief from noggin inhibition [Burstyn-Cohen et al., 2004]. Whereas Wnt1 is likely to be directly regulated by BMPs [Marcelle et al., 1999, Sela-Donenfeld and Kalcheim, 2002, Burstyn-Cohen et al., 2004], the transcription of Wnt3a is not; suggesting that Wnt1 better fits to be involved in crest delamination [Burstyn-Cohen et al., 2004]. Wnt signaling act through the transmembrane receptor Frizzled which is required to modulate the distribution and function of β-catenin [Miller and Moon, 1997]. β-catenin associate directly with the highly conserved cytoplasmic domain of cadherins. The so formed cadherin-catenin complex links to the actin filament network [Ozawa et al., 1989; Hinck et al., 1994; Knudsen et al., 1995;

Weiss et al., 1998]. BMP/Wnt-mediated signals could induce changes in the actin cytoskeleton via rhoB. A role for rhoB in crest delamination has been already suggested based on inhibition experiments in culture [Liu and Jessell, 1998]. A molecular pathway for the activation of Rho by Wnt/frizzled was suggested, which involves the formation of a complex between Rho, dishevelled and Daam1 in the plasma membrane, resulting in the generation of a polarized cytoskeleton [Habas et al., 2002]. Thus, the dynamic association of the catenin-cadherin complex and that of rhoB with the cytoskeleton may be essential for regulating cell-cell interactions leading to neural crest delamination. Notably, Rho GTPases could also be effectors of Wnt signals in this pathway as they were shown to affect morphogenesis by interfering with cell proliferation [Wei et al., 2002].

Later during the development, the induced cells interact to complete neural crest induction by a process that requires *Notch/Delta* signalling. Notch signalling has two roles during neural crest development: first in establishing the neural crest domain within the ectoderm via lateral induction and subsequently in diversifying the fates of cells that arise from the neural crest via lateral inhibition. The first of these roles, specification of neural crest via lateral induction, has been explored primarily in the cranial neural folds from which the cranial neural crest arises. Evidence for such a role has thus far only been obtained from chick and frog; results from these two species differ, but share the feature that Notch signalling regulates genes that are expressed by cranial neural crest through effects on expression of Bmp family members. The second of these roles, diversification of neural crest progeny via lateral inhibition, has been identified thus far only in trunk neural crest. Evidence from several species suggests that Notch-mediated lateral inhibition functions in multiple episodes in this context, in each case inhibiting neurogenesis. In the 'standard' mode of lateral inhibition, Notch promotes proliferation and in the 'instructive' mode, it promotes specific secondary fates, including cell death or glial differentiation [reviewed by Cornell et Eisen, 2005].

Once neural crest formation has been induced, some extracellular factors have been reported to induce the ultimate steps of neural crest differentiation. Bone morphogenetic protein 2 (*BMP2*) was shown to induce neurogenesis in culture, glial growth factor (*GGF*) drives the cells into glial, transforming growth factor-β (*TGFβ*) into smooth muscle differentiation [Shah et al., 1994 and 1996]. Several groups published data on melanocyte differentiation of NC cells [Maxwell et al., 1996; Takano et al., 2002] and demonstrated that Endothelin 3 is an essential factor in that pathway [Lahav et al., 1996 and 1998]. Recent work showed, that chondrogenesis can also be induced in trunk NC cells [McGonnell et Graham, 2002; Oka et Ito, 2007; Maurer et al., 2006].

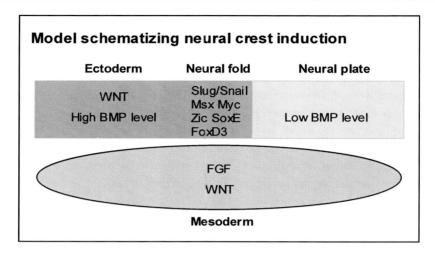

Figure 4. Neural crest induction and its relation to neural plate and neural plate border. Members of the BMP, FGF, and Wnts families of signalling molecules are involved in the formation of the neural plate, the establishment of the neural plate border, and in neural crest induction. These signals can originate from the ectoderm, or the mesoderm.

2) Intrinsic Factors Regulating the Neural Crest Formation

The boundary region between the neural plate and the epidermis is defined by expression of a variety of specific markers, including transcription factors such as *Slug* or *Snail*, *AP-2*, *Foxd3*, *PAX3*, *twist*, *Sox9*, *Zic5*, etc.

Group E Sox genes (Sox8, Sox9 and Sox10) are expressed in the prospective neural crest and *Sox9* expression precedes expression of premigratory neural crest markers. Group E Sox genes act at two distinct steps in neural crest differentiation. Forced expression of Sox9 promotes neural-crest-like properties in neural tube progenitors at the expense of central nervous system neuronal differentiation. Subsequently, in migratory neural crest cells, SoxE gene expression biases cells towards glial cell and melanocyte fate, and away from neuronal lineages. Although SoxE genes are sufficient to initiate neural crest development, they do not efficiently induce the delamination of ectopic neural crest cells from the neural tube consistent with the idea that this event is independently controlled [Reviewed by Cheung et Briscoe 2003]. *Sox10* is expressed by migrating neural crest cells and is required for the survival of neural crest cells before lineage segregation [Southard-Smith et al., 1998; Kapur, 2000; Paratore et al., 2001]. Furthermore, in developing dorsal root ganglia, Sox10 is also required for glial fate acquisition, and Sox10 expression appears to be maintained by differentiating glial cells but not by differentiating neurons [Britsch et al., 2001, Paratore et al., 2001]. Finally, Sox10 heterozygous mutant neural crest cells, survival appears to be normal, while fate specifications are drastically affected. Thereby, the fate chosen by a mutant neural crest cell is context dependent. Several studies indicate that combinatorial signalling by Sox10, extracellular factors such as neuregulin 1, and local cell-cell interactions is involved in fine-tuning lineage decisions by neural crest stem cells [reviewed by Paratore, 2001]. Likewise, the expression of *Sox2* has been proposed to act by maintaining a neural progenitor identity [Graham et al., 2003]. It becomes down-regulated in the neural plate when neural crest cells segregate from the dorsal neural tube, and it remains low during neural crest cell migration. *Sox2* expression is subsequently up-regulated in some crest-derived cells in the developing peripheral nervous system and is later restricted to glial sublineages [Wakamatsu et al., 2004].

Similarities Between Neural Plasticity of MSC and Neural Crest Stem Cells

We recently demonstrated that MSC express the Neural stem cells protein (nestin) [Wislet-Gendebien et al., 2003], an intermediate filament protein predominantly expressed by neural progenitors [Lendahl et al., 1990]. During embryogenesis, nestin is expressed in migrating and proliferating cells (including neural crest stem cells), whereas in adult tissues, nestin is mainly restricted to areas of regeneration [Wiese et al., 2004]. As MSC are able to adopt some neural phenotypes, it appears that the nestin expression is a pre-requisite for the neural differentiation: only nestin-positive MSC are able to differentiate into neuron- and glial-like cells [Wislet-Gendebien et al., 2005]. Moreover, the number of nestin-positive MSC present in culture increase with the number of cell passages suggesting a higher proliferation rate for the MSC with neural abilities. Interestingly, several factors like Sox transcription factors (Sox2 and Sox10); Pax6 transcription factor; ErBb2 and ErBb4 neuregulin receptors; as well as Frizzled Wnt receptors (FZD1, FZD2 and FZD5) are over-expressed by nestin-positive MSC compare to nestin-negative MSC [Wislet-Gendebien et al., 2005].

As previously described, neural crest stem cells are defined by expression of two markers: p75NGFR (low-affinity nerve growth factor receptor) and the transcription factor Sox10 [Stemple et Anderson, 1992; Rao et Anderson, 1997; Paratore et al., 2001; Kim et al., 2003]. Once again, MSC express also those two factors [Wislet-Gendebien et al., 2005].

During the embryonic development, migration and differentiation of neural crest stem cells involved several factors like neuregulins and their receptors ErbB. The *neuregulin* gene encodes various isoforms of a recently identified growth and differentiation factor, which all contain an EGF-like domain. So far, four genes has been described to encode for neuregulin *NRG1*, *NRG2*, *NRG3* and *NRG4* [Burden et Yarden, 1997; Busfield et al., 1997; Carraway et al., 1995; Higashiyama et al., 1997; Harari et al., 1999]. NRG1 gene is the more studied and contains numerous exons that after alternative splicing allow the expression of 14 different proteins that can be classified in 3 groups: (I) type I isoforms (originally identified as *NDF* Neu Differentiation Factor/ *HER* heregulin or *ARIA*, Acetylcholine Receptor Inducing Activity) contain an Ig-like domain, an EGF-like domain that suffices to elicit biological responses [Holmes et al., 1992], a proteolysis site, a hydrophobic domain suggested to act as internal signal sequence for secretion of the factor and additional C-terminal sequences [Holmes et al., 1992]; (II) type II isoforms (originally identified as *GGF* Glial Growth Factor) contain a signal peptide, a kringle-like sequence plus Ig and EGF-like domains [Marchionni et al.,1993]; (III) type III isoforms (originally identified as *SMDF* Sensory and Motor Neuron-derived Factor) share only the EGF-like domain with other isoforms; notable in the N-terminal part is a hydrophobic domain within a cysteine-rich sequence [Ho et al., 1995].

Neuregulin-induced cellular responses are mediated by tyrosine kinase receptors of the erbB family: neuregulin binds erbB3 and erbB4 with high affinity, but not the erbB2 (HER2) and erbB1 (EGF) receptors [Peles et al., 1993; Plowman et al., 1993; Carraway et al., 1995]. Binding affinity of neuregulin to erbB3 is increased by the presence of erbB2 [Sliwkowski et al., 1994]. Moreover, when co-expressed with erbB3 or erbB4, neuregulin induces tyrosine phosphorylation of the erbB2 receptor [Holmes et al., 1992; Wen et al., 1992; Carraway and Cantley, 1994; Beerli et al., 1995]. This is the result of heterodimerization of erbB2 with erbB3 or erbB4 and subsequent receptor cross-phosphorylation.

Meyer et al., [1997] demonstrated that type I neuregulin is expressed in cephalic mesenchyme and cranial ganglia as well as the endocardium and governs development of neural crest-derived neurons. In contrast, type III neuregulin is expressed in differentiating sensory and motor neurons and acts on the Schwann cell precursors, driving their initial development. Concerning the receptors ErbB, distinct receptor combinations are essential in different developmental events: the ErbB2 and ErbB4 receptors cooperate in transmission of neuregulin-1 signals in the heart, whereas ErbB2 and ErbB3 cooperate in neural crest cells [Gassmann et al., 1995; Lee et al., 1995; Erickson et al., 1997; Riethmacher et al., 1997], however, precise developmental event that requires the neuregulin-1 signal and ErbB receptors has not been elucidated. At this point, the lack of ErbB3 expression by the mesenchymal-derived stem cells would not be enough to rule out those cells as potential neural crest stem cells. Indeed, when we look at the functional side, type I neuregulin can interact with both ErbB2/ErbB3 and ErbB2/ErbB4 receptors. Likewise, it seems that ErbB3 expression by neural crest cells is observed early in the development (at the migration stage) or later (at the neural specification stage). Potential neural crest stem cells located in the bone marrow would not express the ErbB3 receptor because they at a post-migration but pre-differentiation stage. Finally, neural crest cells located in the heart express ErbB4 receptor but not ErbB3. However, heart-derived neural crest stem cells are also able to differentiate into mature neural cells under specific conditions [Tomita et al., 2005].

Upon binding to cell surface receptors, Wnts initiate an intracellular cascade that, via several intermediate steps, leads to the translocation of beta-catenin to the nucleus (see above). Ikeya et al., [1997] demonstrated that wnt1 and wnt3a play an important role in the specification of the neural crest derivates and Giarre et al, [1999] demonstrated that the responsiveness to Wnt-1 at the biochemical level is a common property of both epithelial and mesenchymal cells. More recently, Jackson et al., [2005] demonstrated that mesenchymal stem cells express different wnt1- and wnt3a-induced gene that activated the β-catenin dependent pathway. Moreover, wnt3a can activated frizzled receptor Fz1 and Fz2 [Kennell et MacDougald, 2005] which are overexpressed by nestin-positive MSC [Wislet-Gendebien et al., 2005].

CONCLUSION

According to the different studies realised on bone marrow-derived stem cells, it seems that those cells share numerous similarities with the neural crest stem cells. Beside their abilities to differentiate into mesenchymal and neural lineages, bone marrow-derived stem cells are p75NGFr- and Sox10-positives and express some wnt receptors (Frizzled) as well as neuregulin receptors (erbB2 and erbB4), which could activate the intracellular pathways underlying the neural differentiation.

However, if those evidences strongly suggest that neural crest stem cells can be present in the adult bone marrow, the "ultimate" demonstration seems to be missing. This demonstration would involve the tracking of the neural crest stem cells form the early stage of embryonic development to the colonisation of various tissues. Interestingly, Jiang et al. in 2000 developed a two-component genetic system based on Cre/lox recombination to label indelibly the entire mouse neural crest population at the time of its formation, and to detect it at any time thereafter. Briefly, the fate of neural crest cells was mapped *in vivo* by mating *ROSA26* Cre reporter (*R26R*) mice, which express β-galactosidase upon Cre-mediated recombination, with mice expressing Cre recombinase under the control of the *Wnt1* promoter. In *Wnt1-Cre/R26R* double transgenic mice, virtually all neural crest stem cells express β-galactosidase. Using this transgenic model, Sieber-Blum and Grim [2004] demonstrated the presence of pluripotent neural crest stem cells in adult follicle hairs and Wong et al. [2006] recently demonstrated the presence of neural crest cells in the mouse adult skin. This approach could also be useful to look for a possible presence of neural crest-derived cells in bone marrow. These cells keep the ability to differentiation into neurons or astrocytes and as the facility of getting mesenchymal stem cells from bone marrow, could be useful for a cell therapy based on auto-graft. The physiological role of these neural crest derived cells in bone marrow should also be addressed, especially regarding the regulation of haematopoiesis [Katayama et al., 2006].

REFERENCES

Alvarez-Dolado M, Pardal R, Garcia-Verdugo JM, Fike JR, Lee HO, Pfeffer K, Lois C, Morrison SJ, Alvarez-Buylla A: Fusion of bone-marrow-derived cells with Purkinje neurons, cardiomyocytes and hepatocytes. *Nature* 2003, 425:968-973.

Amit M, Carpenter MK, Inokuma MS, Chiu CP, Harris CP, Waknitz MA, Itskovitz-Eldor J, Thomson JA: Clonally derived human embryonic stem cell lines maintain pluripotency and proliferative potential for prolonged periods of culture. *Dev.Biol.* 2000, 227:271-278.

Bang AG, Papalopulu N, Goulding MD, Kintner C: Expression of Pax-3 in the lateral neural plate is dependent on a Wnt-mediated signal from posterior nonaxial mesoderm. *Dev.Biol.* 1999, 212:366-380.

Bastidas F, De Calisto J, Mayor R: Identification of neural crest competence territory: role of Wnt signaling. *Dev.Dyn.* 2004, 229:109-117.

Beerli RR, Graus-Porta D, Woods-Cook K, Chen X, Yarden Y, Hynes NE: Neu differentiation factor activation of ErbB-3 and ErbB-4 is cell specific and displays a differential requirement for ErbB-2. *Mol.Cell Biol.* 1995, 15:6496-6505.

Bianco P, Robey P: Diseases of bone and the stromal cell lineage. *J.Bone Miner.Res.* 1999, 14:336-341.

Brazelton TR, Rossi FM, Keshet GI, Blau HM: From marrow to brain: expression of neuronal phenotypes in adult mice. *Science* 2000, 290:1775-1779.

Britsch S, Goerich DE, Riethmacher D, Peirano RI, Rossner M, Nave KA, Birchmeier C, Wegner M: The transcription factor Sox10 is a key regulator of peripheral glial development. *Genes Dev.* 2001, 15:66-78.

Broxmeyer HE: Biology of cord blood cells and future prospects for enhanced clinical benefit. *Cytotherapy.* 2005, 7:209-218.

Burden S, Yarden Y: Neuregulins and their receptors: a versatile signaling module in organogenesis and oncogenesis. *Neuron* 1997, 18:847-855.

Burstyn-Cohen T, Stanleigh J, Sela-Donenfeld D, Kalcheim C: Canonical Wnt activity regulates trunk neural crest delamination linking BMP/noggin signaling with G1/S transition. *Development* 2004, 131:5327-5339.

Busfield SJ, Michnick DA, Chickering TW, Revett TL, Ma J, Woolf EA, Comrack CA, Dussault BJ, Woolf J, Goodearl AD, Gearing DP: Characterization of a neuregulin-related gene, Don-1, that is highly expressed in restricted regions of the cerebellum and hippocampus. *Mol.Cell Biol.* 1997, 17:4007-4014.

Carraway KL, III, Cantley LC: A neu acquaintance for erbB3 and erbB4: a role for receptor heterodimerization in growth signaling. *Cell* 1994, 78:5-8.

Carraway KL, III, Burden SJ: Neuregulins and their receptors. *Curr.Opin.Neurobiol.* 1995, 5:606-612.

Chen N, Hudson JE, Walczak P, Misiuta I, Garbuzova-Davis S, Jiang L, Sanchez-Ramos J, Sanberg PR, Zigova T, Willing AE: Human umbilical cord blood progenitors: the potential of these hematopoietic cells to become neural. *Stem Cells* 2005, 23:1560-1570.

Cheung M, Briscoe J: Neural crest development is regulated by the transcription factor Sox9. *Development* 2003, 130:5681-5693.

Clegg CH, Hauschka SD: Heterokaryon analysis of muscle differentiation: regulation of the postmitotic state. *J.Cell Biol.* 1987, 105:937-947.

Collo G, Goffi F, Merlo PE, Baldelli P, Benfenati F, Spano P: Immature neuronal phenotype derived from mouse skin precursor cells differentiated in vitro. *Brain Res.* 2006, 1109:32-36.

Crane JF, Trainor PA: Neural crest stem and progenitor cells. *Annu.Rev.Cell Dev.Biol.* 2006, 22:267-286.

Davis AA, Temple S: A self-renewing multipotential stem cell in embryonic rat cerebral cortex. *Nature* 1994, 372:263-266.

De Ugarte DA, Alfonso Z, Zuk PA, Elbarbary A, Zhu M, Ashjian P, Benhaim P, Hedrick MH, Fraser JK: Differential expression of stem cell mobilization-associated molecules on multi-lineage cells from adipose tissue and bone marrow. *Immunol.Lett.* 2003, 89:267-270.

Deng YB, Liu XG, Liu ZG, Liu XL, Liu Y, Zhou GQ: Implantation of BM mesenchymal stem cells into injured spinal cord elicits de novo neurogenesis and functional recovery: evidence from a study in rhesus monkeys. *Cytotherapy.* 2006, 8:210-214.

Dickinson ME, Selleck MA, McMahon AP, Bronner-Fraser M: Dorsalization of the neural tube by the non-neural ectoderm. *Development* 1995, 121:2099-2106.

Domen J, Weissman IL: Self-renewal, differentiation or death: regulation and manipulation of hematopoietic stem cell fate. *Mol.Med.Today* 1999, 5:201-208.

Dunnett SB: Functional analysis of fronto-striatal reconstruction by striatal grafts. *Novartis.Found.Symp.* 2000, 231:21-41.

Erickson SL, O'Shea KS, Ghaboosi N, Loverro L, Frantz G, Bauer M, Lu LH, Moore MW: ErbB3 is required for normal cerebellar and cardiac development: a comparison with ErbB2-and heregulin-deficient mice. *Development* 1997, 124:4999-5011.

Fallahi-Sichani M, Soleimani M, Najafi SM, Kiani J, Arefian E, Atashi A: In vitro differentiation of cord blood unrestricted somatic stem cells expressing dopamine-associated genes into neuron-like cells. *Cell Biol.Int.* 2007, 31:299-303.

Fernandes KJ, Toma JG, Miller FD: Multipotent skin-derived precursors: adult neural crest-related precursors with therapeutic potential. *Philos.Trans.R.Soc.Lond B Biol.Sci.* 2007.

Fernandez CI, Alberti E, Mendoza Y, Martinez L, Collazo J, Rosillo JC, Bauza JY: Motor and cognitive recovery induced by bone marrow stem cells grafted to striatum and hippocampus of impaired aged rats: functional and therapeutic considerations. *Ann.N.Y.Acad.Sci.* 2004, 1019:48-52.

Gage FH: Neurogenesis in the adult brain. *J.Neurosci.* 2002, 22:612-613.

Gandarillas A, Watt FM: c-Myc promotes differentiation of human epidermal stem cells. *Genes Dev.* 1997, 11:2869-2882.

Garcia-Castro MI, Marcelle C, Bronner-Fraser M: Ectodermal Wnt function as a neural crest inducer. *Science* 2002, 297:848-851.

Gassmann M, Casagranda F, Orioli D, Simon H, Lai C, Klein R, Lemke G: Aberrant neural and cardiac development in mice lacking the ErbB4 neuregulin receptor. *Nature* 1995, 378:390-394.

Giarre M, Semenov MV, Brown AM: Wnt signaling stabilizes the dual-function protein beta-catenin in diverse cell types. *Ann.N.Y.Acad.Sci.* 1998, 857:43-55.

Goodwin NC, Ishida Y, Hartford S, Wnek C, Bergstrom RA, Leder P, Schimenti JC: DelBank: a mouse ES-cell resource for generating deletions. *Nat.Genet.* 2001, 28: 310-311.

Gorio A, Torrente Y, Madaschi L, Di Stefano AB, Pisati F, Marchesi C, Belicchi M, Di Giulio AM, Bresolin N: Fate of autologous dermal stem cells transplanted into the spinal cord after traumatic injury (TSCI). *Neuroscience* 2004, 125:179-189.

Graham V, Khudyakov J, Ellis P, Pevny L: SOX2 functions to maintain neural progenitor identity. *Neuron* 2003, 39:749-765.

Gronthos S, Franklin DM, Leddy HA, Robey PG, Storms RW, Gimble JM: Surface protein characterization of human adipose tissue-derived stromal cells. *J.Cell Physiol* 2001, 189:54-63.

Guo L, Yin F, Meng HQ, Ling L, Hu-He TN, Li P, Zhang CX, Yu S, Duan DS, Fan HX: Differentiation of mesenchymal stem cells into dopaminergic neuron-like cells in vitro. *Biomed.Environ.Sci.* 2005, 18:36-42.

Habas R, Kato Y, He X: Wnt/Frizzled activation of Rho regulates vertebrate gastrulation and requires a novel Formin homology protein Daam1. *Cell* 2001, 107:843-854.

Hagg T: Molecular regulation of adult CNS neurogenesis: an integrated view. *Trends Neurosci.* 2005, 28:589-595.

Hall ED: Pharmacological treatment of acute spinal cord injury: how do we build on past success? *J.Spinal Cord.Med.* 2001, 24:142-146.

Harari D, Tzahar E, Romano J, Shelly M, Pierce JH, Andrews GC, Yarden Y: Neuregulin-4: a novel growth factor that acts through the ErbB-4 receptor tyrosine kinase. *Oncogene* 1999, 18:2681-2689.

Herzog EL, Chai L, Krause DS: Plasticity of marrow-derived stem cells. *Blood* 2003, 102:3483-3493.

Higashiyama S, Horikawa M, Yamada K, Ichino N, Nakano N, Nakagawa T, Miyagawa J, Matsushita N, Nagatsu T, Taniguchi N, Ishiguro H: A novel brain-derived member of the epidermal growth factor family that interacts with ErbB3 and ErbB4. *J.Biochem.(Tokyo)* 1997, 122:675-680.

Hinck L, Nelson WJ, Papkoff J: Wnt-1 modulates cell-cell adhesion in mammalian cells by stabilizing beta-catenin binding to the cell adhesion protein cadherin. *J.Cell Biol.* 1994, 124:729-741.

Hochedlinger K, Jaenisch R: Nuclear reprogramming and pluripotency. *Nature* 2006, 441:1061-1067.

Holmes WE, Sliwkowski MX, Akita RW, Henzel WJ, Lee J, Park JW, Yansura D, Abadi N, Raab H, Lewis GD, .: Identification of heregulin, a specific activator of p185erbB2. *Science* 1992, 256:1205-1210.

Ikeya M, Lee SM, Johnson JE, McMahon AP, Takada S: Wnt signalling required for expansion of neural crest and CNS progenitors. *Nature* 1997, 389:966-970.

Isacson O, Bjorklund L, Pernaute RS: Parkinson's disease: interpretations of transplantation study are erroneous. *Nat.Neurosci.* 2001, 4:553.

Itskovitz-Eldor J, Schuldiner M, Karsenti D, Eden A, Yanuka O, Amit M, Soreq H, Benvenisty N: Differentiation of human embryonic stem cells into embryoid bodies compromising the three embryonic germ layers. *Mol.Med.* 2000, 6:88-95.

Jackson A, Vayssiere B, Garcia T, Newell W, Baron R, Roman-Roman S, Rawadi G: Gene array analysis of Wnt-regulated genes in C3H10T1/2 cells. *Bone* 2005, 36:585-598.

Jahoda CA: Cell movement in the hair follicle dermis - more than a two-way street? *J.Invest Dermatol.* 2003, 121:ix-xi.

Johnston LA: Regeneration and transdetermination: new tricks from old cells. *Cell* 2005, 120:288-290.

Kalcheim C: Mechanisms of early neural crest development: from cell specification to migration. *Int.Rev.Cytol.* 2000, 200:143-196.

Kalcheim C, Burstyn-Cohen T: Early stages of neural crest ontogeny: formation and regulation of cell delamination. *Int.J.Dev.Biol.* 2005, 49:105-116.

Kapur RP: Colonization of the murine hindgut by sacral crest-derived neural precursors: experimental support for an evolutionarily conserved model. *Dev.Biol.* 2000, 227:146-155.

Katayama Y, Battista M, Kao WM, Hidalgo A, Peired AJ, Thomas SA, Frenette PS: Signals from the sympathetic nervous system regulate hematopoietic stem cell egress from bone marrow. *Cell* 2006, 124:407-421.

Kawase Y, Yanagi Y, Takato T, Fujimoto M, Okochi H: Characterization of multipotent adult stem cells from the skin: transforming growth factor-beta (TGF-beta) facilitates cell growth. *Exp.Cell Res.* 2004, 295:194-203.

Kennell JA, MacDougald OA: Wnt signaling inhibits adipogenesis through beta-catenin-dependent and -independent mechanisms. *J.Biol.Chem.* 2005, 280:24004-24010.

Kim J, Lo L, Dormand E, Anderson DJ: SOX10 maintains multipotency and inhibits neuronal differentiation of neural crest stem cells. *Neuron* 2003, 38:17-31.

Kim S, Honmou O, Kato K, Nonaka T, Houkin K, Hamada H, Kocsis JD: Neural differentiation potential of peripheral blood- and bone-marrow-derived precursor cells. *Brain Res.* 2006, 1123:27-33.

Kim YM, Jung MH, Song HY, Yang HO, Lee ST, Kim JH, Kim YT, Nam JH, Mok JE: Ex vivo expansion of human umbilical cord blood-derived T-lymphocytes with homologous cord blood plasma. *Tohoku J.Exp.Med.* 2005, 205:115-122.

Knecht AK, Bronner-Fraser M: Induction of the neural crest: a multigene process. *Nat.Rev.Genet.* 2002, 3:453-461.

Knudsen KA, Soler AP, Johnson KR, Wheelock MJ: Interaction of alpha-actinin with the cadherin/catenin cell-cell adhesion complex via alpha-catenin. *J.Cell Biol.* 1995, 130:67-77.

Kokai LE, Rubin JP, Marra KG: The potential of adipose-derived adult stem cells as a source of neuronal progenitor cells. *Plast.Reconstr.Surg.* 2005, 116:1453-1460.

Kondo T, Raff M: Oligodendrocyte precursor cells reprogrammed to become multipotential CNS stem cells. *Science* 2000, 289:1754-1757.

Kondo T, Raff M: Chromatin remodeling and histone modification in the conversion of oligodendrocyte precursors to neural stem cells. *Genes Dev.* 2004, 18:2963-2972.

Kong PY, Luo CJ, Zhou YH, Guo CH: [Promoting effects of stromal cells on hematopoietic reconstitution capability of bone marrow cells expanded under different conditions]. *Zhongguo Shi Yan.Xue.Ye.Xue.Za Zhi.* 2004, 12:265-269.

Kopen GC, Prockop DJ, Phinney DG: Marrow stromal cells migrate throughout forebrain and cerebellum, and they differentiate into astrocytes after injection into neonatal mouse brains. *Proc.Natl.Acad.Sci.U.S A* 1999, 96:10711-10716.

Krause DS, Theise ND, Collector MI, Henegariu O, Hwang S, Gardner R, Neutzel S, Sharkis SJ: Multi-organ, multi-lineage engraftment by a single bone marrow-derived stem cell. *Cell* 2001, 105:369-377.

LaBonne C, Bronner-Fraser M: Neural crest induction in Xenopus: evidence for a two-signal model. *Development* 1998, 125:2403-2414.

LaBonne C, Bronner-Fraser M: Snail-related transcriptional repressors are required in Xenopus for both the induction of the neural crest and its subsequent migration. *Dev.Biol.* 2000, 221:195-205.

Lagenaur C, Schachner M: Monoclonal antibody (M2) to glial and neuronal cell surfaces. *J.Supramol.Struct.Cell Biochem.* 1981, 15:335-346.

Lahav R, Ziller C, Dupin E, Le Douarin NM: Endothelin 3 promotes neural crest cell proliferation and mediates a vast increase in melanocyte number in culture. *Proc.Natl.Acad.Sci.U.S A* 1996, 93:3892-3897.

Lahav R, Dupin E, Lecoin L, Glavieux C, Champeval D, Ziller C, Le Douarin NM: Endothelin 3 selectively promotes survival and proliferation of neural crest-derived glial and melanocytic precursors in vitro. *Proc.Natl.Acad.Sci.U.S A* 1998, 95:14214-14219.

Le Lievre CS, Le Douarin NM: Mesenchymal derivatives of the neural crest: analysis of chimaeric quail and chick embryos. *J.Embryol.Exp.Morphol.* 1975, 34:125-154.

Lechner A, Habener JF: Bone marrow stem cells find a path to the pancreas. *Nat.Biotechnol.* 2003, 21:755-756.

Lee J, Kuroda S, Shichinohe H, Ikeda J, Seki T, Hida K, Tada M, Sawada K, Iwasaki Y: Migration and differentiation of nuclear fluorescence-labeled bone marrow stromal cells after transplantation into cerebral infarct and spinal cord injury in mice. *Neuropathology* 2003, 23:169-180.

Lendahl U, Zimmerman LB, McKay RD: CNS stem cells express a new class of intermediate filament protein. *Cell* 1990, 60:585-595.

Liem KF, Jr., Tremml G, Roelink H, Jessell TM: Dorsal differentiation of neural plate cells induced by BMP-mediated signals from epidermal ectoderm. *Cell* 1995, 82:969-979.

Liu JP, Jessell TM: A role for rhoB in the delamination of neural crest cells from the dorsal neural tube. *Development* 1998, 125:5055-5067.

Mancilla A, Mayor R: Neural crest formation in Xenopus laevis: mechanisms of Xslug induction. *Dev.Biol.* 1996, 177:580-589.

Marcelle C, Ahlgren S, Bronner-Fraser M: In vivo regulation of somite differentiation and proliferation by Sonic Hedgehog. *Dev.Biol.* 1999, 214:277-287.

Marchant L, Linker C, Ruiz P, Guerrero N, Mayor R: The inductive properties of mesoderm suggest that the neural crest cells are specified by a BMP gradient. *Dev.Biol.* 1998, 198:319-329.

Maurer J, Fuchs S, Jager R, Kurz B, Sommer L, Schorle H: Establishment and controlled differentiation of neural crest stem cell lines using conditional transgenesis. *Differentiation* 2007.

Maxwell GD, Reid K, Elefanty A, Bartlett PF, Murphy M: Glial cell line-derived neurotrophic factor promotes the development of adrenergic neurons in mouse neural crest cultures. *Proc.Natl.Acad.Sci.U.S A* 1996, 93:13274-13279.

Mayor R, Guerrero N, Young RM, Gomez-Skarmeta JL, Cuellar C: A novel function for the Xslug gene: control of dorsal mesendoderm development by repressing BMP-4. *Mech.Dev.* 2000, 97:47-56.

McGonnell IM, Graham A: Trunk neural crest has skeletogenic potential. *Curr.Biol.* 2002, 12:767-771.

McGuckin C, Forraz N, Baradez MO, Basford C, Dickinson AM, Navran S, Hartgerink JD: Embryonic-like stem cells from umbilical cord blood and potential for neural modeling. *Acta Neurobiol.Exp.(Wars.)* 2006, 66:321-329.

McKay R: Stem cells in the central nervous system. *Science* 1997, 276:66-71.

McKenzie IA, Biernaskie J, Toma JG, Midha R, Miller FD: Skin-derived precursors generate myelinating Schwann cells for the injured and dysmyelinated nervous system. *J.Neurosci.* 2006, 26:6651-6660.

Meyer D, Yamaai T, Garratt A, Riethmacher-Sonnenberg E, Kane D, Theill LE, Birchmeier C: Isoform-specific expression and function of neuregulin. *Development* 1997, 124:3575-3586.

Mezey E, Chandross KJ: Bone marrow: a possible alternative source of cells in the adult nervous system. *Eur.J.Pharmacol.* 2000, 405:297-302.

Moon RT, Brown JD, Yang-Snyder JA, Miller JR: Structurally related receptors and antagonists compete for secreted Wnt ligands. *Cell* 1997, 88:725-728.

Nagase T, Matsumoto D, Nagase M, Yoshimura K, Shigeura T, Inoue M, Hasegawa M, Yamagishi M, Machida M: Neurospheres from human adipose tissue transplanted into cultured mouse embryos can contribute to craniofacial morphogenesis: a preliminary report. *J.Craniofac.Surg.* 2007, 18:49-53.

Oka K, Oka S, Sasaki T, Ito Y, Bringas P, Jr., Nonaka K, Chai Y: The role of TGF-beta signaling in regulating chondrogenesis and osteogenesis during mandibular development. *Dev.Biol.* 2007, 303:391-404.

Okabe M, Ikawa M, Kominami K, Nakanishi T, Nishimune Y: 'Green mice' as a source of ubiquitous green cells. *FEBS Lett.* 1997, 407:313-319.

Orlic D, Kajstura J, Chimenti S, Limana F, Jakoniuk I, Quaini F, Nadal-Ginard B, Bodine DM, Leri A, Anversa P: Mobilized bone marrow cells repair the infarcted heart, improving function and survival. *Proc.Natl.Acad.Sci.U.S A* 2001, 98:10344-10349.

Ozawa M, Baribault H, Kemler R: The cytoplasmic domain of the cell adhesion molecule uvomorulin associates with three independent proteins structurally related in different species. *EMBO J.* 1989, 8:1711-1717.

Padovan CS, Jahn K, Birnbaum T, Reich P, Sostak P, Strupp M, Straube A: Expression of neuronal markers in differentiated marrow stromal cells and CD133+ stem-like cells. *Cell Transplant.* 2003, 12:839-848.

Paratore C, Goerich DE, Suter U, Wegner M, Sommer L: Survival and glial fate acquisition of neural crest cells are regulated by an interplay between the transcription factor Sox10 and extrinsic combinatorial signaling. *Development* 2001, 128:3949-3961.

Peles E, Yarden Y: Neu and its ligands: from an oncogene to neural factors. *Bioessays* 1993, 15:815-824.

Plowman GD, Green JM, Culouscou JM, Carlton GW, Rothwell VM, Buckley S: Heregulin induces tyrosine phosphorylation of HER4/p180erbB4. *Nature* 1993, 366:473-475.

Potten CS, Booth C, Tudor GL, Booth D, Brady G, Hurley P, Ashton G, Clarke R, Sakakibara S, Okano H: Identification of a putative intestinal stem cell and early lineage marker; musashi-1. *Differentiation* 2003, 71:28-41.

Priller J, Flugel A, Wehner T, Boentert M, Haas CA, Prinz M, Fernandez-Klett F, Prass K, Bechmann I, de Boer BA, Frotscher M, Kreutzberg GW, Persons DA, Dirnagl U: Targeting gene-modified hematopoietic cells to the central nervous system: use of green fluorescent protein uncovers microglial engraftment. *Nat.Med.* 2001, 7:1356-1361.

Rao MS, Anderson DJ: Immortalization and controlled in vitro differentiation of murine multipotent neural crest stem cells. *J.Neurobiol.* 1997, 32:722-746.

Reddy T, Kablar B: Evidence for the involvement of neurotrophins in muscle transdifferentiation and acetylcholine receptor transformation in the esophagus of Myf5(-/-):MyoD(-/-) and NT-3(-/-) embryos. *Dev.Dyn.* 2004, 231:683-692.

Riethmacher D, Sonnenberg-Riethmacher E, Brinkmann V, Yamaai T, Lewin GR, Birchmeier C: Severe neuropathies in mice with targeted mutations in the ErbB3 receptor. *Nature* 1997, 389:725-730.

Rivera FJ, Sierralta WD, Minguell JJ, Aigner L: Adult hippocampus derived soluble factors induce a neuronal-like phenotype in mesenchymal stem cells. *Neurosci.Lett.* 2006, 406:49-54.

Safford KM, Safford SD, Gimble JM, Shetty AK, Rice HE: Characterization of neuronal/glial differentiation of murine adipose-derived adult stromal cells. *Exp.Neurol.* 2004, 187:319-328.

Sanchez-Ramos J, Song S, Cardozo-Pelaez F, Hazzi C, Stedeford T, Willing A, Freeman TB, Saporta S, Janssen W, Patel N, Cooper DR, Sanberg PR: Adult bone marrow stromal cells differentiate into neural cells in vitro. *Exp.Neurol.* 2000, 164:247-256.

Sanchez-Ramos J: Stem cells from umbilical cord blood. *Semin.Reprod.Med.* 2006, 24:358-369.

Sanchez-Ramos JR: Neural cells derived from adult bone marrow and umbilical cord blood. *J.Neurosci.Res.* 2002, 69:880-893.

Scadden DT: The stem-cell niche as an entity of action. *Nature* 2006, 441:1075-1079.

Schuldiner M, Yanuka O, Itskovitz-Eldor J, Melton DA, Benvenisty N: Effects of eight growth factors on the differentiation of cells derived from human embryonic stem cells. *Proc.Natl.Acad.Sci.U.S A* 2000, 97:11307-11312.

Seale P, Rudnicki MA: A new look at the origin, function, and "stem-cell" status of muscle satellite cells. *Dev.Biol.* 2000, 218:115-124.

Sela-Donenfeld D, Kalcheim C: Localized BMP4-noggin interactions generate the dynamic patterning of noggin expression in somites. *Dev.Biol.* 2002, 246:311-328.

Sell S: Is there a liver stem cell? *Cancer Res.* 1990, 50:3811-3815.

Selleck MA, Bronner-Fraser M: Origins of the avian neural crest: the role of neural plate-epidermal interactions. *Development* 1995, 121:525-538.

Shah NM, Marchionni MA, Isaacs I, Stroobant P, Anderson DJ: Glial growth factor restricts mammalian neural crest stem cells to a glial fate. *Cell* 1994, 77:349-360.

Shah NM, Groves AK, Anderson DJ: Alternative neural crest cell fates are instructively promoted by TGFbeta superfamily members. *Cell* 1996, 85:331-343.

Sieber-Blum M, Zhang JM: Growth factor action in neural crest cell diversification. *J.Anat.* 1997, 191 (Pt 4):493-499.

Sieber-Blum M, Grim M, Hu YF, Szeder V: Pluripotent neural crest stem cells in the adult hair follicle. *Dev.Dyn.* 2004, 231:258-269.

Slack WV: Cybermedicine for the patient. *Am.J.Prev.Med.* 2007, 32:S135-S136.

Sliwkowski MX, Schaefer G, Akita RW, Lofgren JA, Fitzpatrick VD, Nuijens A, Fendly BM, Cerione RA, Vandlen RL, Carraway KL, III: Coexpression of erbB2 and erbB3 proteins reconstitutes a high affinity receptor for heregulin. *J.Biol.Chem.* 1994, 269:14661-14665.

Southard-Smith EM, Kos L, Pavan WJ: Sox10 mutation disrupts neural crest development in Dom Hirschsprung mouse model. *Nat.Genet.* 1998, 18:60-64.

Stanford WL, Caruana G, Vallis KA, Inamdar M, Hidaka M, Bautch VL, Bernstein A: Expression trapping: identification of novel genes expressed in hematopoietic and endothelial lineages by gene trapping in ES cells. *Blood* 1998, 92:4622-4631.

Stemple DL, Anderson DJ: Isolation of a stem cell for neurons and glia from the mammalian neural crest. *Cell* 1992, 71:973-985.

Stocum DL: Amphibian regeneration and stem cells. *Curr.Top.Microbiol.Immunol.* 2004, 280:1-70.

Takano N, Kawakami T, Kawa Y, Asano M, Watabe H, Ito M, Soma Y, Kubota Y, Mizoguchi M: Fibronectin combined with stem cell factor plays an important role in melanocyte proliferation, differentiation and migration in cultured mouse neural crest cells. *Pigment Cell Res.* 2002, 15:192-200.

Terada N, Hamazaki T, Oka M, Hoki M, Mastalerz DM, Nakano Y, Meyer EM, Morel L, Petersen BE, Scott EW: Bone marrow cells adopt the phenotype of other cells by spontaneous cell fusion. *Nature* 2002, 416:542-545.

Toma JG, Akhavan M, Fernandes KJ, Barnabe-Heider F, Sadikot A, Kaplan DR, Miller FD: Isolation of multipotent adult stem cells from the dermis of mammalian skin. *Nat.Cell Biol.* 2001, 3:778-784.

Tomita Y, Matsumura K, Wakamatsu Y, Matsuzaki Y, Shibuya I, Kawaguchi H, Ieda M, Kanakubo S, Shimazaki T, Ogawa S, Osumi N, Okano H, Fukuda K: Cardiac neural crest cells contribute to the dormant multipotent stem cell in the mammalian heart. *J.Cell Biol.* 2005, 170:1135-1146.

Tsonis PA: Regeneration of the lens in amphibians. *Results Probl.Cell Differ.* 2000, 31:179-196.

Vassilopoulos G, Russell DW: Cell fusion: an alternative to stem cell plasticity and its therapeutic implications. *Curr.Opin.Genet.Dev.* 2003, 13:480-485.

Wakamatsu Y, Endo Y, Osumi N, Weston JA: Multiple roles of Sox2, an HMG-box transcription factor in avian neural crest development. *Dev.Dyn.* 2004, 229:74-86.

Wei Y, Renard CA, Labalette C, Wu Y, Levy L, Neuveut C, Prieur X, Flajolet M, Prigent S, Buendia MA: Identification of the LIM protein FHL2 as a coactivator of beta-catenin. *J.Biol.Chem.* 2003, 278:5188-5194.

Weimann JM, Charlton CA, Brazelton TR, Hackman RC, Blau HM: Contribution of transplanted bone marrow cells to Purkinje neurons in human adult brains. *Proc.Natl.Acad.Sci.U.S A* 2003, 100:2088-2093.

Weimann JM, Johansson CB, Trejo A, Blau HM: Stable reprogrammed heterokaryons form spontaneously in Purkinje neurons after bone marrow transplant. *Nat.Cell Biol.* 2003, 5:959-966.

Weiss EE, Kroemker M, Rudiger AH, Jockusch BM, Rudiger M: Vinculin is part of the cadherin-catenin junctional complex: complex formation between alpha-catenin and vinculin. *J.Cell Biol.* 1998, 141:755-764.

Wen D, Peles E, Cupples R, Suggs SV, Bacus SS, Luo Y, Trail G, Hu S, Silbiger SM, Levy RB, .: Neu differentiation factor: a transmembrane glycoprotein containing an EGF domain and an immunoglobulin homology unit. *Cell* 1992, 69:559-572.

Wiese C, Rolletschek A, Kania G, Blyszczuk P, Tarasov KV, Tarasova Y, Wersto RP, Boheler KR, Wobus AM: Nestin expression--a property of multi-lineage progenitor cells? *Cell Mol.Life Sci.* 2004, 61:2510-2522.

Wislet-Gendebien S, Leprince P, Moonen G, Rogister B: Regulation of neural markers nestin and GFAP expression by cultivated bone marrow stromal cells. *J.Cell Sci.* 2003, 116:3295-3302.

Wislet-Gendebien S, Bruyere F, Hans G, Leprince P, Moonen G, Rogister B: Nestin-positive mesenchymal stem cells favour the astroglial lineage in neural progenitors and stem cells by releasing active BMP4. *BMC Neurosci.* 2004, 5:33.

Wislet-Gendebien S, Hans G, Leprince P, Rigo JM, Moonen G, Rogister B: Plasticity of cultured mesenchymal stem cells: switch from nestin-positive to excitable neuron-like phenotype. *Stem Cells* 2005, 23:392-402.

Wong CE, Paratore C, Dours-Zimmermann MT, Rochat A, Pietri T, Suter U, Zimmermann DR, Dufour S, Thiery JP, Meijer D, Beermann F, Barrandon Y, Sommer L: Neural crest-derived cells with stem cell features can be traced back to multiple lineages in the adult skin. *J.Cell Biol.* 2006, 175:1005-1015.

Woodbury D, Schwarz EJ, Prockop DJ, Black IB: Adult rat and human bone marrow stromal cells differentiate into neurons. *J.Neurosci.Res.* 2000, 61:364-370.

Woodbury D, Reynolds K, Black IB: Adult bone marrow stromal stem cells express germline, ectodermal, endodermal, and mesodermal genes prior to neurogenesis. *J.Neurosci.Res.* 2002, 69:908-917.

Wu J, Saint-Jeannet JP, Klein PS: Wnt-frizzled signaling in neural crest formation. *Trends Neurosci.* 2003, 26:40-45.

Wu KY, Hong SJ, Lin CP, Lai YH, Wang HZ: Endothelin-induced changes of secondary messengers in cultured corneal endothelial cells. *J.Ocul.Pharmacol.Ther.* 2001, 17:351-361.

Ying QL, Nichols J, Evans EP, Smith AG: Changing potency by spontaneous fusion. *Nature* 2002, 416:545-548.

Zhang H, Wang JZ, Sun HY, Zhang JN, Yang SY: The effects of GM1 and bFGF synergistically inducing adult rat bone marrow stromal cells to form neural progenitor cells and their differentiation. *Chin J.Traumatol.* 2004, 7:3-6.

Zhao LX, Zhang J, Cao F, Meng L, Wang DM, Li YH, Nan X, Jiao WC, Zheng M, Xu XH, Pei XT: Modification of the brain-derived neurotrophic factor gene: a portal to transform mesenchymal stem cells into advantageous engineering cells for neuroregeneration and neuroprotection. *Exp.Neurol.* 2004, 190:396-406.

Zuk PA, Zhu M, Mizuno H, Huang J, Futrell JW, Katz AJ, Benhaim P, Lorenz HP, Hedrick MH: Multilineage cells from human adipose tissue: implications for cell-based therapies. *Tissue Eng* 2001, 7:211-228.

In: Encyclopedia of Stem Cell Research (2 Volume Set)   ISBN: 978-1-61761-835-2
Editor: Alexander L. Greene   © 2012 Nova Science Publishers, Inc.

Chapter XXXIV

CENTRAL NERVOUS SYSTEM LYMPHOMA

Andrew Lister[1], Lauren E. Abrey[2], and John T. Sandlund[3]*
[1]St. Bartholomew's Hospital, West Smithfield, London, United Kingdom
[2]Memorial Sloan-Kettering Cancer Center, New York, NY, US
[3]St. Jude Children's Research Hospital, Memphis, TN, US

ABSTRACT

Central nervous system involvement with malignant lymphoma whether primary or secondary is an uncommon but not rare complication observed in the management. Importance lies in the considerable morbidity and mortality with which it is associated and the inadequacy of therapy.

In Section I, Dr. Lauren Abrey addresses the totality of the problem of primary central nervous system lymphoma, with emphasis on strategies increasingly dependent on systemic chemotherapy.

In Section II, Dr. John Sandlund reviews the success of sequential clinical trials of overall therapy for acute lymphoblastic leukemia in child-hood, identifying those patients at high risk of central nervous system leukemia and the development of a rational therapeutic strategy for prevention.

In Section III, Dr. Andrew Lister discusses the issue of secondary central nervous system involvement with lymphoma and the indications for prophylaxis.

I. PRIMARY CENTRAL NERVOUS SYSTEM LYMPHOMA

Primary central nervous system lymphoma (PCNSL) is a rare form of non-Hodgkin's lymphoma (NHL) arising within and confined to the CNS. It was first described by Bailey [1] in 1929 as a perithelial sarcoma. Subsequent classifications have included reticulum cell

---

* Correspondence concerning this section should be addressed to: Dr. Lauren E. Abrey, Memorial Sloan-Kettering Cancer Center, 1275 York Avenue, New York, NY 10021.

sarcoma and microglioma. Improvements in histopathology and immunohistochemical techniques definitively established the lymphoid nature of PCNSL.

PCNSL is of particular interest for several reasons. First, this tumor has increased in incidence over the past several decades. Therefore, although it remains relatively rare, it is an increasingly important differential diagnosis of intracranial mass lesions. Second, unlike many primary brain tumors PCNSL is very responsive to treatment, and aggressive management may lead to prolonged remission or cure. Finally, the long-term consequences of aggressive therapy may result in significant neurologic dysfunction.

Epidemiology

PCNSL accounts for approximately 1% of all primary brain tumors in large autopsy-based series More recent data suggest that the incidence among immunocompetent patients in the United States is increasing. Data from the National Cancer Institute Surveillance, Epidemiology, and End Result (SEER) database found a threefold increase in PCNSL between 1973-1975 and 1982-1984. Further analysis found a tenfold or greater increase between 1973 and 1992.

The incidence of ocular lymphoma has similarly in-creased by 1.5-fold. There has been a parallel rise in the incidence of all extranodal lymphomas, but the increase has been disproportionate in the brain and eye. This in-creased incidence is not explained by advances in neuroimaging or tumor diagnosis. As PCNSL primarily affects individuals age 60 and older, one possible explanation would be the general aging of the population; however, the data indicate an increase across all age groups.

PCNSL is diagnosed in 1.6% to 9.0% of the human immunodeficiency virus (HIV)-infected population [2,3] and is the second most common intracranial mass lesion. Prior to the introduction of highly active antiretroviral therapy (HAART), the incidence of PCNSL in the HIV-infected population was continuing to rise. However, the impact of these new drug regimens on the CD4 count may result in a decline in PCNSL, as the susceptibility to PCNSL is inversely proportional to the CD4 count [4].

Pathology

Grossly, PCNSL is a soft, granular, ill-defined lesion. Associated necrosis, hemorrhage, and neovascularity are uncommon except in AIDS-related PCNSL. Microscopically, PCNSL is a diffuse lesion with an angiocentric growth pattern; some tumors may even invade the blood vessel wall. In addition to malignant lymphocytes there are varying numbers of small, benign, reactive T lymphocytes infiltrating the tumor, and reactive astrocytes are common. Malignant lymphocytes freely invade normal surrounding brain and autopsy studies have demonstrated widespread infiltration of normal brain.

Immunohistochemical stains are extremely useful in differentiating PCNSL from high-grade glioma and metastatic carcinoma. Leukocyte common antigen clearly identifies the malignant cells as white blood cells but may be negative in a small number of PCNSLs.

Ninety percent or more are B-cell lymphomas (CD20+), usually of diffuse large-cell, large-cell immunoblastic, or lymphoblastic subtype. These tumors can be identified by the immunohistochemical B-cell marker L26. The reactive infiltrating cells are typically T lymphocytes, although primary T-cell lymphomas (CD3+, CD45RO+) are reported.

Histologically, PCNSL is indistinguishable from systemic NHL. Biologically, PCNSL behaves in an aggressive fashion, and it should be considered a high-grade tumor. Genetically, PCNSL has been found to demonstrate clonal abnormalities of chromosomes 1, 6, 7, and 14, identical to those detected in systemic NHL [5]. Analysis of cell surface markers including NCAM and integrins is also identical to that of systemic lymphoma. Kumanishi et al found p15 and p16 deletions in 4 out of 5 PCNSL tumors [6].

Pathogenesis

The pathogenesis of PCNSL in immunocompetent patients is unknown. T lymphocytes normally traffic in and out of the CNS however, there is no normal traffic of B lymphocytes Therefore, several different hypotheses have been proposed. There are no data to support or disprove any of these potential mechanisms.

PCNSL may arise from a systemic lymphoma that seeds multiple organs, including the brain The immune system has the capacity to find and eliminate the systemic tumor, but the brain, an immunologically privileged site, gives sanctuary to the malignant lymphocytes thereby allowing tumor development. This seems unlikely, as there is no evidence of concomitant lymphoma in other immunologically privileged sites, such as the testes, concomitant with PCNSL.

Another theory is that lymphocytes become trapped in the CNS after an inflammatory process and then undergo malignant transformation. However, inflammatory diseases almost exclusively attract T lymphocytes and PCNSL is usually of B-cell origin. Also, the incidence of PCNSL is not increased in patients with inflammatory CNS diseases.

Clinical Features and Evaluation (Table 1)

The typical patient is between 55 and 70 years old; most have had symptoms for only a few weeks prior to seeking medical attention Cognitive and personality changes are the most common initial symptoms, reflecting the predilection of PCNSL to involve the frontal lobes corpus callosum, and deep periventricular structures. PCNSL is multifocal in approximately one third of patients and may present with any focal neurologic finding, such as hemiparesis or aphasia. Seizures are a presenting complaint in about 10% of patients, less frequent than glioma or brain metastasis. Age less than 60 and an excellent performance status are the most important prognostic factors.

In AIDSrelated PCNSL, the typical patient is younger (30-40 years old), and seizures are more common (25%). The median latency from HIV diagnosis is approximately 5 years. Some studies have found a higher incidence of multiple lesions in AIDS-related PCNSL; however, multifocal lesions in AIDS patients may have different etiologies.

More than 40% of patients have evidence of leptomeningeal dissemination, but concomitant clinical findings are uncommon. Primary leptomeningeal lymphoma is rare and typically presents increased intracranial pressure multifocal cranial neuropathies, or multilevel root involvement. Cerebrospinal fluid (CSF should be obtained in all newly diagnosed patients. CSF evidence of PCNSL may also be a poor prognostic indicator. Tumor markers, including lactate dehydrogenase isoenzymes, â-glucuronidase, and â2-microglobulin, may provide circumstantial evidence of leptomeningeal lymphoma. Immunocytochemical analysis and detection of immunoglobulin gene rearrangements by polymerase chain reaction have been used in the diagnosis of lymphomatous meningitis when routine cytologic evaluation is in-conclusive.

Table 1. Initial evaluation for primary central nervous system lymphoma (PCNSL)

Gadolinium-enhanced cranial MRI scan
CSF cytology
Ophthalmologic examination, including slit lamp
HIV serology
CT scan of chest, abdomen, and pelvis
Bone marrow biopsy
Gadolinium-enhanced spinal MRI if spinal symptoms are present

MRI magnetic resonance imaging; CSF cerebrospinal fluid; CT, computed tomography.

About 15% of patients with PCNSL have ocular disease at presentation, while 50% to 80% of patients with isolated ocular lymphoma go on to develop parenchymal brain lymphoma. Ocular symptoms include blurred, cloudy vision, decreased visual acuity or "floaters," but as many as half of affected patients are asymptomatic. Complete ophthalmologic evaluation, including slit lamp examination, is recommended in all patients. Diagnosis is often delayed in patients with isolated ocular lymphoma because of misdiagnosis as chronic vitreitis or uveitis. Systemic lymphoma is an uncommon finding in PCNSL, and there is disagreement as to whether a comprehensive systemic extent of disease evaluation is needed. In a series from the Mayo Clinic, approximately 2% to 3% of PCNSL patients were found to have systemic lymphoma on an abdominopelvic computed tomography (CT) scan or bone marrow biopsy.

The optimal neuroimaging of PCNSL is gadolinium-enhanced magnetic resonance (MR) scanning. Most lesions are supratentorial and periventricular, often involving deep structures such as the corpus callosum and basal ganglia Lesions may be hypo- or hyperintense on pre-contrast T1 imaging. Dense, homogeneous contrast enhancement is seen in immunocompetent patients but may be irregular and heterogeneous in AIDSrelated PCNSL. Peritumoral edema and local mass effect are often less than expected with intracranial lesions of other etiologies. Calcification, hemorrhage, or cyst formation is rare.

Treatment

Surgery

The role of surgery is to establish a histopathologic diagnosis; therefore, a stereotactic needle biopsy is the procedure of choice. Aggressive resection does not improve survival and may result in neurologic deterioration.

Corticosteroids

Corticosteroids are used empirically in the treatment of vasogenic edema caused by any intracranial mass In PCNSL, corticosteroids also have a potent oncolytic effect, causing tumor cell lysis and radiographic regression in up to 40% of patients [7]. The onset of action is quite rapid, with resolution of symptoms and marked reduction in tumor size within 24 to 48 hours. This can be problematic if a tissue diagnosis has not been obtained. Therefore, steroids should be withheld in any patient with a presumptive diagnosis of PCNSL until stereotactic biopsy has been performed.

Radiotherapy

PCNSL is a radiosensitive tumor, and whole-brain radiotherapy (RT) was the standard treatment for many years. Whole-brain RT is necessary because of the diffuse infiltrative nature of this neoplasm and results in median survivals ranging from 10 to 18 months [8,9]. Craniospinal RT does not confer any additional survival benefit and is associated with significant morbidity limiting the administration of subsequent chemotherapy.

The optimal dose of whole-brain RT remains controversial, but the results of several studies suggest a dose between 40-50 Gy. The addition of a boost does not improve local tumor control or survival In patients with evidence of ocular lymphoma the posterior two thirds of the globe should be radiated to a dose of 36-40 Gy. Treatment planning should take into account both intracranial and ocular disease to eliminate overlapping fields and to minimize any toxicity to the optic nerve and retina.

Chemotherapy

The use of chemotherapy has significantly improved the treatment of PCNSL. However, the standard regimens (CHOP, MACOP-B) used in the treatment of systemic lymphoma are not effective in PCNSL because of their inability to penetrate the blood-brain barrier.

High-dose methotrexate (MTX) is the single most active agent in the treatment of PCNSL. While standard-dose MTX does not cross the blood-brain barrier, doses ~ 1 g/m^2 result in tumoricidal levels in the brain and doses ~ 3.5 g/m^2 yield tumoricidal levels in the CSF. Therefore, most treatment regimens now incorporate high-dose MTX (1 to 8 g/m^2) alone or in combination with other chemotherapeutic agents followed by whole-brain RT. This combined-modality approach has resulted in response rates approaching 100% and median survivals ranging between 30 and 60 months (Table 2) [10-14].

There has been increasing interest in using chemotherapy alone in order to minimize long-term effects of treatment. One approach has been to employ hyperosmolar agents to disrupt the blood-brain barrier, followed by intra-arterial MTX [13]. This technique results in similar overall response and survival rates as the combined-modality approach; however, the acute toxicities are more significant and include focal seizures, cerebral ischemia, cerebral edema and local arterial trauma Careful neuropsychological testing of this patient cohort has been performed and indicates that patients who remain in remission are not at increased risk for delayed neurotoxicity.

Table 2. Chemotherapy regimens for PCNSL

Ref	Type	N	Regimen	RT	Result	Other
[35]	Series	10	DHAP	+/–	70% response 40% prolonged remission	4 newly diagnosed, 6 recurrent Several did not receive RT
[36]	Series	10	PCV	+	100% response 30-mo median survival	PCV given post-RT 1 pt received carmustine
[11]	Series	13	MTX 3.5 g/m^2	+	92% response 9+- mo median survival	Survival up to 54+ mos
[10]	Series	25	MTX 3.5 g/m^2	+	88% response 33-mo median survival	59% relapse rate
[37]	Series	74	MTX BBBD	–	65% complete response 40.7-mo median survival	
[38]	Series	31	MTX 1 g/m^2	+	64% response 41-mo median survival	
[23]	Phase II	14	MTV IT Ara-C	–	100% response 16.5-mo PFS	68.8% alive at 54 mos 2 pts with severe leukoencephalopathy
[39]	Prospective	19	BOMES	+	84% response rate 6-mo median PFS	5 pts with concurrent systemic lymphoma
[40]	Series	19	MTX-based 3.5-8 g/m^2	–	94% response rate	
[41]	Phase II	102	MPV Ara-C	+	94% response rate 30+-mo median survival	
[14]	Prospective	52	MPV Ara-C	+/–	60-mo median survival	22 older pts did not receive RT

PCNSL, primary central nervous system lymphoma; DHAP, dexamethasone, high-dose cytarabine, and cisplatin; PCV, procarbazine, CCNU, and vincristine; MTX, methotrexate; BBBD, blood-brain-barrier disruption; MTV, methotrexate, thiotepa, and vincristine; IT, intrathecal; Ara-C, cytarabine; BOMES, BCNU, vincristine, methotrexate, etoposide, and methylprednisolone; MPV, methotrexate, procarbazine, and vincristine; RT, whole-brain radiotherapy; mo, months; PFS, progression-free survival; pt, patient.

Adapted with permission from Abrey LE, Primary central nervous system lymphoma.The Neurologist. 2000;6:245-254.

In our experience, it is possible to treat older patients with MTX-based chemotherapy alone and achieve similar results as those achieved using combined-modality treatment in older patients. Both groups have a median survival of 32-33 months; [14] the difference is that patients treated with chemotherapy alone are more likely to relapse early, while patients treated with combined-modality therapy are more likely to develop delayed neurotoxicity. Importantly, older patients are able to tolerate aggressive chemotherapy without any excess acute morbidity.

High-dose chemotherapy with autologous peripheral blood stem cell support has been used a strategy to dose intensify chemotherapy given to patients with primary CNS lymphoma. Theoretically the administration of high dose consolidation chemotherapy can be used in place of standard cranial radiotherapy in an effort to avoid treatment-related neurotoxicity. There have been two small trials for newly diagnosed patients and the preliminary results indicate that this strategy is feasible [1,2]. Further studies will be needed to identify the optimal induction and high dose chemotherapy regimens [15,16].

AIDS-Related

The treatment of AIDSrelated PCNSL is dictated in large part by the clinical condition of the patient. One of the most critical factors is making a definitive diagnosis early, as delay may result in significant neurologic deterioration, precluding the ability to tolerate aggressive treatment.

Small series suggest that individual patients may benefit from aggressive combined-modality therapy [17-20] HAART was reported to cause a 26-month remission in 1 AIDS patient with PCNSL and may represent an important new treatment alternative [21].

Ocular Lymphoma

There is no standard approach to isolated ocular lymphoma Ocular lymphoma is exquisitely sensitive to corticosteroids (including topical ophthalmic preparations) and focal RT. Unfortunately, in most patients the disease will recur either in the eyes or in the brain at which time the disease may be more refractory to therapeutic intervention Systemic administration of MTX and cytarabine can yield therapeutic levels of drug in the intraocular fluids, and clinical responses have been documented; however, relapse is common [22-24]. Therefore, our current approach is to treat isolated ocular lymphoma with combined-modality therapy [25,26]. Direct intravitreal administration of chemotherapy is being explored as a therapeutic alternative.

Relapse

The risk of relapse for patients treated with combined-modality therapy is about 50%. Most recurrences are observed within 2 years of completing initial therapy, but relapses have been seen as late as 5 years. Patients with ocular or leptomeningeal disease at diagnosis have a higher likelihood of recurrence Relapse primarily occurs in the brain at either the original or distant sites; however, leptomeningeal and ocular relapses are seen, and systemic relapse has been reported to account for as much as 10%.

The prognosis at relapse is generally poor but further treatment often results in transient remission. Pro-longed survival is possible, and some patients continue to be sensitive to salvage therapy despite multiple re-lapses. Success has been reported using high-dose MTX (even in patients previously treated with MTX), high-dose cytarabine, PCV (procarbazine, lomustine, and vincristine), and high-dose cyclophosphamide RT is particularly effective for ocular relapse. Intensive chemotherapy with autologous peripheral blood stem cell sup-port is standard therapy for patients with relapsed, chemosensitive, systemic NHL; this strategy has been used with some success for relapsed PCNSL [3]. However, patients previously treated with whole brain radiotherapy have a higher risk of neurologic toxicity [27].

Treatment-Related Neurotoxicity

The most significant consequence of aggressive combined-modality therapy utilizing MTX followed by cranial RT is delayed neurologic toxicity Older patients are at particularly high risk of developing a progressive neurological syndrome characterized by dementia gait ataxia and urinary dysfunction Up to 90% of patients over 60 who survive 1 year after completion of treatment will be affected [28]. Patients usually become symptomatic within 1 year of treatment, with a significant decline in their performance status necessitating constant supervision and custodial care. Attempts to treat delayed neurotoxicity have been generally unrewarding, although a subset of patients may have transient improvement following placement of a ventriculoperitoneal shunt [29,30]. Other agents, such as methylphenidate, have been utilized with success in individual patients.

Delayed treatment-related cerebrovascular disease has been observed in younger patients 7-10 years after completion of therapy [31,32]. This has been observed in isolation or in conjunction with a progressive leukoencephalopathy. Accelerated atherosclerosis is a known complication of cranial RT that typically develops 10 to 20 years after treatment [33,34]. Stroke-like episodes have been re-ported acutely in children receiving high-dose MTX, but these typically occur days to weeks after chemotherapy and resolve spontaneously. It is also possible that PCNSL may predispose patients to cerebrovascular damage if lysis of angiocentric tumor cells damages neighboring endothelium.

II. LYMPHOMATOUS MENINGITIS: THE ACUTE LYMPHOBLASTIC LEUKEMIA MODEL[*]

CNS involvement among children with acute lymphoblastic leukemia (ALL) has historically been defined at most institutions by either the presence of at least 5 leukocytes per microliter of cerebrospinal fluid (CSF) associated with the presence of leukemic blasts (identified on a cytocentrifuged preparation) or the presence of a cranial nerve; palsy on physical examination [1]. Therapeutic approaches for both CNS prophylaxis and therapy have included the following: (1) intrathecal administration of chemotherapy ranging from single-agent MTX to triple-agent intrathecal therapy consisting of MTX, hydrocortisone and cytarabine; (2) cranial irradiation and (3) the systemic administration of chemotherapeutic

[*] Correspondence concerning this section should be addressed to Dr. John T. Sandlund, 3St. Jude Children's Research Hospital, 332 N. Lauderdale, Box 318, Memphis, TN 38101-0318. Supported by grant CA2 1765 from the National Cancer Institute and by the American Lebanese Syrian Associated Charities (ALSAC).

agents with good CNS penetration (e.g., high-dose MTX, high-dose cytarabine, and dexamethasone). De-spite these measures; there are patients who have been shown to still be at increased risk for CNS treatment failure.

CNS Status Refinement

Mahmoud et al2 challenged the conventional definition by showing that the presence of leukemic blast cells in the CSF, regardless of cell count, increased the risk of CNS relapse. In that study, all 351 children with newly diagnosed ALL were entered on a randomized trial in which each patient received intrathecal therapy throughout the first year. Patients who were considered at in-creased risk for treatment failure because of their clinical or cytogenetic features also received 1 8-Gy cranial irradiation and intrathecal chemotherapy 1 year from the remission date. Those with CNS disease at diagnosis (as defined by at least 5 leukocytes/microliter of CSF with leukemic blasts on a cytocentrifuged prep or by the pres-ence of cranial nerve palsy on physical examination) received 24-Gy cranial irradiation and additional intrathecal chemotherapy. Patients were classified retrospectively into 3 CNS groups based on the CSF findings: 291 patients had CNS-1 status (no blasts in the CSF), 42 had CNS-2 status (blasts present with fewer than 5 leukocytes/microliter), and 18 had CNS-3 status (5 or more leukocytes/microliter of CSF with leukemic blasts on a cytospin sample or cranial nerve palsy). The probability of an isolated CNS relapse in patients with CNS-2 status was higher than in those with CNS-1 status but was not different from that of patients with CNS-3 status. All CNS relapses occurred during the first year of treatment, before scheduled cranial irradiation. In a multivariate analysis, CNS-2 status was independently related to the risk of an isolated CNS relapse, suggesting that these patients require intensification of CNS-directed treatment early in the course of therapy. While a study of the former Pediatric Oncology Group confirmed this result [3], studies by the former Children's Cancer Group and the Dutch Childhood Leukemia Study Group did not find a significant difference in outcome between patients with or without a lower number of blasts in the CSF [4,5]. These seemingly conflicting results may reflect differences in therapy.

Traumatic Lumbar Punctures

Gajjar et al., [6] performed a single-institution retrospective study of children with newly diagnosed ALL in which they demonstrated that a traumatic lumbar puncture (LP) at diagnosis adversely affected outcome. In this study, 546 children were treated on 2 consecutive St. Jude trials in which 2 sequential LPs were performed at presentation—the first for diagnosis and the second for instillation of the first intrathecal chemotherapy treatment, generally 1 to 2 days later. It was demonstrated that patients with 1 CSF sample contaminated with blast cells had an inferior event-free survival compared to those with CNS1 status $(P = 0.026)$. The prognosis for those with 2 consecutive contaminated CSF samples had a particularly poor treatment result (5-year event-free survival = 46% ± 9%); this feature was shown to be the strongest prognostic indicator in a Cox multiple regression analysis, with a hazard ratio of 2.39 (95% confidence interval, 1.36-4.20). It was concluded from this study that contamination of the CSF with circulating leukemic blasts adversely influences treatment outcome and is an indication for early intensification of intrathecal chemotherapy administration. This result was recently con-firmed by the investigators of the Berlin-Frankfurt-Münster group (BFM; M Schrappe, personal communication).

A recent study by Howard et al (unpublished data) examined risk factors associated with the occurrence of traumatic (at least 10 red blood cells per microliter) and/ or bloody (at least 500 red blood cells per microliter) LPs. Risk factors associated with traumatic or bloody taps included the following: (1) age less than 1 year; (2) black race (3) early treatment era during which sedation was used very seldom; (4) a platelet count less than 100×109/L; (5) a short (1 day) time interval since the previous LP; and (6) a less experienced practitioner. On the basis of these findings, the investigators recommended that diagnostic LPs in newly diagnosed patients with ALL should be performed by an experienced practitioner, in a dedicated procedure area with general anesthesia, following platelet transfusion if the platelet count is less than 100×109/L and circulating blasts are present. Using this approach, we have already substantially reduced the rate of traumatic LP with blasts from 11% to 4% to date.

Impact of Intensified CNS Therapy/Prophylaxis

In a St. Jude Children's Research Hospital study per-formed by Pui et al., [7] it was demonstrated that early intensification of intrathecal chemotherapy used in the context of the Total Therapy Study XIII virtually eliminates CNS relapse in children with ALL. Children with any amount of leukemic blasts in the CSF, whether or not the CSF blasts were introduced iatrogenically to the CSF because of a traumatic LP and regardless of the presence or absence of other high-risk clinical features, received additional doses of intrathecal chemotherapy (MTX, hydrocortisone and cytarabine) during induction and throughout the first year of continuation therapy Cranial irradiation at 18 Gy, given during weeks 56 to 59 of the continuation phase, was reserved for only those with certain high-risk features: B-cell progenitor phenotype with a leukocyte count of at least 100×109/L, T - cell phenotype with a leukocyte count of at least 50×109/L, or a karyotype with the Philadelphia chromosome The 5-year cumulative risk of an isolated CNS relapse among the 165 patients studied was 1.2% (95% confidence interval, 0%-2.9%), whereas the risk of any CNS relapse was 3.2% (95% confidence interval, 0.4%-6.0%). It appears from this study that early intensification of intrathecal chemotherapy administration may reduce or eliminate the occurrence of CNS relapse associated with the above-mentioned risk factors (i.e., CNS-2 status at diagnosis, and traumatic or bloody LP at diagnosis). A similar result was obtained in a subsequent St. Jude clinical trial (XIIIB) (unpublished data).

Trend toward Reducing Use of Radiotherapy for CNS Disease/Prophylaxis

Most clinical trials limit the use of cranial irradiation to 5% to 10% of patients at high risk of CNS relapse, in large part because of the concern of late sequelae such as second cancer endocrinopathy, and neuropsychologic defects Moreover, in some protocols, cranial irradiation is given at a reduced dose. For example, the BFM has reduced the dose of prophylactic cranial irradiation to 12 Gy and the dose of therapeutic cranial irradiation for those with overt CNS disease to 18 Gy [8]. Other trials, which have eliminated cranial irradiation in all patients, have not observed an excessive rate of relapse [9-11]. The elimination of cranial irradiation is also being studied in our current St. Jude trial. Thus far, no CNS relapse has been observed among 150 patients treated with median follow-up of 2 years (unpublished data).

CNS Disease in Pediatric NHL

Children with NHL are considered to have CNS involvement if lymphoma cells are identified in the CSF on a cytocentrifuged preparation or if a cranial nerve palsy is identified in a physical exam [12]. These criteria are similar to those used for children with ALL, although there are some differences. For example, children with Burkitt's lymphoma who have any classic L3 blasts in the CSF would be considered to have CNS disease, even if there were fewer than 5 white cells per microliter in the unspun CSF.

In a single-institution study of 445 children with newly diagnosed NHL, 36 (8%) were found to have CNS disease [13]. Among these, 23 had morphologically identifiable lymphoma cells in the CSF 9 had cranial nerve palsies, and 4 had both features. CNS disease at diagnosis was identified in 13%, 7%, and 1% of Burkitt's, lymphoblastic, and large-cell lymphoma cases, respectively. In a multivariate analysis of various risk factors including CNS disease, stage, and LDH, only stage and serum LDH had prognostic significance. Among patients with Burkitt's lymphoma, a multivariate analysis demonstrated that only serum LDH had independent prognostic significance. This review therefore suggested that CNS disease per se was not an independent risk factor. Other studies have made similar observations14, 15] How-ever, in a retrospective study performed by the CCG [16], it was concluded that among patients with Burkitt's lymphoma, the presence of meningeal disease or CNS pa-renchymal masses at diagnosis was associated with a nominally worse outcome independent of initial bone marrow status and LDH level, although this effect was not statistically significant. In the recently published result of the French LMB-89 study for children with B-cell lymphoma and L3 leukemia, CNS involvement was the only adverse prognostic factor identified among group C patients [17].

The modalities used for both CNS prophylaxis and treatment of overt CNS disease are similar to those used for children with ALL. They include high-dose systemic chemotherapy (e.g., MTX, cytarabine), intrathecal instillation of chemotherapy (e.g., single-agent MTX, triple-agent therapy [MTX, hydrocortisone and cytarabine]), and, less frequently, cranial irradiation. The implementation of these approaches does vary with respect to histologic subtype.

1. Burkitt's lymphoma Most centers currently use systemic high-dose MTX, and cytarabine and intrathecal MTX, hydrocortisone and cytarabine for both CNS prophylaxis and treatment. Two of the most successful treatment regimens are the French LMB-89 [17] regimen and the German BFM-90 protocol18] The LMB-89 regimen incorporated cranial irradiation for those with overt CNS disease at diagnosis; however, most current regimens have excluded cranial irradiation. In fact, the current international collaborative French study has excluded cranial irradiation. In the BFM-90 regimen [18], cranial irradiation was not incorporated; however, an intraventricular access device was used for drug delivery to the spinal fluid In this regard, St. Jude is currently piloting a regimen in which an intraventricular access device is used in the context of LMB-89 directed systemic therapy.

2. Lymphoblastic lymphoma Systemic and intrathecal chemotherapy is used for CNS prophylaxis and treatment. For patients with overt CNS involvement at diagnosis, many centers would consider incorporating cranial irradiation. The role of cranial irradiation for CNS prophylaxis is more controversial, although, as in the case for ALL, there is a distinct trend to move away from it. For example, in the highly effective BFM-90 regimen [19], patients with stage III or IV disease receive 12-Gy cranial irradiation as prophylaxis; however, a subsequent study is determining the safety of its omission. Among patients with CNS-2 status at diagnosis, a current St. Jude study incorporates intensified intrathecal treatment without cranial irradiation.

3. Large-cell lymphoma Determining the optimal approach to CNS prophylaxis and treatment for this group is somewhat problematic, in part because the large-cell lymphomas are a more heterogeneous group. Those with a B-cell immunophenotype are often treated with the same regimen used for Burkitt's lymphoma, as described above. The majority of non-B-cell cases are anaplastic large-cell lymphomas for which a spectrum of therapeutic approaches has been reported. The BFM has had great success using a regimen derived from a Burkitt's lymphoma strategy [20]. In the United States the APO regimen has also been shown to be effective; with this approach, CNS prophylaxis includes single-agent intrathecal MTX [21]. The optimal approach to managing overt CNS disease at diagnosis is controversial, primarily because of the low frequency of this clinical presentation.

4. Primary CNS lymphoma PCNSLs in children are very rare. Also, there is little information with respect to clinical trial data in children to guide treatment. For children who are HIV negative, most pediatric oncologists would consider intensive systemic multiagent chemotherapy featuring agents with good CNS penetration (e.g., high-dose MTX/ cytarabine, dexamethasone); cranial radiotherapy would also be a consideration in some cases. Strategies that have been shown to be effective in adults are often used on an individual basis in children.

5. Patients who are HIV positive and develop a PCNSL are considered to have an extremely poor prognosis In an attempt to provide a novel curative approach, Slobod et al [22], treated 2 HIV-positive patients who presented with primary EBV-positive CNS lymphomas with hydroxyurea. This strategy was used based on in vitro studies of an EBV-positive Burkitt's lymphoma cell line in which expo-sure to hydroxyurea resulted in loss of cytoplasmic EBV episomes and subsequent loss of malignant

phenotype. On the basis of this observation, hydroxyurea was given to HIV-positive patients who had EBV-positive PCNSLs with objective clinical and radiographic responses, suggesting that antiviral approaches may have a role in these malignancies.

CNS Prophylaxis in Adult ALL

The approaches most commonly used for CNS prophylaxis in adults are similar to those that have been used in children: (1) intrathecal therapy (e.g., MTX, cytarabine, hydrocortisone); (2) high dose systemic therapy; and (3) cranial irradiation23. These measures have reduced the rate of CNS relapse to < 5-10% from the > 30% rate reported when no prophylaxis is provided [23]. Gökbuget and Hoelzer reviewed the published data on CNS prophylaxis and found that a combination of all three of the above mentioned approaches resulted in the lowest incidence of isolated or combined CNS relapses (5%, range of 1-12%) [23,24]. Nevertheless, the use of cranial irradiation remains controversial. In the GMALL studies, a higher rate of CNS relapses was observed when cranial irradiation was either omitted or delayed [23,24]. However, in Kantarjian et al's study of the Hyper-CVAD regimen, which features high-dose systemic (MTX and cytarabine) and intrathecal therapy (no cranial irradiation) for CNS prophylaxis, the CNS relapse rate was very low (4%) [26].

III. SECONDARY CENTRAL NERVOUS SYSTEM LYMPHOMA: THE CASE FOR PROPHYLAXIS*

"Secondary" lymphomatous involvement of the CNS was first recognized in the 19th century when Murchison [1] described a tumor encroaching on the foramen magnum infiltrating the dura mater at autopsy. The problem of extradural deposits was recognized later [2-4]. By the middle of the 20th century, secondary central nervous system lymphoma (SCNSL) had been the subject of many manuscripts [5-7], representing as closely as possible the natural history, with Sparling et al6 in 1947 reporting an autopsy incidence of only 1 in 118 cases. As the natural history of the lymphomas has been superseded by the clinical course (induced by partially successful therapy not targeting the CNS), survival of some subtypes has been prolonged. In the 1970s, incidence of SCNSL increased to approximately 10% [8,9].

A clear clinical picture, reflecting the outcome of therapy introduced in the late 1960s and early 1970s, emerges from a number of retrospective analyses from both single institutions and groups [10-22], in which symptomatic disease occurred in 4-29%, depending on histology and extent of disease. The commonest features were headache, cranial nerve palsies, spinal cord compression, and altered mental state and affect These problems usually arose within the context of poorly controlled lymphoma elsewhere, although the nervous system was occasionally an isolated site of recurrence In the large majority of cases, the

---

* Correspondence concerning this section should be addressed to Dr. Andrew Lister, MD 1St. Bartholomew's Hospital, 45 Little Britain, West Smithfield, EC1A 7BE London, United Kingdom.

diagnosis was based on the history and the finding of abnormal cells on a cytospin of CSF There was a strong association with bone marrow involvement; a correlation was also drawn between central nervous system lymphoma (CNSL) and involvement of the testis or paranasal sinuses. Likewise, close correlation was found between histological subtype and probability of the occurrence of CNSL; it was common with lymphoblastic lymphoma and Burkitt's and "Burkitt'slike" lymphoma, to the extent that the next generation of treatment included CNS-targeted therapy.

The Problem Today: Incidence, Risk Factors

Twenty years on, the demonstration of new prognostic factors and the introduction of the International Prognostic Index (IPI) have made it possible to identify more closely those patients for whom SCNSL is a high enough risk to warrant specific prophylactic therapy.

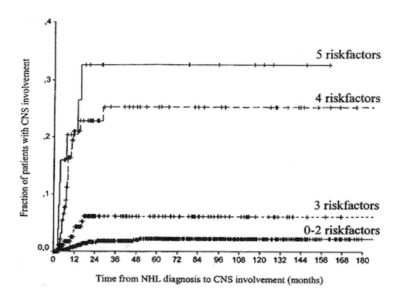

Figure 1. The risk of central nervous system (CNS) recurrence according to the number of risk factors (age, lactate dehydrogenase, albumin, number of extranodal sites, retroperitoneal involvement) in 1220 patients with high-grade non-Hodgkin's lymphoma (NHL). Reprinted with permission from Van Besien K, Ha CS, Murphy S, et al. Risk factors, treatment and outcome of central nervous system recurrence in adults with intermediate-grade and immunoblastic lymphoma. Blood. 1 998;91:1178-1184.

At the M.D. Anderson Hospital [23], 24 of 605 patients with 'large-cell' or immunoblastic lymphoma developed CNS recurrence, with an actuarial risk at 1 year of 4.5%. In 5 cases, the recurrence was concurrent with systemic progression (within 40 days); in 7 others, it preceded systemic progression up to 6 months later. Involvement of more than 1 extranodal site and elevated LDH at presentation were both independently predictive of CNS recurrence on multivariate analysis: if both were present, the actuarial risk was almost 20% at 1 year (Figure1). However, despite intervention with some apparent early benefit, only 1 of 24 patients was alive a year after recurrence.

The Hovon multicenter group [24] reviewed the risk of CNS recurrence in a trial testing the role of high-dose therapy with hematopoietic stem cell rescue, in patients responding "slowly" to 3 cycles of CHOP. One hundred ninety-three of 267 patients entered complete remission CR). Ten patients (5%) developed SCNSL, 8 of them simultaneously with systemic progression. The risk was highest for patients with a high IPI score, but CNS recurrence occurred in all the risk groups. Survival data were not presented.

Zinzani et al. [25] reported an apparently higher incidence of isolated CNS recurrence in an unselected series (excluding Burkitt's and lymphoblastic lymphoma of patients with high-grade NHL (Kiel classification). One hundred seventy-five patients entered CR following therapy with MACOP-B or F MACHOP, both of which include modest doses of MTX intravenously but exclude intrathecal therapy. None had clinical evidence of CNS involvement at presentation. The minimum follow-up at the time of analysis was 3 years. Nine of 175 developed isolated CNS recurrence at a median of 3 months after CR had been documented. Multivariate analysis revealed advanced stage (III and IV) to be the only independent predictor of the likelihood of isolated CNS recurrence, although B symptoms, elevated LDH, and bone marrow involvement were all significant on univariate analysis. The outcome, whether the recurrence was leptomeningeal or parenchymal, was appalling, with all patients having died within 2 years because of CNS progression.

In contrast, Haioun et al., [26] reported the outcome for 1373 patients treated in a GELA study for patients with 'aggressive' NHL; lymphoblastic lymphoma and Burkitt's lymphoma were excluded. CNS prophylaxis included intrathecal MTX with each cycle of systemic chemotherapy and 2 pulses of MTX 2 g/m2 with folinic acid res¬cue. There were 16 isolated CNS recurrences and a further 6 with progression at other sites Initial multivariate analysis confirmed more than one extranodal site and elevated LDH to be independent risk factors predictive of CNS recurrence each with a relative risk (RR) of 5. A further multivariate analysis (in¬corporating IPI score as a unique parameter male gender and B symptoms was subse¬quently performed. IPI score remained the only parameter significantly associated with increased risk (low and low-intermediate ver¬sus high-intermediate and high, RR 7). Once again, the prognosis overall was poor the median survival being 5 months and progres¬sive disease being the predominant cause of death.

A further study from the GELA [27] adds support for the benefit of CNS prophylaxis for this group of patients. Seven hundred eight adults aged 6 1-69 years with at least 1 adverse prognostic factor (IPI) were entered onto a trial comparing a relatively intensive chemotherapy program incorporating both intrathecal MTX and consolidation with systemic MTX, ifosphamide, and cytosine arabino side, with standard CHOP. The CR rates were the same, despite a higher treatment-related mortality in the trial arm; overall survival, however, was better in the latter (P = .002). The frequency of CNS recurrence was also significantly lower in the trial arm (8 versus 25; P = .003). These results have been published in abstract form only to date. They are, however, supported by an earlier analysis from the M.D. Anderson Hospital in which out-come of patients receiving CNS prophylaxis in the form of intrathecal and intravenous MTX was better than that of matched historical controls [16].

The largest body of data defining the extent of the problem at the end of the 20th century comes from the Norwegian Radium Hospital, Oslo [28]. Twenty-five hundred fourteen adults were treated for NHL according to protocols of the day, based on the histological subtype

(Kiel) and the extent of disease at presentation. CNS prophylaxis was given to < 1%, 11%, and 83% of patients with low-grade, high-grade, and Burkitt's or lymphoblastic lymphoma respectively. The analysis addressed only the question of CNS progression, so 30 patients presenting with CNS involvement were excluded.

Overall, the incidence reported for the histological groupings was very similar to that of other series. Less than 3% of those with "low-grade histology" developed SCNSL. Multivariate analysis confirmed B symptoms and involvement of bone marrow and skin as significant prognostic factors, with relative risks of 2.8, 2.8, and 3.7, respectively. The incidence for patients with Burkitt's or lymphoblastic lymphoma was, in contrast, very high, being 24% overall, 78% in those not receiving prophylaxis, and 19% at 5 years in those that did.

As in several other series, the SCNSL rate in 'high-grade' lymphoma was about 4%, the minority having received prophylaxis with intrathecal methotrexate about which no conclusions were drawn. Univariate analysis revealed a multitude of factors, including IPI and ageadjusted IPI, to predict for CNS recurrence Testicular involvement in itself was not significant. Further analysis confirmed 5 factors to have an independent impact on CNS involvement: age, LDH, albumin, retroperitoneal nodes, and number of extranodal sites (Table 3).

Although the hazard ratios are not identical, a general picture may be created by adding the risk factors and correlating increasing numbers with time-to-CNS involvement (Figure 2).

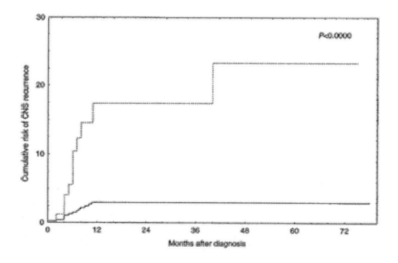

Figure 2. Incidence of central nervous system (CNS) recurrence in patients with increased lactate dehydrogenase (LDH) and involvement of more than 1 extranodal site (n = 93; dotted line) versus all other patients (n = 512; solid line). Reprinted with permission from Hollender A, Kvaloy S, Nome O, et al. Central nervous system involvement following diagnosis of non-Hodgkin's lymphoma: a risk model. Ann Oncol. 2002;1 3:1099-1107.

Table 3. Risk of central nervous system involvement

Variable	Relative Risk	(95% Confidence Interval)	P Value
No. of extranodal sites (>1 vs ≤ 1)	3.0	(1.7-5.4)	< 0.001

Age > 60 vs ≤ 60 yrs	2.8	(1.5-5.4)	0.002
Album in < 3.5 g/L vs > 3.5 g/L	2.5	(1.3-4.6)	0.005
LDH ~ 450 m/L vs < 450 m/L	2.1	(1.0-4.4)	0.049
Retroperitoneal glands:Yes vs no	1.9	(1.0-3.5)	0.037

The Challenge Today

The elimination of CNS involvement with lymphoma is a very important goal, even if it affects only a relatively small proportion of patients, most of whose overall survival will be dictated by uncontrolled disease elsewhere. It is a highly distressing complication, with potentially extensive morbidity which, when established, is very difficult to eliminate. Theoretically, therefore, a prophylactic strategy, analogous to that employed so success-fully for ALL, is indicated. The risk of meningeal involvement in childhood lymphoblastic leukemia has been reduced from more than 50% to very low levels, after painstaking observations, identification of groups with different degrees of risk, and clinical trials to determine the most effective therapy with the lowest acceptable toxicity for each category. Most children now do not develop CNSL, nor do most have excessive long-term morbidity from the therapy.

The first part of the process has been achieved for NHL. Follicular lymphoma and the other lymphocytic lymphomas have been shown to have a less than 1% probability of CNS infiltration, except when transformation has occurred: there can thus be no justification for prophylaxis. Burkitt's lymphoma and lymphoblastic lymphoma (T and B) both have a high incidence of SCNSL: patients therefore now receive both intrathecal chemotherapy and high doses of MTX (and cytosine arabinoside in some instances) or cranial irradiation As a consequence of this strategy, the incidence of CNS involvement is much reduced.

For the remainder of the lymphomas, predominantly diffuse large B-cell lymphoma (DLBCL) and peripheral T-cell lymphoma not otherwise specified (PTCL-NOS), there is still no uniformity of practice, which reflects the complexity of the situation and the fact that the data are open to differing interpretation. However, the picture may be clearer than it was 20 years ago.

There is a recurring theme throughout the recent publications. CNS lymphoma is uncommon but not rare, and when it occurs, devastating. Patients presenting with a high IPI score, particularly reflecting the presence of a high LDH or involvement of more than one extranodal site, are at much higher risk of CNS involvement than the rest. Notwithstanding less impressive statistical proof of their individual significance, patients with testicular and sinus involvement are also at high risk. Some of the data reported above suggest that prophylaxis, with intrathecal therapy and systemic MTX, may reduce the risk.

It could therefore be concluded that all patients with these histological subtypes of lymphoma (DLBCL and PTCL-NOS) should have the CNS evaluated by history, examination, and LP, and that those with a high IPI score, or high LDH and more than one extranodal site, should proceed to prophylaxis. There is a superficial attraction to designing a randomized trial to test the hypothesis. It might be difficult to execute.

If it is difficult to select the appropriate group to receive CNS prophylaxis, it is equally difficult to deter-mine what constitutes the best prophylaxis. Before the introduction of 'high-dose' MTX [29] into combination chemotherapy the only modalities available were intrathecal chemotherapy and irradiation. It may be clear from the above that intrathecal chemotherapy of short duration while probably reducing the risk does not eliminate it. Extrapolation from ALL makes this unsurprising: all treatments relying on intrathecal therapy alone demand much more prolonged treatment. Vital information about the efficacy of systemic MTX and the dose required in the absence of intrathecal therapy will come from the long follow-up analysis of the Southwestern Oncology Group-Eastern Oncology Group (SWOGECOG) study comparing CHOP with M-BACOD, MACOP-B, and PROMACE-CYTABOM, the trial arms including MTX and folinic acid rescue at a dose of 200 mg/m2, 400 mg/m2, and 1500 mg/m2, respectively. It may be anticipated that only the last dose might be effective. Further information accrued from clinical trials incorporating high-dose cytosine arabinoside may be helpful. Given at a dose of 2 g/m2, daily for 5 days, as part of the therapy for adults with ALL, cytosine arabinoside was as effective (compared with historical controls) as cranial irradiation in a small study [30].

It would be foolhardy in the extreme to make didactic statements about optimal CNS prophylaxis: in the light of all that has gone before, recommendations can be made only on the basis of circumstantial evidence and must be seen as part of the best treatment of the disease overall. While none of the third-generation treatments above compared favorably with CHOP, perhaps a treatment for those with a high IPI score incorporating high-dose MTX (> 3 g/m2) and cytosine arabinoside (> 1 g/ m2) might improve outcome. Were that perceived to be the case, a prospective evaluation of the strategy, particularly including long-term toxicity, would be required.

Attention has been focused on reasons in favor of prophylaxis as opposed to against it. Emphasis has been placed on the unpleasant nature of the complication and the difficulty of eliminating it, once established. There are powerful clinical and economic reasons for not giving CNS-directed treatment if it can be avoided. The long-term toxicity of irradiation given for PCNSL has been reviewed above. Even though the long-term sequelae of prophylactic cranial irradiation are less worrying, there are enough data to suggest that high-dose systemic chemotherapy may be as effective and less toxic. It is, however, not without morbidity and mortality which increase with the dose. Conversely, intrathecal therapy is inconvenient and not to be desired, has well-known toxicity, and is costly for both the patient and the hospital. All this must be taken into account in devising the best way to improve therapy, and demonstrate the improvement, while offering the individual the best advice.

For future consideration: What emphasis should be given to the risk at the time of recurrent or progressive lymphoma Do the same risk factors apply? Should more or less attention be directed to the problem? Should it be considered for only those still being treated with curative intent?

REFERENCES

Primary Central Nervous System Lymphoma

[1]   Bailey P. Intracranial sarcomatous tumors of leptomeningeal origin. *Arch. Surg.* 1929;18:1359-1402.

[2]   Rosenblum ML, Levy RM, Bredesen SYT, Wara W, Zeigler JL. Primary central nervous system lymphomas in patients with AIDS. *Ann. Neurol.* 1988;23:S13-S16.

[3]   Welch K, Finkbeiner W, Alpers CE, et al. Autopsy findings in the acquired immune deficiency syndrome. *JAMA.* 1984;252:1 152-1159.

[4]   Sparano JA, Anand K, Desai J, Mitnick RJ, Kalkut GE, Hanau LH. Effect of highly active antiretroviral therapy on the incidence of HIV-associated malignancies at an urban medical center. *J. Acquir. Immune Defic. Syndr.* 1999;21:S18-S22.

[5]   Itoyama T, Sadamori N, Tsutsumi K, et al. Primary central nervous system lymphomas. *Cancer.* 1994;73:455-463.

[6]   Kumanishi T, Zhang S, Ichikawa T, Endo S, Washiyama K. Primary malignant lymphoma of the brain: demonstration of frequent p16 and p15 gene deletions. *Jpn. J. Cancer Res.* 1996;87:691-695.

[7]   Weller M. Glucocorticoid treatment of primary CNS lymphoma. *J. Neurol. Oncol.* 1999;43:237-239.

[8]   DeAngelis LM. Current management of primary central nervous system lymphoma. *Oncology.* 1995;9:63-71.

[9]   Rampen FHJ, van Andel JG, Sizoo W, van Unnik JA. Radiation therapy in non-Hodgkin's lymphomas of the CNS. *Eur. J. Cancer.* 1980;16:177-184.

[10]   Glass J, Gruber ML, Cher L, Hochberg FH. Preirradiation methotrexate chemotherapy of primary central nervous system lymphoma: long-term outcome. *J. Neurosurg.* 1994;81:188-195.

[11]   Gabbai AA, Hochberg FH, Linggood RM, Bashir R, Hotleman K. High-dose methotrexate for non-AIDS primary central nervous system lymphoma. *J. Neurosurg.* 1989;70:190-194.

[12]   Littman P, Wang CC. Reticulum cell sarcoma of the brain. *Cancer.* 1975;35:1412-1420.

[13]   Dahlborg SA, Braziel R, Crossen JR, Tableman M, Petrillo A, Neuwelt EA. Non-AIDS primary CNS lymphoma: first example of a durable response in a primary brain tumor using enhanced chemotherapy delivery without cognitive loss and without radiotherapy. *Cancer J. Sci. Am.* 1996;2:166-174.

[14]   Abrey LE, Yahalom J, DeAngelis LM. Treatment for primary central nervous system lymphoma (PCNSL): the next step. *J. Clin. Oncol.* 2000;18:3144-3150.

[15]   Abrey LE, Moskowitz CH, Mason WP, et al. A phase II study of intensive methotrexate and cytarabine followed by high dose beam chemotherapy with autologous stem cell transplantation (ASCT) in patients with newly diagnosed primary central nervous system lymphoma (PCNSL) [abstract]. *Proc. ASCO.* 2001 ;20:53a.

[16]   Illerhaus G, Marks R, Derigs G, et al. High-dose-chemotherapy with autologous PBSCT and hyperfractionated radiotherapy as first-line treatment for primary CNS lymphoma (PCNSL) – Update of a multicenter Phase II study. *Onkologie.* 200 1;54 (Suppl 6): 14.

[17]   Forsyth PA, Yahalom J, DeAngelis LM. Combined-modality therapy in the treatment of primary central nervous system lymphoma in AIDS. *Neurology*. 1994;44:1473-1479.

[18]   Chamberlain MC, Kormanik PA. AIDS-related central nervous system lymphomas. *J Neurol Oncol*. 1999;43:269-276.

[19]   Jacomet C, Girard P-M, Lebrette M-G, Farese VL, Monfort L, Rozenbaum W. Intravenous methotrexate for primary central nervous system non-Hodgkin's lymphoma in AIDS. *AIDS*. 1997;1 1:1725-1730.

[20]   Corn BW, Trock BJ, Curran WJ Jr. Management of primary central nervous system lymphoma for the patient with acquired immunodeficiency syndrome. *Cancer*. 1995;76(2):163-166.

[21]   McGowan JP, Shah S. Long term remission of AIDS-related primary central nervous system lymphoma associated with highly active antiretroviral therapy. *AIDS*. 1998;12:952-953.

[22]   Baumann MA, Ritch PS, Hande KR, Williams GA, Topping TM, Anderson T. Treatment of intraocular lymphoma with high-dose Ara-C. *Cancer*. 1986;57:1273-1275.

[23]   Sandor V, Stark-Vancs V, Pearson D, et al. Phase II trial of chemotherapy alone for primary CNS and intraocular lymphoma. *J. Clin. Oncol*. 1998;16(9):3000-3006.

[24]   Strauchen JA, Dalton J, Friedman AH. Chemotherapy in the management of intraocular lymphoma. *Cancer*. 1989;63:1918-1921.

[25]   Peterson K, Gordon KB, Heinemann MH, DeAngelis LM. The clinical spectrum of ocular lymphoma. *Cancer*. 1993;72:843-849.

[26]   Valluri S, Moorthy RS, Khan A, Rao NA. Combination treatment of intraocular lymphoma. *Retina*. 1995;15:125-129.

[27]   Soussain C, Suzan F, Hoang-Xuan K, et al. Results of intensive chemotherapy followed by hematopoietic stem-cell rescue in 22 patients with refractory or recurrent primary CNS lymphoma or intraocular lymphoma. *J. Clin. Oncol*. 2001;19:742-9.

[28]   Abrey LE, Yahalom J, DeAngelis LM. Relapse and late neurotoxicity in primary central nervous system lymphoma [abstract]. *Neurology*. 1997;48:A18.

[29]   Abrey LE, Thiessen B, DeAngelis LM. Treatment related neurotoxicity in primary CNS lymphoma. *Society for Neuro-Oncology Annual Meeting*. 1997. [abstract]

[30]   Thiessen B, DeAngelis LM. Hydrocephalus in radiation leukoencephalopathy: results of ventriculoperitoneal shunting. *Arch. Neurol*. 1998;55:705-710.

[31]   DeAngelis LM, Yahalom J, Thaler HT, Kher U. Combined modality therapy for primary CNS lymphoma. *J Clin Oncol*. 1992;10:635-643.

[32]   Abrey LE, DeAngelis LM, Yahalom J. Long-term survival in primary CNS lymphoma. *J. Clin. Oncol*. 1998;16:859-863.

[33]   Duffey P, Chari G, Cartlidge NEF, Shaw PJ. Progressive deterioration of intellect and motor function occurring several decades after cranial irradiation. *Arch. Neurol*. 1996;53:814-818.

[34]   McGuirt WF, Feehs RS, Strickland JL, McKinney WM. Irradiation induced atherosclerosis: a factor in therapeutic planning. *Ann. Otol. Rhinol. Laryngol*. 1992;101:222-228.

[35]   McLaughlin P, Velasquez WS, Redman JR, et al. Chemotherapy with dexamethasone, high-dose cytarabine, and cisplatin for parenchymal brain lymphoma. *J. Natl. Cancer Inst.* 1988;80(17):1408-1412.

[36]   Chamberlain MC, Levin VA. Adjuvant chemotherapy for primary lymphoma of the central nervous system. *Arch. Neurol.* 1990;47:1113-1116.

[37]   McAllister LD, Doolittle ND, Guastadisegni PE, et al. Cognitive outcomes and long-term follow-up after enhanced chemotherapy delivery for primary CNS lymphoma. *Neurosurgery.* In press.

[38]   Nelson DF, Martz KL, Bonner H, et al. Non-Hodgkin's lymphoma of the brain: can high-dose, large-volume radiation therapy improve survival? Report on a prospective trial by the Radiation Therapy Oncology Group (RTOG): RTOG:8315. *Int. J. Radiat. Oncol. Biol. Phys.* 1992;23:9-17.

[39]   Cheng AL, Yeh KH, Uen WC, Hung RL, Liu MY, Wang CH. Systemic chemotherapy alone for patients with non-acquired immunodeficiency syndrome-related central nervous system lymphoma: a pilot study of the BOMES protocol. *Cancer.* 1998;82:1946-1951.

[40]   Cher L, Glass J, Harsh GR, Hochberg FH. Therapy of primary CNS lymphoma with methotrexate-based chemotherapy and deferred radiotherapy: preliminary results. *Neurology.* 1996;46: 1757-1759.

[41]   DeAngelis LM, Seiferheld W, Schold SC, Fisher B, Schultz CJ. Combined modality treatment of primary central nervous system lymphoma (PCNSL) [abstract]. *Proc. ASCO.* 1999;18:140a.

Lymphomatous Meningitis: The Acute Lymphoblastic Leukemia Model

[1]   Pinkel D, Woo S. Prevention and treatment of meningeal leukemia in children. *Blood.* 1994;84:355-366.

[2]   Mahmoud HH, Rivera GK, Hancock ML, et al. Low leukocyte counts with blast cells in cerebrospinal fluid of children with newly diagnosed acute lymphoblastic leukemia. *N. Engl. J. Med.* 1993;329:314-319.

[3]   Lauer S, Shuster J, Kirchner P, et al. Prognostic significance of cerebrospinal fluid (CSF) lymphoblasts (LB) at diagnosis (dx) in children with acute lymphoblastic leukemia (ALL). *Proc. ASCO.* 1994;13:317.

[4]   Gilchrist GS, Tubergen DG, Sather HN, et al. Low numbers of CSF blasts at diagnosis do not predict for the development of CNS leukemia in children with intermediate-risk acute lymphoblastic leukemia: a children's cancer group report. *J. Clin. Oncol.* 1994;12:2594-2600.

[5]   van den Berg H, Vet R, den Ouden E, Behrendt H. Significance of lymphoblasts in cerebrospinal fluid in newly diagnosed pediatric acute lymphoblastic malignancies with bone marrow involvement: possible benefit of dexamethasone. *Med. Pediatr. Oncol.* 1995;25:22-7.

[6]   Gajjar A, Harrison PL, Sandlund JT, et al. Traumatic lumbar puncture at diagnosis adversely affects outcome in childhood acute lymphoblastic leukemia. *Blood.* 2000;96:3381-3384.

[7]   Pui C-H, Mahmoud HH, Rivera GK, et al. Early intensification of intrathecal chemotherapy virtually eliminates central nervous system relapse in children with acute lymphoblastic leukemia. *Blood.* 1998;92:41 1-415.

[8]   Schrappe M, Reiter A, Zimmermann M, et al. Long-term results of four consecutive trials in childhood ALL performed by the ALL-BFM study group from 1981 to 1995. *Leukemia.* 2000;14:2205-2222.

[9]   Manera R, Ramirez I, Mullins J, Pinkel D. Pilot studies of speciesspecific chemotherapy of childhood acute lymphoblastic leukemia using genotype and immunophenotype. *Leukemia.* 2000; 14: 1354-1361.

[10]   Vilmer E, Suciu S, Ferster A, et al. Long-term results of three randomized trials (58831, 58832, 58881) in childhood acute lymphoblastic leukemia: a CLCG-EORTC report. *Leukemia.* 2000;14:2257-2266.

[11]   Kamps WA, Bökkerink JPM, Hakvoort-Cammel FGAJ, et al. BFM-oriented treatment for children with acute lymphoblastic leukemia without cranial irradiation and treatment reduction for standard risk patients: results of DCLSG protocol ALL-8 (1991-1996). *Leukemia.* 2002;16:1099-1111.

[12]   Murphy SB, Fairclough DL, Hutchison RE, et al. Non-Hodgkin's lymphomas of childhood: an analysis of the histology, staging, and response to treatment of 338 cases at a single institution. *J Clin Oncol.* 1989;7:186-193.

[13]   Sandlund JT, Murphy SB, Santana VM, et al. CNS involvement in children with newly diagnosed non-Hodgkin's lymphoma. *J. Clin. Oncol.* 2000;18:3018-24.

[14]   Haddy TB, Adde MA, Magrath IT. CNS involvement in small noncleaved-cell lymphoma: is CNS disease per se a poor prognostic sign? *J. Clin. Oncol.* 1991;9:1973-1982.

[15]   Bowman WP, Shuster JJ, Cook B, et al. Improved survival for children with B-cell acute lymphoblastic leukemia and stage IV small noncleaved-cell lymphoma: a pediatric oncology group study. *J. Clin. Oncol.* 1996;14:1252-1261.

[16]   Gururangan S, Sposto R, Cairo MS, Meadows AT, Finlay JL. Outcome of CNS disease at diagnosis in disseminated small noncleaved-cell lymphoma and B-cell leukemia: a children's cancer group study. *J. Clin. Oncol.* 2000;18:2017-2025.

[17]   Patte C, Auperin A, Michon J, et al. The Société Française d'Oncologie Pédiatrique LMB89 protocol: highly effective multiagent chemotherapy tailored to the tumor burden and initial response in 561 unselected children with B-cell lymphomas and L3 leukemia. *Blood.* 2001;97:337-339.

[18]   Reiter A, Schrappe M, Tiemann M, et al. Improved treatment results in childhood B-cell neoplasms with tailored intensification of therapy: a report of the Berlin-Frankfurt-Münster group trial NHL-BFM 90. *Blood.* 1999;94:3294-3306.

[19]   Reiter A, Schrappe M, Ludwig W-D, et al. Intensive ALL-type therapy without local radiotherapy provides a 90% event-free survival for children with T-cell lymphoblastic lymphoma: a BFM Group report. *Blood.* 2000;95:416-421.

[20] Seidemann K, Tiemann M, Schrappe M, et al. Short-pulse B-non-Hodgkin lymphoma-type chemotherapy is efficacious treatment for pediatric anaplastic large cell lymphoma: a report of the Berlin-Frankfurt-Münster Group Trial NHL-BFM 90. *Blood*. 2001;97:3699-3706.

[21] Laver JH, Mahmoud H, Pick TE, et al. Results of a randomized phase III trial in children and adolescents with advanced stage diffuse large cell non-Hodgkin's lymphoma: a pediatric oncology group study. *Leukemia Lymphoma*. 2001;42:399-405.

[22] Slobod KS, Taylor GH, Sandlund JT, Furth P, Helton KJ, Sixbey JW. Epstein-Barr virus-targeted therapy for AIDS-related primary lymphoma of the central nervous system. *Lancet*. 2000;56: 1493-1494.

[23] Gökbuget N, Hoelzer D. Recent approaches in acute lymphoblastic leukemia in adults. *Rev. Clin. Exp. Hematol*. 2002;6:1 14-40.

[24] Gökbuget N, Hoelzer D. Meingeosis leukaemica in adult acute lymphoblastic leukaemia. *J. Neuro-Oncol*. 1998;38:167-180.

[25] Gökbuget N, Aguion-Freire E, Diedrich H, et al. Characteristics and outcome of CNS relapse in patients with adult acute lymphoblastic leukemia (ALL). Abstract #1287

[26] Kantarjian HM, O'Brien S, Smith TL, et al. Results of treatment with hyper-CVAD, a dose-intensive regimen, in adult acute lympocytic Leukemia. *J. Clin. Oncol*. 2000;18:547-561.

Secondary Central Nervous System Lymphoma: The Case for Prophylaxis

[1] Murchison C. Case of 'lymphadenoma' of the lymphatic system, liver, lungs, heart and dura mater. *Trans Pathol. Soc. Lond*. 1870;21:372-389.

[2] Welch JE. Tumor of the neck showing unusual histologic features. *Proc. NY Pathol. Soc*. 1910;10:161.

[3] Guillan, Alajouanine, Perisson. Lymphosarcoma extradural metastique ayant determine une compression medullaire d'apparence primitive, d'evolution rapidement progressive; laminectomie; extirpation et radiotherapie; guerison. *Bull. Mem. Soc. Med. Hop. Paris*. 1925;49:1057.

[4] Verda DJ. Malignant lymphomas of the spinal epidural space. *Surg. Clin. N. Am*. 1944;24:1228-1244.

[5] Davison C, Michaels JJ. Lymphosarcoma with involvement of the central nervous system. *Arch. Intern. Med*. 1930;45:908-925.

[6] Sparling HJ, Adams RD, Parker F. Involvement of the central nervous system by malignant lymphoma. *Medicine*. 1947;26:285-332.

[7] Williams HM, Diamond DH, Craver LF, Parsons H. Neurological complications of lymphomas and leukaemias. Springfield, IL: Charles C. Thomas; 1959.

[8] Griffin JW, Thompson RW, Mitchinson MJ, de Kiewiet JC, Welland FH. Lymphomatous leptomeningitis. *Am. J. Med*. 1971;51:200-208.

[9]   Law IP, Dick FR, Blom J, Bergevin PR. Involvement of the central nervous system in non-Hodgkin's lymphoma. *Cancer*. 1975;36:225-231.

[10] Gendlemon S, Rizzo F, Moues RJ. Central nervous system complications of leukemic conversion of the lymphomas. *Cancer*. 1969;24:676-682.

[11] Olson ME, Chernik NL, Posner JB. Infiltration of the leptomeninges by systemic cancer: a clinical and pathological study. *Arch. Neurol.* 1974;30:122.

[12] Herman TS, Hammond N, Jones SE, Butler JJ, Byrne GE, McKelvey EM. Involvement of the central nervous system by non-Hodgkin's lymphoma. *Cancer*. 1979;43:390-397.

[13] Young RC, Howser JM, Fisher RI, Jaffe E, DeVita VT. Central nervous system complications of non-Hodgkin's lymphoma. *Am. J. Med.* 1979;68:435-443.

[14] Levitt LJ, Dawson DM, Rosenthal DS, Moloney WC. CNS involvement in the non Hodgkin's lymphomas. *Cancer*. 1980;45:545-552.

[15] Mackintosh FR, Colby TV, Podolsky WJ, et al. Central nervous system involvement in non-Hodgkin's lymphoma: an analysis of 105 cases. *Cancer*. 1982;49:586-595.

[16] Perez-Soler R, Smith TL, Cabanillas F. Central nervous system prophylaxis with combined intravenous and intrathecal methotrexate in diffuse lymphoma of aggressive histologic type. *Cancer*. 1986;57:971-977.

[17] Recht L, Strauss DJ, Cirrincione C, Thaler HT, Posner JB. Central nervous system metastases from non-Hodgkin's lymphoma: treatment and prophylaxis. *Am. J. Med.* 1988;84:425-435.

[18] Liang R, Chiu E, Loke SL. Secondary central nervous system involvement by non Hodgkin's lymphoma: the risk factors. *Hematol Oncol*. 1990;8:141-145.

[19] Bashir RM, Bierman PJ, Vose JM, Weisenburger DD, Armitage OJ. Central nervous system involvement in patients with diffuse aggressive non-Hodgkin's lymphoma. *Am. J. Clin. Oncol.* 1991;14:478-482.

[20] Bunn PA, Schein PS, Banks PM, de Vita VT. Central nervous system complications in patients with diffuse histiocytic and undifferentiated lymphoma. *Blood*. 1976;47:3-10.

[21] Litam JP, Cabanillas F, Smith TL, Bodey GP, Freireich EJ. Central nervous system relapse in malignant lymphomas: risk factors and implications for prophylaxis. *Blood*. 1979;54:1249-1257.

[22] Bollen ELEM, Brouwer RE, Hamers S, et al. Central nervous system relapse in non-Hodgkin's lymphoma. *Arch. Neurol.* 1997;54:854-859.

[23] Van Besien K, Ha CS, Murphy S, et al. Risk factors, treatment and outcome of central nervous system recurrence in adults with intermediate-grade and immunoblastic lymphoma. *Blood*. 1998;91:1178-1184.

[24] Bos GMJ, van Putten WLJ, van der Holt B, van den Bent M, Verdonck LF, Hagenbeek A. For which patients with aggressive non-Hodgkin's lymphoma is prophylaxis for central nervous system disease mandatory? *Ann. Oncol.* 1998;9:191-194.

[25] Zinzani PL, Magagnoli M, Frezza G, et al. Isolated central nervous system relapse in aggressive non-Hodgkin's lymphoma: the Bologna experience. *Leuk. Lymphoma*. 1999;32:571-576.

[26]   Haioun C, Besson C, Lepage E, et al. Incidence and risk factors of central nervous system relapse in histologically aggressive non-Hodgkin's lymphoma uniformly treated and receiving intrathecal central nervous system prophylaxis: a GELA study on 974 patients. *Ann. Oncol.* 2000;11:685-690.

[27]   Tilly H, Coiffier B, Casasnovas O, et al. Survival advantage of ACVBP regimen over standard CHOP in the treatment of advanced aggressive non-Hodgkin's lymphoma (NHL). The LNH 93-5 study [abstract]. *Ann. Oncol.* 2002;13(suppl 2):082a.

[28]   Hollender A, Kvaloy S, Nome O, Skovlund E, Lote K, Holte H. Central nervous system involvement following diagnosis of non-Hodgkin's lymphoma: a risk model. *Ann. Oncol.* 2002;13:1099-1 107.

[29]   Canellos GP, Skarin AT, Ervin T, Weinstein H. A chemotherapeutic approach to CNS lymphoma and leukaemia by the systemic administration of high doses of antimetabolites. In: Whitehouse JMA, Kay HEM, eds. *CNS Complications of Malignant Disease*. Macmillan Press; 1979:142-148.

[30]   Rohatiner AZS, Bassan R, Battista R, et al. High dose cytosine arabinoside in the initial treatment of adults with acute lymphoblastic leukaemia. *Br. J. Cancer.* 1990;62:454.

In: Encyclopedia of Stem Cell Research (2 Volume Set)   ISBN: 978-1-61761-835-2
Editor: Alexander L. Greene   © 2012 Nova Science Publishers, Inc.

Chapter XXXV

BACKGROUND AND LEGAL ISSUES RELATED TO STEM CELL RESEARCH*

Jon O. Shimabukuro

ABSTRACT

In August 2001, President Bush announced that federal funds, with certain restrictions, may be used to conduct research on human embryonic stem cells. Federal research is limited to "the more than 60" existing stem cell lines that were derived (1) with the informed consent of the donors; (2) from excess embryos created solely for reproductive purposes; and (3) without any financial inducements to the donors. No federal funds may be used for the derivation or use of stem cell lines derived from newly destroyed embryos; the creation of any human embryos for research purposes; or cloning of human embryos for any purposes. Legislation that responds to the limitations imposed by the President's 2001 announcement has been introduced in the last two Congresses. During the 110th Congress, at least 10 bills, including the Stem Cell Research Enhancement Act of 2007 (H.R. 3/S. 5/S. 997), have been introduced.

HUMAN EMBRYONIC STEM CELLS

Human embryonic stem cells are "master cells," able to develop into almost any cell in the human body. Building on earlier stem cell research, in 1998, researchers at the University of Wisconsin isolated cells from the inner cell mass of the early human embryo, called the blastocyst, and developed the first human embryonic stem cell lines [1]. Research has focused on the potential that these cells can offer to treat or mitigate diseases and conditions and to generate replacement tissues for disfunctioning cells or organs [2]. Research efforts have focused on spinal cord injury, multiple sclerosis, Parkinson's disease, Alzheimer's disease,

---

* Excerpted from CRS Report RS21044, dated June 21, 2007.

diabetes, and other diseases or conditions. Scientists hope to use specialized cells to replace dysfunctional cells in the brain, spinal cord, pancreas, and other organs [3]. The sources for stem cells include one week old embryos (blastocysts) created via in vitro fertilization (IVF) to treat infertility; five to nine week old embryos or fetuses obtained through elective abortion; embryos created through IVF for research purposes; embryos created through cloning or somatic cell nuclear transfer; and adult tissues (umbilical cord blood, bone marrow). Controversy surrounds the derivation of stem cells from human embryos and fetuses. In order to derive or extract the stem cells found within the embryo, the embryo is destroyed in the removal process. The earliest embryonic stem cells are called totipotent cells, which means they can develop into an entire organism, producing both the embryo and tissues required to support it in the uterus. At a later stage of development, pluripotent embryonic stem cells exist and can develop into almost any type of cell in the body. These stem cells cannot form the supporting tissues, as seen with totipotent cells [4]. Human embryonic stem cells found in the early stage embryo are believed to have a greater ability to become different types of body cells and have more uses than adult stem cells.

BACKGROUND AND RECENT PRESIDENTIAL AND CONGRESSIONAL ACTION

Executive Action

When President Bush took office in January 2001, he announced that he would conduct a review of the stem cell research issue and ordered the Department of Health and Human Services (HHS) to review the National Institutes of Health's (NIH) guidelines issued by the former administration. During the review period, NIH suspended its review of applications from researchers seeking federal funds to perform human embryonic stem cell research. On August 9, 2001, President Bush announced that federal funds would be available to support limited human embryonic stem cell research. The new policy provides that federal funds may be used for research on "the more than 60" existing stem cell lines that have already been derived or were already in existence as of the date of the announcement [5]. In identifying the stem cell lines as being eligible for federal funding, the President said these embryos, from which the existing stem cell lines were created, had been destroyed previously and could not develop as human beings.

Under the new policy, federal agencies, primarily NIH, will consider applications for funding if certain standards or eligibility criteria are met. The White House fact sheet setting forth the President's policy states: federal funds will only be used for research on existing stem cell lines that were derived (1) with the informed consent of the donors; (2) from excess embryos created solely for reproductive purposes; and (3) without any financial inducements to the donors [6]. The President directed NIH to examine the derivation of all existing stem cell lines and create a registry of those lines. Pursuant to this new policy, no federal funds will be used for: (1) the derivation or use of stem cell lines derived from newly destroyed embryos; (2) the creation of any human embryos for research purposes; or (3) cloning of human embryos for any purposes. The new policy replaces previously issued stem cell guidelines and policies. The policy also requires the creation of the President's Council on Bioethics to study stem cells and embryo research as well as other issues. NIH has listed entities that have developed stem cells lines that meet the President's criteria and are eligible for federal funding (the Human Embryonic Stem Cell Registry). The President also stated that in FY2001, the government will spend $250 million on research involving stem cells from other sources (e.g., umbilical cord, placenta, adult, and animal tissues).

Background and Congressional Activity

Prior to President Bush's stem cell announcement, and over the past years, federal law has prohibited HHS from funding human *embryo* research. No federal funds have been used to support research on stem cells derived from human embryos. Research in this area has been done through private funding. Subsequent to several phases of action, in December 1994, President Clinton, through an executive directive, prohibited federal funding on research to support the creation of human embryos for research purposes and directed NIH not to allocate resources for such research [7]. The order banning funding for such research was followed in 1996 by a legislative ban that was enacted in NIH's funding measure [8]. Congress has passed a similar ban annually since that time. The original congressional ban stated that federally appropriated funds could not be used for the creation of a human embryo or embryos for research purposes or for research in which a human embryo or embryos are destroyed, discarded, or knowingly subjected to risk of injury or death greater than that allowed for research on fetuses in utero under 45 C.F.R. § 46.208(a)(2) and 42 U.S.C. § 289g(b). The ban defined "human embryo or embryos" to include any organism, not protected as a human subject under 45 C.F.R. § 46 (Human Subject Protection regulations) that is derived by fertilization, parthenogenesis, cloning, or any other means from one or more human gametes (sperm or egg.) The rider language has not changed significantly over the years. In the subsequent fiscal years after FY1996, the rider was enacted in Title V (General Provisions) of the Labor, HHS and Education appropriations acts. The prohibition does not ban fetal tissue research, although other restrictions apply.

Advances in medical science proceeded and in 1998 critical developments were recognized by scientists at the University of Wisconsin. These researchers were able to isolate human embryonic stem cells and coax them to grow into specialized cells. In light of the presidential and legislative bans, NIH requested a legal opinion from the General Counsel of HHS on whether federal funds could be used to support research on human stem cells derived from embryos or fetal tissue. HHS' General Counsel, Harriet Rabb, concluded that then-current law prohibiting the use of HHS appropriated funds for human embryo research would not apply to research using stem cells "because such cells are not a human embryo within the statutory definition." [9] General Counsel Rabb determined that the statutory ban on human embryo research defines embryo as an "organism" that when implanted in the uterus is capable of becoming a human being. The opinion stated that pluripotent stem cells are not and cannot develop into an organism, as defined in the statute. HHS concluded that NIH could fund research that uses stem cells derived from the embryo by private funds. But, because of the language in the rider, NIH could not fund research that, with federal funds, derived the stem cells from embryos.

Some members of Congress strongly opposed HHS' view and believed that the legislative ban that would continue through FY2001, covered and prohibited such research. Others supported both the administration's position and the funding of such research. In response to those opposed to the HHS opinion, and the subsequently published NIH guidelines, Secretary Shalala stated in a letter that the definition of embryo used in the HHS legal opinion relied on the definition of embryo in the statute and that the ban applied only to research in which human embryos are discarded or destroyed but not to research preceding or following "on such projects."[10] The letter stated: "Moreover ... there is nothing in the legislative history to suggest that the provision was intended to prohibit funding for research in which embryos - organisms - are not involved."

After the HHS legal opinion, and despite expressions of congressional opposition, NIH indicated that it would fund research on pluripotent stem cells derived from human embryos and fetal tissue once guidelines were issued and an oversight committee was established. Draft guidelines were published in the *Federal Register* in December 1999 and final guidelines were issued in August 2000 [11]. The guidelines provided that studies utilizing pluripotent stem cells derived from human embryos may be conducted using NIH funds only if the cells were derived, without federal funds, from human embryos that were created for the purposes of fertility treatment and were in excess of the clinical need of the individuals seeking such treatment. Based upon HHS's interpretation, funds could not be used to extract or derive the stem cells from the embryo, thereby destroying the embryo. NIH initiated the applications process but ultimately funding was not granted to the applications. The prior administration's process was then overtaken by events and the new policy was set.

Congressional interest in stem cell research has continued steadily since the President's announcement in 2001. During the 109th Congress, at least seven bills involving stem cell research were introduced. Two of the measures were enacted. On December 20, 2005, the President signed H.R. 2520, the Stem Cell Therapeutic and Research Act of 2005, a measure that provides for the collection and maintenance of human cord blood stem cells for the treatment of patients and for research (P.L. 109-129).

S. 3504, the Fetus Farming Prohibition Act of 2006, was signed by the President on July 19, 2006 (P.L. 109-242). The act amends the Public Health Service Act (PHSA) to make it unlawful for any person or entity involved or engaged in interstate commerce to either solicit or knowingly acquire, receive, or accept a donation of human fetal tissue knowing that a human pregnancy was deliberately initiated to provide such tissue, or knowingly acquire, receive, or accept tissue or cells obtained from a human embryo or fetus that was gestated in the uterus of a nonhuman animal.

A third measure, H.R. 810, the Stem Cell Research Enhancement Act of 2005, was passed by Congress, but vetoed by the President on July 19, 2006 [12]. H.R. 810 would have amended the PHSA to direct the Secretary of HHS to conduct and support research that utilizes human embryonic stem cells without regard to the date on which the stem cells were derived from a human embryo. To be eligible for use in research conducted or supported by the Secretary, the stem cells would have been required to meet certain conditions. For example, only stem cells derived from human embryos that were donated from in vitro fertilization clinics, were created for the purposes of fertility treatment, and were in excess of the clinical need of the individuals seeking such treatment would have been eligible for use.

In his veto message, the President expressed a need to balance scientific progress with the country's ethical responsibilities:

> H.R. 810 would overturn my Administration's balanced policy on embryonic stem cell research. If this bill were to become law, American taxpayers for the first time in our history would be compelled to fund the deliberate destruction of human embryos. Crossing this line would be a grave mistake and would needlessly encourage a conflict between science and ethics that can only do damage to both and harm our Nation as a whole [13].
> A vote to override the veto was unsuccessful [14].

Finally, S. 2754, the Alternative Pluripotent Stem Cell Therapies Enhancement Act, would have amended the PHSA to direct the Secretary of HHS to conduct and support basic and applied research to develop techniques for the isolation, derivation, production, or testing of stem cells that are not derived from a human embryo. S. 2754 indicated that the research contemplated by the measure would not have affected any policy, guideline, or regulation regarding embryonic stem cell research or human cloning by somatic cell nuclear transfer. S. 2754 was passed by the Senate on July 18, 2006 by a vote 100-0. The House did not vote on the measure.

In the 110th Congress, at least 10 bills involving stem cell research have been introduced [15]. H.R. 3, the Stem Cell Research Enhancement Act of 2007, a measure that is identical in language to the Stem Cell Research Enhancement Act of 2005, was passed by the House on January 11, 2007, by a vote of 253-174. A companion measure, S. 5, was passed by the Senate on April 11, 2007, by a vote of 63-34. S. 5 includes the language of H.R. 3, as well as the language of the Alternative Pluripotent Stem Cell Therapies Enhancement Act from the 109th Congress. On June 7, 2007, the House passed S. 5 by a vote of 247-176.

On June 20, 2007, the President vetoed S. 5. The President observed: "S. 5, like the bill I vetoed last year, would overturn today's carefully balanced policy on stem cell research. Compelling American taxpayers to support the deliberate destruction of human embryos would be a grave mistake."[16] Leaders of the Senate Appropriations Subcommittee on Labor, Health and Human Services, and Education, and Related Agencies have indicated that they will include a provision in the FY2008 Labor-HHS-Education appropriations measure to allow federal funding of a limited number of embryonic stem cells lines above the number at which Bush halted research in 2001 [17].

REFERENCES

[1]   Nat'l Inst. of Health, U.S. Dep't of Health and Hum. Services, *Stem Cells: Scientific Progress and Future Research Directions* 4 (2001), *available at* [*http://stemcells.nih. gov/info/scireport/ 2001report.htm*].

[2]   For additional information on stem cell research, see CRS Report RL33540, *Stem Cell Research: Federal Research Funding and Oversight*, by Judith A. Johnson and Erin D. Williams.

[3]   *Id.* at 4-6.

[4]   Generally, for human development, the term embryo is used for the first eight weeks after fertilization and the term fetus for the 9th week through birth. HHS regulations define fetus as "the product of conception from the time of implantation." 45 C.F.R. § 46.203.

[5]   President's Address to the Nation on Stem Cell Research From Crawford, Texas, 37 Weekly Comp. Pres. Doc. 1149 (August 9, 2001). The number of available embryonic stem cell lines is now understood to be much lower than 60. Although 78 cell lines are listed on the Human Embryonic Stem Cell Registry as eligible for use in federal research, only 22 lines are identified as being available. For additional information on the Human Embryonic Stem Cell Registry, see CRS Report RL33540, *Stem Cell Research: Federal Research Funding and Oversight*, by Judith A. Johnson and Erin D. Williams.

[6]   Id.

[7]   Statement on Federal Funding of Research on Human Embryos, 30 Weekly Comp. Pres. Doc. 2459 (December 2, 1994).

[8]   Balanced Budget Downpayment Act, 1996, P.L. 104-99, § 128, 110 Stat. 26, 34 (1996).

[9]   Letter from HHS Gen. Counsel Harriet Rabb to Harold Varmus, Director, NIH, January 15, 1999.

[10]   Letter from Secretary Shalala to the Honorable Jay Dickey, February 23, 1999.

[11]   64 Fed. Reg.67576 (1999); 65 Fed. Reg. 51,976 (2000), respectively.

[12]   A companion bill, S. 471, was introduced by Sen. Arlen Specter on February 28, 2005.

[13]   152 Cong. Rec. H5435 (daily ed. July 19, 2006) (Stem Cell Research Enhancement Act of 2005 — Veto Message From the President of the United States (H. Doc. No. 109-127)).

[14]   *See* 152 Cong. Rec. H5450 (daily ed. July 19, 2006) (the vote was 235-193).

[15]   For additional discussion of stem cell research legislation in the 110th Congress, see CRS Report RL33540, *supra* note 2.

[16]   Message to the Senate of the United States (June 20, 2007), *available at* [*http://www.whitehouse.gov/news/releases/2007/06/print/20070620-5.html*].

[17]   *See* Anna Edney, *Harkin, Specter to Add Stem-Cell Provision to Spending Bill*, Cong. Daily AM (June 21, 2007), *at* [http://nationaljournal.com/pubs/congressdaily/].

In: Encyclopedia of Stem Cell Research (2 Volume Set)   ISBN: 978-1-61761-835-2
Editor: Alexander L. Greene   © 2012 Nova Science Publishers, Inc.

Chapter XXXVI

BONE MARROW-DERIVED STEM CELLS: HOMING AND RESCUE OF INJURY IN THE LUNG

Donatella Piro,[1] Silvia Lepore,[1]
*Angela Bruna Maffione[1] and Massimo Conese[*1,2]*

[1] Department of Biomedical Sciences, University of Foggia, Foggia, Italy
[2] Institute for the Experimental Treatment of Cystic Fibrosis,
H.S. Raffaele Scientific Institute, Milano, Italy

Bone marrow contains hematopoietic stem cells (HSCs), which differentiate into every type of mature blood cells, endothelial cell progenitors (EPCs), and marrow stromal cells, also called mesenchymal stem cells (MSCs), which can differentiate into mature cells of multiple mesenchymal tissues including fat, bone and cartilage. Moreover, a bone marrow-borne circulating cell with fibroblast-like features, termed fibrocyte, has been described. Numerous studies have demonstrated the ability of HSCs, MSCs, EPCs and fibrocytes to home to the lung and differentiate into a variety of cells types, including epithelial, endothelial, fibroblasts and myofibroblast cells. Injury is an essential catalyst that enables the production of lung cells from bone marrow; however, the degree of organ injury, the mode of injury used, and characteristics of the donor marrow cells may be among the multitude of factors that influence the extent of tissue replacement and the phenotype of newly produced cells. Moreover, engraftment of bone marrow-derived stem cells into the airways is a very inefficient process. Studies on the molecular network (i.e., chemokine/chemokine receptor axis) governing the homing of circulating stem cells to the airways will reveal the mechanism(s) by which stem cells home to the airways. Better knowledge of the local stem cells in the respiratory tract will aid to understand the 'plasticity' of bone marrow-derived stem cells. Some lung disease treatable by stem cell transplantation, like for example cystic

* Corresponding author: Massimo Conese; Department of Biomedical Sciences; University of Foggia; 71100 Foggia; Italy; E-mail: m.conese@unifg.it

fibrosis, will need gene transfer into stem cells, with possible immunological reactions to gene products inserted to replace a deficiency or to down-regulate a hyper-expressed protein. An intensive research effort is therefore necessary before acute and chronic lung diseases can benefit from this stem cell approach.

INTRODUCTION

In many airway diseases, such as asthma, bronchiolitis obliterans, chronic obstructive pulmonary disease, and cystic fibrosis, the pseudostratified airway surface epithelium is severely damaged and must regenerate to restore its defense functions. Other lung diseases originate at the parenchymal level (such as acute respiratory distress syndrome, emphysema, and pulmonary fibrosis) and implicates regeneration of alveolar cells and fibroblasts. One factor involved in these processes must be the ability of local stem or progenitor cells to proliferate and differentiate to replace damaged lung tissues. Although this paradigm has been proven in fast self-renewing tissues, such as skin and intestine, in the lung the search for resident stem/progenitor cells has been challenging for many reasons. The respiratory epithelium displays low rates of cellular proliferation *in vivo* in the normal steady state (for example, the consensus is that the turnover time of the tracheal-bronchial epithelium of adult rodents is more than 100 days) (Blenkinsopp, 1967). Furthermore, the respiratory tract shows cellular and architectural complexity. The mature lung comprises at least 40 morphologically differentiated cell lineages (Engelhardt, 2001). Recent but highly controversial evidence suggests that stem cells from one type of tissue may generate cells typical of other organs. In this fashion, circulating cells derived from bone marrow may augment resident stem cells in the lung, such as epithelial and endothelial cells, fibroblasts and/or myofibroblasts. In view of this, groups have been investigating the possibility of enhancing stem cell repair by the use of exogenous stem cells in chronic lung disease (Gomperts and Strieter, 2007a). In addition, there is hope that recovery and outcome could be improved by the use of stem cells in acute lung conditions (Griffiths *et al.*, 2005). However, homing of circulating cells would augment repair in one setting, whereas contribute to lung fibrosis in another. In the framework of this chapter, we will review evidence for the role of bone marrow-derived stem cells in the repair of lung injury which actually occurs in many respiratory diseases. Hence, we will discuss the potential for these cells in cellular and gene therapy approaches.

STEM CELLS IN THE ADULT LUNG

The lung can be biologically divided into proximal and distal parts. The proximal part of the lung constitutes the major conducting airways, that is, the structures that deliver inspired air to the gas exchange regions in the distal airways. These structures include the nose, trachea, and the bronchi that form the large and small conducting airways. The distal lung contains the bronchioles and alveoli, in which gas exchange occurs. The trachea and bronchi are lined by a pseudostratified ciliated columnar epithelium, with goblet (mucous secreting) cells and submucosal (mucous and liquid secreting) glands also present (Randell, 2006).

More distally in the bronchioles the epithelium changes to a simple ciliated columnar epithelium with submucosal glands, Clara (non-mucous, non-ciliated, liquid secreting) cells, and fewer goblet cells than proximally; and progresses, with further branching, to a non-ciliated simple cuboidal epithelium lacking both goblet cells and submucosal glands, in the terminal bronchioles. The alveoli located here have a simple squamous epithelium, comprised of alveolar type I and II epithelial cells. Although these two epithelial cell types are present in similar numbers, type I cells cover approximately 95% of the alveolar surface. On the other hand, type II are small cuboidal cells which exhibit many functions, among which the synthesis and secretion of surfactant.

Stem cells are pluripotent to generate all cell types in the tissue compartment and usually have adequate growth capacity for the life of the animal. In general, stem cells turn over slowly and display minimal physiologic differentiation. As early descendants of stem cells, transiently amplifying (TA) cells retain significant growth capacity while acquiring differentiated functions. TA cells eventually become incapable of proliferation and enter the terminally differentiated compartment. To conserve growth potential and to prevent genetic injury while vulnerable during mitosis, stem cells are thought to cycle slowly and recruited only as demanded by tissue turnover. Thus, much of the increase in cell number in the staedy state occurs in the TA population, One consequence is that a pulse label of tritiated thymidine or bromodeoxyuridine (BrdU) labeling will mark stem cells that retain the label for an extended period due to slow turnover. Thus, an adequate labeling intensity and a suitable wash-out period of the TA and terminally differentiated compartments will result in so-called label-retaining cells (LCRs) though to represent the stem cell compartment.

It is clear that local stem or TA cells contribute to the repopulation of the injured epithelium in different anatomical regions of the lung (Liu *et al.*, 2006; Otto, 2002; Rawlins and Hogan, 2006). DNA metabolic pulse-labeling studies showed that both basal and columnar secretory cell types in the pseudostratified airway epithelium divide (Breuer *et al.*, 1990; Donnelly *et al.*, 1982; Evans *et al.*, 1986), whereas ciliated cells are considered terminally differentiated (Mason *et al.*, 1997; Rawlins *et al.*, 2007). Both basal and columnar cell types reconstituted a complete epithelium in an *in vivo* model of rat tracheas denuded of their own cells and implanted in immune compatible hosts (Avril-Delplanque *et al.*, 2005; Liu *et al.*, 1994). Colony formation on plastic dishes and lineage tracing studies, as well as more recent analysis of clonal growth and genetic lineage mapping, suggest that mouse tracheal basal cells have enhanced ability to form large differentiated epithelial colonies (see Randell, 2006 and references therein). In mice repeatedly exposed to polidocanol or SO_2, clusters of cells with strong BrdU staining were found along the surface apithelium in the glandless lower trachea, with a ratio of basal to columnar LCRs of approximately 2 to 1 (Borthwick *et al.*, 2001). Recently, human adult basal cells have been shown to retain TA cell properties, as they are capable of proliferating and reconstituting a fully differentiates mucociliary and functional epithelium (Hajj *et al.*, 2007). Thus, there is a consensus that many cells can contribute to repair of injury in the proximal airways, but that basal cells likely represent a compartment enriched for stem cells and/or TA cells. Indeed, concerns exist about the contamination of basal cells in the columnar cell preparations, which were separated by techniques based on cell density (elutriation) or cell shape.

There are suggestions that stem cells are also present in the ducts of submucosal glands. Borthwick et al. have demonstrated a label-retaining cell expansion at submucosal gland ducts in mouse following BrdU labeling, thus supporting the notion that this region may be a stem cell niche in the proximal airways (Borthwick *et al.*, 2001). On the other hand, it has been indicated that basal cells might be involved also in submucosal gland formation (Engelhardt *et al.*, 1995).

In the lower airways Clara cells are thought to provide a stem cell function. After injury by oxidant gases, surviving bronchiolar Clara cells proliferate to restore the bronchiolar epithelium (Evans *et al.*, 1976; Evans *et al.*, 1986). Clara cells have been involved also in the regeneration of the bronchiolar epithelium ensuing after administration of naphthalene, a pollutant that specifically ablates Clara cells (Van Winkle *et al.*, 1995). The naphthalene-resistant progenitor cells represent a subset of Clara cells residing within neuroepithelial bodies, and label retention studies suggest that this unit consitutes a stem cell niche (Hong *et al.*, 2001). After naphthalene injury, pulmonary neuroendocrine cells proliferate (Stripp *et al.*, 1995), but they are thought to provide a niche that regulates expansion of Clara cell secretory protein (CCSP)-expressing stem cell population in mouse distal airways (Hong *et al.*, 2001). A second epithelial stem cell niche has been identified at the junction between the conducting and respiratory epithelium (the bronchioalveolar duct junction [BDJ] in terminal bronchioles (Giangreco *et al.*, 2002). Specific cells in this zone (called bonchioalveolar stem cells, BASCs) coexpress secretoglobin 1a1, a marker of Clara cells also known as CC10 or CCSP, the type II cell marker surfactant protein (SP)-C, CD34, and stem cell antigen-1 (Sca-1) (Kim *et al.*, 2005). BASCs proliferated in response to naphthalene or bleomycin injury, and when purified cells were cultured appropriately, they demonstrated a high clonal growth capacity and differentiation potential to form both Clara cells and distal lung epithelium composed of cells expressing type I and type II cell markers (Kim *et al.*, 2005).

In the gas-exchanging regions of the lung, alveolar type II cells are considered to be the compartment enriched in stem cells. Early studies demonstrated that post-mitotic progeny of type II cells differentiated into type I cells during repair (Evans *et al.*, 1973; Evans *et al.*, 1975). Further studies have confirmed the ability of type II cells to repopulate both type II and type I alveolar cells after injury (Giangreco *et al.*, 2002; Reynolds *et al.*, 2004). Studies using a rat lung injury model have suggested that there may be four groups of type II cells, based on their expression of markers. The E-chaderin-positive subpopulation contained the majority of damaged cells, was quiescent, and expressed low levels of telomerase activity, whereas the E-chaderin-negative subpopulation was undamaged, proliferative, and expressed high levels of telomerase activity. This last subpopulation is thought to harbor the TA progenitor subpopulation of alveolar type II cells responsible for repopulation and repair of damaged alveolar epithelium (Reddy *et al.*, 2004).

Figure 1 depicts the complex structure of the lung as well as the stem cell niches of epithelial lineages in its proximal and distal regions.

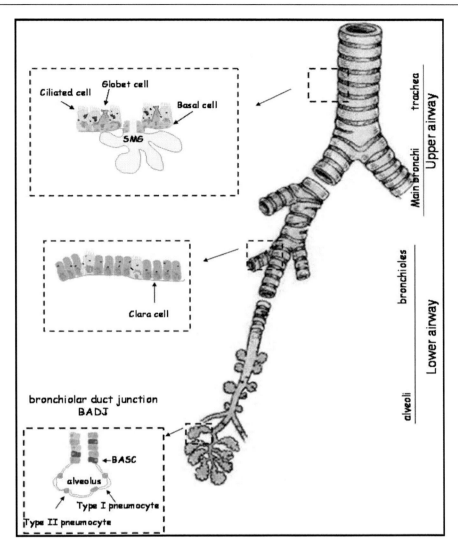

Figure 1. Stem cell niches in the lung. The pseudostratified epithelium of the upper (proximal) airways contains mostly ciliated cells, globet cells and basal cells. Although both basal and columnar secretory cell types divide, there is a consensus that basal cells likely represent a compartment enriched for stem cells and/or TA cells. Basal cells in the ducts of submucosal glands (SMG) also show stem/progenitor cell characteristics. In the more lower (distal) airways, where the epithelium is columnar, Clara cells predominate over ciliated cells. Clara cells in the bronchioles are likely the progenitor of other Clara and ciliated cells, and a variant Clara cell of the bronchiolar-alveolar junction (BASC) appears to regenerate both the bronchiole and the proximal alveoar region. In the distal alveoli, there is evidence that type II cells show stem cell capacity to renew themselves and type I cells.

In contrast to insights regarding candidate stem cells in the respiratory epithelium of adult lung, much less information is vailable regarding stem cells in the vascular compartment of the lung. Side population (SP) cells have been isolated from the lung using their Hoechst 33342 dye efflux properties similar to those of hematopoietic stem cells and other stem cell markers indicative of epithelial and mesenchymal lineages. They comprise 0.03-0.07% of mouse lung cells and are Sca-1 antigen positive, lin negative, heterogeneous for CD45, and express the vascular marker CD31 (Giangreco *et al.*, 2004; Summer *et al.*, 2003). On the basis of the expression of hematopoietic marker CD45, lung SP cells were further subdivided into hematopoietic (CD45-positive) and non-hematopoietic (CD45-negative) subpopulations. Non-hematopoietic SP cells express markers of epithelial and mesenchymal cells and share some characteristics with airway stem cells (Giangreco *et al.*, 2004).

Although MSCs have been detected in adult tissues, including the lung (Sabatini *et al.*, 2005), their origin remains unknown. A recent stydy demonstrates the isolation and characterization of a non-hematopoietic MSC population from the lower respiratory tract of human lung transplant recipients (Lama *et al.*, 2007). Which cells derive from these lung MSCs and their in situ microenvironmental niche within the lung is currently not known. The origin of the primary effector cell of fibrosis in the lung, the myofibroblast, is equally not clearly established (Willis *et al.*, 2006). Two potential sources in the lung resident cells have been hypothesized. The first, and historically most prevalent, hypothesis postulates that preexisting intrapulmonary mesenchymal precursors, such as peribronchiolar and perivascular adventitial fibroblasts, respond to a variety of stimuli during fibrogenic responses and differentiate into myofibroblasts (Phan, 2002; Zhang *et al.*, 1994). TGF-β1, a key regulator of fibrosis, induces transdifferentiation of fibroblasts *in vitro* through a Smad3-dependent mechanism (Hu *et al.*, 2003). A novel second possible source has been recently proposed: that alveolar epithelial cells undergo phenotypic transition to fully differentiated mesenchymal cells, often fibroblasts and myofibroblasts. TGF- β1 causes loss of epithelial cell markers such as aquaporin-5, cytokeratins, and ZO-1 in pure alveolar epithelial cells in culture, while dramatically up-regulating mesenchymal cell markers, including α-smooth muscle actin (α-SMA), vimentin, desmin, and type I collagen, concurrent with transition to a fibroblast-like morphology (Willis *et al.*, 2005). Moreover, tissue examination from patients with advanced idiopathic pulmonary fibrosis revealed that over 80% of the hyperplastic epithelial cells overlying fibroblastic foci coexpressed epithelial (thyroid transcription factor, an epithelial-specific transcription factor, and pro-surfactant protein B) and mesenchymal (α-SMA) markers (Willis *et al.*, 2006), suggesting that they may have been undergoing epithelial-mesenchymal transition (EMT) at the time of tissue sampling.

BONE MARROW-DERIVED STEM CELLS

Because of the easy accessibility of bone marrow and the need to replace hematopoietic cells in many clinical situations, there has been great interest in studying bone marrow stem cells. It is now recognized that the bone marrow contains hematopoietic stem cells (HSCs) as well as stromal cells capable of differentiation into various lineages. HSCs generate all of the blood cells and can reconstitute the bone marrow after depletion caused by disease or irradiation (Orkin and Morrison, 2002; Verfaillie, 2002). Bone marrow stromal cells, also called mesenchymal stem cells (MSCs), depending on the tissue environment, can generate chondrocytes, osteoblasts, adipocytes, myoblasts, and endothelial cell precursors (Pittenger *et al.*, 1999; Prockop, 1997). In addition, circulating endothelial precursor cells have been identified as being derived from BM (Asahara *et al.*, 1997). Finally, a circulating population of hematopoietic origin which displays fibroblast cell characteristics has been described (Abe *et al.*, 2001; Bucala *et al.*, 1994).

A remarkable observation about HSCs is that they may be capable of giving rise to various lineages of cells, such as myocytes (Ferrari *et al.*, 1998; Gussoni *et al.*, 1999), cardiac vascular cells (Orlic *et al.*, 2001), hepatocytes (Lagasse *et al.*, 2000; Petersen *et al.*, 1999; Theise *et al.*, 2000), epithelial cells (Krause *et al.*, 2001), astrocytes (Kopen *et al.*, 1999), and central nervous system neurons (Brazelton *et al.*, 2000; Eglitis and Mezey, 1997), including cerebellar Purkinje neurons (Priller *et al.*, 2001). These results challenge the accepted wisdom that cells of adult organisms, including stem cells, are committed to the generation of restricted lineages, and suggest instead that stem cell differentiation programs are not fixed. A change in stem cell differentiation from one cell type to another is called transdifferentiation, and the multiplicity of stem cell differentiation options is known as developmental plasticity (Korbling and Estrov, 2003; Rosenthal, 2003). More recent studies have raised questions about the plasticity of HSCs (Lemischka, 2002; Wagers *et al.*, 2002). In some situations, transplanted HSCs fuse with host cells and transfer genetic material to them, thus giving the false appearance of having transdifferentiated with generation of new cells in the host (Vassilopoulos *et al.*, 2003; Wang *et al.*, 2003). The relative contribution of true transdifferentiation or cell fusion to the development of various mature cell types from HSC is unclear at present. Also, although BM-derived stem cells (BMSCs) may be able to replace cells in damaged tissues, they do not appear to play a role in the maintenance of these tissues under physiologic conditions (steady state) (Wagers *et al.*, 2002). There is mounting evidence that the generation of tissue cells from BMSCs occurs only at sites of injury, where the response to injury recruits stem cells from the bone marrow for local tissue repopulation. It is also possible that the main contribution of BMSCs to the repair of non-hematopoietic tissues is not the generation of cells for these tissues. Instead, stem cells may produce growth factors and cytokines that act on the cells of the tissue to which they migrate, promoting injury repair and cell replication.

BONE MARROW-DERIVED EPITHELIAL LINEAGES IN THE LUNG

A seminal paper demonstrated that a single bone marrow cell can self-renew *in vivo* as well as into mature cell types of both hematopoietic and non-hematopoietic tissues like cells of the gastro-intestinal (GI) tract, lung and skin. Transplantation with HSCs yielded up to 20% donor-derived pneumocytes and 4% bronchial epithelial cells (Krause *et al.*, 2001). Following this study, transplantation studies in mice were thus performed using whole bone marrow, MSCs, Side Population (SP) cells or preparation enriched for HSCs (table 1). Whole body irradiation, which may determine injury to the lung tissue, is typically used to deplete the host bone marrow. It has been suggested that the lung injury associated with radiation create a milieu that induces marrow progenitors cells to adopt the gene expression pattern of mature pneumocytes and bronchial epithelium, either through differentiation (Harris *et al.*, 2004) or by fusion with mature epithelial cells (Spees *et al.*, 2003). For this reason, different authors have investigated the effect of the recruitment of bone marrow-derived cells following the damage induced by total body irradiation (table 2): Harris and co-workers used the Cre/lox recombinase system (Harris *et al.*, 2004); Grove *et al.* used retrovirally transduced total bone marrow (Grove *et al.*, 2002); Abe *et al.* used a parabiotic mice model (where GFP transgenic mice are surgically joined to wild-type littermates, developing a common circulation) (Abe *et al.*, 2004); others used a sex-mismatched bone marrow transplantation (Herzog *et al.*, 2006; Theise *et al.*, 2002). Since a variable percentage of pneumocytes of donor origin was found, these results show that there is a direct relationship among entity of the damage and the engraftment of BM as lung epithelium (Aliotta *et al.*, 2006; Herzog *et al.*, 2006).

Table 1. Characteristics of adult bone marrow-derived cells used in lung engraftment experiments

Cell type	Phenotype
Hematopoietic Stem Cells (HSCs)	$CD34^{+/-}$, Stem cell antigen (Sca)-1^+, $Thy1^+$, c-kit^+, lineage (lin)$^-$ - characterized by the absence of markers for mature lymphocytes (CD45, CD3, CD4, CD8), myeloid (CD11b/Mac-1), and erythroid (TER-119) cells (Aliotta et al., 2006; Krause et al., 2001; Wagers et al., 2002)
Mesenchymal Stem Cells (MSCs)	no unique phenotype
	isolated mainly by adherence to tissue culture plastic
	$CD34^+$ lin^- MSCs (Theise et al., 2002)
	plastic adherent MSCs (Kotton et al., 2001)
	multi-potent adult progenitor cell (MAPC) (Jiang et al., 2002)
	MSCs immunodepleted for CD34, CD45, and CD11b (Ortiz et al., 2003; Rojas et al., 2005)
Side population (SP) cells	Hoechst dye efflux (Abe et al., 2003; Kotton et al., 2005; Macpherson et al., 2005; MacPherson et al., 2006)
Total bone marrow	(Chang et al., 2005; Grove et al., 2002; Kotton et al., 2005)

The combination of irradiation with other damage has not produced homogeneous data (table 2). The use of NO_2 or endotoxin did not result in significant engraftment of marrow-derived cells in the lung (Beckett *et al.*, 2004). On the other hand, the combination of radiation with intratracheal elastase increased the proportion of BM derived-cells in the lung, including type I pneumocytes (Abe *et al.*, 2004). The use of the cardiotoxin does not increase notably the engraftment of BM derived-type II pneumocites compared with radiation alone (Aliotta *et al.*, 2006).

Other approaches to demonstrate engraftment of BM-derived cells rely on injury after reconstitution of bone marrow in irradiated hosts, including detergent polidocanol (Macpherson *et al.*, 2005; MacPherson *et al.*, 2006) and bleomycin (Kotton *et al.*, 2005). These studies used either whole bone marrow or SP cells, which are isolated by virtue of their ability to exclude the DNA binding dye Hoechst 33342 and are highly enriched in HSC activity (Goodell *et al.*, 1996). Macpherson and associates demonstrated the appearance of BM-derived cells in the tracheal epithelium (Macpherson *et al.*, 2005; MacPherson *et al.*, 2006). On the other hand, Kotton and colleagues reported no evidence of engraftment in type

II pneumocytes (Kotton *et al.*, 2005). It must be emphasized that bleomycin is known to induce lung fibrosis (Xu *et al.*, 2006) and that Kotton *et al.* reported engraftement of donor-derived cells with MSCs (Kotton *et al.*, 2001). This may imply that the type of donor BM-derived cells engrafted into the lung would not be pneumocytes but fibroblasts (Hashimoto *et al.*, 2004 and see below).

Table 2. Injury models used for studying engraftment of bone marrow-derived stem cells into the lung

Injury model	Type of donor stem cells	Lung cell type formed and frequency	Reference
Total body irradiation	Total bone marrow, HSCs (lin$^{+/-}$, cKit$^{+/-}$, Sca-1$^{+/-}$), SP cells, MAPCs, MSCs	Type II alveolar cells (0.025-20%) Bronchial epithelial cells (4-20%)	(Abe et al., 2003; Abe et al., 2004; Aliotta et al., 2006; Beckett et al., 2004; Herzog et al., 2006; Jiang et al., 2002; Kotton and Fine, 2003; Krause et al., 2001; Theise et al., 2002)
Intratracheal bleomycin	MSCs (CD11b$^-$, CD45$^-$)	Type I alveolar cells (1-7%) Type II alveolar cells (1-7%)	(Kotton et al., 2001; Ortiz et al., 2003; Rojas et al., 2005)
Intratracheal elastase	Circulating blood cells	Interstitial monocytes/macrophages, subepithelial fibroblast-like cells, type I alveolar cells	(Abe et al., 2004)
Intranasal LPS	Fetal liver cells	Alveolar epithelium	(Yamada et al., 2004)
Intratracheal LPS	Total bone marrow	No engraftement observed	(Beckett et al., 2004)
Inhalation of NO$_2$	Total bone marrow	No engraftement observed	(Beckett et al., 2004)
Detergent (polidocanol) instillation into the airways	SP (Sca-1$^+$, Gr-1$^-$) cells	Tracheal epithelial cells (0.83%)	(Macpherson et al., 2005; MacPherson et al., 2006)
Intramuscular cardiotoxin	Total bone marrow, HSCs (lin$^{+/-}$, cKit$^{+/-}$, Sca-1$^{+/-}$)	Very modest enhancement of engraftment observed compared to irradiation only	(Aliotta et al., 2006)

HSCs: hematopoietic stem cells; LPS: lipopolysaccharide; MAPCs: multipotential adult progenitor cells; MSCs: mesenchymal stem cells; SP: side population.

To determine whether marrow-derived epithelial cells can function normally, two works have investigated if marrow-derived epithelial cells in the murine GI and upper respiratory tracts (Bruscia *et al.*, 2006) and lung epithelium (Loi *et al.*, 2006) express the cystic fibrosis transmembrane conductance regulator (CFTR) mRNA and protein, and can restore chloride transport through this channel (see below).

Plasticity of adult somatic stem cells has been questioned (Herzog *et al.*, 2003; Wagers and Weissman, 2004). A number of investigators using alternative approaches have found no evidence of BM contribution to epithelial repair in the murine lung (Chang *et al.*, 2005; Kotton *et al.*, 2005; Wagers *et al.*, 2002). These studies relied on a green fluorescent protein (GFP) reporter gene to track marrow-derived cells, and none of them used chromosomal analysis to identify marrow-derived lung epithelium. Because transgene expression has been shown to be relatively insensitive for the identification of marrow-derived epithelial cells, and injury is known to be a critical event for the appearance of these cells, the significance of these negative data is unknown. However, they do illustrate the need for rigorous and consistent study design. Current standards in this field demand either confocal or single-cell analysis of marrow-derived epithelial cells (by deconvolution microscopy) to rule out the possibility of overlay. The addition of hematopoietic antigens to staining protocols is appropriate in many cases. Phenotypic analysis with cell-specific markers is indicated to ensure that the appearance of epithelial cells derived from marrow is not the result of microscopy artifact. Last, where technically feasible, isolation and functional characterization of donor-derived engrafted epithelial cells should be done (Neuringer and Randell, 2006). A greater understanding of how the lung repairs itself after irradiation, including the clearance of apoptotic cells and their replacement with newly formed epithelial cells, will allow us to better understand how marrow-derived cells become epithelial cells in the lung.

The mechanisms about which circulating stem cells are recruited into injured organs are not fully understood. In a mouse model of sex-mismatched tracheal transplantation, Gomperts and colleagues demonstrated that a population of oriented progenitor cells expressing the epithelial marker cytokeratin 5 (CK5) and the chemokine receptor CXCR4 exists in the bone marrow and that CK5$^+$ circulating progenitor epithelial cells contribute to re-epithelialization of the airway and re-establishment of the pseudostratified epithelium (Gomperts et al., 2006). Depletion of CXCL12 prevents precursor recruitment and appropriate epithelial repair and favors squamous metaplasia. These findings demonstrate that CK5$^+$CXCR4$^+$ cells have a crucial role in the re-epithelialization of tracheal transplants and that the CXCL12/CXCR4 axis is involved in epithelial precursor mobilization and recruitment at sites of injury (figure 2). The same axis is though to play an important role also in the recruitment and homing of fibrocystes to the lung (see below).

Sex-mismatched lung and bone marrow transplantation in humans provides a natural model for analysis of donor and recipient cell behaviour. Bronchial epithelial and gland cells (Kleeberger et al., 2003) and type II pneumocytes of host origin (Kleeberger et al., 2003; Zander et al., 2005) were reported in two studies of lung allografts, but not in another (Bittmann et al., 2001). After bone marrow transplantation, epithelial cells of donor origin were not detected in the nasal passages (Davies et al., 2002) while were found in lung epithelium (Albera et al., 2005; Kleeberger et al., 2003; Mattsson et al., 2004; Suratt et al., 2003) and in the lung endothelium (Suratt et al., 2003). Stem cell engraftment in the lung after sex mismatched lung transplantation was studied in two cystic fibrosis patients (Spencer et al., 2005). Evidence of chimerism was found in up to 6.6% of epithelial cells in bronchial and alveolar tissue without apparent evidence of fusion.

One limitation of these studies was that they failed to show evidence of epithelial cell function. Interestingly, in one study (Zander et al., 2005) the number of engrafted type II pneumocytes showed a statistically significant relationship to the cumulative number of episodes of acute cellular rejection, confrming that injury is a necessary token for engraftment of BMSCs into the lung tissue. Many questions remain non answered, including the mechanism whereby cells assume lung cell phenotypes.

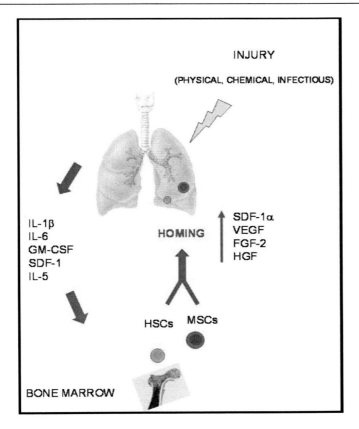

Figure 2. Schematic diagram to show lung injury induced by stimuli, which generates mediators that stimulate the bone marrow to produce and release hematopoietic stem cells (HSCs) and mesenchymal stem cells (MSCs). Mediators are likely secreted by resident macrophages, endothelial cells, and epithelial cells and also regulate HSC and MSC homing to the damaged lung. Once homed, MSCs are though to give rise to fibroblasts/myofibroblasts, endothelial cells and alveolar cells, while HSCs are able to produce, besides granulocyte precursors and antigen presenting cells, epithelial cells of the airways.

Several studies have demonstrated that cell fusion occurs both *in vitro* and *in vivo*, which likely explains why some of the cells contain both donor and lung cell markers (Camargo *et al.*, 2004; Herzog *et al.*, 2003; Spees *et al.*, 2003; Wagers *et al.*, 2002). Harris *et al.* made use of the Cre/lox recombinase system to examine whether fusion occurs between BM-derived stem cells and host cells after BM transplantation (Harris *et al.* 2004). Using this approach, low frequencies of marrow-derived epithelia were detected in the liver, lung, and GI tract. In addition, the donor-derived lung cells were found to contain only one copy of each sex chromosome. Taken together, these data indicate that fusion is not required for the appearance of marrow-derived epithelia at the lung level.

Alternatively, cells may reprogram in the lung environment -a concept termed transdifferentiation (see above). It has been suggested that many of the events previously attributed to transdifferentiation may actually represent cell fusion, particularly due to the influx of fusion-prone myeloid cells into damaged tissues from the repopulated bone marrow (Camargo *et al.*, 2004). Recently, Krause and associates have demonstrated that lung-spcific reprogramming of BMSCs is accompanied by heterokaryon formation and Y chromosome loss after BM transplantation and secondary lung inflammation in SP-C deficient mice, although not therapeutic in this model (Herzog *et al.*, 2007). The presence of chronic inflammation due to SP-C-deficiency and the use of more sensitive techniques used in this work have been invoked as the possible reasons that account different results as compared to previous studies (Harris *et al.*, 2004; Herzog *et al.*, 2006). Thus, new more stringent criteria have been put forth for demonstration of transdifferentiation (Wagers and Weissman, 2004). Bone marrow harbors a generalized pluripotent stem cell (Jiang *et al.*, 2002), called multipotential adult progenitor cells (MAPCs), and the bone marrow cell responsible for lung engraftment has not been identified with certainty. It is possible that rare transdifferentiation events represents migration of a pluripotent bone marrow cell type resembling an embryonic stem or embryonic germ cell still harbored in the adult bone marrow (*e.g.* MAPC). It remains unknown whether bone marrow cells must transit through an intermediate compartment prior to lung colonization or whether circulating stem cells can be mobilized from sources other than bone marrow. It is important to note that bone marrow derived-cells of typical hematopoietic lineage, chimeric cells created by fusion, or lung cells generated by transdifferentiation may all play a role in lung repair by promoting the local production of stem cells or reparative function of lung-specific cell types.

BM-Derived Fibroblasts and Myofibroblasts in the Lung

Studies have shown that BM-derived stromal cells (Prockop, 1997) and hematopoietic precursors (Herzog *et al.*, 2003) engraft and become structural cells, including fibroblasts, particularly following tissue injury. In fact, a unique population of collagen-expressing cells derived from hematopoietic precursors termed "fibrocytes" has been described (Abe *et al.*, 2001; Bucala *et al.*, 1994). Fibrocytes, as defined by collagen$^+$CD45$^+$ and/or CD34$^+$ in expression, only comprise 0.1-0.5% of the nucleated cells in peripheral blood (Metz, 2003; Phillips *et al.*, 2004; Quan *et al.*, 2004). Fibrocytes express mesenchymal markers, such as vimentin, collagens I and III, and fibronectin. In culture, fibrocytes begin to express α-SMA spontaneously, and addition of TGF-β or endothelin increases the levels of α-SMA markedly.

Initial studies have suggested that the bone marrow can potentially contribute to the turnover of myofibroblasts throughout the body (Brittan *et al.*, 2002; Direkze *et al.*, 2003). Following radiation injury, a proportion of myofibroblasts in the lung, stomach, esophagus, skin, kidney, and adrenal capsule were bone-marrow derived. In the lung there was significantly greater engraftment following paracetamol administration (Direkze *et al.*, 2003). On the other hand, the role of fibrocytes in the pathogenesis of pulmonary fibrosis is controversial (recently reviewed in Lama and Phan, 2006 and Gomperts and Strieter, 2007b). In certain studies, fibrocytes home to diseased lungs, express collagen, and contribute to fibrosis (Abe *et al.*, 2004; Epperly *et al.*, 2003; Hashimoto *et al.*, 2004; Phillips *et al.*, 2004; Schmidt *et al.*, 2003). Only in injured lungs, and not in control lungs, it is possible to demonstrate significant numbers of GFP-expressing cells with morphologic characteristics of fibroblasts in areas of active fibrosis, in addition to GFP-positive mononuclear and other leukocytic cells (Abe *et al.*, 2004; Epperly *et al.*, 2003; Hashimoto *et al.*, 2004). Careful analysis of cells isolated and cultured from these injured lungs confirmed that a substantial portion expresses the donor marker gene (GFP). However, none of the GFP-positive cells expresses α-SMA, indicative of failure of the BM-derived fibroblasts to differentiate to myofibroblasts (Hashimoto *et al.*, 2004).

Other investigators have systematically administered mesenchymal stem cells to bleomycin-treated mice (Kotton *et al.*, 2001; Ortiz *et al.*, 2003). In these studies, cells that engrafted into lung tissue displayed characteristics of alveolar epithelial cells. Nevertheless, MSC adminisration reduced the degree of BML-induced inflammation and collagen deposition (Ortiz *et al.*, 2003; Rojas *et al.*, 2005). Although differences in the type of BM-derived mesenchymal stem cells and the protocol of administration might have influenced the different outcome in cell phenotype found in the lung, it could be possible that collagen-producing cells underwent epithelial-mesenchymal transition (Willis *et al.*, 2006).

The biological axis of CXCL2/CXCR4 play a major role in mediating the contribution of fibrocytes to pulmonary fibrosis (figure 2). Fibrocytes express the chemokine receptors CXCR4 and CCR7 and migrate *in vivo* in response to their corresponding ligands, stromal cell-derived factor-1 (SDF-1/CXCL12) and secondary lymphoid-tissue chemokine (SLC) (Abe *et al.*, 2001). The levels of SDF-1 and SLC are increased in the lung following bleomycin treatment (Hashimoto *et al.*, 2004). Phillips *et al.* identified a population of fibrocytes that expressed CCR7, which were distinct from the CXCR4-expressing fibrocyets in bleomycin-induced pulmonary fibrosis (Phillips *et al.*, 2004). They noted that the intrapulmonary recruitment of $CD45^{+}Col\ I^{+}CXCR4^{+}$ fibrocytes was greater than $CD45^{+}Col\ I^{+}CCR7^{+}$ fibrocytes, which correlated with collagen deposition in the lungs of bleomycin-exposed mice. In mice, CXCR4, CCR7, and potentially, CCR2 appear to mediate recruitment of fibrocytes to the lung (Moore *et al.*, 2005; Phillips *et al.*, 2004). In another study of radiation-induced fibrosis (Epperly *et al.*, 2003), influx of bone marrow-derived macrophages preceded that of bone marrow-derived fibroblasts, suggesting that these macrophages may be the source of SDF-1, SLC, or other substances that recruit fibroblast precursors from the bone marrow.

BM-DERIVED ENDOTHELIAL CELLS IN THE LUNG

A key element in repair or regeneration is vasculogenesis, with the endothelial cell being the main component. In addition to proliferation of surviving endothelial cells at the site of injury (angiogenesis), the presence of BM-derived circulating endothelial progenitor cells (EPCs) also has been shown to play a role in vasculogenesis in tissue repair (Asahara *et al.*, 1997; Asahara *et al.*, 1999; Ishizawa *et al.*, 2004; Shi *et al.*, 1998; Zhao *et al.*, 2005). EPCs have the potential to differentiate into mature endothelial cells and display a variety of markers specific for the endothelial lineage, such as CD31, eNOS, and E-selectin (Peichev *et al.*, 2000).

The administration of lipopolysaccharide (LPS) in murine lungs induced a rapid release of EPCs into the circulation and BM-derived cells, including EPCs, contributed to lung repair after LPS-induced lung injury (Yamada *et al.*, 2004). Moreover, these cells appear to be important in vasculogenesis associated with the response to elastase-induced lung injury (Ishizawa *et al.*, 2004). The number of circulating EPCs is significantly higher in patients with acute lung injury (Burnham *et al.*, 2005) and bacterial pneumonia (Yamada et al 2005) as compared with healthy controls. An increased number of EPCs correlates with survival in acute lung injury (Burnham *et al.*, 2005) and patients with low EPC count tended to have persistent fibrotic changes in their lungs even after their recovery from pneumonia (Yamada *et al.*, 2005). When patients with chronic lung disease (obstructive and restricitve) and long-lasting hypoxia were studied, a reduction of circulating EPCs was found (Fadini *et al.*, 2006), suggesting defective mobilization and/or shortened peripheral survival of EPCs in these clinical conditions. These studies would highlight the protective effect of EPCs in helping repair the acute damaged lung. On the other hand, it may be envioned that an exhausted EPC pool may contribute to disease progression and worsening in chronic severe lung disease.

APPLICATION OF BM-DERIVED CELLS TO LUNG DISEASES

The role of BM-borne circulating stem cells in the major lung diseases and their possible therapeutic use is under investigation. The general concept is that augmentation of stem cells in the lung may minimize injury, augment repair, or possibly regenerate lost tissue (Denburg and van Eeden, 2006; Neuringer and Randell, 2004; Stripp and Shapiro, 2006; Yen *et al.*, 2006). However, it should be emphasized that in certain clinical conditions, such as fibrosis, smooth muscle hyperplasia and lung cancer, inihibition of stem cells recruitment and growth could be a valid therapeutic goal. Four options are valid for stem cell-based therapies (Yen *et al.*, 2006). Pharmacological therapy is the application of drugs or cytokines to stimulate endogenous stem cells or recruit exogneous stem cells for tissue regeneration and repair. Cellular therapy is the utilization of exogneous stem cells to help regeneration and repair. It is also possible that stem cells could be used to reconstitute more complex tissues and organs *in vitro*, and then transplanted to replace failed organs. Although tissue engineering is evolving rapidly, only a few stem cell-generated products have entered clinical trials, namely cartilage and skin (Bianco and Robey, 2001; Rahaman and Mao, 2005). Finally, gene therapy with stem cells may be used to correct genetic defect or to introduce exogenous genetic material to modify the function of cells (Grove *et al.*, 2002; Prockop *et al.*, 2003; Wang *et al.*, 2005) (Fang *et al.*, 2004).

In table 3 we summarize major lung diseases likely involving stem cells and the possible interventions based on stem cells as outline above. In the following paragraphs, we discuss the involvement of stem cells in some of these diseases.

Table 3. Major lung disease potentially treatable by stem cell manipulation

Lung disease	Injured, depleted, or deranged cellular compartment	Therapeutic goal	Intervention
Congenital lung hypoplasia	Alveolar epithelium	Generate alveolar septa	Tissue engineering
Bronchopulmonary dysplasia	Alveolar epithelium, alveolar endothelium	Restore or protect the alveolar cells	Tissue, engineering, Cellular therapy
Neonatal RDS	Alveolar epithelium	Enhance surfactant production	Gene therapy
ARDS	Alveolar endothelium, Alveolar epithelium	Reinforce endothelial and epithelial barriers	Pharmacological therapy, Cellular therapy
Pulmonary fibrosis	Interstitial fibroblasts	Inhibit fibroblast proliferation	Gene therapy
COPD	Alveolar epithelium (emphysema), airway epithelium (chronic bronchitis)	Inhibit acinar damage (emphisema), inhibit airway hyperplasia and metaplasia	Gene therapy, Cellular therapy
Asthma	Airway epithelium, myofibroblasts, airway smooth muscle	Inihibit airway wall remodeling. Inhibit smooth muscle hypertrophy and hyperplasia	Pharmacologoical therapy, Cellular therapy, Gene therapy
Cystic fibrosis	Airway epithelium	Deliver functional CFTR	Gene therapy, Cellular therapy
Bronchiolitis obliterans	Airway epithelium	Reinforce the epithelium against toxic, viral or immunologic injury	Gene therapy
Lung cancer	Epithelium	Regulation of stem cell proliferation and differentiation	Gene therapy

ARDS: Acute Respiratory Distress Syndrome; CFTR: Cystic Fibrosis Transmembrane Conductance Regulator; COPD: chronic obstructive pulmonary disease.

In view of the importance of re-epithelialization in successful repair and prevention of fibrosis (Vracko, 1974; Witschi et al., 1981; Yano et al., 1996; Yi et al., 1998), any impairment of this process will likely contribute to formation of fibroblastic foci and progressive fibrosis. Neutralization of CXCL12 results in reduced fibrocytic recruitment to the bleomycin-injured lung, which is accompanied by reduced lung fibrosis (Phillips et al., 2004). This seems to argue for a profibrotic role of the fibrocyte, perhaps by increasing the number of fibroblasts in the lung. In contrast, myelosuppression was shown to cause increased susceptibility to bleomycin, whereas transfer of BM-derived MSCs is protective and accompanied by the presence of MSC-derived fibroblasts in the lung (Rojas et al., 2005). Although there is increasing evidence for extrapulmonary progenitors for the expanded lung fibroblast population in injured and fibrotic lungs (Epperly et al., 2003; Hashimoto et al., 2004; Phillips et al., 2004; Abe et al., 2004; Ortiz et al., 2003; Rojas et al., 2005), their role (protective or not) in the pathogenesis of pulmonary fibrosis is still an open issue.

Emphysema and chronic bronchitis are often clinically grouped together and referred to as chronic obstructive pulmonary disease (COPD), since many patients have overlapping features of damage at both the acinar level (emphysema) and bronchial level (bronchitis).

Since emphysema is characterized by the destruction of alveolar walls, defective repair following injury (by cigarette smoke) has been postulated as a potential mechanism for the development of this disease. It has been found a > 50% decrease in circulating hematopoietic progenitors (CD34$^+$ cells) and AC133$^+$ EPCs in subject with severe COPD (Bonsignore et al., 2006; Palange et al., 2006). These studies also demonstrate an inverse relationship between disease severity (airways obstruction or forced expiratory colume in one second/forced vital capacity ratio) and levels of circulating progenitors, suggesting that this could imply a defective BM-derived stem cell response as critical in the pathogenesis of COPD.

Asthma is characterized by chronic airway inflammation and remodeling of the normal bronchial architecture, whose hallmarks are subepithelial fibrosis, submucosal gland hyperplasia and hypertrophy, hypertrophy of airway epithelial cells, and hypertrophy and hyperplasia of smooth muscle cells (Bousquet et al., 1992; Bousquet et al., 2000; Elias et al., 1999; Redington and Howarth, 1997). Accumulation of eosinophils and basophils in tissues is characteristic of allergic inflammation in rhinitis, nasal polyps and asthma. Cell recruitment is favored, at least in part, by recruitment of progenitors from circulation and bone marrow, under the influence of tissue-elaborated hematopoietic cytokines and chemokines (reviewed in Denburg and van Eeden, 2006). If BM-derived stem cells are recruited in the asthmatic lung to differentiate in nonhematopoietic cells is not known. Schmidt and associates showed that there are significant numbers of CD34$^-$Col I$^+$ cells as well as few CD34$^+\alpha$-SMA$^+$ cells below the basement membrane in the bronchial mucosa of asthmatic patients and that these cells increase dramatically 24 hours after exposure to an allergen (Schmidt et al., 2003). They also confirmed the presence of BM-derived fibrocytes in the tickened bronchial lamina propria in a mouse model of allergic asthma.

In most diffuse obstructive and restrictive lung diseases, progressive pulmonary vascular remodeling and neovascularization may be observed (Hopkins and McLoughlin, 2002; Keane, 2004; Renzoni, 2004). The functional consequence is secondary pulmonary hypertension (PH), which may contribute to premature mortality and added mortality (Barbera et al., 2003; Chaouat et al., 2005). Depletion of circulating EPCs may be involved in altered endothelial homeostasis of pulmonary circulation in chronic lung disorders. Indeed, EPC reduction has been demonstrated to be related to endothelial dysfunction in the systemic circulation (Hill et al., 2003). Animal models of PH have shown that EPC administration prevents anatomical lesions and improves animal survival (Nagaya et al., 2003; Takahashi et al., 2004; Zhao et al., 2005). On the other hand, data are rapidly accumulating in support of the idea that circulating monocytes and/or mononuclear fibrocytes are recruited to the pulmonary circulation of chronically hypoxic animals and that these cells play an important role in the pulmonary hypertensive process (Davie et al., 2004; Frid et al., 2005; Frid et al., 2006; Stenmark et al., 2005). To better understand and take advantage of the therapeutic potential of EPC and/or mononuclear fibrocyte administration and/or modulation in humans with diffuse lung disease and hypoxia is a major challenge for researchers involved in the clinical management of these disorders.

Cystic fibrosis (CF) is an autosomal recessive disorder characterized by alteration in ion and fluid secretion/absorption in many epithelial-lined organs. Despite impressive advances in understanding the molecular basis and pathophysiology of this disorder, it remains the most common life-shortening genetic disorder in the white population with an estimated median survival age of 33.4 years in 2001 (Gibson *et al.*, 2003).

Most of the morbidity and mortality of these patients is associated with chronic obstructive lung disease, whose hallmarks are infection with opportunistic pathogens, exaggerated sputum production, and ongoing inflammation (Mishra *et al.*, 2005). The gene involved in CF, the CF transmembrane conductance regulator (CFTR) is expressed in many cell types in the airways (Engelhardt *et al.*, 1992) (Engelhardt *et al.*, 1994; Kreda *et al.*, 2005) and it might be difficult to target all these cell types at one time by gene or pharmacological therapy. Moreover, CF airways are characterized also by an increased cell turnover (Leigh *et al.*, 1995) and thus CF could be considered for stem cell therapy in view of a regenerative medicine approach (Conese and Rejman, 2006; Spencer and Jaffe, 2004; van Haaften and Thebaud, 2006). CF stem cell therapy would require heterologous or gene corrected autologous stem cells to colonise the airways, proliferate there and differentiate into cells of the surface epithelium and/or of submucosal glands. Some recent studies determined whether transplantation of adult marrow cells containing the gene for wild type Cftr might result in functional Cftr expression in lung epithelium. Loi and colleagues (Loi *et al.*, 2006) transplanted two populations of bone marrow-derived cells (cultured stromal marrow cells and total bone marrow cells) containing the wild type CFTR gene into transgenic CFTR knockout mice. Administration of plastic adherent stromal cells, to naive non-irradiated mice resulted in the engraftment of donor-derived airway epithelial cells, although at very small numbers (approximately 0.025%, of which 0.01% expressed CFTR protein) that is unlikely to affect overall CFTR-dependent chloride transport and other functions in airway epithelium. Nevertheless, Bruscia and colleagues demonstrated that the transplantation of GFP$^+$BMSCs of CFTR+/+ mice into irradiated CFTR-null mice resulted in a partial restoration of CFTR activity of gastrointestinal and nasal epithelium (Bruscia *et al.*, 2006). Most of the CFTR-/- mice had functional CFTR channels in the rectum and nose by 24 weeks. These results correlated with the presence of CFTR-expressing donor derived (GFP$^+$) columnar epithelial cells in the small intestine (with a frequency of <1%). Overall, these results imply that a very low level of cell therapy produced an amplified electrophysiological effect.

BM transplantation was carried out in a mouse model of respiratory infection with *P. aeruginosa* encapsulated in agarose beads (a model to mimic the chronic inflammation in CF) and determined reduced mortality by 50% when CFTR KO mice received wild-type bone marrow (reported in Weiss *et al.*, 2006). Interestingly, epithelial chimerism was not observed since more than 97% of donor origin were confined to CD45$^+$ phenotype and were not epithelial cells, suggesting that BMSCs control pulmonary inflammatory responses in this model of lung inflammation.

The hypothesis that MSCs could be the relevant cell type in the engraftment in the airway epithelium was tested in vitro by Wang and collegaues using human cells (Wang *et al.*, 2005). MSCs obtained from bone marrow of healthy volunteers were mixed with airway epithelial cells (AECs) and grown in air-liquid interface cultures on semi-permeable filters. Almost 10% of the MSCs were induced *in vitro* to acquire an epithelial phenotype of the columnar type, as judged by the expression of cytokeratin 18 and occludin. Moreover, MSCs obtained from CF patients corrected *ex-vivo* with a CFTR-encoding retrovirus and mixed with CF AECs resulted in partial resumption of CFTR-mediated chloride current.

Cellular therapies for immunological mature patients would be susceptible to graft-versus-host-disease, unless the cells were derived from the patient themeselves. The delivery of autologous adult stem cells would prevent immunological rejection by the host (Orkin and Morrison, 2002). Furthermore, BMSCs allow the possibility to expand a patient's own cells before reuse. However, organ transplantation is more likely to be tolerated if a degree of haemotopoietic chimaerism with donor BM-derived stem cells is induced (Weissman, 2000). Moreover, there are reasons to be concerned that exposure of the recipient immune system to engrafted cells and thus to a new protein will be followed by recongnition as nonself and destruction of the expressing cells. Finally, gene therapy could elicit an immune response to delivered therapeutic genes or to proteins which make up the viral vector (Thomas *et al.*, 2003). While immunosuppressants are the only practible answer to these concerns, others are investigating whether administration at a preimmune stage, *i.e.* in the fetal life, would be feasible (Fang *et al.*, 2004).

Another concern about the use of BM-derived stem/progenitor cells in the context of repair/regeneration of lung injury is their fate. After systemic delivery of murine MSCs, cells embolized in lung parenchyma capillaries, trans-migrated and expanded to form tumors resembling well differentiated osteosarcoma. Moreover, this enriched MSC population acquired significant chromosomal abnormalities after *in vitro* passages (Aguilar *et al.*, 2007). These results stress the importance of careful analysis of cells used for cell therapy both before and after transplantation.

CONCLUSION

Promising studies have shown in animal models and in humans that BM-derived stem/progenitor cells can home to different organs, including the lung. Complex chemokine/chemokine receptor axis and inflammatory mediators govern recruitment of BM-borne cells and intervention on these mediators is likely proficient to increase/decrease accumulation of bone marrow-derived cells to the lung. Small numbers of bone marrow–derived multipotent progenitors (CD34+ cells) normally circulate in peripheral blood. Although various kinds of lung injury (chemical, physical, infectious) have been demonstrated to enhance HSCs, EPCs, fibrocytes or MSCs homing to the lung, this happens at low frequency, Neverthelss, certain studies highlighted that some pathological features can be modified/reversed by BM-derived stem/progenitor cells. Then, circulating CD34+ cells indirectly reflect hematopoiesis, but may also be involved in tissue repair processes, either by engrafting in damaged areas, or by promoting angiogenesis and improving oxygen and nutrient supply to damaged tissue.

It is not clear the relative role of these cells as respect to local progenitor cells and further studies should elucidate this issue. Finally, there is mounting evidence that BM-derived stem cells may be useful, if not as true stem cells then at least as vehicles for emerging cell and gene therapies. Regulating and promoting recruitment and homing of BM-derived stem cells offers a novel cell-based therapeutic option for regeneration and repair of lung tissues. Safety issues are still a caveat.

ACKNOWLEDGMENTS

We kindly acknowledge the support received by the European Union (V Framework Programme, Contract #2002-02119) and the Italian Cystic Fibrosis Foundation.

REFERENCES

Abe, R., Donnelly, S. C., Peng, T., Bucala, R. and Metz, C. N. (2001). Peripheral blood fibrocytes: differentiation pathway and migration to wound sites. *J. Immunol. 166*, 7556-7562.

Abe, S., Lauby, G., Boyer, C., Rennard, S. I. and Sharp, J. G. (2003). Transplanted BM and BM side population cells contribute progeny to the lung and liver in irradiated mice. *Cytotherapy. 5*, 523-533.

Abe, S., Boyer, C., Liu, X., Wen, F. Q., Kobayashi, T., Fang, Q., Wang, X., Hashimoto, M., Sharp, J. G. and Rennard, S. I. (2004). Cells derived from the circulation contribute to the repair of lung injury. *Am. J. Respir. Crit. Care Med. 170*, 1158-1163.

Aguilar, S., Nye, E., Chan, J., Loebinger, M., Spencer-Dene, B., Fisk, N., Stamp, G., Bonnet, D. and Janes, S. M. (2007). Murine but not human mesenchymal stem cells generate osteosarcoma-like lesions in the lung. *Stem Cells. 25*, 1586-1594.

Albera, C., Polak, J. M., Janes, S., Griffiths, M. J., Alison, M. R., Wright, N. A., Navaratnarasah, S., Poulsom, R., Jeffery, R., Fisher, C., Burke, M. and Bishop, A. E. (2005). Repopulation of human pulmonary epithelium by bone marrow cells: a potential means to promote repair. *Tissue Eng. 11*, 1115-1121.

Aliotta, J. M., Keaney, P., Passero, M., Dooner, M. S., Pimentel, J., Greer, D., Demers, D., Foster, B., Peterson, A., Dooner, G., Theise, N. D., Abedi, M., Colvin, G. A. and Quesenberry, P. J. (2006). Bone marrow production of lung cells: the impact of G-CSF, cardiotoxin, graded doses of irradiation, and subpopulation phenotype. *Exp. Hematol .34*, 230-241.

Asahara, T., Murohara, T., Sullivan, A., Silver, M., van der Zee, R., Li, T., Witzenbichler, B., Schatteman, G. and Isner, J. M. (1997). Isolation of putative progenitor endothelial cells for angiogenesis. *Science. 275*, 964-967.

Asahara, T., Takahashi, T., Masuda, H., Kalka, C., Chen, D., Iwaguro, H., Inai, Y., Silver, M. and Isner, J. M. (1999). VEGF contributes to postnatal neovascularization by mobilizing bone marrow-derived endothelial progenitor cells. *Embo J. 18*, 3964-3972.

Avril-Delplanque, A., Casal, I., Castillon, N., Hinnrasky, J., Puchelle, E. and Peault, B. (2005). Aquaporin-3 expression in human fetal airway epithelial progenitor cells. *Stem Cells. 23*, 992-1001.

Barbera, J. A., Peinado, V. I. and Santos, S. (2003). Pulmonary hypertension in chronic obstructive pulmonary disease. *Eur. Respir. J. 21*, 892-905.

Beckett, T., Loi, R., Prenovitz, R., Poynter, M., Goncz, K. K., Suratt, B. T. and Weiss, D. J. (2004). Acute lung injury with endotoxin or NO_2 does not enhance development of airway epithelium from bone marrow. *Mol. Ther. 12*, 680-686.

Bianco, P. and Robey, P. G. (2001). Stem cells in tissue engineering. *Nature 414*, 118-121.

Bittmann, I., Dose, T., Baretton, G. B., Muller, C., Schwaiblmair, M., Kur, F. and Lohrs, U. (2001). Cellular chimerism of the lung after transplantation. An interphase cytogenetic study. *Am. J. Clin. Pathol. 115*, 525-533.

Blenkinsopp, W. K. (1967). Proliferation of respiratory tract epithelium in the rat. *Exp. Cell Res. 46*, 144-154.

Bonsignore, M. R., Palange, P., Testa, U., Huertas, A., Antonucci, R., Serra, P. and Bonsignore, G. (2006). Circulating CD34+ cells are decreased in chronic obstructive pulmonary disease. *Proc. Am. Thorac. Soc. 3*, 537-538.

Borthwick, D. W., Shahbazian, M., Krantz, Q. T., Dorin, J. R. and Randell, S. H. (2001). Evidence for stem-cell niches in the tracheal epithelium. *Am. J. Respir. Cell Mol. Biol. 24*, 662-670.

Bousquet, J., Chanez, P., Lacoste, J. Y., White, R., Vic, P., Godard, P. and Michel, F. B. (1992). *Asthma: a disease remodeling the airways. Allergy. 47*, 3-11.

Bousquet, J., Jeffery, P. K., Busse, W. W., Johnson, M. and Vignola, A. M. (2000). Asthma. From bronchoconstriction to airways inflammation and remodeling. *Am. J. Respir. Crit. Care Med. 161*, 1720-1745.

Brazelton, T. R., Rossi, F. M., Keshet, G. I. and Blau, H. M. (2000). From marrow to brain: expression of neuronal phenotypes in adult mice. *Science. 290*, 1775-1779.

Breuer, R., Zajicek, G., Christensen, T. G., Lucey, E. C. and Snider, G. L. (1990). Cell kinetics of normal adult hamster bronchial epithelium in the steady state. *Am. J. Respir. Cell Mol. Biol. 2*, 51-58.

Brittan, M., Hunt, T., Jeffery, R., Poulsom, R., Forbes, S. J., Hodivala-Dilke, K., Goldman, J., Alison, M. R. and Wright, N. A. (2002). Bone marrow derivation of pericryptal myofibroblasts in the mouse and human small intestine and colon. *Gut. 50*, 752-757.

Bruscia, E., Price, J. E., Cheng, E.-C., Weiner, S., Caputo, C., Ferreira, E. C., Egan, M. E. and Krause, D. S. (2006). Assessment of cystic fibrosis transmembrane conductance regulator (CFTR) activity in CFTR-null mice after bone marrow transplantation. *Proc. Natl. Acad. Sci. U S A. 103*, 2965-2970.

Bucala, R., Spiegel, L. A., Chesney, J., Hogan, M. and Cerami, A. (1994). Circulating fibrocytes define a new leukocyte subpopulation that mediates tissue repair. *Mol. Med. 1*, 71-81.

Burnham, E. L., Taylor, W. R., Quyyumi, A. A., Rojas, M., Brigham, K. L. and Moss, M. (2005). *Increased circulating endothelial progenitor cells are associated with survival in acute lung injury. Am. J. Respir. Crit. Care Med. 172*, 854-860.

Camargo, F. D., Chambers, S. M. and Goodell, M. A. (2004). Stem cell plasticity: from transdifferentiation to macrophage fusion. *Cell Prolif. 37*, 55-65.

Chang, J. C., Summer, R., Sun, X., Fitzsimmons, K. and Fine, A. (2005). Evidence that bone marrow cells do not contribute to the alveolar epithelium. *Am. J. Respir. Cell Mol. Biol. 33*, 335-342.

Chaouat, A., Bugnet, A. S., Kadaoui, N., Schott, R., Enache, I., Ducolone, A., Ehrhart, M., Kessler, R. and Weitzenblum, E. (2005). Severe pulmonary hypertension and chronic obstructive pulmonary disease. *Am. J. Respir. Crit. Care Med. 172*, 189-194.

Conese, M. and Rejman, J. (2006). Stem cells and cystic fibrosis. *J. Cyst. Fibros. 5*, 141-143.

Davie, N. J., Crossno, J. T., Jr., Frid, M. G., Hofmeister, S. E., Reeves, J. T., Hyde, D. M., Carpenter, T. C., Brunetti, J. A., McNiece, I. K. and Stenmark, K. R. (2004). Hypoxia-induced pulmonary artery adventitial remodeling and neovascularization: contribution of progenitor cells. *Am. J. Physiol. Lung Cell Mol. Physiol. 286*, L668-678.

Davies, J. C., Potter, M., Bush, A., Rosenthal, M., Geddes, D. M. and Alton, E. W. (2002). Bone marrow stem cells do not repopulate the healthy upper respiratory tract. *Pediatr. Pulmonol. 34*, 251-256.

Denburg, J. A. and van Eeden, S. F. (2006). Bone marrow progenitors in inflammation and repair: new vistas in respiratory biology and pathophysiology. *Eur. Respir. J. 27*, 441-445.

Direkze, N. C., Forbes, S. J., Brittan, M., Hunt, T., Jeffery, R., Preston, S. L., Poulsom, R., Hodivala-Dilke, K., Alison, M. R. and Wright, N. A. (2003). Multiple organ engraftment by bone-marrow-derived myofibroblasts and fibroblasts in bone-marrow-transplanted mice. *Stem Cells. 21*, 514-520.

Donnelly, G. M., Haack, D. G. and Heird, C. S. (1982). Tracheal epithelium: cell kinetics and differentiation in normal rat tissue. *Cell Tissue Kinet. 15*, 119-130.

Eglitis, M. A. and Mezey, E. (1997). Hematopoietic cells differentiate into both microglia and macroglia in the brains of adult mice. *Proc. Natl. Acad. Sci. U S A. 94*, 4080-4085.

Elias, J. A., Zhu, Z., Chupp, G. and Homer, R. J. (1999). Airway remodeling in asthma. *J. Clin. Invest. 104*, 1001-1006.

Engelhardt, J. F., Yankaskas, J. R., Ernst, S. A., Yang, Y., Marino, C. R., Boucher, R. C., Cohn, J. A. and Wilson, J. M. (1992). Submucosal glands are the predominant site of CFTR *expression in the human bronchus. Nat. Genet. 2*, 240-247.

Engelhardt, J. F., Zepeda, M., Cohn, J. A., Yankaskas, J. R. and Wilson, J. M. (1994). Expression of the cystic fibrosis gene in adult human lung. *J. Clin. Invest. 93*, 737-749.

Engelhardt, J. F., Schlossberg, H., Yankaskas, J. and Dudus, L. (1995). Progenitor cells of the adult human airway involved in submucosal gland development. *Development. 121*, 2031-2046.

Engelhardt, J. F. (2001). Stem cell niches in the mouse airway. *Am. J. Respir. Cell Mol. Biol. 24*, 649-652.

Epperly, M. W., Guo, H., Gretton, J. E. and Greenberger, J. S. (2003). Bone marrow origin of myofibroblasts in irradiation pulmonary fibrosis. *Am. J. Respir. Cell Mol. Biol. 29*, 213-224.

Evans, M. J., Cabral, L. J., Stephens, R. J. and Freeman, G. (1973). Renewal of alveolar epithelium in the rat following exposure to NO2. *Am. J. Pathol. 70*, 175-198.

Evans, M. J., Cabral, L. J., Stephens, R. J. and Freeman, G. (1975). Transformation of alveolar type 2 cells to type 1 cells following exposure to NO2. *Exp. Mol. Pathol. 22*, 142-150.

Evans, M. J., Johnson, L. V., Stephens, R. J. and Freeman, G. (1976). Renewal of the terminal bronchiolar epithelium in the rat following exposure to NO2 or O3. *Lab. Invest. 35*, 246-257.

Evans, M. J., Shami, S. G., Cabral-Anderson, L. J. and Dekker, N. P. (1986). Role of nonciliated cells in renewal of the bronchial epithelium of rats exposed to NO2. *Am. J. Pathol. 123*, 126-133.

Fadini, G. P., Schiavon, M., Cantini, M., Baesso, I., Facco, M., Miorin, M., Tassinato, M., de Kreutzenberg, S. V., Avogaro, A. and Agostini, C. (2006). Circulating progenitor cells are reduced in patients with severe lung disease. *Stem Cells. 24*, 1806-1813.

Fang, T. C., Alison, M. R., Wright, N. A. and Poulsom, R. (2004). Adult stem cell plasticity: will engineered tissues be rejected? *Int. J. Exp. Pathol. 85*, 115-124.

Ferrari, G., Cusella-De Angelis, G., Coletta, M., Paolucci, E., Stornaiuolo, A., Cossu, G. and Mavilio, F. (1998). Muscle regeneration by bone marrow-derived myogenic progenitors. *Science. 279*, 1528-1530.

Frid, M. G., Brunetti, J. A., Burke, D. L., Carpenter, T. C., Davie, N. J. and Stenmark, K. R. (2005). Circulating mononuclear cells with a dual, macrophage-fibroblast phenotype contribute robustly to hypoxia-induced pulmonary adventitial remodeling. *Chest. 128*, 583S-584S.

Frid, M. G., Brunetti, J. A., Burke, D. L., Carpenter, T. C., Davie, N. J., Reeves, J. T., Roedersheimer, M. T., van Rooijen, N. and Stenmark, K. R. (2006). Hypoxia-induced pulmonary vascular remodeling requires recruitment of circulating mesenchymal precursors of a monocyte/macrophage lineage. *Am. J. Pathol. 168*, 659-669.

Giangreco, A., Reynolds, S. D. and Stripp, B. R. (2002). Terminal bronchioles harbor a unique airway stem cell population that localizes to the bronchoalveolar duct junction. *Am. J. Pathol. 161*, 173-182.

Giangreco, A., Shen, H., Reynolds, S. D. and Stripp, B. R. (2004). Molecular phenotype of airway side population cells. *Am. J. Physiol. Lung Cell Mol. Physiol. 286*, L624-630.

Gibson, R. L., Burns, J. L. and Ramsey, B. W. (2003). Pathophysiology and management of pulmonary infections in cystic fibrosis. *Am. J. Respir. Crit. Care Med. 168*, 918-951.

Gomperts, B. N., Belperio, J. A., Rao, P. N., Randell, S. H., Fishbein, M. C., Burdick, M. D. and Strieter, R. M. (2006). Circulating progenitor epithelial cells traffic via CXCR4/CXCL12 in response to airway injury. *J. Immunol. 176*, 1916-1927.

Gomperts, B. N. and Strieter, R. M. (2007a). Stem cells and chronic lung disease. *Annu. Rev. Med. 58*, 285-298.

Gomperts, B. N. and Strieter, R. M. (2007b). Fibrocytes in lung disease. *J. Leukoc. Biol.* 82, 449-456.

Goodell, M. A., Brose, K., Paradis, G., Conner, A. S. and Mulligan, R. C. (1996). Isolation and functional properties of murine hematopoietic stem cells that are replicating in vivo. *J. Exp. Med. 183*, 1797-1806.

Griffiths, M. J., Bonnet, D. and Janes, S. M. (2005). Stem cells of the alveolar epithelium. *Lancet. 366*, 249-260.

Grove, J. E., Lutzko, C., Priller, J., Henegariu, O., Theise, N. D., Kohn, D. B. and Krause, D. S. (2002). Marrow-derived cells as vehicles for delivery of gene therapy to pulmonary epithelium. *Am. J. Respir. Cell Mol. Biol. 27*, 645-651.

Gussoni, E., Soneoka, Y., Strickland, C. D., Buzney, E. A., Khan, M. K., Flint, A. F., Kunkel, L. M. and Mulligan, R. C. (1999). Dystrophin expression in the mdx mouse restored by stem cell transplantation. *Nature. 401*, 390-394.

Hajj, R., Baranek, T., Le Naour, R., Lesimple, P., Puchelle, E. and Coraux, C. (2007). Basal cells of the human adult airway surface epithelium retain transit-amplifying cell properties. *Stem Cells. 25*, 139-148.

Harris, R. G., Herzog, E. L., Bruscia, E. M., Grove, J. E., Van Arnam, J. S. and Krause, D. S. (2004). Lack of fusion requirement for development of bone marrow-derived epithelia. *Science. 305*, 90-93.

Hashimoto, N., Jin, H., Liu, T., Chensue, S. W. and Phan, S. H. (2004). Bone marrow-derived progenitor cells in pulmonary fibrosis. *J. Clin. Invest. 113*, 243-252.

Herzog, E. L., Chai, L. and Krause, D. S. (2003). Plasticity of marrow derived stem cells. *Blood .102*, 3483-3493.

Herzog, E. L., Van Arnam, J., Hu, B. and Krause, D. S. (2006). *Threshold of lung injury required for the appearance of marrow-derived lung epithelia. Stem Cells. 24*, 1986-1992.

Herzog, E. L., Van Arnam, J., Hu, B., Zhang, J., Chen, Q., Haberman, A. M. and Krause, D. S. (2007). Lung-specific nuclear reprogramming is accompanied by heterokaryon formation and Y chromosome loss following bone marrow transplantation and secondary inflammation. *Faseb J.*

Hill, J. M., Zalos, G., Halcox, J. P., Schenke, W. H., Waclawiw, M. A., Quyyumi, A. A. and Finkel, T. (2003). Circulating endothelial progenitor cells, vascular function, and cardiovascular risk. *N. Engl. J. Med. 348*, 593-600.

Hong, K. U., Reynolds, S. D., Giangreco, A., Hurley, C. M. and Stripp, B. R. (2001). Clara cell secretory protein-expressing cells of the airway neuroepithelial body microenvironment include a label-retaining subset and are critical for epithelial renewal after progenitor cell depletion. *Am. J. Respir. Cell Mol. Biol. 24*, 671-681.

Hopkins, N. and McLoughlin, P. (2002). The structural basis of pulmonary hypertension in chronic lung disease: remodelling, rarefaction or angiogenesis? *J. Anat. 201*, 335-348.

Hu, B., Wu, Z. and Phan, S. H. (2003). Smad3 mediates transforming growth factor-beta-induced alpha-smooth muscle actin expression. *Am. J. Respir. Cell Mol. Biol. 29*, 397-404.

Ishizawa, K., Kubo, H., Yamada, M., Kobayashi, S., Suzuki, T., Mizuno, S., Nakamura, T. and Sasaki, H. (2004). Hepatocyte growth factor induces angiogenesis in injured lungs through mobilizing endothelial progenitor cells. *Biochem. Biophys. Res. Commun. 324*, 276-280.

Jiang, Y., Jahagirdar, B. N., Reinhardt, R. L., Schwartz, R. E., Keene, C. D., Ortiz-Gonzalez, X. R., Reyes, M., Lenvik, T., Lund, T., Blackstad, M., Du, J., Aldrich, S., Lisberg, A., Low, W. C., Largaespada, D. A. and Verfaillie, C. M. (2002). Pluripotency of mesenchymal stem cells derived from adult marrow. *Nature. 418*, 41-49.

Keane, M. P. (2004). Angiogenesis and pulmonary fibrosis: feast or famine? *Am. J. Respir. Crit. Care Med. 170*, 207-209.

Kim, C. F., Jackson, E. L., Woolfenden, A. E., Lawrence, S., Babar, I., Vogel, S., Crowley, D., Bronson, R. T. and Jacks, T. (2005). Identification of bronchioalveolar stem cells in normal lung and lung cancer. *Cell. 121*, 823-835.

Kleeberger, W., Versmold, A., Rothamel, T., Glockner, S., Bredt, M., Haverich, A., Lehmann, U. and Kreipe, H. (2003). Increased chimerism of bronchial and alveolar epithelium in human lung allografts undergoing chronic injury. *Am. J. Pathol. 162*, 1487-1494.

Kopen, G. C., Prockop, D. J. and Phinney, D. G. (1999). *Marrow stromal cells migrate throughout forebrain and cerebellum, and they differentiate into astrocytes after injection into neonatal mouse brains. Proc. Natl. Acad. Sci. U S A. 96*, 10711-10716.

Korbling, M. and Estrov, Z. (2003). Adult stem cells for tissue repair - a new therapeutic concept? *N. Engl. J. Med. 349*, 570-582.

Kotton, D. N., Ma, B. Y., Cardoso, W. V., Sanderson, E. A., Summer, R. S., Williams, M. C. and Fine, A. (2001). Bone marrow-derived cells as progenitors of lung alveolar epithelium. *Development. 128*, 5181-5188.

Kotton, D. N. and Fine, A. (2003). Derivation of lung epithelium from bone marrow cells. *Cytotherapy. 5*, 169-173.

Kotton, D. N., Fabian, A. J. and Mulligan, R. C. (2005). Failure of bone marrow to reconstitute lung epithelium. *Am. J. Respir. Cell Mol. Biol. 33*, 328-334.

Krause, D. S., Theise, N. D., Collector, M. I., Henegariu, O., Hwang, S., Gardner, R., Neutzel, S. and Sharkis, S. J. (2001). Multi-organ, multi-lineage engraftment by a single bone marrow-derived stem cell. *Cell. 105*, 369-377.

Kreda, S., Mall, M., Mengos, A., Rochelle, L., Yankaskas, J., Riordan, J. R. and Boucher, R. C. (2005). Characterization of wild-type and deltaF508 cystic fibrosis transmembrane regulator in human respiratory epithelia. *Mol. Biol. Cell. 16*, 2154-2167.

Lagasse, E., Connors, H., Al-Dhalimy, M., Reitsma, M., Dohse, M., Osborne, L., Wang, X., Finegold, M., Weissman, I. L. and Grompe, M. (2000). Purified hematopoietic stem cells can differentiate into hepatocytes in vivo. *Nat. Med. 6*, 1229-1234.

Lama, V. N. and Phan, S. H. (2006). The extrapulmonary origin of fibroblasts. *Proc. Am. Thorac Soc. 3*, 373-376.

Lama, V. N., Smith, L., Badri, L., Flint, A., Andrei, A. C., Murray, S., Wang, Z., Liao, H., Toews, G. B., Krebsbach, P. H., Peters-Golden, M., Pinsky, D. J., Martinez, F. J. and Thannickal, V. J. (2007). Evidence for tissue-resident mesenchymal stem cells in human adult lung from studies of transplanted allografts. *J. Clin. Invest. 117*, 989-996.

Leigh, M. W., Kylander, J. E., Yankaskas, J. R. and Boucher, R. C. (1995). Cell proliferation in bronchial epithelium and submucosal glands of cystic fibrosis patients. *Am. J. Respir. Cell Mol. Biol. 12*, 605-612.

Lemischka, I. (2002). A few thoughts about the plasticity of stem cells. *Exp. Hematol. 30*, 848-852.

Liu, J. Y., Nettesheim, P. and Randell, S. H. (1994). Growth and differentiation of tracheal epithelial progenitor cells. *Am. J. Physiol. 266*, L296-307.

Liu, X., Driskell, R. R. and Engelhardt, J. F. (2006). Stem cells in the lung. *Methods Enzymol. 419*, 285-321.

Loi, R., Beckett, T., Goncz, K. K., Suratt, B. T. and Weiss, D. J. (2006). Limited restoration of cystic fibrosis lung epithelium in vivo with adult marrow derived cells. *Am. J. Respir. Crit. Care Med. 173*, 171-179.

Macpherson, H., Keir, P., Webb, S., Samuel, K., Boyle, S., Bickmore, W., Forrester, L. and Dorin, J. (2005). Bone marrow-derived SP cells can contribute to the respiratory tract of mice in vivo. *J. Cell Sci. 118*, 2441-2450.

MacPherson, H., Keir, P. A., Edwards, C. J., Webb, S. and Dorin, J. R. (2006). Following damage, the majority of bone marrow-derived airway cells express an epithelial marker. *Respir. Res. 7*, 145.

Mason, R. J., Williams, M. C., Moses, H. L., Mohla, S. and Berberich, M. A. (1997). Stem cells in lung development, disease, and therapy. *Am. J. Respir. Cell Mol. Biol. 16*, 355-363.

Mattsson, J., Jansson, M., Wernerson, A. and Hassan, M. (2004). Lung epithelial cells and type II pneumocytes of donor origin after allogeneic hematopoietic stem cell transplantation. *Transplantation. 78*, 154-157.

Metz, C. N. (2003). Fibrocytes: a unique cell population implicated in wound healing. *Cell Mol. Life Sci. 60*, 1342-1350.

Mishra, A., Greaves, R. and Massie, J. (2005). The relevance of sweat testing for the diagnosis of cystic fibrosis in the genomic era. *Clin. Biochem. Rev. 26*, 135-153.

Moore, B. B., Kolodsick, J. E., Thannickal, V. J., Cooke, K., Moore, T. A., Hogaboam, C., Wilke, C. A. and Toews, G. B. (2005). CCR2-mediated recruitment of fibrocytes to the alveolar space after fibrotic injury. *Am. J. Pathol. 166*, 675-684.

Nagaya, N., Kangawa, K., Kanda, M., Uematsu, M., Horio, T., Fukuyama, N., Hino, J., Harada-Shiba, M., Okumura, H., Tabata, Y., Mochizuki, N., Chiba, Y., Nishioka, K., Miyatake, K., Asahara, T., Hara, H. and Mori, H. (2003). Hybrid cell-gene therapy for pulmonary hypertension based on phagocytosing action of endothelial progenitor cells. *Circulation. 108*, 889-895.

Neuringer, I. P. and Randell, S. H. (2004). Stem cells and repair of lung injuries. *Respir. Res. 5*, 6.

Neuringer, I. P. and Randell, S. H. (2006). Lung stem cell update: promise and controversy. *Monaldi Arch. Chest Dis. 65*, 47-51.

Orkin, S. H. and Morrison, S. J. (2002). Stem-cell competition. *Nature. 418*, 25-27.

Orlic, D., Kajstura, J., Chimenti, S., Jakoniuk, I., Anderson, S. M., Li, B., Pickel, J., McKay, R., Nadal-Ginard, B., Bodine, D. M., Leri, A. and Anversa, P. (2001). Bone marrow cells regenerate infarcted myocardium. *Nature. 410*, 701-705.

Ortiz, L. A., Gambelli, F., McBride, C., Gaupp, D., Baddoo, M., Kaminski, N. and Phinney, D. G. (2003). Mesenchymal stem cell engraftment in lung is enhanced in response to bleomycin exposure and ameliorates its fibrotic effects. *Proc. Natl. Acad. Sci. U S A. 100*, 8407-8411.

Otto, W. R. (2002). Lung epithelial stem cells. *J. Pathol. 197*, 527-535.

Palange, P., Testa, U., Huertas, A., Calabro, L., Antonucci, R., Petrucci, E., Pelosi, E., Pasquini, L., Satta, A., Morici, G., Vignola, M. A. and Bonsignore, M. R. (2006). Circulating haemopoietic and endothelial progenitor cells are decreased in COPD. *Eur. Respir. J. 27*, 529-541.

Peichev, M., Naiyer, A. J., Pereira, D., Zhu, Z., Lane, W. J., Williams, M., Oz, M. C., Hicklin, D. J., Witte, L., Moore, M. A. and Rafii, S. (2000). Expression of VEGFR-2 and AC133 by circulating human CD34(+) cells identifies a population of functional endothelial precursors. *Blood. 95*, 952-958.

Petersen, B. E., Bowen, W. C., Patrene, K. D., Mars, W. M., Sullivan, A. K., Murase, N., Boggs, S. S., Greenberger, J. S. and Goff, J. P. (1999). Bone marrow as a potential source of hepatic oval cells. *Science. 284*, 1168-1170.

Phan, S. H. (2002). The myofibroblast in pulmonary fibrosis. *Chest. 122*, 286S-289S.

Phillips, R. J., Burdick, M. D., Hong, K., Lutz, M. A., Murray, L. A., Xue, Y. Y., Belperio, J. A., Keane, M. P. and Strieter, R. M. (2004). Circulating fibrocytes traffic to the lungs in response to CXCL12 and mediate fibrosis. *J. Clin. Invest. 114*, 438-446.

Pittenger, M. F., Mackay, A. M., Beck, S. C., Jaiswal, R. K., Douglas, R., Mosca, J. D., Moorman, M. A., Simonetti, D. W., Craig, S. and Marshak, D. R. (1999). Multilineage potential of adult human mesenchymal stem cells. *Science. 284*, 143-147.

Priller, J., Persons, D. A., Klett, F. F., Kempermann, G., Kreutzberg, G. W. and Dirnagl, U. (2001). Neogenesis of cerebellar Purkinje neurons from gene-marked bone marrow cells in vivo. *J. Cell Biol. 155*, 733-738.

Prockop, D. J. (1997). Marrow stromal cells as stem cells for nonhematopoietic tissues. *Science. 276*, 71-74.

Prockop, D. J., Gregory, C. A. and Spees, J. L. (2003). One strategy for cell and gene therapy: harnessing the power of adult stem cells to repair tissues. *Proc. Natl. Acad. Sci. U S A. 100 Suppl 1*, 11917-11923.

Quan, T. E., Cowper, S., Wu, S. P., Bockenstedt, L. K. and Bucala, R. (2004). Circulating fibrocytes: collagen-secreting cells of the peripheral blood. *Int. J. Biochem. Cell Biol. 36*, 598-606.

Rahaman, M. N. and Mao, J. J. (2005). Stem cell-based composite tissue constructs for regenerative medicine. *Biotechnol. Bioeng. 91*, 261-284.

Randell, S. H. (2006). Airway epithelial stem cells and the pathophysiology of chronic obstructive pulmonary disease. *Proc. Am. Thorac. Soc. 3*, 718-725.

Rawlins, E. L. and Hogan, B. L. (2006). Epithelial stem cells of the lung: privileged few or opportunities for many? *Development. 133*, 2455-2465.

Rawlins, E. L., Ostrowski, L. E., Randell, S. H. and Hogan, B. L. (2007). Lung development and repair: contribution of the ciliated lineage. *Proc Natl Acad Sci U S A 104*, 410-417.

Reddy, R., Buckley, S., Doerken, M., Barsky, L., Weinberg, K., Anderson, K. D., Warburton, D. and Driscoll, B. (2004). Isolation of a putative progenitor subpopulation of alveolar epithelial type 2 cells. *Am. J. Physiol. Lung Cell Mol. Physiol. 286*, L658-667.

Redington, A. E. and Howarth, P. H. (1997). Airway wall remodelling in asthma. *Thorax. 52*, 310-312.

Renzoni, E. A. (2004). *Neovascularization in idiopathic pulmonary fibrosis: too much or too little? Am. J. Respir. Crit. Care Med. 169*, 1179-1180.

Reynolds, S. D., Giangreco, A., Hong, K. U., McGrath, K. E., Ortiz, L. A. and Stripp, B. R. (2004). Airway injury in lung disease pathophysiology: selective depletion of airway stem and progenitor cell pools potentiates lung inflammation and alveolar dysfunction. *Am. J. Physiol. Lung Cell Mol. Physiol. 287*, L1256-1265.

Rojas, M., Xu, J., Woods, C. R., Mora, A. L., Spears, W., Roman, J. and Brigham, K. L. (2005). Bone marrow-derived mesenchymal stem cells in repair of the injured lung. *Am. J. Respir. Cell Mol. Biol. 33*, 145-152.

Rosenthal, N. (2003*). Prometheus's vulture and the stem-cell promise. N. Engl. J. Med. 349*, 267-274.

Sabatini, F., Petecchia, L., Tavian, M., Jodon de Villeroche, V., Rossi, G. A. and Brouty-Boye, D. (2005). Human bronchial fibroblasts exhibit a mesenchymal stem cell phenotype and multilineage differentiating potentialities. *Lab. Invest. 85*, 962-971.

Schmidt, M., Sun, G., Stacey, M. A., Mori, L. and Mattoli, S. (2003). Identification of circulating fibrocytes as precursors of bronchial myofibroblasts in asthma. *J. Immunol. 171*, 380-389.

Shi, Q., Rafii, S., Wu, M. H., Wijelath, E. S., Yu, C., Ishida, A., Fujita, Y., Kothari, S., Mohle, R., Sauvage, L. R., Moore, M. A., Storb, R. F. and Hammond, W. P. (1998). Evidence for circulating bone marrow-derived endothelial cells. *Blood. 92*, 362-367.

Spees, J. L., Olson, S. D., Ylostalo, J., Lynch, P. J., Smith, J., Perry, A., Peister, A., Wang, M. Y. and Prockop, D. J. (2003). Differentiation, cell fusion, and nuclear fusion during ex vivo repair of epithelium by human adult stem cells from bone marrow stroma. *Proc. Natl. Acad. Sci. U S A. 100*, 2397-2402.

Spencer, H. and Jaffe, A. (2004). The potential for stem cell therapy in cystic fibrosis. *J. R. Soc. Med. 97 Suppl 44*, 52-56.

Spencer, H., Rampling, D., Aurora, P., Bonnet, D., Hart, S. L. and Jaffe, A. (2005). Transbronchial biopsies provide longitudinal evidence for epithelial chimerism in children following sex mismatched lung transplantation. *Thorax. 60*, 60-62.

Stenmark, K. R., Davie, N. J., Reeves, J. T. and Frid, M. G. (2005). Hypoxia, leukocytes, and the pulmonary circulation. *J. Appl. Physiol. 98*, 715-721.

Stripp, B. R., Maxson, K., Mera, R. and Singh, G. (1995). Plasticity of airway cell proliferation and gene expression after acute naphthalene injury. *Am. J. Physiol. 269*, L791-799.

Stripp, B. R. and Shapiro, S. D. (2006). Stem cells in lung disease, repair, and the potential for therapeutic interventions: State-of-the-art and future challenges. *Am. J. Respir. Cell. Mol Biol 34*, 517-518.

Summer, R., Kotton, D. N., Sun, X., Ma, B., Fitzsimmons, K. and Fine, A. (2003). Side population cells and Bcrp1 expression in lung. *Am. J. Physiol. Lung Cell Mol. Physiol. 285*, L97-104.

Suratt, B. T., Cool, C. D., Serls, A. E., Chen, L., Varella-Garcia, M., Shpall, E. J., Brown, K. K. and Worthen, G. S. (2003). Human pulmonary chimerism after hematopoietic stem cell transplantation. *Am. J. Respir. Crit. Care Med. 168*, 318-322.

Takahashi, M., Nakamura, T., Toba, T., Kajiwara, N., Kato, H. and Shimizu, Y. (2004). Transplantation of endothelial progenitor cells into the lung to alleviate pulmonary hypertension in dogs. *Tissue Eng. 10*, 771-779.

Theise, N. D., Badve, S., Saxena, R., Henegariu, O., Sell, S., Crawford, J. M. and Krause, D. S. (2000). Derivation of hepatocytes from bone marrow cells in mice after radiation-induced myeloablation. *Hepatology. 31*, 235-240.

Theise, N. D., Henegariu, O., Grove, J., Jagirdar, J., Kao, P. N., Crawford, J. M., Badve, S., Saxena, R. and Krause, D. S. (2002). Radiation pneumonitis in mice: A sever injury model for pneumocyte engraftment from bone marrow. *Exp. Hematol. 30*, 1333-1338.

Thomas, C. E., Ehrhardt, A. and Kay, M. A. (2003). Progress and problems with the use of viral vectors for gene therapy. *Nat. Rev. Genet. 4*, 346-358.

van Haaften, T. and Thebaud, B. (2006). Adult bone marrow-derived stem cells for the lung: implications for pediatric lung diseases. *Pediatr. Res. 59*, 94R-99R.

Van Winkle, L. S., Buckpitt, A. R., Nishio, S. J., Isaac, J. M. and Plopper, C. G. (1995). Cellular response in naphthalene-induced Clara cell injury and bronchiolar epithelial repair in mice. *Am. J. Physiol. 269*, L800-818.

Vassilopoulos, G., Wang, P. R. and Russell, D. W. (2003). Transplanted bone marrow regenerates liver by cell fusion. *Nature. 422*, 901-904.

Verfaillie, C. M. (2002). Hematopoietic stem cells for transplantation. *Nat. Immunol. 3*, 314-317.

Vracko, R. (1974). *Basal lamina scaffold-anatomy and significance for maintenance of orderly tissue structure. Am. J. Pathol. 77*, 314-346.

Wagers, A. J., Sherwood, R. I., Christensen, J. L. and Weissman, I. L. (2002). Little evidence for developmental plasticity of adult hematopoietic stem cells. *Science. 297*, 2256-2259.

Wagers, A. J. and Weissman, I. L. (2004). Plasticity of adult stem cells. *Cell. 116*, 639-645.

Wang, G., Bunnell, B. A., Painter, R. G., Quiniones, B. C., Tom, S., Lanson, N. A. J., Spees, J. L., Bertucci, D., Peister, A., Weiss, D. J., Valentine, V. G., Prockop, D. J. and Kolls, J. K. (2005). Adult stem cells from bone marrow stroma differentiate into airway epithelial cells: potential therapy for cystic fibrosis. *Proc. Natl. Acad. Sci. U S A. 102*, 186-191.

Wang, X., Willenbring, H., Akkari, Y., Torimaru, Y., Foster, M., Al-Dhalimy, M., Lagasse, E., Finegold, M., Olson, S. and Grompe, M. (2003). Cell fusion is the principal source of bone-marrow-derived hepatocytes. *Nature. 422*, 897-901.

Weiss, D. J., Berberich, M. A., Borok, Z., Gail, D. B., Kolls, J. K., Penland, C. and Prockop, D. J. (2006). Adult stem cells, lung biology, and lung disease. NHLBI/Cystic Fibrosis Foundation Workshop. *Proc. Am. Thorac. Soc. 3*, 193-207.

Weissman, I. L. (2000). Translating stem and progenitor cell biology to the clinic: barriers and opportunities. *Science. 287*, 1442-1446.

Willis, B. C., Liebler, J. M., Luby-Phelps, K., Nicholson, A. G., Crandall, E. D., du Bois, R. M. and Borok, Z. (2005). Induction of epithelial-mesenchymal transition in alveolar epithelial cells by transforming growth factor-beta1: potential role in idiopathic pulmonary fibrosis. *Am. J. Pathol. 166*, 1321-1332.

Willis, B. C., duBois, R. M. and Borok, Z. (2006). Epithelial origin of myofibroblasts during fibrosis in the lung. *Proc Am Thorac Soc 3*, 377-382.

Witschi, H. R., Haschek, W. M., Klein-Szanto, A. J. and Hakkinen, P. J. (1981). Potentiation of diffuse lung damage by oxygen: determining variables. *Am. Rev. Respir. Dis. 123*, 98-103.

Xu, J., Mora, A. L., LaVoy, J., Brigham, K. L. and Rojas, M. (2006). Increased bleomycin-induced lung injury in mice deficient in the transcription factor T-bet. *Am. J. Physiol. Lung Cell Mol. Physiol. 291*, L658-667.

Yamada, M., Kubo, H., Kobayashi, S., Ishizawa, K., Numasaki, M., Ueda, S., Suzuki, T. and Sasaki, H. (2004). Bone marrow-derived progenitor cells are important for lung repair after lipopolysaccharide-induced lung injury. *J. Immunol. 172*, 1266-1272.

Yamada, M., Kubo, H., Ishizawa, K., Kobayashi, S., Shinkawa, M. and Sasaki, H. (2005). Increased circulating endothelial progenitor cells in patients with bacterial pneumonia: evidence that bone marrow derived cells contribute to lung repair. *Thorax. 60*, 410-413.

Yano, T., Deterding, R. R., Simonet, W. S., Shannon, J. M. and Mason, R. J. (1996). Keratinocyte growth factor reduces lung damage due to acid instillation in rats. *Am. J. Respir. Cell Mol. Biol. 15*, 433-442.

Yen, C. C., Yang, S. H., Lin, C. Y. and Chen, C. M. (2006). Stem cells in the lung parenchyma and prospects for lung injury therapy. *Eur. J. Clin .Invest. 36*, 310-319.

Yi, E. S., Salgado, M., Williams, S., Kim, S. J., Masliah, E., Yin, S. and Ulich, T. R. (1998). Keratinocyte growth factor decreases pulmonary edema, transforming growth factor-beta and platelet-derived growth factor-BB expression, and alveolar type II cell loss in bleomycin-induced lung injury. *Inflammation. 22*, 315-325.

Zander, D. S., Baz, M. A., Cogle, C. R., Visner, G. A., Theise, N. D. and Crawford, J. M. (2005). Bone marrow-derived stem-cell repopulation contributes minimally to the Type II pneumocyte pool in transplanted human lungs. *Transplantation. 80*, 206-212.

Zhang, K., Rekhter, M. D., Gordon, D. and Phan, S. H. (1994). Myofibroblasts and their role in lung collagen gene expression during pulmonary fibrosis. A combined immunohistochemical and in situ hybridization study. *Am. J. Pathol. 145*, 114-125.

Zhao, Y. D., Courtman, D. W., Deng, Y., Kugathasan, L., Zhang, Q. and Stewart, D. J. (2005). Rescue of monocrotaline-induced pulmonary arterial hypertension using bone marrow-derived endothelial-like progenitor cells: efficacy of combined cell and eNOS gene therapy in established disease. *Circ. Res. 96*, 442-450.

In: Encyclopedia of Stem Cell Research (2 Volume Set)   ISBN: 978-1-61761-835-2
Editor: Alexander L. Greene   © 2012 Nova Science Publishers, Inc.

Chapter XXXVII

ROLE OF PLATELET DERIVED FACTORS FOR THE PROTECTION AGAINST GRAFT-VERSUS-HOST DISEASE

Tsuyoshi Iwasaki*

Division of Rheumatology and Clinical Immunology,
Department of Internal Medicine, Hyogo College of Medicine,
1-1 Mukogawa, Nishinomiya, Hyogo, Japan

ABSTRACT

Platelets exhibit the ability to release considerable quantities of secretory products such as proinflammatory mediators and growth factors and to express immune receptors on their membrane. These secretory products and immune receptors play significant roles in inflammation, immune reactions, and tissue regeneration. This review summarizes the secretory products and immune receptors of platelets and their roles for the pathogenesis of graft-versus-host disease (GVHD), focusing on mechanisms responsible for protection against GVHD by platelet derived factors such as hepatocyte growth factor and sphingosine 1-phosphate.

INTRODUCTION

The widespread application of allogeneic hematopoietic stem cell transplantation (HSCT) for treatment of hematological malignancies and other diseases is restricted by the poor availability of suitable donors. Significant barriers to successful major-human leukocyte antigen (HLA) mismatched HSCT include an increased risk of graft failure and the possible induction of severe and refractory acute and/or chronic graft-versus-host disease (GVHD).

* *Tsuyoshi Iwasaki;* Phone:+81-79845-6592; Fax: +81-79845-6593; email: tsuyo-i@hyo-med.ac.jp

Donor T cells play a key role by facilitating engraftment of the allograft and contributing to anti-tumor immunity, but are also primarily responsible for GVHD [1-8]. To date, the approaches to control acute GVHD have employed methods that attempt to remove or suppress the function of all T cells regardless of their immunologic specificity. Although the administration of immunosuppressants achieves an acceptable rate of engraftment with reasonable control of GVHD, these drugs induce a generalized decrease of immunocompetence with its attendant morbidity and mortality. Immunosuppressants may also have significant acute and chronic adverse effects upon organ function [9, 10]. Ex vivo T cell depletion of donor HSCs appears to be more effective at ameliorating or even eliminating GVHD, but this approach is complicated by an unacceptable incidence of graft failure, profound and protracted immunodeficiency and loss of anti-tumor immunity [5-8]. GVHD is a complex process that is unlikely to be controllable by a single agent. Most studies show that partial benefits can be obtained through a variety of approaches including T cell depletion, inhibition of inflammatory cytokines, manipulation of co-stimulation and the use of anti-proliferative agents [5-8, 11, 12]. Therefore, a useful strategy would be to control GVHD by interfering with various steps in the underlying pathophysiology by synergistically employing several approaches.

Platelets are known for their role in haemostasis where they help to prevent blood loss at sites of vascular injury. On activation, platelets exhibit the ability to release considerable quantities of secretory products such as proinflammatory mediators and growth factors and express immune receptors on their membrane, playing significant roles in inflammatory or immune processes and in healing and tissue regeneration processes. This review summarizes the most important findings on the role of platelets in inflammation, immune system, and healing or tissue regeneration during GVHD and will focus on mechanisms responsible for protection against GVHD by platelet derived factors such as hepatocyte growth factor (HGF) and sphingosine 1-phosphate (S1P).

SURFACE MOLECULES ON PLATELETS

P-Selectin

P-Selectin is an integral membrane glycoprotein expressed by platelets [13], endothelial cells [14], and macrophages of atherosclerotic plaques [15]. P-selectin on platelets is an important adhesion molecule for P-selectin glycoprotein ligand-1 (PSGL-1)–bearing immune cells, as it mediates adhesion of activated platelets to monocytes, neutrophils, and lymphocytes, resulting in the formation of platelet/leukocyte complexes and supports leukocyte rolling and arrest on surface-adherent platelets [16-18]. Crosslinking of PSGL-1 on on monocytes by platelet P-selectin induces upregulation and activation of β_1 and β_2 integrins and enhances monocyte recruitment to activated endothelium [19]. It has been proposed that crosslinking PSGL-1 induces clustering of lymphocyte function-associated antigen-1 (LFA-1) 1) on T-helper 1 (Th1) cells [20] and clustering of Mac-1 on neutrophils [21].

Integrins

Platelets express several integrins, but glycoprotein GPIIb/IIIa ($\alpha_{IIb}\beta_3$) is clearly the predominant one [22, 23]. Ligation of $\alpha_{IIb}\beta_3$ through multivalent ligands such as fibrinogen, leads to clustering which is important in cytoskeletal rearrangement in the process of aggregation [24, 25]. Integrin $\alpha_{IIb}\beta_3$ links platelets to sites of injury in vessels through interaction with fibrinogen and von Willebrand factor, which in aggregate form a plug leading leading to hemostasis. Another binding partner of $\alpha_{IIb}\beta_3$ has been shown to be CD40 ligand (CD40L) expressed on the membrane of activated platelets, which is important in stabilizing arterial thrombi [26].

CD40 L

CD40L (also termed CD154) plays a crucial role in pathogen clearance. As a trimeric transmembrane protein, it is structurally related to the cytokine tumor necrosis factor (TNF)-α α and was originally identified on stimulated T cells [27, 28]. Subsequently, platelets were found to upregulate CD40L on activation, which results in stimulation of endothelial cells through its cognate receptor CD40 and in increased expression of adhesion molecules and chemokines enhancing the recruitment of immune cells [29, 30]. Ligation of CD40 by platelet-derived CD40L induces dendritic cell maturation, B-cell isotype switching, and augmentation of CD8$^+$ T cell responses both in vitro and in vivo, causing enhanced protection protection against viral re-challenge [31]. Platelet-derived or even soluble CD40L has recently been found to be sufficient for the initiation and induction of vascularized allograft rejection [32].

CD40

Serving as the receptor for CD40L, CD40 is a trimeric transmembrane protein and belongs to the TNF receptor superfamily. CD40 is displayed by a wide range of immune cells cells including monocytes, dendritic cells, and B cells and contributes to the development of the acquired immune response, depending on its activation and subsequent signal transduction transduction by CD40L [33]. CD40 is not only constitutively expressed on platelets but plays plays an important role in confining the inflammatory response induced by CD40L by inducing the cleavage of CD40L, which results in a 18-kDa soluble form without an inflammatory effect on endothelial cells [34].

Toll-Like Receptors

Initial clearance by innate immune responses is mediated by a group of receptors termed Toll-like receptors (TLRs). Several human and murine TLRs have been characterized, and they recognize a variety of molecular structures found on bacteria, viruses, and fungi [35-37].

Recognition of these molecules leads to TLR signaling primarily through a MyD88-dependent pathway that, in turn, leads to the production of several proinflammatory cytokines [38]. Similar to septicemia in humans, LPS has been shown to induce thrombocytopenia in a mouse mouse model through TLR4-dependent sequestration of platelets to the lungs. This has been attributed to platelet activation via TLR4, which resulted in increased adhesiveness to fibrinogen but was not associated with increased expression of P-selectin, in line with the inability of LPS to induce platelet aggregation or calcium influx [39, 40]. Further support for the functional activity of platelet TLR4 comes from studies showing an in vivo role for LPS-stimulated platelets in triggering TNF-α secretion and confirming the TLR4-dependent thrombocytopenia [41]. Other bacterial pathogens linking platelets to inflammatory responses responses include infections with rickettsia, which can activate platelets via TLR2 and lead to to increased shedding of CD40L [42].

SOLUBLE MEDIATORS IN PLATELETS

Chemokines

Depending on the position of the first N-terminal cysteines that are either adjacent or separated by 1 amino acid residue, chemokines are divided into 2 large subfamilies (CC and CXC chemokines) [43, 44]. In platelets, chemokines synthesized by megakaryocytes are stored within the αgranules and may, in part, be expressed from mRNA transcripts that can be be found in mature platelets [45]. Platelet factor 4 (PF4, CXCL4) together with the ß-thromboglobulins (ß-TGs) are the most abundantly expressed platelet CXC chemokines [46]. PF4 induces exocytosis and firm neutrophil adhesion to endothelium [47, 48]. The CC chemokine RANTES has been found by using a cDNA library enriched for T cell–specific sequences and causes the selective migration of human blood monocytes and T cells [49, 50]. 50]. Later, thrombin stimulation of human platelets was shown to result in the release of RANTES [51]. RANTES play an important role in various immune and allergic disorders. RANTES is a potent chemoattractant for various inflammatory cells such as eosinophils, as well as for memory T cells and monocytes, thus potentially recruiting these cells from the circulation to an inflamed focus.

Cytokines and Growth Factors

Interleukin (IL)-1 is the prototypic cytokine released by inflammatory cells. Whereas IL-1α, because of the lack of a leader sequence, is primarily an intracellular regulator of proinflammatory events, its sibling IL-1ß is a secretable mediator [52-54]. It was demonstrated that platelets do not only contain preformed IL-1ß but that platelet activation induces rapid and sustained synthesis of pro-IL-1ß protein, which is shed in its mature form in in membrane microvesicles and is controlled at the translational level by activation of platelet platelet integrins [55, 56]. There are also various mitogenic factors in platelets essential for wound repair such as platelet-derived growth factor (PDGF), transforming growth factor β

(TGF-β), vascular endothelial growth factor (VEGF), HGF, basic fibroblastic growth factor (bFGF), insulin-like growth factor (IGF-1) [57-65]. It should be noted that some of these growth factors may have both pro and anti-angiogenic properties depending on the situation.

ACTIVE METABOLITES

Platelets provide eicosanoids synthesized from arachidonic acid released from membrane membrane phospholipids. Thromboxian A2 (TXA2) is a powerful vasoconstrictor but is also involved in the injury-induced vascular proliferative response, a process regulated by prostacyclin [66]. S1P is a novel active metabolite able to stimulate mitogenesis. This is liberated from activated platelets during clot formation and stimulates fibronectin matrix assembly through Rho-dependent signaling pathway [67, 68]. Platelet-activating factor (PAF) (PAF) is another platelet-derived bioactive lipid and can play a role in mediating leukocyte arrest and activation on endothelial cells or adherent platelets through P-selectin-dependent mechanisms [69]

BIOLOGICAL EFFECTS OF HGF

HGF was originally identified and cloned as a potent growth factor of hepatocytes and has mitogenic, motogenic, morphogenic and anti-apoptotic effects on various cell types other than hepatocytes [70-74]. HGF is a heparin-binding glycoprotein that is secreted as pro-HGF, a single-chain biologically inert precursor. Under conditions such as tissue damage, pro-HGF is converted by proteolytic digestion to its bioactive heterodimer HGF comprised of a 60,000 Mr α and 30,000 Mr β chain held together by a single disulfide bond (figure 1A).

HGF is expressed in stromal cells such as fibroblasts, smooth muscle cells, mast cells, macrophages, endothelial cells, leukocytes, platelets and megakariocytes but not in epithelial cells. HGF receptor expression, however, is present mainly in epithelial cells. The HGF receptor is encoded by the c-met proto-oncogene and is a heterodimer held together by disulfide bonds. The HGF receptor consists of an α chain which remains entirely extracellular and a β chain which traverses the plasma membrane and contains the intracellular tyrosine kinase domain [75] (figure 1B).

As a result, HGF is an important paracrine mediator of the interaction between the epithelial and stromal compartments of various tissues during development and in the maintenance of tissue homeostasis. Although epithelial cells are one of the major targets of HGF, it is becoming clear that non-epithelial cells such as hematopoietic, endothelial, lymphoid, neural, skeletal muscle cells may also respond to HGF. HGF is highly expressed in the bone marrow, spleen, liver, lung, kidney and skin although other tissues also contain detectable levels of HGF. Plasma HGF levels are elevated in patients with liver and lung damage [76, 77]. In addition, intravenous injection of recombinant HGF enhances liver and kidney regeneration in mice, prevents acute renal failure and suppresses the onset of liver cirrhosis thereby suggesting that HGF plays an important role in tissue repair [78, 79].

A   **B**

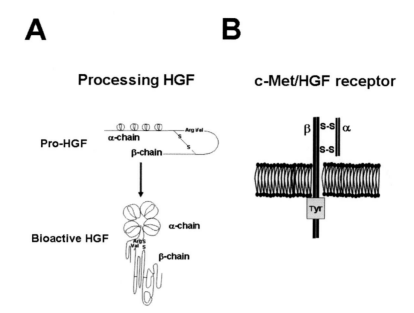

Figure 1. A. Processing HGF. HGF is secreted as an inactive single polypeptide pro HGF that requires proteolytic processing for conversion to the mature bioactive heterodimer HGF. Endoproteolytic processing between Arg[494] and Val[495] results in disulfide-linked α-chain and β-chain. B. c-Met/HGF receptor. The receptor for HGF is the heterodimeric tyrosine kinase encoded by the c-Met proto-oncogene and consists of an α chain which remains entirely extracellular and a β chain which traverses the plasma membrane and contains an intracellular tyrosine kinase domain.

BIOLOGICAL EFFECTS OF S1P

S1P is a cell-derived lysophospholipid growth factor that signals diverse cellular functions. Platelets, mononuclear phagocytes, some epithelial cells and some tumor cells are proven major sources of S1P [80]. S1P is generated by the metabolism of sphingomyelin with S1P levels being tightly regulated by a series of enzymes including sphingosin kinase, S1P phosphatase and S1P lyase. In circulating blood and lymph, S1P binds to albumin and some other proteins and attains blood and lymph concentrations of 0.1-1 µM [67]. Although the biological significance of observed S1P tissue distribution is yet to be determined, S1P is most abundant in the testis and intestine of all rat tissues examined [81-83]. S1P has been reported to have varied functions including platelet aggregation [84], mitogenesis [85] and cytoskeletal remodeling [86]. Such functions are mainly mediated by subfamilies of G protein-coupled receptors (GPCRs), of which the most completely characterized are those encoded by the endothelial differentiation gene (EDG) [87]. To date, five closely related GPCRs of the EDG family, namely S1P$_1$/EDG-1, S1P$_2$/EDG-5, S1P$_3$/EDG-3, S1P$_4$/EDG-6 and S1P$_5$/EDG-8, have been identified as high affinity S1P receptors. They are integral membrane proteins that are probably glycosylated, predicted to have seven transmembrane domains and exhibit approximately 50% amino acid sequence identity (figure 2).

Structures and metabolism of S1P

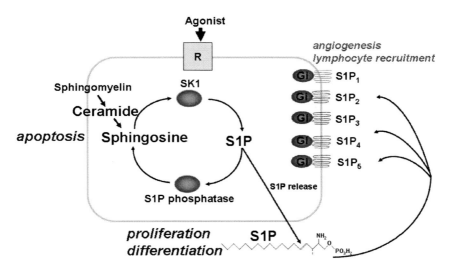

Figure 2. Pathways of S1P metabolism. S1P is generated by metabolism of sphingomyelin with S1P levels being tightly regulated by series of enzymes including sphingosine kinase (SK) and S1P phosphatase. S1P acts as an extracellular mediator by binding to G protein-coupled receptors (GPCRs) and promotes cell proliferation and differentiation, whereas sphingosine and ceramide inhibit cell proliferation and stimulate apoptosis. The balance of these three important lipid signal molecules is critically regulated by SK1, the agonist-inducible isoform that can be activated by a variety of growth factors, cytokines and mitogens. $S1P_1$ is one of the GPCRs of S1P, which promotes angiogenesis and the recruitment of lymphocytes.

$S1P_1$, $S1P_2$ and $S1P_3$ are widely expressed in various tissues whereas expression of $S1P_4$ is confined to lymphoid and hematopoietic tissues and $S1P_5$ expression is largely localized to the central nervous system [88]. S1P was defined as a novel regulator of angiogenesis and is a major bioactive lysophospholipid released from platelets that interacts with endothelial cells under conditions in which critical platelet-endothelial interactions take place such as thrombosis, angiogenesis and atherosclerosis [89].

PLATELETS ARE ACTIVE PLAYERS IN INFLAMMATION AND HEALING

Platelets interact with Gram-positive, Gram-negative bacteria and spirochetes, respond rapidly in the setting of vascular injury, aggregate after contact with bacteria through crossreactive immunodeterminants and plasma proteins, and have the ability to recognize pathogens via TLRs [90, 91]. Because of these rapid responses, platelets accumulate in the setting of endovascular infections such as infectious endocarditis where platelets represent a significant portion of infected cardiac vegetations and emboli and have been traditionally interpreted as contributors to the progression and complications of infectious endocarditis [92, [92, 93]. Besides bacteria, platelets are able to internalize HIV-1 and lentivirus through surface molecules expressed on platelets [94-96]. The capture of HIV-1 by these cells amounts to a considerable threat for the immune system, as platelets can remain infectious over a prolonged time, indicating that platelets might facilitate HIV-1 dissemination.

Autologous platelets can promote healing and wound repair by platelet-derived growth factors. Whitman et al. first used autologous platelets in reconstitutive oral and maxillofacial surgery [97]. Max et al. evaluated the effect of autologous platelets during bone graft reconstruction of mandibular continuity defects and concluded that addition of autologous platelets accelerated the rate and degree of bone formation [98]. Autologous platelets are also also effective for the treatment of skin ulcers, tendon and ligament repair [99, 100].

GVHD PATHOPHYSIOLOGY

Acute GVHD is a pathological state that arises secondary to donor T cell engraftment and manifests as skin rash, diarrhea, jaundice, and wasting; such that the predominant symptoms are related to the skin, liver, and gastrointestinal (GI) tract. The majority of patients with grade III to IV acute GVHD die of their disease (101). Chronic GVHD usually begins at least 100 days after HSCT and can evolve from acute GVHD, follow the resolution of acute GVHD, or even start in patients without any history of acute GVHD. Chronic GVHD can mimic certain autoimmune diseases such as systemic lupus erythematosus, systemic sclerosis, and Sjogren's syndrome [102]. Patients receiving peripheral blood stem cell transplantation have a higher incidence of chronic GVHD than those receiving standard HSCT (103). From the pathophysiological standpoint, the course of acute GVHD can be divided into three phases: (1) damage and cellular activation induced by the preconditioning treatment; (2) donor lymphocyte (T cells) activation; and (3) cellular and inflammatory effectors (104, 105) (figure 3).

Damage to the thymus may allow autoreactive T cells to escape negative selection, which then promote T-helper 2 (Th2) responses and autoreactive B cell activation, leading chronic GVHD (figure 4).

Phase 1 Damage and Cellular Activation Induced by Preconditioning

The first phase of acute GVHD occurs before the donor cells are even infused. Tissue damage caused by factors such as underlying disease, treatment of underlying disease, infection, and transplantation preconditioning can lead to cellular activation and release of inflammatory cytokines, including TNF-α, IL-1, and IL-6. These cytokines induce the up-regulation of host antigens and adhesion molecules, allowing donor T cells to respond to host antigens. Damage to the GI mucosa induced by preconditioning can permit bacteria and bacterial endotoxins to enter the systemic circulation from the GI tract, increasing the secretion of inflammatory cytokines from macrophages [106, 107].

Pathophysiology of acute GVHD

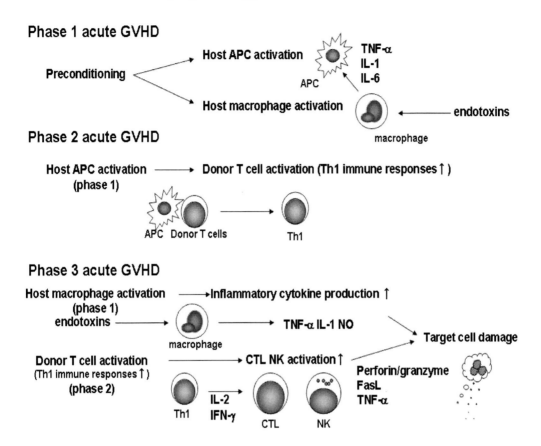

Phase 1 acute GVHD

Preconditioning

Host APC activation

Host macrophage activation

TNF-α
IL-1
IL-6

APC

macrophage ← endotoxins

Phase 2 acute GVHD

Host APC activation (phase 1) → Donor T cell activation (Th1 immune responses ↑)

APC Donor T cells

Th1

Phase 3 acute GVHD

Host macrophage activation (phase 1)
endotoxins → macrophage → Inflammatory cytokine production ↑

TNF-α IL-1 NO

Target cell damage

Donor T cell activation (Th1 immune responses ↑) (phase 2) → CTL NK activation ↑

Th1 IL-2 IFN-γ   CTL   NK

Perforin/granzyme
FasL
TNF-α

Figure 3. The pathophysiology of acute GVHD. Preconditioning, including irradiation and chemotherapy, leads to injury of host tissues, and the activation of host APCs and macrophages. Host tissue injury, involving the intestinal mucosa, allows translocation of endotoxins from the intestinal lumen into the systemic circulation, stimulating the secretion of TNF-α, IL-1, and IL-6 by macrophages. These cytokines increase the expression of MHC antigens and adhesion molecules on host APCs, enhancing the recognition of MHC antigens by mature donor T cells (phase 1). Donor T cells are activated after recognition of MHC antigens on host APCs, differentiate into Th1 cells. Th1 cells secrete IL-2 and IFN-γ, further expanding CTL and NK cell populations (phase 2). CTLs and NK cells expanded in phase 2 damage host tissues by perforin/granzyme and FasL pathways and TNF-α. Macrophages activated in phase 1 are further activated by endotoxins translocated from damaged gastrointestinal lumen, leading to a cytokine storm characteristic of acute GVHD (phase 3). APC: antigen presenting cell; CTL: cytotoxic T lymphocyte; FasL: Fas ligand; IFN: interferon; NK: natural killer; Th1: type 1 helper; TNF: tumor necrosis factor.

Pathophysiology of chronic GVHD

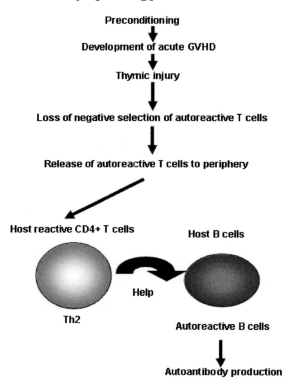

Figure 4. The pathophysiology of chronic GVHD. Chronic GVHD may be the result of autoreactive T cells that escape negative selection in the thymus damaged by preconditioning or acute GVHD. The Th2 immune response of donor CD4+ T cells released from escaped negative selection provide help to host B cells to synthesize autoantibodies.

Phase 2 Activation of Donor Lymphocytes (T Cells)

Donor T cell activation constitute the second phase of acute GVHD. Donor T cells recognize host antigen presenting cells (APCs) and differentiate into Th1 cells that secrete IFN-□ and IL-2 [108, 109].

Phase 3 Cellular and Inflammatory Effectors

In the third phase, target cells are injured. Th1 cells that underwent differentiation during phase 2 induce cytotoxic T cells (CTLs), and activate natural killer (NK) cells. These cells then attack various host target cells via Fas and perforin pathways. Th1 cells can also prime macrophages, which then leads to increased production of inflammatory cytokines, such as TNF-α IL-1, and nitric oxide (NO), in response to stimulation by endotoxins that enter the systemic circulation from the GI tract. These cytotoxic molecules directly attack various host tissues and underlie the clinical manifestations of acute GVHD [110].

Pathophysiology of Chronic GVHD

A murine model of chronic GVHD can be induced by the injection of DBA/2 (H-2^d) spleen cells into immunocompetent (C57BL/6 x DBA/2) F1 (H-$2^{b/d}$) mice, which then show features of a lupus-like disease with renal involvement, including autoantibody formation and polyclonal B cell activation. In this model, the small numbers of donor CD8+ CTL precursors lead to Th2 activation by donor CD4+ T cells and impaired elimination of autoreactive host B cells [111]. The thymus plays a critical role in the prevention of autoimmunity by eliminating autoreactive T cells. It has been suggested that chronic GVHD is caused by autoreactive T cells that escape negative selection in the thymus damaged by conditioning regimens, acute GVHD, and/or age-related atrophy [112]. Murine and human studies of chronic GVHD have revealed involution of the thymic epithelium, lymphocyte depletion, disappearance of Hassal corpuscles, and loss of thymic function [113, 114]. Taken together, these findings suggest that chronic GVHD which can occur months after the allogeneic HSCT may be due to the Th2 immune response of donor CD4+ T cells that escaped the negative thymic selection, and then go on to recognize major histocompatibility complex (MHC) antigens on host APCs. These donor CD4+ T cells then provide help to host B cells to synthesize autoantibodies against various host tissue antigens (figure 4).

ROLE OF HGF IN THE PATHOPHYSIOLOGY OF GVHD

HGF plays an important role in the protection against tissue injury and in tissue repair. Plasma HGF levels are elevated in patients with tissue injury such as liver and lung damage [77, 115]. Plasma HGF levels are also significantly elevated in patients with acute GVHD suggesting that HGF is produced to counteract the resultant tissue damage [116]. This increased plasma HGF may positively benefit patients with GVHD by protecting against tissue injury and enhancing tissue regeneration within injured organs. Experimental therapeutic strategies to protect tissues from injury using HGF have been reported. Recombinant HGF (rHGF) abrogates Fas-induced hepatocyte apoptosis [117] and endotoxin-induced fulminant hepatitis in which TNF-α is involved in the development of hepatic failure [118]. Since HGF protects tissues against injury mediated by FasL [117] and TNF-α[118], HGF may also protect against tissue injury caused by acute GVHD whose major effectors are both FasL and TNF-α [119]. We observed that HGF gene transfection prevented gastrointestinal tract injury caused by acute GVHD and ameliorated systemic GVHD [120]. HGF actively contributes to the recovery of hematopoiesis after HSCT. HGF may contribute both positively and negatively to immunity during acute GVHD by suppressing T cell proliferation [121] or by inducing macrophage activation [122]. Host DCs are crucial for activation of donor T cells and induction of acute GVHD [109]. Although HGF induces maturation of DCs from CD34+ bone marrow cells [123] and enhances the migration of mature DCs [124], its effect upon the antigen presenting functions of DCs is unclear. We observed that HGF gene transfection did not reduce donor T cell expansion in the spleen and thymus and preserved the graft-versus-leukemia (GVL) effect [125].

ROLE OF S1P IN THE PATHOPHYSIOLOGY OF GVHD

The roles of S1P and related lipid mediators for GVHD are not fully understood. However, one of the major features of the pathophysiology of acute GVHD is endothelial and epithelial cell damage caused by increased inflammatory cytokines and cellular effectors. As cytokine stimulation is a major trigger of S1P production from endothelial cells and S1P stimulates endothelial regeneration, the increased plasma level of S1P stimulated by inflammatory cytokines may protect against GVHD-induced endothelial cell damage. Although low concentrations of S1P increase mature T cell functions including chemotaxis, proliferation and cytokine production, high concentrations of S1P inhibit these functions [126]. This action of S1P suggests that the local production of S1P during inflammation could act to inhibit the cellular effector functions of GVHD. Furthermore, increased migratory capacity of hematopoietic progenitor cells by S1P may enhance hematopoietic progenitor cell engraftment. The immunosuppressant agent, FTY720 is structurally homologous to sphingosine and resembles S1P after phosphorylation. FTY720 binds to most of the S1P receptors and inhibits T cell chemotaxis to S1P in vitro [127]. It also suppresses lymphocyte migration out of secondary lymphoid organs in vivo thereby preventing homing to sites of antigen challenge [127, 128]. FTY720 is currently in clinical development but the molecular mechanisms that appear to cause immunosuppression by the sequestration of lymphocytes in secondary lymphoid organs are poorly understood. The suppressing effect of FTY720 on lymphocyte migration out of secondary lymphoid organs could provide an approach to separating GVHD and GVL effects. This was first suggested by the observation of an association between delayed administration of donor lymphocyte infusions to established mixed chimeras and GVHD alloresponses that convert mixed chimeras to full chimeras [129, 130] and mediate GVL effects [131] without causing GVHD. Subsequent experimentation demonstrated that FTY720 markedly reduced GVHD in a clinically relevant, haploidentical strain combination, whilst permitting anti-tumor actions against a T cell lymphoma [132].

PROTECTIVE CYTOKINES AND GROWTH FACTORS FOR GVHD

The usefulness of factors that protect against GVHD has been reported using murine GVHD models. Although IL-7 has been shown to enhance T-cell reconstitution after allogeneic HSCT by thymopoiesis and, in part, by expansion of mature donor T cells, it is currently unresolved whether IL-7 ameliorates or exacerbates GVHD [133-135]. IL-10 is a potent suppressor of TNF-α, IL-1, IL-6, IL-12 and IFN-γ production and may facilitate the induction of tolerance after allogeneic HSCT [136-138]. The administration of IL-10, however, has variable effects in murine models of GVHD [139, 140]. Blazer et al. reported a dose-dependent effect of IL-10 on mice with GVHD. High doses of IL-10 potentiated GVHD whilst lower doses were protective [141]. Clinical studies, however, suggest that elevated levels of endogenous IL-10 may be associated with immunological tolerance. Bacchetta et al. observed an association between increased expression of the IL-10 gene in recipient-derived monocytes and the absence of GVHD after the receipt of HLA-mismatched fetal hematopoietic cells in patients with severe combined immunodeficiency [142]. Holler et al. reported that elevated levels of endogenous IL-10 before transplantation are associated with a reduced risk of GVHD [143]. Lin et al. analyzed single nucleotide polymorphisms in the IL-1□, IL-1Ra, IL-6, IL-10 and TNF-α genes in 570 transplant recipients and their HLA-identical sibling donors and genotypes were tested for an association with GVHD. They showed that the IL-10 promoter region genotype of the recipient was significantly associated with the risk of acute GVHD [144]. IL-12 treatment at the time of HSCT perturbs the activation of donor CD4+ T cells leading to Fas-dependent apoptosis that impedes their expansion and associated GVHD-promoting activity [145]. Serum levels of IL-18 are elevated in clinical and experimental acute GVHD [146, 147]. IL-18 prevents murine chronic GVHD [148], but the effect of IL-18 on the induction of acute GVHD is unclear. The neutralization of IL-18 in non-irradiated HSCT recipients did not alter acute GVHD [147]. Reddy et al. demonstrated that administration of IL-18 reduces the mortality rate by enhancing Fas-mediated donor T cell apoptosis in a lethally irradiated murine BMT model of acute GVHD induced in response to multiple MHC antigens [149]. However, paradoxical effects of IL-18 on the severity of acute GVHD mediated by CD4+ and CD8+ T cells were observed as administration of IL-18 significantly increased survival in CD4+ T cell-mediated GVHD but reduced survival in CD8+ T cell-mediated GVHD [150]. The growth factors IL-11, keratinocyte growth factor (KGF) and HGF have recently been shown to prevent gastrointestinal tract damage and subsequent inflammatory responses induced by endotoxins in the gastrointestinal tract lumen in murine models [120, 151, 152]. Therapy with these growth factors preserved donor T cell responses to host antigens and significantly improved leukemia-free survival and may thus form the basis of novel approaches to separate the GVL effect from GVHD [125, 153, 154]. However, the results of a phase I/II double blind, controlled clinical trial of recombinant IL-11 in the prevention of acute GVHD was unsatisfactory. Patients who received IL-11 exhibited severe fluid retention and early mortality making it impossible to determine whether IL-11 reduced the rate of acute GVHD [155]. Recently, the usefulness of KGF (Palifermin) in combination with tacrolimus and methotrexate for the prevention of acute GVHD in patients at high risk of acute GVHD has been reported [156].

ROLE OF PLATELET DERIVED FACTORS IN THE PATHOGENESIS OF GVHD

The coagulation cascade is initiated when damage to endothelial cells results in exposure of the fibrillar collagen present in the subendothelial matrix. Platelets can also be activated after adhesion to collagen exposed at the site of injury. Platelets adhere to collagen either directly via the collagen receptor or indirectly through von Willebrand factor which binds to both collagen and the platelet receptor. The interaction with collagen stimulates platelet activation, resulting in the formation of platelet aggregates, phospholipase C activation, and the release of the intra-platelet α-granule contents. Both HGF and S1P are abundantly stored in platelets and leukocytes and are released upon activation, thereby regulating angiogenesis, hematopoiesis and immunity. GVHD is a pathological condition initiated by activation of donor T cells recognizing host tissue antigens, with subsequent dysregulation of inflammatory cytokine production by monocytes and macrophages. In this condition, both platelets and leukocytes are activated by injured vascular endothelial cells or inflammatory cytokines, releasing HGF and S1P in the circulation. These platelet derived growth factors may counteract tissue injury caused by GVHD by affording protection against vascular cell injury and enhancing vascular endothelial cell regeneration. Increased HGF and S1P levels may also contribute to the enhancement of hematopoiesis of engrafted HSCs. We and other group have demonstrated that both HGF and FTY720, structurally homologous to sphingosine, protected against acute GVHD after allogeneic HSCT [120, 125, 132]. We further examined the effect of combination therapy of HGF and FTY720 on a murine model of acute GVHD. Combination therapy of HGF and FTY720 significantly reduced the numbers of peripheral blood lymphocytes and CD8+ T cells in the spleen. Furthermore, this treatment significantly inhibited intestinal injuries caused by acute GVHD comparing to the treatment with HGF or FTY720 alone (figure 5).

Effect of combination therapy with HGF and FTY

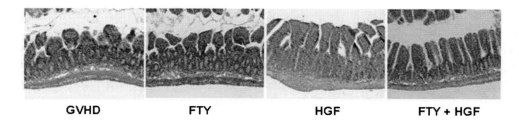

GVHD   FTY   HGF   FTY + HGF

Figure 5. Effect of combination therapy with HGF and FTY720. BDF1 mice were exposed to total body irradiation (TBI) from an x-ray source, after which T-cell–depleted (TCD) BM cells (5 x 10⁶) plus spleen cells (2.5 x 10⁷) were injected. HGF treatment was performed by injection into the gluteal muscle with HVJ liposomes containing 8 μg human *HGF* expression vector (HGF-HVJ liposomes). Gene transfer was repeated once a week after bone marrow transplantation (BMT). The administration FTY720 was performed by daily oral gavage at a dose of 1 mg/kg after BMT. Small-bowel tissues are shown (×50) from one representative animal in each group. Combination therapy with HGF and FTY720 significantly prevented the changes of intestinal morphology observed in GVHD control mice, such as atrophy of the villi, infiltration of lymphocytes, and destruction of crypts in the small intestine.

CONCLUSION

The mechanisms of GVHD have been progressively elucidated over recent years and new treatments have been developed using experimental models. However, both acute and chronic GVHD remain difficult to treat. Many clinical approaches to acute GVHD such as treatment with immunosuppressants or *ex vivo* T-cell depletion of the HSC graft, reduce GVL activity. The most effective approach to treat acute GVHD is likely to be one that disrupts all three phases of the GVHD cascade synergistically. For example, a useful strategy might involve blocking GI tract damage by treatment with IL-11, KGF, or HGF, along with induction of specific anergy using a CTLA-4 monoclonal antibody, and neutralization of TNF-α using Infliximab. Chronic GVHD may be the result of autoreactive T cells that escaped negative selection due to the thymus being damaged by the conditioning regimen, acute GVHD, and/or age related atrophy, and involves increased Th2 immune responses. Therefore, blocking thymic injury using KGF or HGF, or inhibition of Th2 activation by IL-18 may represent useful for the treatments for chronic GVHD. FTY720, structurally homologous to sphingosine, reduces the numbers of effector cells of GVHD by sequestrating lymphocytes in secondary lymphoid organs. Furthermore, FTY720 increases tissue regeneration, thereby may protecting against tissue injuries caused by GVHD. The various new treatment options, including platelet derived factors, currently being examined in animal models should improve the outlook for patients with acute or chronic GVHD.

REFERENCES

[1]   Prentice HG, Blacklock HA, Janossy G, Gilmore MJ, Price-Jones L, Tidman N, Trejdosiewicz LK, Skeggs DB, Panjwani D, Ball S, et al. Depletion of T lymphocytes in donor marrow prevents significant graft-versus-host disease in matched allogeneic leukemic marrow transplant recipients. *Lancet.* 1984, 1, 472-476.

[2]   Thomas ED, Storb R, Clift RA, Fefer A, Johnson L, Neiman PE, Lerner KG, Glucksberg H, Buckner CD. Bone-marrow transplantation (second of two parts). *N. Engl. J. Med.* 1975, 292, 895-902.

[3]   Deeg HJ, Storb R. Graft-versus-host disease: Pathophysiological and clinical aspects. *Annu. Rev. Med.* 1984, 35, 11-24.

[4]   Ferrara JL, Deeg HJ. Graft-versus-host disease. *N. Engl. J. Med.* 1991, 324, 667-674.

[5]   Dobyski WR, Ash RC, Casper JT, McAuliffe T, Horowitz MM, Lawton C, Keever C, Baxter-Lowe LA, Camitta B, Garbrecht F, et al. Effect of T-cell depletion as graft-versus-host disease prophylaxis on engraftment, relapse, and disease-free survival in unrelated marrow transplantation for chronic myelogenous leukemia. *Blood.* 1994, 83, 1980-1987.

[6]   Young JW, Papadopoulos EB, Cunningham I, Castro-Malaspina H, Flomenberg N, Calabasi MH, Gulati SC, Brochstein JA, Heller G, Black P, et al. T-cell-depleted allogeneic bone marrow transplantation in adults with acute nonlymphocytic leukemia in first remission. *Blood.* 1992, 79, 3380-3387.

[7]   Pirsch JD, Maki DG. Infectious complication in adults with bone marrow transplantation and T-cell depletion of bone marrow. Increased susceptibility to fungal infections. *Ann. Intern. Med.* 1986, 104, 619-631.

[8]   Mamont AM, Horowitz MM, Gale RP, Sobocinski K, Ash RC, van Bekkum DW, Champlin RE, Dicke KA, Goldman JM, Good RA, et al. T-cell depletion of HLA-identical transplants in leukemia. *Blood.* 1991, 78, 2120-2130.

[9]   Shulman H, Striker G, Deeg HJ, Kennedy M, Storb R, Thomas ED. Nephrotoxicity of cyclosporin A after allogeneic marrow transplantation; glomerular thrombus and tubular injury. *N. Engl. J. Med.* 1981, 305, 1392-1395.

[10] Kanojia MD, Anagnostou AA, Zander AR, Vellekoop L, Spitzer G., Verma DS, Jagannath S, Dick KA. High-dose methylprednisolone treatment for acute graft-versus-host disease after bone marrow transplantation in adults. *Transplantation.* 1984, 37, 246-249.

[11] Herve P, Flesch M, Tiberghien P, Wijdenes J, Racadot E, Bordigoni P, Plouvier E, Stephan JL, Bourdeau H, Holler E, et al. Phase I-II trial of a monoclonal anti-tumor necrosis factor α antibody for the treatment of refractory severe acute graft-versus-host disease. *Blood.* 1992, 79, 3362-3368.

[12] Guinan EC, Boussiotis VA, Neuberg D, Brennan LL, Hirano N, Nadler LM, Gribben JG. Transplantation of anergic histocompatible bone marrow allografts. *N. Engl. J. Med.* 1999, 340, 1704-1714.

[13] Stenberg PE, McEver RP, Shuman MA, Jacques YV, Bainton DF. A platelet α-granule membrane protein (GMP-140) is expressed on the plasma membrane after activation. *J. J. Cell Biol.* 1985, 101, 880–886.

[14] Bonfanti R, Furie BC, Furie B, Wagner DD. PADGEM (GMP140) is a component of Weibel-Palade bodies of human endothelial cells. *Blood.* 1989, 73, 1109–1112.

[15] Li G, Sanders JM, Phan ET, Ley K, Sarembock IJ. Arterial macrophages and regenerating endothelial cells express P-selectin in atherosclerosis-prone apolipoprotein apolipoprotein E-deficient mice. *Am. J. Pathol.* 2005, 167, 1511–1518.

[16] Diacovo TG, Puri KD, Warnock RA, Springer TA, von Andrian UH. Platelet-mediated lymphocyte delivery to high endothelial venules. *Science.* 1996, 273, 252–255.

[17] Larsen E, Celi A, Gilbert GE, Furie BC, Erban JK, Bonfanti R, Wagner DD, Furie B. PADGEM protein: a receptor that mediates the interaction of activated platelets with neutrophils and monocytes. *Cell.* 1989, 59, 305–312.

[18] Diacovo TG, Roth SJ, Buccola JM, Bainton DF, Springer TA. Neutrophil rolling, arrest, and transmigration across activated, surface-adherent platelets via sequential action of P-selectin and the beta 2-integrin CD11b/CD18. *Blood.* 1996, 88, 146–157.

[19] da Costa Martins PA, van Gils JM, Mol A, Hordijk PL, Zwaginga JJ. Platelet binding to monocytes increases the adhesive properties of monocytes by up-regulating the expression and functionality of beta1 and beta2 integrins. *J. Leukoc. Biol.* 2006, 79, 499–507.

[20] Atarashi K, Hirata T, Matsumoto M, Kanemitsu N, Miyasaka M. Rolling of Th1 cells via P-selectin glycoprotein ligand-1 stimulates LFA-1-mediated cell binding to ICAM-1. *J. Immunol.* 2005, 174, 1424–1432.

[21] Ma YQ, Plow EF, Geng JG. P-selectin binding to P-selectin glycoprotein ligand-1 induces an intermediate state of αMβ2 activation and acts cooperatively with extracellular stimuli to support maximal adhesion of human neutrophils. *Blood.* 2004, 104, 2549–2556.

[22] Shattil SJ, Newman PJ. Integrins: dynamic scaffolds for adhesion and signaling in platelets. *Blood* 2004, 104, 1606–1615.

[23] Bennett JS. Structure and function of the platelet integrin αIIbβ3. *J. Clin. Invest.* 2005, 2005, 115, 3363–3369.

[24] Buensuceso C, de Virgilio M, Shattil SJ. Detection of integrin $\alpha IIb\beta 3$ clustering in living cells. *J. Biol. Chem.* 2003, 278, 15217–15224.

[25] Loftus JC, Albrecht RM. Redistribution of the fibrinogen receptor of human platelets after surface activation. *J. Cell Biol.* 1984, 99, 822–829.

[26] Andre P, Prasad KS, Denis CV, He M, Papalia JM, Hynes RO, Phillips DR, Wagner DD. CD40L stabilizes arterial thrombi by a beta3 integrin-dependent mechanism. *Nat. Med.* 2002, 8, 247–252.

[27] Lederman S, Yellin MJ, Inghirami G, Lee JJ, Knowles DM, Chess L. Molecular interactions mediating T-B lymphocyte collaboration in human lymphoid follicles. Roles of T cell-B-cell-activating molecule (5c8 antigen) and CD40 in contact-dependent help. *J. Immunol.* 1992, 149, 3817–3826.

[28] Armitage RJ, Sato TA, Macduff BM, Clifford KN, Alpert AR, Smith CA, Fanslow WC. Identification of a source of biologically active CD40 ligand. *Eur. J. Immunol.* 1992, 22, 2071–2076.

[29] Henn V, Slupsky JR, Grafe M, Anagnostopoulos I, Forster R, Muller-Berghaus G, Kroczek RA. CD40 ligand on activated platelets triggers an inflammatory reaction of endothelial cells. *Nature.* 1998, 391, 591–594.

[30] Pignatelli P, Sanguigni V, Lenti L, Ferro D, Finocchi A, Rossi P, Violi F. gp91phox-dependent expression of platelet CD40 ligand. *Circulation.* 2004, 110, 1326–1329.

[31] Elzey BD, Grant JF, Sinn HW, Nieswandt B, Waldschmidt TJ, Ratliff TL. Cooperation Cooperation between platelet-derived CD154 and CD4+ T cells for enhanced germinal center formation. *J. Leukoc. Biol.* 2005, 78, 80–84.

[32] Xu H, Zhang X, Mannon RB, Kirk AD. Platelet-derived or soluble CD154 induces vascularized allograft rejection independent of cell-bound CD154. *J. Clin. Invest.* 2006, 2006, 116, 769–774.

[33] Quezada SA, Jarvinen LZ, Lind EF, Noelle RJ. CD40/CD154 interactions at the interface of tolerance and immunity. *Annu. Rev. Immunol.* 2004, 22, 307–328.

[34] Henn V, Steinbach S, Buchner K, Presek P, Kroczek RA. The inflammatory action of CD40 ligand (CD154) expressed on activated human platelets is temporally limited by coexpressed CD40. *Blood.* 2001, 98, 1047–1054

[35] Rock FL, Hardiman G, Timans JC, Kastelein RA, Bazan JF. A family of human receptors structurally related to *Drosophila* Toll. *Proc. Natl. Acad. Sci. U S A.* 1998, 95, 588-593.

[36] Diebold SS, Kaisho T, Hemmi H, Akira S, Reis E, Sousa C. Innate antiviral responses by means of TLR7-mediated recognition of single-stranded RNA. *Science.* 2004,303, 1529-1531.

[37] Takeda K, Kaisho T, Akira S. Toll-like receptors. *Annu. Rev. Immunol.* 2003, 21, 335-376.

[38] Adachi O, Kawai T, Takeda K, Matsumoto M, Tsutsui H, Sakagami M, Nakanishi K, Akira S. Targeted disruption of the *MyD88* gene results in loss of IL-1 and IL-18 mediated function. *Immunity.* 1998, 9, 143-150.

[39] Andonegui G, Kerfoot SM, McNagny K, Ebbert KV, Patel KD, Kubes P. Platelets express functional Toll-like receptor-4. *Blood.* 2005, 106, 2417–2423.

[40] Ward JR, Bingle L, Judge HM, Brown SB, Storey RF, Whyte MK, Dower SK, Buttle DJ, Sabroe I. Agonists of toll-like receptor (TLR)2 and TLR4 are unable to modulate platelet activation by adenosine diphosphate and platelet activating factor. *Thromb. Haemost.* 2005, 94, 831–838.

[41] Aslam R, Speck ER, Kim M, Crow AR, Bang KW, Nestel FP, Ni H, Lazarus AH, Freedman J, Semple JW. Platelet Toll-like receptor expression modulates lipopolysaccharide-induced thrombocytopenia and tumor necrosis factor-α production in vivo. *Blood.* 2006, 107, 637–641.

[42] Damas JK, Jensenius M, Ueland T, Otterdal K, Yndestad A, Froland SS, Rolain JM, Myrvang B, Raoult D, Aukrust P. Increased levels of soluble CD40L in African tick bite fever: possible involvement of TLRs in the pathogenic interaction between Rickettsia africae, endothelial cells, and platelets. *J. Immunol.* 2006, 177, 2699–2706.

[43] Pan Y, Lloyd C, Zhou H, Dolich S, Deeds J, Gonzalo JA, Vath J, Gosselin M, Ma J, Dussault B, Woolf E, Alperin G, Culpepper J, Gutierrez-Ramos JC, Gearing D. Neurotactin, a membrane-anchored chemokine upregulated in brain inflammation. *Nature.* 1997, 387, 611–617.

[44] Bazan JF, Bacon KB, Hardiman G, Wang W, Soo K, Rossi D, Greaves DR, Zlotnik A, Schall TJ. A new class of membrane-bound chemokine with a CX3C motif. *Nature.* 1997, 385, 640–644.

[45] Power CA, Furness RB, Brawand C, Wells TN. Cloning of a full-length cDNA encoding the neutrophil-activating peptide ENA-78 from human platelets. *Gene.* 1994, 151, 333–334.

[46] Brandt E, Ludwig A, Petersen F, Flad HD. Platelet-derived CXC chemokines: old players in new games. *Immunol. Rev.* 2000, 177, 204–216.

[47] Kasper B, Brandt E, Bulfone-Paus S, Petersen F. Platelet factor 4 (PF-4)-induced neutrophil adhesion is controlled by src-kinases while PF-4-mediated exocytosis requires the additional activation of p38 MAP kinase and phosphatidylinositol 3-kinase. kinase. *Blood.* 2004, 103, 1602–1610.

[48] Petersen F, Ludwig A, Flad HD, Brandt E. TNF-α renders human neutrophils responsive to platelet factor 4. Comparison of PF-4 and IL-8 reveals different activity profiles of the two chemokines. *J. Immunol.* 1996, 156, 1954–1962.

[49] Schall TJ, Jongstra J, Dyer BJ, Jorgensen J, Clayberger C, Davis MM, Krensky AM. A human T cell-specific molecule is a member of a new gene family. *J. Immunol.* 1988, 141, 1018–1025.

[50] Schall TJ, Bacon K, Toy KJ, Goeddel DV. Selective attraction of monocytes and T lymphocytes of the memory phenotype by cytokine RANTES. *Nature.* 1990, 347, 669–671.

[51] Kameyoshi Y, Dorschner A, Mallet AI, Christophers E, Schroder JM. Cytokine RANTES released by thrombin-stimulated platelets is a potent attractant for human eosinophils. *J Exp Med* 1992, 176, 587–592.

[52] Stevenson FT, Torrano F, Locksley RM, Lovett DH. Interleukin 1: the patterns of translation and intracellular distribution support alternative secretory mechanisms. *J Cell Physiol* 1992, 152, 223–231.

[53] Dripps DJ, Brandhuber BJ, Thompson RC, Eisenberg SP. Interleukin-1 (IL-1) receptor antagonist binds to the 80-kDa IL-1 receptor but does not initiate IL-1 signal transduction. *J. Biol. Chem.* 1991, 266, 10331–10336.

[54] Schreuder H, Tardif C, Trump-Kallmeyer S, Soffientini A, Sarubbi E, Akeson A, Bowlin T, Yanofsky S, Barrett RW. A new cytokine-receptor binding mode revealed by by the crystal structure of the IL-1 receptor with an antagonist. *Nature.* 1997, 386, 194–194–200.

[55] Lindemann S, Tolley ND, Eyre JR, Kraiss LW, Mahoney TM, Weyrich AS. Integrins regulate the intracellular distribution of eukaryotic initiation factor 4E in platelets. A checkpoint for translational control. *J. Biol. Chem.* 2001, 276, 33947–33951

[56] Lindemann S, Tolley ND, Dixon DA, McIntyre TM, Prescott SM, Zimmerman GA, Weyrich AS. Activated platelets mediate inflammatory signaling by regulated interleukin 1beta synthesis. *J. Cell Biol.* 2001, 154, 485–490.

[57] Reed GL. Platelet secretion. In Platelets (ed: AD Michelson). Elservier Science. San Diego, 2002. pp181-195.

[58] Folkman J, Browder T, Palmblad J. Angiogenesis research: Guidelines for translation to clinical application. *Thromb. Haemost.* 2001, 86, 23-33

[59] Ostman A, Heldin C-H. Involvement of platelet-derived growth factor in disease: Development of specific antagonists. *Adv. Cancer Res.* 2001;80:1-37.

[60] Yu Y, Sweeney M, Zhang S Platoshyn O, Landsberg J, Rothman A, Yuan JX. PDGF stimulates pulmonary vascular smooth muscle cell proliferation by upregulating TRPC6 TRPC6 expression. *Am. J. Cell Physiol.* 2003, 284, C316-330.

[61] Romanashkova JA, Makarov SS. NF-kB is a target of AKT in anti-apoptotic PDGF signaling. *Nature.* 1999, 401, 86-90.

[62] Pintucci G, Form S, Pinnell J, Mignatti P, Rafii S, Green D. Trophic effects of platelets on endothelial cells are mediated by platelet-associated fibroblast growth factor (FGF-2) 2) and vascular endothelial growth factor (VEGF). *Thromb. Haemost.* 2002, 88, 834-842.

[63] Weltermann A, Woltzt M, Petersmann K, Czerni C, Graselli U, Lechner K, Kyrle PA.. Large amounts of vascular endothelial growth factor at the site of hemostatic plug formation in vivo. *Arterioscler. Thromb. Vasc. Biol.* 1999, 19, 1757-1760.

[64] Galvin KM, Donovan MJ, Lynch CA, Meyer RI, Paul RJ, Lorenz JN, Fairchild-Huntress V, Dixon KL, Dunmore JH, Gimbrone MA, Falb D, Huszar D.. A role of Smado in development and hemostasis of the cardiovascular system. *Nature Gen.* 2000, 2000, 24, 171-174.

[65] Matsumoto K, Nakamura T. Hepatocyte growth factor (HGF) as a tissue organizer for organogenesis and regeneration. *Biochem. Biophys. Res. Commun.* 1997, 239, 639-44.

[66] Cheng Y, Austin SC, Rocca B, Koller BH, Coffman TM, Grosser T, Lawson JA, FitzGerald GA.. Role of prostacyclin in cardiovascular response to thromboxian A2. *Science.* 2002, 296, 539-541.

[67] Hla, T. Physiological and pathological actions of sphingosine 1-phosphste. *Semin. Cell Dev. Biol.* 2004, 15, 513-520.

[68] Pyne S, Pyne, N.J. Sphingosine 1-phosphate signaling in mammalian cells. *Biochem. J.* 2000, 349, 385-402.

[69] Weyrich AS, Prescott SM, Zimmerman GA. Platelets, endothelial cells, inflammatory chemokines, and restenosis. Complex signaling in the vascular play book. *Circulation.* 2002, 106, 1433-1435.

[70] Nakamura T, Nawa K, Ichihara A. Partial purification and characterization of hepatocyte growth factor from serum of hepatectomized rats. *Biochem. Biophys. Res. Commun* 1984, 122, 1450-1459.

[71] Russel WE, McGrowan JA, Bucher NL. Partial characterization of a hepatocyte growth factor from rat platelets. *J. Cell Physiol.* 1984, 119, 183-192.

[72] Nakamura T, Nishizawa T, Hagiya M, Seki T, Shimonishi M, Sugimura A, Tashiro, K, Shimizu, S. Molecular cloning and expression of human hepatocyte growth factor. *Nature.* 1989, 342, 440-443.

[73] Rubin JS, Bottaro DP, Aaronson SA. Hepatocyte growth factor/scatter factor and its receptor, the c-met proto-oncogene product. *Biochem. Biophys. Acta.* 1993, 1155, 357-371.

[74] Zarneger R, Michalopoulos G.K. The many faces of hepatocyte growth factor: from hepatopoiesis to hematopoiesis. *J. Cell Biol.* 1995, 129, 1177-1180.

[75] Bottaro DP, Rubin JS, Faletto DL, Chan AM, Kmiecik TE, Van de Wounde G.F, Aaronson SA. Identification of hepatocyte growth factor receptor as the c-met proto-oncogene product. *Science.* 1991, 251, 802-804.

[76] Shiota G, Okano J, Kawasaki H, Kawamoto T, Nakamura T. Serum hepatocyte growth factor levels in liver diseases: clinical implications. *Hepatology.* 1995, 21, 106-112.

[77] Maeda J, Ueki N, Hada T, Higashino K. Elevated serum hepatocyte growth factor/scatter factor levels in inflammatory lung disease. *Am. J. Respir. Crit. Care Med.* 1995, 152, 1587-1591.

[78] Kawaida K, Matsumoto K, Shimazu H, Nakamura T. Hepatocyte growth factor prevents acute renal failure and accelerate renal regeneration in mice. *Proc. Natl. Acad. Sci. USA.* 1994, 91, 4357-4361.

[79] Matsuda Y, Matsumoto K, Yamada A, Ichida T, Asakura H, Komoriya Y, Nishiyama E, Nakamura T. Preventive and therapeutic effects in rats of hepatocyte growth factor infusion on liver fibrosis/cirrhosis. *Hepatology.* 1997, 26, 81-89.

[80] Moolenaar WH. Lysophosphatidic acid, a multiple functional phospholipids messenger. *J. Biol. Chem.* 1995, 270, 12949-12952.

[81] Edsall LC, Spiegel S. Enzymatic measurement of sphingosine 1-phosphate. *Anal. Biochem.* 1999, 272, 80-86.

[82] Igarashi Y, Yatomi Y. Sphingosine 1-phosphaqte is a blood constituent released from activated platelets, possibly playing a variety of physiological and pathological roles. *Acta Biochim. Pol.* 1998, 45, 299-309.

[83] Yatomi Y, Igarashi Y, Yang L, Hisano N, Qi R, Asazumam N, Satoh K, Ozaki Y, Kume S. Sphingosine 1-phosphate, a bioactive sphingolipid abundantly stored in platelets, is a normal constituent of human plasma and serum. *J. Biochem. (Tokyo)* 1997, 121, 969-973.

[84] Yatomi Y, Ruan F, Hakomori S, Igarashi Y. Sphingosine 1-phosphate: a platelet-activating sphingolipid released from agonist-stimulated human platelets. *Blood.* 1995, 86, 193-202.

[85] Olivera A, Spiegel S. Sphingosine 1-phosphate as second messenger in cell proliferation induced by PDGF and FCS mitogens. *Nature.* 1993, 365, 557-560.

[86] Ridley AJ, Hall A. The small GTP-binding protein rho regulates the assembly of focal adhesions and actin stress fibers in response to growth factors. *Cell.* 1992, 70, 389-399.

[87] Hla T, Maciag T. An abundant transcript induced in differentiating human endothelial cells encodes a polypeptide with structural similarities to G-protein-coupled receptors. *J. Biol. Chem.* 1990, 265, 9308-9313.

[88] Sanchez T, Hla T. Structural and functional characteristics of S1P receptors. *J. Cell Biochem.* 2004, 92, 913-922.

[89] Lee MJ, Thangada S, Claffey KP, Ancellin N, Liu CH, Kluk M, Volpi M, Sha'afi RI, Hla, T. Vascular endothelial cell adherence junction assembly and morphogenesis induced by sphingosine 1-phosphate. *Cell.* 1999, 99, 301-312.

[90] Erickson PR, Herzberg MC, Tierney G. Cross-reactive immunodeterminants on Streptococcus sanguis and collagen. Predicting a structural motif of platelet-interactive interactive domains. *J. Biol. Chem.* 1992, 267, 10018–10023.

[91] Scheld WM, Valone JA, Sande MA. Bacterial adherence in the pathogenesis of endocarditis. Interaction of bacterial dextran, platelets, and fibrin. *J. Clin. Invest.* 1978, 1978, 61, 1394–1404.

[92] Durack DT. Experimental bacterial endocarditis. IV. Structure and evolution of very early lesions. *J. Pathol.* 1975, 115, 81–89.

[93] Sullam PM, Bayer AS, Foss WM, Cheung AL. Diminished platelet binding in vitro by Staphylococcus aureus is associated with reduced virulence in a rabbit model of infective endocarditis. *Infect. Immun.* 1996, 64, 4915–4921.

[94] Zucker-Franklin D, Seremetis S, Zheng ZY. Internalization of human immunodeficiency virus type I and other retroviruses by megakaryocytes and platelets. *Blood.* 1990, 75, 1920–1923.

[95] Boukour S, Masse JM, Benit L, Dubart-Kupperschmitt A, Cramer EM. Lentivirus degradation and DC-SIGN expression by human platelets and megakaryocytes. *J. Thromb. Haemost.* 2006, 4, 426–435.

[96] Chaipan C, Soilleux EJ, Simpson P, Hofmann H, Gramberg T, Marzi A, Geier M, Stewart EA, Eisemann J, Steinkasserer A, Suzuki-Inoue K, Fuller GL, Pearce AC, Watson SP, Hoxie JA, Baribaud F, Pohlmann S. DC-SIGN and CLEC-2 mediate human immunodeficiency virus type 1 capture by platelets. *J. Virol.* 2006, 80, 8951–8960.

[97] Whitman DH, Berry RL, Green DM. Platelet gel: an autologous alternative to fibrin glue with applications in oral and maxillofacial surgery. *J. Oral Maxillofac. Surg.* 1997, 55, 1294-1299.

[98] Marx RE, Carson ER, Eichstaedt RN, Schimmele SR, Strauss JE, Georgeff KR. Platelet-rich plasma: growth factor enhancement for bone grafts. *Oral Surg. Oral Med. Oral Pathol. Oral Radiol. Endod.* 1998, 85, 638-646.

[99] Margolis DJ, Kantor J, Santanna J, Strom BL, Berlin JA. Effectiveness of platelet releasate for the treatment diabetic neuropathic foot ulcers. *Diabetes Care.* 2001, 24, 483-488.

[100] Sánchez M, Azofra J, Anitua E, Andía I, Padilla S, Santisteban J, Mujika I. Plasma rich in growth factors to treat an articular cartilage avulsion: a case report. *Med. Sci. Sports Exerc.* 2003, 35, 1648-1652.

[101] Przepiorka D, Weisdorf D, Martin P, Klingemann HG, Beatty P, Hows J, Thomas ED. Consensus Conference on Acute GVHD Grading. *Bone Marrow Transplant.* 1995, 15, 825-828.

[102] Flowers ME, Kansu E, Sullivan KM. Pathophysiology and treatment of graft-versus-host disease. *Hematol. Oncol. Clin. North Am.* 1999, 13, 1091-1112.

[103] Cutler C, Giri S, Jeyapalan S, Paniagua D, Viswanathan A, Antin JH. Acute and chronic graft-versus-host disease after allogeneic peripheral blood stem cell and bone marrow transplantation: a meta-analysis. *J. Clin. Oncol.* 2001, 19, 3685-3691.

[104] Ferrara JL, Levy R, Chao NJ. Pathophysiologic mechanism of acute graft-vs-host disease. *Biol. Blood Marrow Transplant.* 1999, 5, 347-356.

[105] Hill GR, Ferrara JL. The primacy of gastrointestinal tract as a target organ of acute graft-versus-host disease: rationale for the use of cytokine shields in allogeneic bone marrow transplantation. *Blood.* 2000, 95, 2754-2759.

[106] Hill GR, Crawford JM, Cooke KR, Brinson YS, Pan L, Ferrara JL. Total body irradiation and acute graft-versus-host disease: the role of gastrointestinal damage and inflammatory cytokines. *Blood.* 1997, 90, 3204-3213.

[107] Nash RA, Pepe MS, Storb R, Longton G, Pettinger M, Anasetti C, Appelbaum FR, Bowden RA, Deeg HJ, Doney K, Martin PJ, Sullivan KM, Sanders J, Witherspoon RP. Acute graft-versus-host disease: analysis of risk factors after allogeneic marrow transplantation and prophylaxis with cyclosporine and methotrexate. *Blood.* 1992, 80, 1838-1845.

[108] Shlomchik WD, Couzens MS, Tang CB, McNiff J, Robert ME, Liu J, Shlomchik MJ, Emerson SG. Prevention of graft-versus-host disease by inactivation of host antigen-presenting cells. *Science.* 1999, 285, 412-415.

[109] Teshima T, Ordermann R, Reddy P, Gagins S, Liu C, Cooke KR, Ferrara JL. Acute graft-versus-host disease does not require alloantigen expression on host epithelium. *Nat. Med.* 2002, 8, 575-581.

[110] Hill GR, Teshima T, Gerbitz A, Pan L, Cooke KR, Brinson YS, Crawford JM, Ferrara JL. Differential role of IL-1 and TNF-alpha on graft-versus-host disease and graft-versus-leukemia. *J. Clin. Invest.* 1999, 104, 459-467.

[111] Rus V, Svetic A, Nguyen P, Gause WC, Via CS. Kinetics of Th1 and Th2 cytokine production during the early course of acute and chronic murine graft-versus-host disease. *J. Immunol.* 1995, 155, 2396-2406.

[112] Weinberg K, Blazar BR, Wagner JE, Agura E, Hill BJ, Smogorzewska M, Koup RA, Betts MR, Collins RH, Douek DC. Factors affecting thymic function after allogeneic hematopoietic stem cell transplantation. *Blood.* 2001, 97, 1458-1466.

[113] Atkinson K, Incefy GS, Storb R, Sullivan KM, Iwata T, Dardenne M, Ochs HD, Good RA, Thomas ED. Low serum thymic hormone levels in patients with chronic graft-versus-host disease. *Blood.* 1982, 59, 1073-1077.

[114] Seddik M, Seemayer TA, Lapp WS. T cell functional defect associated with thymic epithelial cell injury induced by graft-versus-host reaction. *Transplantation.* 1980, 29, 61-66.

[115] Shiota G, Okano J, Kawasaki H, Kawamoto T, Nakamura T. Serum hepatocyte growth factor levels in liver diseases: clinical implications. *Hepatology.* 1995, 21, 106-112.

[116] Okamoto T, Takatsuka H, Fujimori Y, Wada H, Iwasaki T, Kakishita E. Increased hepatocyte growth factor in serum in acute graft-versus-host disease. *Bone Marrow Transplant.* 2001, 28, 197-200.

[117] Kosai K, Matsumoto K, Nagata S, Tsujimoto Y, Nakamura T. Abrogation of Fas-induced fulminant hepatic failure in mice by hepatocyte growth factor. *Biochem. Biophys. Res. Commun.* 1988, 244, 683-690.

[118] Kosai K, Matsumoto K, Funakoshi H, Nakamura T. Hepatocyte growth factor prevents endotoxin-induced lethal hepatic failure in mice. *Hepatology.* 1999, 30, 151-159.

[119] Hattori K, Hirano T, Miyajima H, Yamakawa N, Tateno M, Oshimi K, Kayagaki N, Yagita H, Okumura K. Differential effects of anti-Fas ligand and anti-tumor necrosis factor alpha antibodies on acute graft-versus-host disease pathologies. *Blood.* 1998, 91, 4051-4055.

[120] Kuroiwa T, Kakishita E, Hamano T, Kataoka Y, Seto Y, Iwata N, Kaneda Y, Matsumoto K, Nakamura T, Ueki T, Fujimoto J, Iwasaki T. Hepatocyte growth factor ameliorates acute graft-versus-host disease and promotes hematopoietic function. *J. Clin. Invest.* 2001, 107, 1365-1373.

[121] Nicola M.D, Carlo-Stella C, Magni M, Longoni PD, Matteucci P, Grisanti S, Gianni AM. Human bone marrow stromal cells suppress T-lymphocyte proliferation induced by cellular or nonspecific mitogenic stimuli. *Blood.* 2002, 99, 3838-3843.

[122] Beilmann M, Odenthal M, Jung W, Vande Woude G.F, Dienes HP, Schirmacher P. Neoexpression of the c-met/hepatocyte growth factor –scatter factor receptor gene in activated monocytes. *Blood.* 1997, 90, 4450-4458.

[123] Ovali E, Ratip S, Kibaroglu A, Tekelioglu Y, Cetiner M, Karti S, Aydin F, Bayik M, Akoglu T. Role of hepatocyte growth factor in the development of dendritic cells from CD34+ bone marrow cells. *Haematologica.* 2000, 85, 464-469.

[124] Kurz SM, Diebold SS, Hieronymus T, Gust T.C, Bartunek P, Sachs M, Birchmeier W, Zenke M. The impact of c-met/scatter factor receptor on dendritic cell migration. *Eur. J. Immunol.* 2002, 32, 1832-1838.

[125] Imado T, Iwasaki T, Kataoka Y, Kuroiwa T, Hara H, Fujimoto J, Sano H. Hepatocyte growth factor preserves graft-versus-leukemia effect and T-cell reconstitution after marrow transplantation. *Blood.* 2004, 104, 1542-1549.

[126] Jin Y, Knudsen E, Wang L, Bryceson Y, Damaj B, Gessani S, Maghazachi A.A. Sphingosin 1-phosphate is a novel inhibitor of T-cell proliferation. *Blood.* 2003, 101, 4909-4915.

[127] Mandala S, Hajdu R, Bergstorm J, Quackenbush E, Xie J, Milligan J, Thompton R, Shei GL, Card D, Keohane C, Rosenbach M, Hale J, Lynch CL, Rupprecht K, Parsons W, Rosen H. Alteration of lymphocyte trafficking by sphingosin-1-phosphate receptor agonists. *Science.* 2002, 296, 346-349.

[128] Brinkmann V, Davis MD, Heise CE, Albert R, Cottens S, Hof R, Bruns C, Prieschl E, Baumruker T, Hiestand P, Foster CA, Zollinger M, Lynch K.R. The immune modulator FTY720 targets sphingosin 1-phosphate receptors. *J. Biol. Chem.* 2002, 277, 21453-21457.

[129] Pelot MR, Pearson DA, Swenson K, Zhao G, Sachs J, Yang YG, Sykes M. Lymphohematopoietic graft-vs-host reactions can be induced without graft-vs-host disease in murine mixed chimeras established with cyclophsphamide-based non-myeloablative conditioning regimen. *Biol. Blood Marrow Transplant.* 1999, 5, 133-143.

[130] Sykes M, Sheard MA, Sachs DH. Graft-versus-host-related immune suppression is induced in mixed chimeras by alloresponses against either host or donor lymphohematopoietic cells. *J. Exp. Med.* 1988, 168, 2391-2396.

[131] Mapara MY, Kim YM, Wang SP, Bronson R, Sachs DH, Sykes M. Donor lymphocyte infusions mediate superior graft-versus-leukemia effects in mixed compared to full allogeneic chimeras: a critical role for host antigen-presenting cells. *Blood.* 2002, 100, 1903-1909.

[132] Kim YM, Sachs T, Asavaroengchai W, Bronson R, Sykes M. Graft-versus-host disease can be separated from graft-versus-lymphoma effects by control of lymphocyte trafficking with FTY720. *J. Clin. Invest.* 2003, 111, 659-669.

[133] Alpdogan O, Muriglan SJ, Eng JM, Willis LM, Greenberg AS, Kappel BJ, van den Brink MR. IL-7 enhances peripheral T cell reconstitution after allogeneic hematopoieric stem cell transplantation. *J. Clin. Invest.* 2003, 112, 1095-1107.

[134] Sinha ML, Fry TJ, Fowler DH, Miller G, Mackall CL. Interleukin-7 worsens graft-versus-host disease. *Blood.* 2002, 100, 2642-2649.

[135] Alpdogan O, Schmaltz C, Muriglan SJ, Kappel BJ, Perales MA, Rotolo JA, Halm JA, Rich BE, van den Brink MR. Administration of interleukin-7 after allogeneic bone marrow transplantation improves immune reconstitution without aggravating graft-versus-host disease. *Blood.* 2001, 98, 2256-2265.

[136] Fiorentino DF, Zlotnik A, Mossmann T.R, Howard M, O'Grra A. IL-10 inhibits cytokine production by activated macrophages. *J. Immunol.* 1991, 147, 3815-3822.

[137] Ding L, Linsley PS, Huang LY, Germain RN, Shevach EM. IL-10 inhibits macrophage costimulatory activity by selectively inhibiting the up-regulation of B7 expression. *J. Immunol.* 1993, 151, 1224-1234.

[138] Taylor PA, Lee CJ, Blazar BR. The infusion of ex vivo activated and expanded CD4(+)CD25(+) immune regulatory cells inhibits graft-versus-host disease lethality. *Blood.* 2002, 99, 3493-3499.

[139] Smith SR, Terminelli C, Pennline KJ, Kenworthy-Bott L, Donkin J, Calzetta A. Inhibitory effects of recombinant human interleukin-10 on disease manifestations in P→F1 model of acute graft-versus-host disease. *Transplantation.* 1995, 59, 890-896.

[140] Blazar BR, Taylor PA, Smith S, Vallera DA. Interleukin-10 administration decreases survival in murine recipients of major histocompatibility complex disparate donor bone marrow grafts. *Blood.* 1995, 85, 842-851.

[141] Blazar, B.R,; Taylor, PA, Panoskaltsis-Mortari A, Narula SK, Smith SR, Roncarolo MG, Vallera DA. Interleukin-10 dose-dependent regulation of CD4+ and CD8+ T cell-mediated graft-versus-host disease. *Transplantation.* 1998, 66, 1220-1229.

[142] Bacchetta R, Bigler M, Touraine JL, Parkman R, Tovo, P.A,; Abrams, J,; de Waal Malefyt, R,; de Vries, J.E,; Roncarolo, M.G. High level of interleukin-10 production in vivo are associated with tolerance in SCID patients with HLA mismatched hematopoietic stem cells. *J. Exp. Med.* 1994, 179, 493-502.

[143] Holler E, Roncarolo MG, Hintermeier-Knabe R, Eissner G, Ertl B, Schulz U, Knabe H, Kolb HJ, Andreesen R, Wilmanns W. Prognostic significance of increased IL-10 production in patients prior to allogeneic bone marrow transplantation. *Bone Marrow Transplant.* 2000, 25, 237-241.

[144] Lin MT, Storer B, Martin PJ, Tseng LH, Gooley T, Chen PJ, Hansen JA. Relation of an interleukin-10 promoter polymorphism to graft-versus-host disease and survival after hematopoietic-cell transplantation. *New England J. Med.* 2003, 349, 2201-2210.

[145] Dey BR, Yang YG, Szot GL, Pearson DA, Sykes M. Interleukin-12 inhibits graft-versus-host disease through an Fas-mediated mechanism associated with alterations in donor T-cell activation and expansion. *Blood.* 1998, 91, 3315-3322.

[146] Fujimori Y, Takatsuka H, Takemoto Y, Hara H, Okamura H, Nakanishi K, Kakishita E. Elevated interleukin-18 levels during acute graft-versus-host disease after allogeneic bone marrow transplantation. *Br. J. Haematol.* 2000, 109, 652-657.

[147] Arnold D, Wasem C, Juillard P, Graber P, Cima I, Frutschi C, Herren S, Jakob S, Alouani S, Mueller C, Chvatchko Y, Brunner T. IL-18 independent cytotoxic T lymphocyte activation and IFN-gamma production during experimental acute graft-versus-host disease. *Int. Immunol.* 2002, 14, 503-511.

[148] Okamoto I, Kohno K, Tanimoto T, Iwaki K, Ishihara T, Akamatsu S, Ikegami H, Kurimoto M. IL-18 prevent the development of chronic graft-versus-host disease in mice. *J. Immunol.* 2000, 164, 6067-6074.

[149] Reddy P, Teshima T, Kukuruga M, Ordermann R, Liu C, Lowler K, Ferrara JL. Interleukin-18 regulates acute graft-versus-host disease by enhancing Fas-mediated donor T cell apoptosis. *J. Exp. Med.* 2001, 194, 1433-1440.

[150] Min CK, Maeda Y, Lowler K, Liu C, Clouthier S, Lofthus D, Weisiger E, Ferrara JL, Reddy P. Paradoxical effects of interleukin-18 on the severity of acute graft-versus-host disease mediated by CD4+ and CD8+ T-cell subsets after experimental allogeneic bone marrow transplantation. *Blood.* 2004, 104, 3393-3399.

[151] Hill G.R, Cooke KR, Teshima T, Crawford JM, Keith JC, Brinson YS, Bungard D, Ferrara JL. Interleukin-11 promotes T cell polarization and prevents acute graft-versus-host disease after allogeneic bone marrow transplantation. *J. Clin. Invest.* 1998, 102, 115-123.

[152] Panoskaltsis-Mortari A, Lancey DL, Vallera DA, Blazar BR. Keratinocyte growth factor administered before conditioning ameliorates graft-versus-host disease after allogeneic bone marrow transplantation in mice. *Blood.* 1998, 92, 3960-3967.

[153] Teshima T, Hill GR, Pan L, Brinson YS, van den Brink MR, Cooke KR, Ferrara JL. IL-11 separates graft-versus-leukemia effects from graft-versus-host disease after bone marrow transplantation. *J. Clin. Invest.* 1999, 104, 317-325.

[154] Krijanovski OI, Hill G.R, Cooke KR, Teshima T, Crawford JM, Brinson YS, Ferrara JL. Keratinocyte growth factor separates graft-versus-leukemia effect from graft-versus-host disease. *Blood.* 1999, 94, 825-831.

[155] Antin JH, Lee SJ, Neuberg D, Alyea E, Soiffer RJ, Sonis S, Ferrara JL. A phase I/II double-blind, placebo-controlled study of recombinant human interleukin-11 for mucositis and acute GVHD prevention in allogeneic stem cell transplantation. *Bone Marrow Transplant.* 2002, 29, 373-377.

[156] Blazar BR, Weisdorf DJ, Defor T, Goldman A, Braun T, Silver S, Ferrara JL. Phase 1/2 randomized, placebo-control trial of palifermin to prevent graft-versus-host disease (GVHD) after allogeneic hematopoietic stem cell transplantation (HSCT). *Blood.* 2006, 108, 3216-3222.

In: Encyclopedia of Stem Cell Research (2 Volume Set)   ISBN: 978-1-61761-835-2
Editor: Alexander L. Greene   © 2012 Nova Science Publishers, Inc.

Chapter XXXVIII

STEM CELL PLASTICITY

Suraksha Agrawal [1,*] Piyush Tripathi [1] and Sita Naik [2]

[1] Department of Medical Genetics, Sanjay Gandhi Post Graduate Institute of Medical Sciences, Raebareli Road, Lucknow (UP) India

[2] Department of Immunology, Sanjay Gandhi Post Graduate Institute of Medical Sciences, Raebareli Road, Lucknow (UP) India

ABSTRACT

Although hematopoetic stem cell (HSC) transplantation has been in practice for almost half a century, the improved understanding of stem cells over past two decades has revolutionized this field making it as most promising aspect of translational medicine. HSC are found in small numbers in peripheral blood as compared to bone marrow. However, use of growth factors has opened new avenues to successfully use peripheral blood as source of CD 34+ HSC. These are pluripotent cells that are competent for self renewal and differentiation to a variety of specialized cells and are replenished with fresh cells every day. Recent understanding about their mobilization, homing and plasticity suggest that they can be useful for the maintenance and regeneration of various specialized tissues. This provides an opportunity to explore the specific niche responsible for stem cell plasticity, their trans-differentiation into specific cellular lineages as well the kinetics of their recovery whenever required. The normal physiological microenvironment may be unable to provide a suitable environment for the rapid regeneration of HSC required for coping with tissue damage and may need some external interventions. The autologous stem –cell transplantation (SCT), has decreased risk of graft –versus –host disease, and provides opportunities of external interventions in terms of ex vivo manipulation. In the diseases of hematopoietic and immune system allogeneic transplant remains a better modality but is associated with grave risk of graft –versus –host disease (GVHD). However, in these cases it is needed to engineer the hematopoietic stem cell (HSC) graft to remove the cells which cause GVHD or relapse to improve graft functions.

* Corresponding Author: Prof. Suraksha Agrawal, Department of Medical Genetics, Sanjay Gandhi Post Graduate Institute of Medical Sciences, Raebareli Road, Lucknow (UP) 226014 India, Phone: 091-522 -2668004-8 Ext 2338, 2346, 2347, Fax No. 091-522 -2668973/2668017, Email: suraksha@sgpgi.ac.in

Hematopoetic stem cell transplantations have been successful in a variety of diseases including leukemia and other hematopoetic disorders. Though results of HSCT are promising, developing a more mechanistic approach to plasticity and improving the external interventions and ex vivo manipulations may lead to improving the efficiency and speed of regeneration of transplanted cells. This could result in better use and wider application of stem cell based therapies.

Keywords: Stem cells, stem cell plasticity, haematopoietic stem cells, transdifferentiation

ABBREVIATIONS

HSC	Haematopoietic Stem Cell
ES cells	Embryonic Stem Cells
MSC	Mesenchymal Stem Cells
HLA	Human Leukocyte Antigen

INTRODUCTION

Stem cell research has got much attention in past decade due to its immense diagnostic and therapeutic potential. Stem cells can be developed into any organ (Smith 2001). It is interesting to note that 5 days old inner cell mass of the blastocyst consist of only 30 -35 cells but hold within it the complex repertoire of instructions that may manifest approximately 100 trillion cells that make up the adult human organism. The procedures based on human stem cells seem to allow new medical treatments for serious diseases like Parkinson's or Alzheimer's disease, leukemia and diabetes etc (Williams 2003). Stem cells remain quiescent (non-dividing) for many years until they are activated by disease or tissue injury. These cells can differentiate to yield the major specialized cell types of the tissue or organ. Some types of adult stem cells have the ability to differentiate into a number of different cell types if given the right environment. Microenvironment around the stem cell is very important as it determines and triggers the cell differentiation into different lineages (figure 1).

Generally stem cell undergo asymmetric cell division (i.e. one stem cell and one differentiated cell), where as a classic progenitor cell divides into two differentiated daughter cells. Embroyonic stem cells are uncommitted and pluripotent in their differential capability, whereas adult stem cells are believed to be committed to differentiate only into specialized cells of the organ or tissue they are derived from. The defining characteristics features of stem cells are:

1. Clonogenicity: The stem cell can give rise to viable clones of dividing cells in all progenies.

Pluripotentiality: The stem cell is able to give rise to a variety of cell lineages, each of which is committed progenitor for a differentiated cell type as shown in figure 2.

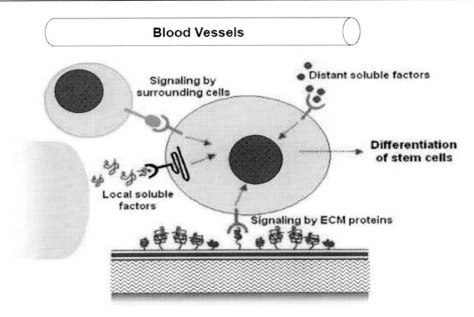

Figure 1. Stem cell niche. Microenvironment around stem cell that trigger the cell division and differentiation into different lineages.

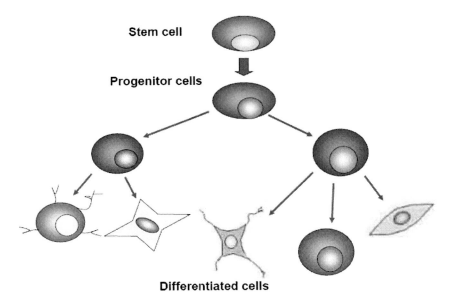

Figure 2. Pluripotency of stem cells: Stem cells are able to give rise to a variety of cell lineages, each of which is committed progenitor for a differentiated cell type.

2. Self renewal: The stem cell clone survives and replicates rather than undergoing irreversible terminal differentiation as do other cell types.

Stem cells are found in a very small populations in the human body i.e. ~1 stem cell in 100,000 cells in circulating blood. The history of research on adult stem cells began about 40 years ago. In 1960s, researchers discovered that the bone marrow contains at least two types of stem cells. One population, called hematopoietic stem cells, which forms all types of blood cells in the body. A second population, called bone marrow stromal cells was discovered a few years later (Dezawa 2007; Dezawa 2006; Gimble and Nuttall 2004). Stromal cells are a mixed cell population that generate bone, cartilage, fat, and fibrous connective tissues. Since its discovery, the most widely studied example of adult stem cells is hematopoietic stem cells (HSCs), which sustain formation of the blood and immune system throughout life. The bone marrow compartment is largely made up of committed progenitor cells, non circulating stromal cells that have the ability to develop into mesenchymal lineages (termed mesenchymal stem cells), and HSCs (Berger and Chassagne 2003; Udagawa et al., 2007). This latter group has been the predominant focus of research examining the stem cell compartment of bone marrow, its identification relying largely on the expression of cell-surface markers to define a subpopulation enriched for HSCs. Although this method of identification can be easily performed in the laboratory, there are several caveats, most notably that there is no assessment of stem cell function inherent to it. However, complete characterization of HSCs before their use invokes the biological equivalent of Heisenberg's uncertainty principle; by the time the cell has been isolated and demonstrated to differentiate into multiple lineages, it is no longer a stem cell. Nevertheless, surface marker expression is used in standard experimental practice to identify a population that is enriched for HSCs.

STEM CELL SURFACE MARKERS

These cells can be differentiated from the other cells on the basis of markers. These markers are specialized proteins called receptors that have the capability of selectively binding or adhering to other "signaling" molecules. There are many different types of receptors that differ in their structure and affinity for the signaling molecules. Normally, cells use these receptors and the molecules that bind to them as a way of communicating with other cells and to carry out their proper functions in the body.

The cell surface that has gathered immense interest is sialomucin CD34, which was initially found to be expressed on a small fraction of human bone marrow cells (Civin et al., 1984). The CD34[+] cells of marrow or mobilized peripheral blood are responsible for most of the hematopoietic activity (Civin et al., 1984; Shpall et al., 1997). CD34 has therefore been considered to be the most critical marker for hematopoietic stem cells (HSCs). CD34 expression on primitive cells is down regulated as they differentiate into mature cells (Sutherland and Keating., 1992). They are cabable of differentiating into different cell types. Recent work on the cell lines has proved that CD34 human progenitor cell line Mutz-3 can be differentiated into functional Osteoclasts (Ciraci et al., 2007). Another surface marker is CD133, which is a 120-kDa glycosylated protein with five transmembrane domains. Recent literature have shown that CD133 expression is not restricted to primitive blood cells, but also present in unique cell populations of non-hematopoietic origin. CD133[+] progenitor cells from peripheral blood can be induced to differentiate into endothelial cells *in vitro* (Gehling et al., 2000, Rountree et al., 2007). ABCG2 was identified in breast cancer cell line by Doyle et al., 1998 it is ATP-binding cassette super family G member 2. It is a determinant of the wide variety of stem cells, including HSC (Kim et al., 2002; Doyle et al., 1998). It is localized to the plasma membrane (Rocchi et al., 2000). Sca-1 (stem cell antigen 1, Ly-6A/E), an 18-kDa phosphatidylinositol-anchored protein is a member of the Ly-6 antigen family. Sca-1 is the most recognized HSC marker in mice with both Ly-6 haplotypes as it is expressed on multipotent HSCs. Sca-1 has also been discovered in several non-hematopoietic tissues, however, can be used to enrich progenitor cell populations other than HSCs.

Most of the stem cell markers are given short names based on the molecules that bind to the stem cell surface receptors. For example, a cell that has the receptor stem cell antigen -1, on its surface, is identified as Sca-1. In many cases, a combination of multiple markers is used to identify a particular stem cell type. For example, a special type of hematopoietic stem cell from blood and bone marrow called "side population" or "SP" is described as ($CD34^{-/low}$, c-Kit^+, Sca-1^+) (Booth and Potten 2000).

The markers on the cells are identified by using fluorescent tags using flow cytometry (Loeffler and Roeder., 2002; Shamblott et al., 1998; Gage, 2000). A second method is based upon stem cell markers and their fluorescent tags to visually assess cells as they exist in tissues by using microscope.

How cells become specialized in the organism's development has been solved by identifying genes and transcription factors which may be unique to stem cells. For example, a gene marker called PDX-1 is specific for a transcription factor protein that initiates activation of the insulin gene. This marker has been used to identify cells that are able to develop islet cells into pancreas.

A gene was inserted into a stem cell a "reporter gene" called green fluorescent protein or GFP (Thomson et al., 1998). The gene is only activated or "reports" when cells are undifferentiated and is turned off once they become specialized. Once activated, the gene directs the stem cells to produce a protein that fluoresces in a brilliant green color.

It was assumed that adult stem cells, unlike ES cells, were lineage restricted, but recent observations demonstrating that bone marrow–derived myogenic progenitors participate in regeneration of damaged skeletal muscle (Ferrari et al., 1998) and ischemic myocardium (Orlic et al., 2001b; Jackson et al., 2001; Orlic et ala., 2001). In addition, presumptive muscle stem cells were also shown to contribute to hematopoiesis (Jackson et al., 1999; Gussoni et al., 1999), although this could relate to their common embryological origin, because both blood and muscle cells derive from the mesoderm. On the basis of the presence of markers the stem cells and the differentiated cells are characterized. The details of markers used for this purpose are shown in table 1.

Using a murine bone marrow stromal cell line, Nakamura et al., (1999) expanded cell fractions that expressed neither CD34 nor lineage markers (CD34- / Lin- cells) and converted these to CD34+ cells. It has been observed that (Pittenger et al., 1999; Horwitz et al., 1999; Kuci et al., 2003; Osawa et al., 1996; Goodell et al., 1996; Morel et al., 1998; Bhatia et al., 1998; Zanjani et al., 1998; Sato et al., 1995), it is conceivable that there is a common precursor cell of HSCs and MSCs giving rise to bone, cartilage, and other mesenchymal organ systems. Thus, CD34- Flk1+ cells, which have been identified as putative "hemangioblasts," (Guo et al., 2003) might, in fact, be more primitive than CD34+ / Flk 1+ cells.

Table 1. Markers used to identify stem cells in differentiated cell types

Marker Name	Cell Type
Blood Vessel	
Fetal liver kinase-1 (Flk1)	Endothelial
Smooth muscle cell-specific myosin heavy chain	Smooth muscle
Vascular endothelial cell cadherin	Smooth muscle
Bone	
Bone-specific alkaline phosphatase (BAP)	Osteoblast
Hydroxyapatite	Osteoblast
Osteocalcin (OC)	Osteoblast
Bone Marrow and Blood	
Bone morphogenetic protein receptor (BMPR)	Mesenchymal stem and progenitor cells
CD4 and CD8	White blood cell (WBC)
CD34	Hematopoietic stem cell (HSC), endothelial progenitor
CD34$^+$Sca1$^+$ Lin$^-$ profile	Mesencyhmal stem cell (MSC)
CD38	Absent on HSC Present on WBC lineages
CD44	Mesenchymal
c-Kit	HSC, MSC
Colony-forming unit (CFU)	HSC, MSC progenitor
Fibroblast colony-forming unit (CFU-F)	Bone marrow fibroblast
Hoechst dye	Absent on HSC
Leukocyte common antigen (CD45)	WBC
Lineage surface antigen (Lin)	HSC, MSC, Differentiated RBC and WBC lineages
Mac-1	WBC
Muc-18 (CD146)	Bone marrow fibroblasts, endothelial
Stem cell antigen (Sca-1)	HSC, MSC
Stro-1 antigen	Stromal (mesenchymal) precursor cells, hematopoietic cells
Thy-1	HSC, MSC
Cartilage	
Collagen types II and IV	Chondrocyte
Keratin	Keratinocyte
Sulfated proteoglycan	Chondrocyte
Fat	
Adipocyte lipid-binding protein (ALBP)	Adipocyte
Fatty acid transporter (FAT)	Adipocyte
Adipocyte lipid-binding protein (ALBP)	Adipocyte
General	
Y chromosome	Male cells

Karyotype	Most cell types
Liver	
Albumin	Hepatocyte
B-1 integrin	Hepatocyte
Nervous System	
CD133	Neural stem cell, HSC
Glial fibrillary acidic protein (GFAP)	Astrocyte
Microtubule-associated protein-2 (MAP-2)	Neuron
Myelin basic protein (MPB)	Oligodendrocyte
Nestin	Neural progenitor
Neural tubulin	Neuron
Neurofilament (NF)	Neuron
Neurosphere	Embryoid body (EB), ES
Marker Name	Cell Type
Noggin	Neuron
O4	Oligodendrocyte
O1	Oligodendrocyte
Synaptophysin	Neuron
Tau	Neuron
Pancreas	
Cytokeratin 19 (CK19)	Pancreatic epithelium
Glucagon	Pancreatic islet
Insulin	Pancreatic islet
Insulin-promoting factor-1 (PDX-1)	Pancreatic islet
Nestin	Pancreatic progenitor
Pancreatic polypeptide	Pancreatic islet
Somatostatin	Pancreatic islet
Pluripotent Stem Cells	
Alkaline phosphatase	Embryonic stem (ES), embryonal carcinoma (EC)
Alpha-fetoprotein (AFP)	Endoderm
Bone morphogenetic protein-4	Mesoderm
Brachyury	Mesoderm
Cluster designation 30 (CD30)	ES, EC
Cripto (TDGF-1)	ES, cardiomyocyte
GATA-4 gene	Endoderm
GCTM-2	ES, EC
Genesis	ES, EC
Germ cell nuclear factor	ES, EC
Hepatocyte nuclear factor-4 (HNF-4)	Endoderm
Nestin	Ectoderm, neural and pancreatic progenitor

Table 1. (Continued)

Neuronal cell-adhesion molecule (N-CAM)	Ectoderm
Oct-4	ES, EC
Pax6	Ectoderm
Pluripotent Stem Cells	
Stage-specific embryonic antigen-3 (SSEA-3)	ES, EC
Stage-specific embryonic antigen-4 (SSEA-4)	ES, EC
Stem cell factor (SCF or c-Kit ligand)	ES, EC, HSC, MSC
Telomerase	ES, EC
TRA-1-60	ES, EC
TRA-1-81	ES, EC
Vimentin	Ectoderm, neural and pancreatic progenitor
Skeletal Muscle/Cardiac/Smooth Muscle	
MyoD and Pax7	Myoblast, myocyte
Myogenin and MR4	Skeletal myocyte
Myosin heavy chain	Cardiomyocyte
Myosin light chain	Skeletal myocyte

In fact, human Flk1+/ CD31- / CD34- cells could not only contribute to hematopoietic and vascular reconstitution, they also readily give rise to epithelial cells of the liver, lung, and gastrointestinal tract of irradiated NOD / SCID mice. No contribution was seen to skeletal, cardiac muscle, skin, and kidney. Just as Krause et al., (2001) described, these differences may be due to less damage induced by iradiation in these tissues or more residual tissue – specific stem cells capable of self –repair within these tissues. Differentiation of FLK1+ / CD31- / CD34 – cells into hematopoietic cells cannot be attributed to the contamination by hematopoietic stem/ progenitor cells. BM cells were depleted of CD45+ and CD34+ cells by magnetic beads sorting before Flk1+/ CD31- / CD34 – cells cultures were initiated. All input Flk1+ / CD31- /CD34- cells were CD11a, CD11b, GlyA, and CD45 negative, and did not express early hematopoietic transcription factors, including GATA -1 and GATA-2 (Weiss and Orkin 1995; Guo et al., 2003). Additionally, culture conditions for Flk1+ / CD31- / CD34- cells are not supportive of hematopoietic stem / progenitor cell differentiation.

Presently the trend is to select the stem cells on the basis of their markers and provide adequate cell culture conditions so that the cells can differentiate in a lineage specific manner. Pruszak et al., 2007 has shown that neural cells are differentiated in vitro from human embryonic stem cells (hESC) which exhibit broad cellular heterogeneity with respect to developmental stage and lineage specification. They have shown that standard conditions for the use and discovery of markers for analysis and cell selection of hESC undergoing neuronal differentiation. To generate better-defined cell populations, they established a working protocol for sorting heterogeneous hESC-derived neural cell populations by fluorescence activated cell sorting (FACS). Using genetically labeled synapsin-GFP (+) hESC-derived neurons as a proof-of-principle they enriched viable differentiated neurons by FACS. Cell sorting methodology using surface markers was developed, and a comprehensive profiling of surface antigens was obtained for immature ES cell types (such as SSEA-3, -4, TRA-1-81, TRA-1-60), neural stem and precursor cells (such as CD133, SSEA-1 [CD15], A2B5, FORSE-1, CD29, CD146, p75 [CD271]) and differentiated neurons (such as CD24 or NCAM [CD56]). At later stages of neural differentiation, the neural cell adhesion molecule NCAM (CD56) was used to isolate hESC-derived neurons by FACS. FACS-sorted hESC-derived neurons survived in vivo after transplantation into rodent brain. These results and concepts provided (1) a feasible approach for experimental cell sorting of differentiated neurons, (2) an initial survey of surface antigens present during neural differentiation of hESC, and (3) a framework for developing cell selection strategies for neural cell-based therapies (Pruszak et al., 2007). Further it has been shown that stem cells with CD133 can follow bilineages if appropriate conditions are provided (Rountree et al., 2007).

STEM CELL PLASTICITY

Recent studies have shown new evidences that several tissues may contain cells capable of generating differentiated cells beyond their own tissue boundaries, defining a process termed stem cell plasticity. The type of cells which show plasticity are bone marrow cells which give rise to blood cells of all lineages, and mesenchymal stem cells which give rise to osteoblasts, adipocytes, and fibroblasts. There are reports showing that bone marrow stem cells can evolve into cells of all dermal lineages, such as hepatocytes, skeletal myocytes, cardiomyocytes, neural, endothelial, epithelial, and even endocrine cells. These findings promise significant therapeutic implications for regenerative medicine. If has been reported that epigenetic alterations some time cause silencing of genes required for HSC's to undergo symmetrical cell divisions. As a result of this there is progressive decline if primitive HSC function (Mahmud et al., 2006). It has been seen that self-renewal capacity of HSC's decreases progressively with HSC differentiation. The mechanisms, which govern stem cell growth, are under tight control but still these are modifiable. The global gene expression of HSC has been described but very little is known about the dynamics of gene expression necessary for HSC fate decisions. Oct-4 gene expression is shown to be regulated by an epigenetic mechanism, which is required for the maintenance of pluripotency of embroyomic stem cells (Hattori et al., 2004). The extrinsic and intrinsic factors for the growth of HSC's are still not known. However, it is thought that growth factors and an adequate microenvironment is crucial for the survival and proliferation of HSC's self renewal/differentiation decisions in HSC appear likely to occur independently of cytokines and are postulated to be determined by the intrinsic properties of HSC. HSC are positive for CD34 and all those cells, which carry the gene P15, are unmethylated but after 7 days of culture the cells undergo the process of methylation and demethylation after 15 days. HSC's can undergo either a symmetric or asymmetric, cell division. Under both the conditions the microenviroment should be such that there is sustenance of long term donor derived hematopoiesis. The methylation machinery in normal hematopoietic development is regulated to allow lineage specific differentiation and control of proliferation, disturbances in methylation lead to gene specific inactivation by promoter silencing (Mahmud et al., 2006). It has been suggested that in combination with demethylating agents with histone deacetylase (HDAC) inhibitors can be used to remove the epigenetic gene inactivation. It has been reported by Maria et al., 2007 that bone marrow cells have the ability to evolve or differentiate into oral and craniofacial tissues, such as the periodontal ligament, alveolar bone, condyle, tooth, bone around dental and facial implants, and oral mucosa (Maria et al., 2007).

If bone marrow cell could give rise to stem cells of another tissue, then they could repopulate whole organs from a few starting cells. This model of dedifferentiation is consistent with recent data from animal models. Genetic analysis of cells of donor origin in vivo and in vitro has brought to light another possible mechanism. The evidences have been gathered from tracking techniques as shown in figure 3.

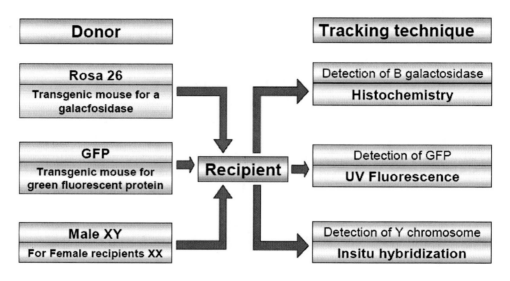

Figure 3. Methods to track the transplanted stem cell.

The heamatopoietic and neural stem cells appear to be the most versatile at cutting across the lineage boundaries. Another component of bone marrow stem cells is mesenchymal stem cells (MSCs), which can be expanded *in vitro* and stimulated to form bone, cartilage, tendon muscle or fat cells. The MSCS in culture may be induced to differentiate into neurons by exposure to beta marcaptoethanol, DMSO or butylated hydrooxyanisole (Woodbury et al., 2000). MSC – derived cells are seen to integrate deep into brain after peripheral injection as well as after direct injection of human MSCs into rat brain, they migrate along pathways used during the migration of neural stem cells developmentally, get distributed and loss of markers take place. In mice model MSCs adopted neural or astrocyte phenolybes with expression of glial fibrillary acidic protein (GFAP) and neurofilament markers (Kopen et al., 1999). Mouse recipients of MSCs prepared from enhanced GFP (eGFP) transgenic mice were found to have a large number of eGFP fluorescent cells in their brain (Brazelton et al., 2000).

The Role of Cell Fusion in Stem Cell Plasticity

The mechanisms involved in cell plasticity are dedifferentiation, transdifferentiation, cell fusion etc. The fusion of host and donor cell can give rise to mature tissue cell without trans– or dedifferentiation. Cell fusion has emerged as a powerful subject of debate in the last few years. Adult stem cell plasticity and the search for mechanisms to explain this process have led to the "rediscovery" of cell fusion. In nature, cell fusion is a normal process involved in sexual reproduction, tissue formation, and immune response (Alvarez-Dolado 2007). Recent studies have identified the specific molecular signals such as SDF-1/CXCR4 complex is required for the interaction of BMC and damaged host tissues (Liu et al., 2006). However, many mechanisms still remain to be unearthed.

Somatic stem cell plasticity has recently been challenged suggesting that any transdifferentiation seen may in fact be the product of cellular fusion between infused stem cells and pre-existing differentiated cells. *In vitro*, mouse bone marrow cells labeled with distinct genetic markers (GFP and puromycin-resistance protein), which have been cultured together with ES cells in a medium containing puromycin showed that surviving colonies were GFP-positive but were similar to ES cells in their morphology and growth kinetics. In addition, they expressed ES-cell proteins and were able to differentiate into various morphologies, including cardiac myocytes (Terada et al., 2002). In a similar approach, neural stem cells have been used, and once again the colonies recovered expressed GFP but had also become ES-like (Ying et al., 2002). However, in the neural cell study, the ES cells had also been labeled with a transgene, which was subsequently expressed on recovered cells (Ying et al., 2002). In addition, genetic analysis in both studies revealed that the derived colonies had supra-diploid DNA content, and the bone marrow –derived progeny were shown to have a hybrid genotype (Terada et al., 2002). This suggests that the alteration in phenotype had arisen through generation of hybrids, which is by cellular fusion.

Subsequent *in vivo* studies have also supported the view that fusion contributes to perceived transdifferentiation. In one study, FAH-expressing liver nodules were generated by transplantation of marrow cells from wild-type males into irradiated FAH-deficient females. A group working on murine model with serial transplantation of bone marrow–derived hepatocytes studied hepatocyte alleles. Analysis of DNA from the tertiary recipients revealed that although massive liver repopulation had occurred, only a fraction of the original donor genotype was preserved in the repopulating cells (Wang et al., 2003), which is less than would have been expected if they had derived solely through transdifferentiation of HSCs.

Differentiation of HSCs into hepatocytes has shown that transdifferentiation takes place upon exposure to the hepatic environment, donor HSCs undergo genetic reprogramming, switch lineage, and generate hepatocytes. The frequency at which this occurs depends on several factors, including the type and extent of liver injury. If fusion of donor HSCs, or indeed other hematopoietic cells such as macrophages, fuse with mature hepatocytes these eventually redifferentiate into terminally differentiated hepatocytes. It should be noted that although most fusion cells contain multiples of the normal karyotypes, approximately 30% of cells are aneuploid. It is a two-step process. Donor HSCs engraft and differentiate into hepatocytes, which then undergo fusion with mature native hepatocytes. All these steps are shown in figure 4.

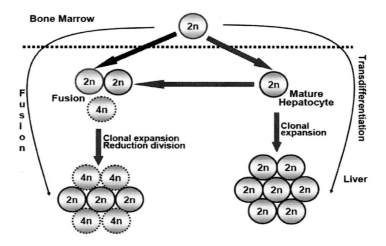

Figure 4. Differentiation stages of HSCs into hepatocytes.

Mobilization of Haematopoietic Stem Cells

Stem cell mobilization is an important phenomenon both in bone marrow transplantation and stem cell therapy. It has been proposed that for mobilization various molecules like adhesion molecule e.g. selectines and integrines, chemokines and their ligands e.g. SDF 1α, CXCR4 and proteolytic enzymes are required (figure 5).

CXCR4 circulate at low levels in the peripheral blood. The concentration increases during tissue damage. The chemoattractants released from the damaged tissue like SDF-1 leads the stem-cells to 'home in' at the site of injury.

Mobilization is important because it protects HSC from toxic injuries. Some times mobilization could be a death pathway a mechanism that can regulate self-cell number. Mobilization mechanisms may be complementing asymmetrical division. Under mobilization if replication event occurs and the microenvironment for the cell is not available, one of the cells will mobilize or die.

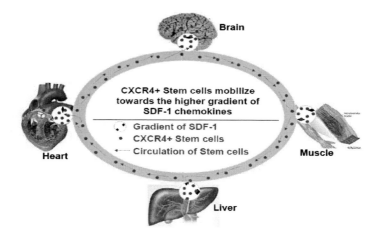

Figure 5. Mobilization of haematopoietic stem cells haematopoietic stem cells express.

The mobilization of stem cells depends on SDF-1α / CXCR4 and VLA-4 / VCAM-1 pathway. VLA-4 / VCAM-1 pathway is important for housing of bone marrow stem cells. It has been demonstrated that $CD34^+$ are involved in lodging in both bone marrow and spleen. Vermeulen et al., 1998 has shown that entry of CFU (colony- forming units) in spleen is highly regulated. Further VLA-4 and CD44 are identified in mobilization of stem cells into blood stream of mice when injected with anti VLA4 or anti CD44. Stem cells mobilized by anti VLA 4 comprise high self renewal potential and can be used for long term reconstitution of tissue (Vermeulen et al., 1998).

It has been shown that bone marrow contains HSC and mesenchymal stem cells (MSC's) both of which may derive from a common primitive blast like cell precursor which are able to differentiate along MSC or HSC potentials (Hall et al., 2001). HSCs return to the bone marrow within 1 day. Different factors are involved in migration and homing the ligand for C kit, B1 integrins, chemokine stromal derived factors (SDF) or its receptors. CXCR4 prevent haematopoiesis transferring from embryonic liver to marrow. SDF1 seems to be chemo attractant for HSC expressing CXCR4. Although CXCR4 cells may also migrate to wards SDF1 and it has been demonstrated in vivo that CXCR4 expression on CD34+ CD38- Lin- cells do not confer any advantage in the rescue of irradiated NOD/ SCID mice (Rosu-Myles et al., 2000). Colony stimulating factor helps in mobilization (Whetton and Graham 1999).

In wound healing the stem cells sense tissue damage and migrate from the distance to the site of injury (Theise et al., 2000; Harraz et al., 2001). Nevertheless, it has been observed that activation of immune response increases regeneration of cells and tissues when transplanted to the host (Krause et al., 2001; Laflamme et al., 2002; Quaini et al., 2002). It has been shown that there is a link between blood and endothetial cell lining in the form of multipotent stem cell, haemangioblast, which give rise to both haematopoietic and endothelial cell lines (Robb and Elefanty 1998). Although this debate still goes on, it seems clear now that stem cells with haemangioblast properties exist in the embryo as well as in the adult (Choi 1998). But the finding that a cell, such as monocyte, which is presumed to be fully committed to myeloid bloodlines, is also capable of generating endothelial cells, has significant consequences for stem cell biology.

Epigenetic Regulation of Hematopoietic Stem Cells (HSC)

The pluripotency of adult stem cells have evoked significant excitement over the possibility of novel functional uses of stem cells, with the final purpose to develop new and more effective treatment strategies (Serafini and Verfaillie 2006). The differentiation can take place under a controlled process by epigenetic alterations (Snykers et al., 2007). It has been reported that neural stem cell can give rise to haematopoietic or myogenous cells (Galli et al., 2000). Neural stem cells help in intrinsic brain repair (Barani et al., 2007). Interestingly, embryonic stem cells spontaneously generate cardiomyocytes that exhibit variety of electrophysiological phenotypes (Franco et al., 2007). It has been reported that phenotype of marrow cell changes with position in the cell cycle. Further, these phenotype changes are reversible. This phenomenon is true for both hematopoietic and non-hematopoietic cells. Stem cell keep on changing with phase of cell cycle presumably based on windows of transcriptional access (Quesenberry et al., 2007). Kim et al., in 2006 have demonstrated that there are set of overlapping genes, 22 are up-regulated and 141 down regulated genes which are involved in the developmental stages of all stem cells (Kim et al., 2006). The genes which are highly up regulated belong to functional category like signaling pathway, transcription factors, transcription regulators, DNA binding, cell cycle, various receptors, genes involved in the metabolic pathways, cytokines and growth factors and some genes with unknown functions. They proposed that functional studies of these genes are required to understand the development of stem cells which may further help in remodeling the different stages of stem cell development into specific adult cell.

Certain chemicals like 5-Azacytine and its analogs as well as HDAC inhibitors have dramatic effect on transcriptional regulation. They can synergistically reactivate the silenced genes. HSC's are slowly cycling cells that are capable of existing G_0/G_1 following exposure to IL1, IL3, IL6, granulocyte stimulating factor (G-CSF), granulocyte macrophage CSF CM-C 3F stem cell factor (SCF), FLT-3 ligand and thrombopvietin (TPO). It has been reported that addition of these compounds into the culture of CD34$^+$ HSCs do not cause reduction in their methylation status, suggesting that hypomethylation induced by these compounds in the culture may promote reactivation of gene critical for maintenance of HSC phenotype and function. It has been shown that 5azaD/TSA treated bone marrow CD34$^+$ cells remained in their primitive cell phenotype (CD34$^+$ CD90$^+$) in spite of nine day long culture. The percentage positivity of these cells was ~ 77%. When the culture was done in the absence of 5azaD/TSA the cells expression CD34$^+$ CD90$^+$ decreased to <1%. When the cell were cultured only in cytokines for nine days there was a dramatic reduction of colony forming cells in comparison of primary bone marrow CD34$^+$ cells (Mahmud et al., 2006).

Better Source of Hematopoietic Stem Cells: PBMCs or Bone Marrow

During autologous Stem Cell Transplantation, source could be bone marrow or peripheral blood as the source of stem cells. Normally collection of stem cells from PBSC is difficult and has fewer stem cells compared to bone marrow. But in case of damaged bone marrow or heavy tumor infiltration, PBMCs remain the only option. In these situations various mobilization regimens can be used to increase the CD34$^+$ concentration in the peripheral blood and thus more CD34+ cells than steady-state bone marrow could be obtained. The infusion of more CD34$^+$ cells not only results in a more rapid engraftment but also of lower risk of being contaminated with tumor cells residing in the bone marrow (Pecora et al., 2002).

However, in allogeneic stem-cell transplantation the engraftment is faster with PBSC than bone marrow thus negating the number of infused CD34$^+$ cells as a critical factor. Another concern in the allogeneic transplantation is graft-versus-host disease (GvHD), caused by lymphocyte subpopulations, particularly T-lymphocytes, thus limiting the use of donor PBSC as the stem-cell graft in allogeneic transplantation (Körbling and Fliedner 1996). However, instead of steady state PBMCs, mobilized PBSC from T lymphocytes depleted bone marrow are used for allogeneic stem-cell grafting, acute GvHD is less frequent. This in part may be due to decreased T cell reactivity after treatment with GCSF used in mobilization regimen.

This is still an ongoing study the use of BM or PBSC as the source of stem cells for allogeneic SCT. Some studies concluded that for good-risk patients (HLA-identical related donor; low or average risk of relapse) bone marrow and peripheral blood is equivalent (Champlin et al., 2000; Horan et al., 2003). However, it has been demonstrated that for good-risk younger patients, bone marrow provides better results. Donor preference is also a critical factor and is the choice of stem cells for match unrelated donor transplants. For allogeneic SCT from partially matched related donors, the number of CD34+ cells infused is very critical (Aversa et al., 1998). As higher number of purified CD34+ cells can only be obtained from PBSCs instead of bone marrow (Aversa et al., 1998) hence use of PBSC appears as a better choice for allogenic HSCT.

Umbilical Cord Blood and Their Ex Vivo Expansion: Source of HSCs

Umbilical cord blood provides an optional therapeutic modality for hematopoietic stem cell therapy. However, it has limitation of fewer numbers of HSCs thus delaying the post transplant engraftment. One of the options to over come this limitation is selective *ex vivo* expansion of primitive progenitor stem cells. A better understanding about the microenvironment of hematopoiesis enabled the expansion of these cells without their differentiation.

However, it has been reported that cellular defects may be acquired during *ex vivo* expansion. This may be due to the defects in the cell cycle abnormalities. It has been demonstrated that once the cells enter G1 phase and are exposed to cytokine these cells reveal reduced engraftment capacity (Glimm et al., 2000). CD34$^+$ cells cultured in the presence of FL, TPO, SCF show increased adhesion hence decreased marrow homing. Further if the cells are exposed to IL3, IL6, SCF, IL11 and FL there is altered expression of VLA -4 and VLA-5, this causes poor engraftment (Ramirez et al., 2001; Zhai et al., 2004). Ex vivo cultures are associated with increased expression of the Fas ligand (CD95) (Liu et al., 2003), this down regulates the expression of the antiapoptosis protein Bct-2 (Domen et al., 2000) and increased caspase activation (Wang et al., 2000) resulting into induction of apoptosis. Various authors demonstrated that cell differentiation was due to cell fusion (Hawley and Sobieski 2002; Wurmser and Gage 2002; Medvinsky and Smith 2003). Stem cells may undergo fusion with other cell types (Terada et al., 2002; Wang et al., 2003).

Recent development in optimization of HSC culture has revealed the choice of cell source, cytokines and stroma used in culture could affect the success in specific expansion of stem cells. The increasing interest has grown about the molecular mechanism that regulates the specific expansion in ex vivo. There are various signaling pathways involved in the HSC proliferation and maintenance. Some examples of these pathways are:

Notch signaling pathway: Notch signaling is involved in cellular differentiation, proliferation, apoptosis, adhesion and epithelial – to-mesenchymal transition. There are five Notch ligands in mammals, Jagged -1/2 and Delta – 1/3/4. Binding of a Notch ligand to a

Notch receptor results into the cleavage which causes release of the interacellular domain of the Notch receptor by a membrane –associated protease complex. The intracellular domain then translocates to the nucleus to join with CBF1/ RBP-J (Schroeter et al., 1998) and mastermind –like (MAML) (Wu et al., 2000) among others. The assembled nuclear complex regulates transcription of several Notch effector genes, including homolog of Drosophila Hairy and Enhancer of Split (Zhou and Hayward 2001). Thus the optimal concentration of Notch ligands in ex – vivo culture has yet to be established and the differing effects of Notch ligands has not yet been fully studied; for instance Delta-1, unlike Jagged-1, inhibits B – cell differentiation (Jaleco et al., 2001) and decreases CFU-GM, CFU-G and CFU-M (Neves et al., 2006).

Wnt signaling pathway: Wnt-mediated signaling involves the binding of Wnt proteins to their receptor-coreceptor complexes, frizzled- LRP, which leads to the accumulation of β-catenin and its translocation to the nucleus. Early studies demonstrated that activation of Wnt signaling induced both mouse fetal liver HSC (AA4$^+$ cKIT$^+$ SCA1) and human bone marrow (Lin)-CD34$^+$ proliferation when HSC were co-cultured on Wnt transduced stromal feeder layers (Austin et al., 1997; Van Den Berg et al., 1998). Interestingly, Wnt-mediated maintenance of HSC immaturity in vitro requires Notch signaling, although HSC survival and entry into the cell cycle is Notch independent (Duncan et al., 2005).

Tie2/ Ag-1 signaling pathway: Tie2 /Ang-1 signaling pathway plays a critical role in the maintenance of HSC in a quiescent state in the BM niche (Arai et al., 2004).

BMP: BMP are members of the TGF-β super family that have long been established to function in the development and regulation of a wide range of biological systems. BMP also play key role in regulating fate choices during stem cell differentiation. Zhang et al, showed that BMP receptor activation of spindle shaped N-cadherin +CD 45- osteoblastic type (SNO) cells maintains the stem cell niche (Zhang et al., 2003).

Bmi-1: B lymphoma Mo-MLV insertion region 1 (Bmi-1), a proto oncogene and member of the Polycomb group repressive complex 1. The importance of Bmi -1 in HSC self-renewal has been demonstrated in mouse models of both genetic gene deletion and transduced overexpression (Park et al., 2003). As a central player in HSC self –renewal, Bmi-1 could be a target for therapeutic manipulation of HSC.

HOXB4: HOX genes encode a large family of transcription factors that have highly conserved DNA –binding motif known as the homeodomain. HOXB4 may be one of the most important regulators of HSC self-renewal. It is expressed in the stem cell fraction of the bone marrow and subsequently down regulated during differentiation in humans (Lawrence and Largman 1992; Sauvageau et al., 1994) and mice (Pineault et al., 2002). HOXB4 –deficient mice have HSC with a reduced proliferative capacity but normal differentiation and lineage pathways (Bjornsson et al., 2003; Brun et al., 2004). Forced expression of HOXB4 also rapidly triggers an increase of human UCB HSC detected by both *in vitro* and *in vivo* assays (Antonchuk et al., 2002). It has been shown that improvement in the culture systems may expand UCB progenitors. Some of these newer manipulations are summarized in table 2.

Table 2. Manipulations in the UCB ex vivo expansion

Target	Description
Epigenetic modification	Epigenetic modification of growth factors by histone methylation inhibition or acetylation (5azaD/ TSA) may slow differentiation.
Cell types	CD34$^+$cells, however, cells with more primitive marker CD133$^+$ provides better engraftment and more accurate functional assays.
Copper chelation	Intracellular copper concentration may be crucial for an immature phenotype and then the engraftment.
Cytokines	SCF, Flt-3 ligand (FL) and thrombopoietin (TPO) are crucial cytokines. FL and TPO may prevent apoptosis.
Retinoids	These are involved in the embryonic development and cellular differentiation. Success has been achieved in using all-trans retinoic acid to increase murine long-term repopulating cells.
Wnt activation	The Wnt pathway is involved in the maintainance of the undifferentiated phenotype in human ebryonic stem cells. Use of Wnt activator to HSC recipient mice improved better recovery.

With a better understanding of the molecular mechanisms of HSC homing, expansion and presentation, a second generation of clinical trials are being initiated and much is based on the enhanced understanding of hematopoiesis. This is occurring at the same time that other clinical trials exploring the use of dual UCB units as the transplant source. Although cord transplants may ultimately supplement our need for HSC expansion, it remains to be determined if this approach will relapse and optimize immune reconstitution as compared to that seen after a living related or unrelated donor transplant. Until this is clarified, expansion studies should continue.

Micro RNA Expression in Stem Cells

It has been reported that micro RNA are expressed specifically dividing embryonic development hence it is thought that their role may be critical for stem cell differentiation and cell proliferation specially at the level of gene regulation. Recently a miRNA microarray technique has helped to study the developmental biology but tissue homeostasis and malignant cell proliferation is still poorly understood. Their role is also demonstrated in model organisms like drosophila, Dicer-1 (DCR-1) which is essential for the formation of mature RNA which is when mutated in Drosophila germline stem cells (GSC) they could not be maintained, suggesting their role is GSC self renewal (Jin and Xie 2007). Their mode of action is hypothesized to regulate various target cells involved in cell differentiation and proliferation.

STEM CELL THERAPY

Experimental biology and medicine have used stem cells in cell therapy for more than 20 years. An *in vitro* method has been developed to culture embryonic stem (EC) cells acquired at abortions or from surplus embryo left after *in vitro* fertilizations, and immediately evoked ideas how to direct the development and differentiation of these cells and utilize them in regeneration of damaged tissues (Filip et al., 2004). Still, the cell therapy faces a difficult task how to detect, harvest and culture stem cells for treatment of several diseases (Lemischka 2005; Lemischka et al., 2003).

Table 3. Diseases Treated with Hematopoietic Stem-Cell Transplantation

Autologous transplantation	Allogeneic transplantation
Multiple myeloma	Multiple myeloma
Non-Hodgkin's lymphoma	Non-Hodgkin's lymphoma
Hodgkin's disease	Hodgkin's disease
Acute myeloid leukemia	Acute myeloid leukemia
Neuroblastoma	Chronic lymphocytic leukemia
Ovarian cancer	Juvenile chronic myeloid leukemia
Germ-cell tumors	Acute lymphoblastic leukemia
Autoimmune disorders	Chronic myeloid leukemia
Amyloidosis	Myelodysplastic syndromes
	Aplastic anemia
	Blackfan–Diamond anemia
	Thalassemia major
	Sickle cell anemia
	Severe combined immunodeficiency
	Inborn errors of metabolism

$CD34^+$ and $FLK-1^+$ stem cells can differentiate into endothelial cells in vivo and in vitro. These can be helpful in ischaemic injury (Arriero et al., 2004). These cells get mobilized after ischaemia or after G-CSF pretreatment. Homing of HSCs has been reported in lung, gastrointestinal tract, liver, pancreas, kidney, skin, skeletal muscle and bone (Quesenberry and Becker 1998). HSCs treatment has been successfully explored in various diseases (table 3).

Animal studies show that transplantation of pluripotent stem cells or fetal cells can successfully treat a number of chronic diseases, such as diabetes, Parkinson's disease, traumatic spinal cord injuries, Purkinje's cellular degeneration, liver failure, heart failure, Duchenne's muscular dystrophy, osteogenesis imperfecta, and others (Horwitz et al., 2001; Soria et al., 2001; Snyder et al., 2004; Kajstura et al., 2005). Although marked progress has been achieved in human transplant therapy, there are still several main setbacks limiting broad application of cells in the routine therapy, such as the need of massive doses of immunosuppressive drugs to prevent rejection of transplanted tissue and also lack of organs from dead donors. Despite all these set-backs, strategy based on human ES cells may allow production of unlimited amounts of cells, eventually tissues, and their sufficient supply from abundant, renewable and quickly available sources. Moreover, ES cells according to their adaptability for stable genetic modification could be treated so as to avoid or inhibit the host immune response. The first step to develop successful therapy is based on human ES cells is to demonstrate their capability to differentiate into certain, cell type, and to purify this line from a mixed population. In the second step, it would be necessary to critically examine that differentiated cell derivatives function in a normal physiologic way, for example, the secretion of insulin in the cells of Langerhans islets is normal and responds to the glucose level. The third step and most important milestone on the route to clinical tests will be the proof of efficiency of model diseases in guinea-pigs and big animals. The fourth step is to exclude formation of tumors developing from derivatives after differentiation of ES cells and transplanted to human recipients.

Considering the progress in these directions goes forward in a big way, however, other problems will certainly show which may limit the therapeutic use of cells. The effort of scientists to treat diseases at present untreatable, the pressure of patients and their families, as well as political pressure may complicate the development of new therapies. Important is to keep a "clear mind", get rid of emotions and respect scientific and ethical rules. Prospective trends in the cell therapy are: therapeutic cloning, ES cells, therapy of the fetus, adult stem cells, use of humoral agents for control of stem cell behavior and, eventually, genetic stem cell modification. At the beginning it appeared that adult stem cells may represent a certain "ethical compromise" to embryonic cells. Today, however, we understand that individual approaches are closely linked together and this, consequently, delays the answers to bioethical issues. Scientists have already shown that a number of cell types, such as neurons and muscle cells (Kehat and Gepstein 2003), pancreatic cells (Soria et al., 2001) and others can be obtained by culture of ES cells. Today, stem cells may be used in quite unexpected cases, such as renal diseases (Mollura et al., 2003; Schachinger and Zeiher 2005) and immunologic repair in AIDS patients (Scadden 2003).

During past three decades, allogeneic stem cell transplantation (ASCT) has developed from being an experimental therapy in patients with end stage leukemia into a well-established therapy in patients with a range of disorders of the immunohematopoietic system. Graft-versus-host disease (GVHD), acute or chronic, attacking host tissue is a major threat. However, donor immunocompetent T cells have a potent graft-versus-leukemia effect. A combination of calcineurin inhibitors and methotrexate is the standard therapy to prevent GVHD. Modulation of the immunosuppressive regimen may induce mild acute and mild chronic GVHD, reduce the risk of relapse, and improve long-term survival. Natural killer cells also play a role in this context. Killer cell immunoglobulin-like receptor incompatibility between recipient and donor may reduce the risk of relapse in patients with myeloid leukemia. Relapse of leukemia is a major cause of death after ASCT. Minimal residual disease and recipient leukemia lineage-specific chimerism are sensitive techniques for early detection of leukemic relapse. Donor lymphocyte infusions can enhance the antitumor effect, especially for patients with molecular relapse. The allogeneic graft-versus-cancer effect has been demonstrated in patients with metastatic breast, renal, colorectal, ovarian, prostatic, and pancreatic carcinoma. Mesenchymal stem cells have immunomodulatory properties and may be used for immunomodulation of GVHD and tissue repair. If all modalities considered, the future looks promising for ASCT (Ringden 2007).

Coronary Artery Disease

One of the diseases where stem cell therapy has been tried is coronary artery disease (CAD), which remains the major cause of morbidity and mortality in the developing countries. In patients with severe CAD, persistent myocardial ischemia in hibernated myocardium results in the progressive loss of cardiomyocytes with development of heart failure. As a result of therapeutic approaches to enhance neovascularization are being under the process of intensive investigations. Recent experimental studies have demonstrated adult bone marrow (BM) can induce neovascularization in ischemic myocardium which can improve heart function. These findings have prompted the development of different cellular transplantation approaches for heart diseases refractory to conventional therapy after myocardial infarction. Although the initial pilot clinical trials have shown potential clinical benefit of BM therapy for therapeutic angiogenesis, the long-term safety, the optimal timing and treatment strategy remains unclear. Furthermore, in order to acquire more optimized quality and quantity of BM derived stem cell for myocardial regeneration, several issues remain to be addressed, such as the development of a more efficient method of stem cells identification, purification and expansion. Emerging, rationally designed, randomized clinical trials are required to assess the clinical implication of BM derived stem cells therapy in treatment of CAD (Tse et al., 2007; Ferrari et al., 1998; Eglitis and Mezey 1997).

The success of transplantation depends on survival, maturation and electro mechanic connection of donor cells with existing heart cells of the recipient and their effect on heart function. There are high requirements for any cell population, so it is not surprising that experiments, until now, brought different results depending on selected cell types. The idea to use bone marrow stem cells for heart regeneration is particularly attractive. They are pluripotent, i.e. able to differentiate into several distinct cell types. As for the heart, these pluripotent cells might be capable of forming heart muscle as well as vessels for alimentation support of the damaged area and for repopulation with muscle cells. Harvesting of cells from bone marrow in adults is easy and routine and does not present any ethical problems connected with the use of embryonic and fetal tissues. The therapy with cells from the patient's own bone marrow eliminates the fear of tissue rejection (a great problem with cells from another donor). Furthermore, it is known that transfer of marrow cells into the scar in the damaged heart improves the heart function if the cells are cultured one week before and then treated to induce expression of muscle proteins (Tomita et al., 1999; Ozbaran et al., 2004). Orlic et al, separated Lin− c-kit+ cells of bone marrow from transgenic mice expressing enhanced green fluorescent protein (EGFP) (Orlic et al., 2001a; Orlic et al., 2001b). Failure to reconstitute infarction was ascribed to difficulties with transplantation of cells into the tissue with high contractile frequency. Also immunologic reaction of female mice to male bone marrow transplant might be the cause for insufficient regeneration in some female recipients. Local transplant of Lin- c-kit+ bone marrow cells showed high capacity for differentiation into cardiac tissue. They led to the formation of new cardiomyocytes, endothelial cells and smooth muscle cells and formed *de novo* myocardium with coronary arteries, arterioles and capillaries.

Partial regeneration of infarcted myocardium means that transplanted cells responded to signals of injured myocardium and induced migration, proliferation and differentiation in the necrotic area of the ventricular wall. Differentiating cardiomyocytes may express nuclear and cytoplasmic proteins typical of heart tissue (Orlic et al., 2001b) but also atypical, such as nestin (Mokrý et al., 2004). The repair of damaged myocardium may be evoked by application of autologous bone marrow cells (Strauer and Kornowski 2003; Eisenberg and Eisenberg 2004), and application of some cytokines such as SCF and G-CSF (Strauer and Kornowski 2003; Deten et al., 2005) and others (Lee and Makkar 2004). Critically evaluating to date published clinical studies on cell therapy of myocardial infarction we have to realize that it will not be easy to find a cell population or cytokine cascade, which would enable us to better, utilize the possibilities that cell therapy offers. The results of these studies are different in both, clinical and biological aspects − numbers of patients are small, application of cells (myocardial injection or intracoronary infusion) is also different and differences in the transplant itself (bone marrow cells, muscle-obtained myoblasts, or separated progenitor cells). Application of bone marrow cells had only minimum complications, such as supraventricular tachycardia and one death, but not due to arrhythmia (Lee et al., 2004). More serious complications were described in patients given muscle-obtained myoblasts. The complications were arrhythmias and ventricular tachycardias, and one death at cell application (Lee et al., 2004). Some other reports preferring the use of marrow cells transdifferentiated into cardiomyocytes with the help of some growth factors, such as G-CSF (Takano et al., 2003) are very interesting and show the possibilities to combine cytokines, for instance. Each of the presented methods has its advantages and disadvantages. With application of bone marrow cells, both, repair of myocardium and its revascularization is presumed. Contrary to this, revascularization is much smaller with muscle cell application. We must not forget to mention late complications of which we do not know much (Abbott and Giordano 2003; Eisenberg and Eisenberg 2004).

Jolicouer et al., have recently assessed the status of cell-based therapies in CAD and have discussed the opportunities to accelerate the process to clinical application (Jolicouer et al., 2007). Further Huber et al, have shown a technique where cardiomyocytes can be selected and identified during human embryonic stem cell differentiation. They generated stable transgenic hESC lines, using lentiviral vectors, and single-cell clones that expressed a reporter gene (eGFP) under the transcriptional control of a cardiac-specific promoter (the human myosin light chain-2V promoter). They have shown that the appearance of eGFP-expressing cells during the differentiation of the hESC as embryoid bodies (EBs) can be identified and sorted using FACS (purity>95%, viability>85%). The eGFP-expressing cells were stained positively for cardiac-specific proteins (>93%), expressing cardiac-specific genes, displayed cardiac-specific action-potentials, and could form stable myocardial cell grafts following *in vivo* cell transplantation (Huber et al., 2007). The generation of these transgenic hESC lines may be helpful to identify and study early cardiac precursors for developmental studies, to robustly quantify the extent of cardiomyocyte differentiation, to label the cells for *in vivo* grafting, and to allow derivation of purified cell populations of cardiomyocytes for future myocardial cell therapy strategies.

It is known that the endothelium has an important regulatory role in the maintenance of vascular homeostasis, vascular tone, blood flow, and in preserving a non-thrombogenic blood-tissue interface. Injury to the vascular wall with subsequent endothelial dysfunction alters these important regulatory functions leading to a state of abnormal endothelial function.

Nossaman et al., 2007 reviewed the athophysiology of endothelial dysfunction and how this disorder is common to the development of erectile dysfunction and of pulmonary arterial hypertension. They have shown that stem cell therapy can be used as a clinical modality for these two disorders of endothelial dysfunction (Nossaman et al., 2007). In conclusion we can say that cell therapy represents a new therapeutic method for myocardial tissue damage.

Autoimmune Diseases

Autoimmune diseases vary in a wide range from mild to severe, intractable diseases. A great development of the therapy has been encountered in the past decades, in particular of formerly incapacitating diseases, such as rheumatoid arthritis or Crohn's disease. While biologic therapy, in particular monoclonal antibodies, offered most new solutions in these disorders, the therapy with many conventional drugs has also been rewritten. Old drugs, such as cyclophosphamid or intravenous immunoglobulin, retained their position in severe forms of autoimmunity. An evolving new area of stem cell transplantation offers benefit for the most severe patients suffering from intractable autoimmune diseases (Kapoor et al., 2007). ESCs under controlled environment can be differentiated into different cell lineages like cartilage and bone. Cultured articular chondrocytes, MSCs have been used for cartilage repair. However, the results are inconsistent. This is because many other factors are also involved like growth factors, tissue scaffolds, diseased microenvironment and alignment of the joint. These are some of the crucial conditions responsible for the success. Presently osteoinductive growth factors that derive MSCs down the osteogenic pathways are under the process of trial in different clinical settings. However, oeteogenic pathway may not be responsible but other factors relating to vascularization of bones may be responsible.

Stem cell therapy has also been used to repair damaged muscles. However, the success rate is not very high. In Osteoarthritis (OA) stem cells have been tried and it has been shown that they are involved in remodeling process including osteophytosis. Most of the time the failure of MSCs therapy is due to inflammatory cytokines that have detrimental effect on bones and cartilages. From these results it appears that the diseased microenvironment plays important role in functioning of osteoarthritis. It is proposed that for degenerative therapy in musculoskeletal diseases the artificial microenvironment may be created which is capable of supporting cell engraftment, committing differentiation, resulting in patterning and maturation of tissue, subsequent anatomy and function. Presently self-assembling in structuring polymers are being used which control the release of bioactive substances oblique morphogenes. These polymers help in cell adherence, proliferation and differentiation as well as biomechanical support. Adipose tissue-derived stromal cells (ADSC) can easily be isolated from human adipose tissue (Zuk et al., 2002, Zuk et al., 2001, Dicker et al., 2005), and they have the potential to differentiate into bone, cartilage, tendons, skeletal muscle, and fat when cultivated under lineage-specific conditions (Wagner et al., 2005, Zuk et al., 2001, Dicker et al., 2005). Tissue engineering of these mesenchymal organs is of major interest in human diseases, such as inherited, traumatic, or degenerative bone, joint, and soft tissue defects (skeletal regeneration and cartilage repair). Schaffler et al., 2007 have proposed that adipose tissue-derived stromal cells (ADSC) have an equal potential to differentiate into cells and tissues of mesodermal origin, such as adipocytes, cartilage, bone, and skeletal muscle (Schaffler et al., 2007).

Chronic Obstructive Pulmonary Disease

To develop a new cell based therapy for chronic obstructive pulmonary disease (COPD), we need to understand 1) the role of tissue-specific and bone marrow-derived stem cells, 2) extracellular matrix, and 3) growth factors. Recently, bronchioalveolar stem cells were identified in distal lungs (Kim et al., 2005). Impairment of these stem cells may cause improper lung repair after inflammation, resulting in pulmonary emphysema. Bone marrow-derived cells are necessary to repair injured lungs. However, the long term role of these cells is not understood yet. Although we need more careful analysis and additional experiments, growth factors, such as hepatocyte growth factor, are good candidates for the new cell based therapy for COPD. Lung was believed as a non-regenerative organ. Based on these recent reports about lung regeneration and stem cells, however, new strategies to treat COPD and a new point of view to understand the pathophysiology of COPD are rising (Randell 2006).

Neurodegenerative Disorders

Lindvall et al., in 2004 has reviewed the generation of neurons from the stem cells in culture in response to injuries (Lindvall et al., 2004). These findings raise hope for the development of stem cell therapies in human neurodegenerative disorders. Neural stem cells are self-removing and pleuripotent, which can differentiate into neurons astrocytes and oligodendrocytes. Due to these properties, MCSs are supposed to be an ideal candidate for clinical purpose. However, there is an effort to develop an efficient method to generate proliferative dopamineargic neurons. Yu et al., 2007 have used a rat model to generate such type of cells in the presence of dFGF, Heparin and Laminin both in vitro and in vivo and have demonstrated that these cells if grafted can survive for at least one month and the migration too of closed tissue was observed on day thirty post transplantation. They have proposed that combination of dFGF, heparin, laminin is advancement in stem cell therapy which can replace lost neuron in injury or neurodegenerative disorders (Yu et al., 2007).

Human adult mesenchymal stem cells have been used in animal models for neurological disorders like cerebral ischemia, Parkinson diseases and spinal chord lesions. It has been reported that transplantation of mesenchymal cells into functional cells (Pisati et al., 2007). They have proposed three mechanisms, which are trans differentiation of the grafted cells with replacement of neurodegenerative cells, cell fusion and neuroprotection of the dying cells. They isolated a restricted number of cells with differentiated astroglial features from human adult mesenchymal stem cells and transplanted into the developing mouse and observed that human mesenchymal cells did not reveal any neuronal trans differentiation but express neurotrophin low affinity {MGFR (p75)} high affinity {trkC} receptors and release now growth factors and neurotrophin3 (Anti-3). The expression was demonstrated even after

45 days of intracerebellar transplantation HMCs into nude mice with surviving astroglial cells. This study is a reflection towards the potential for treating neurological disorders.

As indicated above the human stem cells are capable of generating different types of neurons. However, the cellular mechanisms that underline the development of neurons in vitro are poorly understood. Anisimov et al., 2007 have developed a neuron stem chip which is a highly specialized to characterized the expression of the genes, to show the longitudinal quality control of HSCs population, to see the gene expression after differentiation and confirm the success of differentiation into several neural subtypes (Anisimov et al., 2007).

It has been shown that stem cell therapy can be used in Huntington disease. Huntington disease is a fatal disorder characterized by chorea and progressive dementia. The main pathology of the disease is the loss of medium spinal projection in the stratium due to mutation in Huntington gene. It was thought that cell based therapy may allow the restoration of gain of function by replacing the faulty neuron (Garbuzova- Davis 2002; Garbuzova et al., 2003; Kerr et al., 2003; Dunnett 2000; Kendall et al., 1998; Palfi et al., 1998). Presently a lot of work is going on to explore how to generate and select projection of neurons from stem cells.

As well as replacing cell lost to a degenerative process, stem cells and, in particular, neural stem/ progenitor cells could potentially be used to deliver therapeutic substances such as neurotrophic factors, in the case of neurodegenerative disorders. The aim is to modify the cells to express the protein of interest using *ex vivo* gene therapy and then transplant them into the desired location where they would produce the protein or peptide of interest in a regulated fashion.

In terms of neurotrophic factors, it is well recognized that neurons require adequate tropic support for their growth, development, and maintenance. Substances such as glial cell line – derived neurotrophic factor (GDNF) have been shown to reduce cell death in dopaminergic neurons in vitro (Fan et al., 1998), to promote graft survival in vivo (Ostenfeld et al., 2002), to be reduced in the substantianigra in patients with PD (Chauhan et al., 2001), infusion of GDNF directly into the brain parenchyma via a minipump promoted structural and functional recovery in a primate model of PD (Grondin et al., 2002), and more recently in patents with PD (Gill et al., 2003). Brain-derived neurotrophic factor (BDNF) prevents striatal cell death in excitotoxic models of Huntington's disease (HD) (Bemelmans et al., 1999; Perez-Navarro et al., 2000), and individuals with HD have decreased levels of BDNF compared to age – matched controls (Ferrer et al., 2000). Similar findings are seen with ciliary neurotrophic factor (CNTF) in primate models of HD (Mittoux et al., 2000), which has lead to a pilot study involving the use of CNTF delivered via an encapsulated polymer system in patients with mild to moderate HD (Bachoud Levi et al., 2000). The use of stem cells engineered to release such factors may prove beneficial for the treatment of these neurological disorders.

Stem cells have also been considered for a range of other neurological problems, for example, to deliver chemotherapeutic agents to brain tumors. Aboody et al., demonstrated that transplanted neural stem cells preferentially migrate toward experimentally induced gliomas in vivo, and that when these cells are transfected with the cytosine deaminase gene, which has anti mitotic activity, they decreased the size of the tumor (Aboody et al., 2000). Another study transfected mouse neural progenitor cells with interleukin IL-4, injected them into gliomas of mice and rats, and found that a significant proportion of injected animals survived at 90 days compared to non injected controls (Benedetti et al., 2000). However, injecting the control, non transfected progenitor cells also caused a smaller but significant increase in survival at 90 days.

In addition, certain neurological disorders caused by single gene deficits such as Tay-sachs and mucopoly-saccharidosis type VII (MPS VII) might be amenable to replacement by cell-based approaches. Both are lysosomal storage disorders and caused by a deficiency in the β exosaminidase α subunit gene and the β lucuronidase gene, respectively. Neural cells lines constructed to produce the human β hexosaminidase α subunit and transplanted into the brain of newborn mice were shown to produce therapeutic levels of the protein throughout the brain (Lacorazza et al., 1996). In addition, neural progenitors carrying the β glucuronidase gene transplanted into the lateral ventricle of newborn mice were engrafted along the neuraxis, expressed the protein, and corrected lysosomal storage in neurons and glia of affected mice (Snyder et al., 2002). Finally, stem cells have been used in the treatement of stroke (Kondziolka et al., 2000), and have been considered as treatment for multiple sclerosis (Pluchino et al., 2003), and spinal trauma (Stepanov et al., 2003), as well as a range of other neurological conditions.

Parkinson's Disease

Parkinson's disease (PD) is a neurodegenerative disorder involving a specific neuronal subpopulation that projects to the nucleus striatum. PD is related to the degeneration of dopaminergic fibers, which results in a severe extrapyramidal syndrome. The loss of motor performance (tremor, rigidity, bradykinesia) in PD is partially re-established by oral administration of the dopamine precursor L dopa; however, upon chronic administration of this amino acid, patients develop a fluctuating response to optimal dosage with episodes of complete kinetic block.

The age- dependent and multifactorial nature of Parkinson's pathogenesis allows many strategies of intervention and repair. First, the oxidative stress, protein abnormalities, and cellular inclusions typically seen could be dealt with by antioxidants, trophic factors, and proteolytic enhancements. Second, if the delay of degeneration is not sufficient, the immature dopamine neurons can be placed in the parkinsonian brain by transplantation of dopaminergic neurons taken from human fetuses (Hagell et al., 1999; Lindvall et al., 1990) or highly enriched embryonic stem populations of midbrain neural stem cells. The dopamine neurons generated by the stem cells show electrophysiological and behavioral properties expected of neurons from the midbrain (Kim et al., 2002). Finally, endogenous stem cells can be stimulated to repair the damage of the disease (Isacson 2002; Daadi 2002).

A genetic approach to restore the dopamine levels in PD patients consist of delivery of the gene encoding tyrosine hydroxylase (TH) to boost dopamine production or the delivery of genes encoding neurotrophic factors such as GDNF to promote the survival of dopaminergic neurons (Latchman and Coffin 2001). Studies about the regulation of the expression of the TH gene (Mallet 1996) have shown restoration of dopamine levels in PD animal models, and these results have been achieved either by intracerebral injection of lentiviral vectors carrying the TH gene or by transplantation of cells genetically modified to express TH (Gage 1998).

Moreover, injection of GDNF vectors in the striatum also has a positive effect on the preservation of nigrostriatal projections. Long –term experiments using both AAV (adeno-associated virus) –GDNF and LV (lentivirus)- GDNF have shown that continuous GDNF delivery for a long time (3-6 months) is able to stimulate endogenous self –repair and regeneration activity both in 6 –hydroxi dopamine (OHDA) –lesioned rats and in MPTP (1-methyl-4-phenyl-1, 2,3, 6-tetrahydropyridine)- lesioned monkeys (Bjorklund and Lindvall 2000; Kordower and Sortwell 2000; Bensadoun et al., 2000).

As already mentioned, the use of human primary embryonic tissue raises moral as well as practical issues, mainly related to tissue availability and biosafety. Therefore, the establishment of a technique allowing the continuous production of human catecholaminergic neurons, thus avoiding the systematic use of primary fetal tissue and guaranteeing high biosafety standards, would be of value to the development of therapies for PD. So far, several reports have demonstrated that implantation of precursor –derived dopaminergic neurons from rodents leads to histological, biochemical and functional recovery in animal models of PD (Carvey et al., 2001; Studer et al., 1998; Svendsen et al., 1996), there are few reports on generation of human dopaminergic neurons from any stem cells, using the embryonic midbrain as a tissue source (Studer et al., 1998) and only one study reported *in vitro* generation of human dopaminergic neurons following long –term expansion (Storch et al., 2001).

Previously, it was reported that the isolation of multipotential stem cells from the fetal human brain (Vescovi et al., 1999), their extensive culturing to establish stable cell lines, and the successful engraftment of stem –cell –derived neuronal and glial progeny into mature rodent brain. Previous results from Daadi and Weiss (Daadi and Weiss 1999) described culture conditions under which TH expression is induced in mouse neuronal precursors, deriving directly from the embryonic striatum and adult subependyma of the lateral ventricle or generated from multi potent forebrain stem cells. TH was successfully induced by exposure of these cells to basic FGF2 and B49 glial cell line conditioned medium (B49CM). The epigenetic generation of TH-expressing neurons was also achieved from neuronal multi potential precursor cells obtained from 10.5 post conception week human fetus. Appropriate differentiation of NSCs prior to transplantation is pivotal for the successful engraftment of NSC –derived neurons in the adult rodent striatum. TH induction was gradual, peaked at a value of 4 – 6 % of the total cell number by 5 – 7 days following induction, and occurred in approximately 30% of the differentiated neuronal progeny (Vescovi et al., 1999).

Spinal Cord Injury and Peripheral Nerves Transaction

In spinal cord injury (SCI), the traumatic destruction of nerve fibers that carry motor signals from the brain to the torso and limbs leads to muscle paralysis. In addition, destruction of nerve fibers can lead to loss of sensation, such as touch, pressure, and temperature. SCI pathology is determined not only by the initial mechanical insult, but also by secondary processes, including ischemia, anoxia and free radical formation that occur over hours, days, and weeks following injury. Later, the center of the bruised spine fills with fluid, becoming a cyst, and scar tissue piles up, preventing recovery. CNS intra spinal axonal regeneration appears to be impeded partly by myelin-associated inhibitors and the loss in adult neurons of an intrinsic ability to overcome inhibitory cues.

During the past decade, olfactory ensheathing glia (OEG) transplantation has emerged as a very promising experimental therapy to promote repair of spinal cords after different types of injuries. Transplantation of these cells promoted axonal regeneration and functional recovery after partial and complete spinal cord lesions. Moreover, olfactory ensheathing glia was able to form myelin sheaths around demyelinated axons. The behavior of OECs in two-dimensional (2-D) condition as well as on three-dimensional (3-D) collagen scaffolds has been studied by analyzing their phenotypes such as cell proliferation, apoptosis, morphology, and gene activities of some neurotrophic factors and myelin proteins. OECs proliferation rate was increased on 3-D collagen scaffolds compared to the 2-D culture condition. OECs on 3-D collagen scaffolds also showed less apoptosis (Wang et al., 2006). Olfactory ensheathing glia transplantation might have a future as a therapy for different spinal cord afflictions in humans (Santos-Benito and Ramon Cueto 2003) and can be viewed as a clinically relevant alternative to Schwann cells in the treatment of spinal cord injury.

Three studies (Bradbury et al., 2002; Yick et al., 2000; Moon et al., 2001) have reported an improved regenerative response following treatment of the injured CNS with chondroitinase. Chondroitin sulfate proteoglycans (CSPGs) represent a significant source of inhibition within the injured CNS; these studies indicate that successful CNS regeneration may be brought about by interventions that target these molecules and/or the cells that produce them.

Cells transplanted into the injured spinal cord should be able to survive for extended periods within the injury site, to integrate with host tissue, to rescue injured neurons from cell death and atrophy, to promote axonal regeneration, and, ultimately, to restore function. In addition, because astrocytes have important functions, such as providing substrates for regeneration and trophic supports for surviving neurons, reconstitution of an appropriate glial environment including astrocytes and oligodendrocytes may be essential for promoting functional axonal regeneration and remyelination. NSCs theoretically fit many of the above requirements.

Some of the most promising strategies for regeneration used are peripheral nerves (autologous) or fetal tissue (heterologous) transplants in the visual system and SCI. It has been pointed out (Coumans et al., 2001) that regeneration from supraspinal pathways and recovery of motor function were dramatically increased when ES transplants and neurotrophins were delayed until 2-4 weeks after transection rather than applied acutely. These data suggest that the opportunity for intervention after SCI exists not only in the acute phase but also in chronic phase. Indeed, rat hippocampal NSCs injected into the cerebrospinal fluid throughout the 4th ventricle of 4week-old rats that had been given a contusion spinal cord injury attached to the pial surface at the lesion invaded extensively into the spinal cord tissue as well as into the nerve roots and survived as long as 8 months after transplantation (Wu et al., 2002). A very large part of these cells differentiated into astrocytes and oligodendrocytes and were well integrated with the host tissue inside spinal cord; in the nerve roots, they surrounded myelinated and unmyelinated fibers behaving like Schwann cells of the peripheral nervous system (PNS), suggesting that NSCs may importantly contribute to peripheral nerve regeneration as well.

Another more sophisticated use of the NSCs is to employ genetically modified and grafted NSCs into the lesion site in the spinal cord, which will provide augmented amounts of trophic molecules at the injury site and a potential axonal growth substrate. Particularly, murine NSCs engineered by recombinant retrovirus were induced to secrete NT-3 (Liu et al., 1999; Lu et al., 2003) when transplanted into the injured spinal cord; these cells promote a three-fold increase in axonal growth with respect to unmodified NSCs.

Artificial substrates may be useful for repairing spinal cord and peripheral nerve lesions where bridging is necessary; these substrates have to be easily manipulated, immune tolerant, and contain a porous scaffold for nerve regeneration and cell repopulation biodegradable by the CNS. This tissue engineering approach ought to simulate the architecture of the healthy peripheral nerves and spinal cord through an implant consisting of a polymer scaffold seeded with NSCs. Teng et al, in 2002 have reported that the scaffold's inner portion emulated the gray matter via a porous polymer layer designed for cellular replacement and trophic support, and the outer portion emulated the white matter with long, axially oriented pores for axonal guidance and radial porosity to allow fluid transport while inhibiting in growth of scar tissue. This multi component, degradable, synthetic scaffold (composed of poly-lacticco-glycolic acid) of specified architecture seeded with NSCs directed cell replacement, facilitated regeneration, guided repair to create a more physiologically relevant structure, and, in SCI, mitigated secondary injury impeding glial scar formation. For behavioral recovery, the scaffold alone appears to play a significant role, but the combination of the NSCs and scaffold is critical for the greatest recovery. Lu et al, in 2003 reported that NSCs seemed not to differentiate into neurons and oligodendrocytes; in fact, several donor cells remained largely undifferentiated. Therefore both the major contribution of NSCs to nerve regeneration and the mechanisms by which NSCs and the scaffold interact need to be further investigated.

Multiple Sclerosis

Multiple sclerosis (MS) is an inflammatory disease of the CNS characterized by localized areas of demyelination. MS is believed to be an autoimmune disorder mediated by activated immune cells such as T and B lymphocytes and macrophages/microglia. The impairment of the myelin membrane results in denuded axons that are no longer able to transmit action potentials efficiently within the CNS (in other words there is a lost of saltatory conduction), and results in the production of neurological symptoms.

There are several possible mechanisms of repair of the myelin membrane, including resolution of the inflammatory response followed by spontaneous remyelination, spread of sodium channels from the nodes of Ranvier to cover denuded axon segments and restore conduction, antibody-mediated remyelination, and remyelination resulting from the proliferation, migration, and differentiation of resident oligodendrocyte precursor cells (Noseworthy et al., 2000). So far, experimental cell therapy is based on the transplantation of myelin-forming cells or their precursors at the site of demyelination (Archer et al., 1997; Imaizumi et al., 2000), but the multifocal nature of this chronic inflammatory disease of the CNS raises critical issues regarding the therapeutic use of focal cell transplantation.

It has been shown that, syngeneic adult NSCs cultures, established from the peri ventricular region of the forebrain ventricles of adult mice, have undergone extensive in vitro expansion and successive infection with a lentivirus loading a nuclear-lacZ *(Escherichia coli β-galactosidase)*; these cells were injected into the experimental autoimmune encephalomyelitis (EAE) murine model of MS either intravenously (i.v. systemically) or into the cisterna magna (i.c. intra cerebroventricularly) (Pluchino et al., 2003). Both the systemic and intraventricular injections were performed either before disease onset, at the onset of the disease, or one week later. Ten days after transplantation, independently of the injection type, only EAE mice transplanted after the onset of the disease presented donor cells diffused throughout the neuraxis. Besides the integration, notable changes were observed: significant percentages of the donor cells integrated in demyelinating areas, and both clinical and neurophysiological impairments caused by EAE were almost completely rescued. Forty-five days after transplantation, the central conduction time (CCT), measured by means of motor-evoked potentials (MEPs) in both sham-treated controls and EAE mice transplanted with neural precursors, was significantly reduced in intravenously and intra cerebroventricularly transfused mice. This effect long-lasted up to 80 days post immunization, when CCT in intravenously and intra cerebroventricularly injected mice was closer to a normal value. Clinical recovery was faster in intravenously transplanted mice, but at the end of the follow-up period intravenously and intra cerebroventricularly injected EAE mice were both significantly recovered and these results were also accompanied by a drastic decrease of the extent of demyelination and axonal loss. This study was the first successful attempt to functionally recover a chronic multifocal disease by means the NSCs used therapeutically. Since other approaches such as interferon-β seem to induce the production of antibodies that inhibit or neutralize the biological activity of interferon-β itself (Noseworthy et al., 2000), it seems that stem cell therapy could be the best candidate for the rescue of MS disease.

Brain Ischemic Injury

Extensive ischemic injury is a neurological disorder caused by multiple factors, and one of these, hypoxia, is a common cause of neurological disability in adults and children. This disorder, characterized by extensive damage of cerebral parenchyma, causes a cystic cavity, and consequently important loss of cells and connections that reside there. There are no effective clinical therapies so far.

Two ways of thinking are principally followed in pilot studies: in one of these, the most important aspect is the reconstruction of cerebral tissue by cells and some kind of biocompatible support necessary to structure cellular organization and to direct the growth and the integration with preexisting circuits within the large infarction cavities. A polymeric reasorbable scaffold seeded with NSC was used to reconstruct the cerebral cortex (Park et al., 2002). After an in vitro culturing period of 4 days, NSCs seeded on completely biodegradable fibers made of poly glycolic acid (PGA) were transplanted into 1week-old hypoxic ischemic-induced mice. Some weeks after surgery, NSCs differentiated into oligodendrocytes, astrocytes, and neurons, and migrated into adjacent cortical or hippocampal penumbral areas. Host and donor-derived neurons sent their projections to the PGA scaffold in the "reconstituted" cortical penumbra and to targets in the opposite hemisphere, respectively. Mononuclear cell infiltration and astroglial scarring, physiological processes following CNS injury, seemed to be minimized by and within the ischemic NSC-PGA "regenerated" area. In the control group (PGA alone), none of these effects were significantly appreciable. This work shows an innovative multidisciplinary approach that point out NSCs as the most suitable stable, renewable cell source for a cells replacement method to rescue brain traumatic injuries.

Opposite to this, another group (Veizovic et al., 2001) injected murine immortalized NSCs into the hemisphere contralateral to the ischemic lesion. Their results showed significant functional effects when compared with control groups, including lesion volume reduction mainly by "re-filling" of host cells, NSCs migration, differentiation, and integration. Besides, by testing a lipid transporter (ApoE) distribution associated with ischemic brain damage, they suggested a possible graft-associated neuronal remodeling effect in both the damaged and intact hemispheres. Thus, assuming that these pilot studies need further investigation, new possibilities open for NSCs that, besides cell replacement, may serve to augment constitutive and inducible mechanisms of brain plasticity.

Cellular transplantation therapy is thought to play a central role in the concept of restorative neurosurgery, which aims to restore function to the damaged nervous system. Stem cells represent a potentially renewable source of transplantable cells. However, control of the behavior of these cells, both in the process of clonogenic expansion and post-transplantation, represents formidable challenges. Stem cell behavior is thought to be directed by extracellular signals in their in vivo niches, many of which are protein or peptide based. As only one example, activation of Notch signaling pathway plays an important role in normal development and is the strongest known signal for stem cells to choose glial over neuronal fates. Therefore, artificial extracellular matrix proteins represent a potentially powerful tool to custom design artificial niches to strategically control stem cell behavior. A family of aECM proteins have been developed that incorporate the active domains of the DSL ligands to the Notch receptor into an elastin-based backbone. The development of DSL-elastin artificial proteins demonstrates the strategy and methodology for the production of bioactive artificial extracellular matrix proteins aimed at modulating stem cell behavior, and this method can be used to design other bioactive aECM proteins. A method has been developed for the isolation and characterization of adult human neural stem cells from periventricular tissue harvested from living patients.Which helps in cellular transplantation therapy from the clinical perspective and exploring the intriguing possibility of autologous transplantation, whereby neural stem cells can be harvested from adult patients, expanded or modified *in vitro* in artificial niches, and retransplanted into the original patients (Charles et al., 2003).

HAEMOPOIETIC STEM CELL TRANSPLANTATION FOR GENETIC DISORDERS

Haemopoietic stem cell transplantation has also been employed for the treatment of various genetic disorders. HST has been successfully used in thalassaemia major. The success is higher among young children with lesser iron overload whereas for older patients with significant iron overload, chances of graft failure or toxicity are high. However, SCT is not widely used in sickle cell anaemia. Similarly there are fewer reports about the patients transplanted for red cell and platelet defects. SCT is not routine in any of these conditions and is reserved for patients with severe disease refractory to more conventional therapy. HST in severe combined immune deficiency (SCID) has steadily improved due to better transplant regimes and supportive care. There are also impressive results from haploidentical transplantation, with upto 78% long term survival and no deaths due to GVHD (Buckley et al., 1999). SCID is now classified on a genetic basis and it is becoming clear that some subtypes have better cure rates than others (Buckley 2003). HST has been employed in other disorders of blood cells or bone marrow are shown in table-4.

HST has also been used in the treatment of osteopetrosis and haemophagocytic disorders. Defective osteoclast causes osteopetrosis (Tolar et al., 2004) and uncontrolled histiocytes lead to haemophagocytic disorders. Life threatening haemophagocytosis is mostly initiated by infections in children under the age of 2 years. HST restores normal bone density by replacing cells of monocyte/macrophage lineage.

HST is also useful in treating many metabolic disorders including lysosomal storage diseases (LSD). Infusion of stem cells over enzyme replacement therapy is that it provides lymphocytes producing enzyme and cells that differentiate into microglia, carrying enzyme into the CNS (Peters and Steward 2003). In the success of SCT in metabolic diseases, the degree of tissue damage at the time of transplantation is very critical. Children with the most severe variants of metachromatic leukodystrophy during infancy and type 2 Gaucher's disease is not benefited very well. The benefit of HST also depends on organ systems. The detailed list of conditions where HST has been employed is given in the table-4.

Stem cell transplantation before the onset of disease symptoms could preserve organ function. Stem cell transplantation in adults is highly limited by Graft versus-host disease and thus requires the excessive use of immunosuppression and bone marrow irradiation. In all these cases *in utero* stem cell transplantation offers an alternative to the common postnatal transplantation, where early fetus being immunological immature would have lesser or no immune response against allograft antigens (Billingham et al., 1953) and thus the pretransplantation conditioning regimen could be omitted. The first *in utero* transplantation of haematopoietic stem cells was not successful in a 17-week old fetus. Where maternal T-cell depleted bone marrow injected into the umbilical vein could not result in postnatal engraftment (Linch et al., 1986). Since then intrauterine stem cell transplantation has been attempted in cases of haematopoietic and non-haematopoietic diseases and has been successful in cases with immunodeficiencies (table-4).

The stem cell research has affected the success of tissue regeneration in various branches of medical sciences. In particular the possibilities of trans-differentiation of cells of one lineage into cells of other lineages and also the faster differentiation have augmented the success of this field in the medical sciences. In conclusion, stem cells have enormous potential to be used in therapeutics. The recent developments in this field have enabled us to reveal the mechanism and to use them in various treatment modalities. However, the true success and its routine use in patient treatment would await some safer and *in vivo* intervention in the stem cell differentiation.

Table 4. Haemopoietic stem cell transplantation for genetic disorders

Immunodeficiency diseases	Severe combined immunodeficiency syndromes
	T-cell immunodeficiencies
	Omenn's syndrome
	Purine nucleoside phosphorylase deficiency
	Major histocompatibility complex class II deficiency
	Wiskott-Aldrich syndrome
	CD40 ligand deficiency (X-linked hyper-IgM syndrome)
	Phagocyte disorders
	Agranulocytosis
	Leucocyte adhesion deficiency
	Chronic granulomatous disease
	X-linked lymphoproliferative disease
Bone marrow failure/ cytopenic conditions	Pancytopenia
	Fanconi anaemia
	Shwachman-Diamond syndrome
	Dyskeratosis congenital
	Red cell aplasia
	Diamond-Blackfan anaemia
	Neutropenia
	Severe congenital neutropenia
Disorders of phagocytic cells operating in solid organs	Haemophagocytic conditions
	Haemophagocytic lymphohistiocytosis
	Chediak-Higashi syndrome
	Griscelli syndrome type 2 (due to RAB27A mutations)
	Malignant infantile osteopetrosis
Metabolic disorders	Adrenoleukodystrophy (ALD)
	Aspartylglucosaminuria
	Batten disease (neuronal ceroid lipofuscinosis, NCL)
	Fucosidosis
	Gaucher's disease, types I and III
	Globoid cell leukodystrophy (GLD)
	α-Mannosidosis
	Metachromatic leukodystrophy (MLD)
	Mucolipidosis, type II (I-cell disease)
	Mucopolysaccharidosis
	GM1 and GM2 gangliosidosis
	Niemann-Pick disease types A and C

REFERENCES

Abbott JD, Giordano FJ. Stem cells and cardiovascular disease. *J. Nucl. Cardiol.* 2003, 10:403-12.

Aboody KS, A Brown, NG Rainov, KA Bower, S Liu, W Yang, JE Small, U Herrlinger, V Ourednik, PM Black, XO Breakefield and EY Snyder. Neural stem cells display extensive tropism for pathology in adult brain: Evidence from intracranial gliomas. *Proc. Natl. Acad. Sci. USA.* 2000, 97: 12846-12851.

Alvarez-Dolado M. Cell fusion: biological perspectives and potential for regenerative medicine. *Front Biosci.* 2007,12:1-12.

Anisimov SV, Christophersen NS, Correia AS, Li JY, Brundin P. "NeuroStem Chip": a novel highly specialized tool to study neural differentiation pathways in human stem cells. *BMC Genomics.* 2007, 8:46.

Antonchuk J, Sauvageau G, Humphries RK. HOXB4- induced expansion of adult hematopoietic stem cells ex vivo. *Cell.* 2002, 109:39–45.

Arai F, Hirao A, Ohmura M, Sato H, Matsuoka S, Takubo K et al., Tie2/angiopoietin-1 signaling regulates hematopoietic stem cell quiescence in the bone marrow niche. *Cell.* 2004, 118: 149–161.

Archer DR, PA Cuddon, D Lipsitz and ID Duncan. Myelination of the canine central nervous system by glial cell transplantation: a model for repair of human myelin disease. *Nature Med.* 1997, 3:54-59.

Arriero M, Brodsky SV, Gealekman O, Lucas PA, Goligorsky MS. Adult skeletal muscle stem cells differentiate into endothelial lineage and ameliorate renal dysfunction after acute ischemia. *Am. J. Physiol. Renal. Physiol.* 2004, 287: F621-F627.

Austin TW, Solar GP, Ziegler FC, Liem L, Matthews W. A role for the Wnt gene family in hematopoiesis:expansion of multilineage progenitor cells. *Blood.* 1997, 89:3624–3635.

Aversa F., Tabilio A., Velardi A., Cunningham I., Terenzi A., Falzetti F., Ruggeri L., Barbabietola G., Aristei C., Latini P., Reisner Y., Martelli M.F., Treatment of high-risk acute leukemia with T-cell depleted stem cells from related donors with one fully mismatched HLA haplotype, *N. Engl. J. Med.* 1998, 339: 1186- 1193.

Bachoud_Levi AC, N Deglon, JP Nguyen, J Bloch, C Bourdet, L Winkel, P Remy, M Goddard, JP Lefaucheur, P Brugieres. Neuroprotective gene therapy for Huntington's disease using a polymer encapsulated BHK cell line engineered to secrete human CNTF. *Hum. Gene Ther.* 2000, 11: 1723-1729.

Barani IJ. Benedict SH, Lin PS. Neural stem cells: implications for the conventional radiotherapy of central nervous system malignancies. *Int. J. Radiat. Oncol. Bio Phys.* 2007,

Bemelmans AP, P Horellou, L Pradier, I Brunet, P Colin and J Mallet. Brain-derived neurotrophic factor mediated protection of striatal neurons in a excitotoxic rat model of Huntington's disease, as demonstrated by adenoviral gene transger. *Hum. Gene Ther.* 1999, 10: 2987-2997.

Benedetti S, B Pirola, B Pollo, L Magrassi, MG Bruzzone, D Rigamonti, R Galli, S Selleri, F Di Meco, C De Fraja, A Vescovi, E Cattaneo and G Finocchiaro. Gene therapy of experimental brain tumors using neural progenitor cells. *Nature Med.* 2000, 6: 447-450.

Bensadoun JC, N Deglon, JL Tseng, JL Ridet, AD Zurn and P Aebischer. Lentiviral vectors as a gene delivery system in the mouse midbrain: cellular and behavioral improvements in a 6-OHDA model of Parkinson's disease using GDNF. *Exp. Neurol.* 2000, 164: 15-24.

Berger MG, Chassagne J. Bone marrow mesenchymal stem cells: from characterization to therapeutic use in adults and children. *Bull. Cancer.* 2003, 90:771-8.

Bhatia M, D Bonnet, B Murdoch, OI Gan and JE Dick. A newly discovered class of human hematopoietic cells with SCID-repopulating activity. *Nature Med.* 1998, 4: 1038-1045.

Billingham R, Brent L, Medawar PB. Actively acquired tolerance of foreign cells. *Nature.* 1953, 172:603.

Bjorklund A and O Lindvall. Cell replacement therapies for central nervous system disorders. *Nature Neurosci.* 2000, 3: 537-544.

Bjornsson JM, Larsson N, Brun AC, Magnusson M, Andersson E, Lundstrom P et al., Reduced proliferative capacity of hematopoietic stem cells de.cient in Hoxb3 and Hoxb4. *Mol. Cell Biol.* 2003, 23:3872–3883.

Booth C, Potten CS. Gut instincts: thoughts on intestinal epithelial stem cells. *J. Clin. Invest.* 2000, 105:1493–1499.

Bradbury EJ, LD Moon, RJ Popat, VR King, OS Bennett, PN Patel, JW Fawcett and SB McMahon. Chon- 11 droitinase ABC promotes functional recovery after spinal cord injury. *Nature.* 2002, 416:636--640.

Brazelton TR, Rossi FM, Keshet GI, Blau HM. From marrow to brain: expression of neuronal phenotypes in adult mice. *Science.* 2000, 290:1775-9.

Brun AC, Bjornsson JM, Magnusson M, Larsson N, Leveen P, Ehinger M et al., Hoxb4-de.cient mice undergo normal hematopoietic development but exhibit a mild proliferation defect in hematopoietic stem cells. *Blood.* 2004, 103:4126–4133.

Buckley RH, Schiff SE, Schiff RI, et al., Hematopoietic stem-cell transplantation for the treatment of severe combined immunodeficiency. *N. Engl. J. Med.* 1999, 340: 508–16.

Buckley RH. Treatment options for genetically determined immunodeficiency. *Lancet.* 2003, 361:541–2.

Carvey PM, ZD Ling, CE Sortwell, MR Pitzer, SP McGuire, A Storch and TJ Collier. A clonal line of mesencephalic progenitor cells concerted to dopamine neurons by hematopoietic cytokines: a source of cells for transplantation in Parkinson's disease *Exp. Neurol.* 2001, 171: 98-108.

Champlin R.E., Schmitz N., Horowitz M.M., Chapuis B., Chopra R., Cornelissen J.J., Gale R.P., Goldman J.M., Loberiza F.R., Hertenstain B., Klein J.P., Montserrat E., Zhang M.J., Ringden O., Tomany S.C., Rowlings P.A., Van Hoef M.E.H.M., Gratwohl A., Blood stem cells compared with bone marrow as a source of hematopoietic cells for allogeneic transplantation. *Blood.* 2000, 95: 3702-3709.

Charles Y. Liu, Ulf Westerlund, Mikael Svensson, Morten C. Moe, Mercy Varghese, Jon Berg-Johnsen, Michael L.J. Apuzzo, David A. Tirrell, Iver A. Langmoen. *Journal of Hematotherapy and Stem Cell Research.* 2003, 12: 689-699.

Chauhan NB, GJ Siegel and JM Lee. Depletion of glial cell line–derived neurotrophic factor in substantia nigra neurons of Parkinson's disease. *J. Chem. Neuroanat.* 2001, 21: 277-288.

Choi K. Hemangioblast development and regulation. *Biochem. Cell Biol.* 1998, 76:947-56.

Ciraci E, Barisani D, Parafioriti A, Formisano G, Arancia G, Bottazzo G, Berardi AC. CD34 human hematopoietic progenitor cell line, MUTZ-3, differentiates into functional osteoclasts. *Exp. Hematol.* 2007, 35:967-77.

Civin CI, Strauss LC, Brovall C, Fackler MJ, Schwartz JF, Shaper JH. Antigenic analysis of hematopoiesis. III. A hematopoietic progenitor cell surface antigen defined by a monoclonal antibody raised against KG-1a cells. *J. Immunol.* 1984, 133:157-65.

Coumans JV, IT Lin, HN Dai, L MacArthur, M McAtee, C Nash and BS Bregman. Axonal regeneration and functional recovery after complete spinal cord transection in rats by delayed treatment with transplants and neurotrophins. *J. Neurosci.* 2001, 21 :9334-9344.

Daadi MM and S Weiss. Generation of tyrosine hydroxylas –producing neurons from precursors of the embryonic and adult forebrain. *J. Neurosci.* 1999, 19: 4484-4497.

Daadi MM. Activation and differentiation of endogenous neural stem cell progeny in the rat Parkinson animal model. *Methods Mol. Biol.* 2002, 198: 256-271.

Deten A, Volz HC, Clamors S, Leiblein S, Briest W, Marx G, Zimmer HG. Hematopoietic stem cells do not repair the infarcted mouse heart. *Cardiovasc. Res.* 2005, 65:52-63.

Dezawa M. Insights into auto transplantation: the unexpected discovery of specific induction systems in bone marrow stromal cells. *Cell Mol. Life Sci.* 2006, 63 :2764-72, 2006.

Dezawa M. Insights into auto-transplantation: the unexpected discovery of transdifferentiation systems in bone marrow stromal cells Tanpakushitsu Kakusan Koso. 2007, 52:158-65.

Dicker A, Le Blanc K, Astrom G et al., Functional studies of mesenchymal stem cells derived from adult human adipose tissue. *Exp. Cell Res.* 2005, 308:283–290

Domen J, Cheshier SH, Weissman IL. The role of apoptosis in the regulation of hematopoietic stem cells: overexpression of Bcl-2 increases both their number and repopulation potential. *J. Exp. Med.* 2000, 191: 253–264.

Doyle LA, Yang W, Abruzzo LV, Krogmann T, Gao Y, Rishi AK, Ross DD. A multidrug resistance transporter from human MCF-7 breast cancer cells. *Proc. Natl. Acad. Sci. U S A.* 1998 ,95:15665-70.

Duncan AW, Rattis FM, DiMascio LN, Congdon KL, Pazianos G, Zhao C et al., Integration of Notch and Wnt signaling in hematopoietic stem cell maintenance. *Nat. Immunol.* 2005, 6:314–322.

Dunnett SB, Nathwani F and Bjorklund A. The integration and function of striatal grafts. *Prog. Brain Res.* 2000, 127: 345-380.

Eglitis MA, Mezey E. Hematopoietic cells differentiate into both microglia and macroglia in the brains of adult mice. *Proc. Natl. Acad. Sci. USA.* 1997, 94:4080-5.

Eisenberg LM, Eisenberg CA. An in vitro analysis of myocardial potential indicates that phenotypic plasticity is an innate property of early embryonic tissue. *Stem Cells Dev.* 2004, 13:614-24.

Fan D, M Ogawa, K Ikeguchi, K Fujimoto, M Urabe, A Kume, M Nishizawa, N Matsushita, K Kiuchi, H Ichinose, T Nagatsu, GJ Kurtzman, I Nakano and K Ozawa. Prevention of dopaminergic neuron death by adeno-asso-ciated virus vector –mediated GDNF gene transfer in rat mesencephalic cells in vitro. *Neurosci. Lett.* 1998, 248: 61-64.

Ferrari G, Cusella-De Angelis G, Coletta M et al., Muscle regeneration by bone marrow-derived myogenic progenitors. *Science.* 1998, 279:1528–1530.

Ferrari G, Cusella-De Angelis G, Coletta M, Paolucci E, Stornaiuolo A, Cossu G, Mavilio F. Muscle regeneration by bone marrow-derived myogenic progenitors. *Science.* 1998, 279:1528-30.

Ferrer I, E Goutan, C Marin, MJ Rey and T Ribalta. Brain–derived neurotrophic factor in Huntington disease. *Brain Res.* 2000, 866: 257-261.

Filip S, English D, Mokry J. Issues in stem cell plasticity. *J. Cell Mol. Med.* 2004, 8:572-7.

Franco D, Moreno N, Ruiz–Lozano P. Cardiovascular development: towards biomedical applicability: Non-resident stem cell populations in regenerative cardiac medicine. *Cell Mol. Life Sci.* 2007, 64: 683-91.

Gage FH. Cell therapy. *Nature.* 1998, 392: 18-24.

Gage FH. Mammalian neural stem cells. *Science.* 2000, 287:1433–1438.

Galli V, Olmo N, Barbas C. Development and validation of a capillary electrophoresis method for the measurement of short-chain organic acids in natural rubber latex. *J. Chromatogr. A.* 2000, 894:135-44.

Garbuzova-Davis S, Willing AE, Milliken M, Saporta S, Zigova T, Cahill DW, Sanberg PR. Positive effect of transplantation of hNT neurons (NTera 2/D1 cell-line) in a model of familial amyotrophic lateral sclerosis. *Exp. Neurol.* 2002, 174:169-80.

Garbuzova-Davis S, Willing AE, Zigova T, Saporta S, Justen EB, Lane JC, Hudson JE, Chen N, Davis CD, Sanberg PR. Intravenous administration of human umbilical cord blood cells in a mouse model of amyotrophic lateral sclerosis: distribution, migration, and differentiation. *J. Hematother. Stem Cell Res.* 2003, 12:255-70.

Gehling UM, Ergun S, Schumacher U, Wagener C, Pantel K, Otte M, Schuch G, Schafhausen P, Mende T, Kilic N, Kluge K, Schafer B, Hossfeld DK, Fiedler W. In vitro differentiation of endothelial cells from AC133-positive progenitor cells. *Blood.* 2000, 95:3106-12.

Gill SS, NK Patel, GR Hotton, K O'Sullivan, R McCarter, M Bunnage, DJ Brookes, CN Svendsen and P Heywood. Direct brain infusion of glial cell line-derived neurotrophic factor in Parkinson disease. *Nature Med.* 2003, 9: 589-595.

Gimble JM, Nuttall ME. Bone and fat: old questions, new insights. *Endocrine.* 2004, 23: 183-8.

Glimm, H., J.H. Oh, and C.J. Eaves. Human hematopoietic stem cells stimulated to proliferate in vitro lose engraftment potential during their S/G(2)/M transit and do not reenter G(0). *Blood.* 2000, 96:4185–4193.

Goodell MA, K Brose, G Paradis, AS Conner and RC Mulligan. Isolation and functional properties of murine hematopoietic stem cells that are replicating in vivo. *J. Exp. Med.* 1996, 183: 1797-1806.

Grondin R, Z Zhang, A Yi, WA Cass, N Maswood, AH Andersen, DD Elsberry, MC Klein, GA Gerhardt and DM Gash. Chronic controlled GDNF infusion promotes structural and functional recovery in advanced Parkinsonian mankeys. *Brain.* 2002, 125: 2191-2201.

Guo H, B Fang, L Liao, Z Zhao, J Liu, H Chen, SH Hsu, Q Cui and RC Zhao. Hemangioblastic characteristics of fetal bone marrow–derived Flk 1+ CD31- CD34- cells. *Exp. Hematol.* 2003, 31: 650- 658.

Gussoni E, Soneoka Y, Strickland CD et al., Dystrophin expression in the mdx mouse restored by stem cell transplantation. *Nature.* 1999, 401:390–394.

Hagell P, A Schrag, P Piccini, M Jahanshahi, R Brown, S Rehncrona, H Widner, P Brundin, JC Rothwell, P Odin, GK Wenning, P Morrish, B Gustavii, A Bjorklund, DJ Brooks, CD Marsden, NP Quinn and O Lindvall (1999). Sequential bilateral transplantation in Parkinson's disease: effects of the second graft. *Brain.* 1999, 122: 1121-1132.

Hall FL, Han B, Kundu RK, Yee A, Nimni ME, Gordon EM. Phenotypic differentiation of TGF-beta1-responsive pluripotent premesenchymal prehematopoietic progenitor (P4 stem) cells from murine bone marrow. *J. Hematother. Stem Cell Res.* 2001, 10:261-71.

Harraz M, Jiao C, Hanlon HD, Hartley RS, Schatteman GC. CD34- blood-derived human endothelial cell progenitors. *Stem Cells.* 2001, 19:304-12.

Hattori N, Nishino K, Ko YG, Hattori N, Ohgane J, Tanaka S and Shiota K. Epigenetic control of mouse Oct-4 gene expression in embryonic stem cells and trophoblast stem cells. *Journal of Biological Chemistry.* 2004, 279 17063–17069.

Hawley RG, Sobieski DA. Of mice and men: the tale of two therapies. *Stem Cells.* 2002, 20:275-8.

Horan J.T., Liesveld J.L., Fernandez I.D., Lyman G.H., Phillps G.L., Lerner N.B., Fisher S.G., Survival after HLA-identical allogeneic peripheral blood stem cell and bone marrow transplantation for hematologic malignancies: meta-analysis of randomized controlled trials, *Bone Marrow Transplant.* 2003, 32: 293-298.

Horwitz EM, DJ Prockop, LA Fitzpatrick, WW Koo, PL Gordon, M Neel, M Sussman, P Orchard, JC Marx, RE Pyeritz and MK Brenner. Transplantability and therapeutic effects of bone marrow – derived mesenchymal cells in children with osteogenesis imperfecta. *Nature Med.* 1999, 5: 309 – 313.

Horwitz ME, Barrett AJ, Brown MR, Carter CS, Childs R, Gallin JI, Holland SM, Linton GF, Miller JA, Leitman SF, Read EJ, Malech HL. Treatment of chronic granulomatous disease with nonmyeloablative conditioning and a T-cell-depleted hematopoietic allograft. *N. Engl. J. Med.* 2001, 344:881-8.

Huber I, Itzhaki I, Caspi O, Arbel G, Tzukerman M, Gepstein A, Habib M, Yankelson L, Kehat I, Gepstein L. Identification and selection of cardiomyocytes during human embryonic stem cell differentiation. *FASEB J.* 2007, 13.

Imaizumi T, KL Lankford, WV Burton, WL Fodor and JD Kocsis. Xenotransplantation of transgenic pig olfactory ensheathing cells promotes axonal regeneration in rat spinal cord. *Nature Biotechnol.* 2000, 18:949-953.

Isacson O. Models of repair mechanisms for future treatment modalities of Parkinson's disease. *Brain Res. Bull.* 2002, 57: 839-846.

Jackson KA, Majka SM, Wang H et al., Regeneration of ischemic cardiac muscle and vascular endothelium by adult stem cells. *J. Clin. Invest.* 2001, 107:1395–1402.

Jackson KA, Mi T, Goodell MA. Hematopoietic potential of stem cells isolated from murine skeletal muscle. *Proc. Natl. Acad. Sci. USA.* 1999, 96:14482–14486.

Jaleco AC, Neves H, Hooijberg E, Gameiro P, Clode N, Haury M et al., Differential effects of Notch ligands Delta-1 and Jagged-1 in human lymphoid differentiation. *J. Exp. Med.* 2001, 194:991–1002.

Jin Z, Xie T. Dcr-1 maintains Drosophila ovarian stem cells. *Curr. Biol.* 2007, 17:539-44.

Jolicoeur EM, Granger CB, Fakunding JL, Mockrin SC, Grant SM, Ellis SG, Weisel RD, Goodell MA; National Heart, Lung, and Blood Institute Cell Therapy Working Group Members. Bringing cardiovascular cell-based therapy to clinical application: perspectives based on a National Heart, Lung, and Blood Institute Cell Therapy Working Group meeting. *Am. Heart J.* 2007, 153:732-42.

Kajstura J, Rota M, Whang B, Cascapera S, Hosoda T, Bearzi C, Nurzynska D, Kasahara H, Zias E, Bonafe M, Nadal-Ginard B, Torella D, Nascimbene A, Quaini F, Urbanek K, Leri A, Anversa P. Bone marrow cells differentiate in cardiac cell lineages after infarction independently of cell fusion. *Circ. Res.* 2005, 96:127-37.

Kapoor S, Wilson AG, Sharrack B, Lobo A, Akil M, Sun L, Dalley CD, Snowden JA. Haemopoietic stem cell transplantation--an evolving treatment for severe autoimmune and inflammatory diseases in rheumatology, neurology and gastroenterology. *Hematology.* 2007, 12:179-91.

Karause DS, ND Theise, MI Collector, OHenegariu, S Hwang, R Gardner, S Neutzel and SJ Sharkis. Multi-organ, multi-lineage engraftment by a single bone morrow-derived stem cell. *Cell.* 2001, 105: 369-377.

Kehat I, Gepstein L. Human embryonic stem cells for myocardial regeneration. *Heart Fail Rev.* 2003, 8:229-36.

Kendall AL, Rayment FD, Torres EM, Baker HF, Ridley RM, Dunnett SB. Functional integration of striatal allografts in a primate model of Huntington's disease. *Nat. Med.* 1998, 4:727-9.

Kerr DA, Llado J, Shamblott MJ, Maragakis NJ, Irani DN, Crawford TO, Krishnan C, Dike S, Gearhart JD, Rothstein JD. Human embryonic germ cell derivatives facilitate motor recovery of rats with diffuse motor neuron injury. *J. Neurosci.* 2003, 23:5131-40.

Kim CF, Jackson EL, Woolfenden AE, Lawrence S, Babar I, Vogel S, Crowley D, Bronson RT, Jacks T. Identification of bronchioalveolar stem cells in normal lung and lung cancer. *Cell.* 2005, 121:823-35.

Kim CG, Lee JJ, Jung DY, Jeon J, Heo HS, Kang HC, Shin JH, Cho YS, Cha KJ, Kim CG, Do BR, Kim KS, Kim HS. Profiling of differentially expressed genes in human stem cells by cDNA microarray. *Mol. Cells.* 2006, 21:343-55.

Kim JH, JM Auerbach, JA Rodriguez-Gomez, I Velasco, D Gavin, N Lumelsky, SH Lee, J Nguyen, R Sanchez Pernaute, K Bankiewicz and R McKay. Dopamine neurons derived from embryonic stem cells function in an animal model of Parkinson's disease. *Nature.* 2002, 418: 50-56.

Kondziolka D, L Wechsler, S Goldstein, C Meltzer, KR Thulborn, J Gebel, P Jannetta, S DeCesare, EM Elder, M McGrogan, MA Reitman and L Bynum. Transplantation of culture human neuronal cells for patients with stroke, *Neurology.* 2000, 55: 565-569.

Kopen GC, Prockop DJ, Phinney DG. Marrow stromal cells migrate throughout forebrain and cerebellum, and they differentiate into astrocytes after injection into neonatal mouse brains. *Proc. Natl. Acad. Sci. USA.* 1999, 96:10711-6.

Körbling M., Fliedner T.M., The evolution of clinical peripheral blood stem cell transplantation, *Bone Marrow Transplant.* 1996, 7: 675-678.

Kordower JH and CE Sortwell. Neuropathology of fetal nigra transplants for Parkinson's disease. *Progr. Brain Res.* 2000, 127: 333-344.

Krause DS, Theise ND, Collector MI, Henegariu O, Hwang S, Gardner R, Neutzel S, Sharkis SJ. Multi-organ, multi-lineage engraftment by a single bone marrow-derived stem cell. *Cell.* 2001, 105:369-77.

Kuci S, JT Wessels, HJ Buhring, K Schilbach, M Schumm, G Seitz, J Loffler, P Bader, PG Schlegel, D Niethammer and R Handgretinger. Identifiction of a novel class of human adherent CD34- stem cells that give rise to SCID–repopulating cells. *Blood.* 2003, 101: 869-876.

Lacorazza HD, JD Flax, EY Snyder and M Jendoubi. Expression of human beta-hexosaminidase alpha-subunit gene (the defect of Tay –Sachs disease) in mouse brains upon engraftment of transduced progenitor cells. *Nature Med.* 1996, 2: 424-249.

Laflamme MA, Myerson D, Saffitz JE, Murry CE. Evidence for cardiomyocyte repopulation by extracardiac progenitors in transplanted human hearts. *Circ. Res.* 2002, 90:634-40.

Latchman DS and RS Coffin. Viral vectors for gene therapy in Parkinson's disease. *Rev. Neurosci.* 2001, 12: 69-78.

Lawrence HJ, Largman C. Homeobox genes in normal hematopoiesis and leukemia. *Blood.* 1992, 80:2445–2453.

Lee MS, Makkar RR. Stem-cell transplantation in myocardial infarction: a status report. *Ann. Intern. Med.* 2004, 140:729-37.

Lee S, Bick-Forrester J, Makkar RR, Forrester JS. Stem-cell repair of infarcted myocardium: ready for clinical application? *Am. Heart Hosp. J.* 2004, 2:100-6.

Lemischka IR, Moore KA. Stem cells: interactive niches. *Nature.* 2003, 425:778-9.

Lemischka IR. Stem cell biology: a view toward the future. *Ann. N. Y. Acad. Sci.* 2005, 1044:132-8.

Linch DC, Rodeck CH, Nicolaides K, et al., Attempted bone marrow transplantation in a 17-week fetus. *Lancet.* 1986, 2;1453.

Lindvall O, Kokaia Z, Martinez-Serrano A. Stem cell therapy for human neurodegenerative disorders-how to make it work. *Nat. Med.* 2004, 10 Suppl: S42-50.

Lindvall O, S Rehncrona, P Brundin, B Gustavii, B Astedt, H Widner, T Lindholm, A Bjorklund, KL Leenders, JC Rothwell and et al.. Neural transplantation in Parkinson's disease: the Swedish experience. *Progr. Brain Res.* 1990, 82: 729-734.

Liu B, Buckley SM, Lewis ID, Goldman AI, Wagner JE, van der Loo JC. Homing defect of cultured human hematopoietic cells in the NOD/SCID mouse is mediated by Fas/CD95. *Exp. Hematol.* 2003, 31: 824–832.

Liu DD, Shyu WC, Lin SZ. Stem cell therapy in stroke: strategies in basic study and clinical application. *Acta Neurochir. Suppl.* 2006, 99: 137-9.

Liu Y, BT Himes, J Solowska, J Moul, SY Chow, KI Park, A Tessler, M Murray, EY Snyder and I Fischer. Intraspinal delivery of neurotrophin-3 using neural stem cells genetically modified by recombinant retrovirus. *Exp. Neurol.* 1999, 158:9-26.

Loeffler M, Roeder I. Tissue stem cells: definition, plasticity, heterogeneity, self-organization and models: a conceptual approach. *Cells Tissues Organs.* 2002, 171:8–26.

Lu P, LL Jones, EY Snyder and MH Tuszynski. Neural stem cells constitutively secrete neurotrophic factors and promote extensive host axonal growth after spinal cord injury. *Exp. Neuro.* 2003, I181:115-129.

Mahmud N, Milhem M, Araki H, Hoffman R. Alteration of Hematopoietic Stem Cell Fates by Chromatin-Modifying Agents. *Stem Cell Transplantation.* 2006, 27-42, Wiley-VCH Verlag GmbH and Co. KgaA.

Mallet J. The Tips / TINS Lecture. Catechol-animes: from gene regulation to neuropsychiatric disorder. *Trends Neurosci.* 1996, 19: 191-196.

Maria OM, Khosravi R, Mezey E, Tran SD. Cells from bone marrow that evolve into oral tissues and their clinical applications. *Oral Dis.* 2007, 13:11-6.

Medvinsky A, Smith A. Stem cells: Fusion brings down barriers. *Nature.* 2003, 422:823-5.

Mittoux V, JM Joseph, F Conde, S Palfi, C Dautry, T Poyo, J Bloch, N Deglon, S Ouary, EA Nimchinsky, E Brouillet, PR Hof, M Peschanski, P Aebischer and P Hantraye. Restoration of cognitive and motor functions by ciliary neurotrophic factor in a primate model of Huntingtion's disease. *Hum. Gene Ther.* 2000, 11: 1177-1187.

Mokry J, Cizkova D, Filip S, Ehrmann J, Osterreicher J, Kolar Z, English D. Nestin expression by newly formed human blood vessels. Stem Cells Dev. 2004, 13:658-64.

Mollura DJ, Hare JM, Rabb H. Stem-cell therapy for renal diseases. *Am. J. Kidney Dis.* 2003, 42:891-905.

Moon LD, RA Asher, KE Rhodes and JW Fawcett. Regeneration of CNS axons back to their target following treatment of adult rat brain with chondroitinase ABC. *Nature Neurosci.* 2001, 4:465-466.

Morel F, A Galy, B Chen and SJ Szilvassy. Equal distribution of compertitive long- term reporpulating stem cells in the CD34+ and CD34- fractions of Thy -1 low L in -/lowSca -1+ bone marrow cells. *Exp. Hematol.* 1998, 26: 440-448.

Nakamura Y, K Ando, J Chargui, H Kawada, T Sato, T Tsuji, T Hotta and S Kato. Ex vivo generation of CD34 (+) cells from CD34 (-) hematopoietic cells. *Blood.* 1999, 94: 4053 − 4059.

Neves H, Weerkamp F, Gomes AC, Naber BAE, Gameiro P, Becker JD et al., Effects of Delta1 and Jagged1 on early human hematopoiesis:correlation with expression of Notch signaling-related genes in CD34+ cells. *Stem Cells.* 2006, 24: 1328–1337.

Noseworthy JR, C Lucchinetti, M Rodriguez and BG Weinshenker. Multiple sclerosis. *N. Engl. J. Med.* 2000, 343:938-952.

Nossaman BD, Gur S, Kadowitz PJ. Gene and stem cell therapy in the treatment of erectile dysfunction and pulmonary hypertension; potential treatments for the common problem of endothelial dysfunction. *Curr. Gene Ther.* 2007, 7:131-53.

Orlic D, Kajstura J, Chimenti S et al., Bone marrow cells regenerate infarcted myocardium. *Nature.* 2001a, 410:701–705.

Orlic D, Kajstura J, Chimenti S et al., Mobilized bone marrow cells repair the infarcted heart, improving function and survival. *Proc. Natl. Acad. Sci. USA.* 2001b, 98:10344– 10349.

Osawa M, K Hanada, H Hamada and H Nakauchi. Long-term lymphohematopoietic reconstitution by a single CD34- low / negative hematopoietic stem cell. *Science.* 1996, 273: 242-245.

Ostenfeld T, Y-T Tai, P Martin, N Deglan, P Aebischer and CN Svendsen. Neurospheres modified to produce glial cell line-derived neurotrophic factor increase the survival of transplanted dopamine neurons. *J. Neurosci. Res.* 2002, 69: 955-965.

Ozbaran M, Omay SB, Nalbantgil S, Kulursay H, Kumanlioglu K, Nart D, Pektok E. Autologous peripheral stem cell transplantation in patients with congestive heart failure due to ischemic heart disease. *Eur. J. Cardiothorac. Surg.* 2004, 25:342-50.

Palfi S, Conde F, Riche D, Brouillet E, Dautry C, Mittoux V, Chibois A, Peschanski M, Hantraye P. Fetal striatal allografts reverse cognitive deficits in a primate model of Huntington disease. *Nat. Med.* 1998, 4:963-6.

Park IK, Qian D, Kiel M, Becker MW, Pihalja M, Weissman IL et al., Bmi-1 is required for maintenance of adult self-renewing haematopoietic stem cells. *Nature.* 2003, 423: 302–305.

Park KI, YD Teng and EY Snyder. The injured brain interacts reciprocally with neural stem cells supported by scaffolds to reconstitute lost tissue [comment]. *Nature Biotechno.* 2002, I20:1111-1117.

Pecora A.L., Lazarus H.M., Jennis A.A., Prett R.A., Goldberg S.L., Rowley S.D., Cantwell S., Cooper B.W., Copelan E.A., Herzig R.H., Meagher R., Kennedy M.J., Akard L.P., Jansen J., Ross A., Prilutskaya M., Glassco J., Kahn D., Moss T.J., Breast cancer cell contamination of blood stem cell products in patients with metastatic breast cancer: predictors and clinical relevance, *Biol. Blood Marrow Transplant.* 2002, 8:536-543.

Perez-Navarro E, AM Canudas, P Akerud, J Alberch and E Arenas. Brain-derived neurotropic factor, neurotrophin -3, and neurotrophin – 4/5 prevent the death of striatal projection neurons in a rodent model of Huntington's disease. *J. Neurochem.* 2000, 75: 2190-2199.

Peters C, Steward CG. Hematopoietic cell transplantation for inherited metabolic diseases: an overview of outcomes and practice guidelines. *Bone Marrow Transplant.* 2003, 31:229–39.

Pineault N, Helgason CD, Lawrence HJ, Humphries RK. Differential expression of Hox, Meis1, and Pbx1 genes in primitive cells throughout murine hematopoietic ontogeny. *Exp. Hematol.* 2002, 30:49–57.

Pisati F, Bossolasco P, Meregalli M, Cova L, Belicchi M, Gavina M, Marchesi C, Calzarossa C, Soligo D, Lambertenghi-Deliliers G, Bresolin N, Silani V, Torrente Y, Polli E. Induction of neurotrophin expression via human adult mesenchymal stem cells:

implication for cell therapy in neurodegenerative diseases. *Cell Transplant.* 2007, 16:41-55.

Pittenger MF, AM Mackay, SC Beck, RK Jaiswal, R Douglas, JD Mosca, MA Moorman, DW Simonetti, S Craig and DR Marshak. Multilineage potential of adult human mesenchaymal stem cells. *Science.* 1999, 248: 143- 147.

Pluchino S, A Quattrini, E Brambilla, A Gritti, G Salani, G Dina, R Galli, U Del Carro, S Amadio, R Bergami, R Furlan, G Comi, AL Vescovi and G Martino. In jection of adult neurospheres induces recovery in a chronic model of multiple sclerosis. *Nature.* 2003, 422: 688-694.

Pruszak J, Sonntag KC, Aung MH, Sanchez-Pernaute R, Isacson O. Markers and Methods for Cell Sorting of Human Embryonic Stem Cell-derived Neural Cell Populations. *Stem Cells.* 2007 Jun 22; [Epub ahead of print]

Quaini F, Urbanek K, Beltrami AP, Finato N, Beltrami CA, Nadal-Ginard B, Kajstura J, Leri A, Anversa P. Chimerism of the transplanted heart. *N. Engl. J. Med.* 2002, 346:5-15.

Quesenberry PJ, Becker PS. Stem cell homing: rolling, crawling, and nesting. *Proc. Natl. Acad. Sci. USA.* 1998, 95:15155–7.

Quesenberry PJ, Colvin G, Dooner G, Dooner M, Aliotta JM, Johnson K. The Stem Cell Continuum: Cell Cycle, Injury, and Phenotype Lability. *Ann. N. Y. Acad. Sci.* 2007, [Epub ahead of print]

Ramirez M, Segovia JC, Benet I, Arbona C, Guenechea G, Blaya C et al., Ex vivo expansion of umbilical cord blood (UCB) CD34(+) cells alters the expression and function of alpha 4 beta 1 and alpha 5 beta 1 integrins. *Br. J. Haematol.* 2001, 115: 213–221.

Randell SH. Airway epithelial stem cells and the pathophysiology of chronic obstructive pulmonary disease. *Proc. Am. Thorac. Soc.* 2006, 3:718-25.

Ringden O. Immunotherapy by Allogeneic Stem Cell Transplantation. *Adv. Cancer Res.* 2007, 97C:25-60.

Robb L, Elefanty AG. The hemangioblast--an elusive cell captured in culture. *Bioessays.* 1998, 20:611-4.

Rocchi E, Khodjakov A, Volk EL, Yang CH, Litman T, Bates SE, Schneider E. The product of the ABC half-transporter gene ABCG2 (BCRP/MXR/ABCP) is expressed in the plasma membrane. *Biochem. Biophys. Res. Commun.* 2000, 271:42-6.

Rosu-Myles M, Gallacher L, Murdoch B, Hess DA, Keeney M, Kelvin D, Dale L, Ferguson SS, Wu D, Fellows F, Bhatia M. The human hematopoietic stem cell compartment is heterogeneous for CXCR4 expression. *Proc. Natl. Acad. Sci. U S A.* 2000,97:14626-31.

Rountree CB, Barsky L, Ge S, Zhu J, Senadheera S, Crooks GM. A CD133 Expressing Murine Liver Oval Cell Population with Bi-lineage Potential. *Stem Cells.* 2007 21.

Santos-Benito FF and A Ramon-Cueto. Olfactory ensheathing glia transplantation: a therapy to promote repair in the mammalian central nervous system. *Anat. Rec.* 2003, 271B: 77-85.

Sato T, JH Laver and M Ogawa. GATA transcription factors: key regulators of hematopoiesis. *Exp. Hematol.* 1995, 23: 99- 107.

Sauvageau G, Lansdorp PM, Eaves CJ, Hogge DE, Dragowska WH, Reid DS et al., Differential expression of homeobox genes in functionally distinct CD34+ subpopulations of human bone marrow cells. *Proc. Natl. Acad. Sci. USA.* 1994, 91:12223–12227.

Scadden DT. Stem cells and immune reconstitution in AIDS. *Blood Rev.* 2003, 17:227-31.

Schachinger V, Zeiher AM. Stem cells and cardiovascular and renal disease: today and tomorrow. *J. Am. Soc. Nephrol.* 2005, 16 Suppl 1:S2-6.

Schaffler A, Scholmerich J, Buechler C. Mechanisms of disease: adipokines and breast cancer - endocrine and paracrine mechanisms that connect adiposity and breast cancer. *Nat. Clin. Pract. Endocrinol. Metab.* 2007, 3:345-54.

Schroeter EH, Kisslinger JA, Kopan R. Notch-1 signalling requires ligand-induced proteolytic release of intracellular domain. *Nature.* 1998, 393:382–386.

Serafini M, Verfaillie CM. Pluripotency in adult stem cells: state of the art. *Semin. Reprod Med.* 2006, 24:379-88.

Shamblott MJ, Axelman J, Wang S et al., Derivation of pluripotent stem cells from cultured human primordial germ cells. *Proc. Natl. Acad. Sci. USA.* 1998, 95:13726– 13731.

Shpall EJ, Cagnoni PJ, Bearman SI, Ross M, Nieto Y, Jones RB. Peripheral blood stem cell harvesting and CD34-positive cell selection. *Cancer Treat Res.* 1997, 77:143-57.

Smith AG. Embryo derived stem cells: or mice and men. *Ann. Rev. cell Develop Biol.* 2001, 17: 435 – 462.

Snyder EY, Daley GQ, Goodell M. Taking stock and planning for the next decade: realistic prospects for stem cell therapies for the nervous system. *J. Neurosci. Res.* 2004, 76:157-68.

Snyder EY, RM Taylar and JH Wolfe. Neural progenitor cell engraftment corrects lysosomal storage throughout the MRS VII mouse brain. *Nature.* 2002, 374: 367-370.

Snykers S, Vanhaecke T, De Becker A, Papeleu P, Vinken M, Van Riet I, Rogiers V. Chromatin remodeling agent trichostatin A: a key-factor in the hepatic differentiation of human mesenchymal stem cells derived of adult bone marrow. *BMC Dev. Biol.* 2007, 7:24.

Soria B, Skoudy A, Martin F. From stem cells to beta cells: new strategies in cell therapy of diabetes mellitus. *Diabetologia.* 2001, 44:407-15.

Stepanov GA, DO Karpenko, MA Aleksandrova, OV Podgornyi, RA Poltavtseva, AV Pevishchin, MV Marey and GT Sukhikh. Xenotransplantation of stem/ progenitor cells from human fetal brain to adult rats with spinal trauma. *Bull. Exp. Biol. Med.* 2003, 135: 397-400.

Storch A, G Paul, M Csete, BO Boehm, PM Carvey, A Kupsch and J Schwarz. Long-term proliferation and dopaminergic differentiation of human mesencephalic neural precursor cells. *Exp. Neurol.* 2001, 170: 317-325.

Strauer BE, Kornowski R. Stem cell therapy in perspective. *Circulation.* 2003, 107:929-34.

Studer L, V Tabar and RD McKay. Transplantation of expanded mesencephalic precursors leads to recovery in parkinsonian rats. *Nature Neurosci.* 1998, 1: 290-295.

Sutherland DR, Keating A. The CD34 antigen: structure, biology, and potential clinical applications. *J. Hematother.* 1992, 1:115-29.

Svendsen CN, DJ Clarke, AE Rosser and SB Dunnett. Survival and differentiation of rat and human epidermal growth factor-responsive precursor cells following grafting into the lesioned adult central nervous system. *Exp. Neurol.* 1996, 137: 376-388.

Takano H, Ohtsuka M, Akazawa H, Toko H, Harada M, Hasegawa H, Nagai T, Komuro I. Pleiotropic effects of cytokines on acute myocardial infarction: G-CSF as a novel therapy for acute myocardial infarction. *Curr. Pharm. Des.* 2003, 9:1121-7.

Teng YD, EB Lavik, X Qu, KI Park, J Ourednik, D Zurakowski, R Langer and EY Snyder. Functional recovery following traumatic spinal cord injury mediated by a unique polymer scaffold seeded with neural stem cells. *Proc. Natl. Acad. Sci. USA.* 2002, 99:30243029.

Terada N, Hamazaki T, Oka M et al., Bone marrow cells adopt the phenotype of other cells by spontaneous cell fusion. *Nature.* 2002, 416:542–545.

Theise ND, Badve S, Saxena R, Henegariu O, Sell S, Crawford JM, Krause DS. Derivation of hepatocytes from bone marrow cells in mice after radiation-induced myeloablation. *Hepatology.* 2000,31:235-40.

Thomson JA, Itskovitz-Eldor J, Shapiro SS et al., Embryonic stem cell lines derived from human blastocysts. *Science.* 1998, 282:1145–1147.

Tolar J, Teitelbaum SL, Orchard PJ. Osteopetrosis. *N. Engl. J. Med.* 2004, 351:2839–49.

Tomita S, Li RK, Weisel RD, Mickle DA, Kim EJ, Sakai T, Jia ZQ. Autologous transplantation of bone marrow cells improves damaged heart function. *Circulation.* 1999, 100:II247-56.

Tse HF, Yiu KH, Lau CP. Bone marrow stem cell therapy for myocardial angiogenesis. *Curr. Vasc. Pharmacol.* 2007, 5:103-12.

Udagawa N. Benayahu D, Akavia UD, Shur I. Differentiation of bone marrow stroma-derived mesenchymal cells. *Curr. Med. Chem.* 2007, 14:173-9.

Van Den Berg DJ, Sharma AK, Bruno E, Hoffman R. Role of members of the Wnt gene family in human hematopoiesis. *Blood.* 1998, 92:3189–3202.

Veizovic T, JS Beech, RP Stroemer, WP Watson and H Hodges. Resolution of stroke deficits following contralateral grafts of conditionally immortal neuroepithelial stem cells. *Stroke.* 2001, 32:1012-1019.

Vermeulen M, Le Pesteur F, Gagnerault MC, Mary JY, Sainteny F, Lepault F. Role of adhesion molecules in the homing and mobilization of murine hematopoietic stem and progenitor cells. *Blood.* 1998, 92:894-900.

Vescovi AL, A critti, R Galli and EA Parati. Isolation and intracerebral grafting of nontransformed multipotential embryonic human CNS stem cells. *J. Neurotrauma.* 1999, 16: 689-693.

Wagner W, Wein F, Seckinger A et al., Comparative characteristics of mesenchymal stem cells from human bone marrow, adipose tissue, and umbilical cord blood. *Exp. Hematol.* 2005, 33:1402–1416.

Wang B, Zhao Y, Lin H, Chen B, Zhang J, Zhang J, Wang X, Zhao W, Dai J. Phenotypical analysis of adult rat olfactory ensheathing cells on 3-D collagen scaffolds. *Neurosci. Lett.* 2006, 401:65-70.

Wang LS, Liu HJ, Xia ZB, Broxmeyer HE, Lu L. Expression and activation of caspase-3/CPP32 in CD34(+) cord blood cells is linked to apoptosis after growth factor withdrawal. *Exp. Hematol.* 2000, 28: 907–915.

Wang X,Willenbring H, Akkari Y et al., Cell fusion is the principal source of bone-marrow-derived hepatocytes. *Nature.* 2003, 422:897–901.

Weiss MJ, and SH Orkin. GATA transcription factors: Key regulators of hematopoiesis. *Exp. Hematol.* 1995, 23: 99-107.

Whetton AD, Graham GJ. Homing and mobilization in the stem cell niche. *Trends Cell Biol.* 1999, 9:233-8.

Williams MA. Neural stem cells: one of the keys to everything. *J. of Hemato and stem cell Research.* 2003, 12: 591-594.

Woodbury D, Schwarz EJ, Prockop DJ, Black IB. Adult rat and human bone marrow stromal cells differentiate into neurons. *J. Neurosci. Res.* 2000, 61:364-70.

Wu L, Aster JC, Blacklow SC, Lake R, Artavanis-Tsakonas S, Grif.n JD. MAML1, a human homologue of Drosophila mastermind, is a transcriptional co-activator for NOTCH receptors. *Nat. Genet.* 2000, 26:484–489.

Wu S, Y Suzuki, T Noda, H Bai, M Kitada, K Kataoka, Y Nishimura and C Ide. Immunohistochemical and electron microscopic study of invasion and differentiation in spinal cord lesion of neural stem cells grafted through cerebrospinal fluid in rat. *J. Neurosci. Res.* 2002, 69: 940-945.

Wurmser AE, Gage FH. Stem cells: cell fusion causes confusion. *Nature.* 2002, 416:485-7.

Yick LW, W Wu, KF So, HK Yip and DK Shum. Chondroitinase ABC promotes axonal regeneration of Clarke's neurons after spinal cord injury. *Neuroreport* II: 2000, 1063-1067.

Ying QL, Nichols J, Evans EP et al., Changing potency by spontaneous fusion. *Nature.* 2002, 416:545–548.

Yu Y, Gu S, Huang H, Wen T. Combination of bFGF, heparin and laminin induce the generation of dopaminergic neurons from rat neural stem cells both in vitro and in vivo. *J. Neurol. Sci.* 2007, 255:81-6.

Zanjani ED, G Almeida –porada, AG Livingston, AW Flake and M Ogawa. Human bone marrow CD34- cells engraft in vivo and undergo multilineage expression that includes giving rise to CD34+ cells *Exp. Hematol.* 1998, 26: 353-360.

Zhai QL, Qiu LG, Li Q, Meng HX, Han JL, Herzig RH et al., Short-term ex vivo expansion sustains the homing-related properties of umbilical cord blood hematopoietic stem and progenitor cells. *Haematologica.* 2004, 89: 265–273.

Zhang J, Niu C, Ye L, Huang H, He X, Tong WG et al., Identification of the haematopoietic stem cell niche and control of the niche size. *Nature.* 2003, 425:836–841.

Zhou S, Hayward SD. Nuclear localization of CBF1 is regulated by interactions with the SMRT corepressor complex. *Mol. Cell Biol.* 2001, 21:6222–6232. 115:281–292.

Zuk PA, Zhu M, Ashjian P et al., Human adipose tissue is a source of multipotent stem cells. *Mol. Biol. Cell.* 2002,13:4279–4295.

Zuk PA, Zhu M, Mizuno H et al., Multilineage cells from human adipose tissue: Implications for cell-based therapies. *Tissue Eng.* 2001, 7:211–228.

In: Encyclopedia of Stem Cell Research (2 Volume Set) ISBN: 978-1-61761-835-2
Editor: Alexander L. Greene © 2012 Nova Science Publishers, Inc.

Chapter XXXIX

DENTAL MANAGEMENT BEFORE HEMATOPOIETIC STEM CELL TRANSPLANTATION FOR ADULT AND PEDIATRIC PATIENTS WITH HEMATOLOGICAL DISEASE

Kenji Yamagata, Kojiro Onizawa and Hiroshi Yoshida
Department of Oral and Maxillofacial Surgery, Institute of Clinical Medicine,
University of Tsukuba, Tsukuba, Japan

ABSTRACT

Hematopoietic stem cell transplantation (HSCT) has become an essential treatment for many patients with hematological diseases. Their immunosuppressed status during HSCT makes the patients more susceptible to infection and leads to an increased risk of infectious complications, including the development of severe septicemia, that may be life-threatening. The oral cavity is a potential source for such complications in patients receiving HSCT therapy, because it is an important port of entry for agents that can cause systemic infections. To prevent these oral complications, pre-transplant comprehensive oral care has been incorporated into the preparatory steps for patients scheduled to receive HSCT therapy. Pre-HSCT dental treatments are expected to decrease the risk of local and systemic odontogenic infections during immunosuppression. This approach is supported by the National Institutes of Health consensus statement on oral complications of cancer therapy. Although in the best-case scenario all sources of potential infection would be identified upon pre-HSCT dental screening and treated appropriately, the period available for pre-HSCT dental treatment is limited, sometimes precluding complete treatment. Therefore, we constructed protocols that define the appropriate minimal treatment modality for dental disorders in adults and children scheduled for HSCT to treat hematological malignancies. The protocols were constructed with the intent of preserving the patients' teeth whenever possible, and taking into account the severity of the disorder and the treatment time available.

In this chapter we describe these protocols, their application, and the patient outcomes. We also discuss the treatment modalities chosen for the protocols in the context of findings in the published literature and our own studies.

For our studies, patients scheduled for HSCT were given a pre-treatment clinical and radiological oral examination. Treatment modalities for potentially complicating or conditions were chosen according to the protocols. In adults, these oral conditions were dental caries, pulpitis, periapical and marginal periodontitis, and partially erupted third molars. In pediatric patients, they were dental caries, pulpitis, periapical periodontitis, simple gingivitis, loose primary teeth, and gingivitis associated with tooth eruption. In our studies, following their dental treatment, all the patients received their scheduled HSCT therapy without alteration, interruption, or delay, and none of the patients showed any signs or symptoms of odontogenic infection while they were immunosuppressed. These protocols, therefore, appear to be appropriate for the pre-HSCT dental treatment of adult and pediatric patients with hematological diseases.

INTRODUCTION

Hematopoietic stem cell transplantation (HSCT) has become an essential treatment for many patients with malignant and nonmalignant hematological diseases, including acute and chronic leukemias, aplastic anemia, myelodysplastic syndromes, and lymphomas [1, 2]. Although HSCT is an effective treatment modality for these patients, successful engraftment after HSCT requires adequate immunosuppression of the recipient, which is accomplished by total body irradiation, chemotherapy, or a combination of the two. The patients' immunosuppressed status makes them more susceptible to infection, resulting in an increased incidence of infectious complications, including severe septicemia, that may be life-threatening [2, 3].

The oral cavity is a potential site of origin for such infectious complications in patients receiving HSCT therapy, because it is an important port of entry for agents that can cause systemic infections [4-7] . To prevent these odontogenic complications, comprehensive pre-transplant oral care has been incorporated into the preparatory steps for patients scheduled to receive HSCT therapy. This approach is supported by the National Institutes of Health consensus statement on oral complications of cancer therapy (1989), which states, "All cancer patients should have an oral examination before initiation of cancer therapy, and the treatment of preexisting or concomitant oral disease is essential in minimizing oral complications in all cancer patients. Dental foci are potential sources of systemic infections that need to be eliminated or ameliorated before commencement of anticancer therapy" [8]. Therefore, to prevent significant morbidity, it is very important that patients scheduled to receive HSCT therapy have a pre-transplant dental screening to identify and treat potential sources of infection [2, 9, 10].

This chapter describes our dental management protocols and the detailed treatment criteria for minimal intervention in potentially detrimental dental conditions of adult and pediatric patients scheduled to receive HSCT therapy for hematological malignancies. We describe the outcomes of implementing this protocol, and we explain the basis for choosing the various recommended treatment modalities, which were drawn from the published literature and our previous studies and experience.

1. NECESSITY FOR PRE-HSCT DENTAL TREATMENT

Not all previous studies have supported a need for pre-HSCT dental treatment. Melkos *et al* [11] reported there was no significant difference in the occurrence of infection originating from oral disease during and after HSCT therapy between patients with and without pre-HSCT dental treatments, but they did not describe in detail the severity of the dental diseases of the patients in their study. Toljanic *et al* [12] reported that oncologic treatment outcomes were unaffected by the presence of chronic dental disease or acute exacerbations of these disease states, in a pilot study in which no chronic dental diseases were treated, regardless of severity. However, the great majority of the patients in their study received only chemotherapy, which does not cause the severe immunosuppression required for HSCT therapy. In contrast, Elad et *al.* [13] reported that choosing not to treat dental conditions increases the probability of mortality secondary to dental infections in HSCT patients by an additional 1.8 per 1000, and they stated that dental treatment prior to chemotherapy is the preferred treatment strategy.

Another report indicates that, unlike acute dental pathology, omitting treatment of chronic dental pathology does not add risk to chemotherapy, because chronic dental disease only infrequently converts to an acute state during chemotherapy [12]. This report suggests that not all dental pathologies must be treated. Finally, because any treatment carries its own risk of morbidity and mortality, only the most minimal dental intervention consistent with improving patients' chance of avoiding infection is advisable.

2. AVAILABLE TIME FOR DENTAL TREATMENT

Pre-HSCT dental screening to identify and treat potential oral sources of infection has become standard care for patients scheduled for HSCT therapy [3, 5-7]. Our screening examination consisted of a clinical examination of the hard and soft oral tissues and a radiographic survey, including panoramic and occasionally periapical films for symptomatic teeth. Although, ideally, all potential sources of oral infection should be eliminated by dental treatment before the initiation of the conditioning regimen, which takes place approximately 7-10 days before HSCT, time limitations and the severity of a patient's disease status frequently interfere with comprehensive treatment [3, 6, 7, 14].

Given the time restriction, the removal of potentially preservable diseased teeth may be the only viable treatment option, even though it may not best serve the long-term oral needs of the patient (because the removal of multiple teeth may compromise nutrition during and after HSCT therapy). This situation is further complicated by the fact that complete healing of an extraction socket is considered to require 10 to 14 days [6, 7] and by the associated increased risk of infection, bleeding, or delayed wound healing that could require postponing the scheduled HSCT therapy [15-17]. Thus, it is preferable for dental treatments to be completed by at least 2weeks before the initiation of chemoradiotherapy [6, 7]. Frequent communication between the hematologist and the dentist is therefore desirable if odontogenic infection and delay of HSCT are both to be avoided.

3. POTENTIALLY COMPLICATING ORAL CONDITIONS

We have identified the potentially complicating oral conditions of immunosuppressed adults as follows: dental caries, pulpitis, apical and marginal periodontitis, and partially erupted third molar. Standard dental care for these disorders includes tooth brushing instruction, scaling, restoration, pulpectomy, and endodontic treatment. Tooth extraction is indicated for severe dental disease. In HSCT candidates, such treatments are expected to decrease the risk of local and systemic odontogenic infections during patient immunosuppression [18, 19].

Pediatric HSCT candidates may have any of above-mentioned dental pathologies as well as loose primary teeth and gingivitis associated with erupting permanent teeth; therefore additional dental management modalities are often required for pediatric patients [20-22].

4. DENTAL MANAGEMENT FOR HSCT PATIENTS

Considering the additional morbidity or mortality associated with needless treatment [15, 16] and the limited time period available for pre-HSCT dental treatment [14], minimal dental intervention to treat only sources of potential infected is the current standard of care. To clarify what interventions are most appropriate, protocols that clearly define the best treatment modality for patients undergoing pre-HSCT dental assessments are needed. We previously used retrospective data to construct a brief dental management protocol for patients scheduled to undergo HSCT therapy for hematologic diseases [19]. The protocol was evaluated as significantly beneficial, but it included removing potentially salvageable teeth to lower the risk of infection during immunosuppressive therapy [19]. Based on our experience and the desire to preserve teeth if possible, we designed a new protocol for minimal intervention, in which the treatment modality is decided according to the severity of the dental disease and the time available for dental treatment, and only severely diseased teeth are extracted. The amount of time available for treating dental disorders was discussed between the hematologist and dentist, so that the treatment could be planned for completion before HSCT therapy. Even if minimal dental intervention is adopted, so early dental screening and treatment is essential.

Most studies and our current protocol agree about the best treatment modality for caries, symptomatic periapical lesion, severe advanced marginal periodontitis, and symptomatic partially erupted third molar [3, 7, 16, 23, 24]. However, considerable controversy remains as to the best treatment for asymptomatic periapical lesion, chronic marginal periodontitis, and asymptomatic partially erupted third molar, and practitioners manage these pathologies with approaches that vary from very conservative to aggressive.

1. Our New Dental Treatment Protocol and Its Outcome for Adult HSCT Candidates

The treatment plan described below was designed to preserve diseased teeth whenever possible and to indicate the most minimal dental intervention consistent with a good outcome (figure 1). The results of our study investigating the effectiveness of new dental management protocol was reported previously [18] .The following plan defines the pre-HSCT dental treatment modality for the dental foci identified, taking into account a patient's status and treatment schedule.

- Teeth with mild or moderate caries are restored in patients with sufficient time for dental treatment, but no treatment is given otherwise.
- Decayed teeth with pulpitis are treated by pulpectomy and root canal filling. Residual roots are extracted.
- Teeth with recently symptomatic periapical periodontitis and teeth with asymptomatic periapical periodontitis, including apical radiolucency with a maximal diameter greater than 5 mm, are treated with root canal in patients whose schedule permits. If there is insufficient time for this treatment, these teeth are removed. The symptoms are defined as erythema, swelling, pain, and tenderness of apical gingiva, and tooth sensitivity to percussion.
- Asymptomatic apical periodontitis with periapical radiolucency of less than 5 mm is not treated.
- Teeth affected with marginal periodontitis are removed if the gingiva shows swelling, erythema, pain, tenderness, and purulent discharge, and the probing depth is greater than 8 mm or the teeth have severe mobility.
- Teeth with marginal periodontitis without infectious signs and symptoms are observed, and teeth brushing instruction and/or scaling is provided.
- Partially erupted third molars diagnosed as pericoronitis with symptoms of erythema, swelling, pain, tenderness, and purulent drainage are extracted, and asymptomatic third molars are not treated.

All patients, including those without dental foci, are given tooth-brushing instructions to exfoliate dental plaque.

We reported the outcome of this new dental treatment protocol for adult HSCT patients in an article entitled "A prospective study to evaluate a new dental management protocol before hematopoietic stem cell transplantation." We used this protocol to carry out pre-dental screening and treatment of 71 consecutive patients with hematological malignancies who were candidates for HSCT therapy, between 1998 and 2004. Of the 71 patients, 41 underwent HSCT therapy and 30 did not, because their general condition was too poor or because no appropriate donor could be found. Among the 41 HSCT-treated patients were 22 males and 19 females, ranging in age from 17 to 58 years with a mean of 41.3 years. The hematologic diagnoses were as follows: 14 patients had chronic myeloid leukemia, 11 had malignant lymphoma, 4 had acute myeloid leukemia, 4 had myelodysplastic syndrome, 3 had multiple myeloma, 3 had acute lymphoid leukemia, and 2 had other malignancies. Hematopoietic stem cells were collected from the bone marrow of 28 patients and from the peripheral blood of 13 (table 1).

Table 1. Oncologic diagnosis and medical treatment [18]

Disease	No. of patients
Chronic myeloid leukemia (CML)	14
Malignant lymphoma (ML)	11
Acute myeloid leukemia (AML)	4
Myelodysplastic syndrome (MDS)	4
Multiple myeloma (MM)	3
Acute lymphoid leukemia (ALL)	3
Others	2
Medical treatment	No. of patients
Bone marrow transplant (BMT)	28
Peripheral blood Stem cell transplant (PBSCT)	13

Caries

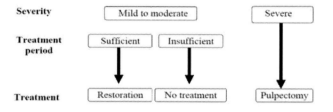

Apical Periodontitis

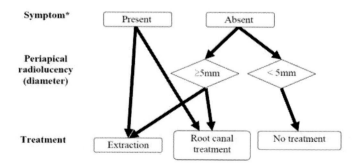

* Erythema, swelling, pain and tenderness of apical gingiva

  Tooth sensitivity to percussion

Marginal Periodontitis

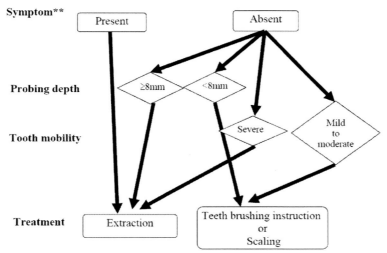

** Gingival erythema, swelling, pain, tenderness, purulent drainage

Partially erupted third molar

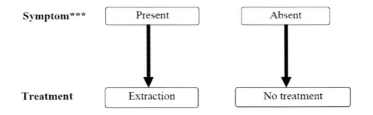

*** Erythema, swelling, pain, tenderness and purulent drainage of the pericoronal
    gingiva

Figure 1. Dental Treatment Protocol for HSCT candidates[18].

The dental status of all the patients was evaluated by an experienced dentist at the initial visit between 7 and 240 days before HSCT (median = 47 days). The screening consisted of a clinical examination of the hard and soft oral tissues and a radiographic survey, including panoramic and occasionally periapical films for symptomatic teeth. All the dental diseases encountered, including caries, apical periodontitis, marginal periodontitis, and impacted third molar, were recorded for each patient. Dental foci were defined as caries, apical and marginal periodontitis, and partially erupted third molar.

The time available for dental treatment was less than 1 month for 13 patients, from 1 to 2 months for 11, from 2 to 3 months for 7, and more than 3 months for 10. Patients who received their dental examination more than 2 months before HSCT were re-examined within 1 month of the scheduled therapy, to check for new dental disease. Thirty-eight of the 41 patients (92.7%) had one or more dental diseases. Caries was discovered in 101 teeth in 26 patients, pulpitis in 5 teeth in 2 patients, apical periodontitis in 43 teeth in 19 patients, marginal periodontitis in 94 teeth in 24 patients, and partially erupted third molar in 21 teeth in 11 patients (table 2). Three patients had no dental disease.

Table 2. Dental diseases of 41 adult patients [18]

Dental Disease	No. of patients	No. of teeth
Caries	26	101
Pulpitis	2	5
Apical periodontitis	19	43
Marginal periodontitis	24	94
Partially erupted third molar	11	21

More than one dental disorder was diagnosed in some patients.

Following dental treatment, each patient was admitted to a sterile room for the HSCT procedure. Episodes of a temperature higher than 38 degrees C and an absolute white blood cell count (WBC) of less than 1,000/ml lasting more than several days, which were manifestations of the patients' immunosuppressed status, were monitored and recorded. The dental follow-up was conducted during the only HSCT hospitalization, which lasted approximately 3 weeks. Any patient with local signs and symptoms consistent with odontogenic infections, such as swelling, pain, erythema, or sensitivity of the gingiva surrounding the teeth had a dental consultation and was given treatment as necessary. The frequency and occurrence of oral complaints and complications were recorded on the patients' medical charts and investigated throughout the course of HSCT therapy, and the effectiveness of the protocol, in which the pre-HSCT dental treatment was defined for the dental foci identified, taking into account the patient's status and treatment schedule, was assessed by the attending dentists and hematologists.

In this prospective study, 36 patients received one or more kinds of dental treatment. Of 101 dental caries in 26 patients, 40 teeth in 12 patients were restored, and the remaining 61 teeth in the other 14 patients were not treated. All five cases of pulpitis were treated with pulpectomy and root canal filling. Of 43 teeth with apical periodontitis in 19 patients, 41 were asymptomatic and 2 were symptomatic. Periapical lesions greater than 5 mm were observed in 10 teeth in 8 patients and lesions smaller than 5 mm in 33 teeth in 11 patients. Seven teeth with asymptomatic lesions greater than 5 mm in 7 patients were removed. Five teeth in 4 patients, including 2 that were symptomatic and 3 that were asymptomatic and had a lesion of over 5 mm, were treated endodontically, and the remaining 31 teeth in 13 patients with asymptomatic apical periodontitis and periapical lesions of less than 5 mm were followed without treatment. Of 94 teeth affected with marginal periodontitis, 6 teeth of 5 patients were removed, and the remaining 88 teeth of 24 patients were preserved with scaling and professional tooth brushing instruction. Only 3 of 21 partially erupted third molars were symptomatic. One patient had 2 symptomatic lower third molars. All 3 symptomatic teeth were extracted, and no treatment was given for the 8 upper and 10 lower asymptomatic third molars (table 3).

Table 3. Dental treatment outcome of adult patients [18]

Dental treatment	No. of patients	No. of teeth
Restoration	12	40
Scaling	24	
Professional tooth brushing instruction	21	
Extraction	10	14
Apical periodontitis	7	7
Marginal periodontitis	5	6
Partially erupted third molar	2	3
Pulpectomy	2	5
Endodontic treatment	4	5

The planned dental treatment was completed at least 10 days before the initiation of the conditioning regimen for all 36 patients. All 41 patients, including the 5 that did not require dental treatment, underwent HSCT therapy without showing signs or symptoms associated with odontogenic infection.

During HCST, the patients' experienced temperatures of more than 38 degrees C for a median of 4 days, ranging from 0 to 60 days, with no significant difference between the 28 patients treated with bone marrow transplantation (BMT) and the 13 treated with peripheral blood stem cell transplantation (PBSCT). The patients had a WBC of less than 1,000/ml for a median of 17 days, ranging from 6 to 75 days for the BMT-treated patients, and from 0 to 12 days for the PBSCT-treated patients; this difference was statistically significant.

Only two of the 41 patients (4.9%) experienced gingival pain before and during HSCT therapy. One was a 31-year-old female who complained of mild pain in the lower anterior gingiva, where gingivitis had been induced by anti-cancer agents. Another was a 30-year-old male who complained of mild pain in the gingiva of the upper third molar, which was under observation as asymptomatic. In both cases, there were no symptoms except pain, and there was no evidence of odontogenic infection. The pain reported by both patients resolved spontaneously without treatment, and the HSCT therapy was carried out as scheduled. Thus, no alteration, interruption, or delay of HSCT therapy was required for any patient.

2. Our Dental Treatment Protocol and Its Outcome for Pediatric HSCT Candidates

The treatment protocol for pediatric patients is the same as for adult patients, for caries, periapical periodontitis, and simple gingivitis. Loose deciduous teeth and gingivitis associated with erupting teeth, which are characteristic of the pediatric population, may increase the risk of oral infection, leading to life-threatening septicemia in immunosuppressed children, but there is little information available regarding optimal dental management of these conditions [21, 25, 26]. In the protocol for pediatric candidates, we established the following treatment criteria for these dental conditions (figure 2).

- Loose deciduous teeth with mild mobility are not treated, but kept under observation. Teeth with bobbing (i.e., severe mobility) and those expected to exfoliate within a few weeks are removed.
- Gingivitis associated with tooth eruption is treated with tooth brushing instruction and kept under observation.

Children who cannot brush their own teeth are assisted by instructed nurses and parents. All the children, including those with no dental pathology, are instructed in tooth brushing, and directed to brush three times daily.

Caries

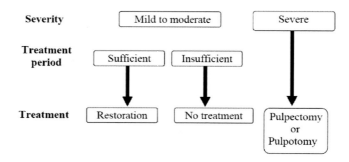

Apical Periodontitis

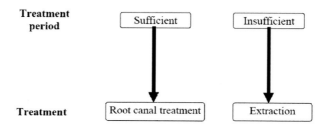

Simple gingivitis

Tooth brushing instruction and scaling

Loose primary teeth

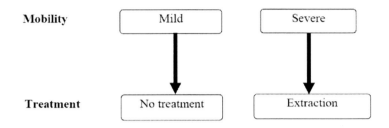

Gingivitis associated with tooth eruption

Tooth brushing instruction and observation

#Children showing no dental pathology were instructed in tooth brushing as daily oral hygiene care.

Figure 2. Dental Treatment Protocol for Pediatric HSCT Candidates [28].

We reported the outcome of this dental treatment protocol for pediatric HSCT candidates in an article entitled "Dental management of pediatric patients undergoing hematopoietic stem cell transplant." The study population was 30 children, consisting of 18 boys and 12 girls, who were referred for pre-HSCT dental assessment from 2000 to 2003. They ranged in age from 2 to 18 years, with a mean of 10.8 years. The hematological malignancies were acute lymphocytic leukemia in 20 patients, acute myelocytic leukemia (AML) in 2, and other malignancies in 8. Bone marrow transplantation (BMT) was performed for 25 patients, umbilical cord blood transplant (UCBT) for 3, and peripheral blood stem cell transplant (PBSCT) for 2.

Each patient received clinical and panoramic radiographic evaluations as needed to search for possible chronic or occult oral infections at the initial visit. Dental pathologies were diagnosed clinically and radiographically, and treated based on the protocol for pediatric patients (figure 2). Three children (10%) had primary dentition, 12 (40%) had mixed dentition, and 15 (50%) had permanent dentition. Nineteen of the 30 children (63.3%) showed one or more dental pathologies or conditions. Mild caries was discovered in 30 teeth in 9 patients, pulpitis in 2 teeth in 2 patients, and periapical periodontitis in 2 teeth in 2 patients. Loose primary teeth were found in 17 teeth in 7 children, and gingivitis associated with erupting permanent teeth in 6 teeth in 4 patients. Simple gingivitis was found in 7 patients. Eleven children showed no dental pathology (table 4).

Table 4. Dental diseases of 30 pediatric patients [28]

Dental pathology	No. of patients	No. of teeth
Mild caries	9	30
Pulpitis	2	2
Periapical periodontitis	2	2
Loose primary teeth		
mild mobility	4	9
severe mobility	3	8
Gingivitis associated with tooth eruption	4	6
Simple gingivitis	7	-

* More than one odontogenic disorder was diagnosed in some patients.

The available time for pre-HSCT dental treatment was less than 2 weeks for 5 children, 2 weeks to 1 month for 14, and more than 1 month for 11. The patients' conditions, the outcomes of the dental management, and any episode of odontogenic complication were evaluated by reviewing their medical records for the first 3 weeks or so following HSCT, while the patients were hospitalized in a clean room and were immunosuppressed.

Of the 19 children with dental pathologies or conditions, 15 received treatment and 4 were observed. Of the 9 children with mild caries, the teeth of 6 children were treated with restoration, and those of 3 children were observed, because there was insufficient time for restoration treatment before HCST. Pulpectomy was performed for 2 children with permanent teeth with pulpitis, and root canal treatment was given to 2 children with permanent teeth with periapical periodontitis. These treatments were finished with temporary root canal fillings of calcium hydroxide paste, because of the limited time available. All 8 severely loose deciduous teeth in 3 children were removed, and all the mildly mobile primary teeth in 4 children were observed. In 7 patients, simple gingivitis was treated with scaling and instruction in oral hygiene care and tooth brushing. Thus, the dental management program was completed for all 19 patients with pathologies or conditions. At the time of the HSCT, mild caries in the teeth of 3 children, 9 loose primary teeth of 4, and 6 permanent teeth associated with erupting gingivitis in 4 patients remained under observation (table 5).

All the children received their scheduled HSCT therapy without alteration, interruption, or delay after completion of the dental treatments, and they did not experience signs or symptoms associated with odontogenic infection during the immunosuppressive stages. None of the 30 children, with or without dental pathologies, complained of tooth pain, swelling, or pain of the gingiva around the teeth, or had a high fever attributable to dental infection before or during the period of immunosuppression. No odontogenic infection occurred in any of the patients treated with our dental management program. Three pediatric patients died from recurrence of hematologic disease and 7 suffered from chronic GVHD during the observation period after HSCT therapy.

Table 5. Dental treatment outcome of pediatric patients [28]

Treatment	No. of patients	No. of teeth
Restoration	6	26
Pulpectomy	2	2
Root canal treatment	2	2
Extraction	3	8
Tooth brushing instruction and scaling	7	-

5. MANAGEMENT OF DENTAL PATHOLOGIES

1. Oral Hygiene

Oral hygiene is a significant factor affecting the need for pre-transplant dental treatment. In fact, one of the most important goals of pre-transplant dental management is to motivate patients to maintain an appropriate level of oral hygiene. Some studies report that systematic oral assessment, regular encouragement of patient self-care, and consistent oral care may be the most important factors related to the prevention or amelioration of oral infection during HSCT therapy [7, 26, 29]. Patient caregivers should be given careful instructions in advance regarding appropriate oral care during the immunosuppressive stages.

Before dental treatment, all the patients in the our study were educated to exfoliate dental plaque, which produces dental caries and marginal periodontitis [18]. Strategies for removing dental plaque from around the teeth and gums are critically important for patient health and for diminishing the risk of a number of oral complications, because the build-up of bacterial plaque increases the risk of local infection and hemorrhage. It is also becoming clear that oral bacteria increase the risk and severity of oral mucositis [26].

The use of mechanical plaque removal techniques is dependent upon the patient's blood count and the presence of oral ulcerations. During periods of severe mucositis, the level of oral hygiene level may drop because of severe pain, resulting in dental caries and periodontal infection. There are several specially designed extra-soft toothbrushes that can be used during periods of mucositis. Some HSCT teams believe that tooth brushing increases the risk of bacteremia and bleeding, and advocate the discontinuation of oral hygiene with a regular brush, particularly during neutropenic periods. However, some studies indicate that infectious problems are more likely to arise when immunosuppressed patients are not compliant with good oral hygiene habits, since tooth brushing is the most effective means for removing plaque and reducing gingival inflammation and dental caries [5, 21, 29]. If patients cannot tolerate brushing, a soft regular toothbrush or sponge can be used. Sponge swabs have been recommended as an alternative to tooth brushes when the platelet count drops below $50,000/mm^3$, although some clinicians suggest not using swabs until the count drops below $20,000/mm^3$ [7, 30-33]. These recommendations are also made for flossing. Because plaque accumulation and gingival inflammation may be more detrimental than the risk associated with brushing and flossing, plaque control measures should be assessed individually for each patient [26].

For pediatric patients, although oral care is almost the same as for adults, an effective approach is to educate not only the children but also their caretakers, such as family members, nurses, and dental hygienist, about the importance of oral care for minimizing discomfort and maximizing the chances of a successful transplant [28]. Preventive measures include the use of fluoridated toothpaste, fluoride supplements if indicated, neutral fluoride gel/rinses, or applications of fluoride varnish for patients at risk for caries [25].

2. Dental Caries

Dental caries should be treated during the pre-HSCT period, whenever possible. It may not be possible to provide restorative dental treatment depending on the time available before transplantation and the general condition of the patient, but without treatment decay can progress significantly and thus severely compromise dental health. While permanent restorations are best, temporary materials can stabilize teeth safely until more definitive therapy is possible [26]. According to our protocol, teeth with mild or moderate caries should be restored in patients with sufficient time for dental treatment, but be observed in all others. Decayed teeth with pulpitis should be treated by pulpectomy and root canal filling [18]. For primary and permanent teeth in pediatric patients, topical fluorides and remineralizing solutions can stabilize incipient caries [26].

3. Periapical Periodontitis

Teeth with symptomatic periapical pathologies should be treated with endodontics or extraction, taking into account the patient's status, treatment schedule, and the condition of the teeth. These treatment modalities are widely accepted. Endodontic treatment of symptomatic periapical periodontitis should be completed at least 1week before the conditioning regimen to allow sufficient time to assess treatment success [25]. Although extraction is the treatment of choice for teeth that cannot be treated by definitive endodontic treatment in single visit [25], to prevent post-extraction complications, extractions should be performed at least two or three weeks before HSCT [19, 26].

As regards asymptomatic periapical periodontitis, one study suggests that there is no increase in the incidence of infectious complications during HSCT therapy when teeth with post-endodontic periapical radiolucencies of greater than 1.5 mm are not treated [23]. Our previous study also showed that untreated periapical periodontitis radiolucencies smaller than 2 mm did not convert to the acute stage during HSCT therapy [19]. However, treatment is commonly required for large periapical lesions in the healthy population. As presented in the protocol for adult patients, we did not treat asymptomatic periapical periodontitis with apical radiolucencies that were smaller than 5 mm, and there was no occurrence of conversion to the acute stage or of infectious complications. The outcomes of our study suggest that it is safe not to treat asymptomatic periapical lesions smaller than 5 mm before immunosuppressive conditioning [18].

4. Pulpitis and Periapical Periodontitis of Pediatrics

The indications for pulpotomy, pulpectomy for pulpitis, and root canal for periapical periodontitis in pediatric patients are controversial. Some reports do not advocate these therapies because a failure of the procedure can lead to infection [21, 26], and because it is difficult to complete the treatment in a single visit [21]. Instead, these reports advise tooth extraction. Although there have been no studies to date that address the safety of performing pulpotomy or pulpectomy in primary teeth prior to the initiation of chemotherapy and/or radiotherapy, many clinicians choose the more radical treatment of extraction, because pulpal, periapical, and furcal infections can have a significant impact on cancer treatment and become life-threatening during periods of immunosuppression [25]. For permanent teeth affected with pulpitis or with small radiolucent periapical periodontitis, many dentists assert that the teeth should not be extracted within the two to three weeks preceding HSCT [12, 19], because serious complications may occur after the extraction during the pancytopenic phase that follows BMT [15, 16].

In our study of pediatric patients, no endodontic treatment of primary teeth was performed. Permanent teeth with pulpitis and teeth with periapical periodontitis were treated and finished with temporary root canal fillings made of calcium hydroxide paste, because of the limited time available, and no periapical infection was subsequently observed in any of the patients during the immunosuppressive period [28]. Consequently, we recommend that severe caries with pulpitis be treated, not by extraction, but by pulpectomy or pulpotomy and temporary root canal fillings.

5. Marginal Periodontitis

Chronic marginal periodontitis is the most common significant dental infection that affects HSCT patients [4, 6, 26]. A retrospective investigation reported that 64% of patients with chronic periodontal disease had positive blood cultures associated with clinical signs of septicemia during the initial 100 days after HSCT [34]. However, because little data are available about the effect treating chronic periodontitis pre-HSCT on the incidence of infectious complications, the treatment modality has varied from observing affected teeth to removing asymptomatic teeth [35-37]. Teeth with a poor periodontal prognosis are generally extracted, but no relationship has been found between radiographic periodontal status and the incidence of septicemia [34]. Potential sites of oral infection are currently defined as a periodontal pocket more than 6 mm apical to junction of crown and root surface, and periodontal disease involving the furcation of the molar roots [6, 7]. In our protocol, only symptomatic teeth with acute conversion, a probing depth greater than 8 mm, or teeth with severe mobility were extracted. Teeth without these symptoms were treated with scaling and instruction in proper brushing technique. There was no occurrence of infectious complications in any of these patients following HSCT. These outcomes indicate that teeth with chronic marginal periodontitis, except severely symptomatic teeth, can be treated conservatively [18].

6. Partially Erupted Third Molar

Dental extraction guidelines for patients scheduled to receive HSCT therapy have been published [6, 26]: extractions should avoid trauma as much as possible, should include alveolectomies as necessary, primary closure should be with multiple interrupted sutures, and the use of hematostatic agents such as microfibrillary collagen, etc., should be considered. When possible, the extraction should be performed 10 to14 days before the start of conditioning. If the platelet count was <40,000/mm^3, platelets should be transfused before surgery. If the absolute granulocyte count was <2,000/mm^3 on the day of extraction, a prophylactic antibiotic should be used (table 6).

Table 6. Guidelines for dental extractions [6, 26]

Primary wound closure with multiple interrupted sutures
10-14 days of healing between extraction and start of conditioning
Consider use of hemostatic agents: microfibrillary collagen, etc.
Platelet transfusions to maintain platelet count < 40,000/mm3
Prophylactic antibiotics if granulocyte count <2,000/mm3

There are two basic treatment options for managing an asymptomatic partially erupted third molar. Some clinicians advocate prophylactic extraction as soon as possible [35, 38], whereas others prefer a more conservative approach [16, 39], because the risk of developing diseases associated with the third molar may be further reduced if the patient has good oral hygiene. A previous study showed that 40% of patients who underwent the prophylactic removal of partially erupted third molars, regardless of whether they were symptomatic or asymptomatic, experienced postoperative complications, such as bleeding, alveolitis, trismus, or infection, in the course of intensive cancer therapy, including HSCT [16]. The complication rate in these patients was also much higher than that reported in the healthy population [27]. Another study reported treating most non-extracted symptomatic third molars with antibiotics and analgesics, but the impact on the outcomes of the scheduled HSCT therapy was not described [16]. In our study, only symptomatic teeth were extracted, and asymptomatic third molars were not treated. None of the patients who underwent HSCT therapy showed signs or symptoms of odontogenic infection. This outcome indicates that extraction for symptomatic third molars and non-surgical intervention for asymptomatic ones is safe [18].

7. Loose Deciduous Teeth

The optimal management of loose deciduous teeth has not been defined. Da Fonseca reported that loose primary teeth should be left to exfoliate naturally because there are no complications in these cases [21]. The guidelines on dental management of pediatric patients recommend that patients should be counseled not to play with loose deciduous teeth, to avoid bacteremia [25]. Others have suggested that very mobile deciduous teeth concomitant with inflammation are infection foci and should be removed [40, 41]. Considering that leaving extremely mobile primary teeth until their natural exfoliation would increase the risk of odontogenic infection, and that the removal of such teeth would be inevitable later because of frequent chewing pain and the risk of bacteremia, we extracted these teeth, but did not treat mildly mobile ones, in our protocol [28]. Subsequent complications did not occur under our management.

Because tooth extraction just before or during HSCT can cause serious complications, such as hemorrhage, infection, and delayed wound healing [16, 42], it is best to remove permanent teeth at least two or three weeks before HSCT [19, 26]. However, the extraction wound caused by removing loose primary teeth is usually quickly covered by epithelium. Therefore, the extraction of extremely loose primary teeth, even a short time before HSCT conditioning is initiated, is considered necessary and sufficiently safe to prevent infection during the immunosuppression following HSCT [28].

8. Gingivitis Associated with Erupting Permanent Teeth

Gingivitis associated with erupting permanent teeth can act as the focus of life-threatening infections in children and adolescents [22], since debris and plaque can collect under the tissue flap [38]. One study reported that patients scheduled for HSCT should receive prophylactic extraction of teeth with gingivitis [36]. However, the removal of permanent teeth, except for the third molar, is not advised because such extraction may compromise nutrition. As an alternative treatment modality to removal, the overlying gingival tissue can be excised if it is believed to present potential risk, and if the patients' hematological status permits [25]; however, the daily removal of dental debris and plaque with brushing prevents the gross accumulation of bacteria on tooth surfaces, reducing the patient's risk for bacteremia [20]. In our study, no odontogenic infection caused by gingivitis of erupting permanent teeth was observed during recovery from HSCT. Because erupting gingivitis is considered a transient pathology before the accomplishment of eruption, good, regular oral hygiene should be performed to prevent serious infection [28].

CONCLUSION

We described recommended treatment modalities for various dental pathologies that have been reported in the literature and that we have experienced in our practice and studies. Incorporating our policy of preserving patients' teeth whenever possible, we established separate protocols defining the appropriate minimal treatment modality according to the severity of each dental disorder, for adult and pediatric patients scheduled for HSCT to treat hematological malignancies. All the patients screened and treated according to our protocols received their scheduled HSCT therapy without alteration, interruption, or delay, and none showed any signs or symptoms of odontogenic infection while they were immunosuppressed. These protocols, therefore, appear to be appropriate for the pre-HSCT dental treatment of patients with hematological diseases. It is worth noting, as well, that the treatment modalities of our protocols are largely non-controversial, and widely accepted: if there is enough time for the dental treatment to be completed before HSCT, the treatment plan is almost the same as for healthy individuals.

REFERENCES

[1]   Bortin, MM; Horowitz, MM; Gale, RP et al. Changing trends in allogeneic bone marrow transplantation for leukemia in the 1980s. *Jama,* 268, 607-12.

[2]   Appelbaum, FR. The use of bone marrow and peripheral blood stem cell transplantation in the treatment of cancer. *CA Cancer J. Clin.* 46, 142-64.

[3]   Prevention, CfDCa. Guidelines for preventing opportunistic infection among hematopoietic stem cell transplant recipients. *MMWR Recomm. Rep.* 49, 1-128.

[4]   Overholser, CD; Peterson, DE; Williams, LT; Schimpff, SC. Periodontal infection in patients with acute nonlymphocyte leukemia. Prevalence of acute exacerbations. *Arch. Intern. Med.* 142, 551-4.

[5]   Sonis, S; Kunz, A. Impact of improved dental services on the frequency of oral complications of cancer therapy for patients with non-head-and-neck malignancies. *Oral Surg. Oral Med. Oral Pathol.* 65, 19-22.

[6]   Peterson, DE. Pretreatment strategies for infection prevention in chemotherapy patients. *NCI Monogr.* 61-71.

[7]   Barker, GJ. Current practices in the oral management of the patient undergoing chemotherapy or bone marrow transplantation. *Support Care Cancer.* 7, 17-20.

[8]   National Institutes of Health Consensus. Development Panel. Consensus statement: oral complications of cancer therapies. *NCI Monogr.* 3-8.

[9]   Heimdahl, A; Mattsson, T; Dahllof, G et al. The oral cavity as a port of entry for early infections in patients treated with bone marrow transplantation. *Oral Surg. Oral Med. Oral Pathol.* 68, 711-6.

[10]   Bergmann, OJ. Oral infections and septicemia in immunocompromised patients with hematologic malignancies. *J. Clin. Microbiol.* 26, 2105-9.

[11]   Melkos, AB; Massenkeil, G; Arnold, R; Reichart, PA. Dental treatment prior to stem cell transplantation and its influence on the posttransplantation outcome. *Clin. Oral Investig.* 7, 113-5.

[12]   Toljanic, JA; Bedard, JF; Larson, RA; Fox, JP. A prospective pilot study to evaluate a new dental assessment and treatment paradigm for patients scheduled to undergo intensive chemotherapy for cancer. *Cancer.* 85, 1843-8.

[13]   Elad, S; Thierer, T; Bitan, M et al. A decision analysis: The dental management of patients prior to hematology cytotoxic therapy or hematopoietic stem cell transplantation. *Oral Oncol.* in press.

[14]   Elad, S; Garfunkel, AA; Or, R et al. Time limitations and the challenge of providing infection-preventing dental care to hematopoietic stem-cell transplantation patients. *Support Care Cancer.* 11, 674-7.

[15]   Barasch, A; Mosier, KM; D'Ambrosio, JA et al. Postextraction osteomyelitis in a bone marrow transplant recipient. *Oral Surg. Oral Med. Oral Pathol.* 75, 391-6.

[16]   Tai, CC; Precious, DS; Wood, RE. Prophylactic extraction of third molars in cancer patients. *Oral Surg. Oral Med. Oral Pathol.* 78, 151-5.

[17]   Overholser, CD; Peterson, DE; Bergman, SA; Williams, LT. Dental extractions in patients with acute nonlymphocytic leukemia. *J. Oral Maxillofac. Surg.* 40, 296-8.

[18]   Yamagata, K; Onizawa, K; Yanagawa, T et al. A prospective study to evaluate a new dental management protocol before hematopoietic stem cell transplantation. *Bone Marrow Transplant.* 38, 237-42.

[19]   Yamagata, K; Onizawa, K; Yoshida, H et al. Dental management of patients before bone marrow transplantation. *Jpn. J. Transplant.* 34, 22-26.

[20]   Berkowitz, RJ; Crock, J; Strickland, R et al. Oral complications associated with bone marrow transplantation in a pediatric population. *Am. J. Pediatr. Hematol. Oncol.* 5, 53-7.

[21]   da Fonseca, MA. Pediatric bone marrow transplantation: oral complications and recommendations for care. *Pediatr. Dent.* 20, 386-94.

[22]   Marques, AP; Walker, PO. Intraoral etiology of a life-threatening infection in an immunocompromised patient: report of case. *ASDC J. Dent. Child.* 58, 492-5.

[23]   Peters, E; Monopoli, M; Woo, SB; Sonis, S. Assessment of the need for treatment of postendodontic asymptomatic periapical radiolucencies in bone marrow transplant recipients. *Oral Surg. Oral Med. Oral Pathol.* 76, 45-8.

[24]   Raut, A; Huryn, JM; Hwang, FR; Zlotolow, IM. Sequelae and complications related to dental extractions in patients with hematologic malignancies and the impact on medical outcome. Oral Surg. *Oral Med. Oral Pathol. Oral Radiol. Endod.* 92, 49-55.

[25]   Clinical Affairs Committee. Guideline on dental management of pediatric patients receiving chemotherapy, hematopoietic cell transplantation, and/or radiation. *Pediatr. Dent.* 27, 170-5.

[26]   Majorana, A; Schubert, MM; Porta, F et al. Oral complications of pediatric hematopoietic cell transplantation: diagnosis and management. *Support Care Cancer.* 8, 353-65.

[27]   Bruce, RA; Frederickson, GC; Small, GS. Age of patients and morbidity associated with mandibular third molar surgery. *J. Am. Dent. Assoc.* 101, 240-5.

[28]   Yamagata, K; Onizawa, K; Yoshida, H et al. Dental management of pediatric patients undergoing hematopoietic stem cell transplant. *Pediatr. Hematol. Oncol.* 23, 541-8.

[29]   Borowski, B; Benhamou, E; Pico, JL et al. Prevention of oral mucositis in patients treated with high-dose chemotherapy and bone marrow transplantation: a randomised controlled trial comparing two protocols of dental care. *Eur. J. Cancer B Oral Oncol.* 30B, 93-7.

[30]   Seto, BG; Kim, M; Wolinsky, L et al. Oral mucositis in patients undergoing bone marrow transplantation. *Oral Surg. Oral Med. Oral Pathol.* 60, 493-7.

[31]   Dahllof, G; Heimdahl, A; Bolme, P et al. Oral condition in children treated with bone marrow transplantation. *Bone Marrow Transplant.* 3, 43-51.

[32]   Poland, J. Prevention and treatment of oral complications in the cancer patient. Oncology. (Williston Park), 5, 45-50; *discussion.* 52, 57, 61-2.

[33]   Ferretti, GA; Ash, RC; Brown, AT et al. Control of oral mucositis and candidiasis in marrow transplantation: a prospective, double-blind trial of chlorhexidine digluconate oral rinse. *Bone Marrow Transplant.* 3, 483-93.

[34]   Akintoye, SO; Brennan, MT; Graber, CJ et al. A retrospective investigation of advanced periodontal disease as a risk factor for septicemia in hematopoietic stem cell and bone marrow transplant recipients. *Oral Surg. Oral Med. Oral Pathol. Oral Radiol. Endod.* 94, 581-8.

[35]   Maxymiw, WG; Wood, RE. The role of dentistry in patients undergoing bone marrow transplantation. *Br. Dent. J.* 167, 229-34.

[36]   Lazarchik, DA; Filler, SJ; Winkler, MP. Dental evaluation in bone marrow transplantation. *Gen. Dent.* 43, 369-71.

[37]   Sonis, ST; Woods, PD; White, BA. Oral complications of cancer therapies. Pretreatment oral assessment. *NCI Monogr.* 29-32.

[38]   Carl, W. Bone marrow transplants and oral complications. *Quintessence Int. Dent. Dig.* 15, 1001-9.

[39]   Mercier, P; Precious, D. Risks and benefits of removal of impacted third molars. A critical review of the literature. *Int. J. Oral Maxillofac. Surg.* 21, 17-27.

[40]   Raber-Durlacher, JE; Abraham-Inpijn, L; van Leeuwen, EF et al. The prevention of oral complications in bone-marrow transplantations by means of oral hygiene and dental intervention. *Neth. J. Med.* 34, 98-108.

[41]   Donker, AE; van Merkesteyn, JP; Bredius, RG; van Weel-Sipman, MH. Value of panoramic radiographs in paediatric pre-bone marrow transplantation oral evaluation. *Int. J. Oral Maxillofac. Surg.* 31, 170-2.

[42]   Williford, SK; Salisbury, PL, 3rd; Peacock, JE, Jr. et al. The safety of dental extractions in patients with hematologic malignancies. *J. Clin. Oncol.* 7, 798-802.

In: Encyclopedia of Stem Cell Research (2 Volume Set)   ISBN: 978-1-61761-835-2
Editor: Alexander L. Greene   © 2012 Nova Science Publishers, Inc.

Chapter XL

Haematopoietic Stem Cell Transplantation and Quality of Life

Ladislav Slovacek[1,2,3] and Birgita Slovackova[4]

[1] University of Defence, Faculty of Military Health Sciences,
Department of Field Internal Medicine, Hradec Kralove, Czech Republic
[2] Charles University Hospital and Medical Faculty,
Department of Clinical Haematology, Hradec Kralove, Czech Republic
[3] Charles University Hospital and Medical Faculty,
Department of Clinical Oncology and Radiotherapy,
Hradec Kralove, Czech Republic
[4] Charles University Hospital and Medical Faculty,
Department of Psychiatry, Hradec Kralove, Czech Republic

Introduction

Haematopoietic stem cell transplantation (HSCT) is a modern therapeutic method used for biomodulation antitumour therapy of haematological malignancies (acute and chronic leukemia, malignant Hodgkin´s and non-Hodgkin´s lymphoma, multiple myeloma, aplastic anaemia, etc.) and of the selected solid tumours (Grawitz´s tumour of the kidney, breast carcinoma, testicular tumours, neuroblastoma, small-cellular lung carcinoma) [1-4]. It is also used for the therapy of non-tumour and hereditary diseases (demyelinization disease – sclerosis multiplex, systemic disease - systemic lupus erythematodes, systemic sclerodermia and hereditary disease – Fanconi´s anaemia) [1, 4]. It is divided into the bone marrow transplantation (BMT), the transplantation of stem (progenitor) cells (PSCT) and the umbilical cord blood transplantation (UCBT) [1, 2, 4]. From a donor´s point of view there are three kinds of transplantations: syngenic transplantation (the donor is a monozygotic twin), allogeneic transplantation (HLA from a compatible sibling or parent or HLA from a compatible donor) and autologous transplantation (patient is the donor). The aim of the

HSCT is to replace a patient's pathological bone marrow which contains tumorous cells with haematopoietic cells from a healthy donor and to restore haematopoiesis which is damaged by an intensive antitumour therapy [1-4].

As well as all the other treatments, HSCT also affects the disease process, and with that also quality of patient life. In the last decade of the 20th century, several studies about quality of life (QoL) in patients after HSCT were undertaken and there was influence at particular dimensions of QoL observed [5]. The QoL is generally defined as "a patient's subjective evaluation of his life situation" [5]. The QoL term contains the information on an individual's physical, psychological, social and spiritual condition [5, 6] (see figure 1). The QoL evaluation is carried out by means of generic and specific questionnaires [5, 6]. Generic questionnaires generally evaluate a patient's overall condition regardless of his disease [5]. Specific questionnaires are designed for the evaluation of a patient's overall condition in a particular type of disease [5]. Modules are often used with these specific questionnaires. These modules are focused on specific symptoms and complaints in a particular type of disease. The areas investigated in QoL questionnaires usually include a patient's physical, psychological and social functions, including his financial situation, his integration into the society, including pain, quality of sleep, spiritual aspects (interests, hobbies) and also symptoms which are specific for a particular disease [5].

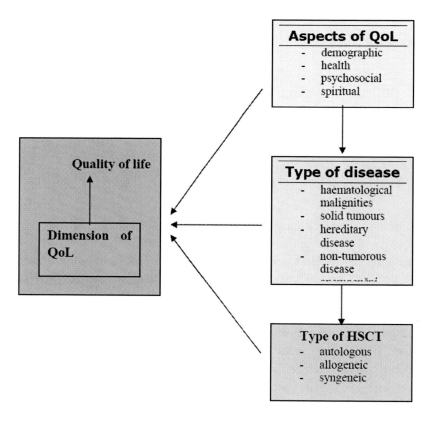

Figure 1. Quality of life of patients treated by means of HSCT [5].

QUALITY OF LIFE OF ADULT PATIENTS TREATED BY MEANS OF HAEMATOPOIETIC STEM CELL TRANSPLANTATION: AN EFFECT OF SELECTED DEMOGRAPHIC, PSYCHOSOCIAL AND HEALTH ASPECTS ON QUALITY OF LIFE

Aims of Study

The study has two main aims:

1) To analyze selected demographic, psychosocial and health aspects on quality of life (QoL) of adult patients treated by means of haematopoietic stem cell transplantation (HSCT).
2) To evaluate the global QoL of adult patients treated by means of HSCT.

Design of Study

The study is retrospective and descriptive and it is based on data obtained during the year 2004 – 2005 in 95 adult patients treated by means of HSCT at the Department of Clinical Haematology of 2nd Internal Clinic of Charles University Hospital and Faculty of Medicine in Hradec Kralove, Czech Republic.

PATIENTS AND METHODS

Group Characteristics

The total number of adult patients treated by means of HSCT from 2001 to 2003 was 171 (135 patients undergoing autologous HSCT and 36 patients undergoing allogeneic HSCT). The total number of respondents was 95. The return rate of questionnaires was 72.1% (71 respondents) and we could evaluate 100% of them. The number of respondents treated by means of HSCT from 2001 to 2003 was the following: in year 2001: 20 respondents (10 male and 10 female), their average age was 55.5 years old, in year 2002: 20 respondents (10 male and 10 female), their average age was 55.0 years old, in year 2003: 31 respondents (19 male and 12 female), their average age was 55.5 years old. Out of the total number of 71 respondents 66 respondents undergoing autologous HSCT and 5 respondents undergoing allogeneic HSCT (in 2001 there was no respondent with allogeneic HSCT, in 2002 there were 2 respondents and in 2003, 3 respondents). In the group of patients undergoing allogeneic HSCT, 3 patients had the mucocutaneous form of chronic Graft-Versus-Host Disease (cGVHD). These were patients with acute myeloid leukaemia. Tables I and II show the representation of respondents undergoing HSCT according to the type of this transplantation and according to the type of disease.

Table I. Number of respondents according to the type of HSCT

Type of HSCT / year	2001	2002	2003	Total number
Autologous HSCT	20	18	28	66
Allogeneic HSCT	0	2	3	5

Table II. Number of respondents according to the type of disease

Type of disease	Number of respondents	Autologous / allogeneic HSCT
Hodgkin´s lymphoma	9	7 / 2
Non-Hodgkin´s lymphoma	15	15 / 0
Acute lymphoblastic leukaemia	2	2 / 0
Acute myeloid leukaemia	12	9 / 3
Chronic myeloid leukaemia	1	1 / 0
Multiple myeloma	32	32 / 0

Measurements

The Czech version of an international generic European Quality of Life Questionnaire – Version EQ-5D (EuroQol – EQ-5D) was used [4, 7-14]. This questionnaire evaluates 2 indicators, objective and subjective indicators [4, 14-16]. The objective indicator includes 5 dimensions of QoL: ability to move, self-sufficiency, usual activity, pain/complaints, anxiety/depression. Three kinds of answers which express the degree of complaints are offered to each question (no complaints, mild complaints, severe complaints). Totally 243 (3^5) combinations of health conditions exist. The outcome is EQ-5D score (dimensions of QoL) which has values from 0 to 1 (0 - the worst health condition, 1 – the best health condition) [4, 14-16]. Subjective indicator includes visual analogous scale (the value of 100 – the best health condition, the value of 0 – the worst health condition). The respondent marks his subjectively perceived health condition at the thermometer scale. The outcome is EQ-5D VAS (a subjective health condition) which has values from 0 to 100 [4, 14-16].

Procedure

The Euro Qol EQ-5D Questionnaire with a covering letter, in which the whole project was explained, together with a stamped envelope were mailed to a respondent's address. The filling in of the questionnaire was voluntary and anonymous.

Data Analysis, Statistical Analysis

The independent variables were age, sex, level of education, marital status, increasing number of associated diseases, smoking abuse, religion, type of HSCT and time lapse from HSCT. We did not monitor the effect of chronic cGVHD on QoL of patients undergoing allogeneic HSCT because of the small amount of patients in the collection. The dependent variables were EQ-5D score (dimensions of QoL) and EQ-5D VAS (a subjective health condition). The basic statistical characteristics were fixed (mean value, standard deviation, maximum and minimum value) for all respondents collection. The effect of selected aspects on QoL of patients was evaluated by means of analysis of variance. The value $P<0.05$ was considered significant. The QoL questionnaires was evaluated by means of descriptive analysis in accordance with European Quality of Life Group method [14]. StatSoft STATISTICA Base Version 7.1 was used for analysis.

Results of Study

The above-mentioned aspects proved statistically significant dependence of QoL (EQ-5D score and EQ-5 VAS) on age (in both cases $p<0.01$), increasing number of associated diseases (in both cases $p<0.01$), religion (in both cases $p<0.01$) and type of disease (in both cases $p<0.05$). EQ-5D score (dimensions of QoL) and EQ-5D VAS (a subjective health condition) significantly decrease with increasing age and with a higher increasing number of associated diseases (see table III, IV). They are significantly higher in patients who believe in God compared to patients without religious beliefs (see table V). They are significantly most high QoL in patients with malignant lymphoma and with acute myeloid leukaemia and most low QoL in patients with multiple myeloma. The mean value of EQ-5D score was 68.9% and mean value of EQ-5D VAS was 66.6% and in patients with malignant lymphoma and acute leukemia the mean value of EQ-5D score was 82.7% and mean value of EQ-5D VAS was 76.7%.

Global QoL of patients treated by means of HSCT is on a very high level, which is seen from EQ-5D score (mean value of EQ-5D score of all respondents was 72.5%) and EQ-5D VAS (mean value of EQ-5D VAS was 76.5%) values.

Table III. Comparison of mean values of EQ-5D score and mean values of EQ-5D VAS in individual age groups

Age range	Number of respondents	Mean values of EQ-5D score (in %)	Standard deviation	Mean values of EQ-5D VAS (in %)	Standard deviation
20-29	6	93.3	11.4	79.2	13.6
30-39	8	96.2	5.3	85.0	8.4
40-49	11	89.6	12.7	76.2	15.6
50-59	23	70.2	15.4	67.0	14.0
60-69	17	65.4	9.5	64.1	13.7
70-79	6	57	9.6	64.5	11.1

Table IV. Comparison of mean values of EQ-5D score and mean values of EQ-5D VAS with an increasing number of associated diseases

Number of diseases	Number of respondents	Mean values of EQ-5D score (in %)	Standard deviation	Mean values of EQ-5D VAS (in %)	Standard deviation
0	30	83.9	16.4	76.3	12.4
1	13	74.7	18.8	71.5	18.4
2	14	70.9	15.2	66.2	13.0
3	7	71.0	12.8	67.1	12.9
>3	7	56.7	11.4	57.1	14.7

Table V. Comparison of mean values of EQ-5D score and mean values of EQ-5D VAS with religion

Religion	Number of respondents	Mean values of EQ-5D score (in %)	Standard deviation	Mean values of EQ-5D VAS (in %)	Standard deviation
Believers	43	85.6	12.9	76.6	12.8
Non-believers	28	60.4	11.9	57.6	12.9

Table VI. Comparison of respondents with multiple myeloma and malignant lymphoma and acute myeloid leukaemia treated by means of HSCT according to the level of troubles

Dimension of quality of life	Level of evaluation	Malignant lymphoma and acute myeloid leukaemia	Multiple myeloma
Number of Respondents		rel	rel.
Mobility	No troubles	70.8%	41%
	with troubles	29.2%	59%
	Immobile	0	0
Self-care	No troubles	91.7%	81.2%
	with troubles	8.3%	18.8%
	Incapable	0	0
Usual activities	No troubles	70.8%	18.8%
	with troubles	25.0%	81.2%
	Incapable	4.2%	0
Pain / Discomfort	None	66.7%	28.1%
	Weighty	33.3%	68.8%
	Extreme	0	3.1%
Anxiety / Depression	None	75.0%	41%
	Weighty	20.8%	59%
	Extreme	4.2%	0
Number of Respondents		38	32

DISCUSSION OF RESULTS

1. The Effect of Age on Qol of Adult Patients Treated by Means of HSCT Has Been Proved

Our results show that a lower QoL correlates with increasing age of patients undergoing HSCT. We think that increasing age correlates with an increasing number of associated diseases. QoL of patients with increasing age should be stressed. Also, we think that increasing overall fatigue and emotional complaints which decrease the QoL correlate with increasing age.

2. The Effect of Increasing Number of Associated Diseases on Qol of Adult Patients Treated by Means of HSCT Has Been Proved

Our results show that a lower QoL correlates with an increasing number of associated diseases. We think that an increasing number of associated diseases correlates with overall fatigue and emotional difficulties and in patients with an increasing number of associated diseases there is a lower overall physical fitness and this causes a lower QoL.

3. The Effect of Religion on Qol of Adult Patients Treated by Means of HSCT Has Been Proved

It is clear from our results that the QoL of patients undergoing HSCT who believed in God was higher than in patients who were non-believers. We think that the non-believing patients have to stop various activities, including his interests and hobbies.

4. The Effect of Type of Disease on Qol of Adult Patients Treated by Means of HSCT Has Been Proved

We confirmed in our retrospective study a statistically significant dependence of QoL of adult patients undergoing HSCT on the type of disease. We found the lowest QoL in the cohort of patients with multiple myeloma and the highest QoL in the cohort of patients with malignant lymphoma and acute leukaemia undergoing HSCT. Prevailing complaints in the cohort of patients with multiple myeloma are: (1). regular activity with complaints 81.2%, (2). medium serious pain/discomfort 68.8%, (3). movement with complaints 59%, (4). medium serious anxiety/depression 59%. Prevailing complaints in the cohort of patients with malignant lymphoma and acute leukaemia are: (1). medium serious pain/discomfort 33.3%, (2). movement with complaints 29.2 %, regular activity with complaints 25 %, medium serious anxiety/depression 20.8%.

ACUTE MYELOID LEUKAEMIA IN ADULT PATIENTS TREATED BY MEANS OF AUTOLOGOUS PROGENITOR STEM CELL TRANSPLANTATION AND QUALITY OF LIFE

Aims of Study

The study has two main aims:

1) To analyse an effect of selected demographic, psychosocial and health aspects on quality of life (QoL) in respondents with acute myeloid leukaemia (AML) treated by means of autologous progenitor stem cell transplantation (PSCT).
2) To evaluate global QoL in respondents with AML treated by means of autologous PSCT.

Design of Study

The study is a cross-sectional, retrospective and descriptive and it is based on dates obtained during the year 2004 – 2005 (from 1st September 2004 to 30st January 2005) in 12 respondents with AML treated by means of autologous PSCT from 2001 to 2003 at the Department of Clinical Haematology of the 2nd Department of Medicine of Charles University Hospital and Faculty of Medicine in Hradec Kralove, Czech Republic.

PATIENTS AND METHODS

Group Characteristics

The total number of respondents with AML treated by means of autologous PSCT was 31. The total number of respondents was 19 (7 patients died and 5 patients underwent retransplantation). The return rate of questionnaires was 63%, i.e. 12 respondents (7 male, 5 female) and we could evaluate 100% of them. The average age of respondents was 47.5 years (age range 27-68 years old).

Measurements

The Czech version of an international generic European Quality of Life Questionnaire – Version EQ-5D (EuroQol – EQ-5D) was used [4, 7-14].

Data Analysis, Statistical Analysis

The evaluation of QoL questionnaires was carried out by means of descriptive analysis in accordance with European Quality of Life Group method [14]. The effect of selected demographic (age, sex), psychosocial (level of education, marital status, religion) and health aspect (increasing number of associated disease, smoking abuse, time lapse from transplantation) on QoL of respondents was determined by means of analysis of variance. The StatSoft STATISTICA Base 7.1 software was used for complete evaluating of dates. The value $p < 0.05$ was considered significant.

Procedure

QoL questionnaire with a covering letter, in which the whole project was explained, together with a stamped envelope were mailed to a respondent's address.

Results of Study

The above-mentioned factors proved statistically significant dependence of QoL (EQ-5D score and EQ-5D VAS) on age (in both cases $p < 0.01$) (see table VII), religion (in both cases $p < 0.05$) (see table VIII), smoking abuse (in both cases $p < 0.01$) (see table IX), level of education (in both cases $p < 0.05$) (see table X) and increasing number of associated disease (in both cases $p < 0.05$) (see table XI). EQ-5D score (dimensions of QoL) and EQ-5D VAS (a subjective health condition) significantly decrease with increasing age, religion, smoking abuse, level of education and increasing number of associated disease in respondents with AML treated by means of autologous PSCT. The effect of other aspects on QoL was not proven as statistically significant.

Table VII. Comparison of mean values of EQ-5D score and
mean values of EQ-5D VAS in individual age groups

Age range	Number of respondents	Mean values of EQ-5D score (in %)	Standard deviation	Mean values of EQ-5D VAS (in %)	Standard deviation
20-29	1	70	0	60	0
30-39	1	98	0	95	0
40-49	5	86.2	15.7	73.6	13.9
50-59	3	60	14.5	58.3	2.4
60-69	2	61	15	56	4

Table VIII. Comparison of mean values of EQ-5D score and mean values of EQ-5D VAS with religion

Religion	Number of respondents	Mean values of EQ-5D score (in %)	Standard deviation	Mean values of EQ-5D VAS (in %)	Standard deviation
Believers	8	83.9	15.9	71	16.6
Non-believers	4	57.5	17.6	60.5	10.2

Table IX. Comparison of mean values of EQ-5D score and mean values of EQ-5D VAS with smoking abusu

Smoking abuse	Number of respondents	Mean values of EQ-5D score (in %)	Standard deviation	Mean values of EQ-5D VAS (in %)	Standard deviation
Non-smokers	6	90.7	11.4	77.2	16.4
Smokers	6	59.5	14.1	57.8	3.5

Table X. Comparison of mean values of EQ-5D score and mean values EQ-5D VAS with level of education

Level of education	Number of respondents	Mean values of EQ-5D score (in %)	Standard deviation	Mean values of EQ-5D VAS (in %)	Standard deviation
Elementary	2	43	4.2	53.5	2.12
Apprentice	3	67	8.5	60	0
Secondary	3	74	4.0	65	8.7
University	4	98	0	82	17.9

Table XI. Comparison of mean values of EQ-5D score and mean values of EQ-5D VAS with an increasing number of associated diseases

Number of associated diseases	Number of respondents	Mean values of EQ-5D score (in %)	Standard deviation	Mean values of EQ-5D VAS (in %)	Standard deviation
0	3	88.7	16.2	71.7	20.2
1	4	83.2	18.7	77	15.7
2	4	64	16.6	58.8	2.5
3 and more	1	46	0	52	0

Global QoL in respondents with AML treated by means of autologous PSCT is on a very good level (mean value of EQ-5D score was 75.1% and mean value of EQ-5D VAS was 67.5%).

DISCUSSION OF RESULTS

1) The effect of age on QoL in respondents with AML treated by means of autologous PSCT has been proved.

2) The results show that a lower QoL correlates with an increasing age.

3) The effect of religion on QoL in respondents with AML treated by means of autologous PSCT has been proved.

4) It is clear from our results that QoL in respondents with AML who believed in God was higher than in respondents who were non-believers. Respondents who believed in God had a higher QoL than non-believers.

5) The effect of smoking abuse on QoL in respondents with AML treated by means of autologous PSCT has been proved.

6) We proved a lower level of QoL in smokers in comparison with non-smokers or former smokers.

7) The effect of level of education on QoL in respondents with AML treated by means of autologous PSCT has been proved.

8) We proved a higher level of QoL in respondents with higher education (secondary and university education).

9) The effect of increasing number of associated diseases on QoL in respondents with AML treated by means of autologous PSCT has been proved.

Our results show that a lower level of QoL correlates with an increasing number of associated diseases. We think that an increasing number of associated diseases correlates with overall fatigue and emotional difficulties, lower overall physical fitness and worse quality of sleep.

QUALITY OF LIFE IN PATIENTS WITH MULTIPLE MYELOMA AND MALIGNANT LYMPHOMA TREATED BY MEANS OF AUTOLOGOUS PROGENITOR STEM CELL TRANSPLANTATION

Aims of Study

The study has two main aims:

1) To analyse an effect of selected demographic, psychosocial and healthy aspects on quality of life (QoL) in patients with multiple myeloma (MM) and malignant lymphoma (ML) treated by means of autologous progenitor stem cell transplantation (PSCT).

2) To evaluate global QoL in patients with MM and ML treated by means of autologous PSCT.

Design of Study

The study is a cross-sectional and retrospective and it is based on data obtained during the year 2004 – 2005 (from 1st September 2004 to 30st January 2005) in 56 patients with MM and ML treated by means of autologous PSCT from 2001 to 2003 at the Department of Clinical Haematology of the 2nd Department of Medicine of Charles University Hospital and Faculty of Medicine in Hradec Kralove, Czech Republic.

PATIENTS AND METHODS

Group Characteristics

The total number of patients with MM and ML treated by means of autologous PSCT from 2001 to 2003 was 122 (70 patients with MM and 52 patients with ML). The total number of respondents was 80 (36 patients died and 6 patients underwent retransplantation). The return rate of questionnaires was 70% (56 respondents: 32 respondents - 18 male and 14 female with MM and 24 respondents - 11 male and 13 female with ML) and we could evaluate 100% of them. The average age of patients with MM was 60 years. The average age of patients with ML was 44,5 years. Table XII shows the representation of respondents with MM and ML treated by means of autologous PSCT from 2001 to 2003.

Measurements

The Czech version of an international generic European Quality of Life Questionnaire – Version EQ-5D (EuroQol – EQ-5D) was used [4, 7-14].

Data Analysis, Statistical Analysis

The evaluation of QoL questionnaires was carried out by means of descriptive analysis in accordance with European Quality of Life Group method [14]. The independent variables were age, sex, level of education, marital status, number of associated diseases, smoking abuse, religion and time lapse from autologous PSCT. The dependent variables were EQ-5D score (dimensions of QoL) and EQ-5D VAS (a subjective health condition). The effect of selected aspects of QoL of patients was evaluated by means of analysis of variance.

**Table XII. Number of respondents with MM and ML treated
by means of autologous PSCT from 2001 to 2003**

Type of disease / year	2001	2002	2003	Total number
Multiple myeloma	10	8	14	32
Malignant lymphoma	8	6	10	24

The StatSoft STATISTICA Base 7.1 software was used for complete evaluating of dates. The value p<0.05 was considered significant.

Procedure

QoL questionnaire with a covering letter, in which the whole project was explained, together with a stamped envelope were mailed to a respondent's address.

Results of Study

The above-mentioned aspects proved a statistically significant dependence of QoL (EQ-5D score and EQ-5 VAS) on age (in both cases p<0.01), on smoking abuse in patients with MM (in both cases p<0.05) and statistically significant dependence of QoL (EQ-5D score and EQ-5 VAS) on type of disease (in both cases p<0.01). EQ-5D score (dimensions of QoL) and EQ-5D VAS (a subjective health condition) significantly decrease with increasing age in both groups patients (see figure 2, 3). They are significantly higher in non-smokers in the MM group (see figure 4). They are significantly higher in patients with ML (see figure 5 and table XIII). The effect of other aspects on QoL (EQ-5D score and EQ-5D VAS) was not proven as statistically significant.

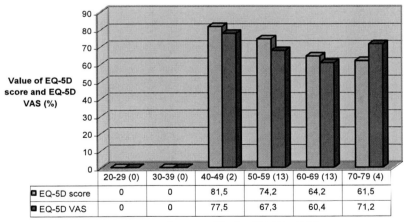

Value of EQ-5D score and EQ-5D VAS (%)	20-29 (0)	30-39 (0)	40-49 (2)	50-59 (13)	60-69 (13)	70-79 (4)
EQ-5D score	0	0	81,5	74,2	64,2	61,5
EQ-5D VAS	0	0	77,5	67,3	60,4	71,2

Age range (Number of respondents)

Figure 2. Dependence of EQ-5D score and EQ-5D VAS on individual age groups in patients with MM treated by means of autologous PSCT from 2001 to 2003 (n = 32, p<0,01).

Global QoL in patients with MM treated by means of autologous PSCT is on a lower level (mean value of EQ-5D score was 68.9% and mean value of EQ-5D VAS was 66.6%) than in patients with ML treated by means of autologous PSCT (mean value of EQ-5D score was 82.7% and mean value of EQ-5D VAS was 76.7%).

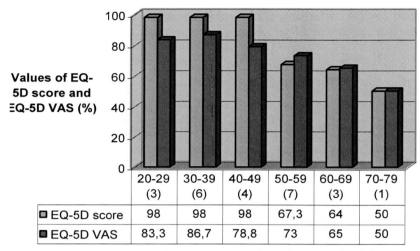

Age range (Number of respondents)

Figure 3. Dependence of EQ-5D score and EQ-5D VAS on individual age groups in patients with ML treated by means of autologous PSCT from 2001 to 2003 (n = 24, p<0.01).

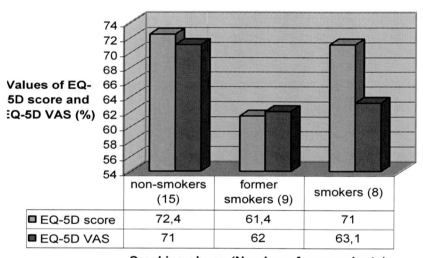

Smoking abusu (Number of respondents)

Figure 4. Dependence of EQ-5D score and EQ-5D VAS on smoking abuse in patients with MM treated by means of autologous PSCT from 2001 to 2003 (n = 32, p<0.01).

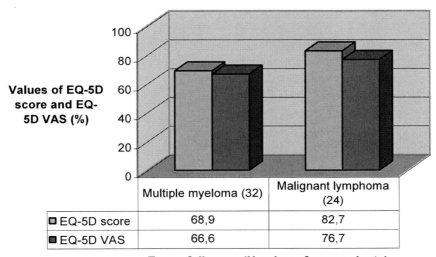

Type of disease (Number of respondents)	Multiple myeloma (32)	Malignant lymphoma (24)
EQ-5D score	68,9	82,7
EQ-5D VAS	66,6	76,7

Figure 5. Dependence of EQ-5D score and EQ-5D VAS on type of disease in patients treated by means of autologous PSCT from 2001 to 2003 (n = 56, p<0,01).

Table XIII. Comparison of respondents with MM and ML treated by means of autologous PSCT according to the level of troubles

Dimension of quality of life	Level of evaluation	Malignant lymphoma	Multiple myeloma
Number of respondents		*abs. rel*	*abs. rel.*
Mobility	No troubles	17 70.8%	13 41%
	with troubles	7 29.2%	19 59%
	immobile	0	0
Self-care	No troubles	22 91.7%	26 81.2%
	with troubles	2 8.3%	6 18.8%
	incapable	0	0
Usual activities	No troubles	17 70.8%	6 18.8%
	with troubles	6 25.0%	26 81.2%
	incapable	1 4.2%	0
Pain/discomfort	none	16 66.7%	9 28.1%
	weighty	8 33.3%	22 68.8%
	Extreme	0	1 3.1%
Anxiety/depression	None	18 75.0%	13 41%
	Weighty	5 20.8%	19 59%
	Extreme	1 4.2%	0
Total number of respondents		24	32

Discussion for Results

1) The effect of age on QoL in both patient groups treated by means of autologous PSCT has been proved.

Our results show that a lower QoL correlates with increasing age of patients who underwent autologous PSCT. We think that the increasing age of patients correlates with an increasing number of associated diseases and it creates a problem of low level of QoL of patients. Also, we think that in patients with an increasing age and an increasing number of associated diseases is a lower overall physical condition and this means a lower QoL.

2) The effect of smoking abuse on QoL in groups of patients with MM treated by means of autologous PSCT has been proved.

In the cohort of patients with MM we proved a lower QoL in smokers in comparison with non-smokers or former smokers.

3) The effect of the type of disease on QoL in patients treated by means of autologous PSCT has been proved.

We confirmed in our cross-sectional follow-up a statistically significant dependence of QoL in patients treated by means of autologous PSCT on the type of disease. We found out a lower global QoL in the cohort of patients with MM in comparison with the cohort of patients with ML. Prevailing complaints in the cohort of patients with multiple myeloma are: (1). regular activity with complaints 81.2% (26/32 respondents), (2). medium serious pain/discomfort 68.8% (22/32 respondents), (3). movement with complaints 59% (19/32 respondents), (4). medium serious anxiety/depression 59% (19/32 respondents). Prevailing complaints in the cohort of patients with malignant lymphoma are: (1). medium serious pain/discomfort 33.3% (8/24 respondents), (2). movement with complaints 29.2 % (7/24 respondents), regular activity with complaints 25 % (6/24 respondents), medium serious anxiety/depression 20.8% (5/24 respondents).

QUALITY OF LIFE IN PATIENTS WITH ACUTE MYELOID LEUKAEMIA AND MULTIPLE MYELOMA UNDERGOING AUTOLOGOUS PROGENITOR STEM CELL TRANSPLANTATION

Aims of Study

The study has two main aims:

1) To analyse the effect of selected psychosocial, health and demographic aspects on QoL in patients with acute myeloid leukaemia (AML) and malignant myeloma (MM) undergoing autologous PSCT.
2) To evaluate the global QoL in patients with AML and MM undergoing autologous PSCT.

Design of Study

The study is a cross-sectional, retrospective and descriptive. It is based on data obtained during the year 2004 - 2005 (from September 1, 2004 to January 31, 2005) in 12 adult patients with AML and 32 patients with MM undergoing autologous PSCT from 2001 to 2003.

PATIENTS AND METHOD

Group Characteristics

The total number of respondents with AML undergoing autologous PSCT was 12 (7 male, 5 female). The average age of patients with AML was 47.5 years (range 27-68 years old). The total number of respondents with MM undergoing autologous PSCT was 32 (18 male and 14 female). The average age of patients with MM was 60 years (range 45-78 years old).

Measurements

The Czech version of an international generic European Quality of Life Questionnaire – Version EQ-5D (EuroQol – EQ-5D) was used [4, 7-14].

Data Analysis, Statistical Analysis

The evaluation of questionnaires was carried out by means of descriptive analysis in accordance with European Quality of Life Group method (14). The independent variables were age, sex, level of education, marital status, increasing number of associated diseases, smoking abuse, religion, type of disease and time lapse from autologous PSCT. The dependent variables were EQ-5D score (dimensions of QoL) and EQ-5D VAS (a subjective health condition). The effect of selected aspects on QoL in patients was evaluated by means of analysis of variance. The StatSoft STATISTICA Base 7.1 software was used for complete evaluation of dates. The value $p<0.05$ was considered significant.

Procedure

The QoL questionnaire with a covering letter, in which the whole project was explained, together with a stamped envelope were mailed to a respondent's address. The filling in of the questionnaire was voluntary and anonymous.

RESULTS OF STUDY

The above-mentioned aspects proved a statistically significant dependence of QoL (EQ-5D score and EQ-5D VAS) on age in both cohorts (p<0.01) (see table XIV and figure 6), religion in AML cohort (p<0.05) (see table XV), smoking abuse in both cohorts (p<0.01) (see table XVI and figure 7), level of education in AML cohort (p<0.05) (see table XVII), increasing number of associated diseases in AML cohort (p<0,05) (see table XVIII) and type of disease (p<0,05) (see table XIX). The effect of other aspects on QoL was not proven as statistically significant.

Table XIV. Comparison of mean values of EQ-5D score and mean values of EQ-5D VAS in individual age groups in respondents with AML (n = 12, p<0.01)

Age range	Number of respondents	Mean values of EQ-5D score (in %)	Standard deviation	Mean values of EQ-5D VAS (in %)	Standard deviation
20-29	1	70	0	60	0
30-39	1	98	0	95	0
40-49	5	86.2	15.7	73.6	13.9
50-59	3	60	14.5	58.3	2.4
60-69	2	61	15	56	4

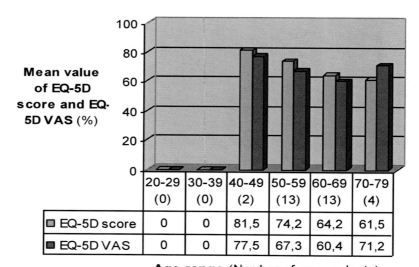

Age range (Number of respondents)	20-29 (0)	30-39 (0)	40-49 (2)	50-59 (13)	60-69 (13)	70-79 (4)
EQ-5D score	0	0	81,5	74,2	64,2	61,5
EQ-5D VAS	0	0	77,5	67,3	60,4	71,2

Age range (Number of respondents)

Figure 6. Comparison of mean values of EQ-5D score and mean values of EQ-5D VAS in individual age groups in respondents with with MM (n = 32, p<0,01).

Table XV. Comparison of mean values of EQ-5D score and mean values of EQ-5D VAS with religion in respondents with AML (n = 12, p<0,05)

Religion	Number of respondents	Mean values of EQ-5D score (in %)	Standard deviation	Mean values of EQ-5D VAS (in %)	Standard deviation
Believers	8	83.9	15.9	71	16.6
Non-believers	4	57.5	17.6	60.5	10.2

Global QoL in patients with AML undergoing autologous PSCT is on a very good level (mean value of EQ-5D score was 75.1%, mean value of EQ-5D VAS was 67.5%) than in patients with MM undergoing autologous PSCT (mean value of EQ-5D score was 68.9%, mean value of EQ-5D VAS was 66.6%).

Table XVI. Comparison of mean values of EQ-5D score and mean values of EQ-5D VAS with smoking abusu in respondents with AML (n = 12, p<0,01)

Smoking abuse	Number of respondents	Mean values of EQ-5D score (in %)	Standard deviation	Mean values of EQ-5D VAS (in %)	Standard deviation
Non-smokers	6	90.7	11.4	77.2	16.4
Smokers	6	59.5	14.1	57.8	3.5

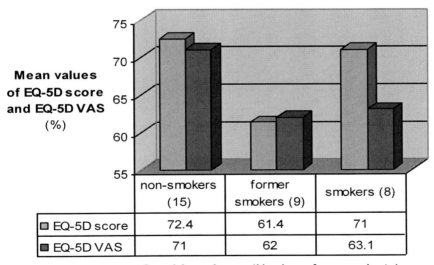

	non-smokers (15)	former smokers (9)	smokers (8)
◼ EQ-5D score	72.4	61.4	71
◼ EQ-5D VAS	71	62	63.1

Smoking abusu (Number of respondents)

Figure 7. Comparison of mean values of EQ-5D score and mean values of EQ-5D VAS with smoking abuse in respondents with MM (n = 32, p<0.01).

Table XVII. Comparison of mean values of EQ-5D score and mean values of EQ-5D VAS with level of education in respondents with AML (n = 12, p<0.05)

Level of education	Number of respondents	Mean values of EQ-5D score (in %)	Standard deviation	Mean values of EQ-5D VAS (in %)	Standard deviation
Elementary	2	43	4.2	53.5	2.12
Apprentice	3	67	8.5	60	0
Secondary	3	74	4.0	65	8.7
University	4	98	0	82	17.9

Table XVIII. Comparison of mean values of EQ-5D score and mean values of EQ-5D VAS with an increasing number of associated diseases in respondents with AML (n = 12, p<0,05)

Number of diseases	Number of respondents	Mean values of EQ-5D score (in %)	Standard deviation	Mean values of EQ-5D VAS (in %)	Standard deviation
0	3	88.7	16.2	71.7	20.2
1	4	83.2	18.7	77	15.7
2	4	64	16.6	58.8	2.5
3 and more	1	46	0	52	0

Table XIX. Comparison of respondents with AML and MM according to the level of troubles (n = 44, p<0.05)

Dimension of quality of life	Level of evaluation	Respondents with AML	Respondents with MM
Number of respondents		abs. rel	abs. rel.
Mobility	No troubles	10 83,3%	13 41%
	with troubles	2 16,7%	19 59%
	immobile	0	0
Self-care	No troubles	10 83,3%	26 81,2%
	with troubles	2 16,7%	6 18,8%
	incapable	0	0
Usual activities	No troubles	9 75%	6 18,8%
	with troubles	3 25%	26 81,2%
	incapable	0	0
Pain / discomfort	none	10 83,3%	9 28,1%
	weighty	2 16,7%	22 68,8%
	Extreme	0	1 3,1%
Anxiety /depression	None	9 75%	13 41%
	Weighty	2 16,6%	19 59%
	extreme	1 8,4%	0
Number of respondents		12	32

DISCUSSION OF RESULTS

1) The effect of age on QoL in both cohorts of patients treated by means of autologous PSCT has been proved.

Our results show that a lower QoL correlates with increasing age of patients who underwent autologous PSCT. We think that with an increasing age of patients correlates with an increasing number of associated diseases and it creates a problem of low level of QoL of patients. Also, we think that in patients with an increasing age and an increasing number of associated diseases is a lower overall physical condition and this means a lower QoL.

2) The effect of religion on QoL in AML cohort treated by means of autologous PSCT has been proved.

It is clear from our results that QoL in respondents with AML who believed in God was higher than in respondents who were non-believers. Respondents who believed in God had a higher QoL than non-believers.

3) The effect of smoking abuse on QoL in both cohorts of patients treated by means of autologous PSCT has been proved.

In both cohorts of patients we proved a lower QoL in smokers in comparison with non-smokers or former smokers.

4) The effect of level of education on QoL in AML cohort treated by means of autologous PSCT has been proved.

In AML cohort we proved higher level of QoL in respondents with higher education (secondary and university education).

5) The effect of increasing number of associated diseases in AML cohort treated by means of autologous PSCT has been proved.

In AML cohort we proved a lower QoL correlates with an increasing number of associated diseases. We think that with increasing number of associated diseases correlate with overall fatigue and emotional difficulties and in patients with an increasing number of associated diseases there is a lower overall physical fitness and this causes a lower QoL.

6) The effect of type of disease has been proved.

QoL in patients with AML undergoing autologous PSCT is on a very good level (mean value of EQ-5D score was 75.1%, mean value of EQ-5D VAS was 67.5%) than in patients with MM undergoing autologous PSCT (mean value of EQ-5D score was 68.9%, mean value of EQ-5D VAS was 66.6%).

CONCLUSION

Own process of HSCT is quite challenging for patients and that's for several reasons [4, 8-10]. First of all there are unwanted effects of systematic chemotherapy, repetitive invasive performances - central and peripheral vein catetrization, diagnostic aspiration of bone marrow and so on. In men it is also sperm taking followed by cryoconservation of seminal fluid because of the possibility of reproductive organs dysfunction caused by intensive antitumorous therapy (permanent or temporary infertility). Hormonal substitutional therapy is indicated in young females, because of the possibility of damaging the reproductive organs. Also we have to consider several weeks of isolation in an aseptic box. There is increased sensibility to opportunistic infections (bacterial, viral, fungal, mycoplasmatic, etc.) as an effect of bone marrow toxicity caused by high-dose chemotherapy. Besides those symptoms the is patient loaded with results of toxicity caused by high dose chemotherapy (mucositis, gastroenteritis, dermatitis, alveolitis, signs of cardiotoxicity and neurotoxicity). Serious complication is acute or chronic GVHD, which is the result of allogeneic transplantation (from relative or non-relative donor). Acute GVHD affects especially the liver, mucosa of the intestinal tract and skin [2, 3]. Serious forms can cause death. Chronic GVHD damage particularly intestinal tract and skin and can handicap the patient [4]. By listing all possible risks and complications it is necessary to mention, that high-dose chemotherapy followed by HSCT cannot 100% insure that all malignant cells will be eliminated. There is a possibility of relapse and as an optional treatment, we can again choose high dose chemotherapy followed by HSCT [4, 8-10].

It is common in clinical medicine practice to evaluate a patient´s health condition and the success of the treatment based only on one type of marker, the most often by means of somatic, laboratory or detecting markers [4, 7-13]. But the trend in modern clinical medicine and especially in clinical oncology, radiotherapy and clinical haematooncology to evaluate a patient´s health condition in a more complex way, using other aspects. The QoL means more dimensional evaluation of a number of life aspects [4, 7-13]. Different aspects can be affected in a different way in a different phase of the disease and its treatment. That is why this information enriches our knowledge concerning a patient´s needs and it can significantly contribute to the medical treatment improvement. It can also help us to reveal the mechanisms which modify the origin and the course of disease [4, 7-13, 17].

We are also aware of the fact that our study can be limited by a few other factors: (1). The study deals only with the effect of selected demographic, psychosocial and healthy aspects on QoL. We could add a few other aspects. But we decided on these aspects because patients were able and willing to provide this information in a retrospectively and anonymously carried out study. (2). In the study we used only a generic European Quality of Life Questionnaire - EQ-5D for evaluation of global QoL in our patients. We decided on its evaluation because our patients were able and willing to complete only this questionnaire. Our patients emphasized that this questionnaire was very intelligible and especially brief. We could use the originally Czech version of FACT–G Questionnaire or EORTC QLQ-C30 Questionnaire, but our patients were negative for completing one of these questionnaires. The patients emphasized that this questionnaire is very comprehensive and exacting for time.

In the future, we would like to continue this study and carry on a prospective study which would longitudinally evaluate health-related quality of life (HRQoL) and which would be more oriented on characteristics of particular diseases, on methods of pretransplantation procedure and on the type of transplantation.

REFERENCES

[1]   Andel, M. Internal Medicine – Part IIIb – Hematology. 1st. edc. Praha: Galen, 2001.

[2]   Atkinson, K. et al. The BMT Data Book: *A Manual for Bone Marrow and Blood Stem Cell Transplantation.* 1st. ed. Cambridge: University Press, 1998.

[3]   Giralt, S., Slavin, S. *New Frontiers in Cancer Therapy: Non-Myeloablative Stem Cell Transplantation (NST).* 1st. edc. Darwin Scientific Publishing, 2000.

[4]   Slovacek, L., Slovackova, B., Jebavy, L. Global Quality of Life in Patients Who Have Undergone the Hematopoietic Stem Cell Transplantation: Finding from Transversal and Retrospective Study. *Exp. Oncol.* 2005, 27 (3): 238-242.

[5]   Slovacek, L., Slovackova, B., Blazek, M., Jebavy, L. Quality of life of oncological patients – definition, conception and measurement. *Journal of Czech and Slovak Society of Clinical Oncology* 2006, 19 (3): 163-166.

[6]   Ferrell, B.R., Grant, M.M. Quality of Life Scale: Bone Marrow Transplant. In.: *Quality of Life from Nursing and Patient Perspectives: Theory, Research, Practice.* 2nd ed. Jones and Bartlett Publishers, 2003.

[7]   Slovacek, L., Slovackova, B., Jebavy, L., Blazek, M. Autologous Progenitor Stem Cell Transplantation in Acute Myeloid Leukemia Survivors: An Effect on Quality of Life. Abstract Book from 18th International Congress on Anti Cancer Treatment, Paris, France, 2007, 389-389.

[8]   Slovacek, L., Slovackova, B., Jebavy, L., Blazek, M. Global Quality of Life in Patients with Multiple Myeloma and Malignant Lymphoma after the Autologous Progenitor Stem Cell Transplantation: Finding from Retrospective Study. Abstract Book from 18th International Congress on Anti Cancer Treatment, Paris, France, 2007, 389-390.

[9]   Slovacek, L., Slovackova, B., Blazek, M., Jebavy, L. Quality of Life and Hematopoietic Stem Cell Transplantation. Abstract Book from 18th International Congress on Anti Cancer Treatment, Paris, France, 2007, 390-390.

[10]   Slovacek, L., Slovackova, B., Jebavy, L., Blazek, M., Horacek, J. Retrospective Assessement of the Global Quality of Life of Patients with Acute Myeloid Leukemia after HSCT from Nurses Perspectives: finding from a cross-sectional and retrospective study. *Haematol – Hematol. J.* 2006, 91 (s1): 402-402.

[11]   Slovacek, L., Slovackova, B., Blazek, M., Jebavy, L., Horacek, J. Global Quality of Life of Patients with Multiple Myeloma and Malignant Lymphoma after the HSCT: A Cross-sectional and Retrospective Study. *Haematol – Hematol. J.* 2006, 91 (s1): 462-462.

[12]   Slovacek, L., Slovackova, B., Jebavy, L., Horacek, J., Blazek, M. Quality of Life of Oncological and Hematooncological Patients after the HSCT: Finding from Cross-sectional and Retrospective Study. *Haematol – Hematol.* J. 2006, 91 (s1): 524-525.

[13] Slovacek, L., Slovackova, B., Jebavy, L. Healthy and psychosocial aspects in patients undergoing autologous progenitor stem cell transplantation. *Cas. Lek. Ces.* 2006, 145 (12): 976-979.

[14] The EuroQol Group. EuroQol – a new facility for the measurement of health-related quality of life. *Health Policy* 1990, 16: 199-208.

[15] Badia, X., Herdman, M., Schiaffino A. Determining correspondence between scores on the EQ-5D "thermometer" and a 5-point categorical rating scale. *Medical Care* 1999, 37 (7): 671-677.

[16] Busschbach, J. J., McDonnell, J., Essink-Bot, M. L. et al. Etimating parametric relationships between health desciption and health valuation with an application to the EuroQol EQ-5D. *J. Health Econ.* 1999, 18 (5): 551-571

[17] Mesanyova, M., Simek, J. Bone Marrow Transplant from Patients Overview. Czech Pract. 2004, 84 (9): 536-40.

In: Encyclopedia of Stem Cell Research (2 Volume Set)   ISBN: 978-1-61761-835-2
Editor: Alexander L. Greene   © 2012 Nova Science Publishers, Inc.

Chapter XLI

RISK FACTORS FOR SURVIVAL IN PEDIATRIC PATIENTS UNDERGOING ALLOGENEIC CORD BLOOD TRANSPLANTATION

Marta Gonzalez-Vicent, Julian Sevilla, Alvaro Lassaletta,
Manuel Ramírez, Luis Madero and Miguel A. Diaz
Hospital Niño Jesús, Madrid, Spain

ABSTRACT

The presence of primitive and committed hematopoietic progenitor cells (HPC) in the cord blood was initially described in the early seventies. Broxmeyer et al, later in experimental studies showed the potential application of umbilical cord blood (UCB) stem cells for clinical transplantation. However it was in the late eighties when for the first time was reported the success of a cord blood transplant (CBT). It was performed in a child with Fanconi anemia, and it provided both hematological and immunological reconstitution after myeloablative therapy. Since then, umbilical cord blood (UCB) is being increasingly used as an alternative source for hematopoietic stem cell transplantation. To further analyze the clinical outcome and survival, we report results of CB transplants performed in our center for both malignant and nonmalignant diseases in 34 pediatric patients. The median follow-up for survivors was 36 months (range:2-96).

Median age was 6 years (range: 1-18). There were nineteen male. Four cases were HLA-identical sibling CB donors and the others were unrelated CB donors. The diagnosis was malignancy in 27 patients and non malignancy in 7 patients. Disease status was early in 5 patients, intermediate in 2 patients and advanced disease in 27 patients. For 13 patients, it was the second stem cell transplant.

The conditioning regimen was chemotherapy based in all cases. Tymoglobulin was added in 28 patients. Graft versus-host disease (GVHD) prophylaxis consisted on cyclosporine A (CsA) and steroids in unrelated and CsA alone in related CB transplants.

The median number of total nucleated cells (TNC) and CD34+ cells infused was 4.64×10^7 /Kg (range:1.4-44) and 1.4×10^5 /Kg (range:0.1-7.5), respectively.

HLA match was as follows: 6/6 in eight patients, 5/6 in eight, 4/6 in fifteen and 3/3 in three.

The cumulative incidence for neutrophil and platelet engraftment at day +60 was 81% and 51% respectively. The probability of develop acute GVHD grade $\geq$ II was 31$\pm$11% and chronic GVHD 19$\pm$10%.

The 3-year event-free survival (EFS) for whole group was 34$\pm$8%. The variables associated with improved survival by multivariate analysis were early disease status at transplant and a higher number of CD34+ cells infused (>1.5×10^5/Kg). If we analyze separately these results, the EFS in children transplanted in early phase of disease and with higher number of CD34+ cells was 100% whereas for patients transplanted in advanced phase of disease and with a lower number of CD34+ cells was of 7$\pm$6%. The patients with only one of these favorable factors had an EFS of 46$\pm$13%.

These results strongly suggest that the main factor to select the CB unit for stem cell transplant should be the CD34$^+$ cell dose.

Available data show that umbilical cord blood offer at least comparable results to other sources of progenitor cells for hematopoietic transplantation. In our experience, the CD34+ cell dose is the main factor related to overall results in this clinical setting.

Keywords: Cord blood transplant, prognostic factors, children and infections.

INTRODUCTION

Umbilical cord blood (CB) is being increasingly used as an alternative source of allogeneic hematopoietic stem cells for patients with malignant and nonmalignant disorders with no suitable bone marrow donor[1-4].

It offers clinical advantages such as rapid availability, ease of procurement and decreased risk of severe acute and chronic graft-versus-host disease (GVHD) despite HLA-disparity. However, these potential benefits may be offset by an insufficient cell dose with a delayed time to engraftment (mainly platelet recovery) and a slower immune reconstitution with an increased incidence of infections, principally viral infections. Moreover, there is concern that graft versus leukemia activity may be diminished after CBT, leading to an increased rate of relapse [5-7].

The majority of previous reports are multicentric and show the results of registries such as Eurocord or International Bone Marrow Transplant Registry (IBMTR)[26,27]. However, there have been few reports of single centers with pediatric patients that use uniform treatment plans and methods of assessment.

We report the results of CBT performed in 34 pediatric patients in a single center over the last 8 years. The main objective of this study was to analyze predictive factors for survival. Secondary objectives were to study hematopoietic recovery, infections, GVHD and relapse.

PATIENTS AND METHODS

Patients

Between January 1996 and May 2004, 34 children (19 boys and 15 girls) underwent CBT for malignant (n=27) and non-malignant diseases (n=7) at the Niño Jesus Children´s Hospital. The median age at transplantation was 6 years (range: 1-18 years). Pretransplantation patient characteristics are shown in Table 1. For purposes of further analysis, patients were categorized for disease status as early, intermediate and advance. Patients with acute leukemia in first complete remission (CR) were considered as early disease and patients in relapse, refractory disease and third or subsequent remission were considered advance disease. Acute leukemia in second CR was considered intermediate disease. All patients with nonmalignant disorders were classified as advanced disease.Written consent was obtained from all patients or their guardians. Protocols were approved by the Institutional Review Board of our institution.

Table 1. Patient characteristics (n=34).

Gender	
• Male	19
• Female	15
Age, median (range)	6 (1-18)
Weight, median (range)	21 (6-73)
CMV serology	
• Negative	11
• Positive	23
Diagnosis	
• ALL	15
• AML	7
• MDS	3
• NHL	2
• SCID	4
• Osteopetrosis	2
• Blackfan-Diamond Anemia	1
Disease status	
• Early	5
• Intermediate	2
• Advance	27
No of transplant	
• First	21
• Second	13

Abbreviations: ALL, acute lymphoblastic leukemia; AML, acute myeloblastic leukemia; MDS, myelodysplasic syndrome; NHL, non-Hodgkin lymphoma; SCID, severe combinated immunodeficiency.

Cord Blood Selection

Four of the 34 patients received transplants using CB from an HLA-compatible sibling. Patients were eligible for unrelated donor CBT if a related or unrelated bone marrow donor was unavailable.

HLA typing for class I HLA-A, HLA-B and HLA-C antigens was determined by means of standard serological methods. Class II, HLA-DRB1 typing was performed with the use of high-resolution DNA techniques. Prior to 1999, HLA-typing was used to select the most closely matched donor-recipient pair. Since 1999, a CB unit was considerable for transplant only when ≤ 2 HLA antigen differences with the recipient were detected and priority was given to the unit with the largest nucleated cell dose and if disposable, a higher CD34+ cell dose.

CB units were obtained from several CB banks around the world. The cryopreserved CB unit was shipped in an appropriate container cooled by liquid nitrogen in vapor phase. The CB progenitors were thawed and washed following the procedure described by Rubinstein et al[8]. CD34+ cell count and TNC dose were determined after washing by means of flow-cytometric analysis.

Cord blood unit characteristics are shown in Table 2.

Table 2. Cord unit characteristics (n=34).

Gender	
• Male	16
• Female	16
• Unknown	2
CMV serology	
• Negative	11
• Positive	18
• Unknown	5
HLA disparity	
• 6/6	8
• 5/6	8
• 4/6	15
• 3/6	3
Nucleated cells/Kg ($x10^7$) infused	
Median (range)	4.64 (1.4-44)
CD34+/Kg ($x10^5$) infused	
Median (range)	1.5 (0.1-7.5)

Abbreviations: CMV, cytomegalovirus.

There is a positive correlation between TNC and CD34+ cell doses (r= 0.82, p < 0.0001).

Conditioning Regimen

16 patients received Eurocord regimen[3] consisted on total body irradiation (TBI), cyclophosphamide and lymphoglobulin; in < 3 years, busulphan was used instead of TBI. Since September 2002, 13 patients received a national protocol[9] based on thiotepa (5mg/Kg, once daily i.v. on days −9 and −8), busulphan (1mg/Kg, four times daily i.v., on days −7, -6 and −5), cyclophosphamide (60mg/Kg, once daily i.v. on days −4 and −3) and rabbit antithymocyte globulin (Thymoglobulin®) (2mg/Kg, once daily by i.v. infusion over 16 hours for 4 consecutive days, starting on day −5). Four patients with non-malignant diseases received busulphan (1mg/Kg, four times daily i.v., over 4 consecutive days, starting on day − 7) and cyclophosphamide (60mg/Kg, once daily i.v. on days −3 and −2). One patient underwent reduced intensity regimen, because of poor performance status at trasplantation, with fludarabine (30mg/m^2, once daily i.v., over 5 consecutive days starting on day −7) and melphalan (140mg/m^2, once daily i.v. on day −2).

Transplant characteristics are shown in Table 3.

Table 3. Transplant characteristics (n=34).

ABO mismatches	
• Yes	14
• No	15
• Unknown	5
CMV patient/donor serology	
• / -	5
• / +	11
• + / +	13
• Unknown	5
Conditioning	
• Eurocord protocol	16
• National protocol	13
• BU-CY	4
• Other	1
GVHD prophylaxis	
• CsA+steroids	30
• CsA alone	4
Thymoglobulin	
• Yes	28
• No	6
G-CSF postinfusion	
• Yes	26
• No	8

Abbreviations: CMV, cytomegalovirus; BU, busulphan; CY, cyclophosphamide; CsA, cyclosporine A; GVHD, graft versus host disease; G-CSF, granulocyte colony-stimulating factor.

GVHD Prophylaxis

Acute GVHD prophylaxis in unrelated CBT consisted of cyclosporine A (CsA) and methylprednisolone (MP). CsA was initiated on day –1 until day +90 and taper thereafter if GVHD was not present. The dosage of CsA was adjusted to maintain therapeutic trough levels at 200-400 ng/mL in whole blood. MP was started on day +7 until 2 mg/Kg/day and tapered on day +28 unless the patient developed acute GVHD. Related CBT used CsA alone as GVHD prophylaxis.

Supportive Care

Patients were nursed in single rooms ventilated with high-efficiency particulate air filtration systems (HEPA). Cytomegalovirus (CMV) serologic status was studied before transplantation in all patients and their donors. Prophylaxis of reactivation of herpes virus and CMV infection consisted of acyclovir (500mg/m^2/day in 3 doses). Documented CMV reactivation or infection demonstrated by antigenemia testing after transplantation was treated with ganciclovir, or in the neutropenic patient, with foscarnet.

All patients received oral cotrimoxazole (5 mg/Kg/day, twice daily) as prophylaxis for Pneumocystis carinii during conditioning. After neutropenia, cotrimoxazole was given 3 days each week, starting from the day of engraftment, for 6 months after transplantation.

Fluconazole was administered for prophylaxis of fungal infections for 100 days or during steroids treatment, whenever later.

Broad-spectrum antibiotics were administered for fever during neutropenia and amphotericin B liposomal(1-3 mg/Kg/day) was added for persistent fever unresponsive to antibiotic therapy. Granulocyte colony-stimulating factor (G-CSF, Neupogen; Amgen, Thousand Oaks, CA, USA) was given at a dose of 10µg/Kg daily from day +7 until engraftment to 26 of the 34 patients. Intravenous immune globulin was administered at a dose of 500 mg/Kg to maintain immunoglobulin G (IgG) levels of 400 mg/dL.

Blood products were infused to maintain the hemoglobin levels of 8 g/dL and platelet count >10-20 x 10^9/L. All transfusions were leukocyte-depleted and irradiated.

Hematopoietic Recovery and Engraftment

Neutrophil engraftment was defined as the first of 3 consecutive days with an ANC >0.5 x 10^9/L and platelet engraftment as the first day to reach a platelet count >20 x 10^9/L without platelet transfusion for 7 consecutive days.

Chimerism status was determined by quantitative PCR analysis of informative polymorphic variable number of tandem repeat (VNTR) regions. Complete chimerism was defined as the presence of donor hematopoietic cells ≥ 99%. It was performed on peripheral blood at engraftment day and on bone marrow at day + 30.

The absence of hematopoietic recovery at 60 days after transplant and the autologous hematopoietic reconstitution were considered as primary graft failure according to Eurocord criteria [10].

Graft versus Host Disease

Acute and chronic GVHD were graded according to previously published criteria [11,12]. Diagnosis of GVHD was based on clinical criteria and histopathologic confirmation when possible. Patients with GVHD were treated initially increasing steroids dose (MP).

Infections

Time to infection was considered from day 0 to the first day of a bacterial, viral or fungal infection.

Infections were analyzed according to incidence, type (bacterial, viral or fungal) and outcome.

Outcome and Survival

Transplant-related mortality (TRM) was defined as all causes of non-relapse death. Event-free survival (EFS) was defined as the time interval from CBT to first event (relapse or death).

Statistical Analysis

Baseline characteristics of all patients were summarized using descriptive statistics. Data are expressed as median and range. The probabilities of neutrophil and platelet recovery, acute and chronic GVHD, treatment related mortality and relapse were calculated with cumulative incidence functions and their 95% confidence intervals (CI) [13]. Kaplan-Meier (KM) method [14] was used to estimate the event-free survival (EFS).

Cox's proportional-hazards regression model [15] was used to correlate each potential prognostic factor with survival in univariate analysis. All variables found to have a P value of less than 0.1 were included in a multivariate analysis, with the use of a stepwise procedure. Survival curves comparison was performed using the log-rank test. Results were considered significant if the p value was < 0.05.

RESULTS

Hematopoietic Recovery and Engraftment

Graft failure occurred in 3 patients (9%); 1 experienced autologous reconstitution and 2 regrowth of leukemia cells. The median number of total nucleated cells (TNC) and CD34+

cells infused are shown in Table 2. About 25% of progenitor cells were lost during the procedure.

The cumulative incidence of neutrophil recovery was $81.1\pm7\%$ at day +60. The median time to neutrophil engraftment was 17 days (range:9-41 days). In univariate analysis, probability of neutrophil recovery was strongly associated with the infused CD34+ cell dose (HR: 2.62, 95%CI: 1.14-6.02, $p < 0.02$) and non-malignant disease (HR: 3.71, 95%CI: 1.26-10.86, $p < 0.01$). Notably, if we grouped patients according to CD34+ cell dose median (1.5×10^5/Kg), probability of engraftment was superior in patients receiving a higher cell dose ($92.5\pm7\%$ at day +60) than in patients receiving a lower cell dose ($74.7\pm11\%$ at day +60) (p=0.02). Moreover, probability of neutrophil engraftment was higher in patients with non-malignant diseases (100% at day +60) than in patients diagnosed of malignancies ($78\pm8\%$ at day +60) (p=0.01).

The cumulative incidence of platelet recovery at day +60 was $51\pm10\%$. The median time to achieve a platelet count $> 20 \times 10^9$/L and $> 50 \times 10^9$/L was 37 days (range: 12-200 days) and 78 days (range: 14-230), respectively. In univariate analysis, platelet engraftment $>20 \times 10^9$/L was associated with infused CD34+ cell dose (HR: 4.3, 95%CI: 1.13-16.29, p <0.03), non-malignant disease (HR: 16.94, 95%CI: 3.47-83.33, $p < 0.0005$) and disease status at transplant (HR: 5.46, 95%CI: 1.61-18.51, $p < 0.006$). According to CD34+ cell dose, probability of platelet engraftment was superior in patients infused a higher cell dose ($72.1\pm14\%$ at day +60) versus a lower cell dose ($33.8\pm12\%$ at day +60), (p=0.08). If we consider diagnosis, probability of platelet engraftment was higher in patients with nonmalignant diseases ($79.2\pm18\%$ at day +60) than in patients diagnosed of malignancies ($46\pm11\%$ at day +60)(p=0.002). Regarding disease status at transplant, probability of engraftment of patients transplanted in early phase was higher ($85.7\pm13\%$ at day +60) than those in advanced phase ($39.7\pm11\%$ at day +60) (p=0.009).

The median time to complete chimerism was 17 days (range: 9-570). The probability of develop complete chimerism was $78\pm8\%$ at day +100.

Supportive Care

The median transfusion requirements was 6 units (range:1-65 units) and 18 units (0-89 units) for red blood cells and platelets, respectively. The median number of hospitalization days was 36 days (range: 1-84 days). Twelve patients needed Intensive Care Unit (ICU) admission.

Graft Versus Host Disease

Acute GVHD was observed in 19 patients at a median time of 13 days (range: 8-80 days). The cumulative incidence of $\geq$ grade II acute GVHD was $31\pm11\%$. In Cox regression analysis, acute GVHD was not associated with any predictor, although there was a trend to less acute GVHD in early disease status at transplant (HR: 5.88, 95% CI: 0.75-45.45, p < 0.09).

Chronic GVHD was developed in 7 patients at a median time of 120 days (range: 73-365 days). It was limited in one patient and extensive in six patients. The cumulative incidence of chronic GVHD was 19±10%. In multivariate analysis, the only factor associated with chronic GVHD was previous acute GVHD (HR: 6.17, 95%CI: 0.71-52.63, p < 0.09). If we analyze separately the probability of develop chronic GVHD according to the grade of acute GVHD, it was of 65.4±18.4 for acute GVHD II-IV and 14.3±13% for acute GVHD 0-I (p < 0.05).

Infections

Virus was the most common cause of infection, mainly BK virus that affected to 18 patients developing hemorrhagic cystitis. Other virus implicated was: cytomegalovirus (CMV) in eight, varicela-zoster virus in five, adenovirus in two and human herpes virus 6 (HHV-6) in two patients. The median time to viral infection was 34 days (range: 19-120 days). The probability of develop viral infection was 59.4±9% at day +100. In multivariate analysis, viral infection was associated with acute GVHD > II (HR: 4.25, 95%CI: 1.48-12.19, p < 0.007) and with not using thymoglobulin (HR: 7.40, 95%CI: 0.96-57.03, p < 0.05).

About bacterial infections, the median time to develop was 24 days (range: 5-102) in 18 patients. The probability of develop bacterial infection was 55.8±9% at day +100. In multivariate analysis, bacterial infection was associated with a lower dose of CNT infused (HR: 10.1, 95%CI: 1.24-83.33, p < 0.03) and with diagnosis of non-malignant disease (HR: 13.15, 95%CI: 1.28-142.8, p < 0.02).

The median time to develop fungal infections was 38 days (range:36-41) in 6 patients, with a probability of 20±7% at day +100. No variables were found associated.

Infection was the main cause of death in 8 patients.

Treatment Related Mortality (TRM)

Twenty two patients died at a median time of 75 days (range: 1-178 days). The cumulative incidence of TRM was 40±9% at day +100 and 57.5±9% at 1 year postransplant. The causes of death in all 22 patients are outlined in Table 4.

Table 4. Causes of death (n=22).

	n
Infection	8
GVHD	6
Relapse	4
Graft failure	2
CNS hemorrhage	1
Interstitial pneumonia	1

Abbreviations: GVHD, graft versus host disease; CNS,central nervous system.

Outcome

At a median follow-up of 36 months (range: 2-96 months) after transplant, 12 patients are alive and disease-free survival. The probability of relapse was 30.2±10.2%. In multivariate analysis, the only factor associated with relapse was the absence of chronic GVHD (HR: 1.05, 95%CI: 1-1.1, p < 0.02). Thus, no patient with chronic GVHD relapsed.

The probability of 3-year EFS for all patients was 34±8%. The variables associated with a significant improvement in EFS in a multivariate analysis were a high number of CD34+ cells infused (>1.5 x 10^5/Kg) (HR: 4.16, 95%CI: 1.28-12.82, p< 0.01) and early disease status at transplant (HR: 10.63, 95%CI: 1.35-83.33, p< 0.02). The 3-year Kaplan-Meier (KM) estimate of EFS was 60±12% for patients infused > $1.5x10^5$ CD34+ cells/Kg and 12.7±8% for patients with ≤ $1.5x10^5$ CD34+ cells/Kg (p<0.01). Regarding disease status at transplant, the KM of EFS was 71.4±17% for early disease and 23.6±8% for advanced disease at transplant (p<0.01).

If we analyze separately these results, the EFS in children transplanted in early phase of disease and with high number of CD34+ cells was 100%, whereas for patients transplanted in advanced phase of disease and with a lower number of CD34+ cells was of 7±6%. The patients with only one of these favorable factors had an EFS of 46±13% (p<0.01).

DISCUSSION

Much of previously reported in children undergoing allogeneic cord blood transplant are registries data analysis or review [28].

Our study was designed to identify clinical factors influencing outcome in pediatric patients undergoing allogeneic cord blood transplantation in a single center. Cell dose measured as the quantities of CD34+ cells infused in the graft was the main factor predictive of survival. Although we found a positive correlation between TNC and CD34+ cell doses such as Wagner et al [19], the TNC infused were not associated with engraftment and survival. Possibly, the number of CD34+ cells reproduces more accurately the potential graft capacity than TNC.

In our series, probability of engraftment was higher in patients receiving >1.5 x10^5 CD34+ cells /Kg (92% vs 74%). Neutrophil engraftment occurred in 81% of patients at day +60 and the median time to engraftment was 17 days, earlier to previously reported data in children[10, 16,17] that was about 27 days. This difference may be explained by the use of methotrexate as GVHD prophylaxis which appears to delay the engraftment or by a slightly lower infused cell dose in the other series. The use of G-CSF postinfusion has not influenced because the majority of patients had regularly received hematopoietic growth factors as part of the transplant procedures. The routine administration of G-CSF is questionable because it may decreases the generation of Th1 responses after CBT, with decreased capacity to control opportunistic viral and fungal infections [23]. We also found that the probability of neutrophil engraftment was higher in patients with nonmalignant diseases in opposite to the work of Styczynski [17] et al that found a decrease in neutrophil engraftment in nonmalignancies. This difference may be due to the majority of our nonmalignancies are severe combinated immunodeficiencies with easier engraftment and there is no hemoglobinopathies where is more frequently the graft failure. The incidence of graft failure in our serie was 9%.

Platelet recovery ($>20 \times 10^9$/L) was achieved in 51% at day +60 comparable to prior reports [16,17]. The most important factors was a higher number of CD34+ cells infused such as in the study of Locatelli et al[10] and early disease status at transplant. Also the probability of platelet engraftment was higher in nonmalignant diseases.

A significant contributing factor to nonrelapse mortality in allogeneic transplantation is both acute and chronic GVHD [16]. A potential advantage of cord blood over bone marrow is a lower risk of GVHD. Rocha et al [20] compared the rates of GVHD in children who received a cord blood or bone marrow from an HLA identical sibling and found a lower incidence of acute and chronic GVHD with the use of cord blood. Later, an Eurocord study [21] comparing the outcomes of unrelated bone marrow and umbilical cord blood transplants in children with acute leukemia support the same results.

Our cumulative probability of grade II or greater GVHD was 31%, similar to results obtained in other studies of CBT [10,16,17,22]. We observed that neither the extent of HLA disparity nor the type of HLA class mismatch influenced the incidence of acute GVHD such as in the study of Styczynski et al [17]. The extent to which HLA disparity between recipient and donor correlates with the frequency and severity of GVHD and with the outcome of CBT is still unclear[6]. Rubinstein´s analysis [4] revealed a correlation between the severity of acute GVHD and the extent of HLA incompatibility.

Gluckman et al [24] found an association between the number or type of HLA disparities with engraftment and acute GVHD grade III-IV but TRM and survival were not associated with HLA disparities.

The cumulative incidence of chronic GVHD is low (19%) such as prior reports [16,17]. This low probability of chronic GVHD may be due to the immunologic properties of CB [16] with a decreased absolute numbers and responsiveness of T lymphocytes contributing to lesser alloreactivity and greater tolerant immune [23]. In fact, cord blood lymphocytes are naïve and produce lower amounts of pro-inflammatory cytokines [5].

The treatment related mortality was 66% at 12 months being infection the main cause of death as previous reports [19]. In comparative studies between bone marrow and cord blood as source of stem cells, deaths related to GVHD were more common after BMT and deaths related to infection from any cause after CBT [20]. The greater incidence of infection after CBT may be due to the immunologic characteristics of immaturity of lymphocytes [6] and the long-lasting period of deep immunosupression.

We report a relapse incidence of 29% similar to other pediatric studies [17] and the only factor associated with relapse was the absence of chronic GVHD such as with other sources of stem cells [29]. Rocha et al demonstrated that the relapse rates are similar after BMT and CBT, suggesting that graft versus leukemia effect of CB is comparable to that of conventional BM [20].

Estimated 3-year EFS in our series was 34%, but its important to remember that the majority of patients was in advanced disease at transplantation and for 13 patients it was the second stem cell transplant. In a multivariate analysis, the variables associated with an improved EFS were: a high number of CD34+ cells infused: $>1.5 \times 10^5$/Kg (p<0.01) and early disease status at transplant (p<0.02). We made a risk score using these 2 pretransplant variables to know EFS in each case. If we analyze separately these results, the EFS in children transplanted in early phase of disease and with high number of CD34+ cells was 100%, whereas for patients transplanted in advanced phase of disease and with a lower number of CD34+ cells was of 7±6%. The patients with only one of these favorable factors had an EFS of 46±13%.

The available data suggest that cell dose, and if its available CD34+ cell dose should be the primary criteria for donor selection, because a higher cell dose infused partially overcomes the negative impact of HLA disparity. In adults, the main obstacles to more widespread use of cord-blood transplantation have been the risks of graft failure and delayed hematopoietic recovery [25] because a high weight and lesser cell dose per kilogram. Recently, two studies have been performed in adults with leukemia to compare outcomes after unrelated BMT or CBT and the incidence of leukemia-free-survival were not significantly different in the two groups [26,27].

To overcome the problem of the cell dose in CBT, several experimental approaches are being investigated. One strategy with encouraging results is the use of two partially HLA-matched UCB units (referred as "double UCB") with the goal of increasing the total cell dose available [30]. Double CBT has led to more rapid neutrophil recovery after a myeloablative therapy and more consistent engraftment (rates of 90%) for adults. Brunstein et al [31] postuled that acute and chronic GVHD might be higher after double CBT. The incidence of grade II but no grade III-IV acute GVHD may be higher. The main reason is that recipients of two partially HLA-matched UCB units are more likely to receive at least one 4 out of 6 HLA-antigen matched unit; in addition, they received larger numbers of CD3+ cells. However, the increased risk of grade II acute GVHD in recipients of double CBT has not resulted in an increased incidence of TRM. Notably, the increased risk of acute GVHD may be associated with a greater graft-versus-leukemia effect. The use of two partially HLA-matched UCB units was also related with a significantly lower risk of relapse [32].

Another promising strategy has been the co-infusion of partially HLA-matched, T-cell depleted peripheral blood stem cells to promote a transient early neutrophil recovery until the engraftment of the CB unit [33].

Wagner et al [31], are investigating the use of intra bone marrow injection of UCB for reducing non-specific losses of hematopoietic stem cells that may get trapped in tissues when are injected intravenously.

Additionally, phase I and II studies of UCB ex vivo expansion have been reported, but there has been no evidence of benefit [34].

Other strategies that are in development phase or in clinical trials include the co-infusion of accessory cells, such as T regulatory cells, a subset of CD4+ T cells that co-express CD25 (interleukin-2 receptor alpha chain) and Fox p3 and mesenchymal stem cells (MSC) [35]. It is hypothesized that such cell populations may promote engraftment either by local host immune suppression or by a "supportive" stromal

CONCLUSION

Allogeneic CBT from either a related or an unrelated donor is as possible procedure as BMT in children with malignant and nonmalignant diseases, especially if transplanted in an early disease status. Furthermore, graft selection should be based mainly on CD34+ cell dose. New strategies are now being explored to address the obstacle of low cell dose, to expand the utilization of UCB as a useful source of hematopoietic stem cells.

REFERENCES

[1]   Gluckman E, Broxmeyer HE, Auerbach AD, et al. Hematopoietic reconstitution in a patient with Fanconi´s anemia by means of umbilical cord blood from an HLA-identical sibling. *N. Engl. J. Med.* 1989; 321: 1174-78.

[2]   Wagner JE, Kernan NA, Steinbuch M, et al. Allogeneic sibling umbilical-cord-blood transplantation in children with malignant and non-malignant disease. *Lancet* 1995; 346: 214-19.

[3]   Gluckman E, Rocha V, Boyer-Chammard A, et al. Outcome of cord-blood transplantation from related and unrelated donors. *N. Engl. J Med* .1997; 337: 373-81.

[4]   Rubinstein P, Carrier C, Scaradavou A, et al. Outcomes among 562 recipients of placental-blood transplants from unrelated donors. *N .Engl. J. Med* .1998; 339: 1565-77.

[5]   Locatelli F, Giorgiani G, Giraldi E, et al. Cord blood transplantation in childhood. *Haematologica* 2000; 85 (suppl to nº11): 26-9.

[6]   Wadlow RC and Porter DL. Umbilical cord blood transplantation: Where do we stand? *Biol. Blood Marrow Transplant* 2002; 8: 637-47.

[7]   Cohen Y and Nagler A. Umbilical cord blood transplantation- how, when and for whom? *Blood Reviews* 2004; 18: 167-79.

[8]   Rubinstein P, Dobrila L, Rosenfield RE, et al. Processing and cryopreservation of placental/umbilical cord blood for unrelated bone marrow reconstitution. *Proc .Natl. Acad. Sci. USA* 1995; 92: 10119-10122.

[9]   Sanz GF, Saavedra S, Planelles D, et al. Standardized unrelated donor cord blood transplantation in adults with hematologic malignancies. *Blood* 2001; 98: 2332-8.

[10]   Locatelli F, Rocha V, Chastang C, et al. Factors associated with outcome after cord blood transplantation in children with acute leukemia. *Blood* 1999; 93: 3662-3671.

[11]   Glucksberg H, Storb R, Fefer A, et al. Clinical manifestations of graft-versus-host disease in human recipients of marrow from HLA-matched sibling donors. *Transplantation* 1974; 18: 295-304.

[12]   Shulman HM, Sullivan KM, Weiden PL, et al. Chronic graft-versus-host syndrome in man: a long-term clinicopathologic study of 20 Seattle patients. *Am. J. Med.* 1980; 69: 204-17.

[13]   Gooley TA, Leisenring W, Crowley J, et al. Estimation of failure probabilities in the presence of competing risks: new representation of old estimator. *Stat. Med.* 1999; 18: 695-706.

[14] Kaplan EL, Meier P. Nonparametric estimation from incomplete observation. *J. Am. Stat. Assoc.* 1958; 53: 457-481.

[15] Cox DR. Regression models and life tables. *J. Royal Stat. Soc.* 1972; 34: 187-220.

[16] Thomson BG, Robertson KA, Gowan D, et al. Analysis of engraftment, graft-versus-host disease, and immune recovery following unrelated donor cord blood transplantation. *Blood* 2000; 96: 2703-11.

[17] Stycynski J, Cheung Y-K, Garvin J, et al. Outcomes of unrelated cord blood transplantation in pediatric recipients. *Bone Marrow Transplant.* 2004; 1-8.

[18] Iori AP, Cerretti R, De Felice L, et al. Pre-transplant prognostic factors for patients with high-risk leukemia undergoing an unrelated cord blood transplantation. *Bone Marrow Transplant* 2004; 33: 1097-1105.

[19] Wagner JE, Barker JN, DeFor TE, et al. Transplantation of unrelated donor umbilical cord blood in 102 patients with malignant and nonmalignant diseases: influence of CD34 cell dose and HLA disparity on treatment-related mortality and survival. *Blood* 2002; 100: 1611-18.

[20] Rocha V, Wagner JE, Sobocinski KA, et al. Graft-versus-host disease in children who have received a cord-blood or bone marrow transplant from an HLA-identical sibling. *N. Engl. J. Med.* 2000; 342: 1846-54.

[21] Rocha V, Cornish J, Sievers EL, et al. Comparison of outcomes of unrelated bone marrow and umbilical cord blood transplants in children with acute leukemia. *Blood* 2001; 97: 2962-2971.

[22] Gluckman E, Rocha V. Cord blood transplantation for children with acute leukemia: a Eurocord registry analysis. Blood cells, molecules and diseases 2004; 33: 271-3.

[23] Chao NJ, Emerson SG and Weinberg KJ. Stem Cell Transplantation (Cord Blood Transplants). *Hematology* 2004: 354-371.

[24] Gluckman E, Rocha V, Arcese W, et al. Factors associated with outcomes of unrelated cord blood transplant: Guidelines for donor choice. *Exp. Hematol.* 2004; 32: 397-407.

[25] Sanz MA. Cord-blood transplantation in patients with leukemia: a real alternative for adults. *N. Engl. J. Med.* 2004; 351: 2328-2330.

[26] Rocha V, Labopin M, Sanz G, et al. Trasplants of umbilical-cord blood or bone marrow from unrelated donors in adults with acute leukemia. *N. Engl. J. Med .*2004; 351: 2276-2285.

[27] Laughlin MJ, Eapen M, Rubinstein P, et al. Outcomes after transplantation of cord blood or bone marrow from unrelated donors in adults with leukemia. *N. Engl. J. Med .*2004; 351: 2265- 2275.

[28] Benito A, González Vicent M, Díaz MA, et al. Hematopoietic Stem Cell Transplantation Using Umbilical Cord Blood Progenitors. Review of Current Clinical Results. Bone *Marrow Transplant.* 2004;33:675-690.

[29] Díaz MA, Vicent MG, González ME, et al. Risk assessment and outcome of chronic graft-versus-host disease after allogeneic peripheral blood progenitor cell transplantation in pediatric patients. *Bone Marrow Transplant.* 2004; 34:433-8.

[30] Barker J,Weisdorf DJ, DeFor TE, et al. Transplantation of 2 partially HLA-matched umbilical cord blood units to enhance engraftment in adults with hematologic malignancy. *Blood* 2005; 105: 1343-7.

[31] Brunstein CG, Setubal DC and Wagner JE. Expanding the role of umbilical cord blood transplantation. *Br. J. Haematol* .2007; 137: 20-35.

[32] Verneris MR, Brunstein C, DeFor TE, et al. Risk of relapse (REL) after umbilical cord blood transplantation (UCBT) in patients with acute leukemia: marked reduction in recipients of two units. *Blood* 2005; 106: 93a.

[33] Fernández MN, Regidor C, Cabrera R et al. Unrelated umbilical cord blood transplants in adults: early recovery of neutrophils by supportive co-transplantation of a low number of highly purified peripheral blood CD34+ cells from an HLA-haploidentical donor. *Experimental Hematology* 2003; 31: 535-44.

[34] Shpall EJ, Quinones R, Giller R, et al. Transplantation of ex vivo expanded cord blood. *Biol. Blood Marrow Transplant.* 2002; 8: 368-76.

[35] Taylor PA, Lees CJ and Blazar BR. The infusion of ex vivo activated and expanded CD4+ CD25+ immune regulatory cells inhibits graft-versus-host lethality. *Blood* 2002; 99: 3493-9.

[36] Kim DW, Chung YJ, Kim TG, et al. Cotransplantation of third-party mesenchymal stromal cells can alleviate single-donor predominance and increase engraftment from double cord transplantation. *Blood* 2004; 103: 1941-8.

[37] MacMillan ML, Ramsay NKC, Atkinson K, et al. Ex-vkivo culture-expanded parental haploidentical mesenchymal stem cells to promote engraftment in recipients of unrelated donor umbilical cord blood: results of a phase I-II clinical trial. *Blood* 2002; 100: 836a.

In: Encyclopedia of Stem Cell Research (2 Volume Set) ISBN: 978-1-61761-835-2
Editor: Alexander L. Greene © 2012 Nova Science Publishers, Inc.

Chapter XLII

MULTIPOPTENT MESENCHYMAL STROMAL CELLS FOR SKIN WOUND HEALING AND SKELETAL MUSCLE REPAIR

Ying Zhu, Chunmeng Shi[*], Xinze Ran,
Yongping Su, Chengji Luo and Tianmin Cheng
Institute of Combined Injury, State Key Laboratory of Trauma,
Burns and combined injury, College of Preventive Medicine,
Third Military Medical University, Chongqing, China

ABSTRACT

Skin and skeletal muscle are frequently damaged tissues after trauma due to their localization and constant turn-over. Large skin or skeletal muscle defects are also sometimes life threatening. Bone marrow-derived multipotent mesenchymal stromal cells have the potential to differentiate into various cell lineages that participating in wound healing and skeletal muscle repair. One of the present goals in our lab is to promote the skin wound healing and skeletal muscle repair after traumatic events, particular for the impaired-healing wounds after radiation. Mesenchymal stromal cells can effectively accelerate the speed and improve the quality of skin wound healing and skeletal muscle repair after topical implantation. Pathological studies confirm that mesenchymal stem cells differentiate into fibroblasts, vascular endothelial cells, epidermal cells and skeletal muscle cells in regenerated tissues. Transplantation of mesenchymal stromal cells over-expressing healing-promoting factors such as vascular endothelial growth factor (VEGF), platelet derived growth factor (PDGF) for skin wound healing and muscle differentiation-initiating gene MyoD for skeletal further improves the therapeutic effects. Taken together,

[*] Correspondence concerning this article should be addressed to Dr. Chunmeng Shi, Institute of Combined Injury, State Key Laboratory of Trauma, Burns and Combined Injury, College of Preventive Medicine, Third Military Medical University, 30 Gaotanyan Street, Shapingba District, Chongqing, 400038, China. E-mail: shicm1010@yahoo.com.cn; Telephone: 86-23-65462263; Fax: 86-23-68752009

bone marrow multipotent mesenchymal stromal cells appear to provide a very promising tool for cell-based therapeutic strategies in skin and skeletal muscle regeneration.

Keywords: bone marrow, mesenchymal stromal cells, wound healing, skeletal muscle, regeneration, radiation.

INTRODUCTION

Multipotent mesenhcymal stromal cells have been extensively investigated in the past decade. This population of cells is described with different terms such as mesenchymal stem cells, marrow stromal cells, marrow mesenchymal stem cells or even multipotent adult progenitor cells in early studies [1, 2]. There is still in debate to define candidate stem cell populations in adult tissues since the potential of stem cells varies with different developmental stages [3, 4]. Recently, there is a trend to notice that the term mesenchymal stem cells is not concise since some of the previous studies did not apply the stringent criteria of adult stem cells (generally defined as clonogenic cell populations with the capabilities of both self-renewal and multilineage differentiation). Consequently, a position statement proposed to use "multipotent mesenchymal stromal cells" to designate the plastic-adherent cells isolated from bone marrow or other tissues with multipotent differentiation capacity [5]. These cells can also be designated by acronym MSC. MSCs are first described from bone marrow, and later, similar cells have been isolated and identified from different species and other adult sources including fat, umbilical cord, dermis, hair follicle, placenta as well as a variety of fetal tissues even amniotic fluids [6-16].

With the early and many subsequent studies on the biological properties of MSCs in the past years, MSCs have shown great potential for the application in regenerative medicine. Although MSCs are present in bone marrow and other adult tissues in low frequency and lack of specific surface markers, it can be easily to obtain plastic-adherent cell populations with spindle-shaped morphological characteristics by a variety of methods in culture media. MSCs have high potential of proliferation and can growth over a 500-fold expansion retained long telomeres and a normal karyotype [17]. Moreover, MSCs have the potential to differentiate into various mesenchymal lineages including bone, cartilage, adipose, stroma, and muscle in response to nonphysiological stimuli. Other studies also show that these cells are more broadly multipotent with the ability to differentiate into cell types representing each embryonic germ layer, including cells of endothelial, neuronal and even hepatic lineages [8]. The differentiated cells derived from MSCs are also confirmed to display specialize functions by both in vitro and in vivo studies [18-20]. In addition to multipotency, MSCs have a unique property of immunological advantage. MSCs are imunologically immature and they can modulate immune responses by suppressing the proliferation of lymphocytes and are able to survive in a xenogeneic environment for a longer time. MSCs have also been successfully used to treat the graft-versus-host disease (GVHD) in clinical patients [21-32]. The advantage of MSCs has attracted great interests and efforts to use them for cellular therapy and is very likely to have an important impact on clinical practice in the near future. So far, MSCs have been used in numerous preclinical models to generate a variety of injured tissues and some clinical trials are also in undergoing. For MSCs from different sources, bone marrow derived multipotent mesenchymal stromal cells (BMMSCs) are most extensively studied in the past years. Skin and skeletal muscle are frequently damaged tissues after trauma due to their localization and constant turn-over. Large skin or skeletal muscle defects are also sometimes life threatening. In this chapter, we will focus on the recent advances of using BMMSCs to improve wound healing and skeletal muscle repair.

BMMSCS AND SKIN WOUND HEALING

With the development of modern science and technology, the treatment of simple wounds is a mature practice, but the treatment of impaired-healing or non-healing chronic wounds still remains difficult [33, 34]. The chronic wounds are usually caused by complicated tissue environmental factors (such as infection, ischemia and poor vascularization) or by accompany with systemic diseases (such as diabetes and total body irradiation). With the appropriate wound care procedures including debridement of the necrotic tissue, removal of edema fluid, decreasing the bacterial burden, and providing the right balance of moisture to the wound bed, some wounds and ulcers are able to heal [35, 36]. However, there are still many chronic wounds that either do not heal at all or do so very slowly. In addition, there is also a need to accelerate the healing of acute wounds with large defects such as severe burns or traffic injures. In recent years, there have been efforts to develop more advanced treatment modalities. In the past ten years, several growth factors have been produced and used in clinic [37, 38]. Platelet-derived growth factor–BB (PDGF-BB) is approved for use in the treatment of diabetic neuropathic ulcers of the foot in the United States. Basic fibroblast growth factor (bFGF) and epidermal growth factor (EGF) have been approved by the State Food and Drug Administrative of China for the treatment of acute wounds and some chronic ulcers. However, when we look back to these studies from different research groups, some results are encouraging while some are not [39, 40]. On the other hand, it has been found that in some chronic ulcers, the endogenous level of some growth factors in the wounds are not decreased, even higher than that in simple wounds. Basing on these evidence, the application of growth factors for the treatment of chronic ulcers still needs further extensively evaluation. Cell-based therapeutic strategies (such as cell transplantation, tissue engineering and gene therapy) have attracted great attention in recent years. Some kinds of bioengineered skin substitutes have been approved by the Food and Drug Administration in the United States and other countries for specific indications. Some gene therapy studies are also in the development phase.

MSCs in Simple Cutaneous Wound Healing

Stem cells that have the high self-renewal potential and multi-lineage differentiation capacity are ideal candidate for cell-based therapy. In this term, stem cell-based therapy has come of age and there is excitement in the use of stem cells to offset impaired healing [34, 41]. It has long been known and emphasized recently that cells derived from bone marrow can act as a source of skin cells during the repair process. The presence of bone-marrow-derived epithelial cells has also been documented. Recent studies strongly suggest that bone marrow-derived keratinocytes can form colonies in the regenerating epidermis in vivo, and the colony-forming capacity of these cells can be recapitulated in vitro [42, 43, 44]. Following transplantation of Flk-(1+) bone marrow mesenchymal stromal cells, obtained from BALB/c mice (H-2Kd, white hair), into lethally irradiated C57BL/6 mice (H-2Kb, black hair), white hairs, which are largely composed of donor-derived H-2Kd cells, are produced in the recipient mice [45]. Analysis of the developmental plasticity of bone marrow-derived cells (BMDCs) is usually complicated by the possibility of cell–cell fusion; however, there is evidence that bone marrow cells can form epidermal keratinocytes without undergoing cell fusion [46, 47]. These results support the use of bone marrow-derived cells in therapeutic applications for epidermis repair. The contribution of wound healing fibroblasts and enthelial cells from BMMSCs is reported. Further studies also indicate that MSCs and circulating fibrocytes can contribute to the myofibroblast population and play a key role in wound closure [48]. A recent study further shows the potential of adult MSCs to the repair of skin appendages after injury [49, 50]. BrdU-labeled MSCs are co-cultured with heat-shocked confluent sweat gland cells (SGCs) in vitro and later intravenously are injected into full-thickness skin wounds in rats. Labeled MSCs are noted in hair follicles, sebaceous glands, blood vessels, and dermis in wounded tissues and the incorporated cells in hair follicles and sebaceous glands are positive for pan-cytokeratin. A subset of adult MSCs is also found to differentiate into SGCs under the regulation by epidermal growth factor and the injured microenvironment. However, whether MSCs can retain the phenotype of skin appendages cells permanently needs additional studies.

MSCs in the Healing of Wounds with Radiation

There is direct evidence that bone marrow-derived cells can give rise to functional skin cells and regenerate skin tissue. Pilot studies further suggest that BMMSCs can accelerate wound repair or even reconstitute the wound bed. But whether BMMSCs can improve the impaired-healing wounds is not clear. It has been known for long time that ionizing irradiation can delay the skin wound healing. Combined radiation and wound injury (CRWI) can occur in nuclear attacks and severe nuclear accidents [51]. The possibility of radiological terrorist attack further emphasizes the significance of studies on CRWI. This kind of skin wound is very complex and difficult to heal since high dose of irradiation can delay the wound healing and cause bone marrow dysplasia. To explore the effects and the mechanisms of BMMSCs on the repair of skin wound combined with local irradiation injury, autologous MSCs are isolated from the adult swine bone marrow and are directly transplanted into the full-thickness skin wounds combined with 20 Gy local irradiation [52]. The results show that direct transplantation of autologous MSCs into skin wounds accelerates the speed of wound healing. The granule tissues are abundant and the content of collagen is increased by MSCs treatment. Moreover, MSCs attracted the inflammatory cells and repairing cells to immigrate into wounds by producing IL-6, IL-8 and G-CSF and thus initiated the repairing processes. The wound microenvironment also induces the proliferation and expression of collagen type I in MSCs. These data show that local transplantation MSC promoted the repair of skin wounds combined with irradiation injury. The promoting effects are achieved by the bi-directional interactions between MSCs and wound microenvironment. In order to further improve the effects of MSCs, a kind of skin equivalent is constructed by co-culture of MSCs and epidermal cells on the human amino membrane in which the cellular components are depleted. When applied to the full-thickness skin wounds combined with radiation injury, the graft of HAM loaded with MSCs and epidermis cells plays a more effective role in promoting the healing of wounds with combined radiation injury [53]. Transplantation of MSCs with exogenous expression of PDGF-BB or VEGF also improves the therapeutic effects. As expected, PDGF-BB and VEGF improve the poor vasculary conditions in the wound bed after radiation and induce better tissue remodeling. In addition, the study on impaired-healing wound by total body irradiation (TBI) has been emphasized in our group since 1990s. The pathological basis of the wound healing process after TBI is also extensively studied. According to our results, the wounds combined with TBI of 5Gy or 6Gy can be a typical impaired-healing wound model for study [34]. In these models, there are very significant changes of the hematopoiesis and wound healing process. With this model, we report for the first time that systemically transplanted multipotent cells can migrate and reside into the injured tissues to improve both wound healing and hematopoietic recovery in animals with combined skin wound and total body irradiation [54].

BMMSCs and Skeletal Muscle Repair

Skeletal muscle satellite cells have long been considered as the only source of stem/progenitor cells for postnatal muscle repair and regeneration [55, 56]. Recent reports suggest that bone marrow derived progenitor cells may also be involved in skeletal muscle regeneration [57-59]. Although there are several candidate stem cell populations which have been identified from bone marrow, there are increasing evidence to show that MSC is likely to be the predominant stem cell population for skeletal muscle repair and regeneration. It is reported that transplantation of the adherent cell fraction (containing MSCs) from bone marrow into regenerating muscle resulted in higher engraftment than that with the nonadherent fraction (containing hemopoietic stem cells, HSCs) [57]. Another study shows that the expression of dystrophin is higher following implantation into dystrophin-null muscle of nonpurified BM compared with marrow enriched for HSCs [60]. More recently, it is demonstrated that the MSCs and not the hemopoietic compartment in human BM is the predominant cell population capable of fusing with myoblasts [61]. Other studies also have confirmed the myogenic potential of MSCs derived from other sources outside of bone marrow [62]. BMMSCs have been confirmed to have the ability to differentiate into smooth muscle and cardiac muscle cells. By these data, BMMSCs may represent as an alternative source of stem/progenitor cells for therapy of skeletal muscular dystrophies. Progenitor cells that contribute to muscle repair appear to enter a program that is similar to that displayed during the embryonic development of skeletal muscle [63, 64]. At a molecular level, myogenesis is controlled by a family of myogenic regulatory factors (MRFs), which includes MyoD, Myf5, myogenin [65, 66]. Moreover, Muscle repair and functional restoration from progenitor cells require an appropriate environment to promote the process of myogenesis, which comprises cell commitment, proliferation, fusion, and terminal maturation.

Modulation of MSCs by Wound Environment

However, it is not known whether local signals released after damage are specific for satellite cells or whether they also promote the myogenic commitment and differentiation of MSCs. It has been proposed that factors released from injured muscle provide the signals that contribute to the establishment of a favorable microenvironment to affect stem cell proliferation, migration and differentiation. However, whether the local signals released after damage can promote the myogenic commitment and differentiation of MSCs are not quite clear. In our group, the wound fluid is collected from the mouse skeletal muscle at the 8 to 72 hours with mechanical incision and freezing injury by liquid nitrogen. When incubated with MSCs, wound fluids show a promotion of cell proliferation, but failed to induce myogenin expression even in 6 days. But in another study, the researchers show that the incubation of rat MSCs with a conditioned medium prepared from chemically damaged but not undamaged muscle resulted in a time-dependent change from fibroblast-like into elongated multinucleated cells, a transient increase in the number of MyoD positive cells, and the subsequent onset of myogenin, α-actinin, and myosin heavy chain expression [67]. These differences may be resulted from the different wound model and in vitro culture systems. However, for in vivo studies, when applied to a mouse skeletal muscle injury model by topical implantation or by systemic transplantation via tail vein injection, MSCs can migrate to the wounded muscle tissue and participate in the repair process [68].

Effects of 5-Azacytidine and MyoDg of MSCs Enic Regulatory Factors

5-azacytidine (5-Aza) is a DNA methylation inhibitor which has the potential to induce myogenic differentiation in immortalized rodent and rabbit MSCs [69, 70]. Our group further established an in vitro system using 5-azacytidine to induce the differentiation of cultured primary mouse bone marrow MSCs into myotubes. The results indicate that MSC proliferation is not affected by 3uM of 5-azacytidine, but 20uM of 5-azacytidine induces the cytotoxicity. When given 10uM 5-azacytidine to MSCs, Myf5 begins to express at 6 hours and reach the peak at 9 hours. Myogenin appear at 24 hours and reach the peak at 48 hours after induction. Some cells express desmin at 7 days and myosin at 14 days. The cell morphology change is observed at days 9 and myotube-like structures can be seen at 14-16 days [71, 72]. The mechanism for the 5-azacytidine to induce MSCs myogenic differentiation is proposed to act through stochastic hypomethylation of random DNA residues, which in turn results in the activation of myogenic regulatory factors [73]. After induction with 5-azacytidine, the phosphorylation p38 activity and phosphoinositide-3 kinase (PI-3K) increase, but when blocking the p38 signaling pathway by SB203580 or blocking the PI-3K pathway by LY294002, the expression of Myf5 and myosin is delayed. Insulin growth factor (IGF-I) can increase the expression of myogenic regulatory factors induced by 5-azacytidine as well as the p38 and PI-3K signaling molecules. These results suggest that p38, PI-3K and IGF-I may have a positive effect in the myogenic differentiation process of MSCs by 5-azacytidine. Although there are no reports of successful myogenic conversion of adult BM-derived MSCs with 5-azacytidine in humans, this approach produces low levels of myogenic conversion of synovial membrane-derived human MSCs [74]. Notwithstanding this, high-efficiency conversion has been achieved with a subpopulation of human BM-derived stem cells called multipotent adult progenitor cells [75]. Further investigation is performed to study the myogenic differentiation of MSCs using in vivo skeletal muscle injury models. Purified MSCs derived from the bone marrow of male mice and MSCs with pre-treatment by 5-azacytidine are transplanted into the normal muscle tissues and injured muscle tissues of female mice. MSCs can differentiate into myoblasts after being implanted into the local injured muscle environment. The myoblast differentiation of MSCs is observed at days 15 in control MSCs group and at day 6 in MSC group treated with 5-azacytidine .

MyoD is a key regulatory gene in the development of skeletal muscles that activates the transcription of myogenic genes and can transform the nonmyogenic cells into muscle cells. It has been documented that MyoD alone can induce muscle stem cells to differentiate into myoblasts. In our group, the eukaryotic expression plasmid vector pIRES2-EGFP-MyoD is constructed by molecular cloning and is introduced into MSCs by lipofetamine-mediated gene transfection. The positive cells are selected by G418 and are confirmed by the expression of MyoD using RT-PCR and immunohistochemical staining. The results show that MyoD trasnfection effectively initiates the expression of myogenic regulatory factors myogenin, myosin, myoglobulin and desmin. Morphological changes with a smaller nucleus/cytoplasma ratio, compacted chromatin, abundant cytoplasmic organelles and microfilaments also support the occurrence of myoblast differentiation of MSCs by MyoD [76, 77]. Galectin-1, a 14–15-kDa lectin, belongs to a family of animal ß-galactoside-binding proteins, has recently been found to induce skeletal muscle differentiation in human fetal mesenchymal stem cells (hfMSCs) and increases muscle regeneration [78]. It has been reported that galectin-1 is a soluble factor responsible for myogenic conversion of dermal fibroblasts [79]. Continuous exposure to galectin-1 resulted in more efficient muscle differentiation than pulsed exposure. When transplanted into regenerating murine muscle, galectin-1-exposed hfMSCs formed four-fold more human muscle fibers than nonstimulated hfMSCs, with similar results obtained in a *scid/mdx* dystrophic mouse model. These data suggest that hfMSCs readily undergo muscle differentiation in response to galectin-1 through a stepwise progression similar to that which occurs during embryonic myogenesis [80]. The high degree of myogenic conversion achieved by MyoD trasnfection and galectin-1treatment has relevance for the development of therapies for muscular dystrophies.

MECHANISMS OF ACTION AND FUTURE DIRECTIONS

The promise of BMMSCs-mediated wound repair and regeneration is an exciting prospect and current indications strongly support the emphasis of these therapeutic strategies. BMMSCs can migrate to the wounded sites and differentiate into target cell types for tissue repair either by local or systemic implantation. BMMSCs can also elicit an indirect paracrine effect to improve tissue repair via production of soluble cytokines and extracelluar matrix. Although early data appear encouraging, much work remains to be done. So far, the MSCs in many studies are mixed cell populations, there is still a need to identify specific markers and to establish more effective methods to isolate pure MSC populations. Wound healing requires a complex interaction between tissue repairing cells and wound environments. Our knowledge is still very limited of the behaviors of MSCs under the modulation by wound environment. It is reported that even MSCs have been confirmed to differentiate into some epithelial cell types, the frequency is very low. How to induce MSCs to efficiently differentiate into specific target cells is still challenging. Furthermore, the malignant transformation of MSCs has been reported recently and the safety of MSCs for clinical application should also be carefully and extensively investigated [81]. Despite of these limitations, it is clear that MSCs will become a useful resource for the therapeutic applications of skin wounds and skeletal muscular dystrophies

ACKNOWLEDGMENTS

This work is supported by general program from National Science Foundation of China (NO. 30400188), "973" program (NO. 2005CB522605) from the Ministry of Science and Technology of China, Foundation for the Author of National Excellent Doctoral Dissertation (NO.200777) and Program for Changjiang Scholars and Innovative Research Team in University of PR China .

REFERENCES

[1]   Keating A. Mesenchymal stromal cells. *Curr. Opin. Hematol.* 2006;13(6):419-425.

[2]   He Q, Wan C, Li G. Concise review: multipotent mesenchymal stromal cells in blood. *Stem Cells.* 2007;25(1):69-77.

[3]   Shi CM, Cheng TM. A hypothesis of adult stem cell plasticity. *Chinese journal of clinical rehabilitation.* 2003;7（23）:3249-3251.

[4]   Weissman IL. Stem cells: units of development, units of regeneration, and units in evolution. *Cell.* 2000;100:157–168.

[5]   Horwitz EM, Le Blanc K, Dominici M, et al. Clarification of the nomenclature for MSC: The International Society for Cellular Therapy position statement. *Cytotherapy.* 2005;7:393–395.

[6]   Liechty KW, MacKenzie TC, Shaaban AF et al. Human mesenchymal stem cells engraft and demonstrate site-specific differentiation after in utero transplantation in sheep. *Nat. Med.* 2000;6:1282–1286.

[7]   Prockop DJ. Marrow stromal cells as stem cells for nonhematopoietic tissues. *Science.* 1997;276:71–74.

[8]   Jiang Y, Jahagirdar BN, Reinhardt RL, et al. Pluripotency of mesenchymal stem cells derived from adult marrow. *Nature.* 2002;418:41–49.

[9]   Mackenzie TC, Flake AW. Multilineage differentiation of human MSC after in utero transplantation. *Cytotherapy.* 2001;3:403–405.

[10] Toma C, Pittenger MF, Cahill KS, et al. Human mesenchymal stem cells differentiate to a cardiomyocyte phenotype in the adult murine heart. *Circulation.* 2002; 105:93–98.

[11] Zuk PA, Zhu M, Ashjian P, De Ugarte DA, et al. Human adipose tissue is a source of multipotent stem cells. *Mol. Biol. Cell.* 2002; 13:4279–4295.

[12] Sarugaser R, Lickorish D, Baksh D, et al. Human umbilical cord perivascular (HUCPV) cells: a source of mesenchymal progenitors. Stem Cells, 2005; 23:220–229.

[13] Shih DT, Lee DC, Chen SC, et al. Isolation and characterization of neurogenic mesenchymal stem cells in human scalp tissue. *Stem Cells.* 2005; 7:1012–1020.

[14] In't Anker PS, Scherjon SA, Kleijburg-van der Keur C, et al. Isolation of mesenchymal stem cells of fetal or maternal origin from human placenta. *Stem cells.* 2004; 22:1338–1345.

[15] Shi C, Cheng T. Effects of acute wound environment on the neo-natal dermal multipotent cells. *Cells Tissues Organs.* 2003; 175(4): 177-185.

[16] De Coppi P et al. Isolation of amniotic stem cell lines with potential for therapy. *Nat. Biotechnol.* 2007;25(1):100-106.

[17] Gregory CA, Prockop DJ, Spees JL. Non-hematopoietic bone marrow stem cells: molecular control of expansion and differentiation. *Exp. Cell Res.* 2005; 306:330–335.

[18] Pochampally RR, Horwitz EM, DiGirolamo CM, et al. Correction of a mineralization defect by overexpression of a wild-type cDNA for COL1A1 in marrow stromal cells (MSCs) from a patient with osteogenesis imperfecta: a strategy for rescuing mutations that produce dominant-negative protein defects. *Gene Therapy.* 2005; 12:1119–1125.

[19] Horwitz EM, Gordon PL, Koo WKK, et al. Isolated allogeneic bone marrow-derived mesenchymal cells engraft and stimulate growth in children with osteogenesis imperfecta: implications for cell therapy of bone. *Proc. Natl. Acad. Sci. USA.* 2002; 99:8932–8937.

[20] Koc ON, Day J, Neider M, et al. Allogeneic mesenchymal stem cell infusion for treatment of metachromatic leukodystrophy (MLD) and Hurler syndrome (MPS-IH). *Bone Marrow Transplant.* 2002; 30:215–222.

[21] Bartholomew A, Sturgeon C, Siatskas M, et al. Mesenchymal stem cells suppress lymphocyte proliferation in vitro and prolong skin graft survival in vivo. *Exp. Hematol.* 2002; 30:42–48.

[22] Le Blanc K, Tammik C, Rosendahl K, et al. HLA expression and immunologic properties of differentiated and undifferentiated mesenchymal stem cells. *Exp. Hematol.* 2003; 31:890–896.

[23] Maitra B, Szekely E, Gjini K, et al. Human mesenchymal stem cells support unrelated donor hematopoietic stem cells and suppress T-cell activation. *Bone Marrow Transplant.* 2004; 33:597–604.

[24] Gotherstrom C, Ringden O, Tammik C, et al. Immunologic properties of human fetal mesenchymal stem cells. *Am. J. Obstet. Gynecol.* 2004; 190:239–245.

[25] Klyushnenkova E, Mosca JD, Zernetkina V, et al. T cell responses to allogeneic human mesenchymal stem cells: immunogenicity, tolerance, and suppression. *J. Biomed. Sci.* 2005; 12:47–57.

[26] Spaggiari GM, Capobiance A, Becchetti S, et al. Mesenchymal stem cell-natural killer cell interactions: evidence that activated NK cells are capable of killing MSCs, whereas MSCs can inhibit IL-2-induced NK-cell proliferation. *Blood.* 2006; 107:1484–1490.

[27] Saito T, Kuang JQ, Bittira B, et al. Xenotransplant cardiac chimera: immune tolerance of adult stem cells. *Ann. Thorac. Surg.* 2002; 74:19–24.

[28] Grinemmo KH, Mansson A, Dellgren G, et al. Xenoreactivity and engraftment of human mesenchymal stem cells transplanted into infarcted rat myocardium. *J. Thorac. Cardiovasc. Surg.* 2004; 127:1293–1300.

[29] Le Blanc K, Tammik L, Sundberg B, et al. Mesenchymal stem cells inhibit and stimulate mixed lymphocyte cultures and mitogenic responses independently of the major histocompatibility complex. *Scand. J. Immunol.* 2003; 57:11–20.

[30] Rasmusson I, Ringden O, Sundberg B, et al. Mesenchymal stem cells inhibit lymphocyte proliferation by mitogens and alloantigens by different mechanisms. *Exp. Cell Res.* 2005; 305:33–41.

[31] Corcione A, Benvenuto F, Ferretti E, et al. Human mesenchymal stem cells modulate B-cell functions. *Blood.* 2006; 107:367–372.

[32] Sudres M, Norol F, Trenado A, et al. Bone marrow mesenchymal stem cells suppress lymphocyte proliferation in vitro but fail to prevent graft-versus-host disease in mice. *J. Immunol.* 2006; 176:7761–7767.

[33] Cheng T, Chen Z, Yan Y, et al. Experimental studies on the treatment and pathological basis of combined radiation and burn injury. *Chin. Med. J.* 2002;115(12):1763-1766.

[34] Shi CM, Su YP, Cheng TM. Recent advances in the pathological basis and experimental management of impaired wound healing due to total-body irradiation. *Med. Sci. Monit.* 2006;12(1):RA1-4.

[35] Dini V, Bertone M, Romanelli M. Prevention and management of pressure ulcers. *Dermatol. Ther.* 2006 19(6):356-364.

[36] Dinh TL, Veves A. Treatment of diabetic ulcers. *Dermatol. Ther.* 2006;19(6):348-355.

[37] Fu X, Li X, Cheng B, et al. Engineered growth factors and cutaneous wound healing: success and possible questions in the past 10 years. *Wound Repair Regen.* 2005;13(2):122-130.

[38] Gharaee-Kermani M and Phan SH. Role of cytokines and cytokine therapy in wound healing and fibrotic diseases. *Curr. Pharm. Des.* 2001; 7:1083–1103.

[39] Suzuki S, Matsuda K, Isshiki N, et al. Experimental study of a newly developed bilayer artificial skin. *Biomaterials.* 1990; 11:356–360.

[40] Sheridan RI and Tompkins RG. Skin substitutes in burns. *Burns.* 1990; 25:97–103.

[41] Shi C, Zhu Y, Su Y, et al. Stem cells and their applications in skin-cell therapy. *Trends Biotechnol.* 2006;24(1):48-52.

[42] Fathke C, Wilson L, Hutter J, et al. Contribution of bone marrow-derived cells to skin: collagen deposition and wound repair. *Stem Cells.* 2004; 22:812–822.

[43] Deng W, Han Q, Liao L, et al. Allogeneic bone marrow-derived flk-1+Sca-1- mesenchymal stem cells leads to stable mixed chimerism and donor-specific tolerance. *Exp. Hematol.* 2004; 32:861–867.

[44] Tran SD, Pillemer SR, Dutra A, et al., Differentiation of human bone marrow-derived cells into buccal epithelial cells in vivo: a molecular analytical study. *Lancet.* 2003; 361: 1084–1088.

[45] Deng W, Han Q, Liao L, et al. Engrafted bone marrow-derived flk-(1+) mesenchymal stem cells regenerate skin tissue. *Tissue Eng.* 2005; 11:110–119.

[46] Harris RG, Herzog EL, Bruscia EM, et al. Lack of a fusion requirement for development of bone marrow-derived epithelia. *Science.* 305 (2004), pp. 90–93.

[47] Brittan M, Braun KM, Reynolds LE, et al. Bone marrow cells engraft within the epidermis and proliferate in vivo with no evidence of cell fusion. *J. Patho.* 2005; 205:1–13.

[48] Yamaguchi Y, Kubo T, Murakami T, et al. Bone marrow cells differentiate into wound myofibroblasts and accelerate the healing of wounds with exposed bones when combined with an occlusive dressing. *Br. J. Dermatol.* 2005;152(4):616-622.

[49] Fu X, Qu Z, Sheng Z. Potentiality of mesenchymal stem cells in regeneration of sweat glands. *J. Surg. Res.* 2006;136(2):204-208.

[50] Li H, Fu X, Ouyang Y, et al. Adult bone-marrow-derived mesenchymal stem cells contribute to wound healing of skin appendages. *Cell Tissue Res.* 2006;326(3):725-736.

[51] Ran XZ, Su YP, Zong ZW, et al. Effects of serum from rats with combined radiation-burn injury on the growth of hematopoietic progenitor cells. *J. Trauma.* 2007;62(1):193-198.

[52] Ai G, Su Y, Yan G, et al. The experimental study of bone marrow mesenchymal stem cells on the repair of skin wound combined with local radiation injury. *Zhonghua Yi Xue Za Zhi.* 2002;82(23):1632-6.

[53] Yan G, Su Y, Ai G. Study on human amniotic membrane loaded with marrow mesenchymal stem cells and epidermis cells in promoting healing of wound combined with radiation injury. *Zhongguo Xiu Fu Chong Jian Wai Ke Za Zhi.* 2004;18(6):497-501.

[54] Shi C, Cheng T, Su Y, et al.Transplantation of dermal multipotent cells promotes survival and wound healing in rats with combined radiation and wound injury. *Radiat Res.* 2004l;162(1):56-63.

[55] Chargé SBP and Rudnicki MA. Cellular and molecular regulation of muscle regeneration. *Physiol. Rev.* 2004; 84:209–238.

[56] Zammit PS and Beauchamp JR. The skeletal muscle satellite cell: stem cell or son of stem cell? *Differentiation.* 2001; 68:193–204.

[57] Ferrari G, Cusella-De Angelis G, Coletta M, et al. Muscle regeneration by bone marrow derived myogenic progenitors. *Science.* 1998; 279:1528–1530.

[58] Bittner RE, Shofer C, Weipolshammer K, et al. Elbe-Burger and F. Wachtlerm, Recruitment of bone marrow derived cells by skeletal and cardiac muscle in adult dystrophic mdx mice. *Anat. Embryol.* 1999;199:391–396.

[59] LaBarge MA and Blau HM. Biological progression from adult bone marrow to mononucleated muscle stem cell to multinucleate muscle fiber in response to injury. *Cell.* 2002; 111:589–601.

[60] Gussoni E, Soneoka Y, Strickland CD et al. Dystrophin expression in the mdx mouse restored by stem cell transplantation. *Nature.* 1999;401:390–394

[61] Shi D, Reinecke H, Murry CE et al. Myogenic fusion of human bone marrow stromal cells, but not hematopoietic cells. *Blood.* 2004;104:290–294.

[62] de Bari C, Dell'Accio F, Vandenabeele F et al. Skeletal muscle repair by adult human mesenchymal stem cells from synovial membrane. *J. Cell Biol.* 2003;160:909–918.

[63] Sabourin LA and Rudnicki MA. The molecular regulation of myogenesis. *Clin. Genet.* 2000; 57:16–25.

[64] Parker MH, Seale P and Rudnicki MA. Looking back to the embryo: defining transcriptional networks in adult myogenesis. *Nat. Rev.* 2003; 4: 495–505.

[65] Smith CK, Janney MJ and Allen RE. Temporal expression of myogenic regulatory genes during activation, proliferation, and differentiation of rat skeletal muscle satellite cells. *J. Cell Physiol.* 1994; 159:379–385.

[66] Cooper RN. Tajbakhsh S. Mouly V, et al. In vivo satellite cell activation via Myf5 and MyoD in regenerating mouse skeletal muscle. *J. Cell Sci.* 1999; 112:2895–2901.

[67] Santa Maria L, Rojas CV, Minguell JJ. Signals from damaged but not undamaged skeletal muscle induce myogenic differentiation of rat bone-marrow-derived mesenchymal stem cells. *Exp. Cell Res.* 2004;300(2):418-26.

[68] Zhou J, Zou Z, Guo C, et al. Engraftment of bone marrow mesenchymal stem cells after systemic transplantation in mouse. *Chin. J. Radiol. Med. Protec.* 2002,22(3):167-169.

[69] Wakitani S, Saito T, Caplan AI. Myogenic cells derived from rat bone marrow mesenchymal stem cells exposed to 5-azacytidine. *Muscle Nerve.* 1995;18:1417–1426.

[70] Rangappa S, Fen C, Lee EH, et al. Transformation of adult mesenchymal stem cells isolated from the fatty tissue into cardiomyocytes. *Ann. Thorac. Surg.* 2003;75:775–779.

[71] Wang J, Luo C, Xu H, et al. Experimental study on the myogenic differentiation of marrow mesenchymal stem cells in the local muscle tissues. *Zhongguo Xiu Fu Chong Jian Wai Ke Za Zhi.* 2005;19(1):70-73.

[72] Wang J, Luo C, Ran X, et al. Effects of wound fluid from injured skeletal muscle on mesenchymal stem cells. *Chin. J. Clinical Rehabilitation.* 2003,7(26):3552-3553.

[73] Santi DV, Norment A, Garrett CE. Covalent bond formation between a DNA-cytosine methyltransferase and DNA containing 5-azacytosine. *Proc. Natl. Acad. Sci. U. S. A.* 1984;81:6993–6997.

[74] de Bari C, Dell'Accio F, Tylzanowski P, et al. Multipotent mesenchymal stem cells from adult human synovial membrane. *Arthritis Rheum.* 2001;44:1928–1942.

[75] Reyes M, Lund T, Lenvik T, et al. Purification and ex vivo expansion of postnatal human marrow mesodermal progenitor cells. *Blood.* 2001;98:2615–2625

[76] Zhang Y, Zou Z, Guo C, et al. Morphological properties of muscle injury by cardiotoxin. *Acta. Academiae. Medicine. Militaris. Tertiae.* 2003; 25(14):1302-1304.

[77] Zhang Y, Zou Z, Guo C, et al. Experimental study on MyoD gene induced to differentiate of bone marrow mesenchymal stem cells into myoblasts in vitro. *J. Med. Coll. PLA.* 2003,18(1):27-31.

[78] Smetana K Jr, Lukas J, Paleckova V et al. Effect of chemical structure of hydrogels on the adhesion and phenotypic characteristics of human monocytes such as expression of galectins and other carbohydrate-binding sites. *Biomaterials.* 1997;18:1009–1014.

[79] Goldring K, Jones GE, Sewry CA et al. The muscle-specific marker desmin is expressed in a proportion of human dermal fibroblasts after their exposure to galectin-1. *Neuromuscul. Disord.* 2002;12:183–186.

[80] Chan J, O'Donoghue K, Gavina M, et al. Galectin-1 induces skeletal muscle differentiation in human fetal mesenchymal stem cells and increases muscle regeneration. *Stem Cells.* 2006;24(8):1879-1891.

[81] Cheng TM, Shi CM, Su YP. Spontaneous malignant transformation of adult stem cell in vitro culture proliferation. *Zhonghua Yi Xue Za Zhi.* 2005;85(27):1883-1884.

In: Encyclopedia of Stem Cell Research (2 Volume Set)   ISBN: 978-1-61761-835-2
Editor: Alexander L. Greene   © 2012 Nova Science Publishers, Inc.

Chapter XLIII

NORMAL AND PATHOLOGICAL DEVELOPMENT OF PLURIPOTENT STEM CELLS

Olga F. Gordeeva

Institute of Developmental Biology of Russian Academy of Sciences, Moscow, Russia

ABSTRACT

Pluripotent cells of the early embryo originate all types of somatic cells and germ cells of adult organism. Pluripotent stem cell lines were derived from mammalian embryos and adult tissues using different techniques and from different sources—inner cell mass of the blastocyst, primordial germ cells, parthenogenetic oocytes, and mature spermatogonia — as well as by transgenic modification of various adult somatic cells. Despite different origin, all pluripotent stem cell lines demonstrate considerable similarity of the major biological properties: unlimited self-renewal and differentiation into various somatic and germ cells in vitro and in vivo, similar gene expression profiles, and similar cell cycle structure. Their malignant counterpart embryonal teratocarcinoma stem cell lines have restricted developmental potentials caused by genetic disturbances that result in deregulation of proliferation and differentiation balance. Numerous studies on the stability of different pluripotent stem cell lines demonstrated that, irrespective of their origin, long-term in vitro cultivation leads to the accumulation of chromosomal and gene mutations as well as epigenetic changes that can cause oncogenic transformation of cells. Our research of signaling pathways and pattern of specific gene expression in pluripotent stem cells and teratocarcinoma cells is focused on discovery of fundamental mechanisms that regulate normal development of pluripotent cells into different lineages and are disrupted in cancer initiating cells. Analysis gene expression profiles, differentiation potentials and cell cycle of normal and mutant pluripotent stem cells provide new data to search molecular targets to eliminate malignant cells in tumors.

INTRODUCTION

The development of higher multicellular animals starts from a totipotent zygote. The developmental potential of blastomeres of mammalian embryos changes during the period of cleavage and pluripotent cells appear in the inner cell mass of the blastocyst, they continue to proliferate in epiblast and then differentiate into multipotent precursor cells of different somatic lineages which will give rise to terminally differentiated specialized cells. Pluripotent cells appear for a short period of mammalian embryonic development—from cleavage to pre-gastrulation stages. This cell type underlies the development of all somatic cell types including extraembryonic structures and germline cells. Pluripotent embryonic cells transferred to in vitro conditions maintain their features and self-renew as undifferentiated cells during long-term culture. Pluripotent stem cell lines were derived from early embryos and they were experimentally converted from adult somatic cells. Today there exist different approaches and methods of pluripotent stem cell line derivation. The traditional ways are isolation of pluripotent cells from preimplantation embryos and conversion of embryonic and adult germ line cells (embryonic germ cells, EGCs, spermatogonial stem cells and partenogenetic and androgenetic embryonic stem cells, PG and AG ESC) into pluripotent cells. Another approach is an experimental alteration of differentiated cell potential using different reprogramming procedures, that is: somatic nuclear transfer to enucleated oocyte, fusion of pluripotent and somatic cells and pluripotency induction by retroviral transduction of pluripotency-related genes into somatic cells or without transgen integration using piggyBack transposon and episomal delivery (Figure 1).

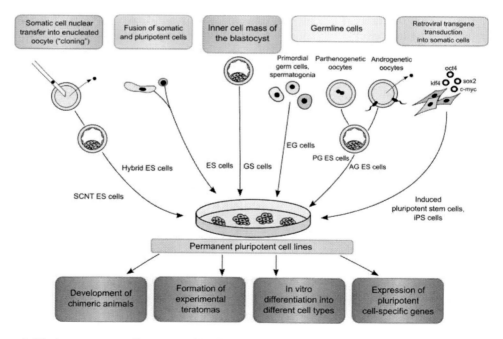

Figure 1. Pluripotent stem cells generated by different technologies.

Despite different origin, all pluripotent stem cell lines demonstrate considerable similarity of the major biological properties: high self-renewal rate and differentiation into various somatic and germ cells in vitro and in vivo, and therefore the nature of pluripotent stem cells make them an ideal source of cell-based products for regenerative medicine. Each pluripotent stem cell line can give rise to multiple somatic cell types that can be used for cell therapy for different diseases treatment and injured tissue recovery. Development of technologies that create an individual patient –specific pluripotent stem cell lines (cloning ES cells and iPS cells) can resolve the histocompatibility problem for transplanted cell derivatives. Establishment of standard model system for research of pluripotent stem cell lines of different origin maintained in strictly defined conditions is very important for development of effective and safe cell-based technologies as well as for drug discoveries.

Pluripotent stem cells can be derived from embryonic and adult somatic cells with diverse epigenetic state and transcriptional and metabolic activity. This initial background may have an influence on proliferation rate maintenance and subsequent differentiation pattern of different pluripotent stem cell lines. Therefore, role of intrinsic cell factors governing pluripotent cell differentiation programme and influence of micro environmental extrinsic factors that present in artificial niche of pluripotent stem cells – culture media - must be determined and clarified.

Utilizing the whole range of pluripotent cell lines of different origin as experimental models can entirely expose the mechanisms of normal and pathological development of various cell types in human and mammalian ontogeny. The models of permanent pluripotent cell lines derived from preimplantation embryos as well as from committed and differentiated cells by experimental manipulations are widely exploited in the research of fundamental problems of developmental biology related to the mechanisms of cell potential realization during embryogenesis and carcinogenesis.

Pluripotent Stem Cell Lines of Different Origin

Pluripotent cells are present only transiently in embryos at early stages of embryogenesis, as they quickly differentiate into various somatic cells through development. During this short period pluripotent cells fall within diverse cell environment and are affected by different extracellular signals that promote subsequent developmental events. To improve the research of early mammalian development there were established permanent embryo-derived cell lines – embryonic stem cells (ES cells), trophoblast stem (TS cells) cells, extraembryonic endoderm cells(XEN) and epiblast stem cells (EpiS cells) [1-6].

First mouse pluripotent ES cell lines were derived from the inner cell mass of blastocyst in 1981 [1, 2]. Isolated inner cell mass of mouse blastocyst was placed onto mitotically inactivated mouse primary embryonic fibroblasts and was grown in media conditioned by teratocarcinoma cells supplemented by fetal bovine serum [2]. At present, these conditions with mouse fibroblast feeder cells are most effective for derivation of ES cell lines of different species including human ES cells and most suitable for the propagation and expansion ES cells in vitro and preservation their stability [4, 7]. Monkey ES cell lines were isolated by Thomson et al. in 1995, and three years later the first human ES cell lines were derived in this laboratory [4, 8]. Initially, human ES cell lines were derived from the blastocysts discarded after in vitro fertilization procedures; later, from the morulae and individual blastomeres in the early embryos [4, 9, 10]. The efficiency of monkey and human ES cell line generation varies (10-25%) largely depending on the blastocysts quality. To date, numerous animal ES cell lines and more than 400 different lines and sublines of human and monkey ES have been derived. These lines are widely used in fundamental and applied research, and the techniques for the production, maintenance, and differentiation of pluripotent cells are still improved [1, 4, 8-13]. More recently, epiblast stem cell lines (EpiS cells) have been established from epiblasts isolated from E5.5 to E6.5 post-implantation mouse and rat embryos that differ significantly from mouse ES cells but share key features with human ES cells [5,6]. For example, EpiSCs derivation failed in the presence of LIF and/or BMP4, the two factors required for the derivation and self-renewal of mouse ES cells. In contrast, similar to human ES and iPS cells, FGF and TGFβ1/Activin/Nodal signaling appear critical for EpiSC derivation. Gene expression profile of EpiS cells closely reflects their post-implantation epiblast origin and is distinct from mouse ES cells. Nevertheless, EpiSCs do share the two key features characteristic of ES cells: prolonged proliferation in vitro and multilineage differentiation. On the other side, EpiSC lines from post-implantation epithelialised epiblast are unable to colonise the embryo even though they express the core pluripotency genes Oct4, Sox2 and Nanog [4, 5, 14]. ES cells can readily become EpiSCs in response to growth factor cues but EpiSCs do not change into ES cells without reprogramming.

The ability to derive pluripotent stem cells from early post-implantation embryos is consistent with early extrauterine embryo transplantation experiments where transplanted mouse embryos at stages ranging from one cell to egg cylinders (E8) are able to form teratocarcinomas, but this ability is quickly lost with further development [15,16].

Mouse embryonic germ cell lines were derived from primordial germ cells of different developmental stages and their pluripotency were confirmed using in vitro and in vivo tests [17-20]. In 1998, the first five human EG cell lines were derived from primordial germ cells of the rudimentary gonads in 5-9-week-old human fetuses and characterized [21]. Human EG cell lines closely resemble human ES cell lines and demonstrate the ability to differentiate into different somatic cells in vitro and in teratomas formed after transplantation into immune-deficient mice.

Pluripotent stem cell lines can be generated from germ line cells of the later stages of development – from spermatogonial cells of newborn and adult mice. Mouse spermatogonial stem cells (GS cells) derived from neonatal and adult mouse testis display ES-like morphology, express pluripotent cell marker, form teratomas after transplantation into immunocompromised mice and give rise to chimerical animals with germ line transmission [22, 23]. Thus, primordial germ cells and spermatogonial cells that are committed unipotent cells can be reprogrammed in vitro without experimental manipulation in cell population which has similar features with ES cells.

Another method to produce pluripotent cells from germline cells is the generation of parthenogenetic and androgenetic ES cell lines. Such lines of mammalian pluripotent stem cells were successfully produced and characterized in several laboratories [24-31]. Although the parthenogenetic and androgenetic embryos die during early postimplantation stages, the parthenogenetic (PG) and androgenetic (AG) ES cell lines can grow in culture and differentiate. Murine PG ES cells and AG ES cells retain the pluripotency in vitro and in vivo conditions and contribute to somatic tissues and germ cells of chimeric embryos as well as in tetraploid embryos but different cell lines show variable developmental potential [31,34]. At the same time, their clinical applicability is limited since the resulting zygote develops from the activated oocytes with uniparental genome and it does not express a number of imprinted genes correctly. Nevertheless, these ES cell lines are interesting models to study the role of genome imprinting in histogenesis of different tissues.

The fundamental research made it possible to develop several major strategies to produce pluripotent cell lines histocompatible with each patient as a biological material for cell therapy. The first approach includes the generation of ES cell lines using somatic cell nuclear transfer into enucleated oocytes (NTES cells). A blastocyst develops from the reconstructed zygote and to give rise to an ES cell line with the genotype of the somatic nuclear donor (therapeutic cloning strategy). In this case, active molecules in the oocyte required for the normal development are the reprogramming factors.

The first successes in generating reconstructed ES-like cell lines from somatic cells via nuclear transfer reported have been performed in the cow, and then the mouse [34-36]. These ES -like cell lines are believed to possess the same capacities for unlimited self-renewal and pluripotency as conventional ES cell lines derived from normal embryos produced by fertilization. Interestingly, NTES cell lines can be established with success rates 10 times higher than reproductive cloning [37-40].

The technique for reconstructed NTES cell line production is laborious and has limitations. First, limited human oocytes number are available for reprogramming manipulations; second, the rate of embryos developed to the blastocyst stage is low due to mechanical and chemical damage of different kinds. These technical problems are supplemented with biological limitations resulting from abnormal reactivation of the genetic and epigenetic programs of development in somatic cell nuclei. The top efficiency of producing reconstructed mouse ES cell lines is 20% for this technique [37, 40]; and if a similar efficiency is reached for human ES cell lines, it will become very promising for cell therapy. The attempts to produce human and monkey reconstructed blastocysts, which are required for ES cell line isolation, failed for a long period. The first progress in the technique development was made in 2007 when two rhesus monkey ES cell lines, CRES1 and CRES2, were obtained [41]. In this case, the technique of pronuclear removal has been improved using the new Oosight Spindle Imaging System, and the rate of viable reconstructed blastocysts increased from 1 to 16%. Attempts to produce human reconstructed cell lines are currently underway [42]. Generation of interspecific cell hybrids using the donor oocytes from monkey (as the closest species to human) and human somatic cell nuclei is also a promising approach to derivation of reconstructed human ES cell lines.

Reprogrammed ES cell lines were derived by the fusion of different somatic cells from the adult tissues and ES cells, which yielded stable human tetraploid ES cell lines with the properties and characteristics of pluripotent cells [43-45]. Nevertheless, despite the relative simplicity of production technique, these lines have not the clinical value, since hybrid cells contain a foreign genome, and differentiated somatic cells are recognized by the recipient immune system. In addition, the instability of the tetraploid genome in hybrid cells can lead to malignant transformation. On the other hand, the reactivation mechanisms of genes controlling the pluripotent status as well as the mechanisms of gene expression inactivation in specialized cells during reprogramming can be successfully studied using this experimental system.

A new revolutionary method to produce pluripotent stem cell lines (iPS cells) by reprogramming somatic cells was proposed by Shinya Yamanaka et al, and it was tested first on mouse cells and then on human cells [46-48]. This technique involves the production of ES cell-like lines from different somatic cells (embryonic and adult fibroblasts, keratinocytes, neural, blood, stomach cells, and other) using transgenic modification of their genome with viral vectors carrying pluripotency-related genes [46-52]. In this case, the integration (or not) of viral vectors into the somatic cell genome and subsequent transient expression of the regulatory genes Oct4, Sox2, C-myc, and Klf4 reprograms the somatic cell genome and reverts terminally differentiated cells to the pluripotent state. After several weeks of culture, about 0.1% of transduced cells demonstrate a dramatic change in their morphology and potential. The experiments with mouse induced pluripotent stem cells showed that they can provide for the development of chimeric animals, which completely confirms their pluripotent state. At the same time, some of these mice had laryngeal cancer, which points to the altered developmental program in pluripotent cells with such transgenic modification [53, 54]. These experiments shed new light on the changes in cell potential and on the mechanisms controlling the cell pluripotent state; however, further studies on induced pluripotent stem cells are needed. Despite a very low rate of reprogramming cells, their number suffices for a relatively rapid production of cell lines with a particular genotype. The safety of such pluripotent cell lines for clinical use remains questionable, since the degree of reprogramming correctness in somatic cells remains unclear. The generation of induced pluripotent cells involves viral vectors, which may cause genetic instability and tumorigenicity; especially if they include the C-myc oncogene that is overexpressed in the most of studied human cancers. The use of such cell lines in cell therapy requires the exclusion of this oncogene from the technique. The experiments in this direction demonstrated that lines of induced pluripotent cells can still be generated after such modification but the method efficiency considerably decreases [48, 55].

Malignant teratocarcinoma cell lines were established in the 70s of 20th century. That was significantly earlier than ES cells were derived [56-61]. These cell lines were the first model system for study mechanisms of early development. Embryonal teratocarcinoma lines (EC cells) were isolated from mouse and human ovarian and testicular tumors and they displayed variable developmental potential therefore they can be considered as malignant pluripotent stem cells. The most of teratocarcinoma cell lines demonstrate restricted differentiation potential and cannot contribute to germ line of chimeric embryos, some of these lines, nullipotent cell lines, completely lost the ability to differentiate into somatic or germ cells with the exception of extraembryonic endoderm cells [60]. Current studies of EC cells provide unique opportunities to dissect mechanisms of cancer initiation at the earliest stages of development and its progression with different spectrum of developmental disturbances.

Pluripotent Stem Cell Characteristics

Irrespective of the cell sources and production techniques, all pluripotent cell lines share the same biological properties but demonstrate individual variation in some culture properties, the capacity to differentiate into different somatic cell types, and maintenance of genetic and epigenetic stability. The revealed differences can be due to genetic background of cell sources that initiate pluripotent stem cell lines, to individual sensitivity to different adaptive effects of in vitro cultivation, and to methodical variations of culture maintenance in different laboratories.

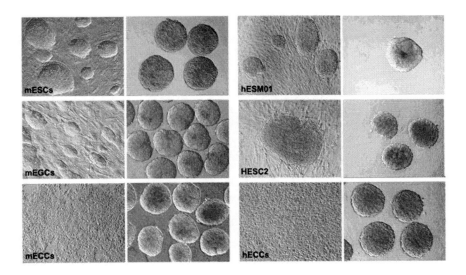

Figure 2. The initial stages of in vitro differentiation of pluripotent mES, mEG, hES cells and their malignant counterparts mEC, hEC cells. These cell lines can form embryoid bodies of similar morphology despite their different origins.

Similar in vitro culture systems are used to generate and maintain ES cells as well as induced pluripotent stem cells. These systems include various feeder cell types or extracellular matrix protein components and fetal serum or serum replacement, various growth factors such as leukemia inhibitory factor basic fibroblast growth factor (bFGF), Activin, and Nodal [62-69]. Routine ES cell cultivation includes enzymatic treatment for passaging. The characteristic feature of monkey and human ES cells is low survival rate of individual cells and accordingly low clonogenic capacity, and therefore, in this case, cultures are separated into cell clusters rather than into individual cells to increase the survival rate and to support the cell growth. Monkey and human ES cells are more prone to in vitro differentiation compared to mouse ones; accordingly, differentiated cells should be removed from the population to maintain the major line properties. To allow in vitro differentiation pluripotent cells are placed in media containing differentiation promoting growth factors or small molecules. In course of spontaneous in vitro differentiation, pluripotent stem cells as well as malignant teratocarcinoma cells form three-dimensional cell aggregates that recapitulate the early pregastrulation stages of mammalian embryo development (Figure 2, 4B).

Several tests were developed to characterized pluripotent cell lines. The "gold standard" of mouse ES cell pluripotency is their capacity to contribute into development of different tissues and organs of chimeric animals developed from the blastocyst injected with ES cells. However, ethical restrictions does not allow this test for human ES cells, and the described and novel ES cell lines of human and primates are assigned to pluripotent cell lines based on other properties that are largely the same for mice, primates, and human.

The pluripotency is primarily evaluated using the teratoma test, i.e., the capacity of ES, EG, and iPS cells to form teratomas in immune-deficient animal models (Nude or SCID mice). The classical teratomas formed from pluripotent cells contain rudiments of different tissues and structures derived from the three germ layers [70, 71]. On the contrary, EC cells being malignant counterparts of pluripotent stem cells demonstrate restricted differentiation potential or undifferentiated tumor cell growth only after transplantation into different tissue sites of immune-deficient mice (Figure 3).

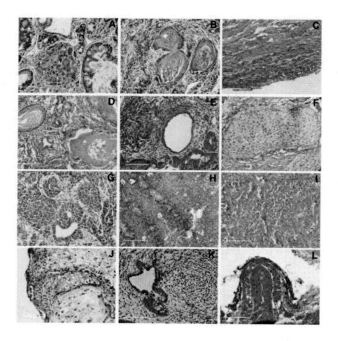

Figure 3. Differentiation of mouse and human pluripotent and teratocarcinoma cells in experimental teratomas formed after transplantation into of immunedeficient mice. Histological sections of teratomas, formed by mESCs (A-C), mEGCs (D-G), hESCs (J-L) and teratocarcinomas, developed by nullipotent mECCs (H) and hECCs (I). Teratomas contained various types of differentiated somatic cells, including ectodermal, mesodermal and endodermal lineages: neural rosettes (G), ciliated epithelium of intestinal type (A,K), striated muscles (C, L), keratinized epithelium (B, D), hyaline cartilage (F, J), and intestinal cysts (D, F). Teratocarcinomas included undifferentiated cells solely (H, I). Bar, 100μm.

All undifferentiated pluripotent cell lines are morphologically identical; they grow in vitro as colonies of small densely packed cells with a high nuclear—cytoplasmic ratio (Fig. 2). All cells in a colony express specific transcription factors (Oct4 and Nanog) and membrane proteins (stage-specific embryonic antigens SSEA3, SSEA4, as well as CD9 and keratin sulfate antigens TRA-160 and TRA-1-81) and demonstrate high telomerase and alkaline phosphatase activities (Figure 4A).

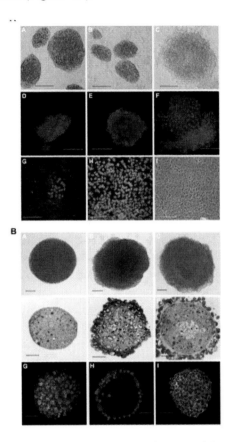

Figure 4. Activity of alkaline phosphatase and expression of Oct4 and GATA4 in mouse ES, EG and EC cells and in embryoid bodies. (A) Alkaline phosphatase (A-C) and Oct4 (D-F) are highly expressed in all undifferentiated ES (A,D), EG (B, E) and EC (C, F) cells. Minor fraction of EC cells expressed marker of extraembryonic endoderm Gata4 (G-I). Bar, 100μm.
(B) Embryoid bodies developed after in vitro differentiation of ES cells on day 1(A, D), 3(B, E, G-I), 5(C, F). Activity of alkaline phosphatase were retained in undifferentiated cells (A-C) but marker of extraembryonic endoderm Gata4 were already expressed in the outer cells of embryoid bodies. Morphological reorganization in embryoid bodies reproduce the early stages of embryogenesis (D-F) and epiblast-like inner cells of embryoid bodies are in contact using adherent cell junction (E-cadherin, I). Bar, 100μm (A-C), 50 μm (D-I).

The transcription profiles of pluripotent cell lines and their differentiated derivatives have been studied in detail using the Microarray technology. The results of these studies demonstrate that the expression level of many genes can vary in different pluripotent stem cell lines; however, all studied mouse, monkey and human stem cell lines showed high expression level of stem cell-specific factors, Pou5f1(Oct4), Sox2, Nanog, Tdgf/Cripto, Lefty2, Dnmt3b, GDF3, and Gabrb3 [41, 47, 72-78]. Comparative analysis of transcriptional profiles of mouse ES and EG cell lines with diverse genetic backgrounds showed that ES cells and EG cells are indistinguishable based on global gene expression patterns alone. All pluripotent cell lines showed similar gene expression patterns, which separated them clearly from other tissue stem cells with lower developmental potency. Differences between pluripotent lines derived from different sources were smaller than differences between lines derived from different mouse strains (129 vs. C57BL/6). Even in the differentiation-promoting conditions, these pluripotent cells showed the same general trends of gene expression changes regardless of their origin and genetic background [77] . Similarly, the study of 59 human ES cell lines obtained and maintained in 17 laboratories worldwide demonstrated expression variations of components of signaling pathways and regulators of proliferation, FGF4, LEFTYB, EBAF(LEFTYA), NODAL, TDGF1, IFITM1, FOXD3, GAL, LIN28, TERT, UTF1, etc. [76]. The causes of the expression variation in different human ES cell lines are unclear. Probably, like in mouse pluripotent stem cells, the revealed heterogeneity of the expression profiles may be attributed to different genotypes of embryonic cell sources. This variation can also be due to the initial events during ES cell line isolation, since cells in the inner cell mass of the blastocyst are to a certain extent a heterogeneous population and adapt differently to the artificial environment. One cannot exclude that the observed variations result from different processing algorithms of experimental data obtained using the microarray technology.

Recently, it was shown that somatic/ES cell hybrid cell lines resemble their pre-fusion ES cell partners in terms of behavior in culture and pluripotency. However, they contain unique expression profiles that are similar but not identical to normal ES cells [45]. A study of gene expression profiles of mouse and human ES cells and iPS cells suggests that, while iPS cells are quite similar to their embryonic counterparts, a recurrent gene expression signature appears in iPS cells regardless of their origin or the method by which they were generated. Upon extended culture, human iPS cells adopt a gene expression profile more similar to human ES cells; however, they still retain a gene expression signature unique from ES cells that extends to miRNA expression. Genome-wide data suggested that the iPS cell signature gene expression differences are due to differential promoter binding by the reprogramming factors. High-resolution array profiling demonstrated that there is no common specific subkaryotypic alteration that is required for reprogramming and that reprogramming does not lead to genomic instability. Based on these data iPS cells can be considered as unique subtype of pluripotent cell [78].

The capacity of ES cell lines of different origin, EG cell lines, and iPS cell lines to in vitro multilineage differentiation is also a pluripotency test for each line. Numerous studies of in vitro differentiation of various mammalian pluripotent cell lines have developed protocols to produce different types of differentiation cells in culture: neurons and glial cells, cardiomyocytes, hematopoietic, endothelial, osteogenic, insulin-producing, and hepatocyte-like cells, adipocytes, melanocytes, keratinocytes, trophoblast and prostate cells [31, 79-85]. The fundamental studies of the mechanisms underlying the regulation of different histogeneses using the pluripotent cell lines of different origins gave an impetus to the development of techniques to produce particular cell types for clinical use.

Self-Renewal and Maintenance of Genomic Integrity in Pluripotent Stem Cells

Pluripotent cells actively self-renew during prolonged cultivation in vitro, and their proliferation rate is comparable to that in immortalized or transformed cells. Studies on the mechanisms of self-renewal of pluripotent cells in different animals demonstrated that the cell cycle regulation in ES, EG and other types of pluripotent cells indeed has some specific properties and considerably differs from that in normal somatic cells. First, mouse, monkey, and human pluripotent stem cells remain in S-phase more than a half of the cell cycle, while the G1 and G2 periods are substantially reduced [86-90]. Analysis of cell cycle stage distribution in ES, EG as well as EC cells demonstrate that the most of undifferentiated cells, 60-70% are in S-phase and only 15-25% cells in G1. This indicates that their cell cycle is specifically regulated so that newly formed cells start new DNA replication nearly immediately after the previous mitosis. However, in contrast to cancer cells, ES cells have mechanisms providing for their high sensitivity to differentiation promoting factors and not preventing death of abnormal cells [86-90]. Characteristics of mouse ES cell cycle regulation are the lack of dependence on serum stimulation and mitogen-activated protein kinase kinase (MEK)–associated signaling [91, 92]. Mouse ES cells rely on phosphatidyl inositol-3 kinase (PI3K) dependent signaling for progression through the G1 phase as well as for inhibition of differentiation [92, 93]. However, PI3K activity is not dependent on persistent serum stimulation but rather largely relies on both on stimulation of the leukemia inhibitory factor (LIF) receptor and on expression of the ESC-specific Eras factor [92, 94].

Studies of mechanisms underlying cell cycle control in ES cells from different mammals demonstrate kind-specific differences in the regulation of pluripotent stem cell self-renewal despite high similarity of cell cycle structure. For instance, hyperphosphorylated Rb and cyclin E (proteins specific for the S and G2/M phases) proved to be present in mouse, monkey and human ES cells throughout their cell cycle; however, in contrast to mouse ES cells, cyclin A is not continuously expressed in monkey ES cells, and Rb protein dynamic is similar in mouse and human ES cells. In mouse ES cells, there is compelling evidence that the G1/S transition is not dependent on a functional cyclin D-Cdk4/6 and RB-E2F pathway [87, 88, 95-97] and that rapid progression through the cell cycle relies largely on constitutively active cyclin E-Cdk2 and cyclin A-Cdk2 complexes [98]. Monkey ES cells also express cyclin E during all phases of the cell cycle, suggesting that ectopic cyclin E-Cdk2 kinase activity may also be a characteristic feature of primate ESCs. However, monkey ES cell line ORMES-1 cells did not express cyclin A in all phases of their cell cycle, in contrast to mouse ESCs [89]. Thus, heterogeneous cell cycle duration that characterizes rhesus ESCs could result from discontinuous expression of cyclin A.

Analysis of the expression profiles of human ES cells demonstrated the absent or low-level expression of the p53 gene as well as of p16, p19 *and* p21 involved in the cell cycle regulation. Conversely, mouse ES cells demonstrated high expression level of these genes and their negative regulators MDM genes [99, 100]. It is assumed that the inactivation of the p53- and Rb-dependent pathways is nevertheless an essential component of the cell cycle regulation in pluripotent cells of different mammals [101]. In addition, the mitotic cycle regulation in ES cells features the independence of the stimulation by serum factors as well as of the mitogen-activated protein kinase kinase pathway [87].

Recently, there was shown that human ES cells express all G1-specific CYCLINs (D1, D2, D3 and E) and cyclin-dependent kinases CDK2, CDK4 and CDK6 at variable levels. In contrast to murine ES cells, most of the cell cycle regulators in hES cells show cell cycle-dependent expression, thus revealing important differences in the expression of cell cycle regulatory components between these two embryonic cell types. Knockdown of CDK2 using RNA interference resulted in hES cells arrest at G1 phase of the cell cycle and differentiation to extraembryonic lineages [102]. Moreover, it was shown that NANOG, a master transcription factor, regulates S-phase entry in human embryonic stem cells via transcriptional regulation of cell cycle regulatory components. Chromatin immunoprecipitation combined with reporter-based transfection assays reveal that the C-terminal region of NANOG binds to the regulatory regions of CDK6 and CDC25A genes under normal physiological conditions. Decreased CDK6 and CDC25A expression in human ES cells suggest that both CDK6 and CDC25A are involved in S-phase regulation. The effects of NANOG overexpression on S-phase regulation are mitigated by the down-regulation of CDK6 or CDC25A alone. Overexpression of CDK6 or CDC25A alone can rescue the impact of NANOG down-regulation on S-phase entry, suggesting that CDK6 and CDC25A are downstream cell cycle effectors of NANOG during the G1 to S transition [103].

The experiments on monkey ES cells demonstrated that gamma-irradiation does not arrest their cell cycle in G1, which points to the absence of the G1/S checkpoint typical of untransformed cells and required for DNA damage repair. On the other side, irradiated human ES cells were accumulated in G1 stage. The apoptotic factors are activated and aberrant cells with damaged DNA are rapidly eliminated in mouse, primate, and human ES cells [88, 89]. Genetically damaged human ES cells demonstrated changed biosynthesis of histone proteins: mRNA transcription and processing are affected and H4 mRNA is destabilized, which disrupts the normal mitotic process [90]. An alternative pathway for damaged cells has been demonstrated: p53 can repress the promoter of the pluripotent cell-specific Nanog gene in mouse ES cells, which induces irreversible differentiation of these cells and, thus, eliminates them from the pool of undifferentiated cells but not from the total cell population [104].

On the other hand, efficient mechanisms of protection from oxidative stress-induced damage and DNA repair are active in undifferentiated mouse and human ES cells. The resistance of ES cells to damage can be due to high activity of multiple drug resistance transporter of verapamil, heat shock proteins, and double-stranded DNA damage repair systems. Interestingly, that high ES cell resistance to active oxygen species mediated by the glutathione/thioredoxin system is observed only in undifferentiated cells, and its efficiency substantially reduces during early differentiation [105, 106]. Analysis of the transcription profiles of human ES cell lines demonstrates high expression levels of various genes including APEX, RAD, MSH, and genes involved in DNA repair, which provides for secure protection of the genetic material. Nevertheless, the data on the control mechanisms of cell cycle and resistance to various stress factors in different pluripotent cell types or their differentiated derivatives are limited, and these problems require further investigation.

Despite the cell cycle similarity in ES cells of different mammals, the mechanisms providing for the unique proliferative potential of pluripotent cells in different species and types of cell lines derived from different sources remain unclear, since almost no published data are available on this problem. In summary, one can propose that the mechanisms controlling the active proliferation of pluripotent cell lines in culture slightly differ from those in the embryo. A high rate of cell division to yield the required cell mass is the priority task during early embryogenesis; however, the extraembryonic structures, trophoectoderm and extraembryonic endoderm, differentiate during this short period, i.e., the mechanisms inhibiting differentiation are not active in them. Self-renewal of pluripotent cell lines in artificial in vitro culture continues over long periods, and the maintenance of this cell status requires external stimuli maintaining high rate of cell divisions and preventing differentiation events at the same time. Under such suboptimal conditions, appearance of genetically transformed cells in population is inevitable within long-term cultivation. Apparently, pluripotent line founder cells that can faster adapt to in vitro conditions, faster proliferate, and don't respond to differentiation signals during their short G1 period are selected during the establishment of pluripotent cell line. Thus, in terms of pluripotent cell adaptation to artificial in vitro conditions as a process of minimum transformation, one can propose that the variants with a shorter cycle and low sensitivity to differentiation and damaging factors have a selective advantage. In other words, artificial conditions of in vitro culture maintaining high growth rate of pluripotent cells are the proper factors initiating the genetic and epigenetic alterations in these cells.

Genetic Mutation and Epigenetic Modification in Pluripotent Stem Cells and Problem of Cancer Transformation

The maintenance of genome stability in pluripotent cells is the crucial factor of their structural and functional integrity, which is manifested as the normal balance between proliferation and differentiation in different cell types in vitro and in vivo. Long-term ES cell cultures can accumulate cells with different genetic aberrations and epigenetic changes. Analysis of the karyotype in long-term cultures of different human ES cell lines (passages 34-140) demonstrated aneuploidy of chromosomes X, 12, and 17 [107-113]. Preferred trisomy of chromosomes 12 and 17 has been revealed in lines HUES, H1, H14, BG01, and BG02 [107, 108, 113-115]. Trisomy of chromosomes 13 and 3 has been revealed in lines SA002 and Miz-hES13, respectively [116-118]. Cytogenetic analysis of 18 ORMES lines of rhesus monkey ES cells using G-banding demonstrated a diploid set of 42 chromosomes in 15 lines; various chromosomal abnormalities including balanced translocations t(11;16), t(5;19), and t(1;18) in three lines (ORMES-1, -2, and -5); and a pericentric inversion in chromosome 1 in one line. However, these aberrations were observed in ES cells at early passages (9) that suggest that these abnormalities could be initially present in the source embryos [81]. Aneuploidy have also been found in one out of seven parthenogenetic lines of human ES cells (karyotype phESC-7, 47,XXX, and 48,XXX+6) at early passages, which also suggests that this mutation was inherited from germ cells [30].

One of two monkey ES cell lines (CRES-1) generated by somatic cell nuclear transfer had normal karyotype 42,XY; while the other line (CRES-2) demonstrated chromosomal aberrations at early passages. The Y chromosomes was missing in 12% of cells, while other cells contained the Y isochromosome with two extra copies of the long arm (karyotype 41,X[3]/42,Xi(Y)q10[17]) [41].

Note that the trend to accumulate chromosomal abnormalities is not observed in all human and primate ES cell lines. Sporadic aneuploidy that can have no selective advantage is sometimes observed. For instance, SA002c cells with trisomy of chromosome 13 had no advantage in clonal growth and disappeared from the population in subsequent passages [118]. Another study demonstrated that seven novel isolated lines of human ES cells from blastocyst-stage embryos diagnosed as aneuploid in preimplantation genetic screening exhibited morphology and markers typical of human ES cells and the capacity for long-term proliferation. The derived hES cell lines manifested pluripotent differentiation potential both in vivo and in vitro. Surprisingly, karyotype analysis of these lines that were derived from aneuploid embryos showed that the cell lines carry a normal euploid karyotype. Because authors showed that the euploidy was not achieved through chromosome duplication, they suggest that the euploid human ES cell lines originated from mosaic embryos consisting of aneuploid and euploid cells, and in vitro selection occurred to favor euploid cells [119].

It remains unclear what gives rise to aberrant cells -- different susceptibility of particular genotypes to mutations or specific ES cell culture conditions. For instance, Mitalipova et al. analyzed the karyotype of two human ES cell lines, BG01 and BG02, at early and late passages using different culture techniques: mechanical and enzymatic (using trypsin or collagenase) dissociation of colonies into clusters [113]. In the case of enzymatic treatment, both ES cell lines contained cells with trisomy of chromosomes 12 and 17 and sometimes extra copies of chromosomes 14, 20, and X; while no abnormalities were observed after mechanical dissociation up to passage 105. In other cases, chromosomal aberrations have been revealed after mechanical passage but not after enzymatic passaging [118, 120, 121]. One can propose that the genetic damage of ES cells can also be promoted by extra cycles of cell cryopreservation and thawing.

Studies of various mutant human ES cell sublines demonstrated no significant changes in the transcriptional profiles in most cases; however, the expression level can vary for some genes [113,115]. Many authors reported that human ES cells carrying extra copies of chromosomes 12 and 17 rapidly become dominant in the population and demonstrate advantages growth and higher clonal activity [108, 115, 122, 123]. The isochromosome 12p has been found previously in some germ cell tumors of the gonads including human teratocarcinomas [109,124,125], while the amplification 17q is associated with some neuroblastomas [126]. These chromosomes contain the genes controlling self-renewal and differentiation, NANOG, STELLAR, GDF3, GRB2, and STAT3, whose altered expression in the case of the corresponding extra copies of chromosomes can modulate the cell potential in ES cell lines [88,125]. A comparative study of human ES cell lines BG01 and BG01V and human hyperpolyploid teratocarcinoma NTERA demonstrated that the properties of the abnormal line BG01V are more similar to the original line BG01 rather than to the teratocarcinoma NTERA. BG01V cells differentiated in experimental teratomas with the formation of various ectodermal, entodermal, and mesodermal structures; however, a higher number of undifferentiated cells was observed compared to the BG01 teratomas [115].

A detailed study of the genetic changes in 10 human ES cell lines in long-term culture demonstrated (passages 22--105) one (or more) genetic damages that are commonly observed in various cancer cells in eight out of nine studied lines [112]. According to these data, the aberrations in ES cells included different changes in the number of gene copies (45%), sequence changes in mitochondrial DNA (22%), and changes in the methylation level in some gene promoters (90%). In particular, some ES cell lines at late passages studied in this work demonstrated the amplification of gene loci containing the C-MYC oncogene that are present in nearly all cancer types including that after spontaneous transformation of mesenchymal stem cells of the bone marrow during in vitro culture (127, 128]. All data available to date indicate that long-term culture of all ES cell lines leads to their genetic damage that can considerably change the cell phenotype and introduce oncogenic properties to mutant cells.

Different epigenetic modifications of chromatin take place together with the structural changes of the genome in long-term in vitro cultures of pluripotent stem cell lines. The epigenetic changes in chromatin structure are the key factors in the regulation of gene imprinting, expression of non-imprinted genes, X chromosome inactivation, and genome stability [129,130]. A set of different epigenetic modifications in DNA and associated histone proteins is known to determine the timing of gene activation in the cell. The epigenetic modifications of chromatin include cytosine methylation in gene promoter regions, repetitive sequences, and imprinted genes as well as histone methylation and acetylation. In most cases, DNA methylation in the promoter or differentially methylated region inactivates the corresponding gene expression. Abnormal DNA methylation pattern in the cells results developmental defects and various pathologies including carcinogenesis [131- 139]. For instance, the inactivation of oncogenesis suppressor genes in some tumors results from the hypermethylation of their promoters, and conversely, the hypomethylation of the regulatory regions of oncogenes can induce their ectopic transcription.

Genomic imprinting is a form of the epigenetic program including the modification of different gene loci, whose expression during development and cell differentiation is monoallelic according to the parental origin of a particular allele. Imprinted genes have a trend to cluster in "imprinting centers" in the genome. One of such centers is located on chromosome 15 (15q11-q13) and is associated with the Prader-Willi and Angelman syndromes; and another one on chromosome 11 (11p15.5), with the Beckwith-Wiedemann syndrome [140-142]. Imprinting in these regions is controlled in *cis* by so-called imprinting centers (ICs) that regulate parent-specific expression of target genes bidirectionally over long distances. ICs are subject to parent-specific epigenetic modifications including DNA methylation and histone changes recognized by specific factors such as DNA-binding proteins that in turn, activate downstream effects leading to appropriate mono-allelic gene expression. These epigenetic modifications must be reprogrammed during development, involving first erasure of old epigenetic marks during germ cell development and establishment of new marks in a gender-specific manner. Methylation of CpG dinucleotides within ICs is proposed to be one of the initial mechanisms differentially marking parental chromosomes in gametes. Once established, locus-specific DNA methylation profiles must be stably maintained in future generations of cells.

During development, DNA methylation is provided by coordinated activity of DNA methyltransferases including Dnmt1 and de novo DNA methyltransferases Dnmt3a and Dnmt3b. DNMT3 deficiency in humans causes substantial demethylation of the centromeric minor satellite repeats, and such individuals demonstrate rare genetic disease, ICF syndrome (or Immunodeficiency, Centromere instability and Facial anomalies syndrome) [143, 144].

The methylation profile alterations in the promoter regions of some genes in pluripotent cell lines of different origin demonstrated that specific in vitro culture conditions can modulate the methylation of imprinted genes, although, not in all human and monkey ES cell lines and largely at late passages [145-147]. Monoallelic expression of imprinted genes H19, KCNQ1, PEG10, and NDNL1 was observed in human ES cell lines SHhES1 and HUES-7 at both early and late passages, and the corresponding methylation status of imprinted genes KCNQ1, IGF2, SCL22A18, NESP55, and SNRPN has also been revealed at early and late passages in lines H9, H7, HUES-3, and HSF6. After a long-term culture of the H9 line, the changes in the methylated region of the H19 gene were recorded without the gametic imprinting loss [146, 147]. It is of interest that the normal methylation profile of the imprinted genes H19, SNRPN, and DLK1/MEG3 was conserved in the genetically abnormal human ES cell line BG01V [115]. A study of expression of 10 imprinted genes SNRPN, IPW, KCNQ10T1, PEG3, IGF2, MEST, H19, NESP55, MEG3, and SCL22A18 in 59 human ES cell lines demonstrated monoallelic expression in 80% of cases and expression from the other parental allele or biallelic expression in the other 20% of samples [76]. Overall, these data indicate high stability of the methylation status in imprinted genes in human ES cell lines.

On the other hand, a study of the methylation status and expression pattern of imprinted genes in primate ES cell lines demonstrated biallelic expression of the IGF2 and H19 genes in all studied lines, while the SNRPN and NDN genes demonstrated normal expression of the parental allele only. Conversely, the normal expression of the parental IGF2 allele and maternal H19 allele was detected in the rhesus monkey blastocysts that were the sources of ES cell lines. These data suggest that the changes in the IGF2 and H19 methylation status in monkey ES cells took place at the initial stages of line isolation [81,148].

As mentioned above, the changes in the DNA methylation of non-imprinted gene loci is associated in many cases with the development of various malignant tumors; that is why analysis of the methylation status stability in oncogenes and tumor suppressor genes in different ES cell lines is important to understand the evolution of these lines in long-term in vitro cultures [149]. DNA hypermethylation in the promoter regions of oncosuppressor genes RASSF1 and PTPN6 has been found in long-term cultures of human ES cell lines BG01, BG02, BG03, HUES-2, HUES-3, H7, H9, SA001, and SA002; while the methylation of the TNFRSF10C promoter was observed only in two of these lines, HUES-2 and SA002 [112].

Significant variation in the expression level of DNA methyltransferase DNMT3B in different human ES cell lines was reported in numerous studies [8, 150-152]. Different levels of this enzyme expression and activity can be the main variation factor of the methylation status and epigenetic stability in different pluripotent cell lines. The ES cell genome is largely hypomethylated (in a 'transcription-ready' state), and the expression of many genes specific for different cell types is basically regulated at the post-transcriptional level [153].

The overexpression of genes located on the X chromosome during cell differentiation is known to be compensated by the inactivation of one of X chromosomes in the cells with the female genotype as a result of DNA methylation, histone modification, and expression of the noncoding XIST mRNA. Several publications demonstrated considerable variation in XIST expression indicative of the X chromosomes inactivation in both undifferentiated and differentiated cells of different ES cell lines with the female genotype [8, 76, 154]. Noteworthily, XIST mRNA was detected at early passages of undifferentiated cells of euploid human ES cell line H7, and it was undetectable at the late passages; while XIST expression was not detected even in differentiated cells of the aneuploid subline of H7 [122]. What underlies such heterogeneity in different ES cell lines remains unclear. Presumably, it can be due to the X chromosome inactivation status in cells of the inner cell mass of the embryo that served as line sources, or it was affected by in vitro culture conditions. Thus, the epigenetic modifications revealed in different human and primate ES cell lines take place during the adaptation to culture conditions at different passages in individual cells of the same line. These changes as well as the genetic aberrations can contribute to genome instability and cell transformation.

Regulation of Pluripotent State Maintenance and the Initial Stage of Differentiation of Pluripotent Stem Cells

Pluripotent stem cells retain their features to differentiate into all cell types of organism including germ line and extraembryonic tissue even after prolonged cultivation in artificial microenvironment which significantly differs from embryonic niche. However, pluripotent stem cell can realize their potential completely only if they are returned to blastocysts which are their natural niche. After injection of pluripotent stem cells into ectopic adult tissue sites they develop teratomas which represent chaotic development of different tissue structure of different degree of maturation. Pluripotent stem cells can recapitulate several elements of developmental program of mammalian embryo during in vitro differentiation but they can reproduce the histogenesis of some somatic tissues only after experimental modulation of signaling and growth factors' gradients. Though, pluripotent stem cells of different origin differentiate asynchronously and incompletely even after step-by-step treatment by different differentiation inductors. One of the challenges of pluripotent stem cell-based technology for regenerative medicine is uncompleted differentiation and as the result - variable percentage of residual undifferentiated cells that can form teratomas. Therefore, role of intrinsic cell factors governing pluripotent cell differentiation programme and influence of extrinsic factors that drive the in vitro differentiation of pluripotent stem cells must be determined and clarified.

The pluripotency is maintained by a complex of extracellular and intracellular factors that set up a specific pattern of the gene expression. Molecular signaling network working in pluripotent cells controls self-renewal and maintenance of the pluripotent cell identity. When the external signals from the environment niche (it is culture media for pluripotent cell lines) do change and the balance of proliferation and differentiation promoting factors alters then the pluripotent cells are involved in the lineages' determination.

One of the core regulator of pluripotent state is octamer-binding homeobox transcriptional factor POU family Oct4 which was the first identified factor that sustained pluripotent phenotype in cells of pre-implantation embryo and in germ cells as well as in ES, EG, iPS cells and expressed in different EC cell lines [46, 75, 155, 156,]. Two other transcriptional factors Sox2 and FoxD3 can interact with Oct4, in particular, Sox2 and Oct4 bind to adjacent cites within the enhancer of several target genes and act cooperatively to stimulate the transcription [157]. The second identified pluripotency-related homeodomain transcription factor Nanog was identified in mouse and human pluripotent and teratocarcinoma cells. Pattern of Nanog expression is differed from Oct4 and detected firstly in late morula stage and then it decreases in epiblast cells. Nanog is detectable in migrating primordial germ cells and in residing early gonocytes but it is not expressed in adult gonads [158-161].

Obviously, Oct4, Nanog and Sox2 function as suppressors of differentiation of inner cell mass into extraembryonic lineages – trophoblast and extraembryonic endoderm but they act cooperatively with many other genes that are elements of developmental programme of pluripotent cells. These core genes control expression of numerous target genes that are involved in cell cycle progression and lineages determination [103, 162]. Expression of Oct4, Nanog and Sox2 was detected in various mouse and human teratocarcinoma cells with different differentiation potential and mRNA Oct4 has been found in some other tumors too (breast, pancreas and colon cancer) [8, 163, 164].

Yamanaka et al, have demonstrated that ectopic expression of four transcription factors Oct4, Sox2, Klf4, and c-Myc can reprogram mouse and human somatic cells to induced pluripotent stem (iPS) cells. As it was mentioned above, Oct4, Sox2 together with Nanog are key genes underlying pluripotency. The fourth gene Kruppel-like factor 4 (Klf4) cooperates with Oct4 and Sox2 to activate Lefty1expression, and that Klf4 acts as a mediating factor that specifically binds to the proximal element of the Lefty1promoter [165]. Recently it was shown, after using PiggyBac transposition to introduce a single reprogramming factor, Klf4, into EpiS cells a fraction of cells formed undifferentiated ES-like colonies. These EpiSC-derived induced pluripotent stem (Epi-iPS) cells activated expression of ES cell-specific transcripts including endogenous Klf4, and down regulated markers of lineage specification. They produced high-contribution chimaeras that yielded germline transmission. These properties were maintained after Cre-mediated deletion of the Klf4 transgene, formally demonstrating complete and stable reprogramming of developmental phenotype. Thus, re-expression of Klf4 in an appropriate environment can regenerate the ground state from EpiSCs [14].

In mouse ES cells, Klf4 is mainly activated by the Jak-Stat3 pathway and preferentially activates Sox2, whereas Tbx3 is preferentially regulated by the phosphatidylinositol-3-OH kinase-Akt and mitogen-activated protein kinase pathways and predominantly stimulates Nanog. In the absence of LIF, artificial expression of Klf4 or Tbx3 is sufficient to maintain pluripotency while maintaining Oct4 expression. Notably, overexpression of Nanog supports LIF-independent self-renewal of mouse ES cells in the absence of Klf4 and Tbx3 activity. Therefore, Klf4 and Tbx3 are involved in mediating LIF signaling to the core circuitry but are not directly associated with the maintenance of pluripotency, because ES cells keep pluripotency without their expression in the particular context [162].

Another component of the regulation of gene expression pattern in mouse and human ES cells is polycomb group (PcG) proteins which directly repress a large cohort of differentiation regulators. Using genome-wide location analysis in murine ES cells, there was found that the Polycomb repressive complexes PRC1 and PRC2 co-occupied 512 genes, many of which encode transcription factors with important roles in development [166, 167]. The polycomb repressor complex PRC2 is involved in the initiation of silencing and contains histone methyltransferases that can methylate histone H3 lysine 9 and 27, which are marks of silenced chromatin. The PRC2 is involved in the initiation of silencing and contains EZH2, the histone methyltransferase that places the histone methylation modification HeK27me. On the other side, the PRC1 complexes contain chromo domain proteins such as the CBX family that recognize the HeK27me mark, and the key stem cell protein Bmi1, which can silence the p16 gene (a key gene epigenetically silenced early in cancers). Enrichment of EZH2 and the H3K27me mark is a property of the promoters of DNA hypermethylated and silenced genes as is the sirtuin deacetylase SIRT1, which has been associated with PRC2 complexes found in stem and cancer cells. Steady-state levels of EZH2, Bmi1, and other PcG complex members are increased in cancer too. Thus, dysregulation of the PcG system potentially links cancer formation to stem cell biology [168].

The investigation of signaling pathways that underlay pluripotent state maintenance demonstrated that there exist several differences between mouse and human ES cells. It was shown that leukemia inhibitory factor (LIF) is essential for self-renewal mouse ES and EG cells but doesn't require for pre-gastrulation mouse development and for derivation and maintenance of EpiS cells [169-172, 5, 6]. LIF is binding to the LIF receptor and activates the signal transducer and activator of transcription 3 (Stat-3). Phosphorilated Stat-3 translocates into nucleus and regulates target genes transcription. Mouse ES cells growing without feeder cells begin to differentiate after several days of LIF withdrawal. On the other hand, human ES cells are not sensitive to LIF absence and the supplement to this factor to culture media does not prevent the differentiation [173]. With the presence of LIF, bone morphogenetic protein 4 (BMP4) enhance the self-renewal of ES cells and activate Id (inhibitor of differentiation) genes. Opposite, without LIF, BMP4 activates other signaling cascades that promote the differentiation of mouse ES cells. BMP4 also stimulates human ES cells to differentiate into trophoblast cells or mesodermal precursors [79, 161, 174, 175].

Nanog and Stat3 were found to bind to and synergistically activate Stat3-dependent promoters, moreover, Nanog binds to NFkappa B proteins and inhibits transcriptional activity of NFkappa B proteins. Endogenous NFkappa B activity and target-gene expression increased during differentiation of ES cells. Overexpression of NFkappa B proteins promoted differentiation, whereas inhibition of NF kappa B signalling, either by genetic ablation of the Ikbkg gene or overexpression of the Ikappa B alpha super-repressor, increased expression of pluripotency markers. Thus, Nanog can repress the pro-differentiation activities of NFkappaB and can cooperate with Stat3 to maintain pluripotency [176].

Although Stat-3 signaling is involved in mouse ES cell self-renewal, stimulation of this pathway does not support self-renewal of human ES cells. However, activation of the canonical Wnt pathway is sufficient to maintain self-renewal of both human and mouse ES cells. Wnt pathway activation by 6-bromoindirubin-3'-oxime (BIO), a specific pharmacological inhibitor of glycogen synthase kinase-3 (GSK-3), maintains the undifferentiated phenotype in both types of ES cells and sustains expression of the specific pluripotentcy-related transcription factors Oct4, Rex-1 and Nanog. Wnt signaling is endogenously activated in undifferentiated mouse ES cells and is downregulated upon differentiation. In addition, BIO-mediated Wnt activation is functionally reversible, as withdrawal of the compound leads to normal multilineage differentiation in human and mouse ES cells [177]. Functional screening identifies Wnt5A and Wnt6 as feeder cell-produced factors that potently inhibit ES cell differentiation in a serum-dependent manner. Furthermore, direct activation of beta-catenin without disturbing the upstream components of the Wnt/β-catenin pathway fully recapitulates the effect of Wnts on ES cells. In addition, the WNT/β-catenin pathway up-regulates the mRNA for Stat3, that suggests that LIF is able to mimic the serum effect to act synergistically with Wnt proteins to inhibit ES cell differentiation [178].

Specific signals that determine the cell fate in early embryogenesis are modulated via interactions of several signaling pathways to form a unique regulatory cell network, essential for differentiation of a certain cell type. Factors of TGFβ family (Activin, Nodal, Lefty, BMP, GDF and TGFβ) are involved in the regulation of specialization of the precursors of ecto-, endo-, and mesoderm, as well as of germline cells [179-182]. These factors are implicated in the regulation of morphogenesis, formation of polarity axes of vertebrate embryos. Factors of the TGFβ family control proliferation, differentiation, migration, adhesion and apoptosis of different cell types in adult tissues and alterations in their activity are often found in various tumors [182,183].

Previously, genetic studies demonstrated that TGFβ family signaling regulates the maintenance of pluripotent cell identity because it was shown that mouse embryos deficient in Smad4 (signal transducer in TGFβ signaling) display defective epiblast proliferation and delayed outgrowth of the inner cell mass and that Nodal-deficient mouse embryos had reduced epiblast cell population which expressed very low level of Oct4 [184-186]. Large-scale gene profiling of ES cells has revealed that TGFβ family signaling has important role in the maintance pluripotency and in cell lineages commitment [99]. Several groups demonstrated that the preserving of undifferentiated state of human ES cells requires Activin and Nodal signaling interaction with FGF2 cascade [68,187]. Inhibition of Activin and Nodal signaling by pharmacological inhibitor of receptor kinases SB-431542 resulted in a decreased expression of pluripotent cell specific genes [188]. On the contrary, hES cell treatment by BMP, TGFβ and Cripto led to the stimulation of their differentiation and the number of Oct4-positive cells was significantly decreased [68, 189]. Inhibition of signals from Activin/Nodal receptors also led to the initiation of differentiation of human ES cells even in the presence of FGF [68; 188].

The developmental fate of differentiating ES cells depends on the complex combination of growth factors and extracellular matrix proteins constituting the developmental niche in which these stem cells exist. The numerous findings suggest important parallels of TGFβ family signaling in germ layer specification between embryogenesis and ES cells in vitro differentiation systems. For instance, embryoid bodies derived from either Lefty or Cerb-S (Nodal antagonists) overexpressing human ES cells showed increased expression of neuroectoderm markers Sox1, Sox3, and Nestin. Conversely, they were negative for a definitive endoderm marker Sox17 and did not generate beating cardiomyocyte structures in conditions that allowed mesendoderm differentiation from WT hESCs. Embryoid bodies derived from either Lefty or Cerb-S expressing hES cells also contained a greater abundance of neural rosette structures as compared to controls and generated a dense network of beta-tubulin III positive neuritis. SB431542 treatments reproduced the neuralising effects of Lefty overexpression in human ES cells. These results show that inhibition of Nodal signaling promotes neuronal specification, indicating a role for this pathway in controlling early neural development of pluripotent cells [190].

On the other side, several lines of evidence have demonstrated the role of TGFβ family signaling in the development of the cardiac lineage from ES cells. BMP2 and Cripto have been shown to promote or improve cardiomiocytes differentiation but they act as stimulators of mesoderm precursor differentiation. Interestingly, transient inhibition of BMP signaling in undifferentiated ES cells by noggin dramatically induces cardiomycyte differentiation of mouse ES cells [191-193].

The embryonic stem cell differentiation system was used to define the roles of the Activin/Nodal, BMP, and canonical Wnt signaling pathways at three distinct developmental stages during hematopoietic ontogeny: induction of a primitive streak-like population, formation of Flk1(+) mesoderm, and induction of hematopoietic progenitors. It was shown that Activin/Nodal and Wnt, but not BMP, signaling is required for the induction of the primitive streak. Although BMP is not required for primitive streak induction, it displays a strong posteriorizing effect on this population. All three signaling pathways regulate induction of Flk1(+) mesoderm. The specification of Flk1(+) mesoderm to the hematopoietic lineages requires VEGF and Wnt, but not BMP or Activin/Nodal signaling. Specifically, Wnt signaling is essential for commitment of the primitive erythroid, but not the definitive lineages. These findings highlight dynamic changes in signaling requirements during different lineages' development from pluripotent stem cells [194].

Our research of the earliest stages of human and mouse ES, EG and EC differentiation is focused on the study of the interaction between different branches of TGFβ family signaling that regulate the pluripotency and specification of different embryonic cell populations and on determining which of them are impaired in malignant teratocarcinoma cells.

Comparative analysis of cell growth dynamic of mouse pluripotent ES, EG and nullipotent EC cells demonstrates that ES and EG cells and EC cells respond to serum factors and LIF in different ways [75, 195]. ES and EG cell growth was insensitive to serum factors but depended on LIF presence. After LIF withdrawal ES and EG cells initiated differentiation and their growth rate was diminished in serum containing and serum-free conditions. Cell cycle distribution test revealed that spontaneous differentiation of ES and EC cells but not EC cells was accompanied by cell accumulation in G1 phase of the cell cycle. Proportion of ES and EG cells l in G1 phase of the cell cycle went up to 11-17% after 5day LIF withdrawal and no changes were found in cell cycle distribution of EC cell population (Figure 5).

Therewith, in spontaneously differentiating ES and EG cells the expression of Oct4, Nanog and alkaline phosphatase activity were down-regulated but the expression of markers of all three germ layers and extraembryonic endoderm GATA4, 6, AFP, Nestin, Pax6, Bry was up-regulated. On the contrary, LIF-independent EC cells reduced their proliferation rate in serum-free conditions more than twice but expression of Oct4 and alkaline phosphatase was invariable in serum and serum-free culture systems (Figure 6). We have found that in course of spontaneous differentiation of ES and EG cells expression level of ActivinA, Nodal, Lefty1, 2 and GDF3 was down regulated together with Oct4 and Nanog expression while expression of other member of TGFβ family, BMP4 and TGFβ1, was at the steady level. Interestingly, that expression of genes that are the components of TGFβ family signaling (receptors Teri, ActrI,ActrII, BmprI and signal transducers Smad2,4,5) was sensibly sensibly constant.

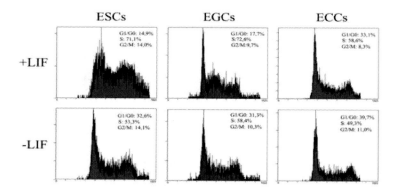

Figure 5. Cell cycle distribution in undifferentiated (+LIF) and differentiating (-LIF) ES, EG, EC cell populations. EC cells don't initiate differentiation after LIF withdrawal within 5 days.

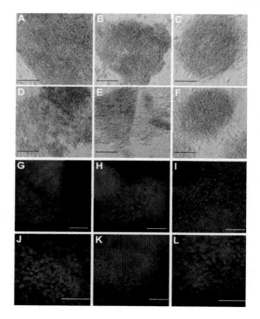

Figure 6. Activity of alkaline phosphatase (A-F) and expression of Oct4 (G-L) in mouse ES (A,D,G,F), EG (B,E,H,K) and EC(C,F,I,L) cells growing in LIF-supplemented media (A-C, G-I) and after LIF withdrawal (D-F, J-L) within 5 days. Bar, 100µm.

On the other side, in teratocarcinoma cells expression of pluripotency-related genes and GATA4, 6, Pax6 as well as signal ligands, receptors and signal transducers has not changed. We have revealed that nullipotent EC cells don't express ActivinA as apposed to pluripoten stem cells. These data indicate that malignant transformation of pluripotent stem cells to teratocarcinoma cells may be conducted with the initiation of new mechanisms regulating self-renew and differentiation which are LIF and ActivinA independent. Disturbed signaling network in EC cells results in deregulation of proliferation and differentiation balance. Note that we have revealed similar trends in transcriptional profiles of human ES and EC cells that argue for the conservative mechanism of malignant teratocarcinoma transformation [196]. However, the origin of these disturbances remains unclear and our study of these defective mechanisms will be continued in future.

CONCLUSION

Numerous pluripotent stem cell lines derived from different sources using different techniques demonstrate their considerable similarity in the basic biological properties as well as individual variations. More than twenty years of intense studies of the stability of different pluripotent stem cell lines demonstrated the accumulation of chromosomal and gene mutations and epigenetic alterations during their long term in vitro culture, which can lead to malignant transformation. It is generally accepted that the line stability maintenance requires continuous monitoring of the line karyotype, epigenetic profile, and carcinogenesis-associated gene mutations. One of the most important lessons that came from the recent studies of stem cells biology postulates that the deregulation of signaling pathways involved in control of self-renewal and differentiation stem cells and progenitors leads to carcinogenesis in embryonic and adult tissues. In the context of clinical use of pluripotent stem cell lines, the maintenance of the genetic and epigenetic stability is crucial for the development of safe and efficient cell technologies. Considering the high risk of carcinogenesis, the outlooks of clinical application of induced pluripotent stem cell lines still remain questionable despite relative simplicity of producing patient-specific lines. Nevertheless, the available data clearly indicate that the elucidation of the evolutionary patterns of cell lines with different genotypes and the development of techniques providing their stability in long-term in vitro cultures are the main goals in the production and application of permanent pluripotent stem cell lines. Correct studies of the basic mechanisms regulating pluripotent cell self-renewal and specialization into different cell types clearly require the validation of the main cell parameters in the model lines. This also applies to the utilization of ES cells as test systems to study the efficiency and toxicity of new drugs.

ACKNOWLEDGMENTS

This work was supported by the Russian Foundation for Basic Research (project no. 08-04-09307).

REFERENCES

[1]   Evans, M. J. and Kaufman, M. H. (1981). Establishment in culture of pluripotential cells from mouse embryos. *Nature*, 292, 154-156.

[2]   Martin, G. R. (1981). Isolation of pluripotent cell line from early mouse embryo cultured in medium conditioned by teratocarcinoma stem cells. *Proc. Natl. Acad. Sci.*

USA., 78, 7634-7638.

[3]   Rossant, J. (2001). Stem cells from mammalian blastocyst. *Stem Cells*, 19, 477-482.

[4]   Thomson, J. A., Itskovitz-Eldor, J., Shapiro, S. S., Waknitz, M. A., Swiergiel, J. J,
      Marshall, V. S. and Jones J. M. (1998). Embryonic stem cell lines derived from human
      blastocysts. *Science*, 282(5391), 1145-1147.

[5]   Brons, I. G., Smithers, L. E., Trotter, M. W., Rugg-Gunn, P., Sun, B., Chuva de Sousa
      Lopes, S. M., Howlett, S. K., Clarkson, A., Ahrlund-Richter, L., Pedersen, R, A. and
      Vallier, L. (2007). Derivation of pluripotent epiblast stem cells from mammalian
      embryos. *Nature*, 448(7150), 191-195.

[6]   Tesar, P. J,, Chenoweth, J. G,, Brook, F. A, Davies, T, J., Evans, E. P., Mack, D. L.,
      Gardner, R. L. and McKay, R. D. (2007). New cell lines from mouse epiblast share
      defining features with human embryonic stem cells. *Nature*, 448(7150), 196-199.

[7]   Mitalipova, M. M., Rao, R. R. and Hoyer, D. M., et al. (2005). Preserving the genetic
      integrity of human embryonic stem cells. *Nat. Biotechnol*, 23, 19-20.

[8]   Thomson, J. A., Kalishman, J. and Golos, T. G. et al. (1995). Isolation of a primate
      embryonic stem cell line. *Proc. Natl. Acad. Sci.* U S A, 92(17), 7844-7848.

[9]   Strelchenko, N., Verlinsky, O., Kukharenko, V., Verlinsky, Y. (2004). Morula-derived
      human embryonic stem cells. *Reprod. Biomed. Online*, 9(6), 623-629.

[10] Klimanskaya, I., Chung, Y. and Becker, S. et al. (2006). Human embryonic stem cell
      lines derived from single blastomeres. *Nature*, 444(7118), 481-485.

[11] Nagy, A., Rossant, J. and Nagy, R. et al. (1993). Embryonic stem cells alone are able to
      support fetal development in the mouse. *Proc. Natl. Acad. Sci.* U S A, 90, 8424-8428.

[12] Suemor, i. H., Tada, T. and Torii, R. et al. (2001). Establishment of embryonic stem
      cell lines from cynomolgus monkey blastocysts produced by IVF or ICSI. *Devel. Dyn.*,
      222, 273-279.

[13] Mitalipov, S., Kuo, H.C., Byrn, e. J. et al. (2006). Isolation and characterization of
      novel rhesus monkey embryonic stem cell lines. *Stem Cells*, 24, 2177-2186.

[14] Guo, G., Yang, J., Nichols, J,, Hall, J. S., Eyres, I., Mansfield, W. and Smith, A.
      (2009). Klf4 reverts developmentally programmed restriction of ground state
      pluripotency. *Development*, 136(7), 1063-9.

[15] Stevens, L.C. (1970). The development of transplantable teratocarcinomas from
      intratesticular grafts of pre- and postimplantation mouse embryos. *Dev. Biol.*, 21, 364-
      382.

[16] Solter, D., Skreb, N. andmjanov, I. (1970). Extrauterine growth of mouse egg-cylinders
      results in malignant teratoma. *Nature*, 227, 503-504.

[17] Matsui, Y., Zsebo, K. and Hogan, B. L. (1992). Derivation of pluripotential embryonic
      stem cells from murine primordial germ cells in culture. *Cell*, 70, 841-847.

[18] Resnick, J. L., Bixler, L. S., Cheng, L. and Donovan, P. J. (1992). Long-term
      proliferation of mouse primordial germ cells in culture. *Nature*, 359, 550-551.

[19] Stewart, C. L., Gadi, I. and Bhatt, H. (1994). Stem cells from primordial germ cells can
      reenter the germ line. *Dev. Biol.*, 161, 626–628.

[20] Labosky, P. A., Barlow, D. P. and Hogan, B.L. (1994). Mouse embryonic germ (EG)
      cell lines: transmission through the germline and differences in the methylation imprint
      of insulin-like growth factor 2 receptor (Igf2r) gene compared with embryonic stem
      (ES) cell lines. *Development*, 120, 3197–3204.

[21] Shamblott, M. J., Axelman, J., Wang. S. et al. (1998). Derivation of pluripotent stem
      cells from cultured human primordial germ cells. *Proc. Natl. Acad. Sci.* U S A, 95,
      13726-13731.

[22] Kanatsu-Shinohara, M., Inoue, K., Lee, J., Yoshimoto, M., Ogonuki, N., et al. (2004). Generation of pluripotent stem cells from neonatal mouse testis. *Cell, 119*, 1001-1012.

[23] Guan, K., Nayernia, K., Maier, L. S., Wagner, S., Dressel, R., Lee, J. H., Nolte, J., Wolf, F., Li, M., Engel, W. and Hasenfuss, G. (2006). Pluripotency of spermatogonial stem cells from adult mouse testis. *Nature*, 440, 1199-1203.

[24] Robertson, E. J., Evans, M. J. and Kaufman, M. H. (1983). X-chromosome instability in pluripotential stem cell lines derived from parthenogenetic embryos. *J. Embryol.* exp. Morph., 74, 297-309.

[25] Mann, J. R., Gadi, I., Harbison, M. L., Abbondanzo, S. J. and Stewart, C. L. (1990). androgenetic mouse embryonic stem cells are pluripotent and cause skeletal defects in chimeras: Implications for genetic imprinting. *Cell,* 62, 251-260.

[26] Mann, J. R. and Stewart, C. L. (1991). Development to term of mouse androgenetic aggregation chimeras. *Development*, 113, 1325-1333.

[27] Cibelli, J. B., Grant, K. A., Chapman, K. B. et al. (2002). Parthenogenetic stem cells in nonhuman primates. *Science*, 295, 819.

[28] Vrana, K. E., Hipp, J. D., Goss, A.M. et al. (2003). Nonhuman primate parthenogenetic stem cells. *Proc. Natl. Acad. Sci.* U S A, 100, 11911-11916.

[29] Lin, G., OuYang, Q., Zhou, X. et al. (2007). A highly homozygous and parthenogenetic human embryonic stem cell line derived from a one-pronuclear oocyte following in vitro fertilization procedure. *Cell Res.*, 17(12), 999-1007.

[30] Revazova, E. S., Turovets, N. A., Kochetkova, O. D. et al. (2007). Patient-specific stem cell lines derived from human parthenogenetic blastocysts. *Cloning Stem Cells*, 9(3), 432-449.

[31] Eckardt, S., Dinger, T. C., Kurosaka, S., Leu, N. A., Müller, A. M. and McLaughlin, K. J. (2008). In vivo and in vitro differentiation of uniparental embryonic stem cells into hematopoietic and neural cell types. *Organogenesis*, 4(1), 33-41.

[32] Dighe, V., Clepper, L., Pedersen, D. et al. (2008). Heterozygous embryonic stem cell lines derived from nonhuman primate parthenotes. *Stem Cells*, 26(3), 756-766.

[33] Allen, N. D., Barton, S. C., Hilton, K., Norris, M. L. and Surani, M. A. (1994). A functional analysis of imprinting in parthenogenetic embryonic stem cells. *Development,* 120(6), 1473-82

[34] Cibelli, J. B., Stice, S. L., Golueke, P. J., et al. (1998). Transgenic bovine chimeric offspring produced from somatic cell-derived stem-like cells. *Nat. Biotechnol.*, 16, 642-646.

[35] Kawase, E., Yamazaki, Y., Yagi, T., et al. (2000). Mouse embryonic stem (ES) cell lines established from neuronal cell-derived cloned blastocysts. *Genesis*, 28, 156-163.

[36] Munsie, M. J., Michalska, A. E., O'Brien, C. M., et al. (2000). Isolation of pluripotent embryonic stem cells from reprogrammed adult mouse somatic cell nuclei. *Curr. Biol.*, 10, 989-992.

[37] Wakayama, T., Tabar, V., Rodriguez, I., et al. (2001). Differentiation of embryonic stem cell lines generated from adult somatic cells by nuclear transfer. *Science*, 292, 740-743.

[38] Wakayama, S., Jakt, M. L., Suzuki, M., et al. (2006). Equivalency of nuclear transfer-derived embryonic stem cells to those derived from fertilized mouse blastocysts. *Stem Cells*, 24, 2023-2033.

[39] Wakayama, S., Mizutani, E. and Kishigami, S., et al. (2005). Mice cloned by nuclear transfer from somatic and ntES cells derived from the same individuals. *J. Reprod. Dev.*, 51, 765-772.

[40] Wakayama, S., Ohta, H., Kishigami, S., et al. (2005). Establishment of male and female nuclear transfer embryonic stem cell lines from different mouse strains and tissues. *Biol. Reprod.*, 72, 932-936.

[41] Byrne, J. A., Pedersen, D. A., Clepper, L. L., et al. (2007). Producing Primate Embryonic Stem Cells by Somatic Cell Nuclear Transfer. *Nature*, 450, 497-505.

[42] French, A. J., Adams, C. A., anderson, L. S. et al. (2008). Development of human cloned blastocysts following somatic nuclear transfer (SCNT) with adult fibroblast. Stem Cells, 26, 485-493.

[43] Cowan, C. A., Atienza, J., Melton, D. A. and Eggan, K. (2005). Nuclear reprogramming of somatic cells after fusion with human embryonic stem cells. *Science*, 309, 1369-1373.

[44] Yu, J., Vodyanik, M. A., He, P., Slukvin, I. I., and Thomson, J. A. (2006). Human embryonic stem cells reprogram myeloid precursors following cell–cell fusion. *Stem Cells*, 24, 168–176.

[45] Ambrosi, D. J., Tanasijevic, B., Kaur, A., Obergfell, C., O'Neill, R. J., Krueger, W., Rasmussen, T. P. (2007). Genome-wide reprogramming in hybrids of somatic cells and embryonic stem cells. *Stem Cells*, 25(5), 1104-13.

[46] Takahashi, K., Yamanaka, S. (2006). Induction of pluripotent stem cells from mouse embryonic and adult fibroblast cultures by defined factors. *Cell*, 126. P. 663–676.

[47] Takahashi, K., Tanabe, K., Ohnuki, V. et al. (2007). Induction of pluripotent stem cells from adult human fibroblasts by defined factors. *Cell*, 131, 861-872.

[48] Yu, J., Vodyanik, M., Smuga-Otoo, K. et al. (2007). Induced pluripotent stem cell lines derived from human somatic cells. *Science*, 318, 1917-1920.

[49] Lowry, W. E., Richter, L., Yachechko, R., et al. (2008). Generation of human induced pluripotent stem cells from dermal fibroblasts. *Proc. Natl. Acad. Sci.,* 105, 2883–2888.

[50] Park, I. H., Zhao, R., West, J. A., et al. (2008). Reprogramming of human somatic cells to pluripotency with defined factors. *Nature*, 451,141–146.

[51] Aoi, T., Yae, K., Nakagawa, M., et al. (2008). Generation of pluripotent stem cells from adult mouse liver and stomach cells. *Science*, 321(5889), 699-702.

[52] Hanna, J., Markoulaki, S., Schorderet, P., et al. (2008). Direct reprogramming of terminally differentiated mature B lymphocytes to pluripotency. *Cell*, 133(2), 250-64.

[53] Maherali, N., Sridharan, R., Xie, W. et al.(2007). Directly reprogrammed fibroblasts show global epigenetic remodeling and widespread tissue contribution. *Cell Stem Cell*, 1, 55–70.

[54] Okita, K., Ichisaka, T. and Yamanaka, S. (2007). Generation of germ-line competent induced pluripotent stem cells. *Nature*, 448, 13–317.

[55] Nakagawa, M., Koyanagi1, M., Tanabe, K. et al. (2008). Generation of induced pluripotent stem cells without Myc from mouse and human fibroblasts. *Nat. Biotech.*, 26, 101-106.

[56] Kleinsmith, L. J. and Pierce, G. B. (1964). Multipotentiality of single embryonal carcinoma cells. *Cancer Res.*, 24, 1544–1552.

[57] Hogan, B., Fellows, M., Avner, P. and Jacob, F. (1977) Isolation of a human teratoma cell line which expresses F9 antigen. *Nature*, 270, 515–518.

[58] Lee, V. M.-Y. and andrews, P. W. (1986). Differentiation of NTERA-2 clonal human embryonal carcinoma cells into neurons involves the induction of all three neuro. Lament proteins. *J. Neurosci.,* 6, 514–521.

[59] Rossant, J. and McBurney, M.W (1982). The developmental potential of a euploid male teratocarcinoma cell line after blastocyst injection. *J Embryol Exp Morphol*, 70, 99-112.

[60] andrews, P. W. (2002). From teratocarcinomas to embryonic stem cells. *Philos Trans R Soc Lond B Biol Sci., 357*, 405-417.

[61] Blelloch, R. H., Hochedlinger, K., Yamada, Y., Brennan, C., Kim, M., Mintz, B., Chin, L. and Jaenisch, R. (2004). Nuclear cloning of embryonal carcinoma cells. *Proc Natl Acad Sci* U S A, 101, 13985-13990.

[62] Xu, C., Inokuma M. S., Denham J. et al. (2001). Feeder-free growth of undifferentiated human embryonic stem cells. *Nat Biotechnol.*, 19(10), 971-974.

[63] Xu, C., Jiang, J., Sottile V. et al. (2004). Immortalized fibroblast-like cells derived from human embryonic stem cells support undifferentiated cell growth. *Stem Cells*, 22(6), 972-980.

[64] Xu, C., Rosler E., Jiang J. et al. (2005). Basic fibroblast growth factor supports undifferentiated human embryonic stem cell growth without conditioned medium. *Stem Cells*, 23(3), 315-323.

[65] Hovatta, O., Mikkola, M., Gertow, K. et al. (2003). A culture system using human foreskin fibroblasts as feeder cells allows production of human embryonic stem cells. *Hum. Reprod.*, 18, 1404-1409.

[66] Rosler, E. S., Fisk, G. J., Ares, X. et al. (2004). Long-term culture of human embryonic stem cells in feeder-free conditions. *Dev. Dyn.*, 229, 259-274.

[67] Beattie, G. M., Lopez, A. D., Bucay, N. et al. (2005) Activin A maintains pluripotency of human embryonic stem cells in the absence of feeder layers. *Stem Cells*, 23, 489-495.

[68] Vallier, L., Alexander, M. and Pedersen, R. A. (2005). Activin/Nodal and FGF pathways cooperate to maintain pluripotency of human embryonic stem cells. *J. Cell Sci.,* 118, 4495-4509.

[69] Bigdeli, N., andersson, M. and Strehl, R. et al. (2008). Adaptation of human embryonic stem cells to feeder-free and matrix-free culture conditions directly on plastic surfaces. *J. Biotechnol.*, 133(1), 146-153.

[70] Przyborski, S. A. (2005). Differentiation of Human Embryonic Stem Cells After Transplantation in Immune-Deficient Mice. *Stem Cells*, 23, 1242-1250.

[71] Gordeeva, O.F. Pluripotent cells in embryogenesis and in teratoma formation. In: Parsons D.W, editor. *Stem cells and cancer.* N.Y.: Nova Sci. Publ. Ink.; 2007; 62-85.

[72] Ramalho-Santos, M., Yoon, S., Matsuzaki, Y., Mulligan, R. C. andFigureMelton, D. A. (2002). «Stemness»: transcriptional profiling of embrionic and adult stem cells. *Science*, 298, 597-600.

[73] Sato, N., Sanjuan, I. M., Heke, M., et al. (2003). Molecular signature of human embryonic stem cells and its comparison with the mouse. *Dev. Biol.,* 260, 404-413.

[74] Gordeeva, O. F., Krasnikova, N. Yu., Larionova, A. V., et al. (2006). Analysis of Expression of Genes Specific for Pluripotent and Primordial Germ Cells in Human and Mouse Embryonic Stem Cell Lines. *Dokl. Akad. Nauk*, 406(6), 835-839.

[75] Gordeeva, O. F., Lifantzeva, N. V. and Nikonova, T. M. (2009). Regulation of in vitro and in vivo differentiation of embryonic stem, embryonic germ and teratocarcinomal cell by factors of TGFβ family. *Ontogenez*, 40(6), 403-418.

[76] Adewumi, O., Aflatoonian, B., Ahrlund-Richter, L. et al. (2007). Characterization of human embryonic stem cell lines by the International Stem Cell Initiative. *Nat. Biotech.*, 25, 803-816.

[77] Sharova, L. V., Sharov, A. A., Piao, Y., et al. (2007). Global gene expression profiling reveals similarities and differences among mouse pluripotent stem cells of different origins and strains. *Dev Biol.* 307(2), 446-59.

[78] Chin, M. H., Mason, M. J., Xie, W., et al. (2009). Induced pluripotent stem cells and

embryonic stem cells are distinguished by gene expression signatures. *Cell Stem Cells*, *5(1)*, 111-23.

[79] Gerami-Naini, B., Dovzhenk, O. V., Durning, M. et al. (2004). Trophoblast differentiation in embryoid bodies derived from human embryonic stem cells. *Endocrinology*, 145, 1517-1524.

[80] Fang, D., Leishear, K., Nguyen,T. K. et al. (2006). Defining the conditions for the generation of melocytes from human embryonic stem cells. *Stem Cells*, 24, 1668-1677.

[81] Mitalipov, S., Kuo, H.C., Byrne, J. et al. (2006). Isolation and characterization of novel rhesus monkey embryonic stem cell lines. *Stem Cells*, 24, 2177-2186.

[82] Schwanke, K., Wunderlich, S., Reppel, M. et al. (2006). Generation and characterization of functional cardiomyocytes from rhesus monkey embryonic stem cells. *Stem Cells*, 24, 1423-1432.

[83] Shin, S., Mitalipova, M., Noggle, S., et al. (2006). Long-term proliferation of human embryonic stem cell–derived neuroepithelial cells using defined adherent culture conditions. *Stem Cells*, 24, 125-138.

[84] Taylor, R. A., Cowin, P. A. and Cunha, G. R. et al. (2006). Formation of human prostate tissue from embryomic stem cells. *Nat. Methods.*, 3, 179-181.

[85] Rajesh, D., Chinnasamy, N., M. Mitalipov, S. M. et al. (2007). Differential Requirements for Hematopoietic Commitment Between Human andRhesus Embryonic Stem Cells. *Stem Cells*, 25, 490-499.

[86] Savatier, P., Huang, S., Szekely, L., et al. (1994). Contrasting patterns of retinoblastoma protein expression in mouse embryonic stem cells and embryonic fibroblasts. *Oncogene*, 9, 809-818.

[87] Savatier, P., Lapillonne, H., Grunsven van, L.A., et al. (1996). Withdrawal of differentiation inhibitory activity/leukemia inhibitory factor up-regulates D type cyclins and cyclin-dependent kinase inhibitors in mouse embryonic stem cells. *Oncogene*, 12, 309-322.

[88] Burdon, T., Smith, A. and Savatier, P. (2002). Signaling, cell cycle and pluripotency in embryonic stem cells. *Trends Cell Biol.*, 12, 432-438.

[89] Fluckiger, A. C., Marcy, G., Marchand, M., et al. (2006). Cell cycle features of primate embryonic stem cells. *Stem Cells*, 24, 547-556.

[90] Becker, K. A., Stein, J. L., Lian, J. B., et al. (2007). Establishment of histone gene regulation and cell cycle checkpoint control in human embryonic stem cells. *J. Cell Physiol.*, 210, 517-526.

[91] Burdon, T., Stracey, C., Chambers, I., et al. (1999). Suppression of SHP-2 and ERK signaling promotes self-renewal of mouse embryonic stem cells. *Dev. Biol.*, 210, 30–43.

[92] Jirmanova, L., Afanassieff, M., Gobert-Gosse, S., et al. (2002). Differential contributions of ERK and PI3-kinase to the regulation of cyclin D1 expression and to the control of the G1/S transition in mouse embryonic stem cells. *Oncogene*, 21, 515–5528.

[93] Paling, N. R., Wheadon, H., Bone, H. K., et al. (2004). Regulation of embryonic stem cell self-renewal by phosphoinositide 3-kinase-dependent signaling. *J. Biol. Chem.*, 279, 48063– 48070.

[94] Takahashi, K., Mitsui, K. and Yamanaka, S. (2003). Role of ERas in promoting tumourlike properties in mouse embryonic stem cells. *Nature*, 423, 541–545.

[95] Dannenberg, J. H., van Rossum, A., Schuijff, L., et al. (2000). Ablation of the retinoblastoma gene family deregulates G(1) control causing immortalization and increased cell turnover under growth-restricting conditions. *Genes Dev.*, 14, 3051–

3064.

[96] Sage, J., Mulligan, G. J., Attardi, L. D., et al. (2000). Targeted disruption of the three Rb-related genes leads to loss of G(1) control and immortalization. *Genes Dev.*, 14, 3037–3050.

[97] White, J., Stead, E. and Faast, R., et al. (2005). Developmental activation of the Rb-E2F pathway and establishment of cell cycle regulated Cdk activity during embryonic stem cell differentiation. *Mol. Biol. Cell*, 16, 2018 –2027.

[98] Stead, E., White, J., Faast, R., et al. (2002). Pluripotent cell division cycles are driven by ectopic Cdk2, cyclin A/E and E2F activities. *Oncogene*, 21, 8320–8333.

[99] Brandenberger, R., Wei, H., Zhang, S. et al. (2004). Transcriptome characterization elucidates signaling networks that control human ES cell growth and differentiation. *Nat. Biotechnol.*, 22(6), 707-716.

[100] Miura, T., Luo, Y., Khrebtukova, I. et al. (2004). Monitoring early differentiation events in human embryonic stem cells by massively parallel signature sequencing and expressed sequence tag scan. *Stem Cells Devel.*, 13, 694–715.

[101] Zeng X. (2007). Human embryonic stem cells: mechanisms to escape replicative senescence? *Stem Cell Rev.*, 3, 270-279.

[102] Neganova, I., Zhang, X., Atkinson, S.and Lako, M. (2009). Expression and functional analysis of G1 to S regulatory components reveals an important role for CDK2 in cell cycle regulation in human embryonic stem cells. *Oncogene*, *28(1)*, 20-30.

[103] Zhang, X., Neganova, I., Przyborski, S., et al. (2009). A role for NANOG in G1 to S transition in human embryonic stem cells through direct binding of CDK6 and CDC25A. *J. Cell Biol.*, 184(1), 67-82.

[104] Lin, T., Chao, C., Saito, S., et al. (2005). p53 induces differentiation of mouse embryonic stem cells by suppressing Nanog expression. *Nat. Cell Biol.*, 7, 165–171.

[105] Saretzki, G., Armstrong, L., Leake, A., et al. (2004). Stress defense in murine embryonic stem cells is superior to that of various differentiated murine cells. *Stem Cells*, 22(6), 962-971.

[106] Saretzki, G., Walter, T., Atkinson, S., et al. (2008). Downregulation of multiple stress defense mechanisms during differentiation of human embryonic stem cells. *Stem Cells*, 26(2), 455-464.

[107] Brimble, S. N., Zeng, X., Weiler, D. A., et al. (2004). Karyotypic stability, genotyping, differentiation, feeder-free maintenance, and gene expression sampling in three human embryonic stem cell lines derived prior to August 9, 2001. *Stem Cells Dev.*, 13, 585-597.

[108] Cowan, C. A., Klimanskaya, I., McMahon, J. et al. (2004). Derivation of embryonic stem-cell lines from human blastocysts. *N. Engl. J. Med.,* 50, 1353-1356.

[109] Draper, J. S., Smith, K., Gokhale, P., et al. (2004). Recurrent gain of chromosomes 17q and 12 in cultured human embryonic stem cells. *Nat. Biotechnol.*, 22, 53-54.

[110] Inzunza, J., Sahlen, S., Holmberg, K., et al. (2004). Comparative genomic hybridization and karyotyping of human embryonic stem cells reveals the occurence of an isodicentric X chromosome after long-term cultivation. *Mol. Hum. Reprod.*, 10, 461-466.

[111] Hanson, C. and Caisander, G.. (2005). Human embryonic stem cells and chromosome stability. *Apmis*, 113, 751-755.

[112] Maitra, A., Arking, D. E. and Shivapurkar, N., et al. (2005). Genomic alterations in cultured human embryonic stem cells. *Nat. Genet.*, 37, 1099-1103.

[113] Mitalipova, M. M., Rao, R. R., Hoyer, D. M., et al. (2005). Preserving the genetic

integrity of human embryonic stem cells. *Nat. Biotechnol.*, 23, 19-20.

[114] Lakshmipathy, U., Pelacho, B., Sudo, K., et al. (2004). Efficient transfection of embronic and adult stem cells. *Stem Cells*, 22, 531-543.

[115] Plaia, T. W., Josephson, R., Liu, Y., et al. (2005). Characterization of a new NIH registers variant human embryonic stem cell line BG01V: a tool for human embryonic stem cell research. *Stem Cells*, 24, 531-546.

[116] Heins, N., Englund, M. C., Sjoblom, C., et al. (2004*). Derivation, characterization, and differentiation of human embryonic stem cells. *Stem Cells*, 22, 367-376.

[117] Kim, S. J., Lee, J. E., Park, J. H. et al. (2005). Efficient derivation of new human embryonic stem cell lines. *Mol. Cells*, 19, 46-53.

[118] Caisander, G., Park, H., Frej, K. et al. (2006). Chromosomal integrity maintained in five human embryonic stem cell lines after prolonged in vitro culture. *Chromosome Res*, 14, 131-137.

[119] Lavon, N., Narwani, K., Golan-Lev, et al. (2008). Derivation of euploid human embryonic stem cells from aneuploid embryos. *Stem Cells*, 7, 1874-82.

[120] Thomson, A., Wojtacha, D., Hewitt, Z., et al. Human embryonic stem Buzzard, J. J., Gough, N. M., Crook, J. M. and Colman A. (2004). Karyotype of human ES cells during extended culture. *Nat. Biotechnol.*, 22, 381-382.

[121] cells passaged using enzymatic methods retain a normal karyotype and express CD30. *Cloning Stem Cells*, 10(1), 89-106.

[122] Enver, T., Soneji, S., Joshi, C., et al. (2005). Cellular differentiation hierarchies in normal and culture-adapted human embryonic stem cells. *Hum. Mol. Genet.*, 14, 3129-3140.

[123] Herszfeld, D., Wolvetang, E., Langton-Bunker, E., et al. (2006). CD30 is a survival factor and a biomarker for tranformed human pluripotent stem cells. *Nat. Biotechnol.*, 24, 351-357.

[124] Skotheim, R. I., Monni, O. and Mousses, S., et al. (2002). New insights into testicular germ cell tumorigenesis from gene expression profiling. *Cancer Res.*, 62, 2359-2364.

[125] Clark, A. T., Rodrigues, R. T. and Bodnar, M. S., et al. (2004). Human STELLAR, NANOG, and GDF3 genes are expressed in pluripotent cellsand map to chromosome 12p13, a hotspot for teratocarcinoma. *Stem Cells*, 22, 169-179.

[126] Westermann, F. and Schwab, M. (2002). Genetic parameters of neuroblastomas. *Cancer Lett.*, 184, 127-147.

[127] Secombe, J., Pierce, S. B. and Eisenman, R. N. (2004). Myc: a weapon of mass destruction. *Cell*, 117, 153-156.

[128] Miura, M., Miura, Y. and Padilla-Nash, H. M. et al. (2005). Accumulated chromosomal instability in murin bone marrow mesenchymal stem cells leads to malignant transformation. *Stem Cells,* 24, 1095-1103.

[129] Onyango, P., Jiang S. and Uejima, H. et al. (2002). Monoallelic expression and methylation of imprinted genes in human and mouse embryonic germ cell lineages. *Proc. Natl. Acad. Sci.* U S A, 99, 10599-10604.

[130] Jaenisch, R., and Bird, A. (2003). Epigenetic regulation of gene expression: how the genome integrates intrinsic and environmental signals. *Nat. Genet.*, 33, 245-254.

[131] van Gurp, R. J., Oosterhuis, J. W. and Kalscheuer, V., et al. (1994). Biallelic expression of the H19 and IGF2 genes in human testicular germ cell tumors. *J. Natl. Cancer Inst.*, 86, 1070-1075.

[132] Szabo, P. E. and Mann, J. R. (1995). Biallelic expression of imprinted genes in the mouse germ line: implications for erasure, establishment, and mechanisms of genomic

imprinting. *Genes Devel.*, 9, 1857-1868.

[133] Nonomura, N., Miki, T. and Nishimura, K., et al. (1997). Altered imprinting of the H19 and insulin-like growth factor II genes in testicular tumors. *J. Urol.,* 157, 1977-1979.

[134] Nakagawa, H., Chadwick, R. B., Peltomaki, P., et al. (2001). Loss of imprinting of the insulin-like growth factor II gene occurs by biallelic methylation in a core region of H19-associated CTCF-binding sites in colorectal cancer. *Proc. Natl. Acad. Sci.* U S A, 98, 591-596.

[135] Takai, D., Gonzales, F.A., Tsai, Y.C., et al. (2001). Large scale mapping of methylcytosines in CTCF-binding sites in the human H19 promoter and aberrant hypomethylation in human bladder cancer. *Hum. Mol. Genet.*, 10, 2619-2626.

[136] Cui, H., Onyango, P., Brandenburg, S., et al. (2002). Loss of imprinting in colorectal cancer linked to hypomethylation of H19 and IGF2. *Cancer Res.,* 62, 6442-6446.

[137] Hernandez, L., Kozlov, S., Piras, G. and Stewar, C. L. (2003). Paternal and maternal genomes confer opposite effects on proliferation, cell-cycle length, senescence, and tumor formation. *Proc. Natl. Acad. Sci.* U S A, 100, 13344-13349.

[138] Ulaner, G. A., Vu, T. H., Li, T., et al. (2003). Loss of imprinting of IGF2 and H19 in osteosarcoma is accompanied by reciprocal methylation changes of a CTCF-binding site. *Hum. Mol. Genet.*, 12, 535-549.

[139] Feinberg, A. P. and Tycko, B. (2004). The history of cancer epigenetics. *Nat. Rev. Cancer*, 4, 143-153.

[140] Nicholls, R. D. and Knepper, J. L. (2001). Genome organization, function, and imprinting in Prader-Willi and Angelman syndromes. *Annu. Rev. Genomics Hum. Genet*, 2, 153-175.

[141] Weksberg, R., Smith, A. C., Squire, J. and Sadowski, P. (2003). Beckwith-Wiedemann syndrome demonstrates a role for epigenetic control of normal development. *Hum. Mol. Genet.*, 12, 61-68.

[142] Soejima, H. and Wagstaff, J. (2005). Imprinting centers, chromatin structure, and disease. *J. Cell Biochem.*, 95, 226-233.

[143] Okano, M., Bell, D. W., Haber and D. A., Li, E. (1999). DNA methyltransferases Dnmt3a and Dnmt3b are essential for de novo methylation and mammalian development. *Cell*, 99(3), 247-257.

[144] Xu, G. L., Bestor, T. H., Bourc'his, D., et al. (1999). Chromosome instability and immunodeficiency syndrome caused by mutations in a DNA methyltransferase gene. *Nature*, 402 (6758), 187-191.

[145] Fujimoto, A., Mitalipov, S. M., Clepper, L. L. and Wolf, D. P. (2005). Development of a monkey model for the study of primate genomic imprinting. *Mol. Hum. Reprod.* , 11, 413-422.

[146] Rugg-Gunn, P. J., Ferguson-Smith, A. C. and Pedersen, R. A. (2005). Epigenetic status of human embryonic stem cells. *Nat. Genet*, 37, 585-587.

[147] Sun, B. W., Yang, A. C., Feng, Y., et al. (2006). Temporal and parental-specific expression of imprinted genes in a newly derived Chinese human embrionic stem cell line and embryoid bodies. *Hum. Mol. Genet.*, 15, 65-75.

[148] Mitalipov, S., Clepper, L., Sritanaudomchai, H., et al. (2007). Methylation status of imprinting centers for H19/IGF2 and SNURF/SNRPN in primate embryonic stem cells. *Stem Cells*, 25, 581-588.

[149] Burbee, D. G., Forgacs, E., Zochbauer-Muller, S., et al. (2001). Epigenetic inactivation of RASSF1A in lung and breast cancers and malignant phenotype suppression. *J. Natl. Cancer Inst.,* 93, 691-699.

[150] Bhattacharia, B., Miura, T., Brandenberger, R., et al. (2004). Gene expression in human embryonic stem cell lines: unique molecular signature. *Blood*, 103(8), 2956-2961.

[151] Rao, R. R., Calhoun, J. D., Qin, X., et al. (2004). Comparative transcriptional profiling of two human embryonic stem cell lines. *Biotech. Bioengin.*, 88(3), 273-286.

[152] Skottman, H., Mikkola, M., Lundin, K., et al. (2005). Gene expression signatures of seven individual human embryonic stem cell lines. *Stem Cells, 23*, 343-1356.

[153] Ohm, J. E., McGarvey, K. M., Yu, X., et al. (2007). A stem cell–like chromatin pattern may predispose tumor suppressor genes to DNA hypermethylation and heritable silencing. *Nat. Genet.*, 39, 237-242.

[154] Hoffman, L. M., Hall, L., Batten, J. L., et al. (2005). X-inactivation status varies in human embryonic stem cell lines. *Stem Cells*, 23, 1468-1478.

[155] Palmieri, S. L., Peter, W., Hess, H. and Scholer, H.R. (1994). Oct-4 transcription factor is differentially expressed in the mouse embryo during establishment of the first two extraembryonic cell lineages involved in implantation. *Dev. Biol.*, 166, 259-267.

[156] Niwa, H., Miyazaki. J. and Smith, A.G. (2000). Quantitative expression of Oct-3/4 defines differentiation, dedifferentiation or self-renewal of ES cells. *Nat. Genet.*, 24, 372-376.

[157] Boiani, M. and Schöler, H. R. (2005). Regulatory networks in embryo-derived pluripotent stem cells. *Nat. Rev. Mol. Cell Biol.*, 6, 872-884.

[158] Chambers, I., Colby, D., Robertson, M., Nichols, J., Lee, S., Tweedie, S. and Smith, A. (2003). Functional expression cloning of Nanog, a pluripotency sustaining factor in embryonic stem cells. *Cell*, 113, 643-655.

[159] Mitsui, K., Tokuzawa, Y., Itoh, H., Segawa, K., Murakami, M., Takahashi, K., Maruyama, M., Maeda, M. and Yamanaka, S. (2003). The homeoprotein Nanog is required for maintenance of pluripotency in mouse epiblast and ES cells. *Cell*, 113, 631-642.

[160] Hart, A. H., Hartley, L., Ibrahim, M. and Robb, L. (2004). Identification, cloning and expression analysis of the pluripotency promoting Nanog genes in mouse and human. *Dev Dyn.*, 230, 187-198.

[161] Chambers, I. and Smith, A. (2004). Self-renewal of teratocarcinoma and embryonic stem cells. *Oncogene*, 23, 7150-7160.

[162] Niwa, H., Ogawa, K., Shimosato, D. and Adachi, K. (2009). A parallel circuit of LIF signalling pathways maintains pluripotency of mouse ES cells. *Nature*, 460(7251), 118-22.

[163] Josefson, R., Ording, J. C., Liu, Y., et al. (2007). Qualification of Embryonal Carcinoma 2102Ep As a Reference for Human Embryonic Stem Cell Research. *Stem Cells*, 25, 437–446.

[164] Monk, M. and Holding, C. (2001). Human embryonic genes re-expressed in cancer cells. *Oncogene, 20*, 8085-8091

[165] Nakatake, Y., Fukui, N., Iwamatsu, Y., et al. (2006). Klf4 cooperates with Oct3/4 and Sox2 to activate the Lefty1 core promoter in embryonic stem cells. *Mol. Cell Biol.*, 20, 7772-82.

[166] Boyer, L. A., Plath, K. and Zeitlinger, J., et al. (2006). Polycomb complexes repress developmental regulators in murine embryonic stem cells. *Nature*, 441, 349-353.

[167] Lee, T. I., Jenner, R. G., Boyer, L. A., et al. (2006). Control of developmental regulators by Polycomb in human embryonic stem cells. *Cell*, 125, 301-313.

[168] Jones, P. A., Stephen B. and Baylin, S. B. (2007). The Epigenomics of Cancer. *Cell*, 128, 683–692.

[169] Smith, A. G., Heath, J. K., Donaldson, D. D., Wong, G. G., Moreau, J., Stahl, M. and Rogers, D. (1988). Myeloid leukaemia inhibitory factor maintains the developmental potential of embryonic stem cells. *Nature*, 336, 684-687.

[170] Boeuf, H., Hauss, C., Graeve, F. D., Baran, N. and Kedinger, C. (1997). Leukemia inhibitory factor-dependent transcriptional activation in embryonic stem cells. *J Cell Biol., 138*, 1207-1217.

[171] . Niwa, H., Burdon, T., Chambers, I. and Smith, A. (1998). Self-renewal of pluripotent embryonic stem cells is mediated via activation of STAT3. *Genes Dev.*, 12, 2048-2060.

[172] Nichols, J., Davidson, D., Taga, T., Yoshida, K., Chambers, I. and Smith, A. (1996). Complementary tissue-specific expression of LIF and LIF-receptor mRNAs in early mouse embryogenesis. *Mech Dev.*, 57, 123-131.

[173] Daheron, L., Opitz, S. L., Zaehres, H., Lensch, W. M., andrews, P. W., Itskovitz-Eldor, J. and Daley, G. Q. (2004). LIF/STAT3 signaling fails to maintain self-renewal of human embryonic stem cells. *Stem Cells*, 22, 770-778.

[174] Ying, Q. L., Nichols, J., Chambers, I. and Smith, A. (2003). BMP induction of Id proteins suppresses differentiation and sustains embryonic stem cell self-renewal in collaboration with STAT3. *Cell*, 115, 281-292.

[175] Schuldiner, M., Yanuka, O., Itskovitz-Eldor, J., Melton, D. A. and Benvenisty, N. (2000). Effects of eight growth factors on the differentiation of cells derived from human embryonic stem cells. *Proc Natl Acad Sci* U S A, 97, 11307-11312.

[176] Torres, J. and Watt, F. M. (2008). Nanog maintains pluripotency of mouse embryonic stem cells by inhibiting NFkappaB and cooperating with Stat3. *Nat Cell Biol.*, 10(2), 194-201.

[177] Sato, N., Meijer, L., Skaltsounis, L., Greengard, P. and Brivanlou, A. H. (2004). Maintenance of pluripotency in human and mouse embryonic stem cells through activation of Wnt signaling by a pharmacological GSK-3-specific inhibitor. *Nat Med.*, 10, 55-63.

[178] Hao, J., Li, T. G., Qi, X., Zhao, D. F. and Zhao, G. Q. (2006). WNT/beta-catenin pathway up-regulates Stat3 and converges on LIF to prevent differentiation of mouse embryonic stem cells. *Dev Biol.*, 290, 81-91.

[179] Saijoh, Y., Adachi, H., Mochida, K., Ohishi, S., Hirao, A. and Hamada, H. (1999). Distinct transcriptional regulatory mechanisms underlie left-right asymmetric expression of lefty-1 and lefty-2. *Genes Dev.*, 13, 259-269.

[180] Tremblay, K. D., Dunn, N. R. and Robertson, E. J. (2001). *Mouse embryos lacking Smad1 signals display defects in extra-embryonic tissues and germ cell formation. Development*, 128, 3609-3621.

[181] Panchision, D. M., Pickel, J. M., Studer, L., Lee, S. H., Turner, P. A., Hazel, T. G. and McKay, R. D. (2001). Sequential actions of BMP receptors control neural precursor cell production and fate. *Genes Dev.*, 15(16), 2094-2110.

[182] Vincent, S. D., Dunn, N. R., Hayashi, S., Norris, D. P., Robertson, E. J. (2003). Cell fate decisions within the mouse organizer are governed by graded Nodal signals. *Genes Dev.,* 17, 1646-1662.

[183] Derynck, R., Akhurst, R. J. and Balmain, A. (2001). TGF-β signaling in tumor suppression anf cancer progression. *Nat. Genet.,* 29, 117-129.

[184] Sirard, C., de la Pompa, J. L., Elia, A., et al. (1998). The tumor suppressor gene Smad4/Dpc4 is required for gastrulation and later for anterior development of the mouse embryo. *Genes Dev.*, 12, 107-119.

[185] Conlon, F. L., Lyons, K .M., Takaesu, N., et al. (1994). A primary requirement for

nodal in the formation and maintenance of the primitive streak in the mouse. *Development*, 120, 1919-1928.

[186] Robertson, E. J., Norris, D. P., Brennan, J. and Bikoff, E. K. (2003). Control of early anterior-posterior patterning in the mouse embryo by TGF-β signaling. *Philos. Trans. R. Soc. Lond. B Biol. Sci.*, 358, 1351-1357.

[187] Beattie, G. M., Lopez, A. D., Bucay, et al. (2005). Activin A maintains pluripotency of human embryonic stem cells in the absence of feeder layers. *Stem Cells*, 23, 489-495,

[188] James D, Levine A, J., Besser, D. and Hemmati-Brivanlou, A. (2005). TGFbeta/activin/nodal signaling is necessary for the maintenance of pluripotency in human embryonic stem cells. *Development*, 132, 1273-1282.

[189] Xu, R. H., Peck, R. M., Li, D. S., et al. (2005). Basic FGF and suppression of BMP signaling sustain undifferentiated proliferation of human ES cells. *Nat. Methods.*, 2, 185-190.

[190] Smith, J. R., Vallier, L., Lupo, G., Alexander, M., Harris, W. A. and Pedersen, R. A. (2008). Inhibition of Activin/Nodal signaling promotes specification of human embryonic stem cells into neuroectoderm. *Dev Biol.*, 313(1), 107-17.

[191] Parisi, S., D'andrea, D., Lago, C. T., Adamson, E. D., Persico, M. G. and Minchiotti, G. (2003). Nodal-depend Cripto signaling promotes cardiomyogenesis and redirects the neural fate of embryonic stem cells. *J. Cell Biol.*, 163, 303-314.

[192] Kawai, T., Takahashi, T., Esaki, M., Ushikoshi, H., Nagano, S., Fujiwara, H. and Kosai, K. (2004). Efficient cardiomyogenic differentiation of embryonic stem cells by fibroblast growth factor 2 and bone morphogenetic proteins 2. *Circ. J.,* 68, 691-702.

[193] Yuasa, S., Itabashi, Y., Coshimizu, U., Tanaka, T., Sugimura, K., Kinoshita, M., Hattori, F., Fukami, S., Shimazaki, T., Okano, H., et al. (2005). Transient inhibition of BMP signaling by Noggin induces cardiomyocyte differentiation of mouse embryonic stem cells. *Nat. Biotechnol.*, 23, 607-611.

[194] Nostro, M. C., Cheng, X., Keller, G. M. and Gadue, P. (2008). Wnt, activin and BMP signaling regulate distinct stages in the developmental pathway from embryonic stem cells to blood. *Cell Stem Cell.*, 2(1), 60-71.

[195] Krasnikova. N. Iu. and Gordeeva, O. F. (2007). Comparative analysis of expression of TGFbeta family factors and their receptors in mouse embryonic stem and embryonic teratocarcinoma cells. *Ontogenez*, 38(2), 126-135.

[196] Krasnikova, N. Y. and Gordeeva, O. F. (2006). Nodal signaling in the regulation of pluripotent state of human and mouse ES and EC cells. *FEBS*, 273(suppl 1), 126.

In: Encyclopedia of Stem Cell Research (2 Volume Set)   ISBN: 978-1-61761-835-2
Editor: Alexander L. Greene   © 2012 Nova Science Publishers, Inc.

Chapter XLIV

MOLECULAR MECHANISM INVOLVED IN THE MAINTENANCE OF PLURIPOTENT STEM CELLS

***Raymond Ching-Bong Wong[1], Peter J Donovan[1,2]
and Alice Pébay[3]***

[1]Department of Biological Chemistry,
[2]Department of Developmental and Cell biology, University of California Irvine,
Irvine, CA, US
[3]Centre for Neuroscience, Department of Pharmacology The University of Melbourne,
Parkville, Australia and Bernard O'Brien Institute, Fitzroy, VIC, Australia

ABSTRACT

The idea of growing human cells *in vitro* to yield a renewable source of cells for transplantation has captured the imagination of scientists for many years. The derivation of human embryonic stem cells (hESC) represented a major milestone in achieving this goal. hESC are pluripotent and can proliferate *in vitro* indefinitely, rendering them an ideal source for cell replacement therapy. Moreover, recent advances in reprogramming somatic cells into induced pluripotent stem cells (iPS cells) have enabled us to unravel some of the key master regulators of stem cell pluripotency. By integrating recent findings of molecular mechanism involved in maintenance of these different pluripotent stem cell types, we aim to present a global picture of how extracellular signals, intracellular signal transduction pathways and transcriptional networks cooperate together to determine the cell fate of pluripotent stem cells. Unraveling the signaling networks that control stem cell pluripotency will be helpful in deriving novel methods to maintain these pluripotent stem cells *in vitro*.

INTRODUCTION

Human embryonic stem cells (hESC) were originally derived from the inner cell mass of human blastocysts (Thomson, Itskovitz-Eldor et al. 1998; Reubinoff, Pera et al. 2000). They possess the remarkable ability to self-renew indefinitely *in vitro* while maintaining the potential to differentiate into cells representative of the three primary germ layers (Pera, Reubinoff et al. 2000). hESC have great potential for regenerative medicine, and serve as a great model to study the underlying mechanisms of self-renewal and differentiation during human embryo development. Recently, several signaling pathways have emerged to be important players in the maintenance of hESC pluripotency. Moreover, the development of induced pluripotent stem cells (iPS cells) has demonstrated that several key 'stemness' transcription factor can be used to reprogram somatic cells to a pluripotent state (Takahashi, Tanabe et al. 2007; Yu, Vodyanik et al. 2007). In this chapter we review current knowledge of the molecular mechanism that defines cell pluripotency, focusing mainly on human pluripotent stem cells. Learning how to control stem cell pluripotency may point to new methods of up-scaling the production of undifferentiated hESC as well as deriving efficient methods to generate patient-specific iPS cells.

SIGNAL TRANSDUCTION PATHWAYS THAT MAINTAIN PLURIPOTENCY

Differences in Signal Transduction Pathways That Maintain Pluripotency in mESC and hESC

Emerging evidence has suggested that growth factor requirements for maintaining mouse embryonic stem cells (mESC) and hESC are rather different. In mESC, a combination of Leukemia inhibitory factor (LIF) and bone morphogenetic factor 4 (BMP4) can alleviate the need for serum and feeder cells to maintain undifferentiated mESC (Ying, Nichols et al. 2003). However, LIF signaling fails to maintain self-renewal in hESC (Daheron, Opitz et al. 2004; Humphrey, Beattie et al. 2004), and BMP signaling promotes differentiation of hESC (Xu, Chen et al. 2002; Pera, Andrade et al. 2004). Wnt signaling has also emerged as a key player in maintaining mESC pluripotency (Sato, Meijer et al. 2004), but many studies have failed to maintain hESC by activating this signaling pathway (Cheon, Kim et al. 2005; Dravid, Ye et al. 2005). Moreover, Fibroblast growth factor (FGF)-4 stimulation of Erk1/2 signaling caused differentiation in mESC (Kunath, Saba-El-Leil et al. 2007), whereas in hESC the same signaling cascades promote self-renewal (Mayshar, Rom et al. 2008). These results highlight the differences in signaling requirement for pluripotency in hESC and mESC. Instead, recent evidence suggested that the signaling requirement for determining cell fate in hESC is more similar to pluripotent cells derived from the mouse epiblast, termed mouse epiblast stem cells (Brons, Smithers et al. 2007; Vallier, Touboul et al. 2009). Since research in mouse epiblast stem cells is still in its early stage, in this section we will focus on reviewing our current knowledge of the role of various signaling pathways in regulating cell pluripotency in hESC.

The STAT3 Pathway and LIF in hESC

LIF belongs to the Interleukin 6 class cytokine and exert its biological effects by binding to its receptor complex constituted of the transmembrane proteins gp130 and LIFRβ. In turn, receptor activation induces the recruitment of the Janus Kinases (JAK), activation of the Signal Transducer and Activator of Transcription 3 (STAT3) pathway, and transcription of self-renewal genes in mESC (Burdon, Chambers et al. 1999; Burdon, Smith et al. 2002). LIF also activates the Mitogen-Activated Protein Kinases (MAPK)-Extracellular Signal-Regulated Kinase (ERK) 1 and 2 pathway which is involved in mESC differentiation but also proliferation (Burdon, Chambers et al. 1999; Burdon, Stracey et al. 1999; Burdon, Smith et al. 2002). In hESC, LIF activates the STAT3 and the ERK pathways but it is not sufficient to maintain hESC (Thomson, Itskovitz-Eldor et al. 1998; Reubinoff, Pera et al. 2000; Daheron, Opitz et al. 2004; Humphrey, Beattie et al. 2004; Sato, Meijer et al. 2004). Similarly, constitutive activation of STAT3 also fails to maintain hESC (Daheron, Opitz et al. 2004; Humphrey, Beattie et al. 2004), indicating a major difference in signaling requirements between mESC and hESC. It has been hypothesized that the fate of hESC is dependent on the phosphorylation site of the transcription factor STAT3 (Androutsellis-Theotokis, Leker et al. 2006), with the JAK-dependent phosphorylation of Tyr705 leading to hESC differentiation and the JAK-independent Ser727 phosphorylation promoting hESC survival (Androutsellis-Theotokis, Leker et al. 2006). However, as LIF promotes hESC differentiation and induces the phosphorylation of both sites (Daheron, Opitz et al. 2004), further study is needed to confirm this hypothesis.

The Smad Pathways and the TGFβ Superfamily

A number of studies converge to suggest that the Transforming Growth Factor (TGF) β superfamily control essential aspects of hESC pluripotency. The TGFβ superfamily consists of two subfamilies: the TGFβ/Activin/Nodal subfamily which activates the downstream Smad 2/3 proteins; and the BMP/GDF/MIS subfamily which activates Smad 1/5/8 proteins (Figure 1; Miyazawa, Shinozaki et al. 2002; Shi and Massague 2003). TGFβ ligands bind to serine/threonine kinase type II receptors which induce the recruitment of the serine/threonine kinase type I receptors, leading to the activation of either Smad2/3 or Smad 1/5/8 signaling pathways. Subsequently, this induces binding with Smad4 and translocation into the nucleus and regulation of gene expression (Letamendia, Labbe et al. 2001). Activin and nodal bind to type I (Alk4/ActR-IB) and type II (ActR-IIB) receptors, and nodal also binds to another type I (Alk7) receptor (Reissmann, Jornvall et al. 2001; Shi and Massague 2003). This signaling pathway can be regulated by Cripto, an extracellular GPI-linked protein which acts as an accessory receptor (Shi and Massague 2003). On the other hand, BMP act through the receptors BMPIα (Alk2, Alk3) BMPI β (Alk6) and BMPII.

Previous studies demonstrated that the feeder layer of MEF express multiple ligands in the TGFβ superfamily, including TGFβ 1, 2, 3, BMP-2, 4 and Activin A (Beattie, Lopez et al. 2005; Wang, Zhang et al. 2005) as well as the BMP antagonists gremlin and noggin (Pera, Andrade et al. 2004; Xu, Peck et al. 2005). On the other hand, hESC express TGFβ 1, 2, 3, activin, nodal, cripto, BMP-2, BMP-4, BMP-7 and the receptors TGFβR1, 2, 3, BMPIα, BMPIβ and BMPII (Besser 2004; Vallier, Reynolds et al. 2004; Vallier, Alexander et al. 2005; Wang, Zhang et al. 2005; Rho, Yu et al. 2006). Therefore, a paracrine signaling circuit between MEF and hESC as well as an autocrine signaling between hESC is likely to occur to maintain hESC undifferentiated. In undifferentiated hESC, the Smad2/3 pathway is active with Smad 2/3 proteins found to be present within the hESC nucleus (James, Levine et al. 2005; Vallier, Alexander et al. 2005), while the Smad 1/5/8 signaling pathway is repressed. Upon hESC differentiation, Smad2/3 signaling is decreased while Smad1/5/8 is activated (James, Levine et al. 2005; Xu, Peck et al. 2005). It was recently described that the transcriptional regulator TAZ is required for the nuclear accumulation of Smad2/3 and thus regulate the maintenance of hESC by TGFβ (Varelas, Sakuma et al. 2008). In this regard, Activin can induces the phosphorylation of Smad2/3 in hESC (Vallier, Alexander et al. 2005; Wong, Tellis et al. 2007), whereas BMP-4 stimulates the Smad1/5/8 pathway and their subsequent nuclear translocation, an effect independent of the ERK1/2 pathway (Vallier, Alexander et al. 2005). Hence, these results suggested that stimulating Smad 2/3 or repressing Smad1/5/8 would be expected to maintain hESC while the opposite would be hypothesized to induce hESC differentiation.

However, although activin is used to promote hESC self-renewal at lower concentration (5-50 ng/ml), it can promotes definite endoderm differentiation of hESC at a high concentration of 100 ng/ml (D'Amour, Agulnick et al. 2005). Whether its sole incubation is sufficient to maintain hESC in culture on the long-term is somewhat controversial. For instance Vallier et al. (2005) reported that activin delays the short term differentiation of hESC and needs to be co-incubated with bFGF to maintain the long-term hESC pluripotency (Vallier, Alexander et al. 2005). Contrary to this result, Xiao et al. (2006) showed that activin A on its own is able to maintain self-renewal and pluripotency of hESC (Xiao, Yuan et al. 2006). Microarray analysis of gene expression showed that the up-regulation of activin A in hESC is correlated with an increase in the expression of Oct4 and Nanog, and of genes involved in the FGF, Nodal/Activin, Wnt and Hedgehog signaling pathways (Xiao, Yuan et al. 2006). Furthermore, activin A stimulation of Smad2/3 nuclear translocation could also cross-talks with the Wnt signaling (Beattie, Lopez et al. 2005; James, Levine et al. 2005). Clearly, further analysis of the role of activin signaling in hESC is required.

Another member of the TGFβ superfamily, Nodal has also been shown to be involved in maintenance of hESC pluripotency. Indeed, its over-expression in hESC is correlated with a prolonged expression of pluripotent markers and an inhibition of neuroectodermal differentiation upon embryoid body formation (Vallier, Reynolds et al. 2004). Moreover, the inhibition of nodal signaling by Lefty-A down-regulates the expression of stem cell marker Oct4 (Xiao, Yuan et al. 2006), whereas inhibition of nodal by cerberus 1 is accompanied by hESC differentiation (Katoh 2006). However, similar to activin, nodal alone is not sufficient to maintain hESC undifferentiated and would require the presence of bFGF for the long-term maintenance of these cells (Vallier, Alexander et al. 2005). The effects of bFGF and nodal on hESC is dependent on the Activin/Nodal receptors as their inhibition by SB431542 reduces the expression of hESC pluripotency markers (Vallier, Alexander et al. 2005).

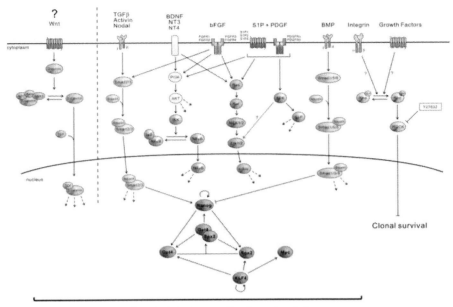

Figure 1. Proposed signaling networks in maintenance of proliferation, survival and pluripotency in hESC. Note that Wnt signaling remains controversial in its role in maintaining undifferentiated hESC. Dotted arrows indicated activation of targets yet to be identified in hESC. Abbreviations not mentioned in the text: MEK: Mitogen-activated protein kinase kinase; SPK: Sphingosine kinase; IκB: Inhibitor of kappa B; IKK: IκB kinase.

On the other hand, BMP have been shown to promote trophoblast differentiation of hESC (Xu, Chen et al. 2002), yet blockage of BMP signaling with noggin does not maintain hESC undifferentiated but promotes neural differentiation (Pera, Andrade et al. 2004; Itsykson, Ilouz et al. 2005). Instead, prolonged culture of undifferentiated hESC can be achieved by a combination of bFGF and blockage of BMP signaling by noggin (Wang, Zhang et al. 2005; Xu, Peck et al. 2005). How bFGF acts in this cooperative effect remains unclear, as it does not inhibit Smad 1/5/8 phosphorylation (Xu, Peck et al. 2005). Taken together, emerging evidence suggested an opposing role of the two Smad pathways in determining the cell fate of hESC: the activation of the Smad2/3 pathway leading to hESC maintenance, while Smad1/5/8 pathway play a pro-differentiation role in hESC (Figure 1).

The ERK, PI3K/Akt and NFκB Pathways in hESC

Various data now point to an important role of constitutively active PI3K/Akt and ERK pathways in the maintenance of hESC. Indeed, these two pathways are active in most culture media used for the maintenance of hESC (Li, Wang et al. 2007). Various pro-maintenance factors activate these signaling pathways in hESC, in particular bFGF, neurotrophins, sphingosine-1-phosphate (S1P) and platelet-derived growth factor (PDGF). The inhibition of the PI3K/Akt pathway has been shown to inhibit hESC proliferation (Li, Wang et al. 2007) and to induce hESC differentiation (Armstrong, Hughes et al. 2006; Li, Wang et al. 2007;

McLean, D'Amour et al. 2007) and apoptosis (Li, Wang et al. 2007; Wong, Tellis et al. 2007). The inhibition of the ERK1/2 pathway induces differentiation and increases cell death in hESC (Armstrong, Hughes et al. 2006; Wong, Tellis et al. 2007), but the latter effect on differentiation is not observed in other study (Li, Wang et al. 2007). Similarly, inhibition of the Nuclear Factor Kappa-light-chain-enhance of activated B cells (NFκB) pathway also leads to differentiation and cell death in hESC (Armstrong, Hughes et al. 2006). How these three pathways crosstalk to each other is not well understood. Some data suggest that the PI3K/Akt pathway is upstream of the ERK1/2 and the NFκB pathways (Armstrong, Hughes et al. 2006) while others suggest that the activation of the ERK1/2 pathway in hESC is independent of the PI3K/Akt pathway (Kang, Kim et al. 2005; Li, Wang et al. 2007; Wong, Tellis et al. 2007). Hence more studies are needed to understand the interaction between these pathways that resulted in maintenance of hESC. Taken together, these results demonstrated the importance of these three pathways in hESC pluripotency, and various culture systems for hESC rely on the addition of growth factors that signal through these three pathways, including bFGF, S1P, PDGF and neurotrophins (Figure 1).

Basic fibroblast growth factor and insulin-like growth factor

bFGF is a member of the FGF family that comprises of at least 22 members in human (Itoh and Ornitz 2004). Alternative splicing of the mRNA results in two different isoforms of bFGF with different cellular effects in human: a low molecular mass isoforms (LMM, 18kDa) and a higher molecular mass isoforms (HMM, 21-24 kDa) (Delrieu 2000). The HMM bFGF isoform is generally localized within the nucleus, while the LMM bFGF isoform is generally cytoplasmic and can also be secreted (Delrieu 2000; Stachowiak, Fang et al. 2003). This secreted form of bFGF can signals through binding to its receptor FGFR1b, 1c, 2c, 3c and 4 (Itoh and Ornitz 2004).. Upon ligand binding, the FGF receptors dimerize and induce phosphorylation of a set of downstream signaling molecules, capable of activating the Erk1/2 pathway, PI3K/Akt pathway and also the phospholipase C (PLC)/protein kinase C (PKC) pathway (Figure 1, Schlessinger 2004).

bFGF is a potent pro-maintenance factor of hESC. bFGF was first used at 4 ng/ml to enhance hESC clonal growth (Amit, Carpenter et al. 2000; Xu, Inokuma et al. 2001) and was subsequently used at higher concentration with unconditioned knockout serum replacement (KSR) to support hESC growth in the absence of feeder cells. Examples of higher concentrations that maintain hESC in culture include: 16 ng/ml bFGF with LIF in a feeder-free system that allowed successful derivation of hESC (Klimanskaya, Chung et al. 2005); and 20-40 ng/ml bFGF to sustain the long-term culture of hESC in some conditions (Wang, Li et al. 2005; Xu, Rosler et al. 2005; Yao, Chen et al. 2006), while 100 ng/ml bFGF is effective in propagating hESC (Levenstein, Ludwig et al. 2005; Ludwig, Levenstein et al. 2006). However, other data showed opposite results, where bFGF (up to 20 ng/ml) decreased hESC colony outgrowth (Dvorak, Dvorakova et al. 2005). The reason why bFGF needs to be added in such high concentration is not fully understood. It is hypothesized that this could be linked to a rapid degradation of bFGF in the culture medium (Levenstein, Ludwig et al. 2005), or high concentration of bFGF can suppresses the pro-differentiation effect of BMP signaling in hESC (Xu, Peck et al. 2005).

The four FGF receptors are expressed by hESC with FGFR1 being dominant, and hESC synthesize multiple members of the FGF family ligand, including FGF-4, FGF-11, FGF-13 and both LMM and HMM isoforms of bFGF (Delrieu 2000; Sato, Sanjuan et al. 2003; Sperger, Chen et al. 2003; Brandenberger, Wei et al. 2004; Ginis, Luo et al. 2004; Itoh and Ornitz 2004; Dvorak, Dvorakova et al. 2005; Kang, Kim et al. 2005; Rho, Yu et al. 2006). The secreted LMM isoform of bFGF could reach a concentration of 80-100 pg/ml in hESC-conditioned medium, suggesting an autocrine and paracrine activation of the FGF receptors within hESC (Dvorak, Dvorakova et al. 2005). It is becoming clear that there is also a paracrine signaling between the feeder layer and hESC involving bFGF. Previous study has shown that bFGF can maintain hESC in the presence of MEF conditioned medium in a feeder-free system (Xu, Inokuma et al. 2001). In a follow up study, Diecke *et al.* (2008) studied the gene expression profile of bFGF-primed MEF to asse   ss whether MEF release pro-maintenance factors. The results showed that upon bFGF treatment MEF up-regulate such as the BMP antagonist gremlin, and molecules involved in the activation of the Smad 2/3 pathway (Diecke, Quiroga-Negreira et al. 2008). Recent study also demonstrated that hESC-derived fibroblasts respond to bFGF and secret insulin-like growth factors (IGF), which acts on hESC to maintain pluripotency by activation of the PI3K/Akt pathway (Bendall, Stewart et al. 2007; McLean, D'Amour et al. 2007). Hence, the effect of bFGF on hESC maintenance can also be indirect, by inducing IGF release from more differentiated cells that in turn signal to maintain hESC undifferentiated (Gotoh 2009).

In hESC, bFGF activates the ERK1/2 pathway with subsequent *c-fos* expression (Dvorak, Dvorakova et al. 2005; Kang, Kim et al. 2005; Li, Wang et al. 2007) but also crosstalks with members of the TGFβ superfamily (such as BMPs, TGFβ1, nodal and activin) (Amit, Shariki et al. 2004; Vallier, Alexander et al. 2005; Wang, Zhang et al. 2005; Xu, Peck et al. 2005). Indeed, addition of the BMP inhibitor noggin, together with bFGF maintain hESC undifferentiated (Wang, Zhang et al. 2005; Xu, Peck et al. 2005), yet bFGF does not inhibit BMP-4 stimulation of Smad 1/5/8 signaling in hESC (Vallier, Alexander et al. 2005), suggesting that bFGF does not act on the Smad 1/5/8 pathway *per se*. As bFGF's impact on pluripotency is dependent on the activin/nodal signaling within hESC, bFGF might be a "competence factor" for the activin/nodal signaling in hESC maintenance   (Vallier, Alexander et al. 2005).

Neurotrophins

The neurotrophin family includes Nerve Growth Factor (NGF), Brain-Derived Neurotrophic Factor (BDNF) and Neurotrophins (NT) 3 and 4 which bind their specific receptors Tropomyosin Receptor Kinases (TRK) A, B and C and the p75 neurotrophin receptor (p75NGFR) (Figure 1, Lu, Pang et al. 2005). Limited research have study the role of neurotrophins in hESC. hESC express high levels of TRKB and TRKC, while MEF express NGF, BDNF, NT3 and NT4 while (Pyle, Lock et al. 2006). Importantly, neurotrophins have been shown to increase hESC clonal survival and viability, an effect that is largely attributed to activation of the PI3K/Akt pathway (Pyle, Lock et al. 2006).

Sphingosine-1-phosphate and platelet-derived growth factor

Sphingosine-1-phosphate (S1P) is a bioactive lysophospholipid that binds its specific receptors $S1P_{1-5}$ which are coupled to at least three G protein families, G_i, G_q and G_{12} (Chun, Goetzl et al. 2002; Takuwa, Takuwa et al. 2002), while Platelet Derived Growth Factor (PDGF) binds to two specific tyrosine kinase receptors PDGFRα and PDGFRß. The two factors can cooperate to activate classical protein kinase signaling pathways, including the sphingosine kinases (SPK) which generate intracellular S1P (Figure 1). Both MEF and hESC express $S1P_{1-3}$, PDGFRα and PDGFRß (Pebay, Wong et al. 2005; Inniss and Moore 2006). Different profiles of lipid content of sphingosine, S1P, sphingomyelin and glucosylceramide were found in hESC than in MEF (Brimble, Sherrer et al. 2007), suggesting that MEF may release bioactive sphingolipids in the culture medium which could account for some of the MEF-mediated effects on hESC. Importantly, S1P and PDGF have been demonstrated to maintain hESC pluripotency and proliferation and inhibit apoptosis (Pebay, Wong et al. 2005; Inniss and Moore 2006; Wong, Tellis et al. 2007), allowing long-term maintenance of hESC in the presence of MEF (Pebay, Wong et al. 2005). However, S1P on its own is not sufficient to maintain hESC (Pebay, Wong et al. 2005). Recently, a micro-array analysis showed that S1P up-regulates anti-apoptotic genes, cell cycle progression and cell adhesion genes and down-regulates pro-apoptotic genes (Avery, Avery et al. 2008). However, S1P also down-regulates pluripotency genes such as *nanog* and *Oct-4* (Avery, Avery et al. 2008), confirming that S1P by itself is not sufficient to maintain hESC undifferentiated. Both S1P and PDGF stimulate the ERK1/2 pathway and PDGF also stimulates the PI3K/Akt pathway, and the two pathways are necessary to the anti-apoptotic effect of S1P and PDGF in hESC (Wong, Tellis et al. 2007; Avery, Avery et al. 2008). Interestingly, neither S1P nor PDGF modifies Smad2 phosphorylation in hESC, even after two hours of incubation, thus raising the possibility that hESC maintenance can be achieved without activation of the Smad2/3 signaling pathway (Wong, Tellis et al. 2007). Moreover, S1P and PDGF also stimulate other branches of the MAPK pathways, p38 and JNK1/2 phosphorylation, with physiological consequences yet to be identified (Pitson and Pebay Submitted).

The Wnt Signaling in hESC

Wnts are lipid modified glycoproteins that bind to their membrane receptor complex constituted of Frizzled and Low-density-Lysoprotein-Related-Protein5/6 (LRP). In the absence of canonical Wnt signaling, cytoplasmic β-catenin is bound in a complex with Glycogen Synthase Kinase (GSK)-3-beta, Axin, and Adenomatosis Polyposis Coli (APC), resulting in its phosphorylation and subsequent degradation via the ubiquitin pathway. Upon Wnt binding to its receptors, the protein Dishevelled mediates the inhibition of GSK-3 phosphorylation of beta-catenin, leading to the accumulation of cytosolic β-catenin, followed by its nuclear translocation where β-catenin acts as a transcriptional cofactor of T cell factor (TCF)/ Lymphoid Enhancer Binding Factor1 (Figure 1, Cadigan and Liu 2006).

MEF express transcripts of Wnt2, Wnt4, Wnt5a, Wnt6 and the Wnt inhibitors Dkk-1 and Dkk-3 (Sato, Meijer et al. 2004; Dravid, Ye et al. 2005; Wang, Zhang et al. 2005). Although Wnt1, Wnt3, and Dkk-1 have been found to be expressed in hESC (Walsh and Andrews

2003; Rho, Yu et al. 2006), other studies found no evidence of Wnt ligands in hESC (Brandenberger, Wei et al. 2004; Davidson, Jamshidi et al. 2007). In addition, in hESC only a low level of β-catenin/TCF mediated activation were detected, suggesting that the canonical Wnt signaling pathway is inactive in undifferentiated hESC (Dravid, Ye et al. 2005). Previous report from Sato et al. (2004) claimed that the activation of the Wnt signaling pathway - by either Wnt3a or the GSK-3 inhibitor, 6-bromoindirubin-3'-oxime (BIO) maintains hESC undifferentiated and pluripotent (Sato, Meijer et al. 2004). Yet, these data were not reproduced with the use of another GSK-3 inhibitor LiCl (Sato, Meijer et al. 2004) and other studies have failed to maintain hESC using either Wnt3a, BIO, or by blocking endogenous Wnt signaling using Frizzled-Related Protein 2 (FRP2) and Dkk-1 (Cheon, Kim et al. 2005; Dravid, Ye et al. 2005). Despite its inability to maintain pluripotency, Wnt3a appears to increase single-cell survival (Hasegawa, Fujioka et al. 2006) and to stimulate proliferation in hESC, an effect that is dependent on the presence of an undefined anti-differentiation factors (Dravid, Ye et al. 2005). Candidates of such factors are hypothesized to be members of the TGFβ superfamily (James, Levine et al. 2005). More research is needed to clarify the role of Wnt signaling in the maintenance of hESC.

The Rho/ROCK Pathway in hESC

The Rho/ROCK pathway is also involved in regulating hESC clonal survival (Figure 1). Indeed, data suggest that the Rho/ROCK pathway is activated in hESC and responsible for cell-cell contacts (Harb, Archer et al. 2008), and the inhibition of ROCK significantly increases hESC single cell survival (Watanabe, Ueno et al. 2007; Damoiseaux, Sherman et al. 2008). These data have allowed the development of new techniques to improve hESC culture and cryopreservation (Li, Meng et al. 2008; Claassen, Desler et al. 2009; Heng 2009; Li, Krawetz et al. 2009). Furthermore, it is hypothesized that ROCK inhibition may not act directly by reducing apoptosis, but rather act by desensitizing cells to their environment thus limiting apoptosis (Krawetz, Li et al. 2009). Further work is now needed to confirm this hypothesis and also identify whether pro- and anti-differentiation factors modulate the Rho/ROCK signaling axis.

TRANSCRIPTIONAL NETWORK GOVERNING PLURIPOTENCY IN MOUSE AND hESC

The signaling pathways discussed previously eventually lead to activation of a transcriptional program that govern cell pluripotency, by activating genes that support self-renewal and repressing genes that promote differentiation. Several transcription factors have been identified as key regulators in this transcriptional network, including Oct4, Sox2 and Nanog. Using genome-wide mapping analysis, previous studies have demonstrated that Oct4, Sox2 and Nanog co-occupy a substantial portion of their target genes in hESC (Boyer, Lee et al. 2005) and mESC (Chen, Xu et al. 2008; Kim, Chu et al. 2008). Furthermore, they are able to regulate each other and effectively forming a core regulatory circuitry regulating stem cell pluripotency, where Oct4, Sox2 and Nanog are proposed to be the master regulators of this transcriptional network.

In addition to Oct4, Sox2 and Nanog, the recent development of iPS cells have also confirmed the important roles of other genes in regulating cell pluripotency. An elegant experiment by Takahashi et al. (2007) demonstrated that mouse somatic cells can be reprogrammed to a pluripotent state using four transcription factors Oct4, Sox2, c-Myc and Klf4 (Takahashi and Yamanaka 2006). Subsequent study by the same group has demonstrated that the same four factors used in mice can be used to generate human iPS cells (Takahashi, Tanabe et al. 2007). These suggested that although the upstream signal transduction pathways regulating pluripotency are different in mESC and hESC (see discussion in previous section), the downstream transcriptional network that defines pluripotency may be similar in mouse and human. In this aspect, studies in early mouse embryos or mESC are helpful in understanding this transcriptional network in defining hESC pluripotency. Subsequently, Nanog and Lin28 have also been used for generation of iPS cells (Yu, Vodyanik et al. 2007). In this section, we will discuss the role of these factors in regulating cell pluripotency in early mouse embryo, mESC and hESC.

Oct4

Oct4, also known as Oct3 or Pou5F1, is one of the most extensively studied transcription factors associated with pluripotent cells of the embryo (Scholer, Balling et al. 1989; Okamoto, Okazawa et al. 1990; Rosner, Vigano et al. 1990). It belongs to a family of transcription factors containing the POU DNA binding domain. In the developing mouse embryo, Oct4 is restricted to the inner cell mass, primitive ectoderm, and later in primordial germ cells (Pesce and Scholer 2001). *In vitro*, Oct4 is expressed in undifferentiated EC cells and ESC and down-regulated upon differentiation (Rosner, Vigano et al. 1990; Assou, Le Carrour et al. 2007). This restricted expression of Oct4 renders it a useful marker for stem cell pluripotency. However, this simplistic view should be treated cautiously, as Oct4 seems to regulate pluripotency in a dosage-dependent manner. Transient increase in Oct4 expression has been observed in mESC during mesodermal differentiation (Zeineddine, Papadimou et al. 2006). In support of this, previous studies have demonstrated that transgene-mediated increase of Oct4 level in mESC drives differentiation into extraembryonic endoderm, mesoderm or neuroectoderm under different conditions (Niwa, Miyazaki et al. 2000; Shimozaki, Nakashima et al. 2003; Zeineddine, Papadimou et al. 2006). Therefore, a precise level of Oct4 is required in maintaining cell pluripotency.

Pluripotency in early embryo or ESC depends on the tight control of Oct4 expression. Knockout of Oct4 in mice resulted in embryonic lethality due to failure to form the inner cell mass, and *in vitro* culture of Oct4 knockout embryos showed that the inner cell mass cells loss pluripotency and differentiate into trophectoderm cells (Nichols, Zevnik et al. 1998). Subsequent studies have shown that Oct4 can directly inhibit Cdx2, Eomes and hCG, three important regulators in trophectoderm differentiation (Liu and Roberts 1996; Liu, Leaman et al. 1997; Niwa, Toyooka et al. 2005). Therefore, Oct4 is generally viewed as a repressor for trophectoderm differentiation as well as required for maintaining pluripotency in the inner cell mass. Consistent with this idea, siRNA mediated knockdown of Oct4 resulted in trophectoderm differentiation in both hESC and mESC (Niwa, Miyazaki et al. 2000; Matin, Walsh et al. 2004; Zaehres, Lensch et al. 2005; Fong, Hohenstein et al. 2008; Hohenstein, Pyle et al. 2008).

In human, several splice variants of Oct4 are reported, including Oct4a, Oct4b and recently Oct4b1 (Takeda, Seino et al. 1992; Atlasi, Mowla et al. 2008). While Oct4a and Oct4b1 are restricted to pluripotent cells, Oct4b is expressed in many nonpluripotent cell types (Atlasi, Mowla et al. 2008). Importantly, Oct4a is expressed in the nucleus and confers stem cell pluripotency, while Oct4b is expressed in the cytoplasm and cannot sustains stem cell self-renewal (Lee, Kim et al. 2006). On the other hand, the function of Oct4b1 is not well understood. These facts point out the importance of choosing the right tools for the study of Oct4 in human, and it also suggest a more complex picture of how Oct4 act to maintain cell pluripotency.

To date, all protocols for generating iPS cells require the addition of Oct4, suggesting its importance as a master regulator in governing cell pluripotency (Feng, Ng et al. 2009). However, it is apparent that Oct4 on its own is not sufficient to induce pluripotency and the presences of binding partners determine whether the target genes are activated or repressed. For example, when Oct4 binds to FoxD3, it functions as a corepressor to inhibit FoxD3 activation of the endodermal genes FoxA1 and FoxA2, effectively preventing ESC from differentiation (Guo, Costa et al. 2002). On the other hand, Sox2 represents an important binding partner for Oct4 to activate stem cell specific genes, such as Sox2, Fbx10, FGF4 and UTF1 (Yuan, Corbi et al. 1995; Ambrosetti, Basilico et al. 1997; Okuda, Fukushima et al. 1998; Tomioka, Nishimoto et al. 2002; Tokuzawa, Kaiho et al. 2003).

Sox2

The SRY-related HMG box (Sox) gene family encodes transcription factors with a single HMG DNA-binding domain. In the developing mouse embryo, Sox2 is expressed in pluripotent cells of the inner cell mass and epiblast, primodial germ cells as well as multipotent cells of extraembryonic ectoderm (Avilion, Nicolis et al. 2003). Unlike Oct4, Sox2 expression is persistent in neural stem cells throughout development (Ellis, Fagan et al. 2004). Sox2 knockout mice die shortly after implantation due to defects in epiblast formation (Avilion, Nicolis et al. 2003). *In vitro*, Sox2 is expressed in undifferentiated ESC and can be use as a marker to select for neural progenitor cells upon embryoid bodies formation (Li, Pevny et al. 1998). Consistent with this idea, Sox2 overexpression in mESC biased the cells towards neural differentiation (Zhao, Nichols et al. 2004; Kopp, Ormsbee et al. 2008).

On the other hand, siRNA-mediated knockdown of Sox2 in hESC resulted in trophectoderm differentiation (Fong, Hohenstein et al. 2008). Similar results are seen in mESC using a dominant negative form of Sox2 (Li, Pan et al. 2007) or an inducible knockout system (Masui, Nakatake et al. 2007). However, ectopic expression of Oct4 can rescue this phenotype in mESC, suggesting that the essential function of Sox2 is to maintain Oct4 expression (Masui, Nakatake et al. 2007). Surprisingly, the expression of many Oct4/Sox2 target genes was not affected by the loss of Sox2. This suggested that the role of Sox2 may be compensated by other Sox family members, such as Sox4, Sox11 and Sox15 present in ESC.

Sox2 is involved in defining distinct cell fates that is largely dependent on its binding partner: Pax6 for lens differentiation, Brn2 for neural differentiation, and Oct4 for maintaining pluripotency in ESC (Kondoh, Uchikawa et al. 2004). In the latter case, the interaction between Sox2 and Oct4 had been implicated in stimulating expression of FGF4 (Ambrosetti, Basilico et al. 1997), UTF1 (Nishimoto, Fukushima et al. 1999; Nishimoto, Miyagi et al. 2005) and Nanog (Kuroda, Tada et al. 2005; Rodda, Chew et al. 2005), all of which are important in maintenance of ESC. Moreover, the Oct4-Sox2 complex can stimulate the expression of Oct4 and Sox2 itself, effectively forming a positive feedback loop to maintain pluripotency in ESC (Figure 1, Chew, Loh et al. 2005).

Nanog

Nanog is a homeodomain protein that was recently identified as a new master regulator for maintenance of stem cell pluripotency (Chambers, Colby et al. 2003; Mitsui, Tokuzawa et al. 2003). Similar to Oct4, Nanog is restricted to the inner cell mass, epiblast and primodial germ cells in the developing embryo. *In vitro*, Nanog is highly enriched in a number of pluripotent cells lines such as ESC, EC cells and embryonic germ (EG) cells (Chambers, Colby et al. 2003). Previous reports demonstrated an important role of Nanog in maintaining pluripotency. Overexpression of Nanog prevents mESC from differentiation (Chambers, Colby et al. 2003; Ivanova, Dobrin et al. 2006). However, in the absence of Oct4, Nanog alone is not enough to sustain self-renewal in mESC (Chambers, Colby et al. 2003). Similarly in hESC, overexpression of Nanog enables hESC to stay undifferentiated in conditions that favour differentiation (Darr, Mayshar et al. 2006).

On the other hand, Nanog-null mouse embryos fail to form inner cell mass, and *in vitro* culture has shown that the mutant inner cell mass differentiates into parietal endoderm-like cells (Mitsui, Tokuzawa et al. 2003). Moreover, reduction of Nanog drives differentiation to multi-lineage cells in mESC (Mitsui, Tokuzawa et al. 2003; Hatano, Tada et al. 2005; Ivanova, Dobrin et al. 2006) and hESC (Hyslop, Stojkovic et al. 2005; Zaehres, Lensch et al. 2005; Fong, Hohenstein et al. 2008). All of these studies point to an indispensible role of Nanog in safeguarding pluripotency. However, this view is being challenged by a recent experiment from Chambers et al. (2007), where the authors demonstrated that in the absence of Nanog undifferentiated mESC can persist with normal self-renewal and differentiation potentials (Chambers, Silva et al. 2007). Moreover, the authors show that down-regulation of Nanog expression is reversible, and transient down-regulation of Nanog does not mark commitment to differentiate unless the extrinsic conditions favour differentiation (Chambers, Silva et al. 2007). Taken together, Nanog is presented as an important regulator in pluripotency, but unlike Oct4 and Sox2, it is not essential in housekeeping stem cell pluripotency.

Nanog can physically interact with Oct4 (Wang, Rao et al. 2006) and cooperates extensively with Oct4 and Sox2 in the core-transcriptional network both in human (Boyer, Lee et al. 2005) and mESC (Chen, Xu et al. 2008; Kim, Chu et al. 2008). In this aspect, Oct4,

Sox2 and Nanog can also bind to their own promoters, thus forming an autoregulation loop to maintain ESC self-renewal (Figure 1, Boyer, Lee et al. 2005). Moreover, in mESC it has been demonstrated that Nanog can also interact with Smad1 to block BMP-induced differentiation (Suzuki, Raya et al. 2006).

Klf4

The role of *Klf4* and its family members in the maintenance of pluripotency have not been realized until recently. Klf4 belongs to the Krüppel-like factor family of zinc finger transcription factors, whose members have important roles in regulating different physiological processes (McConnell, Ghaleb et al. 2007; Evans and Liu 2008). Klf4 can be an oncogene or a tumor suppressing gene depending on the cell context (Rowland and Peeper 2006). Together with Oct4, Sox2 and c-Myc, Klf4 have demonstrated its ability to reprogram somatic cells back to a pluripotent state (Takahashi and Yamanaka 2006; Takahashi, Tanabe et al. 2007). Overexpression of Klf4 also prevents differentiation into erythroid progenitors in mESC, indicating it is an important regulator of cell pluripotency (Li, McClintick et al. 2005).

Klf4 knockout mice die soon after birth due to dehydration caused by defects in the epidermal barrier of the skin (Segre, Bauer et al. 1999). However, these knockout mice are normal during early embryo development in their pluripotent stem cell populations. Similarly, although Klf4 is an abundant transcript in mESC, knocking down Klf4 does not generate an obvious phenotype (Nakatake, Fukui et al. 2006; Jiang, Chan et al. 2008). One explanation is that there may be functional redundancy among other Klf family members in ESC. Indeed, triple knockdown of the Klf2, Klf4 and Klf5 resulted in rapid differentiation in mESC (Jiang, Chan et al. 2008). Consistent with this idea, other Klf family members (Klf1, Klf2 or Klf5) can substitute for Klf4 in the generation of iPS cells (Nakagawa, Koyanagi et al. 2008).

However, not all Klf factors have totally redundant functions. A recent study by Ema et al. (2008) demonstrated that knockout of Klf5 in mice resulted in early embryo lethality due to defects in implantation, a result in sharp contrast to Klf4 knockout mice. Furthermore, knockout of Klf5 in mESC leads to rapid differentiation whereas Klf5 overexpression confers resistance to differentiation and increase in proliferation (Ema, Mori et al. 2008). Importantly, ectopic expression of Klf4 can rescue the differentiation phenotype in Klf5-null mESC, but proliferation is markedly decreased. These results suggested that although Klf4 and Klf5 have a similar function in suppressing differentiation, they may play an opposing role in proliferation as observed in other cell types (Ghaleb, Nandan et al. 2005).

The precise mechanism of how Klf4 contributes to somatic cell reprogramming or maintaining pluripotency remains unclear. Previous studies have demonstrated that Klf4 is not essential in iPS cell generation (Yu, Vodyanik et al. 2007). But rather, Klf4 serves as a secondary factor to enhance iPS cell generation. One hypothesis is that Klf4 may act synergistically with Oct4, Sox2 and Nanog to restart the pluripotent stem cell-specific gene expression program. In mESC, Klf4 can cooperate with Oct4 and Sox2 to activate a subset of ESC specific genes (Nakatake, Fukui et al. 2006). Through global mapping of promoter analysis, in mESC Klf4 has been demonstrated to bind to the promoter of Oct4, Sox2, Nanog, Myc and Klf4 itself (Figure 1, Chen, Xu et al. 2008; Kim, Chu et al. 2008). Whether the same interaction is conversed in hESC is not confirmed yet, but in hESC Klf4 can directly bind and activate expression of Nanog (Chan, Zhang et al. 2009). Furthermore, many Klf family members share similar target genes with Nanog, suggesting Klf proteins are important components of the transcriptional network regulating cell pluripotency (Jiang, Chan et al. 2008). Another hypothesis is that Klf4 acts as an inhibitor of apoptosis which in turn help somatic cell reprogramming. Klf4 is a negative regulator of p53 (Rowland, Bernards et al. 2005), therefore this could counteract the effect of c-Myc in inducing p53-mediated apoptosis during reprogramming (Adhikary and Eilers 2005). Studies that address whether p53 depletion in somatic cells can enhance iPS cell generation will be particularly interesting in this context.

Lin28

Lin28 was first identified as a heterochronic gene that regulates the developmental timing pathway in *Caenorhabditis Elegans*, where mutation of Lin28 leads to precocious development and gain of function allele leads to retarded development (Moss, Lee et al. 1997). Lin28 encodes for a cytoplasmic RNA binding protein that contains a cold shock domain and retroviral type zinc finger motifs and has been implicated as a translational enhancer (Polesskaya, Cuvellier et al. 2007).

Lin28 was identified as a hESC-specific gene in transcriptome study by serial analysis of gene expression (SAGE) (Richards, Tan et al. 2004). However, functional studies of Lin28 in hESC and mESC have yielded opposing results. Overexpression of Lin28 resulted in accelerated cell proliferation in mESC (Xu, Zhang et al. 2009), but seemed to slow down proliferation and cause extraembryonic endoderm differentiation in hESC (Darr and Benvenisty 2009). Conversely, knockdown of Lin28 resulted in decreased cell proliferation in mESC (Xu, Zhang et al. 2009), while in hESC there is no obvious phenotype (Darr and Benvenisty 2009). Whether Lin28 play a different role in human and mouse is unclear at the moment. However in human, Lin28 seemed to be dispensable for ESC self-renewal but is involved in differentiation commitment (Darr and Benvenisty 2009). At this point, it is worth noting that although Lin28 is used in conjunction with Nanog, Oct-4, and Sox2 to reprogram human fibroblast to pluripotency, it only has a modest effect on reprogramming (Yu, Vodyanik et al. 2007). Moreover, Lin28 can be replaced by other combinations of transcription factors (Takahashi, Tanabe et al. 2007). Together, this suggests that Lin28 may not be a core component of the transcriptional network governing ESC pluripotency, but rather an enhancer to induce pluripotency much like Klf4. Clearly, a complete understanding of the role of Lin28 in ESC self-renewal and iPS cell reprogramming awaits further study.

How Lin28 contributes to maintain ESC pluripotency is intriguing at the moment. One proposed mechanism is that Lin28 acts to block the processing of let7 microRNA family members, a group of microRNA associated with differentiation (Viswanathan, Daley et al. 2008). Moreover, let7 has been suggested to act as tumor suppressor by repressing oncogene expression such as c-Myc and Ras, therefore Lin28 may be promoting oncogenic proliferation by down-regulating let7 (Peter 2009). Another proposed mechanism of Lin28 is that it may acts to stabilize and enhance translation of certain mRNAs that are critical for pluripotency. A previous study have demonstrated that Lin28 can reside in both polysomal ribosome fractions, in which mRNA is translated, and also P-bodies, in which mRNA is degraded (Balzer and Moss 2007). Therefore, Lin28 may regulate pluripotency by selectively enhancing translation for certain mRNA while degrading other mRNA.

Myc

The Myc gene family has been intensively studied for more than two decades. c-Myc have a well documented role in cancer biology. Deregulated levels of c-Myc have been observed in human cancers and demonstrated to promote cell transformation and tumor progression (Kendall, Adam et al. 2006). c-Myc is believed to regulate the expression of 15% of all genes, including genes involved in cellular apoptosis, cell cycle control, protein biosynthesis and metabolism (Patel, Loboda et al. 2004). c-Myc has been shown to regulate its target genes through interactions with chromatin remodeling complexes, histone modifying enzymes, DNA methyltransferases and general components of the transcription machinery (Eilers and Eisenman 2008).

Research addressing the role of Myc in pluripotent cells in the pre-implantation embryo has yielded contradictory results. In mouse embryo, c-Myc expression is initiated at the four-cell stage and is highly expressed during the blastocyst stage (Paria, Dey et al. 1992). Knockdown of c-Myc using antisense DNA leads to developmental arrest before the blastocyst stage, suggesting a critical role of c-Myc in early mouse embryo (Paria, Dey et al. 1992; Naz, Kumar et al. 1994). However, knockout studies of c-Myc or another family member N-Myc in mice resulted in embryo lethality but die at a much later time at E9.5-E12.5 (Charron, Malynn et al. 1992; Stanton, Perkins et al. 1992; Davis, Wims et al. 1993). The reason for this contradiction in previous studies is unclear at this stage, and further study is needed to clarify the role of Myc in pluripotent cells in early embryo.

Previous studies have demonstrated that c-Myc play a critical role in mESC. Sustained expression of c-Myc renders mESC resistant to differentiation, whereas expression of a dominant negative form of c-Myc antagonizes self-renewal and promotes differentiation (Cartwright, McLean et al. 2005). Surprisingly, c-Myc behaves quite differently in hESC. Overexpression of c-Myc drives hESC to apoptosis and differentiation into extraembryonic endoderm and trophectoderm (Sumi, Tsuneyoshi et al. 2007). In this latter study, the authors also demonstrated that blockage of p53 and caspase signaling effectively prevent the apoptosis phenotype evoked by c-Myc, but the differentiation phenotype still occurs in c-Myc overexpressing cells. Therefore, it is unlikely that c-Myc-driven apoptotic signals are driving hESC to differentiate (Sumi, Tsuneyoshi et al. 2007).

c-Myc was identified as one of four factors able to generate both mouse and human iPS cells (Takahashi and Yamanaka 2006; Takahashi, Tanabe et al. 2007). However, subsequent studies demonstrated that somatic cell reprogramming can be achieved without addition of c-Myc, although with significantly reduced efficiency and kinetics (Nakagawa, Koyanagi et al. 2008; Wernig, Meissner et al. 2008). Moreover, Klf4 and c-Myc can be replaced by a combination of Nanog and Lin28, suggesting that c-Myc is not essential for induced pluripotency (Yu, Vodyanik et al. 2007). How c-Myc contributes to induced pluripotency is an area under intense study right now. Recent evidence suggest that c-Myc play an important part during early reprogramming by down-regulating somatic gene expressions, a process that occurs before the activation of the pluripotency gene networks (Sridharan, Tchieu et al. 2009). Genome-wide analysis of promoter binding demonstrated that c-Myc regulates a different set of target genes compared to other pluripotency factors Oct4, Sox2 and Klf4 in mESC (Chen, Xu et al. 2008; Kim, Chu et al. 2008). This suggests that the function of c-Myc in ESC maybe very different to other 'stemness' transcription factors. One proposed function of c-Myc is that it may induce a cell cycle program that is necessary for self-renewal of stem cells. Previous studies have demonstrated that c-Myc can activate proliferation-associated genes (i.e. cyclin A, cyclin E or E2F) and suppresses genes associated with growth arrest (i.e. p21, p27) (Vermeulen, Berneman et al. 2003). Moreover, Myc has a documented role in maintaining the epigenetic status of chromatin (Knoepfler, Zhang et al. 2006). Thus another proposed mechanism for c-Myc is that it can modify the chromatin structure to allow expression of genes that promote self-renewal and inhibit expression of pro-differentiation genes.

CONCLUSION

As summarized in Figure 1, this chapter has provided a detailed review of the signal transduction pathways and the transcriptional network regulating self-renewal in ESC. Emerging evidence suggests that no one signaling pathways is sufficient to maintain hESC undifferentiated on its own. Instead, multiple signaling pathways cooperate together to achieve self-renewal, such as activin and bFGF signaling. The interactions between these signaling pathways are still poorly understood. Similarly, in the transcriptional network not one transcription factor is sufficient to maintain ESC pluripotency, but the important genes such as Oct4, Sox2, Nanog and Klf4 often cooperate together to activate a gene expression program that governs stem cell self-renewal. As limited studies have attempted to link the upstream signaling pathways to the downstream transcriptional network that regulate cell pluripotency, this remains a major challenge for future research in hESC. For instance, in hESC activin stimulation of Smad2/3 binds and activates Nanog, whereas BMP stimulation of Smad1 binds and represses Nanog (Xu, Sampsell-Barron et al. 2008). Future research that bridges the gap between the upstream signaling pathways with the downstream transcriptional network will help to unravel this complex molecular mechanism governing stem cell pluripotency. These studies in turn will help in the goal of using human pluripotent stem cells to develop mew treatments for human disease as well as provide critical insigits into early human development.

ACKNOWLEDGMENTS

The authors wish to thank Dr. Sandy S.C. Hung for proof reading the manuscript and helping with generating the figure. The authors are also grateful to supports from California Institute of Regenerative Medicine (Grant T1-00008 to Raymond C.B. Wong, RCI-00110 to Peter J. Donovan), National Institute of Health (Grant HD49488 and HD47675 to Peter J. Donovan), University of Melbourne, National Health and Medical Research Council of Australia (Grant 454723 to Alice Pébay) and Friedreich Ataxia Research Association.

REFERENCES

Adhikary, S. and Eilers, M. (2005). "Transcriptional regulation and transformation by Myc proteins." *Nat Rev Mol Cell Biol* 6(8): 635-45.

Ambrosetti, D. C., Basilico, C., et al. (1997). "Synergistic activation of the fibroblast growth factor 4 enhancer by Sox2 and Oct-3 depends on protein-protein interactions facilitated by a specific spatial arrangement of factor binding sites." *Mol Cell Biol* 17(11): 6321-9.

Amit, M., Carpenter, M. K., et al. (2000). "Clonally derived human embryonic stem cell lines maintain pluripotency and proliferative potential for prolonged periods of culture." *Dev Biol* 227(2): 271-8.

Amit, M., Shariki, C., et al. (2004). "Feeder layer- and serum-free culture of human embryonic stem cells." *Biol Reprod* 70(3): 837-45.

Androutsellis-Theotokis, A., Leker, R. R., et al. (2006). "Notch signalling regulates stem cell numbers in vitro and in vivo." *Nature* 442(7104): 823-6.

Armstrong, L., Hughes, O., et al. (2006). "The role of PI3K/AKT, MAPK/ERK and NFkappabeta signalling in the maintenance of human embryonic stem cell pluripotency and viability highlighted by transcriptional profiling and functional analysis." *Hum Mol Genet* 15(11): 1894-913.

Assou, S., Le Carrour, T., et al. (2007). "A meta-analysis of human embryonic stem cells transcriptome integrated into a web-based expression atlas." *Stem Cells* 25(4): 961-73.

Atlasi, Y., Mowla, S. J., et al. (2008). "OCT4 spliced variants are differentially expressed in human pluripotent and nonpluripotent cells." *Stem Cells* 26(12): 3068-74.

Avery, K., Avery, S., et al. (2008). "Sphingosine-1-phosphate mediates transcriptional regulation of key targets associated with survival, proliferation, and pluripotency in human embryonic stem cells." *Stem Cells Dev* 17(6): 1195-205.

Avilion, A. A., Nicolis, S. K., et al. (2003). "Multipotent cell lineages in early mouse development depend on SOX2 function." *Genes Dev* 17(1): 126-40.

Balzer, E. and Moss, E. G. (2007). "Localization of the developmental timing regulator Lin28 to mRNP complexes, P-bodies and stress granules." *RNA Biol* 4(1): 16-25.

Beattie, G. M., Lopez, A. D., et al. (2005). "Activin A maintains pluripotency of human embryonic stem cells in the absence of feeder layers." *Stem Cells* 23(4): 489-95.

Bendall, S. C., Stewart, M. H., et al. (2007). "IGF and FGF cooperatively establish the regulatory stem cell niche of pluripotent human cells in vitro." *Nature* 448(7157): 1015-21.

Besser, D. (2004). "Expression of nodal, lefty-a, and lefty-B in undifferentiated human embryonic stem cells requires activation of Smad2/3." *J Biol Chem* 279(43): 45076-84.

Boyer, L. A., Lee, T. I., et al. (2005). "Core transcriptional regulatory circuitry in human embryonic stem cells." *Cell* 122(6): 947-56.

Brandenberger, R., Wei, H., et al. (2004). "Transcriptome characterization elucidates signaling networks that control human ES cell growth and differentiation." *Nat Biotechnol* 22(6): 707-16.

Brimble, S. N., Sherrer, E. S., et al. (2007). "The cell surface glycosphingolipids SSEA-3 and SSEA-4 are not essential for human ESC pluripotency." *Stem Cells* 25(1): 54-62.

Brons, I. G., Smithers, L. E., et al. (2007). "Derivation of pluripotent epiblast stem cells from mammalian embryos." *Nature* 448(7150): 191-5.

Burdon, T., Chambers, I., et al. (1999). "Signaling mechanisms regulating self-renewal and differentiation of pluripotent embryonic stem cells." *Cells Tissues Organs* 165(3-4): 131-43.

Burdon, T., Smith, A., et al. (2002). "Signalling, cell cycle and pluripotency in embryonic stem cells." *Trends Cell Biol* 12(9): 432-8.

Burdon, T., Stracey, C., et al. (1999). "Suppression of SHP-2 and ERK signalling promotes self-renewal of mouse embryonic stem cells." *Dev Biol* 210(1): 30-43.

Cadigan, K. M. and Liu, Y. I., (2006). "Wnt signaling: complexity at the surface." *J Cell Sci* 119(Pt 3): 395-402.

Cartwright, P., McLean, C., et al. (2005). "LIF/STAT3 controls ES cell self-renewal and pluripotency by a Myc-dependent mechanism." *Development* 132(5): 885-96.

Chambers, I., Colby, D., et al. (2003). "Functional expression cloning of Nanog, a pluripotency sustaining factor in embryonic stem cells." *Cell* 113(5): 643-55.

Chambers, I., Silva, J., et al. (2007). "Nanog safeguards pluripotency and mediates germline development." *Nature* 450(7173): 1230-4.

Chan, K. K., Zhang, J., et al. (2009). "KLF4 and PBX1 Directly Regulate NANOG Expression in Human Embryonic Stem Cells." *Stem Cells* 27(9): 2114-25.

Charron, J., Malynn, B. A., et al. (1992). "Embryonic lethality in mice homozygous for a targeted disruption of the N-myc gene." *Genes Dev* 6(12A): 2248-57.

Chen, X., Xu, H., et al. (2008). "Integration of external signaling pathways with the core transcriptional network in embryonic stem cells." *Cell* 133(6): 1106-17.

Cheon, S. H., Kim, S. J., et al. (2005). "Defined Feeder-Free Culture System of Human Embryonic Stem Cells." *Biol Reprod* 74(3): 611.

Chew, J. L., Loh, Y. H., et al. (2005). "Reciprocal transcriptional regulation of Pou5f1 and Sox2 via the Oct4/Sox2 complex in embryonic stem cells." *Mol Cell Biol* 25(14): 6031-46.

Chun, J., Goetzl, E. J., et al. (2002). "International Union of Pharmacology. XXXIV. Lysophospholipid Receptor Nomenclature." *Pharmacol Rev* 54(2): 265-9.

Claassen, D. A., Desler, M. M., et al. (2009). "ROCK inhibition enhances the recovery and growth of cryopreserved human embryonic stem cells and human induced pluripotent stem cells." *Mol Reprod Dev* 76(8): 722-32.

D'Amour, K. A., Agulnick, A. D., et al. (2005). "Efficient differentiation of human embryonic stem cells to definitive endoderm." *Nat Biotechnol* 23(12): 1534-41 .

Daheron, L., Opitz, S. L., et al. (2004). "LIF/STAT3 signaling fails to maintain self-renewal of human embryonic stem cells." *Stem Cells* 22(5): 770-8.

Damoiseaux, R., Sherman, S. P., et al. (2008). "Integrated Chemical Genomics Reveals Modifiers of Survival in Human Embryonic Stem Cells." *Stem Cells* 27(3): 533-42.

Darr, H. and Benvenisty N. (2009). "Genetic analysis of the role of the reprogramming gene LIN-28 in human embryonic stem cells." *Stem Cells* 27(2): 352-62.

Darr, H., Mayshar, Y., et al. (2006). "Overexpression of NANOG in human ES cells enables feeder-free growth while inducing primitive ectoderm features." *Development* 133(6): 1193-201.

Davidson, K. C., Jamshidi, P., et al. (2007). "Wnt3a regulates survival, expansion, and maintenance of neural progenitors derived from human embryonic stem cells." *Mol Cell Neurosci* 36(3): 408-15.

Davis, A. C., Wims, M., et al. (1993). "A null c-myc mutation causes lethality before 10.5 days of gestation in homozygotes and reduced fertility in heterozygous female mice." *Genes Dev* 7(4): 671-82.

Delrieu, I. (2000). "The high molecular weight isoforms of basic fibroblast growth factor (FGF-2): an insight into an intracrine mechanism." *FEBS Lett* 468(1): 6-10.

Diecke, S., Quiroga-Negreira, A., et al. (2008). "FGF2 signaling in mouse embryonic fibroblasts is crucial for self-renewal of embryonic stem cells." *Cells Tissues Organs* 188(1-2): 52-61.

Dravid, G., Ye, Z., et al. (2005). "Defining the Role of Wnt/{beta}-Catenin Signaling in the Survival, Proliferation, and Self-Renewal of Human Embryonic Stem Cells." *Stem Cells* 23(10): 1489-1501.

Dvorak, P., Dvorakova, D., et al. (2005). "Expression and potential role of fibroblast growth factor 2 and its receptors in human embryonic stem cells." *Stem Cells* 23(8): 1200-11.

Eilers, M. and Eisenman, R. N. (2008). "Myc's broad reach." *Genes Dev* 22(20): 2755-66.

Ellis, P., Fagan, B. M., et al. (2004). "SOX2, a persistent marker for multipotential neural stem cells derived from embryonic stem cells, the embryo or the adult." *Dev Neurosci* 26(2-4): 148-65.

Ema, M., Mori, D., et al. (2008). "Kruppel-like factor 5 is essential for blastocyst development and the normal self-renewal of mouse ESCs." *Cell Stem Cell* 3(5): 555-67.

Evans, P. M. and Liu, C., (2008). "Roles of Krupel-like factor 4 in normal homeostasis, cancer and stem cells." *Acta Biochim Biophys Sin* (Shanghai) 40(7): 554-64.

Feng, B., Ng, J. H., et al. (2009). "Molecules that promote or enhance reprogramming of somatic cells to induced pluripotent stem cells." *Cell Stem Cell* 4(4): 301-12.

Fong, H., Hohenstein, K. A., et al. (2008). "Regulation of self-renewal and pluripotency by Sox2 in human embryonic stem cells." *Stem Cells* 26(8): 1931-8.

Ghaleb, A. M., Nandan, M. O., et al. (2005). "Kruppel-like factors 4 and 5: the yin and yang regulators of cellular proliferation." *Cell Res* 15(2): 92-6.

Ginis, I., Luo, Y., et al. (2004). "Differences between human and mouse embryonic stem cells." *Dev Biol* 269(2): 360-80.

Gotoh, N. (2009). "Control of stemness by fibroblast growth factor signaling in stem cells and and cancer stem cells." *Curr Stem Cell Res Ther* 4(1): 9-15.

Guo, Y., Costa, R., et al. (2002). "The embryonic stem cell transcription factors Oct-4 and FoxD3 interact to regulate endodermal-specific promoter expression." *Proc Natl Acad Sci U S A* 99(6): 3663-7.

Harb, N., Archer, T. K., et al. (2008). "The Rho-Rock-Myosin signaling axis determines cell-cell integrity of self-renewing pluripotent stem cells." *PLoS ONE* 3(8): e3001.

Hasegawa, K., Fujioka, T., et al. (2006). "A method for the selection of human embryonic stem cell sub-lines with high replating efficiency after single cell dissociation." *Stem Cells* 24(12): 2649-60.

Hatano, S. Y., Tada, M., et al. (2005). "Pluripotential competence of cells associated with Nanog activity." *Mech Dev* 122(1): 67-79.

Heng, B. C. (2009). "Effect of Rho-associated kinase (ROCK) inhibitor Y-27632 on the post-thaw viability of cryopreserved human bone marrow-derived mesenchymal stem cells." *Tissue Cell* 41(5): 376-80.

Hohenstein, K. A., Pyle, A. D., et al. (2008). "Nucleofection mediates high-efficiency stable gene knockdown and transgene expression in human embryonic stem cells." *Stem Cells* 26(6): 1436-43.

Humphrey, R. K., G. M. Beattie, et al. (2004). "Maintenance of pluripotency in human embryonic stem cells is STAT3 independent." *Stem Cells* 22(4): 522-30.

Hyslop, L., Stojkovic, M., et al. (2005). "Downregulation of NANOG induces differentiation of human embryonic stem cells to extraembryonic lineages." *Stem Cells* 23(8): 1035-43.

Inniss, K. and Moore, H., (2006). "Mediation of apoptosis and proliferation of human embryonic stem cells by sphingosine-1-phosphate." *Stem Cells Dev* 15(6): 789-96.

Itoh, N. and Ornitz, D. M. (2004). "Evolution of the Fgf and Fgfr gene families." *Trends Genet* 20(11): 563-9.

Itsykson, P., Ilouz, N., et al. (2005). "Derivation of neural precursors from human embryonic stem cells in the presence of noggin." *Mol Cell Neurosci* 30(1): 24-36.

Ivanova, N., Dobrin, R., et al. (2006). "Dissecting self-renewal in stem cells with RNA interference." *Nature* 442(7102): 533-8.

James, D., Levine, A. J., et al. (2005). "TGFbeta/activin/nodal signaling is necessary for the maintenance of pluripotency in human embryonic stem cells." *Development* 132(6): 1273-82.

Jiang, J., Chan, Y. S., et al. (2008). "A core Klf circuitry regulates self-renewal of embryonic stem cells." *Nat Cell Biol* 10(3): 353-60.

Kang, H. B., Kim, J. S., et al. (2005). "Basic fibroblast growth factor activates ERK and induces c-fos in human embryonic stem cell line MizhES1." *Stem Cells Dev* 14(4): 395-401.

Katoh, M. (2006). "CER1 is a common target of WNT and NODAL signaling pathways in human embryonic stem cells." *Int J Mol Med* 17(5): 795-9.

Kendall, S. D., Adam, S. J., et al. (2006). "Genetically engineered human cancer models utilizing mammalian transgene expression." *Cell Cycle* 5(10): 1074-9.

Kim, J., Chu, J., et al. (2008). "An extended transcriptional network for pluripotency of embryonic stem cells." *Cell* 132(6): 1049-61.

Klimanskaya, I., Chung, Y., et al. (2005). "Human embryonic stem cells derived without feeder cells." *Lancet* 365(9471): 1636-41.

Knoepfler, P. S., Zhang, X. Y., et al. (2006). "Myc influences global chromatin structure." *EMBO J* 25(12): 2723-34.

Kondoh, H., Uchikawa, M., et al. (2004). "Interplay of Pax6 and SOX2 in lens development as a paradigm of genetic switch mechanisms for cell differentiation." *Int J Dev Biol* 48(8-9): 819-27.

Kopp, J. L., Ormsbee, B. D., et al. (2008). "Small increases in the level of Sox2 trigger the differentiation of mouse embryonic stem cells." *Stem Cells* 26(4): 903-11.

Krawetz, R. J., Li, X., et al. (2009). "Human embryonic stem cells: caught between a ROCK inhibitor and a hard place." *Bioessays* 31(3): 336-43.

Kunath, T., Saba-El-Leil, M. K., et al. (2007). "FGF stimulation of the Erk1/2 signalling cascade triggers transition of pluripotent embryonic stem cells from self-renewal to lineage commitment." *Development* 134(16): 2895-902.

Kuroda, T., Tada, M., et al. (2005). "Octamer and Sox elements are required for transcriptional cis regulation of Nanog gene expression." *Mol Cell Biol* 25(6): 2475-85.

Lee, J., Kim, H. K., et al. (2006). "The human OCT-4 isoforms differ in their ability to confer self-renewal." *J Biol Chem* 281(44): 33554-65.

Letamendia, A., Labbe, E., et al. (2001). "Transcriptional regulation by Smads: crosstalk between the TGF-beta and Wnt pathways." *J Bone Joint Surg* Am 83-A Suppl 1(Pt 1): S31-9.

Levenstein, M. E., Ludwig, T. E., et al. (2006). "Basic FGF Support of Human Embryonic Stem Cell Self-Renewal." *Stem Cells* 24(3): 568-74.

Li, J., Pan, G., et al. (2007). "A dominant-negative form of mouse SOX2 induces trophectoderm differentiation and progressive polyploidy in mouse embryonic stem cells." *J Biol Chem* 282(27): 19481-92.

Li, J., Wang, G., et al. (2007). "MEK/ERK signaling contributes to the maintenance of human embryonic stem cell self-renewal." *Differentiation* 75(4): 299-307.

Li, M., Pevny, L., et al. (1998). "Generation of purified neural precursors from embryonic stem cells by lineage selection." *Curr Biol* 8(17): 971-4.

Li, X., Krawetz, R., et al. (2009). "ROCK inhibitor improves survival of *cryopreserved serum/feeder-free single human embryonic stem cells.*" *Hum Reprod* 24(3): 580-9.

Li, X., Meng, G., et al. (2008). "The ROCK inhibitor Y-27632 enhances the survival rate of human embryonic stem cells following cryopreservation." *Stem Cells Dev* 17(6): 1079-85.

Li, Y., McClintick, J., et al. (2005). "Murine embryonic stem cell differentiation is promoted by SOCS-3 and inhibited by the zinc finger transcription factor Klf4." *Blood* 105(2): 635-7.

Liu, L., Leaman, D., et al. (1997). "Silencing of the gene for the alpha-subunit of human chorionic gonadotropin by the embryonic transcription factor Oct-3/4." *Mol Endocrinol* 11(11): 1651-8.

Liu, L. and Roberts, R. M., (1996). "Silencing of the gene for the beta subunit of human chorionic gonadotropin by the embryonic transcription factor Oct-3/4." *J Biol Chem* 271(28): 16683-9.

Lu, B., P. Pang, T., et al. (2005). "The yin and yang of neurotrophin action." *Nat Rev Neurosci* 6(8): 603-14.

Ludwig, T. E., Levenstein, M. E., et al. (2006). "Derivation of human embryonic stem cells in defined conditions." *Nat Biotechnol* 24(2):185-7.

Masui, S., Nakatake, Y., et al. (2007). "Pluripotency governed by Sox2 via regulation of Oct3/4 expression in mouse embryonic stem cells." *Nat Cell Biol* 9(6): 625-35.

Matin, M. M., Walsh, J. R., et al. (2004). "Specific knockdown of Oct4 and beta2-microglobulin expression by RNA interference in human embryonic stem cells and embryonic carcinoma cells." *Stem Cells* 22(5): 659-68.

Mayshar, Y., Rom, E., et al. (2008). "Fibroblast growth factor 4 and its novel splice isoform have opposing effects on the maintenance of human embryonic stem cell self-renewal." *Stem Cells* 26(3): 767-74.

McConnell, B. B., Ghaleb, A. M., et al. (2007). "The diverse functions of Kruppel-like factors 4 and 5 in epithelial biology and pathobiology." *Bioessays* 29(6): 549-57.

McLean, A. B., D'Amour, K. A., et al. (2007). "Activin a efficiently specifies definitive endoderm from human embryonic stem cells only when phosphatidylinositol 3-kinase signaling is suppressed." *Stem Cells* 25(1): 29-38.

Mitsui, K., Tokuzawa, Y., et al. (2003). "The homeoprotein Nanog is required for maintenance of pluripotency in mouse epiblast and ES cells." *Cell* 113(5): 631-42.

Miyazawa, K., Shinozaki, M., et al. (2002). "Two major Smad pathways in TGF-beta superfamily signalling." *Genes Cells* 7(12): 1191-204.

Moss, E. G., Lee, R. C., et al. (1997). "The cold shock domain protein LIN-28 controls developmental timing in C. elegans and is regulated by the lin-4 RNA." *Cell* 88(5): 637-46.

Nakagawa, M., Koyanagi, M., et al. (2008). "Generation of induced pluripotent stem cells without Myc from mouse and human fibroblasts." *Nat Biotechnol* 26(1): 101-6.

Nakatake, Y., Fukui, N., et al. (2006). "Klf4 cooperates with Oct3/4 and Sox2 to activate the Lefty1 core promoter in embryonic stem cells." *Mol Cell Biol* 26(20): 7772-82.

Naz, R. K., Kumar, G., et al. (1994). "Expression and role of c-myc protooncogene in murine preimplantation embryonic development." *J Assist Reprod Genet* 11(4): 208-16.

Nichols, J., Zevnik, B., et al. (1998). "Formation of pluripotent stem cells in the mammalian embryo depends on the POU transcription factor Oct4." *Cell* 95(3): 379-91.

Nishimoto, M., Fukushima, A., et al. (1999). "The gene for the embryonic stem cell coactivator UTF1 carries a regulatory element which selectively interacts with a complex composed of Oct-3/4 and Sox-2." *Mol Cell Biol* 19(8): 5453-65.

Nishimoto, M., Miyagi, S., et al. (2005). "Oct-3/4 maintains the proliferative embryonic stem cell state via specific binding to a variant octamer sequence in the regulatory region of the UTF1 locus." *Mol Cell Biol* 25(12): 5084-94.

Niwa, H., Miyazaki, J., et al. (2000). "Quantitative expression of Oct-3/4 defines differentiation, dedifferentiation or self-renewal of ES cells." *Nat Genet* 24(4): 372-6.

Niwa, H., Toyooka, Y., et al. (2005). "Interaction between Oct3/4 and Cdx2 determines trophectoderm differentiation." *Cell* 123(5): 917-29.

Okamoto, K., Okazawa, H., et al. (1990). "A novel octamer binding transcription factor is differentially expressed in mouse embryonic cells." *Cell* 60(3): 461-72.

Okuda, A., Fukushima, A., et al. (1998). "UTF1, a novel transcriptional coactivator expressed in pluripotent embryonic stem cells and extra-embryonic cells." *EMBO J* 17(7): 2019-32.

Paria, B. C., Dey, S. K., et al. (1992). "Antisense c-myc effects on preimplantation mouse embryo development." *Proc Natl Acad Sci* U S A 89(21): 10051-5.

Patel, J. H., Loboda, A. P., et al. (2004). "Analysis of genomic targets reveals complex functions of MYC." *Nat Rev Cancer* 4(7): 562-8.

Pebay, A., Wong, R. C., et al. (2005). "Essential roles of sphingosine-1-phosphate and platelet-derived growth factor in the maintenance of human embryonic stem cells." *Stem Cells* 23(10): 1541-8.

Pera, M. F., Andrade, J., et al. (2004). "Regulation of human embryonic stem cell differentiation by BMP-2 and its antagonist noggin." *J Cell Sci* 117(Pt 7): 1269-80.

Pera, M. F., Andrade, J., et al. (2004). "Regulation of human embryonic stem cell differentiation by BMP-2 and its antagonist noggin." *J Cell Sci* 117(Pt 7): 1269-80.

Pera, M. F., Reubinoff, B., et al. (2000). "Human embryonic stem cells." *J Cell Sci* 113 (Pt 1): 5-10.

Pesce, M. and Scholer, H. R., (2001). "Oct-4: gatekeeper in the beginnings of mammalian development." *Stem Cells* 19(4): 271-8.

Peter, M. E. (2009). "Let-7 and miR-200 microRNAs: guardians against pluripotency and cancer progression." *Cell Cycle* 8(6): 843-52.

Pitson, S. M. and Pebay, A., (2009). "Regulation of stem cell pluripotency and neural differentiation by lysophospholipids." *Neurosignals* 17(4): 242-54.

Polesskaya, A., Cuvellier, S., et al. (2007). "Lin-28 binds IGF-2 mRNA and participates in skeletal myogenesis by increasing translation efficiency." *Genes Dev* 21(9): 1125-38.

Pyle, A. D., Lock, L. F., et al. (2006). "Neurotrophins mediate human embryonic stem cell survival." *Nat Biotechnol* 24(3): 344-50.

Reissmann, E., Jornvall, H., et al. (2001). "The orphan receptor ALK7 and the Activin receptor ALK4 mediate signaling by Nodal proteins during vertebrate development." *Genes Dev* 15(15): 2010-22.

Reubinoff, B. E., Pera, M. F., et al. (2000). "Embryonic stem cell lines from human blastocysts: somatic differentiation in vitro." *Nat Biotechnol* 18(4): 399-404.

Rho, J. Y., Yu, K., et al. (2006). "Transcriptional profiling of the developmentally important signalling pathways in human embryonic stem cells." *Hum Reprod* 21(2): 405-12.

Richards, M., Tan, S. P., et al. (2004). "The transcriptome profile of human embryonic stem cells as defined by SAGE." *Stem Cells* 22(1): 51-64.

Rodda, D. J., Chew, J. L., et al. (2005). "Transcriptional regulation of nanog by OCT4 and SOX2." *J Biol Chem* 280(26): 24731-7.

Rosner, M. H., Vigano, M. A., et al. (1990). "A POU-domain transcription factor in early stem cells and germ cells of the mammalian embryo." *Nature* 345(6277): 686-92.

Rowland, B. D., Bernards, R., et al. (2005). "The KLF4 tumour suppressor is a transcriptional repressor of p53 that acts as a context-dependent oncogene." *Nat Cell Biol* 7(11): 1074-82.

Rowland, B. D. and Peeper, D. S., (2006). "KLF4, p21 and context-dependent opposing forces in cancer." *Nat Rev Cancer* 6(1): 11-23.

Sato, N., Meijer, L., et al. (2004). "Maintenance of pluripotency in human and mouse embryonic stem cells through activation of Wnt signaling by a pharmacological GSK-3-specific inhibitor." *Nat Med* 10(1): 55-63.

Sato, N., Sanjuan, I. M., et al. (2003). "Molecular signature of human embryonic stem cells and its comparison with the mouse." *Dev Biol* 260(2): 404-13.

Schlessinger, J. (2004). "Common and distinct elements in cellular signaling via EGF and FGF receptors." *Science* 306(5701): 1506-7.

Scholer, H. R., Balling, R., et al. (1989). "Octamer binding proteins confer transcriptional activity in early mouse embryogenesis." *EMBO J* 8(9): 2551-7.

Segre, J. A., Bauer, C. et al. (1999). "Klf4 is a transcription factor required for establishing the barrier function of the skin." *Nat Genet* 22(4): 356-60.

Shi, Y. and Massague, J. (2003). "Mechanisms of TGF-beta signaling from cell membrane to the nucleus." *Cell* 113(6): 685-700.

Shimozaki, K., Nakashima, K., et al. (2003). "Involvement of Oct3/4 in the enhancement of neuronal differentiation of ES cells in neurogenesis-inducing cultures." *Development* 130(11): 2505-12.

Sperger, J. M., Chen, X., et al. (2003). "Gene expression patterns in human embryonic stem cells and human pluripotent germ cell tumors." *Proc Natl Acad Sci U S A* 100(23): 13350-5.

Sridharan, R., Tchieu, J., et al. (2009). "Role of the murine reprogramming factors in the induction of pluripotency." Cell 136(2): 364-77.

Stachowiak, M. K., Fang, X., et al. (2003). "Integrative nuclear FGFR1 signaling (INFS) as a part of a universal "feed-forward-and-gate" signaling module that controls cell growth and differentiation." *J Cell Biochem* 90(4): 662-91.

Stanton, B. R., Perkins, A. S., et al. (1992). "Loss of N-myc function results in embryonic lethality and failure of the epithelial component of the embryo to develop." *Genes Dev* 6(12A): 2235-47.

Sumi, T., Tsuneyoshi, N., et al. (2007). "Apoptosis and differentiation of human embryonic stem cells induced by sustained activation of c-Myc." *Oncogene* 26(38): 5564-76.

Suzuki, A., Raya, A., et al. (2006). "Nanog binds to Smad1 and blocks bone morphogenetic protein-induced differentiation of embryonic stem cells." *Proc Natl Acad Sci* U S A 103(27): 10294-9.

Takahashi, K., Tanabe, K., et al. (2007). "Induction of pluripotent stem cells from adult human fibroblasts by defined factors." *Cell* 131(5): 861-72.

Takahashi, K. and Yamanaka, S., (2006). "Induction of pluripotent stem cells from mouse embryonic and adult fibroblast cultures by defined factors." *Cell* 126(4): 663-76.

Takeda, J., Seino, S., et al. (1992). "Human Oct3 gene family: cDNA sequences, alternative splicing, gene organization, chromosomal location, and expression at low levels in adult tissues." *Nucleic Acids Res* 20(17): 4613-20.

Takuwa, Y., Takuwa, N., et al. (2002). "The edg family g protein-coupled receptors for lysophospholipids: their signaling properties and biological activities." *J Biochem* (Tokyo) 131(6): 767-71.

Thomson, J. A., Itskovitz-Eldor, J., et al. (1998). "Embryonic stem cell lines derived from human blastocysts." *Science* 282(5391): 1145-7.

Tokuzawa, Y., Kaiho, E., et al. (2003). "Fbx15 is a novel target of Oct3/4 but is dispensable for embryonic stem cell self-renewal and mouse development." *Mol Cell Biol* 23(8): 2699-708.

Tomioka, M., Nishimoto, M., et al. (2002). "Identification of Sox-2 regulatory region which is under the control of Oct-3/4-Sox-2 complex." *Nucleic Acids Res* 30(14): 3202-13.

Vallier, L., Alexander, M., et al. (2005). "Activin/Nodal and FGF pathways cooperate to maintain pluripotency of human embryonic stem cells." *J Cell Sci* 118(Pt 19): 4495-509.

Vallier, L., Reynolds, D., et al. (2004). "Nodal inhibits differentiation of human embryonic stem cells along the neuroectodermal default pathway." *Dev Biol* 275(2): 403-21.

Vallier, L., Touboul, T., et al. (2009). "Early cell fate decisions of human embryonic stem cells and mouse epiblast stem cells are controlled by the same signalling pathways." *PLoS One* 4(6): e6082.

Varelas, X., Sakuma, R., et al. (2008). "TAZ controls Smad nucleocytoplasmic shuttling and regulates human embryonic stem-cell self-renewal." *Nat Cell Biol* 10(7): 837-48.

Vermeulen, K., Berneman, Z. N., et al. (2003). "Cell cycle and apoptosis." *Cell Prolif* 36(3): 165-75.

Viswanathan, S. R., Daley, G. Q., et al. (2008). "Selective blockade of microRNA processing by Lin28." *Science* 320(5872): 97-100.

Walsh, J. and Andrews, P. W., (2003). "Expression of Wnt and Notch pathway genes in a pluripotent human embryonal carcinoma cell line and embryonic stem cell." *Apmis* 111(1): 197-210; discussion 210-1.

Wang, G., Zhang, H., et al. (2005). "Noggin and bFGF cooperate to maintain the pluripotency of human embryonic stem cells in the absence of feeder layers." *Biochem Biophys Res Commun* 330(3): 934-42.

Wang, J., Rao, S., et al. (2006). "A protein interaction network for pluripotency of embryonic stem cells." *Nature* 444(7117): 364-8.

Wang, L., Li, L., et al. (2005). "Human embryonic stem cells maintained in the absence of mouse embryonic fibroblasts or conditioned media are capable of hematopoietic development." *Blood* 105(12): 4598-603.

Watanabe, K., Ueno, M., et al. (2007). "A ROCK inhibitor permits survival of dissociated human embryonic stem cells." *Nat Biotechnol* 25(6): 681-6.

Wernig, M., Meissner, A., et al. (2008). "c-Myc is dispensable for direct reprogramming of mouse fibroblasts." *Cell Stem Cell* 2(1): 10-2.

Wong, R. C., Tellis, I., et al. (2007). "Anti-apoptotic effect of sphingosine-1-phosphate and platelet-derived growth factor in human embryonic stem cells." *Stem Cells Dev* 16(6): 989-1001.

Xiao, L., Yuan, X., et al. (2006). "Activin A maintains self-renewal and regulates FGF, Wnt and BMP pathways in human embryonic stem cells." *Stem Cells* 24(6): 1476-86.

Xu, B., Zhang, K., et al. (2009). "Lin28 modulates cell growth and associates with a subset of cell cycle regulator mRNAs in mouse embryonic stem cells." *RNA* 15(3): 357-61.

Xu, C., Inokuma, M. S., et al. (2001). "Feeder-free growth of undifferentiated human embryonic stem cells." *Nat Biotechnol* 19(10): 971-4.

Xu, C., Rosler, E., et al. (2005). "Basic fibroblast growth factor supports undifferentiated human embryonic stem cell growth without conditioned medium." *Stem Cells* 23(3): 315-23.

Xu, R. H., X. Chen, et al. (2002). "BMP4 initiates human embryonic stem cell differentiation to trophoblast." *Nat Biotechnol* 20(12): 1261-4.

Xu, R. H., Peck, R. M., et al. (2005). "Basic FGF and suppression of BMP signaling sustain undifferentiated proliferation of human ES cells." Nat *Methods* 2(3): 185-90.

Xu, R. H., Sampsell-Barron, T. L., et al. (2008). "NANOG is a direct target of TGFbeta/activin-mediated SMAD signaling in human ESCs." *Cell* Stem Cell 3(2): 196-206.

Yao, S., Chen, S., et al. (2006). "Long-term self-renewal and directed differentiation of human embryonic stem cells in chemically defined conditions." *Proc Natl Acad Sci* U S A 103(18): 6907-12.

Ying, Q. L., Nichols, J., et al. (2003). "BMP induction of Id proteins suppresses differentiation and sustains embryonic stem cell self-renewal in collaboration with STAT3." *Cell* 115(3): 281-92.

Yu, J., Vodyanik, M. A., et al. (2007). "Induced pluripotent stem cell lines derived from human somatic cells." *Science* 318(5858): 1917-20.

Yuan, H., Corbi, N., et al. (1995). "Developmental-specific activity of the FGF-4 enhancer requires the synergistic action of Sox2 and Oct-3." *Genes Dev* 9(21): 2635-45.

Zaehres, H., Lensch, M. W., et al. (2005). "High-efficiency RNA interference in human embryonic stem cells." *Stem Cells* 23(3): 299-305.

Zeineddine, D., Papadimou, E., et al. (2006). "Oct-3/4 dose dependently regulates specification of embryonic stem cells toward a cardiac lineage and early heart development." *Dev Cell* 11(4): 535-46.

Zhao, S., Nichols, J., et al. (2004). "SoxB transcription factors specify neuroectodermal lieage choice in ES cells." *Mol Cell Neurosci* 27(3): 332-42.

In: Encyclopedia of Stem Cell Research (2 Volume Set)   ISBN: 978-1-61761-835-2
Editor: Alexander L. Greene   © 2012 Nova Science Publishers, Inc.

Chapter XLV

GENERATION OF CLINICALLY RELEVANT "INDUCED PLURIPOTENT STEM" (IPS) CELLS

Corey Heffernan[1], Huseyin Sumer[1] and Paul J. Verma[1]*

[1]Reprogramming and Stem Cell Laboratory, Monash Institute of Medical Research, Monash University, Clayton, Australia

ABSTRACT

Proviral expression of early development genes Oct4 and Sox2, in concert with cMyc and Klf4 or Nanog and Lin28, can induce differentiated cells to adopt morphological and functional characteristics of pluripotency indistinguishable from embryonic stem cells. Termed induced pluripotent stem (iPS) cells, in mice the pluripotency of these cells was confirmed by altered gene/surface antigen expression, remodeling of the epigenome, ability to contribute to embryonic lineages following blastocyst injection and commitment to all three germ layers in teratomas and liveborn chimeras. Importantly, *in vitro* directed differentiation of iPS cells yield cells capable of treating mouse models of humanized disease. Despite these impressive results, iPS cell conversion is frustratingly inefficient. Also, the unpredictable and random mutagenesis imposed on the host cell genome, inherent with integrative viral methodologies, continues to hamper use of these cells in a therapeutic setting. This has initiated exploration of non-integrating strategies for generating iPS cells. Here, we review mechanisms that drive conversion of somatic cells to iPS cells and the strategies adopted to circumvent integrative viral strategies. Finally, we discuss practical, ethical and legal considerations that require addressing before iPS cells can realize their potential as patient-specific cells for treatment of degenerative disease.

* Corresponding author: Paul J. Verma Ph.D.; c/o Reprogramming and Stem Cell Laboratory, Centre for Reproduction and Development, Level 2, Monash Institute of Medical Research, Monash University, 27-31 Wright Street, Clayton, VIC 3168, Australia. Tel: 61 3 9594 7000, Fax: 61 3 9594 7100, Email: paul.verma@med.monash.edu.au

1. INTRODUCTION: GENERATION OF INDUCED PLURIPOTENT STEM (IPS) CELLS

The process of reversing the genetic program of a somatic cell to one characteristic of embryonic cells, so elegantly demonstrated by cloning of *Dolly* the sheep by somatic cell nuclear transfer (SCNT), is referred to as 'nuclear reprogramming' (Wilmut et al., 1997). The subsequent excitement in the possibility of deriving patient-specific stem cells for autologous cell replacement therapy was counterbalanced with moral ethical concerns surrounding oocyte donation and embryo destruction. The search for alternative methodologies that successfully induce pluripotency in differentiated somatic cells lead to the development of ES-somatic cell fusion, and treatment of somatic cells with cell extracts (for review, see Hochedlinger & Jaenisch, 2007). Takahashi & Yamanaka (2006) invigorated the reprogramming field when they successfully reprogrammed somatic cells by retroviral delivery and forced expression of four key transcription factors Oct4, Sox2, cMyc and Klf4. These cells were coined 'induced pluripotent stem' (iPS) cells. The reversal of the biological safeguards maintaining the stability of lineage committed cells to pluripotent, colony-forming iPS cells was confirmed collectively by gene/surface antigen expression, epigenetic remodeling, contribution to embryonic lineages in liveborns following diploid and tetraploid blastocyst injection and commitment to all three germ layers in teratomas generated in SCID mice (Takahashi & Yamanaka, 2006; Takahashi et al., 2007; Wernig et al., 2007; Maherali et al., 2007; Okita et al., 2008; Kang at el., 2009; Zhao et al., 2009). Originally demonstrated in mouse, iPS cells have been generated in rat (Li et al., 2008), rhesus monkey (Liu et al., 2008[a]) and pig (Esteban et al., 2009; Ezashi et al., 2009), as well as from a range of human cells including keratinocytes (Aasen et al., 2008; Maherali et al., 2008), dermal fibroblasts (Maherali et al., 2008) and peripheral blood (Loh et al., 2009). Interestingly, mouse sequences for the four reprogramming factors can effectively reprogram human somatic cells (Woltjen et al., 2008). Subsequent to the original reports from the Yamanaka lab, a reprogramming cocktail similarly incorporating Oct4 and Sox2, with two alternative factors Nanog and Lin28 was shown to reprogram human cells to pluripotency (Yu et al., 2007). However, low efficiency of conversion from somatic to iPS cells continues to hamper either methodology.

1.1   The Mainstays of the Reprogramming Cocktail: Oct4 & Sox2

Collectively, Oct4 and Sox2 play crucial roles in maintaining pluripotency and self-renewal in ES cells *in vivo* and *in vitro*, and in inducing pluripotency in somatic cells (Takahashi & Yamanaka, 2006; Yu et al., 2007). Expression of the POU domain transcription factor Oct4 from the *POU5F1* locus is a well documented feature of early embryogenesis and ES cells *in vitro*. Oct4 incorporates a POU specific domain (POU_s) and POU homeobox domain (POU_h) coupled by a variable linker sequence (reviewed Pan et al., 2002). The POU_s domain of Oct4 interacts with one of at least two known (sequence dependent) binding sites in the HMG domain of Sox2, an SRY-related HMG domain-box transcription factor (Remenyi et al., 2003). The proximity of POU and HMG DNA recognition sequences, which often reside immediately adjacent to or in close proximity to each other, may dictate assembly of distinct structural confirmations of the Oct4/Sox2 dimer at individual genomic loci, thus mediating diverse regulatory affects of numerous target genes (Tomioka et al., 2002; Remenyi et al., 2003; Catena et al., 2005; Chew et al., 2005; Rodda et al., 2005). However, recent experimental evidence questions the essential nature of Sox2 in Oct4/Sox2 enhancer function. Although Sox2 null ES cells repress Oct4 expression and differentiate into trophectoderm, forced expression of Oct4 in these cells reinstates the ability to contribute to all germ layers of mid-gestation chimeras (Masui et al., 2007). In addition, Nanog expression is maintained in (differentiating) Sox2 null ES cells and Oct4-rescued, Sox2 null ES cells. Surprisingly, Sox2 may regulate Oct4 expression indirectly through regulation of several Oct4 enhancer- and promoter-binding factors, namely nuclear receptor family proteins (Masui et al., 2007). Despite binding regulatory elements as a monomer, Sox2 primarily regulates target genes in concert with co-factor binding. Indeed, DNA binding of Sox2 is enhanced through HMG/POU domain interactions (Remenyi et al., 2003). In contrast to other Octomer family members, fluctuations of Oct4 expression beyond critical upper or lower thresholds induce differentiation into endoderm and mesoderm, or trophectoderm, respectively (Niwa et al., 2000). Intriguingly, recent reports highlight non-transcriptional roles for Oct4 in female cells, primarily X-X chromosome pairing and binding of accessory factors for random X chromosome deactivation (Donohue et al., 2009). In ES cells, transcriptional repression of genes elicited by binding of the Oct4/Sox2 ternary complex is relieved upon detachment of the complex at initiation of differentiation (Boyer et al., 2005). Unsurprisingly, Oct4 and Sox2 null embryos die through lack of ES cell maintenance.

1.2   Alternative Reprogramming Factors: cMyc & Klf4

cMyc is a proto-oncogene with an expanding list of genomic target genes. This factor influences cell proliferation through (i) transcriptional control through co-factor binding or localized chromatin modification, and (ii) pre-replication fork assembly/DNA replication during the G1/S transition (Dominguez-Sola et al., 2007; Martinato et al., 2008; reviewed Eilers & Eisenman, 2009). Myc exerts a combinatorial affect on cell growth; it readily heterodimerizes with the bHLHZ protein Max on *E-box* recognition sequence, (CACGTG)-containing DNA to promote metabolism, translation and mitochondrial processes. Recruitment of cMyc to regulatory elements by Myc-interacting zinc-finger protein (Miz-1) represses expression of factors involved in cell cycle arrest, eg. cyclin-dependent kinase inhibitors; a process that is reversed by TGFβ (Seoane et al., 2001; reviewed Eilers & Eisenman, 2009). Occupancy of cMyc at target promoters results in major, localized chromatin modifications, namely recruitment of histone methyltranferases and acetylases for assembly of regulatory histone marks, and exchange of regular histones for euchromatic histone variants at Myc target promoters (Martinato et al., 2008). In mES cells, Myc occupies one-fifth of all promoters and target gene expression occurs regardless of co-binding with Oct4, Sox2 or Klf4 (Liu et al., 2008[c]). Interestingly, cMyc is the only factor in the cocktail that can't autoregulate in ES cells (Liu et al., 2008[c]).

Structurally, family members of the Kruppel-like transcription factors (Klf) share a C-terminal, zinc finger coupled with a conserved linker sequence. In particular, Klf4 is a tumor-suppressor that can perform transcriptional co-activator or repressor functions in a number of embryonic and adult tissues. The considerable functional redundancy of Kruppel-like factors in ES cell self-renewal perhaps highlights this gene family's importance in maintenance of pluripotency (Jiang et al., 2008). Simultaneous knockdown of Klf2, Klf4 and Klf5 in ES cells initiates loss of pluripotency and upregulation of a number of differentiation genes, including the trophectoderm marker *Cdx2* (an antagonist of Oct4 expression; Jiang et al., 2008). Although these three Klf family members collectively bind a DNA recognition sequence in the Nanog distal enhancer to upregulate its activity, loss of any individual protein can be compensated for by the remaining Klf family members. iPS cells can be induced in neural stem cells with Klf4 omitted from the reprogramming cocktail, however formation of reporter gene[+] colonies is delayed compared to four factor, and three factor (Myc omitted) induction (Kim et al., 2008).

Occupancy of many transcriptional regulators at the promoters of transcriptionally active and silent genes in somatic and ES cells, leading to transcriptional initiation and interrupted transcript elongation, suggests a genetic program representative of pluripotency is potentially permissive to activation (Guenther et al., 2007). Collectively, the four Yamanaka factors regulate 16 developmental pathways in ES cells, including the *p53,* Wnt and TGF-β pathways (Liu et al., 2008[c]). Binding of individual factors, in the absence of co-binding with the other factors, more often elicits transcriptional repression; conversely, co-binding more often associates with transcriptional permissiveness (Liu et al., 2008[c]). Interestingly, excess concentrations of all reprogramming factors are not required to kickstart the reprogramming process; forced expression of Oct4 and Sox2 to levels comparable to that observed in ES cells are sufficient to mediate reprogramming (Carey et al., 2009).

Deciphering levels of cMyc and Klf4 required for reprogramming is more challenging given considerable expression of these factors in many somatic cells (Nakagawa et al., 2007; Segre et al., 1999). Similarly for Oct4 and Sox2, collective exogenous and endogenous cMyc expression that exceeds required concentrations may be detrimental to the specificity of reprogramming, a notion supported by a greater proportion of reporter gene positive colonies in cells reprogrammed with cMyc omitted (Nakagawa et al., 2007). However, augmentation of the Oct4/Sox2/Nanog regulatory network is more rapidly established when cMyc is expressed (Wernig et al., 2008). Future experiments inducing pluripotency in cMyc null somatic cells, or malignant/transformed cells over-expressing cMyc, may elucidate the role this factor has in the reprogramming process.

Despite sharing a conserved Octomer binding motif, Oct4 is not functionally redundant with Octomer family members in an iPS setting, perhaps due to protein stability (Nakagawa et al., 2007). However, Oct4 can be replaced with application of a chemical agent, albeit at the expense of reprogramming efficiency (Shi et al., 2008[a]; Shi et al., 2008[b]; discussed later). However, cMyc can be substituted with (i) less teratogenic Myc family members N-Myc and L-Myc, (ii) a cMyc mutant or (iii) even an alternative transcriptional coactivator, the latter even resulting in markedly increased reprogramming efficiency (Nakagawa et al., 2007; Blelloch et al., 2007; Zhao et al., 2008[b]).

1.3   Alternative Reprogramming Factors: Nanog & Lin28

Klf4 (±Myc) is functionally redundant to Nanog and Lin28, perhaps in part reflective of the many shared regulatory targets of Nanog and Klf4, and potential upregulation of Nanog expression through Klf4-mediated p53 transcriptional repression (Yu et al., 2007; Takahashi & Yamanaka, 2006; Rowland et al., 2005). Nanog is a homeobox domain protein expressed in embryonic lineage committed cells of the morula and ES blastocyst (Mitsui et al., 2003). Nanog expression can maintain pluripotency in the absence of LIF/gp130/Stat3 pathway. Although overexpression of Nanog is beneficial for cell fusion-based reprogramming (Silva et al., 2006), targeted ablation of Nanog in ES cells initiates expression of endoderm transcription factors, parietal and visceral endoderm (Mitsui et al., 2003). Lin28 is highly expressed in ES cells, binding cytosolic RNA to regulate mechanisms such as RNA translation and stability, and cell proliferation. Forced expression or knockdown of Lin28 exerts corresponding affects on cell proliferation. Knockdown of Lin28 in ES cells retards cell proliferation (Xu et al., 2009). During S-phase, the different cell-specific demand for individual core histone monomers is regulated by Lin28 at the RNA level, either by enhancing translation or through RNA stabilization (Xu et al., 2009). Yu et al., (2007) demonstrated reprogramming of human fibroblasts from lentiviral expression of Oct4, Sox2, Nanog and Lin28. Considerable reductions in colony number result from omission of Nanog and/or Lin28 from the reprogramming cocktail, with total loss of colony formation with individual omission of Oct4 or Sox2 (Yu et al., 2007; Nakagawa et al., 2007).

1.4   Early Events in iPS Reprogramming

iPS experiments utilizing somatic cells harboring antibiotic-responsive promoters that drive expression of each reprogramming factor have proved an invaluable tool in revealing the temporal and sequential molecular events that regulate derivation of iPS cells (Stadtfeld et al., 2008; Mikkelsen et al., 2008; Brambrink et al., 2008). To date, experiments investigating the mechanisms of iPS-based reprogramming have focused on those induced by the 'Yamanaka' factors, with little known of the mechanisms that direct Nanog/Lin28-mediated reprogramming.

iPS cell derivation commences with progressive down-regulation of lineage associated genes (eg. Thy1.1, Col5a2, Fibrillin2 in fibroblasts), a phenomenon primarily coordinated directly or indirectly by cMyc ± Klf4 (Stadtfeld et al., 2008; Sridharan et al., 2009; Heffernan et al., manuscript in preparation). Three days of exclusive cMyc expression initiates upregulation of genes implicated in metabolism, translational control, RNA splicing, cell cycle and energy production, whilst repressing collagens, signaling and organ development (Sridharan et al., 2009). In concert with the other 3 reprogramming factors, expression of alkaline phosphatase (AP), an indicator of early reprogramming and marker of stem cells, becomes evident in 3-4% of cells after three days of induction. Although a direct link between cMyc and AP expression has not been demonstrated, the critical role played by cMyc in the initial days of reprogramming is highlighted by reductions in the frequency of alkaline phosphatase (AP)[+] colonies when cMyc expression is extinguished at three days post-induction (Sridharan et al., 2009), and may also explain reductions in reprogramming efficiency when cMyc is omitted from the reprogramming cocktail (Nakagawa et al., 2007). The progressive increase in AP expression to almost half of all cells after 12 days of induction renders it an unreliable prospective indicator of cells destined for complete conversion to the iPS phenotype, or marker for late-stage/fully reprogrammed cells (Brambrink et al., 2008). Indeed, a screen of over 150 AP-positive hiPS colonies at day 17-post infection revealed considerable heterogeneity in their transcriptional profile (Masaki et al., 2008). Nanog-driven drug selection is possible many days before Nanog-driven GFP expression is observed (Okita et al., 2007). Interestingly, expression of Fbx15, an Oct4 downstream target gene, is detectable a number of days preceding detectable Oct4 expression (Stadtfeld et al., 2008), in contrast to Oct4 representing an initial activator of transcriptional cascade in pluripotent ES cells *in vivo*. Since minimal improvement in AP^+ colonies results from cMyc expression past the initial 5 days of reprogramming, and well documented links between cMyc and chromatin modification and proliferative responses, the primary role of cMyc appears to be deactivating expressed lineage genes and preparation for initiation of the embryonic genetic program, through resetting of histone marks (Nakagawa et al., 2007; Sridharan et al., 2009).

1.5   The Partially Reprogrammed Phenotype

A transitional period between days 5-12 days post infection/induction in mouse demarks the partially reprogrammed cell phenotypically lineage gene $(Thy1)^-/AP^+/$stage specific embryonic antigen-1 $(SSEA1)^+$. Partially reprogrammed cells account for between 5-10% of a previously homogenous $Thy1^+$ population (Stadtfeld et al., 2008; Brambrink et al., 2008). The majority of partially reprogrammed cells remain partially reprogrammed, never converting to a fully reprogrammed phenotype. Although genes associated with ES cell self-renewal and maintenance are reactivated in partially reprogrammed cells, genes strictly associated with pluripotency are incompletely activated (Mikkelsen et al., 2008). Seemingly, repression of the host cell expression profile is more readily accomplished than activation of silenced genes, with only cells capable of undertaking both progressing to a fully reprogrammed phenotype. Notably, histone methylation at the promoters of OSK targets is partially reset in the transitional/partially reprogrammed cell. Partially reprogrammed cells appear incapable of reactivating the silent X chromosome in female cells and inept at reactivating Nanog, both characteristic of the ES cells (Sridharan et al., 2009). Incomplete silencing of transgenes may be a feature of partially reprogrammed cells; indeed, expression of the four factors is 3-8-fold higher in partially reprogrammed cells than iPS or ES cells (Sridharan et al., 2009). Also, ES specific metabolic regulators are more completely reprogrammed than transcriptional regulators (Sridharan et al., 2009). Partially reprogrammed cells express a defined panel of genes and remain hypermethylated at loci for pluripotency genes (Mikkelsen et al., 2008). Promoter binding profiles are less conserved between (i) partially reprogrammed cells and (ii) fully reprogrammed iPS or ES cells, particularly in genes co-bound by Oct4, Sox2 and Klf4 with is largely lacking in partially reprogrammed cells. Genes lacking ES-like binding are more often targets of Nanog, a feature that is unsurprising since partially reprogrammed cells lack Nanog expression (Sridharan et al., 2009).

1.6   The Fully Reprogrammed Phenotype

The conversion to a fully reprogrammed mouse iPS cell state occurs between 1-2 weeks from induction/infection, and requires 10-16 days of transgene expression to be fully realized (Stadtfeld et al., 2008; Brambrink et al., 2008). In comparison to partially reprogrammed cells, fully reprogrammed iPS cell lines undergo reactivation of the silent X chromosome (in case of female cells), promoter de-methylation and expression of endogenous Oct4 and Nanog loci (confirmed by knock-in reporter gene expression), widespread resetting of histone methylation marks, mTert activation (albeit with a heterogeneous pattern of expression) and endogenous Sox2 expression (Maherali et al., 2007; Stadtfeld et al., 2008; Sridharan et al., 2009). Activation of endogenous Oct4 and Nanog is temporally correlated with down-regulation of the reprogramming transgenes (Wernig et al., 2007; Brambrink et al., 2008). DNA methyltransferase expression increases over the reprogramming period, with maximal expression in Oct4-GFP expressing cells late in the reprogramming process, and is speculated to mediate gradual ransgene silencing (Stadtfeld et al., 2008). However, specific knockdown of Dnmt1, or *de novo* demethylation with a chemical agent at defined periods of transgene expression, presumably leading to demethylation of the Oct4 and Nanog promoter, increases reprogramming efficiency (Mikkelsen et al., 2008).

ES cells and iPS cells share demethylation of pluripotency gene promoters, high expression of pluripotent and self renewal genes and low expression of some, but not all, lineage specific genes (Mikkelsen et al., 2008). Both cell types self-renew, give rise to germ layers in teratomas and contribute to chimeric development. Genome wide analysis of promoter binding and expression shows strong overlap in iPS cells and ES cells (Sridharan et al., 2009); two-thirds of genes in ES cells co-bound by three or four iPS factors binds the same loci in iPS cells. It is noteworthy that very few promoters co-bound by 3 or 4 factors in ES cells are not bound by any key factor in iPS cells (Sridharan et al., 2009). In loci bound by 1 or 2 factors, the similarity between ES cells and iPS cells increases to 87%. However, some genes are bound by fewer factors in iPS than ES cells, although differences may be insignificant to affect transcription. Total Oct4 and Nanog protein expression in numerous iPS cell lines are comparable to ES cells by qRT-PCR and Western Blot (Wernig et al., 2007). In addition, bivalent histone lysine methylation is noted in iPS cell lines, a characteristic of ES cells that are lacking in somatic cells. Although proviral expression of Oct4, Sox2, and Klf4 is sufficient to mediate upregulation of telomerase activity to similar levels as each other and ES cells, iPS cells also expressing viral cMyc comprise longer telomeres (Marion et al., 2009).

Conceptually, initiation/reactivation of transcriptionally silent genes in terminally differentiated cells during iPS induction is possible since most genes in ES and somatic cells experience transcriptional initiation and suspended elongation regardless of transcriptional status (Guenther et al., 2007). Transcriptionally permissive histone methyl and acetyl marks and occupancy of RNA polymerase II at most promoters initiate transcription, although only a subset of genes produces full-length transcript. However, translated protein levels are likely to be crucial for successful iPS conversion, particularly in the case of Oct4. As discussed, over- and under-expression of Oct4 in ES cells leads to differentiation, and is at least partially regulated by optimal levels of Sox2 (Masui et al., 2007). The majority of Oct4 targets in ES cells are targets of Nanog and Sox2, therefore activation of endogenous Nanog expression is a likely prerequisite for reprogramming progression and may explain low efficiency (Boyer et al., 2005). Perhaps differential expression levels of all factors applicable to viral technologies ensure a cohort of cells will have the right combination of factors at desired concentrations. Knowledge of precise levels of each factor would benefit protein delivery strategies and potentially improve reprogramming efficiency. From 16 days of induction, a small proportion of SSEA1[+] cells/colonies express endogenous Oct4 and/or Nanog, however Nanog[+] hiPS cells are heterogeneous for numerous ES associated genes (Brambrink et al., 2008; Masaki et al., 2008).

Comparisons of the *temporal efficiency*, ie length of time to reverse the epigenotype and phenotype of the somatic genome, and the *reprogramming efficiency*, ie number of fully reprogrammed cells as a proportion of the starting cells, are difficult to elucidate between the various reprogramming methods due to differences in starting cell populations, mechanism of reprogramming, cell proliferation rates and outcomes. In the case of SCNT, the time from transfer of the donor nucleus to harvest of ES cells is constrained by the temporal requirements of embryonic development to blastocyst, typically 5-7 days for many mammals. Although conversion of murine somatic cells to full pluripotency by iPS technology occurs within similar a timeframe, antibiotic selection driven by Nanog has been demonstrated as early as three days post-infection, although there is a delay in observable GFP expression from the same promoter (Okita et al., 2007). Somatic Oct4 reporter gene expression in mES-thymocyte hybrids is observable much sooner (<48 hours from hybridization; Tada et al., 2001), suggesting complete erasure of the somatic cell epigenotype and reactivation of pluripotency markers is possible within shorter timeframes than that observed with SCNT and iPS induction. Viral reprogramming in human cells, and reprogramming with non-viral methods (eg. protein delivery), is more protracted. It should be remembered that the pluripotent partner in SCNT and hybrids, namely the oocyte and ES cell respectively, delivers the entire compliment of factors to induce pluripotency in the somatic cell, whereas iPS technology takes a minimalist approach in respect to number of factors utilized. In addition, the reprogramming efficiency of SCNT continues to be low, where initially 440 oocyte manipulations were required to generate just 29 sheep blastocysts (Wilmut et al., 1997). Similarly, initial iPS experiments could convert only 0.02% of infected human fibroblasts to a pluripotency phenotype (Takahashi & Yamanaka., 2007). Suggestions that differential integrations within a population of infected cells account for the low reprogramming efficiency were dispelled when no improvement in reprogramming efficiency was achieved in iPS experiments utilizing clonal lines of somatic cells harboring inducible transgenes of each key reprogramming factor at identical loci (Brambrink et al., 2008).

Lentivirus, adenovirus and transient plasmid transfection circumvent the requirement of target somatic cells to proliferate for virally-delivered, transgene integration (Stadtfeld et al., 2008[b]; Okita et al., 2008; discussed later). Nonetheless, 80% retroviral infection efficiency (as judged by GFP transgene integration and expression) equates to estimations of 40% of cells receiving all four factors. This method assumes that 20% of cells that are permissive to infection and receive one factor fail to receive one additional factor. Hence, this method is likely to underestimate the number of cells that receive all four factors since cells permissive for viral integration would conceivably receive atleast one copy of all factors during the infection period, generally overnight or 24 hours in duration.

2. EXPLORED / PROPOSED ALTERNATIVE STRATEGIES TO VIRAL DELIVERY OF KEY FACTORS

The unpredictable and random modifications to the host cell genome inherent with retroviral and lentiviral infection methodologies hamper use of these cells in a therapeutic setting and provoked exploration of non-mutagenic expression strategies (figure 1C-G; Carey et al., 2009; Kaji et al., 2009; Woltjen et al., 2009). Although reprogramming factors expressed from monkey moloney leukemia viral (MMLV) promoters are highly expressed in fibroblast, and selectively silenced in ES cells, insertional mutagenesis could activate oncogenes or silence/disrupt key genes. Efforts have also been directed towards improving the poor reprogramming efficiency documented thus far. Alternative reprogramming methods include (i) substituting key factors with chemical agents known to upregulate endogenous loci of key factors, or chromatin modifiers that enhance reprogramming efficiency (Shi et al., 2008[a]; Shi et al., 2008[b]; Huangfu et al., 2008[a]; Huangfu et al., 2008[b]), (ii) use of cells that naturally express combinations of the key iPS factors (Kim et al., 2008; Eminli et al.2008; Kim et al., 2009[a]), (iii) use of excisable transgenes (Kaji et al., 2009; Woltjen et al., 2009), (iv) delivery of protein of each reprogramming factor (Zhou et al., 2009; Kim et al., 2009[b]), and (v) delivery and expression of microRNA to compliment viral-mediated reprogramming or microRNA to knockdown specific factors (Judson et al., 2009; Zhao et al., 2008[b]). Each of these approaches is outlined diagrammatically in figure 1 and further described in the following text.

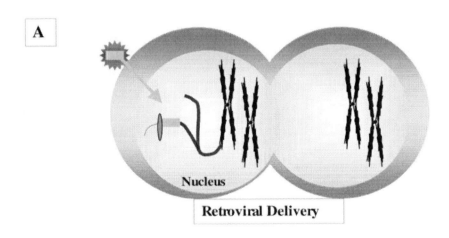

Figure 1. (Continued).

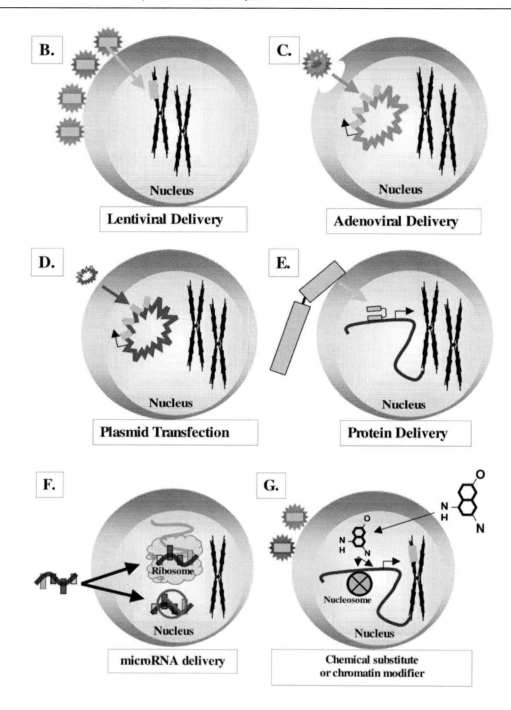

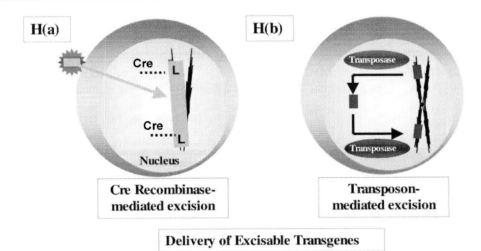

(A) Retroviral Delivery: retrovirus can deliver DNA sequence for each reprogramming factor to proliferating cells where they integrate into target cell DNA, (B) Lentiviral Delivery: the lentiviral pre-integration complex can transduce across the plasma membrane of proliferating and non-proliferating cells to deliver transgenes for each reprogramming factor before integrating into host DNA, (C) Adenoviral Delivery: adenoviral attachment to the host cell initiates invagination of the membrane and packaging into endocytotic vesicles for release into the cytosol. Expression of each reprogramming factor from episomal expression can induce pluripotency before being diluted from the cell population, (D) Plasmid Transfection: plasmids carrying each reprogramming factor can be directly transfected to target cells to drive reprogramming, (E) Protein Delivery: Recombinant proteins incorporating each of reprogramming factor and a plasma membrane transduction domain can transduce to the nuclei of target cells to drive target gene expression, (F) microRNA: microRNA can be delivered to target cells to induce expression of factors favorable to reprogramming, or to knockdown RNA's in the host cell to improve reprogramming efficiency, (G) Chemical Substitute or Chemical Modifier: chemical agents that upregulate endogenous loci of key reprogramming factors, or modify histone or DNA methyl and acteyl patterns, can be added to target cell culture media to improve reprogramming efficiency or replace integrative viral transgenes, (H) Delivery of Excisable Transgenes: (a) Cre Recombinase-mediated excision: floxed, integrated transgenes can be excised from genomic DNA with the application or expression of Cre-recombinase before DNA recombination, L: lox-P site flanking proviral sequences, (b) Transposase-mediated excision: transposase enzyme can integrate and excise transposon DNA elements comprising the reprogramming factors, followed by recombination of the host DNA.

Figure 1. The Numerous Methods for Deriving "Inducing Pluripotent Stem" iPS Cells.

2.1   Treatment of Target Cells with Chemical Agents: (i) to Replace Individual Transgenes, or (ii) Used in Concert with Viral Strategies to Improve Reprogramming Efficiency

The application of chemical agents that activate expression of endogenous loci of key factors (thus eliminating these individual factors from the reprogramming cocktail) remains an attractive alternative to viral-based iPS strategies (figure 1G). Although chemical inducers are readily reversible and allow temporal control over target gene regulation (Xu et al., 2008), chemicals that activate individual reprogramming factors, with minimal secondary affects on other factors or processes, are rare. Since Octamer family members are not functionally redundant and expression of Oct4 is rare in somatic cells, finding a suitable chemical substitute for Oct4 is imperative. Oct4 deactivation in differentiating ES cells is mediated by the histone methyltransferase G9a through direct methylation of histone lysines, or successive recruitment of epigenetic modifiers to chromatin (Tachibana et al., 2002; Feldman et al., 2005; Ikegami et al., 2006; Esteve et al., 2006). Unsurprisingly, G9a is expressed at significantly higher levels in somatic cells than ES cells. Chemical inhibition of G9a with BIX-01294 (BIX) eases the antagonism on histone 3, lysine 9 methylation (H3K9me)-mediated Oct4 expression and can fully substitute virally-delivered Oct4 for derivation of iPS cells from neural progenitor cells (in concert with proviral expression of remaining factors), albeit with dramatically reduced efficiency (Shi et al., 2008[a]). Short-hairpin RNA (shRNA) knockdown of G9a in adult NSC results in demethylation of Oct4 promoter and partial reactivation (~10% of ES cells) of Oct4 expression Ma et al., 2008). Addition of BIX compliments Oct4 and Klf4 retroviral reprogramming in NPC and maintains colony formation efficiency in NPC to four factor levels (Shi et al., 2008[a]). Interestingly, this implies that permanent Oct4 deactivation in differentiated cells is an active and not a permanently static process which can be disrupted some time after terminal differentiation. In concert with BIX, addition of an L-channel calcium agonist (Bayk8644) can substitute for Sox2 and cMyc in fibroblasts, cells that do not express appreciable levels of any reprogramming factor (Shi et al., 2008[b]). However, this compound exerts little affect in the absence of BIX. As noted for ES cells, inhibition of extracellular regulated kinase (ERK) signaling by chemically inhibiting ERK-activating (MEK) enzymes, seven to nine days after Oct4/Klf4 infection to NPC (and continually for 5 days) results in enhanced growth of reprogrammed iPS colonies with higher Oct4 expression (Burdon et al., 1999; Shi et al., 2008[a]). Extracellular Wnt3a can stimulate β–catenin-mediated induction of endogenous cMyc expression in target cells, producing a dramatic improvement in reprogramming efficiency (Marson et al., 2008). These results are not surprising considering Oct4, Sox2 and Nanog collectively activate components of Wnt signalling (Boyer et al., 2005). Another possible and undocumented substitute for cMyc is Okadaic acid (OA), a potent inhibitor of protein serine/threonine phosphatase 2A (PP2A). PP2A dephosphorylates specific serine residues in cMyc and targets it for rapid ubiquitin-regulated degradation. PP2A repression results in accumulated cMyc through upregulation of RNA production and protein sythesis (Zhang et al., 2007). OA also elicits increased Klf4, which in turn binds OA-responsive elements in the cMyc promoter eliciting upregulation of cMyc gene expression (Zhang et al., 2007). OA's additional inhibitory effect on translation, through repression of EIFα, may lead to an initial accumulation of mRNA transcript and subsequent delivery of bolus amounts of translated protein upon OA withdrawal. Replacement of Klf4 with Kenpaullone, a broad spectrum protein kinase inhibitor, to Oct4/Sox2/cMyc retrovirus expressing MEF generates Oct4 selectable iPS cells (albeit at reduced efficiency) able to contribute to germline-competent chimeras (Lyssiotis et al., 2009). Despite these impressive results, deriving iPS cells exclusively through chemical treatment, eg. BIX± Bayk8644+PD0325901+Wnt3a+Kenpaullone, may prove challenging due to only modest induction of target genes, and numerous potential secondary affects due to their broad spectrum of affects.

Treatment with chemical chromatin modifiers, disrupting methyl or acetyl patterns to core histones or DNA, that compliment viral iPS strategies can enhance reprogramming efficiency. High expression of jumonji-domain containing H3K9 demethylase Jhdm2a in ovum and early embryo reflects a critical role in pluripotency and reprogramming (Ma et al., 2008). Reflective of fold-differences between ES cells and somatic cells, overexpression of Jhdm2a in NSC caused global loss of H3K9me and promotes ES-NSC fusion based reprogramming (Ma et al., 2008). Deacetylation of N-terminal histone residues, associated with transcriptional deactivation, can be chemically inhibited to promote transcriptional permissiveness. Indeed, histone deacetylase (HDAC) inhibitor trichostatin A (TSA) increases cloning efficiency by SCNT (Kishigami et al., 2006). One hundred-fold improvements in iPS reprogramming efficiency of murine fibroblasts to (4 viral factor) iPS cells have been observed through chemical inhibition of histone deacetylase activity (Huangfu et al., 2008[a]; 2008[b]). Huangfu et al., (2008[a]; 2008[b]) tested a suite of HDAC inhibitors and found Valproic acid to improve reprogramming efficiency of 2,3 and 4 factor iPS. SCNT cloning efficiency can be improved using somatic cell nuclei genetically deficient in Dnmt1 (Blelloch et al., 2007). It is therefore of little surprise that transient, *de novo* DNA demethylation following retroviral infection increases numbers of AP[+] colonies and/or proportion of reporter gene[+] colonies (Mikkelsen et al., 2008; Huangfu et al., 2008; Shi et al., 2008[b]). Dnmt inhibition can also enhance reprogramming of Oct4/Klf4 mediated reprogramming in the presence of BIX (Shi et al., 2008[b]).

2.2   Elimination of Transgenes by Utilizing Somatic Cells that (i) Express High Concentrations of the Key iPS Factors from Endogenous Loci, or (ii) are Readily Accessible

Sox2, cMyc and Klf4 are each expressed from endogenous loci in a number of somatic cell types. Utilizing somatic cell populations that express high levels of these factors for iPS conversion enables elimination of individual, or combinations, of transgenes. Since endogenous Oct4 expression occurs rarely in adult tissues, it remains the single factor most difficult to substitute or omit. When used as nuclear donors for SCNT, neural stem cells increase the rate of blastocyst formation compared with terminally differentiated neural cells (Blelloch et al., 2007). The unusually high expression of Sox2 and cMyc, as well as pluripotency related factors alkaline phosphatase and SSEA1, in cranial neural progenitor cells (NPC) can be exploited to generate iPS cell viral delivery of Oct4 alone, or in concert with Klf4 (Kim et al., 2008; Eminli et al.2008; Kim et al., 2009[a]). Expression of OSMK from endogenous loci is comparable to that of ES cells in Oct4/Klf4 induced iPS cells by qRT-PCR (Kim et al., 2008). However, differences in Oct4 and Nanog promoter methylation were noted between Oct4 alone, NPC-derived iPS cell and (i) ES cells, and (ii) iPS cells generated from Oct4/Kf4 infection (Kim et al., 2008; Kim et al., 2009[a]). Endogenous Sox2 in NPC is higher than most cells but insufficient to reprogram in the absence of Oct4 (substituted with BIX; Shi et al., 2008[a]). Omission of Sox2 and cMyc from the reprogramming cocktail in NPC doesn't delay conversion to iPS cell as compared to four factor controls (Shi et al., 2008). Addition of BIX with Oct4/Klf4 maintains reprogramming efficiency as observed in four factor reprogramming (Shi et al., 2008a), and reprogrammed cells still commit to the germline in chimeras. However, since NPC's are harvested from crude brain cell extracts, they are not ideal for generating human iPS cells in a therapeutic setting.

Human foreskin represents an abundant source of cells for generating male iPS cells (Yu et al., 2007; Maherali et al., 2008). Human epidermal cells are not only readily accessible, they express high levels of Klf4, are similarly infectable as human interstitial fibroblasts whilst having less viral integrations (Segre et al., 1999; Aasen et al., 2008). Furthermore, human keratinocytes (from human hair follicles) express endogenous Klf4 and cMyc and readily reprogram in less time than other human cells, however improvements in reprogramming efficiency have not been achieved to date (Aasen et al., 2008; Maherali et al., 2008). However, when differentiated, fibroblastic outgrowths from plated hiPS-derived embryoid bodies were picked and re-induced, 'secondary' Oct4[+]/Tra-1-81[+] iPS cells were derived at 100-fold greater efficiency with reduced background iPS-like colonies (Maherali et al., 2008).

2.3   Non-Integrating Virus, Self-cleaving/Excisable Constructs and Direct Transfection of Plasmid to Target Somatic Cells

Random, insertional mutagenesis is neither required nor desirable for reprogramming (Stadfeld et al., 2008[b]). The particular site of retroviral and lentiviral integration could possibly disrupt host genes, influence proviral silencing and/or disrupt host gene expression. In addition, basal proviral expression suspends development of reprogramming cells in a partially reprogrammed phenotype. To facilitate, transient expression of key genes from transient and largely non-integrative adenoviral and plasmid transfection is markedly less likely to result in genomic integration (figure 1C&D). Adenoviral infection of mouse fibroblast, fetal liver and hepatocytes generated iPS cells with high degree chimerism in newborns following blastocyst injection (Stadfeld et al., 2008[b]). However, the markedly reduced efficiency could at least in part be due to reduced infectability. Although episomal adenovirus does integrate rarely (Harui et al., 1999), viral vectors progressively dilute as resultant iPS cells proliferate. Although high degree chimeras can form without evidence of tumour formation, a high incidence (almost a quarter) of tetraploidy has been noted in reprogrammed cells, through unpredictable cell fusion or selective infection of tetraploid cells in original population (Stadtfeld et al., 2008[b]).

Expression of all four factors simultaneously from polycistronic expression cassettes, incorporating 'self-cleaving' 2A peptides, causes 'ribosomal skipping' to enable comparable expression of each factor from a single promoter (Sommer et al., 2008; Carey et al., 2009). With an IRES sequence separating pairs of factors, infected MEF and tail-tip fibroblasts (TTF) expressed a Sox2/GFP reporter and required only 1-3 copies of each factor for complete reprogramming (Sommer et al., 2008). Carey et al., (2009) subsequently constructed doxycycline-inducible factors separated by self-cleaving 2A peptides, without IRES technology. Induced expression of Oct4 and Sox2 from a single polycistronic construct was comparable to that in ES cells and, in addition to Myc and Klf4 expression, sufficient to reprogram murine fibroblast and postnatal human fibroblasts. Reprogramming efficiency of MEF was estimated at 0.0001%, a reduction when compared to alternative viral methods (Carey et al., 2009).

DNA transposons are genetic elements that are excised and re-integrated throughout the genome by specific 'transposase' enzymes, a phenomenon referred to a transposition. *piggyBac* is one such transposon capable of harboring a multiple-gene payload that preferentially inserts in transcriptional DNA units harboring TTAA sequences (Ding et al., 2005). Induction of individual or polycistronic, doxycycline-inducible constructs, delivered to murine and human fibroblasts by transposase-mediated integration and subsequent excision, generated iPS cells exhibiting all the hallmarks of pluripotency, including contribution to mid-gestation embryos by tetraploid complementation assay (figure 1Hb; Woltjen et al., 2009). Although the efficiency of transgene excision by transient transposase expression was variable, proficient recombination of insertion sites to wild type resulted following excision and endogenous pluripotency genes continued to be expressed.

Additionally, floxed proviral constructs can be excised through subsequent infection with transient Cre-recombinase expressing adenovirus (figure Ha; Kaji et al., 2009). Recombined MEF convert to AP$^+$ colonies 9 days post-infection and undergo endogenous gene expression and demethylation of Nanog and Oct4 promoters. A single insertion of multi-expression cassette was enough to induce complete reprogramming. Concurrent and repeated plasmid transfection of two polycistronic plasmids expressing (i) Oct4, Sox2, Klf4, and (ii) cMyc to mouse embryonic fibroblasts also induced pluripotency and produced chimeras, however reprogramming efficiency was compromised compared to retroviral methodologies (Okita et al., 2008). Plasmid construction of the polycistronic plasmid appeared to alter reprogramming efficiencies in some clones, suggesting unexpected and differential expression levels of each factor. This approach is further hampered by rare integration events in some clones (although not detected in chimeras), and a 10-fold reduction in efficiency when cMyc is not transfected with the major construct. In addition, integrative technologies may express higher levels of each factor.

2.4   Protein Delivery as an Alternative to Viral Strategies

Like use of small molecule compounds, protein delivery is an attractive approach to iPS cell generation due to its reversibility (figure 1E). However, the hydophobicity of the cellular lipid bilayer core represents a significant barrier to passive movement of proteins from surrounding milieu to the cellular interior. The inevitable progression to non-viral, non-DNA delivery was first demonstrated by Zhou et al., (2009)[c]. Expressed in *E.coli* and subsequently purified, recombinant proteins incorporating a poly-arginine targeting sequence linked to the four human iPS factors were capable of converting MEF to protein-iPS (piPS) cells with global gene expression patterns similar to ES cells. It should be noted that modifying host cell histone aceytlation patterns was required to yield stable cell lines, and contrary to viral strategies, omission of cMyc protein induced colony formation without reporter gene expression. These results were soon extrapolated to human cells, although this study expressed proteins in transfected human cells and applied whole protein extracts to targets cells without purification (Kim et al., 2009[b]). Importantly, supplementation with chemical agent/s was not required. In addition to being the first demonstration of non-DNA mediated iPS reprogramming, these reports highlight some interesting points. Efficiencies in retroviral reprogramming are calculated on assumptions that around half of the infected cells receive all four viral factors. Yet immunocytochemical stains confirm nuclear localization of each fusion protein in treated cells (Zhou et al., 2009[c]; C.Heffernan, manuscript in preparation). Significant improvements in reprogramming efficiency did not result from protein delivery, regardless of histone deacetylation modulation. Protein delivery circumvents the lag in transcription and translation of critical factors to levels required for reprogramming, yet ES-like colonies were observed much later than in viral strategies. It is unclear whether the thresholds of Oct4 expression that are critical in maintaining pluripotency in ES cells are also applicable in somatic cell conversion to iPS cells.

An arginine-rich basic domain ([49]**RKKRRQRRR**[57]) of trans-activating transcriptional-activator (TAT) of HIV binds heparan sulfate proteoglycans before trans-membrane import through caveolar ('lipid raft') endocytosis (Green & Loewenstein, 1988; Frankel & Pabo, 1988; Rusnati et al., 1999; Tyagi et al., 2001; Fittipaldi et al., 2003). Over 60 TAT-fusion proteins have been used to delivery proteins to nucleus (Becker-Hapak et al., 2001). This domain also mediates importin-independent translocation to the nuclear compartment (Efthymiadis et al., 1998). The rapid (in the order of minutes; Fittipaldi et al., 2003) and efficient translocation to the nuclear compartment renders TAT an ideal fusion partner for delivery of recombinant transcriptional activators to nuclear chromatin (Efthymiadis et al., 1998; Yun et al., 2008). Due to their wide range of biological functions and ligands, heparan sulfate proteoglycans are ubiquitously expressed within and between cell populations, a feature that could be exploited for future experimental and therapeutic applications in piPS.

2.5   RNA Delivery Strategies

Introduction of either (i) miRNA transcripts that mimic those expressed in ES cells, or (ii) siRNAs that interfere with expression of endogenous factors, are both approaches that can be applied to derive iPS cells (figure 1F; Mikkelsen et al., 2008; Zhao et al., 2008[b]; Judson et al., 2009). ES cell-specific cell cycle-regulating (ESCC) miRNA's of the miR290 cluster are expressed in ES cells and accelerate transition through G1/S. Hence, cMyc and nMyc both target mIR-290 cluster, and Oct4 binds five known promoters for miRNA in ES cells (Boyer et al., 2005). Since the miR-290 cluster is a target of cMyc, it is perhaps unsurprising that transfection of miR-294 on days 0 and 6 post-retroviral infection can replace cMyc to 75% efficiency, but not enhance 4 factor iPS (Judson et al., 2009). However, it is noteworthy that replacement of cMyc with miR-294 yielded a greater proportion of Oct4-GFP[+] colonies (Judson et al., 2009).

siRNA knockdown of Dnmt1 can aid cells transgress from partially to fully reprogrammed and increase reprogramming efficiency (Mikkelsen et al., 2008). Similarly, short-hairpin RNA (shRNA) knockdown of G9a, a histone methyltransferase involved in Oct4 deactivation in post-implantation embryos *in vivo*, results in demethylation of the Oct4 promoter and partial reactivation (Feldman et al., 2005; Ma et al., 2008). Addition of p53 siRNA to adult human fibroblasts, in concert with Oct4/Sox2/Klf4 infection, increased efficiency to varying degrees, alone or in combination with additional treatments (Zhao et al., 2008[b]).

3. EXPERIMENTAL APPLICATION OF iPS CELLS FOR THERAPY

Original reports demonstrating induction of iPS cells in human cells confirmed their potential to be differentiated into a number of cell types (Takahashi et al., 2007). Since the therapeutic potential of human differentiated iPS cells cannot be ascertained *in vivo*, mouse models of humanized disease represent an invaluable resource in exploring therapeutic applicability of iPS technology. Hanna et al., (2007) infected adult mouse cells harboring a defective human sickle hemoglobin allele with retrovirus for OSK plus lentivirus for floxed cMyc cDNA. Following adenoviral expression of Cre recombinase and excision of the cMyc sequence, one clone engrafted to peripheral blood and rescued the disease phenotype in the absence of tumor formation (Hanna et al., 2007).

For experimental iPS technology to be translated into therapeutic application, diseased and aged donor cells firstly need to readily convert to iPS cells (Dimos et al., 2008; Soldner et al., 2009). Dimos et al., (2008) was first to demonstrate the feasibility of generating iPS cells in aged, amyotrophic lateral scleroris (ALS) sufferers. Embryoid bodies actively differentiated into glia and neural cells, cell types defective in ALS sufferers. In addition, lentiviral integration of floxed reprogramming factors to fibroblasts from Parkinsons disease sufferers, followed by Cre recombinase-mediated excision of transgenes, generates iPS cells that display molecular signatures closer to ES cells than non-excised iPS cells (Soldner et al., 2009). Dopaminergic neuronal-marker positive neural cells could be derived from these cells by directed differentiation. However, systemic genetic polymorphisms will require correction prior to transplantation, either in the pluripotent state or potentially in the post-iPS differentiated cell. To facilitate, Zou et al., (2009) elegantly demonstrated sequence-specific DNA targeting of a non-specific endonuclease domain in hES and hiPS cells. Digestion of DNA with subsequent homologous recombination can be utilized for gene deletion, or site-specific insertion of wild-type gene sequences.

4. APPLICABILITY OF iPS IN THERAPEUTIC SETTING

It is now indisputable that iPS cells acquire many morphological and functional characteristics reminiscent of ES cells. iPS technology enables retrospective study of disease, once pathology has been identified in sufferers, instead of studying cells of expected sufferers of known pedigree (Nishikawa et al., 2008). Although stem cells generated by nuclear transfer and iPS technology are autologous for donor nuclear DNA, only iPS cells are homoplasmic for mitochondrial DNA (Condic & Rao, 2008). This is an important point when considering the transmission of numerous mitochondrial dysfunctions due to the inherent mixing of mitochondria in NT-derived cells. Thankfully, the US President's Council of Bioethics states "there would seem to be nothing to object to ethically if procedures were developed to turn somatic cells into pluripotent stem cells, non-embryonic functional equivalents of embryonic stem cells", and "...no obstacle to, or reason to oppose, federal funding of research on dedifferentiation of somatic cells" (White Paper: Alternative Sources of Pluripotent Stem Cells, http://www. bioethics.gov/reports/ white_ paper/text.html).

However, despite circumventing the concerns associated with SCNT and animal/human hybrids, significant practical, legal and ethical concerns will impede a smooth transition of iPS cells from lab-bench to clinic. With the recent development of non-integrative methods of iPS generation, it seems timely to consider (i) practical issues associated with generating iPS cells, and (ii) the legal and ethical considerations for using these cells for therapy. Due to familiarity, we focus on regulations under USA and Australian law. Alternative sources of autologous, differentiated cells for therapy are also outlined below.

4.1   Practical Pitfalls of iPS cells for Human Therapy

From the outset, it was evident that integrating viral-based generation of autologous cells was undesirable for human therapeutic applications. Now, micromolar concentrations of recombinant protein transduced into somatic cells is sufficient to reverse their development fate (Zhou et al., 2009^c; Kim et al., 2009^b). In the absence of reporter gene expression, we require stringent criteria for selection of desirable clones from human iPS cultures (Blelloch et al., 2007; Meissner et al., 2007). Although serum starvation of reprogrammed (murine) cells reportedly accelerates reprogramming and also aids selection of desirable clones (Blelloch et al., 2007), such success has not been demonstrated in human iPS. Hence, partially reprogrammed, colony forming units that share many characteristics with fully reprogrammed cells require exclusion from the transplantable cell pool. We need to ensure a homogenously differentiated population of cells is transplanted, and cells remain differentiated following transplantation. Mouse iPS cells initiate tumor formation as prevalent as ES cells when transplanted to brains of immune suppressed mice (Miura et al., 2009). When transplanted to mice following differentiation into neural cells, tumorgenicity is depended on the original cells used for reprogramming and all tumors examined contained variable levels of undifferentiated cells. It is noteworthy that considerably higher tumor formation was observed when adult cells were used. Interestingly, tumor formation occurrence did not correlate with retroviral cMyc expression (Miura et al., 2009).

Since pluripotent cells are inherently teratogenic *in vivo*, complete and universal differentiation of a pool of pluripotent cells to the desired cell type is required for transplantation. It remains an important consideration when potentially treating non-life threatening injury such as spinal cord injury in young sufferers, who are likely to benefit from such a procedure. Will/should spinal cord injury patients accept risks of malignancy with untimely and premature death for greater mobility? The inefficient and protracted isolation, derivation and expansion of iPS cells also limits the swift treatment required of a spinal cord injury, not to mention the related regulatory approval of patient-specific iPS cell lines (Cyranoski, 2008).

Due to differential expression patterns, the cells able to be reprogrammed with the fewest reprogramming factors are perhaps the least accessible in therapeutic settings (Kim et al., 2008; Kim et al., 2009^a). Indeed, standard protocols for human iPS include two extra factors for reprogramming (Park et al., 2008). In light of results shown in the mouse, a logical step forward will be to generate iPS cells in cranial NPC with Oct4 recombinant protein alone. Although impressive in an experimental sense, is it really therapeutically relevant due to their relatively inaccessibility? Isolation of neural progenitors from olfactory mucosa may be more applicable due to greater accessibility, however generation of iPS cell from this cell population has yet to be demonstrated (Murrell et al., 2008). Although hES-like colonies appear 21-30 days post-infection and demonstrate many of hallmarks of ES cells, long term studies are required to ensure malignancy doesn't result from this transient, intracellular over-expression of reprogramming factors. Importantly, dysregulation of each individual iPS factor is causative, or a feature of, malignancy (Liu, 2008).

4.2   Legal and Ethical Considerations of iPS cells for Human Therapy

In the absence of a universal pluripotent cell line for therapy, each individual iPS cell line would likely be classified a "Class 4 *in vitro* device (IVD)" under Australia Federal law, of "high public health risk ... intended to be used to screen for transmissible agents ... or transplantation (Australian Government Department of Health and Aging, Therapeutic Goods Administration http://www.tga.gov.au/ivd/overview.htm). The American equivalent would be Code of Federal Regulations (CFR) governing transplantation of laboratory processed human cells and tissues (Condic & Rao, 2008). Class 4 IVD materials are subject to numerous *in vitro* testing and evaluation before transplantation, a point that may render iPS cells cost inhibitive for many people if not subsidized by Governmental Agencies. Since long term culture of converted iPS cells are almost universally reliant on culture on irradiated fibroblast feeder layer, regulatory authorities are likely to insist on feeder layer-free technologies to eliminate possibility of cross-species or allogenic contamination. Also, random genomic recombination events following (*Cre*-mediated) excision of polycistronic expression cassettes, are likely to attract attention from regulatory authorities, and non-excisable remnants still render the resultant cells genetically modified (Kaji et al., 2009). Although *piggyBac* transposon/transposase based excision of expression cassettes is reportedly 'seamless (Woltjen et al., 2009), similar concerns surrounding unpredictable recombination events in the resultant cell still apply. Incomplete conversion of the epigenome to that of the adopted transplantable cell (from iPS to desired differentiated cell type) may result in regression of transplanted cells to iPS cell *in vivo* or even to that of the original cell type (Miura et al., 2009). These issues will need to be addressed and satisfied for regulatory body approval of such technologies.

Without strict authoritative guidelines, the simplicity of iPS cell derivation may also be its ethical downfall; renegade practitioners may easily undertake transplantation in vulnerable human patients without approval. Consensus will need to be reached between the scientific and lay-communities on what is deemed acceptable. Do the notable differences between iPS cells and ES cells preclude them from being utilized in the clinic? Do we really need to generate iPS cells that are identical, or near identical, to ES cells? Or should the ultimate criteria be direct comparisons between differentiated iPS cells and their *in situ* equivalents?

The use of aged fibroblasts for iPS conversion and subsequent gamete production and IVF could potentially pass on imprinting and DNA damage acquired over time to offspring, and also challenges sensitivities surrounding reproduction for infertile couples (Cyranoski, 2008; Condic & Rao, 2008). However, sperm require a Y-chromosome to form, therefore lesbian couples would be unable to produce genetically-related offspring. Such concerns even provoked Yamanaka himself to lobby for regulation (Cyranoski, 2008). In a therapeutic sense, is it ethically sound to risk the potential teratogenicity of cell transplantation to treat more imminent disease, eg. Parkinson's or Alzheimer's diseases, if death is imminent?

4.3   Potential Alternatives to iPS Cells

The lineage commitment of *in vivo* progenitor cells can be re-directed down a related, but alternative, developmental lineage. Referred to as transdetermination (TDE), this differs from transdifferentiation (TDI) whereby somatic cells substitute their differentiated genetic program with an unrelated other. Utilizing either method for the derivation of cells for therapy circumvents the requirement of a pluripotent intermediate, and represents a possible alternative to the two stage iPS method.

Transdetermination of permissive, hepatic progenitor cells to islet cells can be achieved through transfer of a single transcription factor (Yechoor et al., 2009). Furthermore, adenovirus expressing single pancreatic transcription factor re-directs differentiation to insulin expressing cells (Ferber et al., 2000). Alternatively, TDI has now demonstrated in mesoderm and endoderm lineage cells (Zhou et al., 2008[a]; Takeuchi & Bruneau, 2009). A screen of lineage regulators identified factors that directing pancreatic development *in vivo* (Zhou et al., 2008). Pancreatic exocrine cells derive from pancreatic endoderm. Directed adenoviral delivery of three key factors to pancreatic exocrine cells to immune deficient adult mice *in* vivo resulted in >20% conversion to insulin+ cells. As shown in iPS, one factor can be replaced with alternative factor with accompanying loss in efficiency. Resultant cells were functionally similar to endogenous insulin-secreting β–cells and remained throughout assessment period. They express and suppress relevant markers and recruit vasculature to the local milieu. Adenoviral infection of mice chemically rendered diabetic by ablation of β–cell population caused reprogramming to islet cells and resulted in improved glucose tolerance and serum insulin after 8 weeks. Transgene expression was extinguished within 2 months (Zhou et al., 2008).

Cultured mouse embryos transiently transfected with two transcription factors (Gata4 and Tbx5) and a chromatin modifier (Baf60c) transformed non-cardiac mesoderm to beating cardiomyocytes (Takeuchi & Bruneau, 2009). This pattern is reflective of 4 factor iPS cells, if you consider cMyc a chromatin modifier allowing expression of repressed genes, and experiments using chemical chromatin modifier. As for iPS, redundancy with Gata and Baf family members reduced efficiency. Cardiac gene expression can be induced with Gata4 and Baf60c alone, but Tbx5 is required to achieve beating tissue in half of embryos. Importantly, converted cells did not arise from specific targeting of undifferentiated Isl1[+] progenitor cells. Although this study demonstrates conversion of non-cardiac mesoderm to myocytes, it remains conversion of lineages in the same germ layer.

TDE and TDI represents a preferable method for cell derivation; reprogramming can be achieved with minimal number of factors (Takeuchi & Bruneau, 2009), alleviation of the teratogenicity associated with pluripotent cells, and rapid conversion of intra-lineage cells, suggested to be a result of less epigenetic remodeling (Zhou et al., 2008). Such rapidity of conversion may be attractive for treatment of spinal cord injury, provided suitable methods for trans-differentiating between neural cells *in vitro* are developed. Although demonstrated *in vivo*, efficiency of TDI is reportedly many orders of magnitudes higher that iPS conversion (Zhou et al., 2008), and alleviates the requirement for pre-transplantation, *in vitro* differentiation protocols. Although TDE can be achieved with transfection with a one or two exogenous factor (Ferber et al., 2000; Yechoor et al., 2009), a related progenitor (lineage committed but partially differentiated) cell pool is required which may not be possible or accessible for all cell types/lineages.

Finally, HLA antigen null hES cells could conceivably constitute a 'universal' cell for widespread therapy (Vogel, 2002). These cells could be differentiated in numerous cell types for transplantation and would evade detection of any host immune system due its $HLA^{-/-}$ status. Obvious advantages include (i) evasion of concerns surrounding iPS and alternative technologies, (ii) alleviates the continued derivation of donor cells from each patient, (iii) cells would not have pre-existing mutations or be aged cells, and (iv) and only an initial approval from FDA/TGA agencies before widespread use. However, attempts have proved as yet unsuccessful as HLA molecules are represented by multiple genetic loci. In addition, unpredictable transformations in the transplanted cells would similarly evade detection by the host immune system and may continue unheeded.

CONCLUSION

A considered approach should be employed before clinical trials initiate to avoid the adverse publicity following adverse outcomes of gene therapy trials (Raper et al., 2003). Even if the aforementioned concerns are insurmountable, this methodology is no less revolutionary and remains a radical change in thinking for cellular reprogramming. Indeed, application of iPS-based approaches has initiated development of alternative technologies for cellular therapy, namely transdifferentiation. Whether iPS, transdifferentiation or transdetermination translate to the therapeutic arena remain to be determined.

REFERENCES

Aasen et al., (2008). Efficient and rapid generation of induced pluripotent stem cells from human keratinocytes. *Nat Biotech.* 26: 1272-1284

Becker-Hapak et al., (2001). TAT-mediated protein transduction into mammalian cells. *Methods.* 24:247-256.

Blelloch et al., (2007). Generation of induced pluripotent stem cells in the absence of drug selection. *Cell Stem Cell.* 1: 245-247

Boyer et al., (2005). Core transcriptional regulatory circuitry in human embryonic stem cells. *Cell.* 122: 947-956

Brambrink et al., (2008). Sequential expression of pluripotency markers during direct reprogramming of mouse somatic cells. *Cell Stem Cell.* 2: 151-159.

Burdon et al., (1999). Suppression of SHP-2 and ERK signalling promotes self-renewal of mouse embryonic stem cells. *Dev. Biol.* 210: 30-43.

Carey et al., (2009). Reprogramming of murine and human somatic cells using a single polycistronic vector. *PNAS.* 106(1): 157-162

Catena et al., (2004). Conserved POU binding DNA sites in the Sox2 upstream enhancer regulate gene expression in embryonic and neural stem cells. *J. Biol. Chem.* 279(40): 41846-41857

Chew et al., (2005). Reciprocal trasncriptional regulation of Pou5f1 and Sox2 via the Oct4/Sox2 complex in embryonic stem cells. *Mol. Cell Biol.* 25(14): 6031-6046.

Condic ML. & Rao M. (2008). Regulatory issues for personalized pluripotent cells. *Stem Cells.* 26(11): 2753-2758

Cyranoski, D. (2008). Stem Cells: 5 Things to know before jumping on the iPS bandwagon. *Nature.* 452(7186): 406-408.

Dimos et al., (2008). Induced pluripotent stem cells generated from patients with ALS can be differentiated into motor neurons. *Science.* 321:1218-1221

Ding et al., (2005). Efficient transposition of the piggyBac (PB) transposon in mammalian cells and mice. *Cell.* 122:473-483.

Dominguez-Sola et al., (2007). Non-transcriptional control of DNA replication by c-Myc. *Nature.* 448: 445-452.

Donohue et al., (2009). The pluripotency factor Oct4 interacts with Ctcf and also controls X-chromosome pairing and counting. *Nature.* In press.

Efthymiadis et al., (1998). The HIV-1 Tat nuclear localization sequence confers novel nuclear import properties. *J Biol.Chem.* 273(3): 1623-1628.

Eilers & Eisenman (2009). Myc's broad reach. *Genes Dev.* 22(20): 2755-2766.

Ema et al., (2008). Kruppel-like factor 5 is essential for blastocyst development and the normal self-renewal of mouse ESCs. *Cell Stem Cell.* 3: 555-567.

Esteban et al., (2009). Generation of induced pluripotent stem cell lines from Tibetan miniature pig. *J.Biol.Chem.* 284(26): 17634-17640.

Esteve et al., (2006). Direct interaction between DNMT1 and G9a coordinates DNA and histone methylation during replication. *Genes Dev.* 20: 3089-3103.

Ezashi et al., (2009). Derivation of induced pluripotent stem cells from pig somatic cells. *PNAS.* 106(27): 10993-10998

Feldman et al., (2005). G9a-mediated irreversible epigenetic inactivation of Oct3/4 during early embryogenesis. *Nat. Cell Biol.* 8(2): 188-194.

Ferber et al., (2000). Pancreatic and duodenal homeobox gene 1 induces expression of insulin genes in liver and ameliorates streptozotocin-induced hyperglycemia. *Nat Med.* 6(5): 568-572.

Fittipaldi et al., (2003). Cell membrane lipid rafts mediate caveolar endocytosis of HIV Tat fusion proteins. *J. Biol. Chem.* 278(36): 34141-34149.

Frankel & Pabo, (1988). Cellular uptake of the Tat protein from human immunodeficiency virus. *Cell.* 55:1189-1193.

Green & Loewenstein, (1988). Autonomous functional domains of chemically synthesized human immunodeficiency virus tat trans-activator protein. *Cell.* 55(6): 1179-88.

Guenther et al., (2007). A chromatin landmark and transcription initiation at most promoters in human cells. *Cell Stem Cell.* 130: 77-88

Hanna et al., (2007). Treatment of sickle cell anemia mouse model with iPS cells generated from autologous skin. *Science.* 318(5858): 1920-1923.

Harui et al., (1999). Frequency and stability of chromosomal integration of adenovirus vectors. *J Virol.* 73: 6141-6146

Hochedlinger & Jaenisch. (2007). Nuclear reprogramming and pluripotency. *Nature.* 441: 1061-1067

Huangfu et al., (2008)[a]. Induction of pluripotent stem cells by defined factors is greatly improved by small-molecule compounds. *Nat Biotech.* 26(7): 795-797.

Huangfu et al., (2008)[b]. Induction of pluripotent stem cells from primary human fibroblasts with only Oct4 and Sox2. *Nat Biotech.* 26(11): 1269-1275.

Ikegami et al., (2006). Genome-wide and locus-specific DNA hypomethylation in G9a deficient mouse embryonic stem cells. *Genes to Cells.* 12(1): 1-11.

Jiang et al., (2008). The core Klf circuitry regulates self-renewal of embryonic stem cells. *Nat Cell Biol.* 10(3): 353-360.

Judson et al., (2009). Embryonic stem cell-specific microRNAs promote induced pluripotency. *Nat. Biotech.* 27(5): 459-461.

Kaji et al., (2009). Virus-free induction of pluripotency and subsequent excision of reprogramming factors. *Nature.* 458(7239): 771-775.

Kang et al., (2009). iPS cells can support full-term development of tetraploid blastocyst-complemented embryos. *Cell Stem Cell.* 5: in press.

Kim et al., (2008). Pluripotent stem cells induced from adult neural stem cells by reprogramming with two factors. *Nature.* 454(7204): 646-650.

Kim et al., (2009)[a]. Oct4-induced pluripotency in adult neural stem cells. *Cell.* 136(3): 411-419.

Kim et al., (2009)[b]. Generation of human induced pluripotent stem cells by direct delivery of reprogramming proteins. *Cell Stem Cells.* 4: 472-476.

Kishigami et al., (2006). Significant improvement of mouse cloning technique by treatment with trichostatin A after somatic nuclear transfer. Biochem. *Biophys. Res. Commun.* 340(1): 183-189.

Li et al., (2008). Generation of rat and human induced pluripotent stem cells by combining genetic reprogramming and chemical inhibitors. *Cell Stem Cell.* 4:16-19.

Liu et al., (2008)[a]. Generation of induced pluripotent stem cells from adult rhesus monkey fibroblasts. *Cell Stem Cell.* 3:587-590

Liu, (2008): iPS cells: a more critical review. *Stem Cell Dev.* 17(3): 391-397.

Liu et al., (2008)[c]. Yamanaka factors critically regulate the developmental signaling network in mouse embryonic stem cells. *Cell Res.* 18:1177-1189

Loh et al., (2009). Generation of induced pluripotent stem cells from human blood. *Blood.* 113(22): 5476-5479.

Lyssiotis et al., (2009). Reprogramming of murine fibroblasts to induced pluripotent stem cells with chemical complementation of Klf4.*PNAS.* 106(22): 8912-8917.

Ma et al., (2008). G9a and Jhdm2a regulate embryonic stem cell fusion-induced reprogramming of adult neural stem cells. *Stem Cells.* 26(8): 2131-2141.

Maherali et al., (2007). Directly reprogrammed fibroblasts show global epigenetic remodeling and widespread tissue contribution. *Cell Stem Cell.* 1:55-70.

Maherali et al., (2008). *A* high-efficiency system for the generation and study of human induced pluripotent stem cells. *Cell Stem Cell.* 3(3):340-345.

Marion et al., (2009). Telomeres acquire embryonic stem cell characteristics in induced pluripotent stem cells. *Cell Stem Cell.* 4: 141-154.

Marson et al., (2008). Wnt signalling promotes reprogramming of somatic cells to pluripotnecy. *Cell Stem Cell.* 7: 132-135.

Martinato et al., (2008). Analysis of Myc-induced histone modifications on target chromatin. *PLoS ONE.* 3(11): e3650

Masaki et al., (2008). Heterogeneity of pluripotent marker gene expression in colonies generated in human iPS cell induction culture. *Stem Cell Res.* 1: 105-115

Masui et al., (2007). Pluripotency governed by Sox2 via regulation of Oct3/4 expression in mouse embryonic stem cells. *Nat Cell Biol.* 9(6): 625-635

Meissner et al., (2007). Direct reprogramming of genetically unmodified fibroblasts into pluripotent stem cells. *Nature Biotech.* 25(10): 1177-11

Mikkelsen et al., (2008). Dissecting direct reprogramming through integrative genomic analysis. *Nature.* 454: 49-55.

Mitsui et al., (2003). The homeoprotein Nanog is required for maintenance of pluripotency in mouse epiblast and ES cells. *Cell.* 113:631-642

Miura et al., (2009). Variation in the safety of inducd pluripotent stem cell lines. *Nat. Biotech.* In press.

Murrell et al., (2008). Olfactory mucoase is a potential source for autologous stem cell therapy for parkinson's disease. *Stem Cells.* 26: 2183-2192.

Nakagawa et al., (2007). Generation of induced pluripotent stem cells without Myc from mouse and human fibroblasts. *Nat. Biotech.* 26(1): 101-106.

Nishikawa et al., (2008). The promise of human induced pluripotent stem cells for research and therapy. *Nat Rev. Mol Cell. Biol.* 9(9): 725-729.

Niwa et al., (2000). Quantitative expression of Oct3/4 defines differentiation, dedifferentiation or self-renewal of ES cells. *Nat Genet.* 24: 372-376

Okita et al., (2007). Generation of germline-competent induced pluripotent stem cells. *Nature.* 448(7151): 313-317.

Okita et al., (2008). Generation of mouse induced pluripotent stem cells without viral vectors. *Science.* 322: 949-953.

Pan et al., (2002). Stem cell pluripotency and transcription factor Oct4. *Cell Res.* 12(5-6): 321-329.

Park et al., (2008). Generation of human-induced pluripotent stem cells. *Nat. Protocols.* 7: 1180-1186.

Raper et al. (2003). Fatal systemic inflammatory response syndrome in a orthinine transcarbamylase deficient patient following adenoviral gene transfer. *Mol. Genet. Metab.* 80: 148–58.

Remenyi et al., (2003). Crystal structure of a POU/HMG/DNA ternary complex suggests differential assembly of Oct4 and Sox2 on two enhancers. *Genes Dev.* 17: 2048-2059.

Rodda et al., (2005). Transcriptional regulation of Nanog by Oct4 and Sox2. *J. Biol. Chem.* 280(26): 24731-24737

Rowland et al., (2005). The Klf4 tumour suppressor is a transcriptional repressor of p53 that acts as a context-dependent oncogene. *Nat. Cell Biol.* 7(11): 1074-82.

Rusnati et al., (1999). Multiple interactions of HIV-1 Tat protein with size-defined heparin oligosaccharides. *J. Biol. Chem.* 274(40): 28198-28205.

Segre et al., (1999). Klf4 is a transcription factor required for establishing the barrier function of the skin. *Nat Genetics.* 22: 356-360.

Seoane et al., (2001). TGF influences Myc, Miz-1 and Smad to control the CDK inhibitor $p15^{INK4b}$. *Nat Cell. Biol.* 3:400-408.

Shi et al., (2008)[a]. A combined chemical and genetic approach for the generation of induced pluripotent stem cells. *Cell Stem Cell.* 2: 525-528.

Shi et al., (2008)[b]. *Induction of pluripotent stem cells from mouse embryonic fibroblasts by Oct4 and Klf4 with small-molecule compounds. Cell Stem Cell*. 3: 568-574.

Silva et al., (2006). Nanog promotes transfer of pluripotency after cell fusion. *Nature*. 441(7096): 997-1001.

Soldner et al., (2009). Parkinson's disease patient-derived induced pluripotent stem cells free of viral reprogramming factors. *Cell*. 136: 964-977.

Sommer et al., (2008). iPS cell generation using a single lentiviral stem cell cassette. *Stem Cells*. 27(3): 543-549.

Sridharan et al., (2009). Role of the murine reprogramming factors in the induction of pluripotency. *Cell*. 136:364-377

Stadtfeld et al., (2008)[a]. Defining molecular cornerstones during fibroblast to iPS cell reprogramming in mouse. *Cell Stem Cell*. 2: 230-240.

Stadtfeld et al., (2008)[b]. Induced pluripotent stem cells generated without viral integration. *Science*. 322(5903): 945-949.

Tachibana et al., (2002). G9a histone methyltransferase plays a dominant role in euchromatic histone H3 lysine 9 methylation and is essential for early embryogenesis. *Genes Dev*. 16: 1779-1791.

Tada et al., (2001). Nuclear reprogramming of somatic cells by in vitro hybridization with ES cells. *Curr. Biol*. 11(19): 1553-1558

Takahashi & Yamanaka, (2006). *Induction of pluripotent stem cells from mouse embryonic and adult fibroblasts by defined factors. Cell*. 126:1-14.

Takahashi et al., (2007). Induction of pluripotent stem cells from adult human fibroblasts by defined factors. *Cell*. 131:861-872.

Takeuchi & Bruneau, (2009). Directed transdifferentiation of mouse mesoderm to heart tissue by defined factors. *Nature*. 459(7247): 708-711.

The President's Council on Bioethics. *White Paper: Alternative Sources of Human Pluripotent Stem Cells*. In. Washington, D.C.; 2005.

Tomioka et al., (2002). Identification of Sox-2 regulatory region which is under control of Oct3/4-Sox2 complex. *Nuc. Acids Res*. 30(14): 3202-3213.

Tyagi et al., (2001). Internalization of HIV-1 tat requires cell surface heparan sulfate proteoglycans. *J.Biol.Chem*. 276(5): 3254-3261.

Vogel, (2002). *In the Midwest, pushing back the stem cell frontier. Science*. 295: 1818-1820.

Wilmut et al., (1997). Viable offspring derived from fetal and adult mammalian cells. *Nature*. 385: 810-813

Wernig et al., (2007). In vitro reprogramming of fibroblasts into a pluripotent ES-cell-like state. *Nature*. 448: 318-324.

Wernig et al., (2008). c-Myc is dispensable for direct reprogramming of mouse fibroblasts. *Cell Stem Cell*. 2:10-12.

Woltjen et al., (2009). piggyBac transposition reprograms fibroblasts to induced pluripotent stem cells. *Nature*. 458(7239): 766-770

Xu et al., (2008). A chemical approach to stem-cell biology and regenerative medicine. *Nature*. 453: 338-344.

Xu et al., (2009). Histone H2a mRNA interacts with Lin28 and contains a Lin28-dependent posttranscriptional regulatory element. *Nuc. Acids*. Res. In press.

Yechoor et al., (2009). Neurogenin 3 is sufficient for transdetermination of hepatic progenitor cells into neo-islets in vivo but not transdifferentiation of hepatocytes. *Dev. Cell*. 16: 358-373.

Yu et al., (2007). Induced pluripotent stem cell lines derived from human somatic cells. *Science*. 318:1917-1920

Yu et al., (2009). Human induced pluripotent stem cells free of vector and transgene sequences. *Science*. 324(5928): 797-801.

Yun et al., (2008). Transduction of artificial transcriptional regulatory proteins into human cells. *Nuc. Acids*. Res. 36(16): 103

Zhao et al., (2009). iPS cells produce viable mice through tetraploid complementation. *Nature*. In press.

Zhou et al., (2008)[a]. In vivo reprogramming of adult pancreatic exocrine cells to β–cells. *Nature*. 455(7213): 627-632.

Zhou et al., (2008)[b]. Two supporting factors greatly improve the efficiency of human iPSC generation. *Cell Stem Cell*. 3(5):475-479.

Zhou et al., (2009)[c]. Generation of induced pluripotent stem cells using recombinant proteins. *Cell Stem Cell*. 4(5): 381-384.

In: Encyclopedia of Stem Cell Research (2 Volume Set)   ISBN: 978-1-61761-835-2
Editor: Alexander L. Greene   © 2012 Nova Science Publishers, Inc.

Chapter XLVI

AMNIOTIC FLUID AND PLACENTAL STEM CELLS

Emily C. Moorefield, Dawn M. Delo, Paolo De Coppi
and Anthony Atala [*]

ABSTRACT

Human amniotic fluid has been used in prenatal diagnosis for more than 70 years. It has proven to be a safe, reliable, and simple screening tool for a wide variety of developmental and genetic diseases. However, there is now evidence that amniotic fluid may be used as more than simply a diagnostic tool. It may be the source of a powerful therapy for a multitude of congenital and adult disorders. A subset of cells found in amniotic fluid and placenta has been isolated and found to be capable of maintaining prolonged undifferentiated proliferation as well as able to differentiate into multiple tissue types encompassing the three germ layers. It is possible that in the near future, we will see the development of therapies using progenitor cells isolated from amniotic fland and placenta for the treatment of newborns with congenital malformations, as well as adults with various disorders, using cryopreserved amniotic fluid and placental stem cells. In this chapter, we describe a number of experiments that have isolated and characterized pluripotent progenitor cells from amniotic fland and placenta. We also discuss various cell lines derived from amniotic fluid and placenta and future directions for this area of research.

[*] Corresponding author: W. Boyce Professor and Chair, Department of Urology, Director, Wake Forest Institute for Regenerative Medicine, Wake Forest University Health Sciences, Medical Center Boulevard, Winston-Salem, NC 27157 USA, Telephone: 336-716-5701, Fax: 336-716-0656, Email: aatala@wfubmc.edu

INTRODUCTION

Amniotic fluid-derived progenitor cells can be obtained from a small amount of fluid during amniocentesis, a procedure that is already often performed in many pregnancies in which the fetus has a congenital abnormality. Placenta-derived stem cells can be obtained from a small biopsy of the chorionic villi. Observations of cell cultures from these two sources provide evidence that they may represent new sources for the isolation of cells with the potency to differentiate into different cell types, suggesting a new source of cells for research and treatment.

AMNIOTIC FLUID AND PLACENTA IN DEVELOPMENTAL BIOLOGY

Gastrulation is a major milestone in early postimplantation development (Snow and Bennett, 1978). At about embryonic day6.5 (E6.5), gastrulation begins in the posterior region of the embryo. Pluripotent epiblast cells are allocated to the three primary germ layers of the embryo (ectoderm, mesoderm, and endoderm) and germ cells, which are the progenitors of all fetal tissue lineages as well as the extraembryonic mesoderm of the yolk sac, amnion, and allantois (Downs and Harmann, 1997; Downs et al., 2004; Gardner and Beddington, 1988; Loebel et al., 2003). The latter forms the umbilical cord as well as the mesenchymal part of the labyrinthine layer in the mature chorioallantoic placenta (Downs and Harmann, 1997; Moser et al., 2004; Smith et al., 1994). The final positions of the fetal membranes result from the process of embryonic turning, which occurs around day 8.5 of gestation and "pulls" the amnion and yolk sac around the embryo (Kinder et al., 1999; Parameswaran and Tam, 1995). The specification of tissue lineages is accomplished by the restriction of developmental potency and the activation of lineage-specific gene expression (Parameswaran and Tam, 1995; Rathjen et al., 1999). This process is strongly influenced by cellular interactions and signaling (Dang et al., 2002; Li et al., 2004).

The amniotic sac is a tough but thin transparent pair of membranes that holds the developing embryo (and later, the fetus) until shortly before birth. The inner membrane, the amnion, contains the amniotic fluid and the fetus. The outer membrane, the chorion, contains the amnion and is part of the placenta (Kaviani et al., 2001; Kinder et al., 1999; Robinson et al., 2002). Amnion is derived from ectoderm and mesoderm, and as it grows itbegins to fill with a fluid composed mainly of water (Robinson et al., 2002). Originally, it is isotonic, containing proteins, carbohydrates, lipids and phospholipids, urea, and electrolytes. Later, urine excreted by the fetus increases its volume and changes the concentrations of these components (Bartha et al., 2000; Heidari et al., 1996; Sakuragawa et al., 1999; Srivastava et al., 1996). The fetus can breathe in the water, allowing normal growth and the development of lungs and the gastrointestinal tract. The fluid is swallowed by the fetus and passes via the fetal blood into the maternal blood. The amniotic fluid ensures symmetrical structural development and growth, cushions and protects the embryo, helps maintain consistent pressure and temperature, and permits freedom of fetal movement, which is important for proper musculoskeletal development and blood flow (Baschat and Hecher, 2004).

Different origins have been suggested for the mixture of cells within amniotic fluid (Medina-Gomez and del Valle, 1988). The heterogeneous cell population comprising the amniotic fluid has been reported to contain cells of all three germ layers (In 't Anker et al., 2003; Prusa et al., 2004). These cells are thought to be sloughed from the fetal amnion, skin, and alimentary, respiratory, and urogenital tracts. The cell population found within the amniotic fluid changes with time and reflects the changes in the developing fetus (Torricelli et al., 1993). In addition, observations of cells cultured from amniotic fluid as well as placenta provide evidence that some of the cells may represent new stem cell sources with the potential to differentiate into different cell types (Prusa and Hengstschlager, 2002 and DeCoppi et al., 2007). Interestingly, it has been demonstrated that a subpopulation of cells in amniotic fluid expresses high levels of Oct-4, a transcription factor that preserves the undifferentiated state and the pluripotency of ES cells (Prusa et al., 2003 and DeCoppi et al., 2007). Although research is still in early stages, these cells may be used to find treatments or even cures for many diseases in which irreplaceable cells are damaged.

AMNIOTIC FLUID AND PLACENTA FOR CELL THERAPY

Pluripotent stem cells are ideal for regenerative medicine applications because they have the capability to differentiate in stages into a huge number of different types of human cells. Amniotic fluid cells can be obtained from a small amount of fluid during amniocentesis at the second trimester. This procedure is already performed in many pregnancies in which the fetus has a congenital abnormality and is used to determine characteristics such as sex (Hoehn et al., 1975). Kaviani and co-workers reported that just 2 milliliters of amniotic fluid can provide up to 20,000 cells, 80% of which are viable (Kaviani et al., 2001, 2003). Because many pregnant women already undergo amniocentesis to screen for fetal abnormalities, cells can be isolated from this test fluid and saved for future use. Amniotic fluid cells will double in number in about 20 to 24 h, which is faster than umbilical cord stem cells (28 to 30 h) and bone marrow stem cells (more than 30 h) (Tsai et al., 2004). This phenomenon is important and suggests amniotic fluid stem cells might be a better choice for treatment of urgent medical conditions in the future.

In addition, while scientists have been able to isolate and differentiate, on average, only 30% of the mesenchymal stem cells (MSCs) extracted from a child's umbilical cord shortly after birth, the success rate for amniotic fluid-derived MSCs is close to 100% (In 't Anker et al., 2003; Tsai et al., 2004; DeCoppi et al., 2007). Another advantage of extracting cells from from amniotic fluid or placenta is that it allows for autologous reimplantation, effectively bypassing the problems associated with a technique called donor-recipient HLA matching and and minimizing the chances of cell rejection (Tsai et al., 2004). An additional characteristic which makes AFS cells an ideal candidate for cell therapy is their ability to readily take up retroviral, lentiviral, adenoviral and baculoviral vectors without altering the differentiation potential of the cells (DeCoppi et al., 2007, Grisafi et al., 2008 and Liu et al., 2009). This aids aids in the ability to track cells both in vitro and in vivo by infecting cells with a viral vector carrying a GFP or LacZ tag, and it also suggests that the cells could eventually be used in cell-based gene therapy applications.

ISOLATION AND CHARACTERIZATION OF PROGENITOR CELLS

Amniotic fluid progenitor cells are isolated by centrifugation of amniotic fluid obtained via amniocentesis. Placental cells are isolated from single chorionic villi under light microscopy. Amniotic fluid cells and placental cells are allowed to proliferate *in vitro* and are maintained in culture for 4 weeks. The culture medium consists of modified alpha-modified Earl's medium (18% Chang medium B, 2% Chang medium C with 15% embryonic stem cell certified fetal bovine serum, antibiotics, and L-glutamine) (DeCoppi et al, 2007).

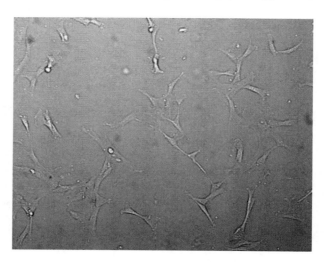

Figure 1. Morphology of amniotic fluid-derived stem cells (AFSCs) in culture.

A pluripotential subpopulation of progenitor cells present in the amniotic fluid and placenta can be isolated through positive selection for cells expressing the membrane receptor c-kit (CD117) (Figure 1) (DeCoppi et al., 2007; DeCoppi, 2001; Siddiqui and Atala, 2004). C-kit is a protein tyrosine-kinase receptor that specifically binds to the ligand stem cell factor (SCF) and it is this complex which has critical functions in gametogenesis, melanogenesis and hematopoiesis (Chabot et al., 1988; Fleischman et al., 1993). In addition, c-kit is expressed on a variety of stem cells including embryonic stem (ES) cells (Hoffman et al., 2005), primordial germ cells and many somatic stem cells (Guo et al., 1997 and Crane et al., 2006). About 0.8 to 1.4% of cells present in amniotic fluid and placenta have been shown to be c-kit positive in analysis by fluorescence-activated cell sorting (FACS) (DeCoppi et al., 2007). Progenitor cells maintain a round shape for 1 week post isolation when cultured in nontreated culture dishes. In this state, they demonstrate low proliferative capability. After the first week the cells begin to adhere to the plate and change their morphology, becoming more elongated and proliferating more rapidly, reaching 80% confluence and a need for passage every 48 to 72 h (DeCoppi et al., 2007). The doubling time of the undifferentiated cells under growth conditions is 36 h, with little variation with passages. No feeder layers are required for maintenance or expansion. The progenitor cells show a high self-renewal capacity with over 250 population doublings. This far exceeds Hayflick's limit, which is defined as 50 doublings for most cultured somatic cells (DeCoppi et al., 2007).

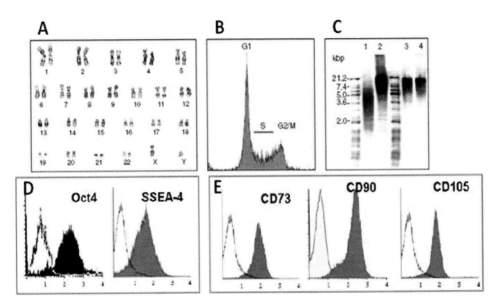

Figure 2. Consistent phenotype of hAFSCs in long term culture. A. Clonal human AFS cells maintain a normal karyotype after 250 pds. B. AFS cells passaged in culture show normal cell cycle control. C. Telomere length is conserved in AFS cells between early passage (20 p.d., lane 3) and late passage (250 p.d., lane 4). Lane 1: short length telomere standards, Lane 2: high length telomere standards. D. AFS cells express markers characteristic of ES cells, Oct4 and SSEA4. E. AFS cells express markers characterisitc of MSCs, CD73, CD90, CD105.

AFS cells have been shown to maintain a normal karyotype at late passages and display normal G1 and G2 cell cycle checkpoints (Figure 2A, 2B). They demonstrate telomere length conservation while in the undifferentiated state as well as telomerase activity even in late passages (Figure 2C). Analysis of protein expression shows that progenitor cells from amniotic fluid express human embryonic stage-specific marker SSEA-4, and the stem cell marker Oct-4, supporting the idea that these cells are able to maintain their pluripotentiality (Figure 2D). Further surface marker analysis demonstrated the presence of the mesenchymal and/or neuronal markers CD29, CD44, CD73, CD90 and CD105 (Figure 2E). AFS cells are also characterized by the absence of a variety of surface molecules, including the hematopoetic lineage marker CD45, hematopoietic stem cell markers CD34, CD133 and ES cell markers SSEA3 and Tra-1-81. This expression profile is of interest as it demonstrates expression of some key markers of the embryonic stem cell phenotype, but not the full complement of markers expressed by ES cells. This indicates that these amniotic cells are not quite as primitive as ES cells, yet they maintain greater potential than most adult stem cells.

Other behaviors showing similarities and differences between these amniotic fluid-derived cells and blastocyst-derived cells exist as well. For example, amniotic fluid progenitor cells do form embryoid bodies *in vitro*, which stain positive for markers of all three germ layers. However, unlike ES cells, when implanted into immunodeficient mice *in vivo*, AFS cells do not form teratomas, an essential consideration for potential cell therapy (DeCoppi et al., 2007). AFS cells have a high clonal capacity based on a technique involving retrovirally tagged cells (DeCoppi et al., 2007). In this assay, a tagged single cell gave rise to a population that was able to be differentiated along six distinct lineages from all three germ layers: adipogenic, osteogenic, myogenic, endothelial, neurogenic and hepatic (DeCoppi et al., 2007). This broad differentiation capability, along with their high proliferation rate, gives gives AFS cells and placental derived stem cells a clear advantage over other known adult stem cell sources.

In Vitro Differentiation of Amniotic Fluid and Placenta Derived Progenitor Cells

Cell populations derived from amniotic fluid and placenta can be selected for c-kit expression, and the c-kit expressing cells are then cloned. The selected cells have been shown to be pluripotent and able to differentiate into osteogenic, adipogenic, myogenic, neurogenic, endothelial, hepatic and chondrocytic phenotypes *in vitro*. Each differentiation has been performed through proof of phenotypic and biochemical changes consistent with the differentiated tissue type of interest (Figure 3). We discuss each set of differentiations separately as reported in DeCoppi et al. (2007) unless otherwise noted.

Adipocytes

To promote adipogenic differentiation, progenitor cells can be induced in dexamethasone, 3-isobutyl-1-methylxanthine, insulin, and indomethacin. Progenitor cells cultured with adipogenic supplements change their morphology from elongated to round within 8 days. This coincides with the accumulation of intracellular droplets. After 16 days in culture, more than 95% of the cells have their cytoplasm filled with lipid-rich vacuoles. Adipogenic differentiation also induces the expression of peroxisome proliferation-activated receptor 2 (PPAR-2), a transcription factor that regulates adipogenesis, and of lipoprotein lipase, as measured by reverse transcription-polymerase chain reaction (RT-PCR) analysis (Cremer et al., 1981; Medina-Gomez and del Valle,1988). Expression of these genes is noted in progenitor cells under adipogenic conditions but not in undifferentiated cells.

Osteocytes

Osteogenic differentiation was induced in progenitor cells with the use of dexamethasone, beta-glycerophosphate, and ascorbic acid 2-phosphate (Jaiswal et al., 1997). Progenitor cells maintained in this medium demonstrated phenotypic changes within 4 days, including a loss of spindle-shape phenotype and development of an osteoblast-like appearance with finger-like excavations into the cytoplasm. At 16 days, the cells aggregated, showing typical lamellar bone-like structures. In terms of functionality, these differentiated cells demonstrate a major feature of osteoblasts, which is to precipitate calcium. Differentiated osteoblasts from the progenitor cells are able to produce alkaline phosphatase (AP) and to deposit calcium, consistent with bone differentiation. Undifferentiated progenitor progenitor cells lack this ability. Progenitor cells in osteogenic medium also express specific genes implicated in mammalian bone development [AP, core-binding factor A1 (CBFA1), and osteocalcin] in a pattern consistent with the physiological analog. In addition, cells grown grown in osteogenic medium show activation of the AP gene at each time point. Expression of CBFA1, a transcription factor specifically expressed in osteoblasts and hypertrophic chondrocytes and that regulates gene expression of structural proteins of the bone extracellular matrix, is highest in cells grown in osteogenic inducing medium on day 8 and decreases slightly on days 16, 24, and 32. Osteocalcin is expressed only in progenitor cells under osteogenic conditions at 8 days (Karsenty, 2000; Komori et al., 1997).

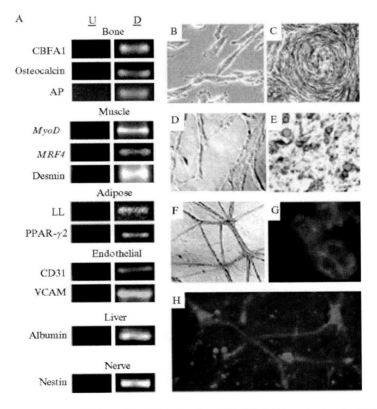

Figure 3. Multilineage differentiation of hAFSCs *in vitro*. (A) RT-PCR analysis of mRNA. Left: Control undifferentiated cells. Right: Cells maintained under conditions for differentiation to bone (8 days), muscle (8 days), adipocyte (16 days), endothelial (8 days), hepatic (45 days), neuronal (2 days) lineages. (B) Phase-contrast microscopy of control, undifferentiated cells. (b–h) Differentiated progenitor cells. (C) Bone: Histochemical staining for alkaline phosphatase. (D) Muscle: Phase contrast microscopy showing fusion into multinucleated myotube-like cells. (E) Adipocyte: Staining with oil red O (day 8) shows intracellular oil aggregation. (F) Endothelial: Phase-contrast microscopy of capillary-like structures. (G) Hepatic: Fluorescent antibody staining (FITC, green) for albumin. (H) Neuronal: Fluorescent antibody staining of nestin (day 2).

Endothelial Cells

Amniotic fluid progenitor cells can be induced to form endothelial cells through culture in endothelial basal medium on gelatin-coated dishes. Full differentiation is achieved by 1 month in culture; however, phenotypic changes are noticed within 1 week of initiation of the protocol. Human-specific endothelial cell surface marker (P1H12), factor VIII (FVIII), and kinase insert domain receptor (KDR) are specific for differentiated endothelial cells. Differentiated cells stain positively for FVIII, KDR, and P1H12. Progenitor cells do not stain for these endothelial-specific markers. Amniotic fluid progenitor-derived endothelial cells, once differentiated, are able to grow in culture and form capillary-like structures *in vitro*. These cells also express platelet endothelial cell adhesion molecule1 (PECAM-1 or CD31) and vascular cell adhesion molecule (VCAM), which are not detected in the progenitor cells on RT-PCR analysis.

Hepatocytes

For hepatic differentiation, progenitor cells are seeded on Matrigel or collagen-coated dishes at different stages and cultured in the presence of hepatocyte growth factor, insulin, oncostatin M, dexamethasone, fibroblast growth factor 4 and monothioglycerol for 45 days (Dunn et al., 1989; Schwartz et al., 2002). After 7 days of the differentiation process, cells exhibit morphological changes and shift from an elongated to a cobblestone-like appearance. The cells stain positively for albumin on day 45 post differentiation and also express the transcription factor hepatocyte nuclear factor 4 (HNF4), the c-Met receptor, the multidrug resistance (MDR) membrane transporter, albumin, and alpha-fetoprotein. RT-PCR analysis further supports albumin production. In addition, AFS cells differentiated to hepatocytes using this method were able to secrete urea, a characteristic liver-specific function that requires coordinated expression of several enzymes and specific mitochondrial amino acid transporters (Morris et al., 2002).

Myocytes

Myogenic differentiation is induced in amniotic fluid-derived progenitor cells by culture in medium containing horse serum and chick embryo extract on a thin coat of Matrigel (Rosenblatt et al., 1995). To initiate differentiation, the presence of 5-azacytidine in the medium for 24 h is necessary. Phenotypically, the cells tend to organize themselves into bundles that fuse to form multinucleated cells. These cells express sarcomeric tropomyosin and desmin, both of which are not expressed in the original progenitor population.

The development profile of cells differentiating into myogenic lineages interestingly mirrors a characteristic pattern of gene expression reflecting that seen with embryonic muscle muscle development (Bailey et al., 2001; Rohwedel et al., 1994). With this protocol, myogenic factor 6 (Myf6) is expressed on day 8 and suppressed on day 16. MyoD expression expression is detectable at 8 days and suppressed at 16 days in progenitor cells. Desmin expression is induced at 8 days and increases by 16 days in progenitor cells cultured in myogenic medium (Hinterberger et al., 1991; Patapoutian et al., 1995).

Neuronal Cells

For neurogenic induction, amniotic progenitor cells are cultured in dimethylsulfoxide (DMSO), butylated hydroxyanisole, and neuronal growth factor (Black and Woodbury, 2001; 2001; Woodbury et al., 2000). Progenitor cells cultured under neurogenic conditions change their morphology within the first 24 h. Two different cell populations become apparent: morphologically large flat cells and small bipolar cells. The bipolar cell cytoplasm retracts toward the nucleus, forming contracted multipolar structures. Over subsequent hours, the cells display primary and secondary branches and cone-like terminal expansions. Induced progenitor cells show a characteristic sequence of expression of neural-specific proteins. At an early stage in differentiation conditions, AFS cells express high levels of the intermediate filament protein nestin, which is expressed in neuroepithelial stem cells. A 2-step process is utilized to differentiate AFS cells to dopaminergic neuron like cells. Induction begins with seeding cells onto fibronectin coated dishes and supplementing the culture medium with N2 and bFGF. During this stage, cells begin to express nestin and, by 8 days of induction, about 80 percent of the culture is positive for nestin protein (Figure 4A). At this stage the cells are then transferred to conditions that have been shown to bias toward the production of dopaminergic neurons (Perrier et al., 2004). Under these conditions a fraction of the cells begin to have a distinct pyramidal morphology (Figure 4B). In addition to the morphologic change, the cells also express a gene which is a member of the G-protein-gated inwardly rectifying potassium (GIRK) channel family, GIRK2, a known marker of dopaminergic neurons (Figure 4C).

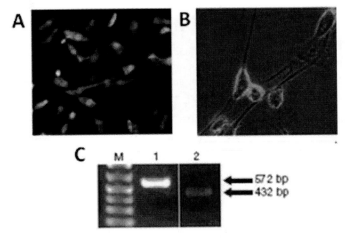

Figure 4. Neuronal differentiation of hAFS cells *in vitro* A. Immunocytochemical detection of nestin after 8 d in the first stage of dopaminergic neuron differentiation. B. Phase contrast image of pyramidal morphology of cells after the second stage of differentiation. C. RT-PCR analysis of cells at the end of the 2 stage dopaminergic neuron differentiation. M: size marker, lane 1: GAPDH, lane 2: GIRK2.

Chondrocytes

Chondrogenic differentiation has been induced in progenitor cells *in vitro* by supplementing medium with members of the transforming growth factor-beta (TGF-β) superfamily in a three-dimensional culture system (Kolambkar et al., 2007). In this effort to test the chondrogenic potential of AFS cells in both pellet and hydrogel systems, many growth factors were tested including TGF-β1, TGF-β3, bone morphogenetic protein 2 (BMP2) and insulin-like growth factor 1 (IGF1), all of which have been previously shown to induce chondrogenic differentiation (Iwasaki eat al., 1993; Johnstone et al., 1998; Kramer et al., 2000; Awad et al., 2003; Sekiya et al., 2005). The system which gave the most robust chondrogenic differentiation of AFS cells as assayed by sGAG synthesis and type II collagen staining was the medium supplemented with TGF-β1. The amount of sGAG production is an indicator of the formation of a cartilaginous matrix and was tested by both biochemical and histological techniques at 3 week time points after the start of differentiation (Figure 5A). These recent experiments provide further evidence of the broad differentiation capabilities of AFS cells.

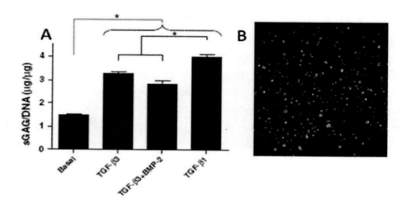

Figure 5. Chondrogenic differentiation of AFS cells *in vitro*. A. sGAG production normalized to the total amount of DNA present in pellet cultures under differentiation conditions after 21 days. B. Immunofluorescent staining for type II collagen deposited by AFS cells in alginate constructs at 21 days.

PRECLINICAL STUDIES IN ANIMAL MODELS

More recent reports have examined the utility of progenitor cells within both *ex vivo* and *in vivo* environments. Undifferentiated c-kit selected and clonally derived AFS cells have been shown to contribute to renal and epithelial lung generation while partially differentiated AFS cells have the ability to contribute to the production of osteocytes and neurons. These important studies are significant for the long term clinical applications of these cells, including tissue engineering as well as gene therapy.

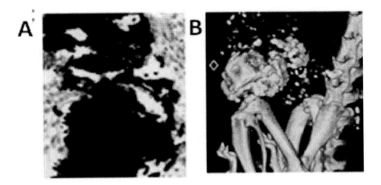

Figure 6. Production of tissue-engineered bone by AFS cells. A. von Kossa staining of AFS cell derived osteocyte seeded scaffold recovered 8 weeks after implantation, black staining indicates strong mineralization. C. Close up view of micro CT scan of seeded scaffold site in mouse 8 weeks post implantation.

Bone repair

In order to determine whether AFS cells have the ability to contribute to bone formation *in vivo*, cells were partially differentiated within a three dimensional scaffold and then implanted subcutaneously into immunodeficient mice (DeCoppi et al., 2007). Following the *in vitro* induction period as described above, the cells expressed genes consistent with the osteoblastic lineage and secreted alkaline phosphatase (AP), but did not yet show calcium deposition. After 8 weeks *in vivo*, the implanted constructs contained highly mineralized tissue as visualized by von Kossa's stain (Figure 6A). Micro CT scanning analysis of constructs at 18 weeks post implantation further confirmed the presence of hard tissue within the hAFSC-seeded constructs (Figure 6B). Additionally, the density of the tissue-engineered bone found at the sites of implantation was found to be somewhat greater than that of mouse femoral bone, demonstrating that AFS cells do contribute to *in vivo* bone formation and may be a valuable tool in future therapies.

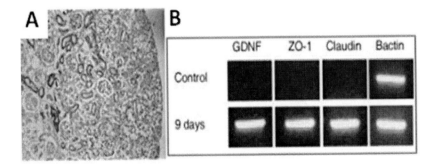

Figure 7. Undifferentiated human AFS cells are able to contribute to renal structures when injected into normal mouse kidneys. A. Chromogenic in situ hybridization for Y chromosome of male hAFS cells injected into a female mouse shows integration into embryonic kidney structures. B. Presence of early kidney markers is detected by RT-PCR 9 days after hAFS cell injection into mouse kidney.

Cardiac Repair

To examine the ability of these progenitor cells to integrate into and repair cardiac tissue, undifferentiated AFS cells shown to be capable of differentiation down the cardiomyocyte linage *in vitro* were injected directly into the wall of the heart in a rat model of myocardial infarction (Chiavegato et al., 2007). Myocardial infarction (MI) causes tissue death, and the ability to replace that lost myocardial tissue has previously been accomplished by transplanting stem cells from various sources (Davani et al., 2005). Surprisingly, transplantation of AFS cells into the heart wall of a xenogeneic host lead to an acute rejection of the cells within 15 days after injection, whether or not an MI had occurred (Chiavegato et al., 2007). This rejection is likely due to the recruitment of immune cells including CD4+ T cells, CD8+ T cells, B lymphocytes, NK cells and macrophages.

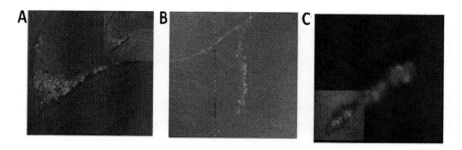

Figure 8. Neurogenically differentiated human AFS cells are able to integrate into the injured mouse brain. Immunohistochemistry performed on samples collected 1month after cell injection into *twitcher* mice. Red: human specific mitochondrial protein, Blue: DAPI. A. Lateral ventrical, B. Periventricular area and hippocampus, C. Olfactory bulb.

Renal Repair

Perin et al. (2007) have shown that AFS cells can contribute to renal development both *ex vivo* and *in vivo*. In their *ex vivo* experiment, labeled hAFS cells were injected into the primordia of the developing kidney, which was maintained in a transwell culture system for 2 to 10 days. Immediately after injection, the AFS cells could be found only at the injection site in the center of the murine embryonic kidney. After just 4 days of culture, however, the AFS cells had divided and spread throughout the organ. In addition, the AFS cells were shown by immunohistochemistry and *in situ* hybridization to have contributed to the embryonic tubular and glomerular structures (Figure 7A). After 9 days of culture, RT-PCR was performed and the expression of several human-specific kidney genes was detected, including Zona occludins-1, claudin, and glial-derived neurotrophic factor (GDNF) (Figure 7B). GDNF is a particularly important factor in renal development and is known to be expressed only in the earliest stages of renal development (Basson et al., 2006; Costantini and Shakya, 2006), so GDNF upregulation at day 9 suggests the initiation of renal differentiation by the AFS cells. To follow up on these results, the same group tested the AFS cells in a mouse model of acute tubular necrosis (ATN). One million labeled AFS cells were injected directly into the damaged kidney and allowed to incubate for 1 day to 6 months. Histological and molecular results suggest that AFS cells were not only able to survive in this environment, but they were also able to integrate into the damaged tubules.

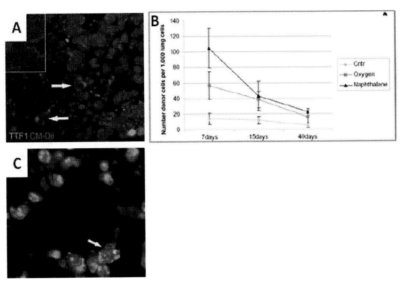

Figure 9. Undifferentiated hAFS cells can engraft and differentiate to epithelial cells in a mouse model of lung injury. A. hAFS cells injected into the embryonic lung ex vivo integrate into the lung epithelium and mesenchyme and express the early differentiation marker TTF1 7 days post injection, Red: CM-Dil-labeled hAFS cells, Green: TTF1, Blue: DAPI. B. Lung injury increases the degree of engraftment of hAFS within the mouse lung. C. Immunohistochemistry of lung 15 days after hAFS cell injection showing that cells can achieve a type II pneumocyte, Red: CM-Dil-labeled hAFS cell, Green: pro-SPC, Blue: DAPI.

Neural Repair

Survival and engraftment abilities of AFS cells within the rodent brain were also examined by DeCoppi et al. (2007). The *twitcher* mouse model of neurological disease, in which endogenous neurons undergo massive degeneration, was used in these studies. Neurogenic induction of AFS cells began *in vitro* by incubation with NGF, resulting in upregulation of the neural stem cell-related gene nestin. These cells were then implanted directly into the lateral ventricles of the developing brain of a newborn mouse in both normal and *twitcher* models, as had been done previously with neural stem cells (Taylor et al., 2006). Lateral ventricle implantation was selected to allow cell penetration into the subventricular zone, an area which contains endogenous, proliferating neural progenitors that have been shown to easily migrate into and integrate throughout the rest of the brain (Taylor and Snyder, 1997). Migration and integration of AFS cells were examined two months after implantation by immunohistochemistry (Figure 8). Both the normal and *twitcher* mice showed similar patterns of cell migration, suggesting that this process is not random. However, the number of cells that were able to engraft was dramatically different in the two groups, with the *twitcher* mice engrafting about 70% of the injected cells into the brain, while only about 30% of the injected cells engrafted in the normal mouse brain. These findings confirm that AFS cells are able to survive and integrate into the fetal mouse brain and may be a useful tool for future therapies for neurodegenerative disorders.

Repair of Lung Epithelium

Studies show that undifferentiated AFS cells have the ability to engraft into developing lung and injured lung tissues and to contribute to epithelial lung lineages (Carraro et al., 2008). *Ex vivo* injection of AFS cells into mouse embryonic lung demonstrated the ability of the cells to engraft and to express the early lung marker thyroid transcription factor 1(TTF1) within 1 week (Figure 9A). Further *in vivo* experimentation illustrated the ability of AFS cells injected into the mouse tail vein to home to the lung and differentiate into epithelial cells. AFS cells labeled with luciferase were injected into both normal and injured immunocompromised mice and their presence was detected 3 to 6 weeks later. In the absence of injury the cells were able to engraft into the recipient lung within 3 weeks after injection; however, no differentiation to epithelial cells was detected. The engraftment potential of hAFS cells was enhanced following lung injury induced either by hypoxia or the aromatic hydrocarbon naphthalene (Figure 9B). Integrated cells continued to show expression of TTF1 up to 7 months after injection as detected by RT-PCR and immunohistochemistry, suggesting the ability of the AFS cells to self-renew and preserve the expression of this early differentiation marker. Additionally, few engrafted cells expressed the mature type II pneumocyte lineage marker SPC as detected by immunohistochemistry. However gene expression was not detected by human specific RT-PCR. This evidence suggests that AFS differentiation to type II pneumocytes is a rare event *in vivo*.

The *in vivo* applications of fetally derived stem cells are still in the initial stages but based on these results, it appears that AFS cells are a pluripotential source of stem cells with the potential for alternative clinical treatment for a variety of diseases in the future. Importantly, AFS cells do not form teratomas when implanted into any of these *in vivo* environments. This fact is critically significant when considering future clinical applications and is an advantage over ES cells. AFS cells are at a stage between ES and adult stem cells, possessing the most advantageous characteristics of both groups.

CONCLUSION

Pluripotent progenitor cells isolated from amniotic fluid and placenta present an exciting possible contribution to the field of stem cell biology and regenerative medicine. These cells are an excellent source for research and therapeutic applications. The ability to isolate progenitor cells during gestation may also be advantageous for babies born with congenital malformations. Furthermore, progenitor cells can be cryopreserved for future self-use. Compared with embryonic stem cells, c-kit positive, cloned progenitor cells isolated from amniotic fluid have many similarities: they can differentiate into all three germ layers, they express common markers, and they preserve their telomere length. However, progenitor cells isolated from amniotic fluid and placenta have considerable advantages. They easily differentiate into specific cell lineages and they avoid the current controversies associated with the use of human embryonic stem cells. The discovery of these cells has been recent, and and a considerable amount of work remains to be done to fully characterize these cells. In the the future, cells derived from amniotic fluid and placenta may represent an attractive and abundant, noncontroversial source of cells for regenerative medicine.

REFERENCES

Bailey, P., Holowacz, T. and Lassar, A. B. (2001). The origin of skeletal muscle stem cells in the embryo and the adult. *Curr.Opin.CellBiol.* 13,679–689.

Bartha, J. L., Romero-Carmona, R., Comino-Delgado, R., Arce, F. and Arrabal, J. (2000). Alpha-Fetoprotein and hematopoietic growth factors in amniotic fluid. *Obstet.Gynecol.* 96,588–592.

Baschat, A. A. and Hecher, K. (2004). Fetal growth restriction due to placental disease. *Semin.Perinatol.* 28,67–80.

Basson, M. A., Watson-Johnson, J., Shakya, R., Akbulut, S., Hyink, D., Costantini, F. D., Wilson, P. D., Mason, I. J. and J. D. Licht. (2006). Branching morphogenesis of the ureteric epithelium during kidney development is coordinated by the opposing functions of GDNF and Sprouty1. *Dev.Biol.* 299, 466–477.

Black, I. B. and Woodbury, D. (2001). Adult rat and human bone marrow stromal stem cells differentiate into neurons. *Blood Cells Mol.Dis.* 27,632–636.

Carraro, G., Perin, L., Sedrakyan, S., Giuliani, S., Tiozzo, C., Lee, J., Turcatel, G., De Langhe, Langhe, S. P., Driscoll, B., Bellusci, S., Minoo, P., Atala, A., De Filippo, R. E. and D. Warburton. (2008). Human amniotic fluid stem cells can integrate and differentiate into epithelial lung lineages. *Stem Cells.* 26(11):2902-11.

Chabot, B., Stephenson, D. A., Chapman, V. M., Besmer, P. and Bernstein, A. (1988). The protooncogene c-kit encoding a transmembrane tyrosine kinase receptor maps to the mouse W locus. *Nature* 335, 88–89

Costantini F. and Shakya. R., (2006). GDNF/Ret signaling and the development of the kidney. *Bioessays* 28, 117–127.

Crane, J. F. and Trainor, P. A. (2006). Neural crest stem and progenitor cells. Annu. Rev. *Cell Dev.Biol.* 22, 267–286.

Cremer, M., Schachner, M., Cremer, T., Schmidt, W. and Voigtlander, T. (1981). Demonstration of astrocytes in cultured amniotic fluid cells of three cases with neural-tube defect. *Hum.Genet.* 56,365–370.

Dang, S. M., Kyba, M., Perlingeiro, R., Daley, G. Q. and Zandstra, P. W. (2002). Efficiency of embryoid body formation and hematopoietic development from embryonic stem cells in different culture systems. *Biotechnol.Bioeng.* 78,442–453.

Davani, S., Deschaseaux, F., Chalmers, F., Tiberghien P. and Kantelip. J. P. (2005). Can stem cells mend a broken heart? *Cardiovasc.Res.* 65:305–16.

DeCoppi, P., Bartsch, G., Siddiqui, M. M., Xu, T., Santos, C. C., Perin, L., Mostoslavsky, G., Serre, A. C., Snyder, E. Y., Yoo, J. J., Furth, M. E., Soker, S. and Atala, A. (2007). Isolation of amniotic stem cell lines with potential for therapy. *Nature Biotechnology* 25, 100-106.

Downs, K. M. and Harmann, C. (1997). Developmental potency of the murine allantois. *Development* 124,2769–2780.

Downs, K. M., Hellman, E. R., McHugh, J., Barrickman, K. and Inman, K. E. (2004). Investigation into a role for the primitive streak in development of the murine allantois. *Development* 131,37–55.

Dunn, J. C., Yarmush, M. L., Koebe, H. G. and Tompkins, R. G. (1989). Hepatocyte function and extracellular matrix geometry: Long-term culture in a sandwich configuration. *FASEBJ.* 3,174–177.

Fleischman, R. A. (1993). From white spots to stem cells: the role of the Kit receptor in mammalian development. *Trends Genet.* 9, 285–290.

Gardner, R. L. and Beddington, R. S. (1988). Multi-lineage "stem" cells in the mammalian embryo. *J.CellSci.Suppl.*10,11–27.

Grisafi, D. Piccoli, M., Pozzobon, M., Ditadi, A., Zaramella, P., Chiandetti, L., Zanon, G. F., Atala, A., Zacchello, F., Scarpa, M., De Coppi, P. and Tomanin, R. (2008). High transduction efficiency of human amniotic fluid stem cells mediated by adenovirus vectors. *Stem Cells Dev.* Oct;17(5):953-62.

Guo, C. S., Wehrle-Haller, B., Rossi, J. and Ciment, G. (1997). Autocrine regulation of neural crest cell development by steel factor. *Dev. Biol.* 184, 61–69.

Heidari, Z., Isobe, K., Goto, S., Nakashima, I., Kiuchi, K. and Tomoda, Y. (1996). Characterization of the growth factor activity of amniotic fluid on cells from hematopoietic and lymphoid organs of different life stages. *Microbiol.Immunol.* 40,583–589.

Hinterberger, T. J., Sassoon, D. A., Rhodes, S. J. and Konieczny, S. F. (1991). Expression of the muscle regulatory factor MRF4 during somite and skeletal myofiber development. *Dev.Biol.* 147,144–156.

Hoehn, H., Bryant, E. M., Fantel, A. G. and Martin, G. M. (1975). Cultivated cells from diagnostic amniocentesis in second trimester pregnancies. III. The fetal urine as a potential source of clonable cells. *Humangenetik.* 29,285–290.

Hoffman, L. M. and Carpenter, M. K. (2005). Characterization and culture of human embryonic stem cells. Nat. *Biotechnol.* 23, 699–708.In 't Anker, P. S., Scherjon, S. A., Kleijburg-van der Keur, C., Noort, W. A., Claas, F. H., Willemze, R., Fibbe, W. E. and Kanhai, H. H. (2003). Amniotic fluid as a novel source of mesenchymal stem cells for therapeutic transplantation. *Blood.* 102,1548–1549.

Jaiswal, N., Haynesworth, S. E., Caplan, A. I. and Bruder, S. P. (1997). Osteogenic differentiation of purified, culture-expanded human mesenchymal stem cells invitro. *J.Cell.Biochem.* 64,295–312.

Karsenty, G. (2000). Role of Cbfa1 in osteoblast differentiation and function. Semin. *CellDev.Biol.* 11,343–346.

Kaviani, A., Perry, T. E., Dzakovic, A., Jennings, R. W., Ziegler, M. M. and Fauza, D. O. (2001). The amniotic fluid as a source of cells for fetal tissue engineering. *J.Pediatr.Surg.* 36,1662–1665.

Kaviani, A., Guleserian, K., Perry, T. E., Jennings, R. W., Ziegler, M. M. and Fauza, D. O. (2003). Fetal tissue engineering from amniotic fluid. *J.Am.Coll.Surg.* 196,592–597.

Kinder, S. J., Tsang, T. E., Quinlan, G. A., Hadjantonakis, A. K., Nagy, A. and Tam, P. P. (1999). The orderly allocation of mesodermal cells to the extraembryonic structures and the anteroposterior axis during gastrulation of the mouse embryo. *Development* 126,4691–4701.

Kolambkar, Y., K., Peister, A., Soker, S., Atala, A. and R. E. Guldberg. (2007). Chondrogenic differentiation of amniotic fluid-derived stem cells. *J Mol Hist* 38:405–413

Komori, T., Yagi, H., Nomura, S., Yamaguchi, A., Sasaki, K., Deguchi, K., Shimizu, Y., Bronson, R. T., Gao, Y. H., Inada, M., Sato, M., Okamoto, R., Kitamura, Y., Yoshiki, S. and Kishimoto, T. (1997). Targeted disruption of Cbfa1 results in a complete lack of bone formation owing to maturational arrest of osteoblasts. *Cell.* 89,755–764.

Li, L., Arman, E., Ekblom, P., Edgar, D., Murray, P. and Lonai, P. (2004). Distinct GATA6-and laminin-dependent mechanisms regulate endodermal and ectodermal embryonic stem cell fates. *Development* 131,5277–5286.

Liu, Z. S., Xu, Y. F., Feng, S. W., Li, Y., Yao, X. L., Lu, X.L. and Zhang, C. Baculovirus-transduced mouse amniotic fluid-derived stem cells maintain differentiation potential. (2009). *Ann Hematol.* 88(6):565-72.

Loebel, D. A., Watson, C. M., De Young, R. A. and Tam, P. P. (2003). Lineage choice and differentiation in mouse embryos and embryonic stem cells. *Dev.Biol.* 264,1–14.

Medina-Gomez, P. and del Valle, M. (1988). The culture of amniotic fluid cells: An analysis of the colonies, metaphase and mitotic index for the purpose of ruling out maternal cell contamination. *Ginecol.Obstet.Mex.* 56,122–126.

Moser, M., Li, Y., Vaupel, K., Kretzschmar, D., Kluge, R., Glynn, P. and Buettner, R. (2004). Placental failure and impaired vasculogenesis result in embryonic lethality for neuropathy neuropathy target esterasedeficient mice. *Mol.Cell.Biol.*24,1667–1679.

Morris, S. M., Jr. (2002). Regulation of enzymes of the urea cycle and arginine metabolism. *Annu. Rev. Nutr.* 22, 87–105.

Parameswaran, M. and Tam, P. P. (1995). Regionalisation of cell fate and morphogenetic movement of the mesoderm during mouse gastrulation. *Dev.Genet.*17,16–28.

Patapoutian, A., Yoon, J. K., Miner, J. H., Wang, S., Stark, K. and Wold, B. (1995). Disruption of the mouse MRF4 gene identifies multiple waves of myogenesis in the myotome. *Development*121,3347–3358.

Perin, L., Giuliani, S., Jin, D., Sedrakyan, S., Carraro, G., Habibiat, R., Warburton, D.,Atala, A. and R. E. De Filippo. (2007). Renal differentiation of amniotic fluid stem cells. *Cell Prolif.* 40, 936–948.

Perrier, A. L., Tabar, V., Barberi, T., Rubio, M.E., Bruses, J., Topf, N., Harrison, N. L. and L. Studer. (2004). Derivation of midbrain dopamine neurons from human embryonic stem cells. *Proc. Natl. Acad. Sci.* 101, 12543–12548.

Prusa, A. R. and Hengstschlager, M. (2002). Amniotic fluid cells and human stem cell research: A new connection. *Med.Sci.Monit.*8,RA253–RA257.

Prusa, A. R., Marton, E., Rosner, M., Bernaschek, G. and Hengstschlager, M. (2003). Oct-4-expressing cells in human amniotic fluid: A new source for stem cell research? *Hum.Reprod.*18,1489–1493.

Prusa, A. R., Marton, E., Rosner, M., Bettelheim, D., Lubec, G., Pollack, A., Bernaschek, G. and Hengstschlager, M. (2004). Neurogenic cells in human amniotic fluid. *Am.JObstet.Gynecol.*191,309–314.

Rathjen, J., Lake, J. A., Bettess, M. D., Washington, J. M., Chapman, G. and Rathjen, P. D. (1999). Formation of a primitive ectoderm like cell population, EPL cells, from ES cells in response to biologically derived factors. *J.CellSci.*112,601–612.

Robinson, W. P., McFadden, D. E., Barrett, I. J., Kuchinka, B., Penaherrera, M. S., Bruyere, H., Best, R. G., Pedreira, D. A., Langlois, S. and Kalousek, D. K. (2002). Origin of amnion and implications for evaluation ofthe fetal genotype in cases of mosaicism. *Prenat.Diagn.*22,1076–1085.

Rohwedel, J., Maltsev, V., Bober, E., Arnold, H. H., Hescheler, J. and Wobus, A. M. (1994). Muscle cell differentiation of embryonic stem cells reflects myogenesis invivo: Developmentally regulated expression of myogenic determination genes and functional expression of ionic currents. *Dev.Biol.*164,87–101.

Rosenblatt, J. D., Lunt, A. I., Parry, D. J. and Partridge, T. A. (1995). Culturingsatellite cells from living single muscle fiber explants. *InVitroCellDev.Biol.Anim.*31,773–779.

Sakuragawa, N., Elwan, M. A., Fujii, T. and Kawashima, K. (1999). Possible dynamic neurotransmitter metabolism surrounding the fetus. *J.Child.Neurol.*14,265–266.

Chiavegato, A., Bollini, S., Pozzobon, M., Callegari, A., Gasparotto, L., Taiani, J., Piccoli, M., Lenzini, E., Gerosa, G., Vendramin, I., Cozzi, E., Angelini, A., Iop, L., Zanon, G.F., Atala, A., DeCoppi, P. and S. Sartore. Human amniotic fluid-derived stem cells are rejected after transplantation in the myocardium of normal, ischemic, immuno-suppressed or immuno-deficient rat. (2007). *Journal of Molecular and Cellular Cardiology* 42(4): 746–759.

Schwartz, R. E., Reyes, M., Koodie, L., Jiang, Y., Blackstad, M., Lund, T., Lenvik, T., Johnson, S., Hu, W. S. and Verfaillie, C. M. (2002). Multipotent adult progenitor cells from bone marrow differentiate into functional hepatocyte-like cells. *J.Clin.Invest.*109,1291–1302.

Siddiqui, M. J. and Atala, A. (2004). Amniotic fluid-derived pluripotentialcells. In"*Handbook of Stem Cells,*" Vol. 2, pp. 175–179. Elsevier Academic Press, San Diego, CA.

Smith, J. L., Gesteland, K. M. and Schoenwolf, G. C. (1994). Prospective fate map of the mouse primitive streak at 7.5 days of gestation. *Dev.Dyn.*201,279–289.

Snow, M. H. and Bennett, D. (1978). Gastrulation in the mouse: Assessment of cell populations in the epiblast of tw18/tw18 embryos. *J.Embryol.Exp.Morphol.* 47,39–52.

Srivastava, M. D., Lippes, J. and Srivastava, B. I. (1996). Cytokines of the human reproductive tract. *Am.J.Reprod.Immunol.*36,157–166.

Taylor, R. M. and Snyder, E. Y. (1997). Widespread engraftment of neural progenitor and stem-like cells throughout the mouse brain. *Transplant. Proc.* 29, 845–847.

Taylor, R. M., Lee, J. P., Palacino, J. J., Bowker, K. A., Li, J., Vanier, M. T., Wenger, D. A., Sidman, R. L. and E. Y. Snyder. (2006). Intrinsic resistance of neural stem cells to toxic metabolites may make them well suited for cell non-autonomous disorders: evidence from a mouse model of Krabbe leukodystrophy. *J. Neurochem.* 97, 1585–1599.

Tsai, M. S., Lee, J. L., Chang, Y. J. and Hwang, S. M. (2004). Isolation of human multipotent mesenchymal stem cells from second-trimester amniotic fluid using a novel two-stage culture protocol. *Hum.Reprod.*19,1450–1456.

Torricelli, F., Brizzi, L., Bernabei, P. A., Gheri, G., Di Lollo, S., Nutini, L., Lisi, E., Di Tomasso, M. and Cariati, E. (1993) Identification of hematopoietic progenitor cells in human amniotic fluid before the 12th week of gestation. Ital. *J. Anat. Embryol.* 98:119-126.

Woodbury, D., Schwarz, E. J., Prockop, D. J. and Black, I. B. (2000). Adult rat and human bone marrow stromal cells differentiate into neurons. *J.Neurosci.Res.*61,364–370.

In: Encyclopedia of Stem Cell Research (2 Volume Set)   ISBN: 978-1-61761-835-2
Editor: Alexander L. Greene   © 2012 Nova Science Publishers, Inc.

Chapter XLVII

EXPLORING A STEM CELL BASIS TO IDENTIFY NOVEL TREATMENT FOR HUMAN MALIGNANCIES

Shyam A. Patel[1, 2] *and Pranela Rameshwar*[2*]

[1]Graduate School of Biomedical Sciences, University of Medicine and Dentistry of New Jersey, Newark, NJ, US
[2]Department of Medicine – Division of Hematology/Oncology, New Jersey Medical School, University of Medicine and Dentistry of New Jersey, Newark, NJ, US

ABSTRACT

Research investigations on various sources of stem cells have been conducted for potential to exert tissue regeneration, reverse immune-enhancement, and protect against tissue insult. At a more distant goal, it is likely that stem cells could be applied to medicine via organogenesis. However, the field of stem cells is not new since immune replacement via bone marrow transplantation is considered a successful form of cell therapy. There is evidence that stem cell therapies are close for several disorders such as neurodegeneration, immune hyperactivity, and functional insufficiencies such as Type I diabetes mellitus. The field of stem cell biology is gaining a strong foothold in science and medicine as the molecular mechanisms underlying stem cell behavior are gradually being unraveled. Although stem cells have tremendous therapeutic applicability in the aforementioned conditions, their uniqueness may also confer adverse properties, rendering them a double-edged sword. The discovery that stem cells have immortal and resilient characteristics has shed insight into the link between stem cells and tumorigenesis. Specifically, recent advancements in cancer research have implicated that a stem cell may be responsible for the refractoriness of cancers to conventional treatment

[*] Corresponding author: Pranela Rameshwar, Ph.D., UMDNJ-New Jersey Medical School, MSB, Rm. E-579, 185 South Orange Ave, Newark, NJ 07103, Tel. (973) 972-0625; Fax (973) 972-8854; E-mail: rameshwa@umdnj.edu

such as chemotherapy and radiation. Here, we summarize the recent advancements in the cancer stem cell hypothesis and present the challenges associated with targeting resistant cancers in the context of stem cell microenvironments.

TRADITIONAL VIEWS ON TUMORIGENESIS

For years, cancer has been viewed as a stochastic process in which random genetic alterations lead to deregulation of cellular division [1]. Among the stochastic events a cell undergoes that ultimately lead to transformation include amplification or overexpression of proto-oncogenes, loss of function of tumor suppressors, and translocations of important cell cycle regulatory genes. In this model, genomic instability can predispose cells to attain mutations [2]. Furthermore, the model holds that all cancer cells from the same tumor are homogeneous and harbor equal malignant capabilities [3,4]. The underlying assumption of the traditional model is that any transformed cell can form new tumors limitlessly [5].

Although this non-hierarchal model is still accepted among scientists, it does not clearly explain the recurrence of cancer after years of disease-free or event-free survival. For example, approximately 30% of patients with breast cancer show micrometastatic foci in the bone marrow, and these sites may be able to serve as origins of relapse after many years from the time of diagnosis [6]. The original belief that that each transformed cell can form tumors indefinitely has been met with opposition on numerous occasions for many types of cancers [5]. For instance, malignant cells from Ewing's sarcoma fail to form tumors when serially transplanted into immunodeficient mice [5]. Therefore, the recurrence of cancer years following initial treatment has led to investigations into identifying resistant subpopulations of cells with indefinite tumor renewability. From these ideas arose the cancer stem cell hypothesis, which we will now discuss in detail.

AMBIGUITY ABOUT THE ORIGIN OF CANCER STEM CELLS

The cancer stem cell hypothesis, sometimes referred to as the tumor-initiating cell hypothesis, is based on a hierarchal model of cancer and holds that hematological and solid organ cancers arise from dysregulation of resident stem cells of normal tissue [4,7] (Figure 1). On the contrary, some groups believe that cancer stem cells arise first from transient amplifying cells that undergo de-differentiation while acquiring self-renewal characteristics [7,8] (Figure 1). It is likely that aspects of both of these theories are responsible for tumor initiation, drug and radiation resistance, dormancy, and recurrence of cancers. It is estimated that as few as 0.0001% of cells within heterogeneous tumors are stem-like in nature [9]. Common to most definitions of the cancer stem cell is that it must be able to self-renew and demonstrate multipotency [10]. Among the broader biological processes that are thought to be regulated by cancer stem cells are angiogenesis, invasion, and metastasis [11,12]. A hallmark of these cells is that they retain sphere-forming ability *in vitro* from single cells. The precise phenotype of tumor-initiating cells is unclear, but specific cluster designation (CD) markers have been attributed to particular tissues from which the cancer stem cells are thought to arise.

Although a functional definition of the cancer stem cell does not include drug resistance, this characteristic is well-recognized by many groups [13]. Normally, cancer treatment modalities such as chemotherapy and radiation can induce apoptosis in cancer cells in a p53-dependent manner [13]. Resistance has been attributed to many molecular events, such as the induction of xenobiotic transporters of the ATP-binding cassette family. This phenotype is discussed in the *Side Populations* section. In addition, although cellular quiescence is not a defining feature of stem cells, cells from tumor-initiating populations may harbor some degree of cell cycle arrest or slow-cycling ability [8].

Despite the unclear nature of the origin of cancer stem cells, it is commonly accepted that these cells have an indefinite ability to self-renew while giving rise to some cells with finite renewability [7]. The cells with finite renewal may include committed progenitors and transient amplifying populations [8]. Acute promyelocytic leukemia, for example, is thought to arise from committed progenitors that acquire self-renewal characteristics [14]. This phenomenon of asymmetric division appears to be partly responsible for resurgence of cancer after years of disease-free survival. Cancer stem cells appear to have limitless tumor-forming ability, unlike other cancer cells which fail to indefinitely repopulate tumors [7].

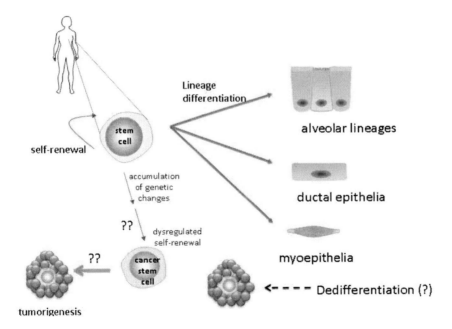

Figure 1. The cancer stem cell hypothesis. Shown is a normal mammary stem cell that differentiates along lineages to generate various epithelial types. Two hypotheses are shown. Firstly, genetic dysregulation can occur in mammary epithelial stem cells to form cancer stem cells, which then produce metastatic tumors through the formation of cancer progenitors (blue cells). Secondly, specialized cells can de-differentiate to form cancer stem cells, which similarly cause metastasis.

THE RELEVANCE OF EPITHELIAL-TO-MESENCHYMAL TRANSITION IN CANCER BIOLOGY

During embryogenesis, unique phenomena occur at the cellular and molecular levels that permit the development of an intact organism [15]. Epithelial and mesenchymal morphologies predominate at different points in development, and both of these states may transition between one another [15]. The epithelial-to-mesenchymal transition is defined as the attainment of increased cellular invasiveness due to the acquisition of a fibroblast-like phenotype by differentiated epithelial cells [16]. In addition to morphological changes, the theory holds that junctional interactions between epithelial cells are lost [16]. Specifically, E-cadherin loss is a central feature of this dynamic process [17]. Cytoskeletal elements undergo re-organization to accommodate the mesenchymal appearance with loss of the apical-basal polarity [16]. These morphological changes have been suggested to underlie the tumor-initiating characteristics and cancer stem cell behavior, and this has been shown clearly for many carcinomas. The correlation between malignancy and the epithelial-to-mesenchymal transition is evident from data suggesting that a mesenchymal phenotype imparts increased motility to cells [15]. Differentiated epithelial cells do not possess invasive tendencies and rarely disseminate to distant sites [15]. Moreover, upon transition to a mesenchymal morphology, cells become less susceptible to apoptosis, a hallmark of tumor-initiating cells [15].

The stimuli for epithelial-to-mesenchymal transition in carcinomas have been investigated, and various growth factors such as transforming growth factor-β (TGF-β) are implicated. In pancreatic adenocarcinoma, TGF-β allows for loss of E-cadherin expression, thereby promoting increased invasiveness of these cancers [17]. This cytokine also promotes conversion to the spindle-shaped morphology [17]. Interestingly, TGF-β signaling is vital in breast cancer cell proliferation and embryogenesis, supporting the idea that undifferentiated cells may be driving tumor growth [18].

A few stem cell signaling pathways appear to mediate the events occurring in the epithelial-to-mesenchymal transition and may function in resistance of cancer to chemotherapy. Resistance to gemcitabine in advanced stage pancreatic adenocarcinoma has been attributable to Notch-2 signaling [16]. Increased expression of both the Notch-2 ligand and its receptor Jagged-1 has been reported in drug resistance cells [16]. Knockdown of Notch in pancreatic cancer appears to partially eliminate the epithelial-to-mesenchymal transition and reduce the invasiveness of pancreatic cancer [16]. The interaction between cancers and the underlying stroma likely plays a critical role in transition to a mesenchymal phenotype [15].

In colon adencarcinoma, the Wnt signaling pathway is important for induction of epithelial cells into a mesenchymal phenotype [19]. β-catenin-mediated gene transcription may be the reason for the dynamic changes in the epithelial-to-mesenchymal transition in these cancers [19]. Inhibitors of this pathway have been suggested for treatment of colon cancer, but the clinic has yet to experience success for these molecular targets. Hypoxia has also been suggested as a stimulus of the transition by some groups [15]. Nonetheless, the evidence is still somewhat ambiguous as most reports on cancer stem cells do not allude to the epithelial-to-mesenchymal transition [16].

As with any other theory, some scientists are wary of the validity of the epithelial-to-mesenchymal transition. Nonetheless, evidence from experiments on mesenchymal stem cells provides a foundation on which the theory may be based [20]. Mesenchymal stem cells have been consistently shown to harbor malignant potential when faced with environmental stressors [20]. Treatment of mesenchymal stem cells with low-dose ionizing radiation in the range representative of cancer radiotherapy has been shown to transform these cells. Irradiated mesenchymal stem cells demonstrate increased numbers of unbalanced translocations and loss of genomic integrity to the point of tumor development [20]. Among sarcomas, mesenchymal stem cells are thought to be the origin of tumors [21]. Fibrosarcoma and malignant histiocytomas are among the tumors with suspected mesenchymal stem cell origin based on recent reports [21] [22].

TUMOR-INITIATING CELLS OF THE BREAST

The idea that resident stem cells can undergo transformation arose not so long ago. Studies of the mammary gland from various specimens have indicated on multiple occasions that stem cells can become cancerous, contrary to the traditional belief that a terminally differentiated epithelial cell of the breast is the origin of tumors [23]. The seminal experiments on identification of the putative breast cancer stem cell demonstrated that the CD44+/CD24^{low}/lin- phenotype allows for the recapitulation of tumors in immunodeficient mice [6]. This subpopulation of cells is able to drive the growth of breast tumors far more successfully than other cancer cells of the breast, which have limited proliferation potential upon serial transplantation [6]. Nevertheless, there are limitations to accepting the CD44+/CD24^{low}/lin- phenotype as the profile for breast cancer stem cells. The phenotype does not correlate with prognosis and may only be applicable to certain type of breast cancers, such as hormone-resistant cancers of the basal type and cancers harboring the familial *BRCA1* mutation [24]. Hence, generalized judgments about breast cancer based on subtype-specific evidence should be cautioned [24].

Numerous ligand/receptor interactions have been suggested for breast cancer maintenance, such as the interaction between the TGF-β superfamily member Nodal and its receptor Cripto-1 [18]. This interaction is important for embryonic development [18]. The interaction between Notch-1 and survivin, a regulator of mitosis in cancer cells and stem cells, has been noted in estrogen receptor-negative basal breast cancers, which have worse prognoses than hormone-responsive cancers [25]. Notch-1 is becoming an important player in breast cancer in relation to the tumor-initiating cell phenotype [25].

Perhaps the most well-recognized ligand/receptor interaction involves chemokines of hematopoiesis. Chemokines involved in stem cell signaling have been implicated in cancer metastasis, especially stage IV breast cancer [26]. Elevated levels of stromal cell-derived factor 1 (SDF-1), the endogenous ligand for chemokine receptor 4 (CXCR4), have been found in metastatic breast cancer sites [27]. A positive correlation exists between CXCR4 expression and the aggressiveness of breast cancer [27]. Regarding highly aggressive breast cancer cells, the SDF-1/CXCR4 axis may be supporting a breast cancer stem cell niche in the bone marrow in addition to its endogenous role in hematopoiesis [28]. Aside from SDF-

1/CXCR4 signaling, chemokine ligand 2 (CCL2) secretion by mesenchymal stem cells of the bone marrow also facilitates the homing of breast cancer cells towards osteoblasts [29]. Based on these findings, specific antagonists have been designed to target homing of cancer cells during stage IV breast cancer.

Clearly, determining the role of chemokines and growth factors in bone marrow stromal microenvironment is critical to understanding the behavior of invasive tumors [30]. The prospect of stem cell therapy for breast cancer has been brought forth recently by a study demonstrating the interactions between stroma and cancerous epithelia [31]. The current theory holds that the tumor stroma may be an impediment to the delivery of effective therapy [31]. Inducible expression of relaxin in hematopoietic stem cells has been proposed to cause degeneration of tumor stroma while promoting infiltration of beneficial immune cells that target the tumor [31]. This phenomenon emphasizes the role of the surrounding stroma in protecting tumors from immune effector mechanisms [31]. Hence, the use of stem cells, particular hematopoietic stem cells in this case, can serve as vehicle for delivery of anti-cancer genes to breast tumors.

The aforementioned evidence pertains mostly to ductal adenocarcinomas of the breast, which represent the most common types of breast cancers. There has been an upsurge of interest, however, in inflammatory breast cancer, which differs from ductal carcinoma in that it confers worse prognosis and invades the subdermal lymphatics [32]. Notch-3 signaling has been implicated in inflammatory breast cancer [32]. Emboli from this breast cancer subtype can obstruct lymphatic flow, and cells from the emboli have been found to possess stemness characteristics, although the existence of tumor-initiating cells from inflammatory breast cancers is not thoroughly supported to date [32].

STEMNESS PROPERTIES IN OTHER EPITHELIAL MALIGNANCIES

Cancers of the breast and prostate, although causing fewer deaths than carcinoma of the lung, are a significant cause of morbidity [33]. CD44 positivity is shared between both breast and neuroendocrine small cell carcinomas of the prostate tumor-initiating cells [33]. The normal function of CD44 is to help maintain cellular adhesions to adjacent cells and to the extracellular matrix [33]. Particular variants of CD44 have been correlated with increased invasiveness, even though CD44 is negatively correlated with invasive potential for many cases of prostate cancers [33,34]. Furthermore, a greater fraction of CD44+ cells in prostate cancer demonstrate aggressive behavior compared to CD44- cells, and they are more likely to form prostatospheres [34].

The commonality between breast and prostate tumors is that they are both modulated by hormonal activity: estrogen for breast cancer and androgens for prostate cancer. This prospect makes these two cancers unique from other malignancies and may explain the disparity in the phenotypes for organ-specific cancer stem cells. Recent studies in prostate cancer biology have shown that prostate tumor-initiating cells fail to express the androgen receptor and lineage-specific antigens [4]. Integrins are also thought to play a role in the prostate cancer stem cell phenotype [4]. Hormone sensitivity does not appear intact among CD44+ cells of the prostate, implying refractoriness of prostate cancer stem cells to treatment [34].

The most common cause of cancer-related death is carcinoma of the lung [35]. The reasons for sustenance and recurrence of lung cancer have been partially elucidated, yet the evidence is not as well-supported in comparison to other solid tumors [36]. Aldehyde dehydrogenase (ALDH1), a stem cell marker, has been found in lung carcinoma cells demonstrating stemness. The significance of this finding is that ALDH1 correlated positively with the tumor grade and stage, suggesting that ALDH1 may serve as a prognostic marker in these cancers [36] [37]. From these discoveries on the cancer stem cell hypothesis for epithelial cancers, it is reasonable to conclude that gaining insights into the molecular phenotypes of various cancers can lead to improvements in clinical decision-making [36].

THE CD133 PHENOTYPE: GROWING EVIDENCE AMONG CENTRAL NERVOUS SYSTEM TUMORS

Tumors of the central nervous system have among the worst prognoses of all solid organ cancers and are refractory to conventional treatment in many cases [11]. Tumor-initiating cells of the central nervous system have received much attention in the recent years and are perhaps the most well-characterized cancer stem cells among solid organs.

The origin of brain tumor stem cells is also elusive, but current theories suggest that they may arise from either [1] dedifferentiation of committed glial progenitors or [2] transformed neural stem cells [38]. Medulloblastomas and glioblastomas have been shown to harbor stemness characteristics [39]. The presence of multiple distinct areas of differentiation among neurological tumors has helped support the brain tumor stem cell hypothesis [39]. Primary tissue from cancers of the central nervous system demonstrated stem-like properties before the findings were discovered in cell lines, but the evidence in human and rat glioma cell lines is gradually accruing [10,40]. The hallmark of sphere formation has been repeatedly demonstrated by the CD133+ phenotype [41].

The radiotherapy resistance of some medulloblastomas has prompted investigations into the reasons for this behavior. Among cerebellar medulloblastomas in children, radiation resistant stem cell compartments have been identified near blood vessels and have been shown to express the intermediate filament protein Nestin [13]. Nestin expression confers increased survivability through PI3K activation and p53-mediated cell cycle arrest [13]. Inhibition of components of the PI3K pathway results in re-establishment of radiosensitivity [13].

The putative phenotype for brain tumor-initiating cells involves CD133, also known as prominin-1, a well-known marker of hematopoietic stem cells, neural stem cells, and endothelial precursors [40]. CD133 positivity is not specific for cancer stem cells of neurological origin, however, as an important report on the characterization of stem cells from Ewing's sarcoma has delineated the role of CD133 in tumor-forming ability [5]. The repopulating ability of CD133+ cells is far superior to that of CD133- cells; the minimal threshold for tumor regeneration *in vivo* is two orders of magnitude less for CD133 positivity compared to negativity [40]. Similar findings have been associated with the putative breast tumor-initiating cell [3]. CD133 positivity is correlated with radiotherapy resistance in gliomblastoma and platinum-based chemotherapy resistance in ovarian cancer [42]. Surprisingly, CD133 has also been suggested to be the marker for pancreatic adenocarinoma stem cells and ovarian cancer stem cells [43,44]. CD133 positive cells have been shown to divide asymmetrically, producing both CD133+ cell daughter and a CD133- daughter, whereas parent cells lacking CD133 fail to produce any CD133+ progeny [44]. Thus, self-renewal has been demonstrated by these cells.

EVIDENCE FOR SIDE POPULATIONS IN CANCER

Side populations, defined by their ability to exclude DNA-binding dyes via ATP-dependent transporters, consist of early progenitors and their parent stem cells [45]. Side populations are also characteristic of endothelial cells [46]. Cells from side populations demonstrate increased ability to generate tumors compared to other cells [47]. The growth capacity of side population cells is superior to cells that are not from side populations, and they demonstrate higher levels of invasiveness [47]. Side populations are typically identified by flow cytometric analysis, and this technique is becoming an increasingly important tool for studying stem cells [48].

The key proteins that are characteristic of side populations are members of the ATP-binding cassette superfamily, such as the multidrug resistance transporter ABCB1 and the breast cancer resistance protein ABCG2. These transmembrane proteins function in ATP-dependent efflux of DNA-binding dyes such as Hoechst 33342 [45]. ATP-binding cassette transporters can be found on resident stem cells of various tissues [8]. ABCG2 expression in particular has been reported in both solid and hematological malignancies, including the lung cancer, prostate cancer, breast cancer, and leukemia [49]. Expression of a whole array of multidrug resistant transporters has been confirmed in a population of liver cell progenitors in patients with hepatocellular carcinoma [50]. The significance of these findings is that presence of particular transporters, such as the multidrug resistance-associated protein MRP1, is correlated with unfavorable prognosis in hepatocellular carcinoma [50]. Although these studies have not definitely demonstrated that a side population is responsible for the resistance of liver cancer to treatment, the possibility should be kept in mind as insights into the cancer stem cell hypothesis are gained.

Methods for the selection of cancer stem cells have been attempted and frequently involve the use of chemotherapeutic agents. In glioma, the alkylating agent temozolomide has been used to isolate a population of stem-like glioma cells [46]. Resistance in this population may be partly attributed to increased expression of O^6-methylguanine DNA methyltransferase. Temozolamide can also induce expression of ABCG2, thereby contributing to chemotherapy resistance [46]. In the case of osteogenic sarcoma, the use of the poly(A) polymerase inhibitor 3-aminobenzamide over a period of nearly four months allowed for the selection of transformed stem cells from these tumors [49]. The resultant population was heterogeneous and harbored the spindle-shaped appearance of mesenchymal stem cells [49]. Characterization of this population from osteosarcoma confirmed phenotypic and functional characteristics of stem cells, namely expression of Oct4 and Nanog and ability to efflux drugs via the ATP-binding cassette members [49].

Uroepithelial side populations have been isolated in cancers of the genitourinary tract based on Hoechst 33342 dye exclusion [48]. Cancers of the bladder, kidney, and prostate appear to entertain small populations of dye-excluding cells in the midst of large tumors. ABCG2 is the transporter responsible for dye exclusion in prostate cancer side populations [48].

Current efforts are geared towards identifying the link, if any, between side population characteristics and cancer quiescence. Some groups have suggested that tumor-initiating cells may be found within side populations, while other groups have shown distinct origins [17]. Side populations in pancreatic cancer may be enriched in cancer stem cells and cells with predilection to undergo the epithelial-to-mesenchymal transition [17]. In fact, both side populations and cells undergoing epithelial-to-mesenchymal transition have increased invasive capability compared to normal cells, and the bridge between these two populations may be closer than previously believed [17].

FUTURE INSIGHTS

It has long been recognized that the efficacy of cancer treatment has been limited by resistance of cells to chemotherapy and radiation. Investigations in the recent years have culminated in the theory that a distinct subpopulation may be responsible for the maintenance and metastasis of tumors. Analysis of the integrity of the human genome in cancers is becoming an important factor in identifying resistant subpopulations [2]. The genomic stability of normal cells is maintained by various cellular repair processes and permits proper regulation of cellular division [2]. Maintenance of the genomic integrity of tumor-initiating cells, however, is not completely understood. Genomic instability has been suggested to promote heterogeneity in cancer as well as the development of cancer stem cells [2]. The origin of cancer stem cells and the underlying mechanisms that lead to development and sustenance of tumors have not been thoroughly explored and remain open to debate.

Differential gene expression may underlie the basis for the behavior of cancer stem cells in comparison to non-stem cancer cells and normal tissue [51]. Gene expression profiling has been proposed for identifying key players in the tumor-initiating populations [51]. Among the most important methods by which genomic profiles can be assessed is the use of microarray. For example, cDNA microarrays have been employed for comparison of high-grade astrocytomas with neural stem cells, and unique expression patterns have been identified in these cancers [38]. Identification of genes involves in tumor proliferation were specific to astrocytoma cells when compared with surrounding tissue, providing evidence for uniqueness of the putative astrocytoma stem cell population [38]. Such high-throughput studies can be followed by gene-specific and targeted studies; this approach may shed insight onto the molecular bases for the chemotherapeutic resistance and subsequent resurgence of cancer.

Only recently has the epithelial-to-mesenchymal transition been associated with the cancer stem cell phenotype, and much evidence is lacking on this dynamic process. Nonetheless, the data appears to support a stem cell basis for cancer. With further investigations into the cellular changes that confer resistance to chemotherapy and radiation, the link between cancer stem cells and epithelial-to-mesenchymal transition may be elucidated.

As scientists gain insight into the molecular mechanisms underlying tumor survival, the development of targeted therapy appears promising. Thus far, targeted therapy has been proposed in the context of cellular signaling. Arguably the most critical pathway involved in cellular survival, proliferation, differentiation, and growth is the phosphoinositide-3-kinase (PI3K)/Akt/mTOR pathway [12]. Inhibition of the PI3K pathway in gliomas has been studied well, and the data shows that small molecule inhibitors specific for Akt in glioma may hinder resistant cancer cell survival and invasiveness without affecting the untransformed resident tissue [11]. Cells of the CD133+ are more susceptible to Akt inhibition that CD133- cells, indicating the specificity towards the putative stem cell population in glioma. Such effects have been demonstrated *in vivo* for immunodeficient mice for glioma and may eventually translate to patients [11]. Aside from the use of Akt inhibitors, PI3K and mTOR inhibition has demonstrated anti-proliferative effects [12].

Targeted therapy for cancer stem cells has been studied by a few groups with some *in vitro* success. For instance, stem cells of glioblastoma multiforme express the chloride channel CLIC1, which mediates efflux of nitrosureas commonly used in cancer chemotherapy [52]. Antagonism of this channel has been shown to help induce apoptosis in glioma cancer stem cells while restoring chemosensitivity to nitrosureas [52]. As another example, viral-mediated therapy has been attempted for breast cancer stem cells [53]. Cells of the CD44+/CD24- phenotype were targeted by a lytic virus of the Reovirus family [53]. Nonetheless, specificity was not established, as the reovirus induced apoptosis in both the CD44+/CD24- and the non-stem cancer cells [53]. Lack of specificity leaves behind the possibility that normal resident tissue can destroyed. Attempts at targeted therapy for breast cancer have resulted in successful elimination of CD44+/CD24^{low} cells by cytotoxic T cells primed with the Numb-1 peptide [54]. This suggests that sensitization of lymphocytes by particular antigens may be gear the immune towards attacking particular phenotypes [54]. Findings such as these give field hope to prospects on targeted therapy.

Although targeted therapy geared at cancer stem cells has not successfully reached the clinic thus far, the prospects for targeted therapy may become favorable as the science advances [11]. The outlooks on targeted therapy are encouraging based on accumulating evidence on the cancer stem cell phenotype. Important benefits for such therapy include increased effectiveness at eliminating refractory tumors and decreased risk of cytotoxic side effects [11]. Central to all therapeutic endeavors is that the molecular mechanisms governing the tumor-initiating phenotype must be determined before success is achieved in the clinic.

Challenges to the cancer stem cell hypothesis are well recognized. Two of the foremost challenges include the successful culturing of these cells *in vitro* and the identification of a targetable phenotype [10]. Phenotypes may be tissue-specific, so attempts at universal characterization are unlikely to be successful. Once a phenotype is established, isolation of these cells is critical for characterization of the subpopulations. Downstream applications may include molecular and functional characterization of the subpopulations, which will ultimately allow for development of targeted therapy [6]. As studies continue on the cancer stem cell hypothesis, science may hold promising therapies for the treatment of the chemo-resistant and radio-resistant tumors that are responsible for the high mortality rates in cancer.

REFERENCES

[1]   Tomasson, MH. Cancer stem cells: a guide for skeptics. *J Cell Biochem* 2009; 106:745-9.

[2]   Li, L, Borodyansky, L and Yang Y. Genomic instability en route to and from cancer stem cells. *Cell Cycle* 2009; 8:1000-2.

[3]   Kakarala, M. and Wicha MS. Implications of the cancer stem-cell hypothesis for breast cancer prevention and therapy. *J Clin Oncol* 2008; 26:2813-20.

[4]   Palapattu, GS, Wu, C, Silvers, CR, Martin, HB, Williams, K, Salamone, L, Bushnell, T, Huang, LS, Yang, Q, Huang and J. Selective expression of CD44, a putative prostate cancer stem cell marker, in neuroendocrine tumor cells of human prostate cancer. *Prostate* 2009. [In press]

[5]   Suva, ML, Riggi, N, Stehle, JC, Baumer, K, Tercier, S, Joseph, JM, Suvà, D, Clément, V, Provero, P, Cironi, L, Osterheld, MC, Guillou, L and Stamenkovic I. Identification of cancer stem cells in Ewing's sarcoma. *Cancer Res* 2009; 69:1776-81.

[6]   Al-Hajj, M, Wicha, MS, Benito-Hernandez, A, Morrison, SJ and Clarke, MF. Prospective identification of tumorigenic breast cancer cells. *Proc Natl Acad Sci* U S A 2003; 100:3983-8.

[7]   Santisteban, M, Reiman, JM, Asiedu, MK, Behrens, MD, Nassar, A, Kalli, KR, Haluska, P, Ingle, JN, Hartmann, LC, Manjili, MH, Radisky, DC, Ferrone, S and Knutson, KL. Immune-Induced Epithelial to Mesenchymal Transition In vivo Generates Breast Cancer Stem Cells. *Cancer Res* 2009. [In press]

[8]   Oates, JE, Grey, BR, Addla, SK, Samuel, JD, Hart, CA, Ramani, V, Brown, MD and Clarke, NW. Hoechst 33342 side population identification is a conserved and unified mechanism in urological cancers. *Stem Cells Dev* 2009. [In press]

[9]   Quintana, E, Shackleton, M, Sabel, MS, Fullen, DR, Johnson, TM and Morrison, SJ. Efficient tumour formation by single human melanoma cells. *Nature* 2008; 456:593-8.

[10]   Yu, SC, Ping, YF, Yi, L, Zhou, ZH, Chen, JH, Yao, XH, Gao, L, Wang. JM and Bian, XW. Isolation and characterization of cancer stem cells from a human glioblastoma cell line U87. *Cancer Lett* 2008; 265:124-34.

[11]   Eyler, CE, Foo, WC, LaFiura, KM, McLendon, RE, Hjelmeland, AB and Rich, JN. Brain cancer stem cells display preferential sensitivity to Akt inhibition. *Stem Cells* 2008; 26:3027-36.

[12]   Endersby, R and Baker, SJ. PTEN signaling in brain: neuropathology and tumorigenesis. *Oncogene* 2008; 27:5416-30.

[13]   Hambardzumyan, D, Becher, OJ, Rosenblum, MK, Pandolfi, PP, Manova-Todorova, K and Holland, EC. PI3K pathway regulates survival of cancer stem cells residing in the perivascular niche following radiation in medulloblastoma in vivo. *Genes Dev* 2008; 22:436-48.

[14]   Wojiski, S, Guibal, FC, Kindler, T, Lee, BH, Jesneck, JL, Fabian, A, Tenen, DG and Gilliland, DG. PML-RARalpha initiates leukemia by conferring properties of self-renewal to committed promyelocytic progenitors. *Leukemia* 2009. [In press]

[15]   Polyak, K. and Weinberg, RA. Transitions between epithelial and mesenchymal states: acquisition of malignant and stem cell traits. Nat *Rev Cancer* 2009; 9:265-73.

[16] Wang, Z, Li, Y, Kong, D, Banerjee, S, Ahmad, A, Azmi, AS, Ali, S, Abbruzzese, JL, Gallick, GE and Sarkar, FH. Acquisition of epithelial-mesenchymal transition phenotype of gemcitabine-resistant pancreatic cancer cells is linked with activation of the notch signaling pathway. *Cancer Res* 2009; 69:2400-7.

[17] Kabashima, A, Higuchi, H, Takaishi, H, Matsuzaki, Y, Suzuki, S, Izumiya, M, Iizuka, H, Sakai, G, Hozawa, S, Azuma, T and Hibi, T. Side population of pancreatic cancer cells predominates in TGF-beta-mediated epithelial to mesenchymal transition and invasion. *Int J Cancer* 2009 [In press]

[18] Strizzi, L, Postovit, LM, Margaryan, NV, Seftor, EA, Abbott, DE, Seftor, RE, Salomon, DS and Hendrix MJ. Emerging roles of nodal and Cripto-1: from embryogenesis to breast cancer progression. *Breast Dis* 2008; 29:91-103.

[19] Vincan, E and Barker, N. The upstream components of the Wnt signalling pathway in the dynamic EMT and MET associated with colorectal cancer progression. *Clin Exp Metastasis* 2008; 25:657-63.

[20] Christensen, R, Alsner, J, Brandt Sorensen F, Dagnaes-Hansen, F, Kolvraa S and Serakinci N. Transformation of human mesenchymal stem cells in radiation carcinogenesis: long-term effect of ionizing radiation. *Regen Med* 2008; 3:849-61.

[21] Rodriguez. R, Rubio. R, Masip. M, Catalina, P, Nieto, A, de la Cueva T, Arriero, M, San, Martin N, de la Cueva, E, Balomenos, D, Menendez, P and García-Castro, J. Loss of p53 induces tumorigenesis in p21-deficient mesenchymal stem cells. *Neoplasia* 2009; 11:397-407.

[22] Yamate, J, Ogata, K, Yuasa, T, Kuwamura, M, Takenaka, S, Kumagai, D, Itoh K, LaMarre J. Adipogenic, osteogenic and myofibrogenic differentiations of a rat malignant fibrous histiocytoma (MFH)-derived cell line, and a relationship of MFH cells with embryonal mesenchymal, perivascular and bone marrow stem cells. *Eur J Cancer* 2007; 43:2747-56.

[23] Stingl, J. Detection and analysis of mammary gland stem cells. *J Pathol* 2009; 217:229-41.

[24] Dontu, G. Breast cancer stem cell markers - the rocky road to clinical applications. *Breast Cancer Res* 2008; 10:110.

[25] Lee, CW, Simin, K, Liu, Q, Plescia, J, Guha, M, Khan, A, Hsieh, CC and Altieri DC. A functional Notch-survivin gene signature in basal breast cancer. *Breast Cancer Res* 2008; 10:R97.

[26] Civenni, G and Sommer, L. Chemokines in neuroectodermal development and their potential implication in cancer stem cell-driven metastasis. *Semin Cancer Biol* 2009; 19:68-75.

[27] Liang, Z, Wu, T, Lou, H, Yu, X, Taichman, RS, Lau, SK, Nie, S, Umbreit, J. and Shim, H. Inhibition of breast cancer metastasis by selective synthetic polypeptide against CXCR4. *Cancer Res* 2004; 64:4302-8.

[28] Corcoran, KE, Malhotra, A, Molina, CA and Rameshwar, P. Stromal-derived factor-1alpha induces a non-canonical pathway to activate the endocrine-linked Tac1 gene in non-tumorigenic breast cells. *J Mol Endocrinol* 2008; 40:113-23.

[29] Molloy, AP, Martin, FT, Dwyer, RM, Griffin, TP, Murphy, M, Barry FP, O'Brien, T. and Kerin, MJ. Mesenchymal stem cell secretion of chemokines during differentiation into osteoblasts, and their potential role in mediating interactions with breast cancer cells. *Int J Cancer* 2009; 124:326-32.

[30] Liang, X, Huuskonen, J, Hajivandi, M, Manzanedo, R, Predki, P, Amshey, JR and Pope, RM. Identification and quantification of proteins differentially secreted by a pair

of normal and malignant breast-cancer cell lines. *Proteomics* 2009; 9:182-93.

[31]   Li, Z, Liu, Y, Tuve, S, Xun, Y, Fan, X, Min, L, Feng, Q, Kiviat, N, Kiem, HP, Disis, ML and Lieber, A. Towards a stem cell gene therapy for breast cancer. *Blood* 2009 [In press]

[32]   Xiao, Y, Ye, Y, Yearsley, K, Jones, S, Barsky, SH. The lymphovascular embolus of inflammatory breast cancer expresses a stem cell-like phenotype. *Am J Pathol* 2008; 173:561-74.

[33]   Simon, RA, di Sant'Agnese, PA, Huang, LS, Xu, H, Yao, JL, Yang, Q, Liang, S, Liu, J, Yu, R, Cheng, L, Oh, WK, Palapattu, GS, Wei, J and Huang, J. CD44 expression is a feature of prostatic small cell carcinoma and distinguishes it from its mimickers. *Hum Pathol* 2009; 40:252-8.

[34]   Patrawala, L, Calhoun, T, Schneider-Broussard, R, Li H, Bhatia, B, Tang, S, Reilly, JG, Chandra, D, Zhou, J, Claypool, K, Coghlan, L, Tang, DG. Highly purified CD44+ prostate cancer cells from xenograft human tumors are enriched in tumorigenic and metastatic progenitor cells. *Oncogene* 2006; 25:1696-708.

[35]   Huang, CH, Millenson, MM, Sherman, EJ, Borghaei, H, Mintzer, DM, Cohen, RB, Staddon, AP, Seldomridge, J, Treat, OJ, Tuttle, H, Ruth, KJ and Langer CJ. Promising survival in patients with recurrent non-small cell lung cancer treated with docetaxel and gemcitabine in combination as second-line therapy. *J Thorac Oncol* 2008; 3:1032-8.

[36]   Jiang, F, Qiu, Q, Khanna, A, Todd, NW, Deepak, J, Xing, L, Wang, H, Liu, Z, Su, Y, Stass, SA and Katz RL. Aldehyde dehydrogenase 1 is a tumor stem cell-associated marker in lung cancer. *Mol Cancer Res* 2009; 7:330-8.

[37]   Balicki, D. Moving forward in human mammary stem cell biology and breast cancer prognostication using ALDH1. *Cell Stem Cell* 2007; 1:485-7.

[38]   Yang, Y, Qiu, Y, Ren, W, Gong, J and Chen, F. An identification of stem cell-resembling gene expression profiles in high-grade astrocytomas. *Mol Carcinog* 2008; 47:893-903.

[39]   Nern, C, Sommerlad, D, Acker, T and Plate, KH. Brain tumor stem cells. *Recent Results Cancer Res* 2009; 171:241-59.

[40]   Wu, A, Oh, S, Wiesner, SM, Ericson, K, Chen, L, Hall, WA, Champoux, PE, Low, WC and Ohlfest, JR. Persistence of CD133+ cells in human and mouse glioma cell lines: detailed characterization of GL261 glioma cells with cancer stem cell-like properties. *Stem Cells Dev* 2008; 17:173-84.

[41]   Annabi, B, Lachambre, MP, Plouff,e K, Sartelet, H and Béliveau, R. Modulation of invasive properties of CD133(+) glioblastoma stem cells: A role for MT1-MMP in bioactive lysophospholipid signaling. *Mol Carcinog* 2009. [In press]

[42]   Diaz Miqueli, A, Rolff, J, Lemm, M, Fichtner, I, Perez, R, Montero, E. Radiosensitisation of U87MG brain tumours by anti-epidermal growth factor receptor monoclonal antibodies. *Br J Cancer* 2009; 100:950-8.

[43]   Bednar, F and Simeone, DM. Pancreatic cancer stem cells and relevance to cancer treatments. *J Cell Biochem* 2009 [In press]

[44]   Baba, T, Convery, PA, Matsumura, N, Whitaker, RS, Kondoh, E, Perry T, Huang, Z, Bentley, RC, Mori, S, Fujii, S, Marks, JR, Berchuck, A and Murphy, SK. Epigenetic regulation of CD133 and tumorigenicity of CD133+ ovarian cancer cells. *Oncogene* 2009; 28:209-18.

[45]   Cabana, R, Frolova, EG, Kapoor, V, Thomas, RA, Krishan, A and Telford, Wg. The Minimal Instrumentation Requirements for Hoechst Side Population Analysis: Stem Cell Analysis on Low-Cost Flow Cytometry Platforms. *Stem Cells* 2006; 24: 2573-

2581.

[46] Bleau, AM, Hambardzumyan, D, Ozawa, T, Fomchenko, EI, Huse, JT, Brennan, CW
      and Holland, EC. PTEN/PI3K/Akt pathway regulates the side population phenotype
      and ABCG2 activity in glioma tumor stem-like cells. *Cell Stem Cell* 2009; 4:226-35.

[47] Ho, MM, Ng, AV, Lam, S and Hung, JY. Side population in human lung cancer cell
      lines and tumors is enriched with stem-like cancer cells. *Cancer Res* 2007; 67:4827-33.

[48] Mathew, G, Timm, EA Jr, Sotomayor, P, Godoy, A, Montecinos, VP, Smith, GJ and
      Huss, WJ. ABCG2-mediated DyeCycle Violet efflux defined side population in benign
      and malignant prostate. *Cell Cycle* 2009; 8:1053-61.

[49] Di Fiore, R, Santulli, A, Ferrante, RD, Giuliano, M, De Blasio, A, Messina, C, Pirozzi,
      G, Tirino, V, Tesoriere, G and Vento, R. Identification and expansion of human
      osteosarcoma-cancer-stem cells by long-term 3-aminobenzamide treatment. *J Cell
      Physiol* 2009; 219:301-13.

[50] Vander Borght, S, Komuta, M, Libbrecht, L, Katoonizadeh, A, Aerts, R, Dymarkowski,
      S, Verslype, C, Nevens, F and Roskams, T. Expression of multidrug resistance-
      associated protein 1 in hepatocellular carcinoma is associated with a more aggressive
      tumour phenotype and may reflect a progenitor cell origin. *Liver Int* 2008; 28:1370-80.

[51] Krivtsov, AV, Wang, Y, Feng, Z and Armstrong, SA. Gene Expression Profiling of
      Leukemia Stem Cells. *Methods Mol Biol* 2009; 538:1-16.

[52] Kang, MK and Kang, SK. Pharmacologic blockade of chloride channel synergistically
      enhances apoptosis of chemotherapeutic drug-resistant cancer stem cells. *Biochem
      Biophys Res Commun* 2008; 373:539-44.

[53] Marcato, P, Dean, CA, Giacomantonio, CA and Lee, PW. Oncolytic Reovirus
      Effectively Targets Breast Cancer Stem Cells. *Mol Ther* 2009. [In press]

[54] Mine, T, Matsueda, S, Li, Y, Tokumitsu, H, Gao, H, Danes, C, Wong, KK, Wang, X,
      Ferrone, S and Ioannides, CG. Breast cancer cells expressing stem cell markers
      CD44(+) CD24 (lo) are eliminated by Numb-1 peptide-activated T cells. *Cancer
      Immunol Immunother* 2008. [In press]

In: Encyclopedia of Stem Cell Research (2 Volume Set)   ISBN: 978-1-61761-835-2
Editor: Alexander L. Greene   © 2012 Nova Science Publishers, Inc.

Chapter XLVIII

OUTSTANDING QUESTIONS REGARDING INDUCED PLURIPOTENT STEM (IPS) CELL RESEARCH

Miguel A. Esteban, Jiekai Chen, Jiayin Yang, Feng Li, Wen Li, and Duanqing Pei

Chinese Academy of Sciences Key Laboratory of Regenerative Biology, South China Institute for Stem Cell Biology and Regenerative Medicine, Guangzhou Institutes of Biomedicine and Health, Guangzhou, China

ABSTRACT

Terminal somatic cell differentiation is not irreversible. The same route that transforms embryonic stem cells (ESCs) into specific lineages can be walked backwards, e.g. by means of the "induced pluripotent stem (iPS) cell" technology discovered by Shinya Yamanaka in 2006. The implications of iPS are out of proportion and its ease and reproducibility has made it a favorite option compared to other existing approaches including cell fusion or somatic cell nuclear transfer (SCNT). iPS allows the generation of patient specific embryonic-like stem cells that are devoid of ethical concerns and may be used for transplantation. iPS has also proven useful to create *in vitro* models that mimic human diseases and this could be used for high throughput drug screening. Besides, thanks to iPS we are now compelled to think of differentiation processes in a bidirectional way, which may be as well cell type and transcription factor specific. Therefore, knowledge is flourishing that will benefit Stem Cell Biology as much as unrelated disciplines. But the pace of discovery has been so quick that every technical advance has raised new issues, creating confusion. Here we will briefly define and try to answer some key questions that in our opinion will shape iPS research and application in following years.

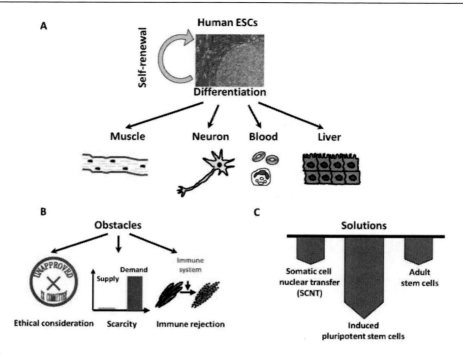

Figure 1. A, Pluripotency and self renewal of ESCs. A capture of human ESCs is shown. B, Some concerns surrounding human ESC research. C, Some solutions to human ESC research and application.

1.   INTRODUCTION TO iPS TECHNOLOGY

ESCs were first isolated (mouse ESCs) in 1981 [1] and are defined by two main characteristics: pluripotency, which means that they have the potential to give rise to all cell types of the adult body, and self renewal, which implies that if cultured under specific conditions they can be maintained undifferentiated indefinitely (Figure 1A). Ever since the discovery of human ESCs (1998) [2], the idea of inducing differentiation "a la carte" to repair damaged tissue has fostered our imagination and stimulated the development of a new branch of Medicine based on tissue regeneration. But on one side the risk of immune rejection, and on the other very important ethical considerations, have hampered human ESC research and application (Figure 1B) [3]. Experiments over the past 50 years have established that, despite the decrease in differentiation potential associated with development, the nuclei of most, if not all, adult cells retain plasticity and can be reset to an ESC-like state. This culminated in 1996 with the birth of Dolly the sheep thanks to SCNT [4]. This technique is founded on the inoculation of somatic cell genomic DNA into an enucleated oocyte that retains the nucleoplasm (nuclear content excluding DNA). The latter may seem irrelevant but indicated that the nucleoplasm contains factors (transcription factors or DNA binding proteins) that drive the nuclear reprogramming. Remarkably, not only whole individuals can be produced this way, the resulting blastocyst may also be broken on feeder layers and cell lines then generated that are similar to ESCs. Despite sheep, mice, pigs, and dogs, have been produced this way, the technique is rather inefficient and the reprogramming usually incomplete.

Moreover, the procedure is not exempt of ethical considerations either, oocytes are scarce, and SCNT has not yet been achieved in humans [5]. A trendy alternative has been autologous transplantation using cell lineages derived from adult stem cells, for example adipose and bone marrow mesenchymal stem cells (MSCs) [6]. But these cells are not pluripotent, can be obtained in very scarce numbers, and are difficult to expand (self renewal is limited) [7]. With these premises, a major scientific goal of recent years has been to achieve a relatively simple method that can reprogram somatic cells into pluripotent ESC-like cells (Figure 1C). The revolution came in 2006 when Yamanaka and collaborators showed that mouse fibroblasts acquire properties similar to ESCs after retroviral transduction of 4 transcription factors, namely Oct4, Sox2, Klf4, and c-Myc (SKOM), abundant in the nuclei of ESCs [8] (Figure 2A). These cells were called induced pluripotent stem (iPS) cells (Figure 2B). The first generation iPS cells were similar to mouse ESCs in morphology and proliferation, had a normal karyotype, and formed teratomas (Figure 3A-C). However, their global gene expression pattern differed significantly from ESCs and they failed to produce mixed color chimeric mice when injected into blastocysts from a different type of mice. In 2007, chimera competence and germline transmission was achieved [9-11] (Figure 3D), and later on iPS was produced from human fibroblasts [12,13]. Moreover, the technique has been reproduced in multiple laboratories and ever since the pace of discovery has been exponential. Potentially, iPS technology can overcome 2 of the most important problems associated with human ESC application (ethical considerations and immune rejection), but still faces many obstacles, some of which are shared with ESCs (e.g. the bona fide and easy differentiation into given lineages) and others that are unique.

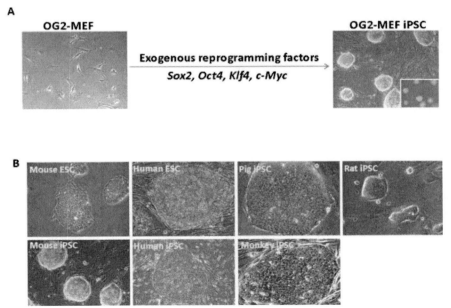

Figure 2. A, Schematic representation of iPS cell colony generation from mouse embryonic fibroblasts. Mouse embryonic fibroblasts (MEFs) from mice (OG2 mice) that bear a transgenic Oct4 promoter driving GFP expression were used, the colonies became GFP positive after reactivation of the endogenous ESC program. B, Captures of ESCs and iPS cell colonies (iPSC) from different species. All cell lines were generated in our laboratory.

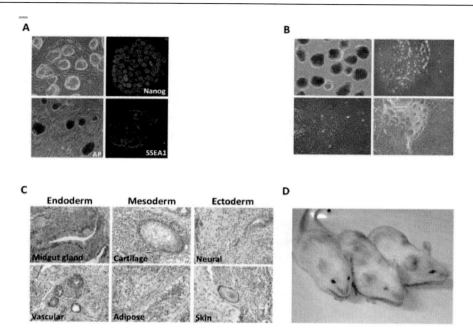

Figure 3. A, Immunofluorescence microscopy captures of mouse iPS cells using antibodies against ESC markers. Alkaline phosphatase (AP) staining is also shown. B, Embryonic bodies formed from human iPS colonies. iPS cells were first cultured in suspension in non adherent culture dishes, after a week of culture in suspension the embryonic bodies were adhered to coverslips and this progressively resulted in differentiation into cells with many shapes and characteristics. Mouse embryonic bodies have similar appearance and behavior (not shown). C, Teratomas derived from mouse iPS cells formed tissues corresponding to the 3 germ layers. D, Captures of chimeric mice produced by injection of iPS cells from black mice into blastocysts from white mice. All experiments in Figure 2 and 3 are unpublished and were performed in our laboratory.

2.   SOME ESSENTIAL QUESTIONS SURROUNDING iPS

2.1   Is iPS Originated From Adult Stem Cells Present in the Starting Population? Can iPS be Induced from Cells of Multiple Tissues?

Like it happened with SCNT [14], one of the first tests for iPS was to find out whether any cell is susceptible to this form of reprogramming or only a small minority of cells with inherent stem cell characteristics that are present in skin biopsias. This was particularly important in light of the extremely low efficiency of the initial iPS reports. We know now that besides fibroblasts, also stomach and liver cells, B lymphocytes, pancreatic beta cells, meningeal membrane cells (meningiocytes), keratinocytes, hair follicle cells, and several others, are susceptible to iPS [15-20]. However, this does not imply that stem cells are not easier to reprogram, as this is for example the case of neural stem cells (NSCs) [21]. The exact reason underlying NSC amenability to iPS is unclear but may be related to basal expression of the complementary factors Sox2, Klf4, and c-Myc. It is also interesting to note that like NSCs other cell types derived from the ectoderm, such as meningiocytes and keratinocytes, are more prone to iPS [18,20]. The ectoderm is the first germ layer to appear during development and this may perhaps imply less extended reorganization of the chromatin relative to ESCs and compared to mesoderm and endoderm.

2.2 Can iPS be Induced With Alternative Combinations of Factors or Using Fewer Factors? Can iPS be Produced Using Different Delivery Methods Apart from Retroviruses? Can it be Enhanced Using Chemicals?

The initial approach of Takahashi and Yamanaka included 24 factors expressed by retroviral vectors and then by substitution this narrowed into 4 magic transcription factors [8,22]. Because c-Myc is an oncogene, SKOM iPS resulted in significant risk of tumor formation and decreased life span in the chimeric mice [10]. Several groups then reported mouse and human iPS excluding c-Myc, albeit with a very poor efficiency of colony formation that makes it unpractical [23,24]. In parallel, Thomson *et al.* produced human iPS using an alternative combination (Sox2, Oct4, Nanog, Lin28) [13]. The choice of Nanog seemed logic given its key role in controlling ESC behavior, as for how Lin28 favors iPS it is yet unclear but may be related to its ability to regulate the microRNA let7. By that time chemical enhancers of iPS were discovered, in particular the histone deacetylase inhibitors (HDACi) valproic acid (VPA) and trichostatin (TSA) [25]. Histone modifications, including acetylation and methylation, alter nucleosomes and facilitate or reduce access of transcription factors to their DNA cognate sequences [26]. HDACi not only allowed significant increase of iPS efficiency using fibroblasts and SKOM or SKO, but also iPS using even fewer factors [27]. Whether HDACi also act at least in part through mechanisms independent of their impact on histone acetylation is not known but remains possible. Substitution of Klf4 using chemicals has also been achieved in mouse iPS by means of high throughput screening [28]. Likewise, iPS has been produced using 1 factor (Oct4 in NSCs), and although use of retroviruses still remains the most widespread delivery system other approaches have proliferated recently: excisable piggyBac transposons [29,30], lox-p flanked factors (polycystronic vectors producing factors linked in tandem by means of 2A autocleavable sequences) [31], adenoviruses [32], episomal vectors [33], and recombinant proteins [34,35]. The last three approaches, in particular the proteins, are very appealing but also extremely unproductive and thus may be difficult to reproduce. Moreover, although the general view is that iPS with fewer factors or without transgene integration will result in safer cell lines, things may not be that easy and it is perhaps difficult to achieve complete reprogramming in such conditions, at least in the human model. On the other hand, several groups have increased the number of factors (by combining Yamanaka's and Thomson's combinations and also with other additions) and used lentiviruses to increase human iPS efficiency [36,37]. Likewise, Sox2 can be replaced by Sox1, Klf4 by Klf2 or Klf5 and by estrogen related receptor beta (Esrrb), and c-Myc by n-Myc or l-Myc [38].

2.3   Can iPS be Produced from other Mammals in Addition to Mouse and Human?

The demonstration that SKOM can reprogram 2 highly unrelated species transmitted optimism regarding universality of the pluripotency network in mammals and stimulated iPS research on other species. Recently, several groups produced iPS cell lines from Rhesus monkey fibroblasts [39], rat fibroblasts and MSCs [40], and fibroblasts and MSCs from Tibetan [41] and farm pig [42,43]. Rat is a far better model than mouse for physiology and disease-orientated studies, and the generation of rat iPS coincided in time with the discovery of chimera competent and germ line competent ESCs [44,45]. Interest in genetic manipulation of rats has consequently been boosted and many surprises lie ahead. It must be noted however that pluripotency of rat iPS cell lines is reduced compared to ESCs, possibly reflecting partial reprogramming. The same can be said for the pig, but for this animal ESCs haven't been isolated yet despite decades of intense effort [46]. Very likely soon we will see reports on iPS from other non human primates like the marmoset (whose reduced size is an advantage), and domestic animals including dog, cat, rabbit or sheep, as well as subsequent improvements of the respective methodologies. Nevertheless, at some point a standard will need to be set for comparison with humans in the form of preclinical trials. In many countries phylogenetic similarity between monkeys and humans poses a barrier towards research, and in addition monkeys may need to be imported, are expensive, and difficult to breed. Given striking parallelisms with humans, the pig, which is an agricultural commodity in most places, may dominate except for cases such as Parkinson or Huntington disease in which neurological evaluation is easier in primates [47]. In the near future, it is also probable that countries will try to show national pride producing iPS from icon animals such as panda in China or kangaroo in Australia. Besides being a curiosity, one might argue that this could be a way to protect endangered species [48].

2.4.   Are iPS Cells Produced from Different Tissues Identical? What Requisites must Fulfill an iPS Cell Line to be Considered Fully Reprogrammed? Are Human iPS Cells Truly Pluripotent?

After the generation of chimera competent mouse iPS, all emphasis was put on the idea that iPS cells and ESCs, either mouse or human, are almost indistinguishable. This was shown using DNA arrays, histone methylation profiling, telomere length, and ultrastructural features, among others [49-51]. However, is the story as simple as this, or iPS is like a make-up, the conversion of a somatic cell to another somatic cell that has the ability to mimic almost all aspects of ESCs? Supporting the idea of some kind of make-up and based on more detailed analysis of data, the paradigm is now emerging that iPS cells differ from ESCs, and iPS from different tissues or generated with different methods are different as well [52-54]. The latter is of particular interest because iPS from a given tissue may retain some epigenetic memory and that could make it more easily differentiated back into the same tissue than other iPS cell lines or even human ESCs. However, caution is needed when comparing iPS cell lines between themselves and with ESCs, as differences could be only reflection of partial reprogramming in spite of the ability to form teratomas. An extra consideration is that human ESCs from varied sources are not identical and the same applies to mouse ESCs [55]. Numbers, in terms of genes going up or down or other differences, are not vital to answer this question, many genes could be changed and this not mean anything, while differences in one gene could have profound consequences. Besides, it is very important that when iPS cell lines are compared, they have been cultured using the same protocols and have been split for a roughly similar number of times. When profiling iPS cell lines from diverse individuals their ethnic background should also be considered. Whole genome DNA methylation analysis of iPS and ESCs may hold the key to reach a conclusion concerning the identity of iPS cells. But to make it affordable (sequencing each base of the genome at least 5 to 10 times on average) new generation sequencing technologies must be developed further. Moreover, in the near future specific regions will need to be selected and standardized so that the epigenetic characteristics of iPS cell lines can be tested quickly.

2.5. Can iPS be Used to Model Human Diseases in Vitro? Are There Any Ethical Concerns to be Considered for iPS Cell Generation and Distribution?

iPS provides an outstanding model to study human genetic diseases in vitro, any hereditary disease in general but in particular those for which animal models don't exist. For example [56], we can generate iPS from a patient with a neurological genetic syndrome, we then characterize those iPS cell lines and make sure that they are truly pluripotent, and finally we differentiate those iPS cells into neurons and compare their functionality with neurons from iPS cell lines derived from unaffected individuals. In the case of monogenic diseases the mutation could be corrected and the neurons from the original or the corrected iPS cell line exhaustively compared. This kind of approach offers the possibility of studying the underlying functional defect at a molecular level, and if properly optimized also high throughput drug screening for compounds that correct the abnormality. For diseases which are not monogenic, like chromosomal abnormalities, the genetic correction is not feasible but the model is no less interesting. In those cases in which the disease has a very complex genetic background the utility is more arguable, and some diseases are not result of one single cell type being affected but very many. For example Alzheimer disease has in cases a familiar history suggestive of genetic predisposition. However, differentiation of iPS cells from these patients into neurons may not yield any conclusion because of the fundamental contribution of the environment and the fact that the disease is consequence of accumulated beta amyloid over many years. One might then argue that challenging those neurons with specific compounds could accelerate the kinetics and this would indeed prove invaluable. Even if this is the case, the analysis of a significant number of patients and comparison with iPS cell lines from unaffected people of the similar social status, age and gender, will be necessary. Likewise, collection of samples from members of one same family, including affected and unaffected is important. Before collecting samples, the individuals should be carefully informed and confidentiality maintained, as these cells may be distributed to other laboratories or even pharmaceutical companies, and they could end up having economic value. The latter would happen if standardized iPS cell lines owned by pharmaceutical companies are commercially distributed for therapeutic purposes in immunologically compatible patients. At this point the Ethics and regulations concerning iPS have not yet been defined [57], but this will likely start soon. In any case, ethical considerations that now apply to human ESCs should not be present in iPS research. Finally, we would like to state the fact that some still argue that iPS must be banned for the simple reason that it might stimulate scientists to do exhaustive comparisons with human ESCs.

2.6   What are the Mechanisms of iPS? Is Insertional Mutagenesis a Requisite? Do Barriers Exist that Limit the Reprogramming and can They be Overcome Through Manipulation?

The mechanisms of iPS remain largely unknown and have been defined as a "black box" [58]. Despite everyone agrees that understanding the molecular machinery will improve the methodology, researchers have so far focused on rather more empirical studies. The quick pace of the field imposed this direction and more laborious mechanistic analysis was set aside with the exception of DNA arrays and ChIP-on-Chip analysis [51,59]. It is known that iPS is a slow process, taking around 15-20 days in the mouse and around 1 month in the human [60]. During this process the first noticeable changes are morphological, cells cluster and start forming aggregates since the first days of reprogramming. Afterwards, alkaline phosphatase staining and suface markers including SSEA1 are progressively acquired. In the last instance, the endogenous ESC program becomes reactivated and the transgenes (at least in the case of retroviruses) become silenced [61]. The latter has been accepted as a criterion for full reprogramming and is based on a self defense reaction of ESCs: methylation of the invading genome [10]. A barrier for exploring iPS has been the low efficiency. Because the population is highly heterogeneous, changes observed in the early phases or reprogramming may not be representative of the internal engine. Low efficiency also raised possibility that the transgenes may need to integrate in specific regions of the genome, and perhaps introduce mutations that activate or silence nearby genes that are in turn critical modulators of iPS. This has not yet been excluded formally but at least it is clear that the integration pattern differs very significantly between different iPS cell lines [62]. Moreover, a single integration of a polycistronic vector can induce iPS [63,64], and iPS can as well be achieved without exogenous insertions [32-35,65]. One might then argue that it is imperative to do single cell analysis using newly developed technologies. But on which basis do we select those cells and how can we be sure they are the "good" ones? If on the top of that we add the fact that time course analysis is needed, then the task is immense, perhaps impossible. DNA arrays produced from time course iPS experiments using secondary fibroblasts generated with doxycicline inducible lentiviruses did not provide clear answers [51]. Addition of the antibiotic produces reactivation of the vectors (lentiviruses are less efficiently silenced than retroviruses) and iPS colonies appear with higher efficiency and quicker kinetics than under standard protocols. Although such approach is powerful, acceleration of the process and biased expression of the integrated factors may alter the whole chain of events that happen in primary cells, and therefore provide wrong conclusions. In the immediate future it is expected that mechanistic investigations will be sorted in three ways: first, use of higher efficiency methods based on previous empirical observations, which may also be coupled to isolation of enriched populations; second, use of high throughput screening assays based on siRNA oligos or vectors; and third, meticulous analysis of pathways relevant to ESCs or to somatic cell functioning in general. Regarding the latter, early stages of reprogramming share similitude with the process of tumorigenesis, as among other things both involve immortalization [66]. Looking at cell cycle check points or tumor suppressor pathways like p21 or p53 will likely shed light into how iPS is accomplished. Manipulating these pathways may as well increase iPS efficiency but since these are guardians of the genome it may also introduce mutations or other abnormalities. This raises the question as to whether the iPS process itself introduces risk of acquiring genomic abnormalities by changing these pathways before the ESC-like identity (and the associated self defense mechanisms) has been achieved. From a different perspective, pre-iPS cell lines, which represent the major part of colonies produced with standard iPS protocols, can be fully reprogrammed by means of chemical additions and this is an outstanding tool to understand iPS mechanisms.

CONCLUSION

Only 3 years ago, what it seemed impossible became real, the fate of somatic cells was changed *in vitro* using a relatively simple methodology. Shinya Yamanaka's approach to induced pluripotency has demolished barriers that politicians could not break with bare talk in over a decade of tense debate surrounding human ESCs. Now everyone talks about iPS, and even if detractors exist, they cannot hide their astonishment. Although many questions remain present, the most difficult step, which is producing the technology, has been accomplished and the rest is only a matter of time. In following years the field is likely to specialize in multiple branches: on one side mechanistic studies coupled to screening of highly susceptible (and easily accessible) cell types and different factor delivery protocols, will converge into a consensus regarding "clinical grade" iPS in humans. On the other, iPS disease models will not rely so much on technical issues or safety, and will look more for ease and robustness. For clinical use of iPS, we will first need to establish adequate large animal models, and the pig will arguably be the reference. Once clinical trials are approved, it is unlikely that autologous transplantation will be a preferred choice, as it is too time consuming and expensive. Creation of an iPS cell bank matching thousands of HLA haplotypes will be instrumental to bring iPS to the general public. Among other things, this would allow use of exhaustively tested iPS cell lines (e.g. teratomas, transcriptome, microRNAs, multilineage differentiation, etc) that with the arrival of new generation sequencing technologies may be studied for existence of insertional or not insertional mutations and their DNA methylation status (other epigenetic marks as well) at a genome wide level. But random banking of iPS cell lines will be unproductive and it is necessary to take advantage of already well established and well characterized cell banks, e.g. of cord blood. iPS from cord blood has not yet been achieved but many laboratories are pursuing this objective and we anticipate a breakthrough soon. Even after this happens, creating an iPS cell bank is an out of dimension enterprise that would benefit from interaction between institutes and countries. An added problem is that pharmaceutical companies will try to purchase large stock of iPS cell lines from laboratories worldwide, and protect the intellectual property; like it happens nowadays with drugs, iPS will at some point move billions. As for the disease models, access to cell banks containing tens or hundreds of well diagnosed patients for every possible disease is equally relevant to achieve effectiveness. So far iPS studies have centered on a very limited number of affected individuals, in occasions 1 or 2, and this is a serious handicap for making serious conclusions. Comparisons between patients of different ethnic groups or countries will be especially valuable to expand credibility. Nevertheless, the study of many genetic diseases will likely be revitalized thanks to iPS. In our opinion, iPS from autosomal recessive diseases is particularly interesting: using homologous recombination techniques the remaining intact allele could be spliced out in a conditional manner that is lineage specific. This could be applied in hereditary cancer syndromes in which the second hit is organ specific (e.g. von Hippel-Lindau syndrome, adenomatous polyposis coli, etc) [67,68]. Apart from all the above considerations, new concepts/approaches may arise from iPS research that could be used to slow down ageing, as this is also in essence a programmed process [69].

REFERENCES

[1]   Evans, M.J. and Kaufman, M.H. (1981). Establishment in culture of pluripotential cells from mouse embryos. *Nature,* 292, 154-6.

[2]   Thomson, J.A., Itskovitz-Eldor, J., Shapiro, S.S., Waknitz, M.A., Swiergiel, J.J., Marshall, V.S. and Jones, J.M. (1998). Embryonic stem cell lines derived from human blastocysts. *Science,* 282, 1145-7.

[3]   Daley, G.Q. et al. (2007). Ethics. The ISSCR guidelines for human embryonic stem cell research. *Science,* 315, 603-4.

[4]   Wilmut, I., Schnieke, A.E., McWhir, J., Kind, A.J. and Campbell, K.H. (1997). Viable offspring derived from fetal and adult. *Science,* 385, 810-3.

[5]   Hwang, W.S. et al. (2004). Evidence of a pluripotent human embryonic stem cell line derived from a cloned blastocyst. *Science,* 303, 1669-74.

[6]   Kern, S., Eichler, H., Stoeve, J., Kluter, H. and Bieback, K. (2006). Comparative analysis of mesenchymal stem cells from bone marrow, umbilical cord blood, or adipose tissue. *Stem Cells,* 24, 1294-301.

[7]   Basem M. Abdallah, Hamid Saeed and Kassem, M. (2009). Human Mesenchymal Stem Cells: Basic Biology and Clinical Applications for Bone Tissue Regeneration. Trends in Stem Cell Biology and Technology, pp. 177-190

[8]   Takahashi, K. and Yamanaka, S. (2006). Induction of pluripotent stem cells from mouse embryonic and adult fibroblast cultures by defined factors. *Cell ,*126, 663-76.

[9]   Maherali, N. et al. (2007). Directly reprogrammed fibroblasts show global epigenetic remodeling and widespread tissue contribution. *Cell Stem Cell,* 1, 55-70.

[10] Okita, K., Ichisaka, T. and Yamanaka, S. (2007). Generation of germline-competent induced pluripotent stem cells. *Nature,* 448, 313-7.

[11] Wernig, M., Meissner, A., Foreman, R., Brambrink, T., Ku, M., Hochedlinger, K., Bernstein, B.E. and Jaenisch, R. (2007). In vitro reprogramming of fibroblasts into a

pluripotent ES-cell-like state. *Nature,* 448, 318-24.

[12] Takahashi, K., Tanabe, K., Ohnuki, M., Narita, M., Ichisaka, T., Tomoda, K. and Yamanaka, S. (2007). Induction of pluripotent stem cells from adult human fibroblasts by defined factors. *Cell,* 131, 861-72.

[13] Yu, J. et al. (2007). Induced pluripotent stem cell lines derived from human somatic cells. *Science,* 318, 1917-20.

[14] Hochedlinger, K. and Jaenisch, R. (2002). Monoclonal mice generated by nuclear transfer from mature B and T donor cells. *Nature,* 415, 1035-8.

[15] Aoi, T., Yae, K., Nakagawa, M., Ichisaka, T., Okita, K., Takahashi, K., Chiba, T. and Yamanaka, S. (2008). Generation of pluripotent stem cells from adult mouse liver and stomach cells. *Science,* 321, 699-702.

[16] Stadtfeld, M., Brennand, K. and Hochedlinger, K. (2008). Reprogramming of pancreatic beta cells into induced pluripotent stem cells. *Curr Biol,* 18, 890-4.

[17] Hanna, J. et al. (2008). Direct reprogramming of terminally differentiated mature B lymphocytes to pluripotency. *Cell,* 133, 250-64.

[18] Qin, D. et al. (2008). Mouse meningiocytes express Sox2 and yield high efficiency of chimeras after nuclear reprogramming with exogenous factors. *J Biol Chem,* 283, 33730-5.

[19] Eminli, S., Utikal, J., Arnold, K., Jaenisch, R. and Hochedlinger, K. (2008). Reprogramming of neural progenitor cells into induced pluripotent stem cells in the absence of exogenous Sox2 expression. *Stem Cells*, 26, 2467-74.

[20] Aasen, T. et al. (2008). Efficient and rapid generation of induced pluripotent stem cells from human keratinocytes. *Nat Biotechnol,* 26, 1276-84.

[21] Silva, J., Barrandon, O., Nichols, J., Kawaguchi, J., Theunissen, T.W. and Smith, A. (2008). Promotion of reprogramming to ground state pluripotency by signal inhibition. *PLoS Biol*, 6, e253.

[22] Qi, H. and Pei, D. (2007). The magic of four: induction of pluripotent stem cells from somatic cells by Oct4, Sox2, Myc and Klf4. *Cell Res,* 17, 578-80.

[23] Nakagawa, M. et al. (2008). Generation of induced pluripotent stem cells without Myc from mouse and human fibroblasts. *Nat Biotechnol,* 26, 101-6.

[24] Wernig, M., Meissner, A., Cassady, J.P. and Jaenisch, R. (2008). c-Myc is dispensable for direct reprogramming of mouse fibroblasts. *Cell Stem Cell,* 2, 10-2.

[25] Huangfu, D., Maehr, R., Guo, W., Eijkelenboom, A., Snitow, M., Chen, A.E. and Melton, D.A. (2008). Induction of pluripotent stem cells by defined factors is greatly improved by small-molecule compounds. *Nat Biotechnol*, 26, 795-7.

[26] Bernstein, B.E. et al. (2006). A bivalent chromatin structure marks key developmental genes in embryonic stem cells. *Cell,* 125, 315-26.

[27] Huangfu, D., Osafune, K., Maehr, R., Guo, W., Eijkelenboom, A., Chen, S., Muhlestein, W. and Melton, D.A. (2008). Induction of pluripotent stem cells from primary human fibroblasts with only Oct4 and Sox2. *Nat Biotechnol,* 26, 1269-75.

[28] Lyssiotis, C.A. et al. (2009). Reprogramming of murine fibroblasts to induced pluripotent stem cells with chemical complementation of Klf4. *Proc Natl Acad Sci U S A,* 106, 8912-7.

[29] Kaji, K., Norrby, K., Paca, A., Mileikovsky, M., Mohseni, P. and Woltjen, K. (2009).

Virus-free induction of pluripotency and subsequent excision of reprogramming factors. *Nature*, 458, 771-5.

[30] Woltjen, K. et al. (2009). piggyBac transposition reprograms fibroblasts to induced pluripotent stem cells. *Nature*, 458, 766-70.

[31] Soldner, F. et al. (2009). Parkinson's disease patient-derived induced pluripotent stem cells free of viral reprogramming factors. *Cell*, 136, 964-77.

[32] Stadtfeld, M., Nagaya, M., Utikal, J., Weir, G. and Hochedlinger, K. (2008). Induced pluripotent stem cells generated without viral integration. *Science*, 322, 945-9.

[33] Yu, J., Hu, K., Smuga-Otto, K., Tian, S., Stewart, R., Slukvin, II and Thomson, J.A. (2009). Human induced pluripotent stem cells free of vector and transgene sequences. *Science*, 324, 797-801.

[34] Zhou, H. et al. (2009). Generation of induced pluripotent stem cells using recombinant proteins. *Cell Stem Cell*, 4, 381-4.

[35] Kim, D. et al. (2009). Generation of human induced pluripotent stem cells by direct delivery of reprogramming proteins. *Cell Stem Cell*, 4, 472-6.

[36] Liao, J. et al. (2008). Enhanced efficiency of generating induced pluripotent stem (iPS) cells from human somatic cells by a combination of six transcription factors. *Cell Res*, 18, 600-3.

[37] Mali, P., Ye, Z., Hommond, H.H., Yu, X., Lin, J., Chen, G., Zou, J. and Cheng, L. (2008). Improved efficiency and pace of generating induced pluripotent stem cells from human adult and fetal fibroblasts. *Stem Cells*, 26, 1998-2005.

[38] Yamanaka, S. (2009). A fresh look at iPS cells. *Cell*, 137, 13-7.

[39] Liu, H. et al. (2008). Generation of Induced Pluripotent Stem Cells from Adult Rhesus Monkey Fibroblasts. *Cell Stem Cell*, 3, 587-590.

[40] Liao, J. et al. (2009). Generation of Induced Pluripotent Stem Cell Lines from Adult Rat Cells. *Cell Stem Cell*, 4, 11-15.

[41] Esteban, M.A. et al. (2009). Generation of induced pluripotent stem cell lines from tibetan miniature pig. *J Biol Chem*, 284, 17634.

[42] Wu, Z. et al. (2009). Generation of Pig-Induced Pluripotent Stem Cells with a Drug-Inducible System. *J Mol Cell Biol*, 1, 46-54.

[43] Ezashi, T., Telugu, B., Alexenko, A.P., Sachdev, S., Sinha, S. and Roberts, R.M. (2009). Derivation of induced pluripotent stem cells from pig somatic cells. *Proc Natl Acad Sci U S A*, 106, 10993-8.

[44] Li, P. et al. (2008). Germline competent embryonic stem cells derived from rat blastocysts. *Cell*, 135, 1299-1310.

[45] Buehr, M. et al. (2008). Capture of authentic embryonic stem cells from rat blastocysts. *Cell*, 135, 1287-1298.

[46] Hall, V. (2008). Porcine embryonic stem cells: a possible source for cell replacement therapy. *Stem Cell Rev*, 4, 275-82.

[47] Yang, S.H. et al. (2008). Towards a transgenic model of Huntington's disease in a non-human primate. *Nature*, 453, 921-4.

[48] Trounson, A. (2009). Rats, cats, and elephants, but still no unicorn: induced pluripotent stem cells from new species. *Cell Stem Cell*, 4, 3-4.

[49] Zeuschner D., Mildner K. , Zaehres, H. and Scholer H,. (2009). Induced Pluripotent

Stem Cells at Nano Scale. Stem cells and development. *Epub ahead of print.*

[50] Marion, R.M., Strati, K., Li, H., Tejera, A., Schoeftner, S., Ortega, S., Serrano, M. and Blasco, M.A. (2009). Telomeres acquire embryonic stem cell characteristics in induced pluripotent stem cells. *Cell Stem Cell*, 4, 141-54.

[51] Mikkelsen, T.S. et al. (2008). Dissecting direct reprogramming through integrative genomic analysis. *Nature,* 454, 49-55.

[52] Chin, M.H. et al. (2009). Induced pluripotent stem cells and embryonic stem cells are distinguished by gene expression signatures. *Cell Stem Cell*, 5, 111-23.

[53] Deng, J. et al. (2009). Targeted bisulfite sequencing reveals changes in DNA methylation associated with nuclear reprogramming. *Nat Biotechnol*, 27, 353-60.

[54] Miura, K. et al. (2009). Variation in the safety of induced pluripotent stem cell lines. *Nat Biotechnol*, 27, 743-5.

[55] Sharova, L.V., Sharov, A.A., Piao, Y., Shaik, N., Sullivan, T., Stewart, C.L., Hogan, B.L. and Ko, M.S. (2007). Global gene expression profiling reveals similarities and differences among mouse pluripotent stem cells of different origins and strains. *Dev Biol,* 307, 446-59.

[56] Ebert, A.D., Yu, J., Rose, F.F., Jr., Mattis, V.B., Lorson, C.L., Thomson, J.A. and Svendsen, C.N. (2009). Induced pluripotent stem cells from a spinal muscular atrophy patient. *Nature*, 457, 277-80.

[57] Aalto-Setala, K., Conklin, B.R. and Lo, B. (2009). Obtaining consent for future research with induced pluripotent cells: opportunities and challenges. *PLoS Biol*, 7, e42.

[58] Sridharan, R. and Plath, K. (2008). Illuminating the black box of reprogramming. *Cell Stem Cell*, 2, 295-7.

[59] Sridharan, R., Tchieu, J., Mason, M.J., Yachechko, R., Kuoy, E., Horvath, S., Zhou, Q. and Plath, K. (2009). Role of the murine reprogramming factors in the induction of pluripotency. *Cell*, 136, 364-77.

[60] Maherali, N. and Hochedlinger, K. (2008). Guidelines and techniques for the generation of induced pluripotent stem cells. *Cell Stem Cell*, 3, 595-605.

[61] Hotta, A. and Ellis, J. (2008). Retroviral vector silencing during iPS cell induction: an epigenetic beacon that signals distinct pluripotent states. *J Cell Biochem,* 105, 940-8.

[62] Hawley, R.G. (2008). Does retroviral insertional mutagenesis play a role in the generation of induced pluripotent stem cells? *Mol Ther*, 16, 1354-5.

[63] Carey, B.W., Markoulaki, S., Hanna, J., Saha, K., Gao, Q., Mitalipova, M. and Jaenisch, R. (2009). Reprogramming of murine and human somatic cells using a single polycistronic vector. *Proc Natl Acad Sci U S A,* 106, 157-62.

[64] Sommer, C.A., Stadtfeld, M., Murphy, G.J., Hochedlinger, K., Kotton, D.N. and Mostoslavsky, G. (2009). Induced pluripotent stem cell generation using a single lentiviral stem cell cassette. *Stem Cells*, 27, 543-9.

[65] Okita, K., Nakagawa, M., Hyenjong, H., Ichisaka, T. and Yamanaka, S. (2008). Generation of mouse induced pluripotent stem cells without viral vectors. *Science*, 322, 949-53.

[66] Hanahan, D. and Weinberg, R.A. (2000). The hallmarks of cancer. *Cell*, 100, 57-70.

[67] Kaelin, W.G., Jr. (2002). Molecular basis of the VHL hereditary cancer syndrome. *Nat Rev Cancer*, 2, 673-82.

[68] Vogelstein, B. and Kinzler, K.W. (2004). Cancer genes and the pathways they control. *Nat Med,* 10, 789-99.

[69] Kirkwood, T.B. (2005). Understanding the odd science of aging. *Cell,* 120, 437-47.

In: Encyclopedia of Stem Cell Research (2 Volume Set)   ISBN: 978-1-61761-835-2
Editor: Alexander L. Greene   © 2012 Nova Science Publishers, Inc.

Chapter XLIX

LEPIDOPTERAN MIDGUT STEM CELLS IN CULTURE: A NEW TOOL FOR CELL BIOLOGY AND PHYSIOLOGICAL STUDIES

Gianluca Tettamanti[1] and Morena Casartelli[2]

[1]Dipartimento di Biotecnologie e Scienze Molecolari,
Università degli Studi dell'Insubria, Varese, Italia
[2]Dipartimento di Biologia, Università degli Studi di Milano,
Milano, Italia

ABSTRACT

Holometabolous insects recruit a wide array of stem cell types to fulfil the growth of larval organs at moulting and their remodelling at metamorphosis, thus achieving the final body organization of the adult.

Over the years a large number of different stem cells, with specific roles in growth and renewal of insect tissues, have been identified in Lepidoptera and Diptera. A particular interest for the stem cells residing within the insect gut is now emerging and the early morphological studies that analyzed the behaviour of these cells are progressively supported by new cellular and molecular data.

After a brief summary of the current knowledge on insect intestinal stem cells, here we will focus on some characteristics of the stem cells in culture of the larval midgut of *Bombyx mori*. These cells can be released from the midgut just before the fourth moult and, once placed in an appropriate medium, they multiply and differentiate in mature cells that are able to perform normal absorptive and digestive functions *in vitro*.

Thereafter we will discuss the use of this reliable *in vitro* system as a tool to study intestinal morphogenesis and differentiation, to investigate the specific roles and reciprocal relationships of autophagy and apoptosis during midgut remodelling, and to analyze physiological functions of midgut cells, such as their ability to internalize different substrates and the mechanisms involved. Studies on midgut stem cells appear of key importance in consideration of the extensive similarities evidenced among mammalian and insect intestinal epithelia in their development, organization and molecular regulatory mechanisms.

Different types of stem cells have been described in several insect organs, where they give rise to a repertoire of tissues during the embryonic, larval and adult stages (for a complete review see [1]). The insect gut makes no exception and an increasing amount of evidence on stem cell behaviour in this organ has been gathered for a long time. More recently, the molecular mechanisms underlying the regulation of these cells have been partially unfolded in species belonging to Diptera and Lepidoptera, the two most widely used *taxa* for the analysis of intestinal stem cell biology. *Drosophila melanogaster* has lately represented a model to analyze stem cells in the adult gut, while in lepidopteran species efforts have been devoted to the larval midgut. The main part of the information reported below will refer to these two systems.

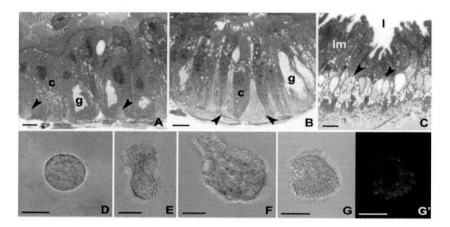

A-C. Cross sections of *B. mori* midgut at different larval stages. A. Fourth larval instar. Stem cells (arrowheads) are localized at the base of the midgut epithelium. B. Fourth larval moult. Stem cells (arrowheads) proliferate and differentiate into new cells that intercalate among columnar (c) and goblet (g) cells. C. Fifth instar. In the prepupal period, stem cells (arrowheads) proliferate underneath the degenerating larval midgut epithelium (lm) and form the new pupal epithelium. l: midgut lumen. Scale bar: 10 µm. D-G. Brightfield and confocal laser scanning micrographs of midgut cells in culture. D. Typical rounded stem cell. E. Mature columnar cell characterized by an apical membrane with well developed microvilli, a centrally placed nucleus and a cylindrical shape. F. Mature goblet cell with the typical flask-like shape, the wide cavity, and a basally located nucleus. G and G'. Brightfield and confocal laser scanning micrographs (optical sections), respectively, of a columnar cell incubated for 1 h at 25 °C in the presence of 1.4 µM FITC-albumin. The punctuate distribution of FITC-albumin inside the cytoplasm is consistent with a vesicular compartmentalization, which is expected for a protein that is internalized by endocytosis and follows a precise intracellular pathways (Casartelli et al., 2008). Scale bars: 5 µm (D); 10 µm (E-G).

The alimentary canal of insects can be divided into three regions: the foregut, the midgut and the hindgut. The foregut and the hindgut are of ectodermal origin and are covered by a cuticle that is continuous to the epidermal layer one, while the midgut, which has a primary role in nutrient digestion and absorption, is an endodermal derivative devoid of cuticle but lined by a specialized peritrophic membrane. In adult *Drosophila*, the midgut is a pseudostratified epithelium composed mostly of large cells with absorptive function, the enterocytes, and of enteroendocrine cells [2], while the midgut of Lepidopteran larvae consists of a highly folded monolayered epithelium formed by columnar, goblet and endocrine cells [3]. In both cases a further cell type, the stem cells (recently called intestinal stem cells (ISCs) in Diptera and previously indicated as regenerative cells in Lepidoptera and other insects), are located at the base of the midgut epithelium. Following appropriate stimuli, these cells are capable to proliferate and differentiate into the other gut cell types [3].

In adult *Drosophila* ISCs are set in motion to maintain midgut homeostasis: when the midgut epithelial cells become damaged by ingested food, pathogens or toxins, ISCs divide, become enteroblasts, and differentiate into enterocytes or enteroendocrine cells, thus replacing lost cells [2]. While the role of stem cells in midgut homeostasis in the adult fly has been well described *in vivo* [4, 5], the molecular mechanisms by which these cells originate and differentiate into other cell types during development are poorly studied.

Like in *Drosophila,* in lepidopteran larvae midgut stem cells repair the damaged midgut by replacement [6], maintaining the tissue functional integrity [7]. In addition, it has been long demonstrated that these cells, normally present as single cells during the larval feeding periods (Figure A), proliferate extensively before each moult, forming large nests, or "nidi", and then intercalate between the mature cells of the intestinal monolayer, differentiating into mature columnar and goblet cells during the moult (Figure B) [8, 9]. Besides repair and increase of midgut size along larval growth, stem cells have a key role in the generation of a functional adult midgut. We have recently shown that during the prepupal stage of *Heliothis virescens* larvae, Programmed Cell Death (PCD) events lead to the degradation of the larval midgut monolayer, providing a supply of nutrient molecules that will be readily exploited by the new pupal midgut developing underneath, generated by the massive proliferation and differentiation of stem cells (Figure C) [10].

Although a full comprehension of the mechanisms involved in proliferation and differentiation of midgut stem cells in Lepidoptera is still lacking, in the last fifteen years studies on cultured stem cells derived from the midgut of different lepidopteran species provided several clues on the regulatory factors involved in their proliferation and differentiation, with important outcomes for the setup of primary cultures of midgut cells. Just considering only the most important factors, 20-hydroxyecdysone (20E), that triggers metamorphosis in insects, stimulates the differentiation *in vitro* of stem cells isolated from *Spodoptera littoralis*, while the inactive prohormone ecdysone (E) is very active on their proliferation [11]. 20E also induces the production by the fat body of a Multiplication Factor (MF), a protein that induces the multiplication of stem cells in culture [12]. In Loeb's lab, four different polypeptides that promote differentiation of midgut stem cells have been isolated from midgut cell-conditioned media or pupal hemolymph [13]. These factors, called Midgut Differentiation Factors 1-4 (MDFs 1-4), seem to have partially overlapping functions on midgut stem cells of various Lepidoptera, although the pivotal factor exerting control over stem cell differentiation *in vitro* should be MDF4. The complex interplay of factors regulating proliferation of these stem cells comprehends also α-arylphorin [14], an active mitogen isolated from the fat body, and Bombyxin [15], a member of the insulin family whose source *in vivo* is still unidentified, that acts in concert with α-arylphorin.

Loeb et al. [16] have shown that the administration of these growth factors and insect hormones to stem cells can induce their differentiation towards cell phenotypes identical or similar to those described in larval or pupal midguts *in vivo* and, even more interesting, showed that the cells were sensitive to vertebrate factors like PDGF, EGF and Retinoic Acid, all fundamental for differentiation processes in mammals. These indications are a strong incentive to the identification of insect genes and molecules whose vertebrate counterparts regulate intestinal stem cells.

B. mori can be considered a representative model among Lepidoptera, because of indisputable advantages as a large number of information gathered on its developmental biology, physiology and endocrinology, the availability of numerous genetics and molecular biology tools and a completely sequenced genome.

We have developed a protocol to maintain in culture *B. mori* larval midgut cells, from stem cells to mature cells (Figures D-F). The protocol is described in detail in Cermenati et al. [9], in which all the modifications of the original procedure of Sadrud-Din et al. [17] are specified. Just before the last (fourth) larval-larval moult, stem cells are located in numerous nidi at the base of the epithelium, while during the feeding periods they are few and singly dispersed in the epithelium; therefore, the largest number of stem cells can be isolated in the period just preceding the fourth moult. The stem cells can be easily removed from the surrounding tissue because they are not linked to the other cells by junctions. Following the indications of Sadrud-Din *et al.* [17, 18], with addition of α-arylphorin to the culture medium [14] and the presence of stimulating factors produced by the mature and differentiating cells [13], stable primary cultures of isolated cells in suspension were obtained. A detailed analysis of their evolution with time was performed by counting the different cell types (stem cells, differentiating cells, mature columnar and globlet cells) present since the initial stem cell isolation [9].

Midgut stem cell models *in vivo* are a potent tool to unveil the mechanisms of cell proliferation, differentiation and tissue homeostasis, as recently emphasized by Illa-Bochaca and Montuenga [19]. We believe that the *in vitro* cultured stem cell system from *B. mori* midgut represents a versatile tool to tackle complex issues in different biological contexts that will complement the information acquired by *in vivo* models (*Drosophila, Locusta* and several lepidopterans*)*, exploiting the high degree of conservation of biological processes evidenced to date between these insect species.

Here we will dwell on three topics, that we expect will be of crucial interest in the forthcoming years:

1. *Gut morphogenesis and differentiation.* The presence of ISCs in *Drosophila* has been unambiguously assessed only in recent years, being characterized first in adult fly midgut (mgISCs) [4, 5] and later on in hindgut (hgISCs) [20]. While in the midgut the differentiation of stem cells into enterocytes proceeds from the basal membrane towards the lumen, in the hindgut this renewal process occurs along the antero-posterior axis, with the cells migrating and differentiating from the portion termed hindgut proliferation zone. This latter pattern of proliferation presents large similarities to that occurring within the crypts of mammalian intestine [21]. Subsequent analyses of the signalling molecules that regulate proliferation and differentiation of stem cells revealed that the similitude of the two systems goes far beyond. In fact, in a fashion similar to the mammalian counterpart, the balance

between self-renewal and differentiation of mgISCs is controlled by canonical Wnt and Notch signalling pathways: while Wingless (Wg) is required for the maintenance and proliferation of ISCs, Notch actively controls the determination of the cell fate of ISCs daughter cells. Interestingly, a peculiarity of fly ISCs is that lineage selection and differentiation seem to occur without relying on any identifiable anatomic niche, thus highlighting an active role of stem cells in the cell fate decision of their daughters [22]. These results shed a new light on the importance of this new invertebrate stem cell system. In fact an in depth dissection of the regulatory mechanisms that control crucial phenomena in development will surely benefit from the availability of primary cultures of insect midgut cells, a powerful tool to study biological processes in a simplified experimental context: it will be possible to get further insights into some aspects of Wnt signalling in mammalian crypts [2], to understand the relationships between tissue damage and control of stem cell proliferation [23], and to address some questions about tissue aging and tumour insurgence in the intestine [24].

2. *Dissection of Programmed Cell Death (PCD) processes.* Although the first evidence of the occurrence of PCD processes in midgut cells of insects can be dated back to the '60s, today it is well known that in this tissue two PCD mechanisms are responsible for the disappearance of larval cells at metamorphosis. Besides apoptosis, a second mechanism, namely autophagy, has attracted scientists' attention, making the insect midgut an appealing experimental model to study the regulation of this cell self-eating process. Further, one of the most intriguing and relevant issue that still needs to be addressed is the overlap between apoptosis and autophagy, and more efforts need to be spent to identify the specific regulatory mechanisms and those in common between these two processes. In fact, although some typical apoptotic markers, such as DNA fragmentation and caspase 3 activation, are present in midgut cells at metamorphosis, autophagy represents the most prominent process responsible for the loss of the large majority of cells, as indicated by the increase in lysosomal enzymes, the presence of autophagic compartments [10] and the expression of autophagy specific genes (Cao Y., personal communication). If a co-occurrence of two distinct PCD processes or an overlap between their signalling pathways occur in this tissue is still an unanswered problem and its solution could serve as a reference for comparative analyses in related biological models. The efficacy of an *in vitro* system to disentangle such an intricate network has been demonstrated in the study of PCD processes in the fat body of Lepidoptera [25]. In the IPLB-LdFB cell line derived from this tissue, it is possible to selectively address cells towards either apoptosis or autophagy, an approach of great help to clarify the dynamics of these two processes. In the literature are reported studies on cultured midgut stem cells from other Lepidoptera, that show perturbations of apoptotic processes induced by 20E [11, 26], a hormone that triggers *in vivo* an increase of the number of lysosomes in midgut stem cells of *B. mori* [26], as well as autophagic processes in *Drosophila* [27]. An appropriate use of activators (e.g. ecdysteroids) and inhibitors of apoptosis and autophagy (e.g. 3-methyladenine and Bafilomycin A1) [28], will allow the manipulation of the two processes also in *B. mori* cultured midgut cells.

Another interesting topic concerns insulin. In fact, members of the insulin family peptides affect the proliferation of lepidopteran cultured stem cells [15] and in *Drosophila* the insulin signalling pathway is critical for ISCs division *in vivo* [23]; moreover, in insects the insulin signalling pathway controlling the nutrition-dependent growth of the cell is strictly coupled to the autophagic process via Target Of Rapamycin (TOR) and Autophagy Gene 1 (ATG1) [29]. We think that these data will be a key starting point for analyzing the links between stem cell proliferation and occurrence of autophagy in midgut cells in culture, derived from stem cell differentiation, under variable nutrient conditions.

3. *Study of midgut cells barrier function.* The movement of orally delivered intact proteins across the digestive system has been shown in numerous insect species (reviewed by Jeffers and Roe [30]). In recent years this field of research has become of particular interest, because a number of proteins with potential insecticide activity has been identified from different biological sources, like viruses, microorganisms, fungi, plants, arthropods (reviewed by Whetstone and Hammock [31]). In most cases, these biopesticides have haemocoelic targets and must pass undegraded the gut barrier to exert their activity when orally administrated. Therefore, an in depth characterization of the mechanisms involved in protein absorption is undoubtedly necessary to develop efficient delivery methods, that would help in reducing the use of broad spectrum chemical pesticides. As in mammals, the mechanism involved in protein absorption in the midgut of lepidopteran larvae is transcytosis [32, 33], a complex sequence of intracellular events in which the protein is internalized at one pole of the cell membrane and transported by vesicles within the cytoplasm to the plasma membrane at the opposite side. The complete transcellular pathway, i.e. the mechanisms of protein endocytosis, the receptors involved, the cellular compartments implicated in the migration of vesicles along the cytoplasm and the role of cytoskeleton in the entire process, need to be carefully investigated, in order to define possible strategies that would increase the rate of protein permeation across the midgut epithelium. The endocytic mechanism responsible for the internalization of albumin, a protein that crosses the insect midgut by transcytosis [32] has been recently characterized in *B. mori* midgut columnar cells in culture (Figure G-G') [34]. This novel information sheds light on the functional mechanisms of protein absorption in the insect midgut and suggests new opportunities for developing suitable molecular strategies to increase the permeation of proteins through the midgut epithelium. Development of delivery systems to enhance protein movement across the insect digestive system is in its infancy and primary cultures of lepidopteran midgut cells will be a major experimental preparation to improve this field of study.

As highlighted by Whetstone and Hammock [31], viruses have been used for biological control purposes. The arthropods' parvoviruses, named densoviruses, are studied with a renewed interest as potential pest control agents since they are lethal for several insects at larval stages, including agronomical pests and insects vector-borne diseases [35, 36, 37]. However, little is known of the route followed for insect invasion. Since the midgut represents the first barrier that the virus must cross to reach the internal tissues, midgut cells in culture will be an helpful tool to study the infection mechanisms and to optimize the development of viral pesticides.

Finally, isolated midgut cells in culture can also represent a simplified experimental context to study the signalling pathways responsible for mediating and coordinating complex physiological function. It has been recently shown that in the isolated midgut of *Bombyx mori* larvae an increment of cAMP or Ca^{2+} concentration in the cytosol induces the opening of the septate junctions, with a consequent increase of the paracellular permeability [38]. The manipulation of this route may be particularly interesting for the delivery of virulence factors of low molecular weight targeting hemocoelic receptors and therefore the clarification of the signalling cascade and the intracellular effector molecules involved in this process are surely intriguing.

ACKNOWLEDGMENTS

The authors are grateful to Prof. Barbara Giordana (Università degli Studi di Milano, Milano, Italia) and Prof. Magda de Eguileor (Università degli Studi dell'Insubria, Varese, Italia) for critically reviewing this manuscript and for their helpful comments. They also thank Prof. Raziel S. Hakim (Howard University, Washington DC, USA) for his support and advise on the preparation of midgut cell cultures and Eleonora Franzetti for image production. G.T.'s work was supported by F.A.R. 2007-2009 grants from the University of Insubria; M.C.'s work was supported by the Italian Ministry of University and Research (PRIN 2006, project n°2006079417).

REFERENCES

[1]   Corley, L.S. and Lavine, M.D. (2006). A review of insect stem cell types. *Semin Cell Dev Biol*, 17, 510-517

[2]   Casali, A. and Batlle, E. (2009). Intestinal stem cells in mammals and Drosophila. *Cell Stem Cell,* 4, 124-127

[3]   Wigglesworth, V.B. (1972). The principles of insect physiology: Digestion and nutrition. *Chapman & Hall.* London, UK; pp 476-552

[4]   Micchelli, C.A. and Perrimon, N. (2006). Evidence that stem cells reside in the adult Drosophila midgut epithelium. *Nature*, 439, 475-479

[5]   Ohlstein, B. and Spradling, A. (2006). The adult Drosophila posterior midgut is maintained by pluripotent stem cells. *Nature*, 439, 470-474

[6]   Hakim, R.S.; Baldwin, K.; Smagghe, G. (2010). Regulation of midgut growth, development and metamorphosis. *Annu Rev Entomol*, 55, 593-608

[7]   Spies, A.G.; Spence, K.D. (1985). Effect of sublethal Bacillus thuringiensis crystal endotoxin treatment on the larval midgut of a moth, Manduca: SEM study. *Tissue Cell*, 17, 379-394

[8]   Baldwin, K.M. and Hakim, R.S. (1991). Growth and differentiation of the larval midgut

epithelium during molting in the moth Manduca sexta. *Tissue Cell*, 23, 411-422

[9]   Cermenati, G.; Corti, P.; Caccia, S.; Giordana, B. and Casartelli, M. (2007). A morphological and functional characterization of Bombyx mori larval midgut cells in culture. *Invert Survival J 4*, 119-126

[10] Tettamanti, G.; Grimaldi, A.; Casartelli, M.; Ambrosetti, E.; Ponti, B.; Congiu, T.; Ferrarese, R.; Rivas-Pena, M.L.; Pennacchio, F. and de Eguileor, M. (2007). Programmed cell death and stem cell differentiation are responsible for midgut replacement in Heliothis virescens during prepupal instar. *Cell Tissue Res*, 330, 345-359

[11] Smagghe, G.; Vanhassel, W.; Moeremans, C.; De Wilde, D.; Goto, S.; Loeb, M.J.; Blackburn, M.B.; Hakim, R.S. (2005). Stimulation of midgut stem cell proliferation and differentiation by insect hormones and peptides. *Ann N Y Acad Sci*, 1040, 472-475

[12] Smagghe, G.J.; Elsen, K.; Loeb, M.J.; Gelman, DB; Blackburn, M (2003). Effects of a fat body extract on larval midgut cells and growth of lepidoptera. *In Vitro Cell Dev Biol Anim*, 39, 8-12

[13] Loeb, M.J.; Coronel, N.; Natsukawa, D. and Takeda, M. (2004). Implications for the functions of the four known midgut differentiation factors: an immunohistologic study of Heliothis virescens midgut. *Arch Insect Biochem Physiol*, 56, 7-20

[14] Hakim, R.S.; Blackburn, M.B.; Corti, P.; Gelman, D.B.; Goodman, C.; Elsen, K.; Loeb, M.J.; Lynn, D.; Soin, T. and Smagghe, G. (2007). Growth and mitogenic effects of arylphorin in vivo and in vitro. *Arch Insect Biochem Physiol*, 64, 63-73

[15] Goto, S.; Loeb, M.J.; Takeda, M. (2005). Bombyxin stimulates proliferation of cultured stem cells derived from Heliothis virescens and Mamestra brassicae larvae. *In Vitro Cell Dev Biol Anim*, 41, 38-42

[16] Loeb, M.J.; Clark, E.A.; Blackburn, M.; Hakim, R.S.; Elsen, K. and Smagghe, G. (2003). Stem cells from midguts of Lepidopteran larvae: clues to the regulation of stem cell fate. *Arch Insect Biochem Physiol*, 53, 186-198

[17] Sadrud-Din, S.Y.; Loeb, M.J. and Hakim, R.S. (1996). In vitro differentiation of isolated stem cells from the midgut of Manduca sexta larvae. *J Exp Biol* 199, 319-325

[18] Sadrud-Din, S.Y.; Hakim, R.S. and Loeb, M.J. (1994). Proliferation and differentiation of midgut cells from Manduca sexta, in vitro. *Invert Reprod Dev* 26, 197-204

[19] Illa-Bochaca, I. and Montuenga, L.M. (2006). The regenerative nidi of the locust midgut as a model to study epithelial cell differentiation from stem cells. *J Exp Biol*, 209, 2215-2223

[20] Takashima, S.; Mkrtchyan, M.; Younossi-Hartenstein, A.; Merriam, J.R. and Hartenstein, V. (2008). The behaviour of Drosophila adult hindgut stem cells is controlled by Wnt and Hh signalling. *Nature*, 454, 651-655

[21] Pitsouli, C and Perrimon, N. (2008). Our fly cousins' gut. *Nature*, 454, 592-593

[22] Ohlstein, B. and Spradling, A. (2007). Multipotent Drosophila intestinal stem cells specify daughter cell fates by differential notch signaling. *Science*, 315, 988-992

[23] Amcheslavsky, A.; Jiang, J. and Ip, Y.T. (2009). Tissue damage-induced intestinal stem cell division in Drosophila. *Cell Stem Cell*, 4, 49-61

[24] Biteau, B.; Hochmuth, C.E. and Jasper, H. (2008). JNK activity in somatic stem cells causes loss of tissue homeostasis in the aging Drosophila gut. *Cell Stem Cell,* 3, 442-

455

[25] Tettamanti, G.; Malagoli, D.; Marchesini, E.; Congiu, T.; de Eguileor, M. and Ottavini, E. (2006). Oligomycin A induces autophagy in the IPLB-LdFB insect cell line. *Cell Tissue Res*, 326, 179-186

[26] Tanaka, Y. and Yukuhiro, F. (1999). Ecdysone has an effect on the regeneration of midgut epithelial cells that is distinct from 20-hydroxyecdysone in the silkworm Bombyx mori. *Gen Comp Endocrinol*, 116, 382-395

[27] Lee, C.Y.; Cooksey, B.A. and Baehrecke, E.H. (2002). Steroid regulation of midgut cell death during Drosophila development. *Dev Biol*, 250, 101-111

[28] Rubinsztein, D.C.; Gestwicki, J.E.; Murphy, L.O. and Klionsky, D.J. (2007). Potential therapeutic applications of autophagy. *Nat Rev Drug Discov*, 6, 304-312

[29] Scott, R.C.; Schuldiner, O.; Neufeld T.P. (2004). Role and regulation of starvation-induced autophagy in the Drosophila fat body. *Dev Cell*, 7, 167-178

[30] Jeffers, L.A. and Roe, R.M. (2008). The movement of proteins across the insect and tick digestive system. *J Insect Physiol 54*, 319-332

[31] Whetstone, P.A. and Hammock, B.D. (2007). Delivery methods for peptide and protein toxins in insect control. *Toxicon*, 49, 576-596

[32] Casartelli, M.; Corti, P.; Leonardi, M.G.; Fiandra, L.; Burlini, N.; Pennacchio, F. and Giordana, B. (2005). Absorption of albumin by the midgut of a lepidopteran larva. *J Insect Physiol, 51*, 933-940

[33] Casartelli, M.; Corti, P.; Cermenati, G.; Grimaldi, A.; Fiandra, L.; Santo, N.; Pennacchio, F. and Giordana B. (2007). Absorption of horseradish peroxidase in Bombyx mori larval midgut. *J Insect Physiol, 53*, 517-525

[34] Casartelli, M.; Cermenati, G.; Rodighiero, S.; Pennacchio, F. and Giordana, B. (2008). A megalin-like receptor is involved in protein endocytosis in the midgut of an insect (Bombyx mori, Lepidoptera). *Am J Physiol, 295*, R1290-R1300

[35] Bergoin, M. and Tijssen, P. (2008) *Encyclopedia of Virology: Parvoviruses of Arthropods*. (B.W.J. Mahy and M.H.V. Van Regenmortel, Editors). Elsevier; Oxford, UK; pp 76-85

[36] Carlson, J.; Suchman, E. and Buchatsky, L. (2006). Densoviruses for control and genetic manipulation of mosquitoes. *Adv Virus Res*, 68, 361-392

[37] El-Far, M.; Li, Y.; Fediere, G.; Abol-Ela, S. and Tijssen, P. (2004). Lack of infection of vertebrate cells by the densovirus from the maize worm Mythimna loreyi (MlDNV). *Virus Res*, 99, 17-24

[38] Fiandra, L.; Casartelli, M. and Giordana, B. (2006). The paracellular pathway in the lepidopteran larval midgut: modulation by intracellular mediators. *Comp Biochem Physiol*, 144A, 464-473

In: Encyclopedia of Stem Cell Research (2 Volume Set)   ISBN: 978-1-61761-835-2
Editor: Alexander L. Greene   © 2012 Nova Science Publishers, Inc.

Chapter L

ARE EMBRYONIC STEM CELLS REALLY NEEDED FOR REGENERATIVE MEDICINE?

*David T. Harris**

Department of Immunobiology, The University of Arizona, Tucson, AZ, US

ABSTRACT

It is estimated that as many as 1 in 3 individuals in the United States might benefit from regenerative medicine therapy. Most regenerative medicine therapies have been postulated to require the use of embryonic stem (ES) cells for optimal effect. Unfortunately, ES cell therapies are currently limited by ethical, political, regulatory, and most importantly biological hurdles. These limitations include the inherent allogenicity of this stem cell source and the accompanying threat of immune rejection. Even with use of the rapidly developing iPS technology, the issues of low efficiency of ES/iPS derivation and the threat of teratoma formation limit ES applications directly in patients. The time and cost of deriving and validating mature, differentiated tissues for clinical use further restricts its use to a small number of well-to-do patients with a limited number of afflictions. Thus, for the foreseeable future, the march of regenerative medicine to the clinic for widespread use will depend upon the development of non-ES cell therapies. Current sources of non-ES cells easily available in large numbers can be found in the bone marrow, adipose tissue and umbilical cord blood. Each of these types of stem cells has already begun to be utilized to treat a variety of diseases.

For the past decade a political debate has raged regarding the derivation and use of embryonic stem cells for regenerative medicine. The fervour and seriousness of the debate has led the public to believe that their government was deliberately keeping life-saving medical advances from them, thanks to the influence of a small partisan group of conservative advocates. Regardless of one's political persuasion, this long-running debate has at least served to increase awareness of the medical potential of stem cells. Hopefully, this increased awareness will also lead to increased funding, which remains to be seen. Unfortunately, the debate (much of which was led by non-scientists on both sides) has also unreasonably raised expectations of wonder treatments and cures that cannot be readily met.

Embryonic stem (ES) cells (including induced pluripotent stem [or iPS] cells) have been touted as the holy grail of regenerative medicine therapies, while other viable alternatives have been overlooked and disregarded. Now, with many of the political and funding obstacles for ES cell use recently removed from the scientific arena (due to a change in political regime and the development of iPS technology), the question remains as to whether there will be a significant role for non-ES cells in such regenerative therapies? To answer that question, one should be cognizant of the fact that ES and iPS cells have numerous biological roadblocks and limitations that significantly hinder their passage to the clinic and rapid access to patients in need.

The first such limitation is the inherent allogenicity for many versions of this stem cell source and the accompanying threat of immune rejection. To date, most ES cells have been derived by methods that utilize donor oocytes or embryos. Even after nuclear transfer or therapeutic cloning, the derived ES cell is allogeneic to the patient being treated. As life-long immunosuppression is neither desirable nor therapeutically possible in many instances, the need to create patient-specific (i.e., "tissue-matched") ES cells has recently been addressed by the development of induced pluripotentcy methods (i.e., iPS cells) (Byrne et al, 2007; Park et al, 2008). Although the threat of immune rejection can be overcome by derivation of iPS cells directly from patients, the threat of teratoma formation is omnipresent as shown in a recent clinical report (Amariglio et al, 2009). It seems that any type of ES (or iPS) cell that is used directly in patients without prior differentiation of the ES/iPS cells into the desired tissue poses a significant chance of tumor induction. Stem cell tumorigenicity represents the major obstacle to safe regenerative medicine when using either ES or iPS cells. Even with iPS cells, the malignant tumor incidence in chimeric mice constructed with such iPS cells has been observed to be 20% or higher. Recent studies have also shown that construction of iPS cells without the use of Myc still results in tumor formation, implying that the reprogramming process may also activate endogenous oncogenes. It seems that the greater the pluripotency and self-renewal potential of a cell, the greater the potential for tumorigenicity. In fact, the probability of tumor formation is higher for iPS cells than with typical ES cells due to the lack of immune mismatch that might trigger some rejection (reviewed in Knoepfler, 2009). Further, this derivation (and the accompanying validation) process involves large amounts of time and monies, as well as invoking multiple regulatory issues.

It is important to note that for many patients not only will autologous cells and tissues be required, but these tissues must be delivered in a timely fashion for optimal therapeutic benefit. For example, it does little good to wait 2-6 months after a stroke to attempt to replace or rescue damaged nervous tissue and brain function. The requirement for "autologous" stem cells and the inability to derive differentiated cell lines or tissues from newly created patient-specific ES/iPS cells in time to meet the treatment "window" required for successful therapies does not seem to have an answer at this time. At its best, derivation of iPS cell lines requires approximately 1 month of time, differentiation of those iPS cells into a desired tissue requires another month of time, and expansion, validation and purification of those tissues will require

---

* Email address: davidh@email.arizona.edu

an additional 1-3 months of time (Condic and Rao, 2008). Once again, it cannot be overemphasized that when a patient suffers a heart attack or a stroke, these patients require therapy within days if not hours. As most patients will present with a limited time to treat, and as creation of patient-specific ES or iPS cell lines can be expected to require months of effort at best, such an ES/iPS-based therapy should have significant limitations.

There really is a "golden hour" of treatment for most patients, similar to what is seen in stroke patients. Although this "golden hour" may actually be a "golden" day or week or even a year, it is not forever. One must generally treat patients within a confined window of time for the therapy to be effective. That is, once tissue has died and scar tissue has formed, there is very little than can be accomplished. At this time stem cells cannot make their way into the damaged tissue to replace the portion that has been affected or stimulate endogenous repair. Further, reintegration of new tissue at this time would also seem to be problematic. Re-integration of "new" nervous tissue would not necessarily mean re-establishment of memory, personality, etc. as these qualities come from personal experience. Therefore, the most optimal therapeutic approach would seem to be a rescue, or minimal tissue replacement, early on after injury mediated by timely stem cell delivery.

Finally, the overall costs of overcoming each of these limitations must be passed on to either the patient or third-party payers, which ultimately will be the major limiting factor for the progress of ES/iPS cell therapies to the clinic and access to the population in general. It has been conservatively estimated that derivation of each patient-specific ES/iPS cell line/differentiated tissue will cost in the neighborhood of $50,000. A portion of these costs is due to the inherent low efficiency in both ES and iPS derivation. ES cell derivation may require as many as 200 oocytes to derive a single ES cell line (I. Rogers, University of Toronto, personal communication). In general, somatic cell reprogramming by non-viral means occurs at frequencies that are 100-fold lower than with integrating viral vectors. However, recent use of transposons has raised the frequencies to 0.1-1% (similar to viral vectors). The problem remains that one must perform clonal analyses afterwards to identify integration-free, correctly excised clones and insure that no chromosomal rearrangements or point mutations have occurred (Stadtfeld & Hochedlinger, 2009). Directed differentiation is also a very inefficient process and is never 100% successful in driving all the iPS cells to differentiate. It is very difficult to fully and completely differentiate ES/iPS cells to mature cells and tissues, such that the possibility of tumor formation is completely eliminated. Multiple studies in animals have shown tumor formation after implantation of differentiated ES/iPS cells. (Condic & Rao, 2008.). Therefore, even using the transposon approach for iPS generation, all iPS cell lines would need to be cloned and tested for the effects of DNA damage, changes in imprinting and epigenetic changes. (Condic & Rao, 2008.). These stem cells would then require differentiation, followed by some method of additional purification in order to pass FDA and RAC regulatory hurdles; again adding to the time and costs involved. Due to the costs, it is difficult to believe that very many patients would be able to afford to create and bank their own ES or iPS cells, and tissues, in advance of future needs.

It has been postulated that to economize the process it might be possible to create iPS cell banks representing most HLA haplotypes (i.e., tissue types) in the population at large. These banks would then be financed by the nation as a national inventory for anyone's use. However, one must realize, based on the last 30 years of stem cell and organ transplants in a variety of patients, that perfect matching is essential to prevent rejection (and other side-effects). The odds of identifying any two individuals with a 6/6 HLA (i.e., tissue) match ranges from 1 in 40,000 to 1 in 80,000 depending on the ethnicity of the two individuals (Harris, 1998). Therefore, to assure a high probability of locating matches for most patients in need, one would require multi-ethnic iPS banks containing upwards of 1-million total samples (at a cost of $50,000 each, a total of more than 1 trillion dollars). Finally, it is not assured that minor histocompatability antigens that would not typed or considered for matching, would not be capable of eliciting immune reactions as observed for many organ transplant patients (Yamanaka, 2009). The estimate that a million ES lines would be needed to eliminate the need for lifelong immunosuppression would be far in excess of the number of spare embryos approved for use, thus making ES cell derivation impractical (not to mention the fact that ES cells created by SCNT would still express histocompatability genes derived from mitochondrial DNA of the egg donor, and serve as a rejection molecule; Condic & Rao, 2008.). Thus, iPS cells would be the only recourse and the only pluripotent cells that would be truly autologous and might be amenable to such tissue banking, but costs again make this approach impractical. Thus, ES and iPS cell banks are not the answer to making regenerative medicine readily available to the public.

In order for regenerative medicine therapies to be successfully transitioned to the general public, one must identify an autologous source of stem cells that can be obtained from the patient, which is easily and economically harvested or derived, and contains large numbers of stem cells. The stem cells could be either multipotent or pluripotent, depending upon the desired use. Finally, the stem cell based therapy must be as successful as current therapy and must be significantly less expensive. Otherwise, "big pharma" and third-party payers will not agree to fund the development and reimbursement of such therapies, even if such treatments hold greater promise than currently used approaches. Thus, it seems that non-embryonic (and non-iPS) stem cells are the only stem cells that meet these requirements. Stem cells found in umbilical cord blood, bone marrow and adipose tissue seem to be ideal solutions to these problems. Each of these stem cell sources can be harvested directly from patients, in a technically simple and economical fashion, in large stem cell numbers. Bone marrow stem cells have been used in clinical trials for patients with cardiovascular disease and for patients with brain injury. Adipose-derived stem cells have also been used in patients with cardiovascular disease as well as in orthopedic applications. In particular, umbilical cord blood stem cells and umbilical cord blood-based therapies seem to be the most ideal source to meet these requirements as compared to the other two stem cell sources. We believe that cord blood stem cells are the best alternative to ES and iPS cells in that these stem cells appear poised between embryonic and adult stem cells, capable of being utilized in many of the same applications claimed for ES and iPS cells, including cardiac, neurological, orthopedic and ophthalmic applications. Further, cord blood stem cells have already make their way into the clinic, being utilized in regenerative medicine approaches to type 1 diabetes, cerebral palsy and brain injury (Harris & Rogers, 2007; Harris et al, 2008; Harris, 2008; Harris, 2009). For additional information on this topic please see the recent reviews by Harris and colleagues (Harris & Rogers, 2007; Harris et al, 2008; Harris, 2008; Harris, 2009).

REFERENCES

Amariglio, N., Hirshberg, A., Scheithauer, B.W., Cohen, Y., Loewenthal, R., Trakhtenbrot, L., Paz, N., Koren-Michowitz, M., Waldman, D., Leider-Trejo, L., Toren, A., Constantini, S., and G Rechavil, G. Donor-Derived Brain Tumor Following Neural Stem Cell Transplantation in an Ataxia Telangiectasia Patient. *PLoS Medicine*, 6(2), 1-11, 2009.

Byrne, J., Pedersen, D., Clepper, L., Nelson, M., Sanger, W., Gokhale, S., Wolf, D., and Mitalipov, S. Producing primate embryonic stem cells by somatic cell nuclear transfer. *Nature*, 450 (7169), 497-502, 2007.

Condic, ML and Rao, M. Regulatory issues for personalized pluripotent cells. *Stem Cells* 26: 2753-2758, 2008.

Harris, D.T. Cord Blood Banking: The University of Arizona Experience : Successes, Problems and Cautions. *Cancer Research Therapy and Control.* 7:63-67, 1998

Harris, D.T. and Rogers, I. Umbilical cord blood: a unique source of pluripotent stem cells for regenerative medicine. *Current Stem Cell Research and Therapy*, 2: 301-309, 2007.

Harris, D.T., Badowski, M, Ahmad, N and Gaballa, M. The Potential of Cord Blood Stem Cells for Use in Regenerative Medicine. *Expert Opinion on Biological Therapy* 7(9): 1311-1322, 2008.

Harris, D.T. Cord Blood Stem Cells: A Review of Potential Neurological Applications. *Stem Cell Reviews* 4(4), 269-274, 2008.

Harris, D.T. Non-Haematological Uses of Cord Blood Stem Cells, *British Journal of Haematology,* In Press, 2009.

Knoepfler, P.S. Deconstructing stem cell tumorigenicity: a roadmap to safe regenerative medicine. *Stem Cell.* 27: 1050-1056, 2009.

Park, I.H., Lerou, P.H., Zhao, R., Huo, H. and Daley, G.Q. Generation of human-induced pluripotent stem cells. *Nature Protocols*, 3, 1180–1186, 2008.

Stadtfeld, M and Hochedlinger, K. Without a trace? PiggyBac-ing towards pluripotency. *Nature Methods* 6(5): 329-330, 2009.

Yamanaka, S. A fresh look at iPS cells. *Cell* 137: 13-17, 2009.

In: Encyclopedia of Stem Cell Research (2 Volume Set)   ISBN: 978-1-61761-835-2
Editors: Alexander L. Greene   © 2012 Nova Science Publishers, Inc.

Chapter LI

GENETIC STABILITY OF MURINE PLURIPOTENT AND SOMATIC HYBRID CELLS MAY BE AFFECTED BY CONDITIONS OF THEIR CULTIVATION

Shramova Elena Ivanovna, Larionov Oleg Alekseevich,
Khodarovich Yurii Mikhailovich and Zatsepina Olga Vladimirovna
Shemyakin and Ovchinnikov Institute of Bioorganic Chemistry,
Russian Academy of Sciences

Abstract

Using mouse pluripotent teratocarcinoma PCC4aza1 cells and proliferating spleen lymphocytes we obtained a new type of hybrids, in which marker lymphocyte genes were suppressed, but expression the *Oct-4* gene was not effected; the hybrid cells were able to differentiate to cardiomyocytes. In order to specify the environmental factors which may affect the genetic stability and other hybrid properties, we analyzed the total chromosome number and differentiation potencies of hybrids respectively to conditions of their cultivation. Particular attention was paid to the number and transcription activity of chromosomal nucleolus organizing regions (NORs), which harbor the most actively transcribed – ribosomal – genes. The results showed that the hybrids obtained are characterized by a relatively stable chromosome number which diminished less than in 5% during 27 passages. However, a long-term cultivation of hybrid cells in non-selective conditions resulted in preferential elimination of some NO-chromosomes, whereas the number of active NORs per cell was increased due to activation of latent NORs. On the contrary, in selective conditions, i.e. in the presence of hypoxanthine, aminopterin and thymidine, the total number of NOR-bearing chromosomes was not changed, but a partial inactivation of remaining NORs was observed. The higher number of active NORs directly correlated with the capability of hybrid cells for differentiation to cardiomyocytes.

Keywords: PCC4aza1 cells, mouse splenocytes, tetraploid hybrids, chromosomes, nucleolus organizing regions, FISH, Ag-NOR, reprogramming, differentiation, cardiomyocytes.

*Corresponding Address: ul. Mikluho-Maklaya, 16/10, Moscow 117997, Russia;
Tel: +7-495-3306465; Fax: +7-495-3350812

1. Introduction

The term 'nuclear reprogramming' is currently understood as the process of modification of the gene expression pattern specific for a cell that leads to a change of the cell properties and phenotype [1]. Reprogramming can be induced by transfer of a somatic cell nucleus to an enucleated oocyte (the nuclear transfer method) [2], by introduction in the differentiated cells of specific factors responsible for the nuclear reprogramming by the use of retroviruses [3, 4], or by *in vitro* hybridization of a pluripotent or a multipotent cell with a differentiated somatic cell [5]. In the last case, embryonic stem (ES) cells and embryonal carcinoma (EC) cells are the most often used as the starting material for fusion with somatic cells. Fusion of the parental cells is achieved in the presence of polyethylene glycol, inactivated Sendai virus or by electric pulses, and is followed by cultivation of the cells in selective medium. The choice of selective conditions is directed by the properties of parental cells and is aimed to eliminate non-fused cells within the first 3–5 days after fusion [6, 7]. During the last years, various types of reconstructed hybrids between ES or EC cells and somatic cells have been obtained [6-13]. In such hybrids the key somatic genes become repressed, whereas the majority of pluripotent or multipotent cell genes, including *Oct-4*, remain expressed.

EC cells belong to the tumor-forming stem cells which possess a significant similarity to cells of early (preimplantation) embryos [14]. They are capable to develop teratocarcinomas in isogenic animals, are included in various tissues of an adult organism [15], and in the presence of inducers can differentiate into embryoid bodies, neuronal cells and cardiomyocytes *in vitro* [16]. Unlike ES cells, EC cells do not demand special culture conditions and thus are more convenient for obtaining intercellular hybrids and analyzing their properties. The study of EC cells hybrids provides many new insights into the mechanisms of differentiation, relationship between pluripotency and tumor genesis, to examine the fundamental mechanisms of the somatic genome reprogramming, and to analyze the impact of environmental conditions on stability and other properties of hybrid cells.

In the present work, we obtained for the first time the stable hybrids between a proliferating mouse spleen lymphocyte and an EC PCC4aza1 cell. We showed that the genetic stability and differentiation potencies of PCC4aza1lymphocyte hybrid cells may be affected by conditions of their cultivation. A few parameters, including the total number of chromosomes and the number and activity of chromosomal nucleolus organizing regions (NORs) have been evaluated. NORs are specific chromosomal loci, where ribosomal genes (rDNA) encoding 18S, 5.8S and 28S rRNA are harbored, in interphase NORs give rise to the functional nucleoli. Ribosomal genes belong to the most actively transcribed genes in eukaryotes, and the level of rDNA transcription is strictly dependent on accessibility of cells to growth factors and cell ploidy [17]. One may expect therefore that the genome reprogramming will result in some assignable changes in the status of chromosomal NORs. However, to the best of our knowledge, the activity and number of NORs as a function of conditions and duration of hybrid cells culturing so far have not been studied.

In the genotype of *Mus musculus* several NO-bearing chromosomes, 12, 15, 16, 18 and 19, are present, but generally only three NORs are transcriptionally active [18]. Active NORs differ from inactive ones by their tight association with the RNA polymerase I transcription complex which has a high affinity to Ag^+ ions and can therefore be revealed by chromosome staining with $AgNO_3$ [19]. The number of active Ag-NORs is used as a measure of activity of rRNA synthesis and cellular metabolism in general [20]. In our study we determined the total number of NO-chromosomes by fluorescence hybridization *in situ* (FISH) with mouse rDNA probes, and compared it with the number of Ag-positive (i.e., active) NORs in PCC4aza1lymphocyte hybrids at various passages and upon different conditions of cell culturing. Our results show that selective conditions (medium with hypoxantin, aminopterin and thymidine (HAT)) promote inactivation of NORs, but do not affect the number of NO-bearing chromosomes. In contrary, in non-selective medium (i.e. medium without HAT) NO-chromosomes are eliminated, but the total number of active NORs is increased. Noteworthy, differentiation potencies of the hybrids were directly correlated with the number of active NORs.

2. Materials and Methods

2.1. Cells Cultures

All cells used in this study were cultured at 37C, 5% CO_2 and in humid atmosphere. Murine embryonal teratocarcinoma PCC4aza1 cells (*hprt*$^-$) were purchased from the Institute of Cytology of the Russian Academy of Sciences (the Russian Cell Culture Collection, St. Petersburg, Russia). The cells of this line have normal mouse karyotype (2n=40). Cells were grown in DMEM medium (PanEco, Russia) containing 8% bovine fetal serum (HyClone, USA) and antibiotics at standard concentrations. To prevent spontaneous differentiation the cells were reseeded every 48 hours.

Mouse spleen cells were isolated from CBAC57BL/6 F_1 one-and-a half year old male following the standard procedure [21]. Lymphocytes were placed in α-MEM medium (Sigma, USA) containing 15% fetal bovine serum (HyClone) at concentration 10^6 cell/ml. To activate proliferation, the medium was supplemented with 3 μg/ml concanavalin A (PanEco) and 5 μM 5-azacytidine (Sigma) for 5 days.

2.2. Obtaining of Hybrid Cells

PCC4aza1 cells and activated lymphocytes were mixed in a ratio of 1:5 in the presence of 45% polyethylene glycol (PEG, MW 1450, Sigma), 10% dimethyl sulfoxide (DMSO, PanEco) and DMEM medium for 1 min. The cells were then transferred to a HAT-containing medium (10^{-4} M hypoxantine, 710^{-7} M aminopterin and 10^{-5} M thymidine, Flow Laboratories, UK) for 24 hours, and then transferred to a medium without HAT. Incubation of PCC4aza1 cells in HAT-containing medium resulted in death of all the cells within 24 hours.

2.3. Polymerase Chain Reaction (PCR)

Genome DNA for PCR was isolated using SiO_2-coated magnetic particles by the usage of approximately 10^6 cells per isolation. PCR was carried out in 10 μl of a reaction mix containing 2 mM $MgCl_2$, 1 unit of Taq DNA-polymerase, 200 μM of each dNTP, primers (for microsatellite markers D1Mit155, D2Mit30, D6Mit15, D6Mit102, D7Mit145, D7Mit178, D8Mit4; for RT-PCR Oct4_(F/R), Act_(F/R), CD11_(F/R), CD45_(F/R)) in the final concentration of 1 pmol/μl and 0.2-1 μg DNA or cDNA. The annealing temperature and elongation time were optimized for the each primer pair used. Parameters for denaturation and elongation reactions were adjusted based on the standard parameters for Taq polymerase functioning. The primer sequences used for PCR microsatellite analysis are listed in Table 1.

Table 1. Primers* used for the microsatellite analysis of PCC4aza1×lymphocyte hybrids, PCC4aza1 cells (originated from the mouse strain 129/Ola) and of mouse spleen lymphocytes (obtained from a CBA×C57BL/6 F$_1$ mice).

Microsatellite marker (chromosome)	Primers sequences (from 5' to 3' ends)	Lengths of the PCR-fragments for the 129/Ola line, CBA line or C57BL/6 line, respectively, bp
D1Mit155 (1)	ATGCATGCATGCACACGT ACCGTGAAATGTTCACCCAT	252 and 216 (CBA), 252 (C57BL/6)
D2Mit30 (2)	CATCCAAGCAGTAACGTAGACG AAATGTTACACCCTCTGCGG	280 and 136 (CBA), 320 (C57BL/6)
D6Mit15 (6)	CACTGACCCTAGCACAGCAG TCCTGGCTTCCACAGGTACT	170 and 195 (CBA)
D6Mit102 (6)	CCATGTGGATATCTTCCCTTG GTATACCCAGTTGTAAATCTTGTGTG	177 and 145 (C57BL/6)
D7Mit145 (7)	CAGGTGACCTTGGTCATGG AGAGCCCAGGGGTTTTAAGA	148 and 200 (C57BL/6)
D7Mit178 (7)	ACCTCTGATTTCAGAACCCTTG TAGAGAGCCACTAGCATATCATAACC	165 and 210 (C57BL/6)
D8Mit4 (8)	CCAACTCATCCCCAAAGGTA GTATGTTCAAGGCTGGGCAT	156 and 195 (CBA), 156 (C57BL/6)

*The primer sequences were selected using the data base provided by Jackson Laboratory, Bar Harbor, Maine, USA (www.informatics.jax.org).

Expression of *Oct4* and β-*actin* genes was analyzed using the following pairs of primers: Oct4_F (5'-GGAGCTAGAACAGTTTGC-3'), Oct4_R (5'-CTTCCTCCACCC-ACTTC-3') and Act_F (5'-GAAATCGTGCGTGACATCAAAG-3'), Act_R (5'-TGTAGT-TTCATGGATGCCACAG-3'), respectively. To analyze the expression of *CD11* and *CD45* genes which are markers of T-lymphocytes the following primer pairs were used: CD11_F (5'-ACACTGTGGCCTGGATGACCTC-3'), CD11_R (5'-GGTAAGTGAACACTCGGC-CTCC-3') and CD45_F (5'-GCGAAGGAAAGCAGACTTATGGAG-3'), CD45_R (5'-CGAGGATGGATGCATGCTTGTG-3').

Total RNA was isolated from 10^6 cells using the YellowSolve kit (Sileks, Russia). The RT-PCR reaction was carried out using a kit for the first cDNA chain synthesis and a mixture of random hexaprimers (Sileks).

2.4.   Isolation of Metaphase Plates

Adhesive cells were synchronized at metaphase by incubation with 50 ng/ml nocodazol (Sigma) for 1–2 hours, treated with 0.56% KCl for 10 min at 37C and fixed in a mixture of absolute methanol and glacial acetic acid (3:1) at -20C for 3 hours. Spleen lymphocytes were also synchronized at metaphase by means of nocodazol, collected by centrifugation, incubated with 0.56% KCl and fixed by the same way as adhesive cells. The cells were dropped onto wet microscope slides, and the quality of metaphase plates was controlled under an ICM 405 (Opton, Germany) microscope. The preparations were stored at room temperature for up to one month.

2.5.   Probes used for Fluorescent *in situ* Hybridization

Two probes for murine rDNA used in the study are depicted in Fig. 1. Probe 1 (the *Eco*RI-*Eco*RI fragment of rDNA, 6.6 kbp, from +5.635 to +12.235) contains a part of the 18S rDNA sequence, the first internal transcribed spacer (ITS1), 5.8S rDNA, the second internal transcribed spacer (ITS2) and about 80% of the 28S rDNA sequence. Probe 2 (an *Eco*RI-*Eco*RI fragment of rDNA, 4.3 kbp, from +12.235 to +16.535) encodes the remaining part of the 28S rDNA and the 3' external transcribed spacer (3'ETS). The rDNA fragments were labeled with digoxigenin by nick translation using the Dig-Nick-Translation Mix (Roche, France) following the manufacturers recommendations.

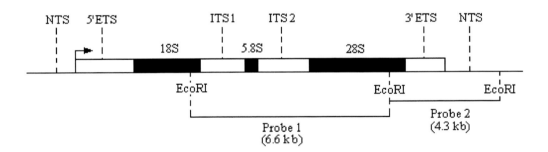

Figure 1. The scheme of the mouse ribosomal repeat and rDNA probes used for fluorescence *in situ* hybridization. NTS – intergenic non-transcribed spacer; 5'ETS – 5'-external transcribed spacer; ITS1 and ITS2 – the first and second internal transcribed spacers correspondingly; 3'ETS – 3'-external transcribed spacer; *Eco*RI – sites of *Eco*RI restriction.

2.6.   Fluorescence *in situ* Hybridization

Fluorescence *in situ* hybridization was performed as described earlier [22]. Chromosome preparations were treated with 100 μg/ml RNase A in a 2 SSC-buffer (0.3 M NaCl; 0.03 M sodium citrate, pH 7.3) for 1 h at 37C, and then with 0.01% pepsin in 0.05 M sodium citrate, (pH 2.0) for 2–4 min at ambient temperature. Preparations were washed in PBS, dried and incubated with hybridization mixture containing 10–25 ng/μl labeled rDNA, 50% deionized formamide and 10% dextransulfate in 2 SSC. Denaturation of the rDNA probes and specimens was made simultaneously at 85C for 10 min. *In situ* hybridization was performed at 37C for 16–18 hours. Specimens were washed in 50% formamide in 4 SSC/Tween 20 buffer at 42C for 10 min, then in 2 SSC for 10 min at room temperature, incubated with rhodamine-conjugated antibodies to digoxigenin, stained with 1 μg/ml Hoechst 33342 for 10 min at room temperature and mounted in Mowiol (Calbiochem, USA). Samples were examined under an Axiovert 200 microscope (Carl Zeiss, Germany) equipped with a 100 PlanApochromat objective (numerical aperture 1.3). The images were recorded by means of a 12-bit monochrome CCD camera CoolSnap$_{cf}$ (Roper Scientific, USA) and processed using Adobe Photoshop software (version 7.0).

2.7. Ag-NOR Staining of Chromosomes

Revealing active NORs of chromosomes was performed according Howell and Black [19]. Two parts of 50% AgNO$_3$ in bidistilled water and one part of 2% gelatin containing 1% formic acid were placed onto a slide with cells. Specimen incubated at 37C for 15 min, thoroughly washed in distilled water, counterstained with 1 μg/ml Hoechst 33342 and mounted in Mowiol. The preparations were then studied as described above.

2.8. Differentiation of Hybrid Cells *in vitro*

For differentiation the hybrid cells were seeded in Petri dishes at about 10^5 cells/ml and cultivated during 5 days with 1% DMSO and then without DMSO. Medium was changed every two days. Endodermal-like cells revealed on 6–7 days after differentiation starting. After 7–8 days after DMSO removal isles of beating cells appeared on substrate. Mitochondria were stained by adding to culture media 6 ng/ml rhodamine 6G for 15 min. The cells were then examined under a light microscope BH2 (Olympus, Japan) using a 60 water-immersion objective U PlanApochromat (Olympus, model UPLAPO60W/1.2, numerical aperture 1.2).

2.9. Statistical Analysis

Correlations were evaluated by simple linear regression analysis. A P value $<0.05\%$ was considered to be significant.

3.   Results

3.1. Hybridization of Cells

The hybrids described in this study have been obtained by fusion of mouse EC teratocarcinoma PCC4aza1 cells with proliferating spleen cells of a (CBAC57BL/6) F$_1$ mouse adult male. They maintained the morphology of PCC4aza1 cells but were lager in size (Fig. 2A, B). In nuclei of the hybrid cells up to ten nucleoli were clearly seen; PCC4aza1 cells and activated spleen lymphocytes generally contained one or two nucleoli (Fig. 2A,

B). PCR analysis of the marker microsatellite sequences for several chromosomes (numbers 1, 2, 6, 7 and 8) showed that at early passages PCC4aza1lymphocyte hybrids contain chromosomes of the both parental cell types (Fig. 3).

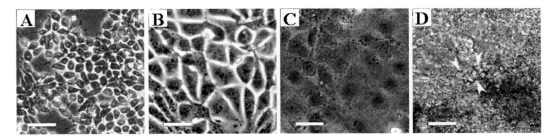

Figure 2. The phenotype of PCC4aza1 cells (A) and PCC4aza1×lymphocyte hybrids in non-selective conditions at the 25th passage of growth (B, C, D). B — non-differentiated hybrid cells; C, D — hybrid cells differentiated to endodermal-like cells (C) or cardiomyocytes (D) in the presence of 1% DMSO. Size bar, 50 μm.

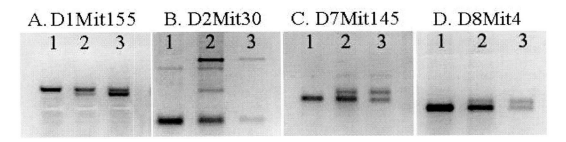

Figure 3. The microsatellite PCR analysis of the chromosomes number 1 (A), 2 (B), 7 (C) and 8 (D) in the mouse strains used to obtain PCC4aza1 cells (129/Ola) and spleen lymphocytes (CBA×C57BL/6). DNA was isolated from PCC4aza1 cells (1), PCC4aza1×lymphocyte hybrids (2), and spleen lymphocytes (3). The length of PCR products for the marker D1Mit155 microsatellite: 252 bp (129/Ola), 216 bp (CBA) and 252 bp (C57BL/6); for the D2Mit30 microsatellite: 280 bp (129/Ola), 136 bp (CBA), and 320 bp (C57BL/6); for the D7Mit145 microsatellite: 148 bp (129/Ola), 148 bp (CBA) and 200 bp (C57BL/6); for the D8Mit4 microsatellite: 156 bp (129/Ola), 195 bp (CBA), and 156 bp (C57BL/6).

It is known that conditions of culturing have a profound impact on the properties EC cells and EC cells hybrids [6, 23, 24]. To examine whether this regularity is also true for our hybrids, at the 17th passage (i.e., about three weeks) after fusion a portion of hybrid cells were transferred to culture medium supplemented with HAT, and the other cells were continued growing in non-selective medium.

In selective medium the morphology of hybrid cells remained similar to that of hybrids which were cultured without HAT. However, under selective conditions the time period for duplication of the cell number was equal to 24 h, whereas without HAT — to 16 h; the duplication rate of PCC4aza1 cells was about 11 h. The mitotic index of hybrids cultured without HAT was $11.3\pm1.6\%$, but with HAT it was diminished to $7.8\pm2.2\%$. These observations showed that selective medium inhibits proliferation activity of the obtained hybrid cells.

3.2. Reprogramming of Somatic Genes in Hybrid Cells

Analysis of expression of the lymphocyte marker genes *CD11* and *CD45* in PCC4aza1 lymphocyte hybrids showed that these genes remained not functional in the presence of HAT and without HAT (Fig. 4). These observations evidenced in favor of reprogramming of the lymphocyte nucleus under exposure to factors present in a PCC4aza1 cell. However, similar to teratocarcinoma PCC4aza1 cells, hybrid cells continued to express *Oct4* that is a gene marker of pluripotent cells [11] (Fig. 4).

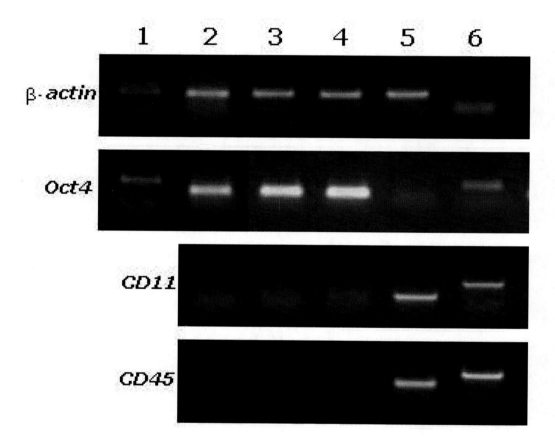

Figure 4. Expression of the β-*actin*, *Oct4*, *CD11* and *CD45* genes in hybrid and parental cells as observed by RT-PCR analysis. The following templates were used: genomic DNA isolated from PCC4aza1 cells (1); cDNA from PCC4aza1 cells (2), cDNA from PCC4aza1 ×lymphocyte hybrids at the 27th passage (nonselective conditions) (3) or from hybrids at the 30th passage (selective conditions) (4), cDNA from mouse spleen lymphocytes (5); genomic DNA from spleen lymphocytes (6).

3.3. Influence of Selective Medium on the Chromosome Stability in Hybrid Cells

Assessment of the total chromosome number in metaphase plates of PCC4aza1lymphocyte hybrids grown in non-selective medium showed that at late (25–27th) passages hybrid cells contained an average of 74 (74.4±2.2) chromosomes (Table 2). At the late (26–30th) passages in selective conditions hybrid cells contained an average of 76 (76.1±1.7) chromosomes. As far as these values do not differ statistically significantly, we concluded that conditions of cell culturing have a low impact on the total number of chromosomes in the obtained hybrids. However, the karyotype of the obtained hybrids was not entirely stable: during three months hybrid cells lost four (in selective conditions) or six (in non-selective conditions) chromosomes that is equal to 5–8% of the total chromosome number expected in PCC4aza1lymphocyte hybrids (Table 2).

Table 2. The average number of chromosomes, FISH-NORs and Ag-NORs in the parental cells and PCC4aza1×lymphocyte hybrid cells. Hybrid cells were cultured for various time periods in non-selective (medium without HAT) or selective (medium with HAT) conditions.

Cell types	Stage	Number of chromosomes	Number of FISH-NORs	Number of Ag-NORs
PCC4aza1	Befor fusion	40	$8(7.9 \pm 0.1)^{\dagger}$	$7(7.0 \pm 0.4)$
Mouse spleen lymphocytes	5th day of activation	40	$7(7.0 \pm 0.1)^{\dagger}$	$6(6.2 \pm 0.5)$
Expected values		80	15	13
350ptHybrids grown in medium without HAT	6th passage	$78(77.2 \pm 2.4)$	$14(13.9 \pm 0.7)$	$10(10.3 \pm 0.9)$
	17th passage	$76(76.0 \pm 0.8)$	n/d	n/d
	25–27th passage	$74(74.4 \pm 2.2)$	$12(12.0 \pm 0.8)$	$10(10.4 \pm 0.8)^{\ddagger}$
Hybrids grown in medium with HAT	26–30th passage	$76(76.1 \pm 1.7)$	$14(13.9 \pm 0.8)$	$9(8.8 \pm 1.1)^{\ddagger}$

M±m are the mean value and standard deviation from the mean value;
n/d – no data, †, ‡ — data that differ statistically significantly.

3.4. The Number of NORs Observed by FISH

In laboratory mice *Mus musculus* the number of chromosomal NORs is known to be the strain specific [18, 25], although in all mouse strains, fluorescence *in situ* hybridization

(FISH) reveals NORs as singular or double spots located close to the centromeric regions [e.g., 22].

The count of the total number of NORs by FISH was first performed in metaphase plates obtained from the parental cells — PCC4aza1 and proliferating spleen lymphocytes. PCC4aza1 cells were found to contain eight NORs per cell. In metaphase plates of activated lymphocytes seven FISH-NORs were present. Thus, the expected total number of NORs in the hybrid cells was 15.

Fig. 5 illustrates the typical metaphase chomosomes of PCC4aza1lymphocyte hybrids obtained in non-selective conditions at an early (6th) (Fig. 5A, D, G) and late (25 –27th) passages (Fig. 5B, E, H). In the majority of metaphase plates from the early passage an average of 14 NO-chromosomes (13.9±0.7) were revealed. At the late passages metaphase plates contained on average of twelve NORs (12.0±0.8). These results showed that cultivation of hybrid cells in non-selective conditions promotes elimination of NO-bearing chromosomes (Table 2).

In contrary, at the late passages 26–30th in selective conditions, PCC4aza1lymphocyte hybrids contained 13.9±0.8 FISH-NORs (Fig. 5C, F, I; Table 2), and regardless of the total chromosome number about 36% of the metaphase plates analyzed contained 15 NO-chromosomes. These results suggest that cultivation of hybrids under selective pressure favors retaining the NO-bearing chromosomes. The data on the FISH-NOR number at different passages and under various cultivation conditions are summarized in Table 2.

3.5.   The Total Number of Ag-NORs

Metaphase plates of the parental PCC4aza1 cells had an average of 7.0±0.4 Ag-NORs per cell and activated lymphocytes — 6.2±0.5 Ag-NORs. Therefore, the expected number of active NORs in hybrid cells was 13. However, in early hybrids (at the 6th passage) only about ten active NORs (10.3±0.9) were present. This value remained almost unchanged in non-selective medium — at the later (25–27th) passages an average of 10.4±0.8 Ag-NORs were revealed in hybrid cells. That is, the loss of three NO-bearing chromosomes during hybrid growth under non-selective conditions was not accompanied by any noticeable change in the number of active Ag-NORs (Table 2).

Different results have been obtained in hybrid cells cultivated under selective conditions: at the late (26–30th) passages they had 8.8±1.1 Ag-NORs. Processing the data by means of the Student criterion showed that the average numbers of Ag-NORs at the late passages under non-selective (10.4±0.8) and selective (8.8±1.1) conditions differed statistically significantly ($p < 0.05$) (Table 2). It may be concluded that selective media promotes preservation of NO-bearing chromosomes, but favour the inactivation of their NORs.

3.6.   Differentiation of PCC4aza1×lymphocyte hybrids *in vitro*

The differentiation capability of hybrids was studied by adding 1% DMSO to the culture medium at the early (6th) or late (25–30th) passages. Irrespectively to the growth conditions hybrid cells were able to differentiate to endodermal-like cells (Fig. 2C). However, only in non-selective conditions hybrids were able to differentiate to cardiomyocytes as well (Fig. 2D). Differentiation to cardiomyocytes was evidenced by the appearance of clusters of

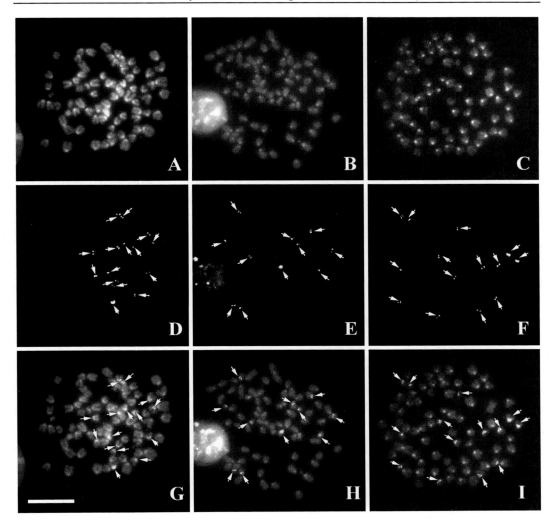

Figure 5. Fluorescence *in situ* hybridization of PCC4aza1×lymphocyte hybrid chromosomes with rDNA probes (D–F) and staining with Hoechst 33342 (A–C) at the 6th (A, D, G) and 27th (B, E, H) passages of cell cultivation in non-selective conditions, and at the 30th passage (C, F, I) of cell cultivation in selective conditions. G–I — overlay of the images. FISH-NORs are indicated by arrows. Size bar, 10 μm.

beating cells, in which numerous mitochondria were revealed after staining with rhodamine 6G. It should be noted that PCC4aza1 did not differentiate either along the endodermal path or to cardiomyocytes under the same conditions. Based on these observations we concluded that the ability of hybrid cells for differentiation depends on their cultivation conditions.

4. Conclusion

It is known that some organs (e.g., liver and heart) of mammals and human contain polyploid cells [26, 27]. Therefore, analysis of regularities of the genome reprogramming in tetraploid hybrids that are capable for differentiation has a fundamental and applied significance.

To obtain hybrids between PCC4aza1 and lymphocytes we used mouse spleen cells activated by concanavalin A and treated with 5-azacytidine for 5 days. To our knowledge, hybrids between EC cells and lymphocytes activated for proliferation are described here for the first time. Since cultivation of primary spleen lymphocytes with concanavalin A *in vitro* leads to activation of only T-lymphocytes [28], it is highly likely that the obtained hybrid cells were resulted from fusion of a PCC4aza1 cell and a T-lymphocyte.

5-azacytidine is known to promote demethylation of DNA and to inhibit activity of DNA methyltransferases [29–31]. It has been shown that treatment of cells with 5-azacytidine induces reprogramming of the somatic genome in hybrids between somatic and ES cells [7] and after nuclei transfer to enucleated oocytes [32, 33]. DNA methylation is known to influence regulation of expression of ribosomal genes, and incubation of cells with 5-azacytidine increases the number of active NORs [34]

In hybrids PCC4aza1lymphocyte expression of the genes specific to T-lymphocytes, *CD11* and *CD45*, ceased whereas expression of *Oct4*, a gene marker of pluripotent cells, was not repressed. Down regulation of *CD11* and *CD45* expression was not due to a loss of the chromosomes bearing these genes (chromosomes 7 and 1 respectively), that was confirmed by microsatellite analysis of DNA isolated from the hybrid cells (Fig. 3).

During the last years a number of works have been published, where was shown that the long-lasting cultivation of ES cells lead to the chromosome aberrations and the genetic instability [35–39]. For maintenance of chromosome stability, hybrid cells are routinely cultivated in selective media, for example, in media containing HAT [23, 24, 40]. Without selective pressure chromosomes are readily lost in intraspecific hybrids between mouse teratocarcinoma and thymus cells [40], EC cells and lymphocytes [24], ES cells and spleenocytes [6] as well as in interspecies hybrids between mouse EC and rat intestinal villus cells [41]. However, in hybrid cells obtained in the present work, the chromosome number was rather stable and diminished only in 5–8% in various conditions of hybrid cultivation (Table 2).

Predominant elimination of NO-chromosomes in PCC4aza1lymphocyte hybrids grown in non-selective conditions has been described here for the first time. To the best of our knowledge, similar phenomena have so far been described only in hybrids of a plant origin. For example, in hybrids of the somatic potato cells chromosomes with more active NORs were eliminated preferentially [42, 43]. The authors the cited works supposed that elimination of NO-chromosomes was genetically controlled and resulted from their spatial associations [42]. This assumption can explain the predominant elimination of NO-chromosomes observed in our hybrids under non-selective conditions, where metabolic activity of cells appeared to be higher than that in HAT-containing medium.

Fusion of PCC4aza1 cells with lymphocytes resulted in partial inactivation of NORs. Indeed, if all NORs of the parental cells used in the study would remain active, the total number of Ag-NORs in PCC4aza1lymphocyte hybrids should be 13. However, the maximal number of Ag-NORs observed in hybrid cells was always less (Table 2). This observation is a good line with literature data on the hybrids between mouse and human somatic cells, which show that respectively to the line of somatic cells used, activity of either human or mouse NORs was suppressed so that in hybrids the total number of active Ag-NORs was less than the sum of the Ag-NORs present in the parental cells [44, 45].

Suppression of NOR activity in PCC4aza1lymphocyte hybrids occurred by one of the two ways — either by elimination of NO-bearing chromosomes (in non-selective conditions) or by inactivation of some NORs (in selective conditions). We concluded that elimination of NO-chromosomes is the most radical mechanism controlling the overall activity of ribosomal genes and synthesis of ribosomes in hybrid cells.

By now the question of relationship between activity of ribosomal genes and differentiation remains to be elucidated. Results of the present work show that hybrid cells possessing a higher number of active NORs (in non-selective conditions; Table 2) also have a higher potencies for differentiation *in vitro* as compared with the parental PCC4aza1 cells or hybrid cells grown in the presence of HAT. Since the amount of Ag-binding material associated with NORs in mitosis directly correlates with transcriptional activity of ribosomal genes in interphase [46, 47], one may assume that lower differentiation potencies of hybrid cells observed in HAT-containing medium are resulted from down-regulation of rDNA transcription and ribosome production and finally lead to depletion of protein factors responsible for differentiation.

Acknowledgments

The study was supported by the Russian Academy of Sciences (the program Molecular and Cell Biology) and in part by the Russian Foundation for Basic Researches (grant 08-04-00854).

References

[1] Sullivan, S., Pells, S., Hooper, M., Gallagher, E. & McWhir, J. (2006). Nuclear reprogramming of somatic cells by embryonic stem cells is affected by cell cycle stage. *Cloning Stem Cells, 8*, 174-188.

[2] Gurdon, J. B. (2006). From nuclear transfer to nuclear reprogramming: the reversal of cell differentiation. *Annu Rev Cell Dev Biol, 22*, 1-22.

[3] Takahashi, K. & Yamanaka, S. (2006). Induction of pluripotent stem cells from mouse embryonic and adult fibroblast cultures by defined factors. *Cell, 126*, 663-676.

[4] Yu, J., Vodyanik M. A., Smuga-Otto, K., Antosiewicz-Bourget, J., Frane, J. L., Tian, S., Nie, J., Jonsdottir, G. A., Ruotti, V., Stewart, R., Slukvin, I. I. & Thomson, J A. (2007). Induced pluripotent stem cell lines derived from human somatic cells. *Sceince, 318*, 1917-1920.

[5] Serov, O., Matveeva, N., Kuznetsov, S., Kaftanovskaya E. & Mittmann, J. (2001). Embryonic hybrid cells: a powerful tool for studying pluripotency and reprogramming of the differentiated cell chromosomes. *An Acad Bras Cienc, 73*, 561-568.

[6] Matveeva, N. M., Shilov, A. G., Kaftanovskaya, E. M., Maximovsky, L. P., Zhelezova, A. I., Golubitsa, A. N., Bayborodin, S. I., Fokina, M. M. & Serov, O. L. (1998). In vitro and in vivo study of pluripotency in intraspecific hybrid cells obtained by fusion of murine embryonic stem cells with splenocytes. *Mol Reprod Dev, 50*, 128-138.

[7] Do, J. T. & Schler, H. R. (2004). Nuclei of embryonic stem cells reprogram somatic cells. *Stem Cells, 22*, 941-949.

[8] Mittmann, J., Kerkis, I., Kawashima, C., Sukoyan, M., Santos, E. & Kerkis, A. (2002). Differentiation of mouse embryonic stem cells and their hybrids during embryoid body formation. *Genet Mol Biol, 25*, 103-111.

[9] Pells, S., Di Domenico, A. I., Gallagher, E. J. & McWhir, J. (2002). Multipotentiality of neuronal cells after spontaneous fusion with embryonic stem cells and nuclear reprogramming in vitro. *Cloning Stem Cells, 4*, 331-338.

[10] Terada, N., Hamazaki, T., Oka, M., Hoki, M., Mastalerz, D. M., Nakano, Y., Meyer, E. M., Morel, L., Petersen, B. E. & Scott, E. W. (2002). Bone marrow cells adopt the phenotype of other cells by spontaneous cell fusion. *Nature, 416*, 542-545.

[11] Flasza, M., Shering, A. F., Smith, K., Andrews, P. W., Talley, P. & Johnson, P. A. (2003). Reprogramming in inter-species embryonal carcinoma-somatic cell hybrids induces expression of pluripotency and differentiation markers. *Cloning Stem Cells, 5*, 339-354.

[12] Tada, M., Takahama, Y., Abe, K., Nakatsuji, N. & Tada, T. (2001). Nuclear reprogramming of somatic cells by in vitro hybridization with ES cells. *Curr Biol, 11*, 1553-1558.

[13] Cowan, C. A., Atienza, J., Melton, D. A. & Eggan, K. (2005). Nuclear reprogramming of somatic cells after fusion with human embryonic stem cells. *Science, 309*, 1369-1373.

[14] Martin, G. R. (1975). Teratocarcinomas as a model system for the study of embryogenesis and neoplasia. *Cell, 5*, 229-243.

[15] Mintz, B. & Illmensee, K. (1975). Normal genetically mosaic mice produced from malignant teratocarcinoma cells. *Proc Natl Acad Sci USA, 72*, 3585-3589.

[16] Martin, G. R., Wiley, L. M. & Damjanov, I. (1977). The development of cystic embryoid bodies in vitro from clonal teratocarcinoma stem cells. *Dev Biol, 61*, 230-244.

[17] Mayer, C. & Grummt, I. (2005). Cellular stress and nucleolar function. *Cell Cycle, 4*, 1036-1038.

[18] Long, E. O. & Dawid, I. B. (1980). Repeated genes in eukaryotes. *Annu Rev Biochem, 49*, 727-764.

[19] Howell, W. M. & Black, D. A. (1980). Controlled silver-staining of nucleolus orga-nizer regions with a protective colloidal developer: a 1-step method. *Experientia, 36,* 1014-1015.

[20] Hadjiolov, A. A. (1985). *The nucleolus and ribosome biogenesis. In: Cell Biology Monographs,* Vol. 12, New York: Springer-Verlag, 1-263.

[21] StGroth, S. F., de & Scheidegger, D. (1980). Production of monoclonal antibodies: strategy and tactics. *J Immunol Methods, 35,* 1-21.

[22] Romanova, L. G., Anger, M., Zatsepina, O. V. & Schultz, R. M. (2006). Implica-tion of nucleolar protein SURF6 in ribosome biogenesis and preimplantation mouse development. *Biol Reprod, 75,* 690-696.

[23] Mise, N., Sado, T., Tada, M., Takada, S. & Takagi, N. (1996). Activation of the inac-tive X chromosome induced by cell fusion between a murine EC and female somatic cell accompanies reproducible changes in the methylation pattern of the Xist gene. *Exp Cell Res, 223,* 193-202.

[24] Forejt, J., Saam, J. R., Gregorova, S. & Tilghman, S. M. (1999). Monoallelic expres-sion of reactivated imprinted genes in embryonal carcinoma cell hybrids. *Exp Cell Res, 252,* 416-422.

[25] Savino, T. M., Gebrane-Younes, J., De Mey, J., Sibaritac, J. B. & Hernandez-Verduna, D. (2001). Nucleolar assembly of the rRNA processing machinery in living cells. *J Cell Biol, 153,* 1097-1110.

[26] Adler, C. P., Friedburg, H., Herget, G. W., Neuburger, M. & Schwalb, H. (1996). Variability of cardiomyocyte DNA content, ploidy level and nuclear number in mam-malian hearts. *Virchows Arch, 429,* 159-164.

[27] Gupta, S. (2000). Hepatic polyploidy and liver growth control. *Semin Cancer Biol, 10,* 161-171.

[28] Stobo, J. D. (1972). Phytohemagglutin and concanavalin A: probes for murine 'T' cell activation and differentiation. *Transplant Rev, 11,* 60-86.

[29] Taylor, S. M. & Jones, P. A. (1979). Multiple new phenotypes induced in 10T1/2 and 3T3 cells treated with 5-azacytidine. *Cell, 17,* 771-779.

[30] Cheng, X. (1995). DNA modification by methyltransferases. *Curr Opin Struct Biol, 5,* 4-10.

[31] Fukuda, K. (2001). Development of regenerative cardiomyocytes from mesenchymal stem cells for cardiovascular tissue engineering. *Artif Organs, 25,* 187-193.

[32] Jones, K. L., Hill, J., Shin, T. Y., Lui, L. & Westhusin, M. (2001). DNA hypomethyla-tion of karyoplasts for bovine nuclear transplantation. *Mol Reprod Dev, 60,* 208-213.

[33] Enright, B. P., Kubota, C., Yang, X. & Tian, X. C. (2003). Epigenetic characteristics and development of embryos cloned from donor cells treated by trichostatin A or 5-aza-2'-deoxycytidine. *Biol Reprod, 69,* 896-901.

[34] Ferraro, M. & Lavia, P. (1983). Activation of human ribosomal genes by 5-azacytidine. *Exp Cell Res, 145,* 452-457.

[35] Brimble, S. N., Zeng, X., Weiler, D. A., Luo, Y., Liu, Y., Lyons, I. G., Freed, W. J., Robins, A. J., Rao, M. S. & Schulz, T. C. (2004). Karyotypic stability, genotyping, differentiation, feeder-free maintenance, and gene expression sampling in three human embryonic stem cell lines derived prior to August 9, 2001. *Stem Cells Dev*, *13*, 585-597.

[36] Draper, J. S., Smith, K., Gokhale, P., Moore, H. D., Maltby, E., Johnson, J., Meisner, L., Zwaka, T. P., Thomson, J. A. & Andrews, P. W. (2004). Recurrent gain of chromosomes 17q and 12 in cultured human embryonic stem cells. *Nat Biotechnol*, *22*, 53-54.

[37] Inzunza, J., Sahln, S., Holmberg, K., Strmberg, A. M., Teerijoki, H., Blennow, E., Hovatta., O. & Malmgren, H. (2004). Comparative genomic hybridization and karyotyping of human embryonic stem cells reveals the occurrence of an isodicentric X chromosome after long-term cultivation. *Mol Hum Reprod*, *10*, 461-466.

[38] Hanson, C. & Caisander, G. (2005). Human embryonic stem cells and chromosome stability. *APMIS*, *113*, 751-755.

[39] Maitra, A., Arking, D. E., Shivapurkar, N., Ikeda, M., Stastny, V., Kassauei, K., Sui, G., Cutler, D. J., Liu, Y., Brimble, S. N., Noaksson, K., Hyllner, J., Schulz, T. C., Zeng, X., Freed, W. J., Crook, J., Abraham, S., Colman, A., Sartipy, P., Matsui, S., Carpenter, M., Gazdar, A. F., Rao, M. & Chakravarti, A. (2005). Genomic alterations in cultured human embryonic stem cells. *Nat Genet*, *37*, 1099-1103.

[40] Rousset, J. P., Bucchini, D. & Jami, J. (1983). Hybrids between F9 nullipotent teratocarcinoma and thymus cells produce multidifferentiated tumors in mice. *Dev Biol*, *96*, 331-336.

[41] Kamp, van der, A. W., Roza-de Jongh, E. J., Houwen, R. H., Magrane, G. G., van Dongen, J. M. & Evans, M. J. (1984) Developmental characteristics of somatic cell hybrids between totipotent mouse teratocarcinoma and rat intestinal villus cells. *Exp Cell Res*, *154*, 53-64.

[42] Pijnacker, L. P., Ferwerda, M. A., Puite, K. J. & Roest, S. (1987). Elimination of Solanum phureja nucleolar chromosomes in S. tuberosum + S. phureja somatic hybrids. *Theor Appl Genet*, *73*, 878- 882.

[43] Pijnacker, L. P., Ferwerda, M. A., Puite, K. J. & Schaart, J. G. (1989). Chromosome elimination and mutation in tetraploid somatic hybrids of Solanum tuberosum and Solanum phureja. *Plant Cell Reports*, *8*, 82-85.

[44] Miller, D. A., Dev, V. G., Tantravahi, R. & Miller, O. J. (1976a). Suppression of human nucleolus organizer activity in mouse-human somatic hybrid cells. *Exp Cell Res*, *101*, 235-243.

[45] Miller, O. J., Miller, D. A., Dev, V. G., Tantravahi, R. & Croce, C. M. (1976b). Expression of human and suppression of mouse nucleolus organizer activity in mouse-human somatic cell hybrids. *Proc Natl Acad Sci USA*, *73*, 4531-4535.

[46] Derenzini, M., Sirri, V., Pession, A., Trer, D., Roussel, P., Ochs, R. L. & Hernandez-Verdun, D. (1995). Quantitative changes of the two major AgNOR proteins, nucleolin

and protein B23, related to stimulation of rDNA transcription. *Exp Cell Res, 219*, 276-282.

[47] Sirri, V., Roussel, P. & Hernandez-Verdun, D. (2000). The AgNOR proteins: qualitative and quantitative changes during the cell cycle. *Micron, 31*, 121-126.

In: Encyclopedia of Stem Cell Research (2 Volume Set)   ISBN: 978-1-61761-835-2
Editor: Alexander L. Greene   © 2012 Nova Science Publishers, Inc.

Chapter LII

RECENT ADVANCEMENTS TOWARDS THE DERIVATION OF IMMUNE-COMPATIBLE PATIENT-SPECIFIC HUMAN PLURIPOTENT STEM CELL LINES

Micha Drukker [*]

Institute for Stem Cell Biology and Regenerative Medicine, Beckman Center,
Stanford, CA, US

ABSTRACT

The derivation of human embryonic stem cell lines from blastocyst stage embryos, first achieved almost a decade ago, demonstrated the potential to prepare virtually unlimited numbers of therapeutically beneficial cells *in vitro*. Assuming that large-scale production of differentiated cells is attainable, it is imperative to develop strategies to prevent immune responses towards the grafted cells following transplantation. This paper presents recent advances in the production of pluripotent cell lines using three emerging techniques: somatic cell nuclear transfer into enucleated oocytes and zygotes, parthenogenetic activation of unfertilized oocytes and induction of pluripotency in somatic cells. These techniques have a remarkable potential for generation of patient-specific pluripotent cells that would be tolerated by the immune system.

Keywords: Human embryonic stem cells (hESCs); Immunogenicity; Parthenogenesis; Somatic cell nuclear transfer (SCNT); Induction of pluripotent stem (iPS) cells.

[*] Email address: dmicha@stanford.edu

INTRODUCTION

Human embryonic stem cells (hESCs) have the capacity perpetuate themselves indefinitely in culture conditions while maintaining the potential to differentiate to all cell types of the body upon induction [1, 2]. These cells offer a considerable therapeutic advantage over the lineage-committed adult stem cell types such as hematopoietic stem cells (HSCs) and neuronal stem cells, since they may serve as virtually an infinite source for all cell lineages. Therefore, the isolation of hESCs has lead to numerous studies that aim to isolate beneficial cells for therapeutics [1]. The goal now remains to develop methodologies for harnessing the potential of hESCs in tissue replacement, repair, maintenance, and/or enhancement of function.

As a first step towards this goal, multiple laboratories have developed an array of differentiation protocols to derive specialized cell types, such as neuronal cells, cardiomyocytes, endothelial cells, hematopoietic precursors and hepatocytes (reviewed in [3]). Yet, other aspects of cellular therapeutics should be addressed before successful therapeutic application of hESC-derived cells is possible. For example, differentiation protocols need to improve to the point that homogenous preparations of particular cell types can be produced without any remaining undifferentiated (and potentially teratogenic) cells. In addition, derivation, propagation and differentiation of hESCs should be carried out in animal product-free culture conditions to prevent cross-specie contaminations. Finally, implanted cells must successfully integrate into the patient's tissue without prompting immune responses towards the graft. This review summarizes the current knowledge about the immune properties of hESCs and their differentiated derivatives (for detailed review see [4]) followed by an discussion of novel strategies that could potentially generate histocompatible patient-specific hESC lines.

IMMUNOGENICITY OF HUMAN EMBRYONIC STEM CELLS AND DIFFERENTIATED CELLS

The two arms of the immune system, innate and adaptive, can interact with transplanted allogeneic cells (from genetically non-identical individual) leading to their rejection. Clearly, the major assaults on allogeneic tissues are mediated either directly through the action of cytotoxic T cells or by alloantibodies that are produced by alloreactive B cells against graft-derived antigens (reviewed in [5]). Class I and II MHC proteins (MHC-I and MHC-II, respectively), which are encoded by a highly variable set of human leukocyte antigens (HLA), lie at the heart of these acute allogeneic responses (reviewed in [6]). Following transplantation, foreign MHC molecules, which are expressed on grafted cells, can interact with the recipient's T cells leading to their sensitization and maturation into cytotoxic T cells that attack the transplant (direct recognition) [7]. In addition, host professional antigen presenting cells can processes foreign MHC molecules and present them to host T and B cells leading to alloantibodies secretion by B cells (indirect recognition) [6]. When alloantibodies enter circulation, they bind to transplanted cells and target them for destruction by phagocytosis and the complement system.

To evaluate whether hESCs and their derivatives could potentially induce allogeneic responses, the expression of MHC molecules on these cells was tested in a number of studies [8, 9]. It was found that undifferentiated hESCs express low levels of MHC-I proteins and that differentiation and application of interferons (IFNs) induces 100-fold increase to somatic levels. In contrast, MHC-II proteins seem to be absent under all tested conditions probably due to minimal differentiation towards hematopoietic fate (MHC-II expression is largely restricted to this lineage). Furthermore, together with colleagues, we tested the immunogenicity of hESCs *in vitro* by incubating the cells with pre-stimulated human T cells. We found that following MHC-I induction by IFNs kT cells specifically recognize and lyse hESCs. In contrast, human T-cell response against differentiated hESCs in mice was very weak most probably due to low expression of co-stimulatory signals (CD80 and CD86) that are necessary for T activation [10]. These data indicate that hESCs express sufficient levels of of MHC-I molecules to elicit rejection by primed cytotoxic T cells, but have a reduced potential to stimulate T cells.

Another line of immune defense that can potentially reject foreign grafts is natural killer (NK) cells. Theses are cytotoxic lymphocytes that lyse cells based on the balance between stimulating and inhibiting signals that are provided by target cells. It is possible that low expression of MHC-I in hESCs and their derivatives could result in their targeting by NK cells since these molecules serve as ligands for NK-cell inhibitory receptors [11]. When we examined the NK-cell response towards hESCs *in vitro*, we found that irrespective of MHC expression NK cells do not readily lyse hESCs [9]. Additional studies are required to determine whether hESCs are sensitive to NK-mediated rejection *in vivo*, and whether NK cells might pose a significant obstacle to hESC therapeutics. At least in one case, it has been shown that hematopoietic progenies of mouse ES are rejected by NK cells *in vivo* [12].

Based on the existing data regarding antigenicity and immunogenicity of hESCs, a complex picture of their immunological status can be drawn. Differentiation to specialized somatic cell types is likely to induce moderate levels of MHC-I expression and in the case of hematopoietic differentiation MHC-II and co-stimulatory molecules will also be expressed [13-15]. Thus, T-cell mediated immune responses are likely to be directed at differentiated hESCs, and in the case of hematopoietic transplantation this reaction may be even more severe. Also, alloantibodies and NK cells may play a role in graft rejection. Therefore, these immune factors must be considered when designing strategies for preventing rejection of hESC-derived transplants.

STRATEGIES FOR IMMUNE PROTECTION OF DIFFERENTIATED HUMAN EMBRYONIC STEM CELLS

Excluding immunosuppression, currently five major approaches may be used to diminish or abolish the immune response against transplanted hESCs (i-iv were reviewed in [4, 16]). These options include: *i)* transplantation of differentiated therapeutic cells to natural environments that restrict immune responses (immune-privileged sites), such as the brain and testis. *ii*) Generation of large hESC line banks will allow matching MHC haplotypes between patients and cell lines. *iii*) Genetic manipulation of the genes that encode for MHC antigens and other immune modulators in hESC. *iv*) Induction of hematopoietic chimerism – a state that allows acceptance of allografts from the donor cell line that is used for hematopoietic stem cell transplantation. *v*) Generation of genetically identical hESC lines specifically for each patient. The latter approach would alleviate most immunological considerations, but until very recently seemed improbable due to technical and ethical issues. This view is changing now as several seminal advancements made within the last two years have indicated that tailored derivations of patient specific syngeneic (genetically close or identical) hESC lines could be done in the near future. I will discuss these developments hereafter (summarized in table 1).

Table 1. Proposed pathways for derivation of patient specific hESC lines

Method	Cell sources		Gender specificity	Immunological considerations for transplantation	Demonstrated in:	
					Mouse	Human
Parthenogenesis	Metaphase II oocytes [19]		Yes, female	Preferentially, MHC heterozygous cells should be used	+	+
Somatic cell nuclear transfer	Oocytes [28] Zygotes [30]	+ Somatic nucleus	No	Mitochondrial mHAgs might induce immune responses	+	-
Fusion with hESCs	Fibroblasts [34]		No	Should be used only as diploid cells	+	+
			No			
Induced pluripotency	Embryonic and adult fibroblasts [36-41]		No	Unknown	+	+

PARTHENOGENETICALLY ACTIVATED OOCYTES GIVE RISE TO SYNGENEIC ES CELL LINES

Parthenogenesis is the process of embryonic development without male fertilization. Mammals do not reproduce by parthenogenesis, but for many species activation of arrested metaphase oocytes by chemical regents can lead to development into diploid blastocyst stage embryos. Protocols for ESC-derivation from pseudo-zygotes were developed for mouse [17], macaque monkey [18] and recently human embryos by Revazova et al., [19]. Quite strikingly, this study showed that about half of the human oocytes that were chemically activated (23 of 46 embryos) progressed to the blastocyst stage, and of these, six parthenogenetic ESC (pESCs) lines were successfully produced. In mice and presumably also in humans, parthenogenetic embryos do not develop past the early limb bud stage as embryonic development require expression from the two parental genomes [20]. Still, the differentiation capacity of mouse, macaque monkey and human pESCs is striking; for example, mouse pESCs differentiate *in vitro* and contribute to multiple tissues in chimeric mice. When transplantation compatibility of these cells was tested, it was found that differentiated pESC lines engrafted only in MHC matched animals, meaning that they are histocompatible with the nucleus donor [21]. Similarly, human pESCs (phESCs) form embryoid bodies (EBs) in culture and teratomas that include cell types of the three embryonic germ layers, however, their immunological properties are yet to be determined [19].

The extent of homozygosity in parthenogenetic cells depends on oocyte activation stage, metaphase-I or metaphase-II and on recombination events. Activation of metaphase-I arrested oocytes (before first polar body extrusion) gives rise to pESC lines that are identical to the donor as they contain the two maternal chromosome homologs. However, it is unlikely that these cells would be used for therapeutics since experiments in mice showed that they were tetraploid or aneuploid. Metaphase-II arrested mouse and human oocytes (before second polar body extrusion) give rise to pESC lines containing duplicated hemizygote genome and have normal karyotype [17]. Therefore, the latter may be clinically applicable.

Although phESC lines are histocompatible with the oocyte donor, NK cells may actually respond against the cells if they lack one set of MHC genes. This phenomenon is thought to be relevant mainly to rejection of bone marrow by NK cells following transplantation (reviewed in [22]) and therefore should be examined carefully prior clinical application. It seems that all metaphase-II derived phESC lines that were reported by Revazova et al., contained full heterozygosity in the MHC region [19]. This means that during oocyte development, recombination occurred between the centromere and the MHC region on chromosome 6 homologs, and the resulting recombinant sister chromatids contain the whole MHC milieu. Therefore, NK-cell response against differentiated phESCs that retain heterozygosity seems unlikely.

It should be noted that phESCs were probably also derived in experiments carried out by Hwang's group in South Korea. Although the team reported the derivation of "cloned" embryo-derived hESCs they could not provide definitive proof to show that the cell lines were not result of parthenogenesis. Recently, Kim et al., found that the most of the genes in pESCs are heterozygous, but close to the centromere the gene copies show predominant homozygosity [23]. In contrast, nuclear transfer-derived ESCs (ntESCs) contain heterozygosity throughout the genome. Analysis of a hESC line that was claimed to be derived from a cloned embryo [24] showed that the cells contain extensive homozygosity in the MHC loci indicating that this cell line is actually parthenote [23].

PhESC lines that carry only one set of MHC genes (when recombination does not occur) could potentially prove beneficial not only for the oocyte donor but also for genetically related individuals. For example, there is a 50% chance that a cell line that is derived for a patient will be histocompatible to any of her children. Moreover, if a sizable depository of MHC homozygous phESC lines that carry MHC alleles that are common in the population were to be generated, it may serve as a hESC MHC matching bank [25]. In summary, if it would be possible to produce phESC lines as effectively as reported, such cells may become a major source of therapeutic histocompatible cell lines for fertile women, genetically related individuals and the general public. It is important to note that the extent of the NK-cell response against such transplants remains unclear and must be further examined. Immune responses against minor histocompatibility antigens and mitochondrial antigens may jeopardize grafted cells from genetically non-identical hESC lines (discussed below). It is likely that additional factors such as the tissue in question, the transplantation site and the extent of donor-derived vasculature would also influence transplantation outcomes.

DERIVATION OF EMBRYONIC STEM CELLS FROM SOMATIC CELL NUCLEAR TRANSFERRED OOCYTES AND ZYGOTES

The seminal experiment of producing live sheep from oocytes that had their nucleus replaced by somatic nucleus (somatic cell nuclear transfer - SCNT) proved for the first time that the genetic information in the somatic mammalian nucleus could be reprogrammed to the embryonic state [26]. Since then, this technique has been successfully translated to other species, including mouse, rabbit, cat, pig, cow and goat (reviewed in [27]). Cloned mouse embryos can give rise to ESC lines with a relatively high success rate [28]. Since the nucleus donor and the ESC line are genetically identical, except for mitochondrial antigens (discussed below), it has been suggested that differentiated tissues derived from human reprogrammed cell lines would not be rejected by the immune system of the donor.

Currently, there is still no proof for isolation of ntESCs from cloned humans oocytes and previous publications that described the derivation of such lines have been retracted [29, 24]. Nevertheless, these studies were probably the first to report derivation of hESCs from parthenogenetic embryos. If SCNT into human oocytes and the generation of histocompatible ESC lines could be achieved, a significant obstacle lies in acquiring the large numbers of oocytes that would be necessary for the clinical application of this technique. A novel approach that may alleviate this issue utilizes mitotically arrested zygotes to reprogram injected mitotic somatic nuclei, following chromosome removal [30]. After release from mitotic arrest, ~20% of the mouse cloned embryos developed to the blastocyst stage, and of these, ~5% developed to full term following transfer to pseudopregnant recipients (no live births were recorded). Cloned blastocysts could give rise to ESC lines that were shown to contribute extensively to chimeric embryos following injection into recipient blastocysts. The authors went on to prove that murine aneuploid zygotes (containing more than 2 polar bodies) could also serve as recipients to chromosome transfer following zygotic chromosome removal. This means that abnormal human embryos containing more than two nuclei and are therefore discarded following in vitro fertilization (about 5% of the embryos), could potentially be used to generate patient specific hESC lines. Still, it is important to note that SCNT into human oocytes or zygotes was not demonstrated to date.

One final immunological issue not addressed by derivation of hESC lines through SCNT is the potential immune response directed towards mitochondrial histocompatibility antigens. It is known that in mouse and rats certain amino acid substitutions in mitochondrial proteins can lead to generation of specific alloreactive cytotoxic T cells [31]. Therefore, it is possible that certain mitochondrial protein polymorphisms might become antigenic and initiate immune responses following transplantation of differentiated hESCs that were generated following SCNT. But, the small number of encoded proteins in mitochondria and the relatively small number of mitochondrial single nucleotide polymorphisms (~170), suggests that the risk of immune response towards donor-derived mitochondrial antigens would be considerably smaller than mismatched genomes. In accordance, it has been shown in cows that transplantation of organs derived from cloned embryos to the adult nuclear donor did not lead to immune response even though they express different mitochondrial haplotypes [32].

REPROGRAMMING OF SOMATIC CELLS BY FUSION WITH EMBRYONIC STEM CELLS

Similarly to the reprogramming effects of oocytes and zygotes, ESCs also have the capacity to reprogram somatic nucleus to the ESC-state. Since ESCs are small and have a high nucleus-to-cytoplasm ratio, reprogramming by SCNT into these cells is technically challenging and has not been reported to date. Still, fusion of somatic cells with ESC partners has a similar reprogramming effect on the somatic nucleus leading to reactivation of embryonic genes [33]. This concept has been proven recently for human somatic cells fused with hESCs in two studies that used foreskin fibroblasts and hESC-derived myeloid progenitors as fusion partners [34, 35]. In both cases, the resulting hybrid cell lines could gave rise to EBs in vitro and teratomas in vivo. Therefore, fusion of patient's somatic cells with hESCs could potentially circumvent the need for oocytes or embryos as vehicles to reprogram somatic cells to the ESC-stage.

Still, it seems unlikely that tetraploid hybrid cells would be considered suitable as therapeutic reagents due to their genomic instability. Moreover, such cell lines contain 4 copies of the MHC region and therefore, MHC matching is improbable. It is possible that in the future technical advancements will allow elimination of the ESC chromosomes before or after cell fusion. Alternatively, enucleated hESCs may preserve the capacity to reprogram the somatic genome. If these techniques will be developed, issues such as the extent of somatic reprogramming and full differentiation capacity of hESC/somatic cell fusions will have to be investigated further.

REPROGRAMMING SOMATIC CELLS BY DEFINED FACTORS

Successful experiments showing nuclear reprogramming by SCNT and by fusion of somatic cells with ESCs have led to the realization that oocytes, early zygotes and ESCs contain reprogramming factors. Successful reprogramming by fusion is of particular importance in trying to isolate these factors since measurements of gene expression can be carried out reliably in ESCs but not in oocytes and zygotes. Using this rationale, Shinya Yamanaka and colleagues have recently examined the ability of 24 genes that are preferentially expressed in mouse ESCs to reprogram somatic cells [36]. Introduction of the genes was carried out by retroviral transduction and then selection of cells that obtained the pluripotent state was carried out by a knock-in of drug resistance cassette into a gene that is specifically expressed in ES cells. They found that co-transfecting all the 24 factors into murine fetal fibroblasts could induce pluripotent state and colonies that had ESC morphology and expressed pluripotency markers were formed. They went on to determine which of 24 factors are necessary for the process and found that the four transcription factors that are critical for induction of pluripotent stem (iPS) cells are Oct3/4, Klf4, Sox2 and c-Myc. The authors also showed that iPS cells can differentiate into EBs, teratomas and contribute to all cell lineages including germline by generating adult chimeras [37].

During the past year, additional two independent laboratories have confirmed these results [38, 39] and very recently Yamanaka [40] and Thomson [41] groups showed that induction of pluripotency is also applicable to human cells. Yamanaka's group used the same four factors to induce pluripotency in human cells whereas Thomson group used Nanog and Lin28 instead of Klf4 and c-Myc. Furthermore, Yamanaka's group showed that iPS colonies could be isolated just by morphological criteria without the use of gene selection [40]. This elegant investigation showed for the first time that pluripotency can be induced using a relatively simple method of over-expressing transcription factors in somatic cells. From the immunological perspective, iPS cells would be fully compatible with the donor since there is no addition of genetic information to the cells.

Since induction of pluripotency by transcription factors is a very recent development it is still undetermined whether introduction of transgenes expressing Oct3/4, c-Myc and Klf4 is safe for clinical use. For example, as a result of c-Myc reactivation, tumors were found in about a fourth of the F1 offspring that were born to iPS cell injected chimeras [37]. Therefore, Therefore, strategies to induce pluripotency without stable integration of oncogenes and retroviruses must be developed. If these issues can be met, iPS cells will be generated per patient needs and it is very likely that they will become the primary source of differentiated cells.

CONCLUSION

The extent to which hESC-derived tissues will be used for therapeutics depends first and foremost on the capacity to develop differentiation protocols and methods for isolation of therapeutically relevant cells free from hazardous undifferentiated cells. Once that is successfully achieved, the immunological response represents the next obstacle that will strongly influence transplantation outcomes and hence the feasibility of such treatments. Our current knowledge indicates that following differentiation, hESCs express MHC-I and possibly MHC-II molecules and therefore might be rejected by adaptive immune responses. Circumventing this hurdle depends on the capacity to either actively prevent the immune response, for example by genetic manipulation of the MHC genes, or by the generation and use of patient specific hESC lines. Until very recently, it seemed that generating patient specific hESC lines would be possible only by SCNT into donated oocytes but the scarcity of donated oocytes, as well ethical issues regarding their obtainment and use, represent considerable obstacles for implementation of this technique.

Outlined in the review, several new key developments may now enable derivation of patient specific "tailor made" hESC lines. Parthenogenetic hESC lines that have the full donor MHC repertoire may be derived, but still their derivation and use is likely to be practical only for fertile women. In contrast, SCNT into genetically abnormal zygotes may be used to produce genetically identical hESC lines for virtually any nucleus donor (although mitochondrial antigens may still vary). It seems that the ethical and religious considerations using these two options would be minimal since parthenogenetic embryos cannot fully develop and abnormal zygotes are routinely discarded. Perhaps the most significant breakthrough, however, is the demonstration that human pluripotent stem cells can be induced in somatic cells by the introduction of four pluripotency-inducing genes. Adaptation of this technique for derivation of transplantation-safe patient-specific human pluripotent cell lines would bypass significant technical, as well as ethical issues that are associated with oocyte and zygote usage [42]. Relevant to all these derivation pathways, is the fact that *in vitro* differentiated hESCs might have somewhat modified expression signature of immunological antigens and other molecules that participate in immune responses. Hence, analysis of their immune properties will need to be further pursued prior to clinical use.

ACKNOWLEDGMENTS

I would like to thank Mr. C. Tang and Drs. T. Serwold, R. Ardehali and Y. Mayshar for critical reading of the manuscript. M.D. is supported by a Human Frontier Science Program postdoctoral fellowship.

REFERENCES

[1] Thomson, J. A. Itskovitz-Eldor, J. Shapiro, S. S. Waknitz, M. A. Swiergiel, J. J. Marshall, V. S. and Jones, J. M. (1998). Embryonic stem cell lines derived from human human blastocysts. *Science,* 282, 1145-1147.

[2] Reubinoff, B. E. Pera, M. F. Fong, C. Y. Trounson, A. and Bongso, A. (2000). Embryonic stem cell lines from human blastocysts: somatic differentiation in vitro. *Nat. Nat. Biotechnol.,* 18, 399-404.

[3] Hyslop, L. A. Armstrong, L. Stojkovic, M. and Lako, M. (2005). Human embryonic stem cells: biology and clinical implications. *Expert Rev. Mol. Med,* 7, 1-21.

[4] Drukker, M. and Benvenisty, N. (2004). The immunogenicity of human embryonic stem-derived cells. *Trends. Biotechnol.,* 22, 136-141.

[5] Rogers, N. J. and Lechler, R. I. (2001). Allorecognition. *Am. J. Transplant.,* 1, 97-102.

[6] Lechler, R. I. Sykes, M. Thomson, A. W. and Turka, L. A. (2005). Organ transplantation--how much of the promise has been realized? *Nat. Med,* 11, 605-613.

[7] Suchin, E. J. Langmuir, P. B. Palmer, E. Sayegh, M. H. Wells, A. D. and Turka, L. A. (2001). Quantifying the frequency of alloreactive T cells in vivo: new answers to an old old question. *J. Immunol,* 166, 973-981.

[8] Draper, J. S. Pigott, C. Thomson, J. A. and Andrews, P. W. (2002). Surface antigens of human embryonic stem cells: changes upon differentiation in culture. *J. Anat.,* 200, 249-258.

[9] Drukker, M. Katz, G. Urbach, A. Schuldiner, M. Markel, G. Itskovitz-Eldor, J. Reubinoff, B. Mandelboim, O. and Benvenisty, N. (2002). Characterization of the expression of MHC proteins in human embryonic stem cells. *Proc. Natl. Acad. Sci.* U. S. A., 99, 9864-9869.

[10] Drukker, M. Katchman, H. Katz, G. Even-Tov Friedman, S. Shezen, E. Hornstein, E. Mandelboim, O. Reisner, Y. and Benvenisty, N. (2006). Human embryonic stem cells and their differentiated derivatives are less susceptible to immune rejection than adult cells. *Stem Cells*, 24, 221-229.

[11] Raulet, D. H. (2006). Missing self recognition and self tolerance of natural killer (NK) cells. *Semin. Immunol*, 18, 145-150.

[12] Rideout, W. M., 3rd Hochedlinger, K. Kyba, M. Daley, G. Q. and Jaenisch, R. (2002). Correction of a genetic defect by nuclear transplantation and combined cell and gene therapy. *Cell*, 109, 17-27.

[13] Anderson, J. S. Bandi, S. Kaufman, D. S. and Akkina, R. (2006). Derivation of normal macrophages from human embryonic stem (hES) cells for applications in HIV gene therapy. *Retrovirology*, 3, 24.

[14] Kaufman, D. S. Hanson, E. T. Lewis, R. L. Auerbach, R. and Thomson, J. A. (2001). Hematopoietic colony-forming cells derived from human embryonic stem cells. *Proc. Natl. Acad. Sci. U. S. A.*, 98, 10716-10721.

[15] Slukvin, II Vodyanik, M. A. Thomson, J. A. Gumenyuk, M. E. and Choi, K. D. (2006). Directed differentiation of human embryonic stem cells into functional dendritic cells through the myeloid pathway. *J. Immunol,* 176, 2924-2932.

[16] Bradley, J. A. Bolton, E. M. and Pedersen, R. A. (2002). Stem cell medicine encounters encounters the immune system. *Nat. Rev. Immunol*, 2, 859-871.

[17] Allen, N. D. Barton, S. C. Hilton, K. Norris, M. L. and Surani, M. A. (1994). A functional analysis of imprinting in parthenogenetic embryonic stem cells. *Development*, 120, 1473-1482.

[18] Cibelli, J. B. Grant, K. A. Chapman, K. B. Cunniff, K. Worst, T. Green, H. L. Walker, S. J. Gutin, P. H. Vilner, L. Tabar, V. Dominko, T. Kane, J. Wettstein, P. J. Lanza, R. P. Studer, L. Vrana, K. E. and West, M. D. (2002). Parthenogenetic stem cells in nonhuman primates. *Science,* 295, 819.

[19] Revazova, E. S. Turovets, N. A. Kochetkova, O. D. Kindarova, L. B. Kuzmichev, L. N. Janus, J. D. and Pryzhkova, M. V. (2007). Patient-Specific Stem Cell Lines Derived from Human Parthenogenetic Blastocysts. *Cloning Stem Cells*.

[20] Kaufman, M. H. Barton, S. C. and Surani, M. A. (1977). Normal postimplantation development of mouse parthenogenetic embryos to the forelimb bud stage. *Nature*, 265, 53-55.

[21] Kim, K. Lerou, P. Yabuuchi, A. Lengerke, C. Ng, K. West, J. Kirby, A. Daly, M. J. and and Daley, G. Q. (2007). Histocompatible embryonic stem cells by parthenogenesis. *Science*, 315, 482-486.

[22] Hoglund, P. Sundback, J. Olsson-Alheim, M. Y. Johansson, M. Salcedo, M. Ohlen, C. Ljunggren, H. G. Sentman, C. L. and Karre, K. (1997). Host MHC class I gene control of NK-cell specificity in the mouse. *Immunol. Rev*, 155, 11-28.

[23] Kim, K. Ng, K. Rugg-Gunn, P., G. Shieh, J. Kirak, O. Jaenisch, R. Wakayama, T. Moore, M., A. Pedersen, R., A. and Daley, G., Q. (2007). Recombination Signatures Distinguish Embryonic Stem Cells Derived by Parthenogenesis and Somatic Cell Nuclear Transfer. *Cell Stem Cell*, 1, 1-7.

[24] Hwang, W. S. Ryu, Y. J. Park, J. H. Park, E. S. Lee, E. G. Koo, J. M. Chun, H. Y. Lee,

B. C. Kang, S. K. Kim, S. J. Ahn, C. Hwang, J. H. Park, K. Y. Cibelli, J. B. and Moon, S. Y. (2004). Evidence of a Pluripotent Human Embryonic Stem Cell Line Derived from a Cloned Blastocyst. *Science.*

[25] Taylor, C. J. Bolton, E. M. Pocock, S. Sharples, L. D. Pedersen, R. A. and Bradley, J. A. (2005). Banking on human embryonic stem cells: estimating the number of donor cell lines needed for HLA matching. *Lancet,* 366, 2019-2025.

[26] Campbell, K. H. McWhir, J. Ritchie, W. A. and Wilmut, I. (1996). Sheep cloned by nuclear transfer from a cultured cell line. *Nature,* 380, 64-66.

[27] Gurdon, J. B. and Byrne, J. A. (2003). The first half-century of nuclear transplantation. *Proc. Natl. Acad. Sci.* U. S. A, 100, 8048-8052.

[28] Hochedlinger, K. and Jaenisch, R. (2003). Nuclear transplantation, embryonic stem cells, and the potential for cell therapy. *N. Engl. J. Med,* 349, 275-286.

[29] Hwang, W. S. Roh, S. I. Lee, B. C. Kang, S. K. Kwon, D. K. Kim, S. Kim, S. J. Park, S. W. Kwon, H. S. Lee, C. K. Lee, J. B. Kim, J. M. Ahn, C. Paek, S. H. Chang, S. S. Koo, J. J. Yoon, H. S. Hwang, J. H. Hwang, Y. Y. Park, Y. S. Oh, S. K. Kim, H. S. Park, J. H. Moon, S. Y. and Schatten, G. (2005). Patient-specific embryonic stem cells derived from human SCNT blastocysts. *Science,* 308, 1777-1783.

[30] Egli, D. Rosains, J. Birkhoff, G. and Eggan, K. (2007). Developmental reprogramming after chromosome transfer into mitotic mouse zygotes. *Nature,* 447, 679-685.

[31] Loveland, B. Wang, C. R. Yonekawa, H. Hermel, E. and Lindahl, K. F. (1990). Maternally transmitted histocompatibility antigen of mice: a hydrophobic peptide of a mitochondrially encoded protein. *Cell,* 60, 971-980.

[32] Lanza, R. P. Chung, H. Y. Yoo, J. J. Wettstein, P. J. Blackwell, C. Borson, N. Hofmeister, E. Schuch, G. Soker, S. Moraes, C. T. West, M. D. and Atala, A. (2002). Generation of histocompatible tissues using nuclear transplantation. *Nat. Biotechnol,* 20, 689-696.

[33] Tada, M. Takahama, Y. Abe, K. Nakatsuji, N. and Tada, T. (2001). Nuclear reprogramming of somatic cells by in vitro hybridization with ES cells. *Curr. Biol,* 11, 1553-1558.

[34] Cowan, C. A. Atienza, J. Melton, D. A. and Eggan, K. (2005). Nuclear reprogramming of somatic cells after fusion with human embryonic stem cells. *Science,* 309, 1369-1373.

[35] Yu, J. Vodyanik, M. A. He, P. Slukvin, II and Thomson, J. A. (2006). Human embryonic stem cells reprogram myeloid precursors following cell-cell fusion. *Stem Cells,* 24, 168-176.

[36] Takahashi, K. and Yamanaka, S. (2006). Induction of pluripotent stem cells from mouse embryonic and adult fibroblast cultures by defined factors. *Cell,* 126, 663-676.

[37] Okita, K. Ichisaka, T. and Yamanaka, S. (2007). Generation of germline-competent induced pluripotent stem cells. *Nature,* 448, 313-317.

[38] Maherali, N. Sridharan, R. Xie, W. Utikal, J. Eminli, S. Arnold, K. Stadtfeld, M. Yachechko, R. Tchieu, J. Jaenisch, R. Plath, K. and Hochedlinger, K. (2007). Directly Reprogrammed Fibroblasts Show Global Epigenetic Remodeling and Widespread Tissue Contribution. *Cell Stem Cell,* 1, 55-70.

[39] Wernig, M. Meissner, A. Foreman, R. Brambrink, T. Ku, M. Hochedlinger, K.

Bernstein, B. E. and Jaenisch, R. (2007). In vitro reprogramming of fibroblasts into a pluripotent ES-cell-like state. *Nature*, 448, 318-324.

[40] Takahashi, K. Tanabe, K. Ohnuki, M. Narita, M. Ichisaka, T. Tomoda, K. and Yamanaka, S. (2007). Induction of pluripotent stem cells from adult human fibroblasts by defined factors. *Cell*, 131, 861-872.

[41] Yu, J. Vodyanik, M. A. Smuga-Otto, K. Antosiewicz-Bourget, J. Frane, J. L. Tian, S. Nie, J. Jonsdottir, G. A. Ruotti, V. Stewart, R. Slukvin, II and Thomson, J. A. (2007). Induced Pluripotent Stem Cell Lines Derived from Human Somatic Cells. *Science*.

[42] Green, R. M. (2007). Can we develop ethically universal embryonic stem-cell lines? *Nat. Rev. Genet*, 8, 480-485.

In: Encyclopedia of Stem Cell Research (2 Volume Set)   ISBN: 978-1-61761-835-2
Editor: Alexander L. Greene   © 2012 Nova Science Publishers, Inc.

Chapter LIII

PLURIPOTENT CELLS IN EMBRYOGENESIS AND IN TERATOMA FORMATION

O. F. Gordeeva

Institute of Developmental Biology Russian Academy of Sciences,
Moscow, Russia

ABSTRACT

Pluripotent cells of the early preimplantation embryo originate all types of somatic cell and germ cells of the adult organism. Permanent pluripotent cell lines (ES and EG cells) that were derived from an inner cell mass of blastocysts and primordial germ cells have a high proliferative potential and ability to differentiate in vitro into a wide variety of somatic and extraembryonic tissues as well as germ cells and to contribute to different organs of chimeric animals. In some cases pluripotent cells and primordial germ cells can generate teratomas, teratocarsinomas and some kinds of seminomas as the results of damages of differentiation programme of these cells. Experimental teratomas which formed after transplantation of undifferentiated ES and EG cells into immunocompromiced mice may provide a unique opportunity to study pluripotent cell specification and to develop novel approaches in carcinogenesis investigations. Research of signaling and metabolic pathways regulating the pluripotent cell maintenance and their multilineage differentiation are essential to search molecular targets to eliminate undifferentiated cells in tumors. Analysis of interactions between pluripotent cells and differentiated cells of the recipient animals, identification of the factors that may drive differentiation ES and EG cells in vivo contribute in understanding the mechanisms involved in the determination of cell fate during normal development and tumorigenesis. These data are important for development of effective and safe stem cell based technologies for prospective clinical treatment.

INTRODUCTION

Stem cells of adult animals have remarkable features: the ability to self-renew throughout all life generating new stem cells and to produce cells which can differentiate into various cell types. Strict control of the balance between proliferation and differentiation processes provides the maintenance of morphological stability and homeostasis in tissues with high cell turnover. The capacity of stem cells to reproduce themselves gives them the potential for unlimited life span and proliferation. When mechanisms underlying control proliferation rate in stem cells is injured they transit to abnormal tumor growth without terminal differentiation into appropriate somatic cells. Cancer stem cells arise from normal stem cells as a result of a direct genetic insult in themselves and disrupting cross talk between stem cells and their environmental niche. It was shown that abnormal stem cells are "the real culprits in cancer" in different tissues [1-5].

Pluripotent cells in early embryo as rapidly dividing and undifferentiated cells, similar with adult stem cells, potentially, can become cancer initiating cells in defined conditions and results in failure of the animal developmental program. Pluripotent cells can originates special kind of tumor called teratoma and teratocarcinoma. Teratoma tumor resembles disintegrated embryogenesis with a set of different immature histological structures that develop anisochronously whereas teratocarcinoma represented by undifferentiated cell mass displays the inability of pluripotent cells to start the differentiation [6]. Mechanisms that prevent tumor progression in the developing organism exist and lead to different malformations and then loss of vitality of embryos, but sometimes embryonic cancer cells survive and expand. Pluripotent cell lines of ES and EG cells represent a novel and interesting experimental system for fundamental research of the regulatory mechanisms that control stem cell pluripotency to understand and appreciate how stem cells orchestrate generation and maintenance different tissues and how to prevent and suppress abnormal growth and differentiation.

Embryo-Derived Pluripotent Stem Cell Lines

Pluripotent cells in a developing embryo appear in the late morula stage (at E3.0 for mouse) and are present until pre-gastrulating stages as early epiblast cells (E5.5). According to their spatial position the outer cell layer of morula becomes the trophoblast and the internal layer becomes the inner cell mass – a tiny little cell cluster that gives rise toall cell types of the adult organism and certain extraembryonic tissues. Pluripotent cells of inner cell mass generate parietal and visceral extraembryonic endoderm as well as a primitive ectoderm also called epiblast. At the start of gastrulation (egg cylinder, E6.5) pluripotent state terminates after segregation of the founders of primordial germ cells from other epiblast cells that originate ectodelmal, mesodermal and endodermal lineage. During this short period pluripotent cells fall within a diverse cell environment and are affected by different extracellular signals that promote subsequent developmental events (Figure 1). Interestingly, pluripotent cells have similar molecular profiles with primordial germ cells (PGC) exceptionally, despite the fact that PGCs are the committed cell population [7-10]. In particular, it was shown, that octamer-binding transcription factor Oct4 is crucial for the regulation of the pluripotent state and viability of germ cells [11].

To improve the research of early mammalian development were established permanent embryo-derived cell lines – embryonic stem cells (ES cells), trophoblast stem (TS cells) cells and extraembryonic endoderm cells(XEN) [12-14] were established. Pluripotent ES cell lines were derived from the inner cell mass of the blastocyst and early epiblast cells (Figure 2). At first, inner cell mass of mouse blastocyst was placed onto mitotically inactivated mouse primary embryonic fibroblasts and was grown in media conditioned by teratocarcinoma cell supplemented by fetal bovine serum. [13] At present, these conditions with mouse fibroblast feeder cells are most effective for derivation of ES cell lines of different species including human ES cells and most suitable for the propagation and expansion ES cells in vitro and preservation their stability [15].

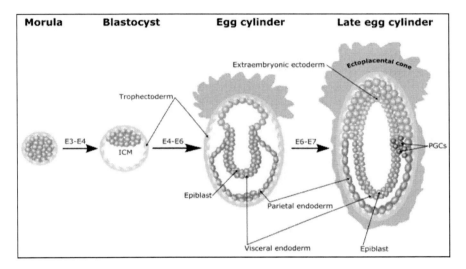

Figure 1. Pluripotent cells in early mammalian development. Pluripotent cells in developing embryo appear in late morula stage and are present until pre-gastrulating stages as early epiblast cells. Founders of primordial germ cells are recognized in distal epiblast prior to gastrulation.

Later, cell lines ehich possessed similar properties were derived from the primordial germ cells of post-implantation stage embryos and called embryonic germ cells (EG cells). ES and EG cells retain pluripotency during prolonged cultivation in vitro and can incorporate into embryoblasts and participate in development of all somatic tissues as well as germ line cells after transplantation into donor blastosysts [14,16-18]. EG cells distinguish from ES cells in their origin but after propagation in artificial culture conditions they take on similar characteristics and become capable to differentiate into somatic cells too (Figure 3). Recently, spermatogonial stem cells (GS cells) were derived from neonatal and adult mouse testis [19,20]. They display ES-like morphology, express a pluripotent cell marker, form teratomas after transplantation into immunocompromised mice and give rise chimerical animals with germ line transmission. Thus, primordial germ cells and spermatogonial cells can be reprogrammed in vitro in a cell population which has identical features with ES cells. No convincing and reproducible evidence about the derivation from the pluripotent cell line from the fetal or adult somatic cells without reprogramming procedure were presented yet (Figure 2).

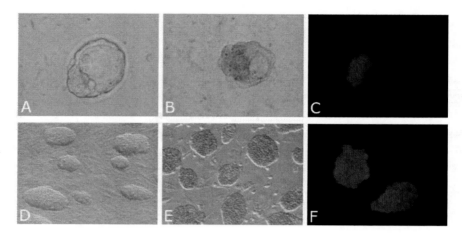

Figure 2. Pluripotent cells in mouse blastocyst (A-C) and in colonies of ES cells (D-F). Pluripotent ES cell lines were derived from the inner cell mass of blastocyst and retained similar features and expression of specific markers: alkaline phosphatase (B,E) and transcriptional factors Oct4 (C, F). Magnification 300x.

Embryonal teratocarcinoma cell (EC) lines are malignant counterparts of ES and EG cells that were derived from different genital tumors. However, EC cell lines unlike ES and EG cells vary in their differentiation potential, pluripotent cell lines have the ability to differentiate into derivatives of three germ layers and nullipotent cell lines have restricted capacity for self-renewal only [21,22]. This distinction is tightly connected with the features and lineage of tumor initiating cells which were the founders of the EC cell line. Mintz and Illmensee injected METT1 teratocarcinomal cells into mouse blastocysts and produced viable chimerical mice, that contained cells with donor genotype in somatic tissues and germ cells. Tumorigenesis rate in the adult mosaic animals was insignificantly higher than in the reference group. This experiment demonstrated the opportunity of the EC cells to contribute in embryogenesis and the transmission of teratocarcinomal genotype to germ line and then to the next generation [23-25] but it indicated that the successful result can be achieved only in the case of using euploid teratocarcinomal cell lines. Authors hypothesized that the changes in gene expression due to tissue disorganization and may apply to some malignancies of stem cells of certain tissues. Unfortunately, these data were not reproduced in other laboratories and question about normalization of malignant teratocarcinomal cells in embryogenesis is still open [26].

At present, ES, EG, and EC cell pluripotency is evaluated by producing chimeric animal with germ line transmission and generation of experimental teratomas in adult immunocompromised mice. It is well known that mammalian ES, EG and EC cells form teratomas and teratocarcinomas when they engraft into an immuno-deficient host (Nude and SCID/Beige mouse strain). Furthermore, it is the only way to test the pluripotency of human and primate ES cells because there are ethical limitations. Teratomas formed by pluripotent cells consist of the variety of differentiated tissues representative of three germ layers.

Undoubtedly, histological analysis of teratomas is more reliable for estimation of developmental potential than immunofluorescent assays of differentiating cells in vitro [27].

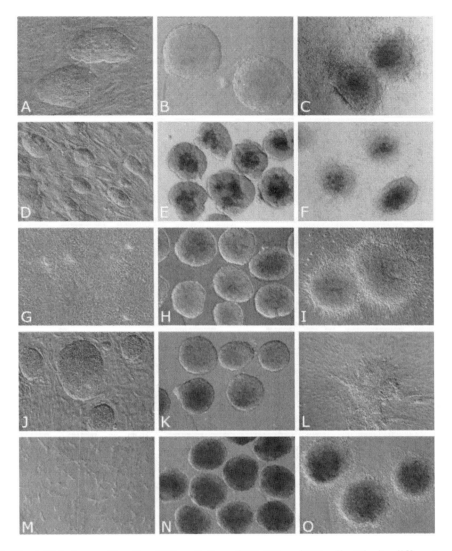

Figure 3. The initial stages of in vitro differentiation of ES, EG and EC cells. Dispite different origins all cell lines can form embryoid bodies of similar morphology. Mouse ES R1 cells (A-C), mouse EGC-10 cells (D-F), mouse EC F9 (G-I), human ES M1 (J-L), human EC PA-1 (M-O). Magnification: A, B 300x, rest 200x.

Reconstructed ES cells or NTES cells generated by somatic nuclear transfer and by fusion ES cells with differentiated cells have the similar developmental potentials with wild type ES cells. These results prove the postulate that nuclei from terminal differentiated cells didn't restrict their potential to support the animal development. In case of multiple genetic and epigenetic changes in the donor nucleus or resulted from nuclear injuries during manipulation procedures cloned mice are dying during early development and the surviving clones have different defects whereas ES cell lines can be derived successfully. Efficiency of cloned mice generation is significantly lower than rate of reconstructed ES establishment (2% vs. 20%) [28].

The crucial question about capacity of cancer cell nucleus to support normal development was investigated recently [29,30]. Nuclear transplantation of tumor cells into oocytes resulted in generation cloned fetus and adult animals only in the case of medulloblastoma, melanoma and three pluripotent teratocarcinoma cell lines. Interestingly, F9 NT ES cells showed neither differentiation into teratomas nor contribution to mosaic embryos while several P19 NT ES chimeras developed into term but pups were afflicted with head and neck teratocarcinomas and were unviable, furthermore differentiation this line in teratomas was limited. METT-1 NT ES chimeric adult animals were morphologically normal [29]. Strikingly, teratoma analysis of corresponding EC and EC NT ES cell lines displayed an identical potential of parental and NT ES cell lines. R. Jaenisch and colleagues show that nuclei of leukemia, lymphoma and breast cancer cells can support the development to the blastocyst stage but they failed to produce NT ES cell lines. However, NTES cells and chimerical animals can be generated from RAS-inducible melanoma cell clone blastocysts. Note, that all chimeras produced from melanoma NT ES cells developed multiple primary melanoma lesions [30].

Study of reprogramming of somatic cells by fusion between ES or EG cells and differentiated cells demonstrated the dominance of pluripotent partner phenotype over a differentiated cell one. In most stable tetraploid hybrids somatic cell chromosomes undergo reprogramming via demethylation, reactivation of pluripotency-associated gene expression and activation of the silent somatic X-chromosome [31-35].

Together, these results suggest the following conclusions:

1) Pluripotency as a capacity of cells to differentiate into various cell type including germ cells with equal probability, can be realized only in genetically and epigenetically stable ES, EG and some EC cell lines maintaining the characteristic gene expression profile of pluripotent cells

2) Chimerical animals producing and experimental teratoma generation may be used for measuring of pluripotency tests

3) In the most cases NT ES cell developmental potential depends on the corrected genetic and epigenetic state of the donor nucleus and the absence of genome abnormalities that hinder their differentiation into various cell types.

Molecular Mechanisms Underlying Pluripotency of ES, EG and EC Cells

The pluripotency is maintained by a complex of extracellular and intracellular factors that set up a specific pattern of the gene expression. Molecular signaling network that working in pluripotent cells controls self-renewal and maintenance of the pluripotent cell identity. When the external signals from the environment niche (culture media for pluripotent cell lines) do change and the balance of proliferation and differentiation promoting factors alters then the pluripotent cells are involved in the lineages' determination.

Octamer-binding homeobox transcriptional factor POU family Oct4 was the first identified factor that sustained the pluripotent phenotype in ES and EC cells as well as in pluripotent cells of pre-implantation embryo and in germ cells [11,36]. Two other transcriptional factors Sox2 and FoxD3 can interact with Oct4, in particular, Sox2 and Oct4 bind to adjacent cites within the enhancer of several target genes and act cooperatively to stimulate the transcription [37]. Recently, the second homeodomain transcription factor Nanog that regulate the plutipotent state was identified in the mouse and human. Nanog expression is detected firstly in late morulae stage and then it decreases in epiblast cells. Nanog is detectable in migrating primordial germ cells and residing in early gonocytes but it is not expressed in adult gonads [38-41].

Obviously, Oct4, Nanog and Sox2 function as suppressors of differentiation of inner cell mass into extraembryonic lineages – trophoblast and extraembryonic endoderm but they act cooperatively with many other genes that are elements of developmental programme of pluripotent cells. Another component of the regulation of gene expression pattern in mouse and human ES cells is the polycomb group (PcG) proteins that directly repress a large cohort of differentiation regulators. Using genome-wide location analysis in murine ES cells, there was found that the Polycomb repressive complexes PRC1 and PRC2 co-occupied 512 genes, many of which encode transcription factors with important roles in development [42, 43].

The investigation of signaling pathways that underlay pluripotent state maintenance in ES cells demonstrated that several differences exist between mouse and human ES cells. It was shown that leukemia inhibitory factor (LIF, and differentiation inhibitory factor Dia) is essential for self-renewal mouse ES and EG cells but it is not necessary for pre-gastrulating mouse development [44-47]. LIF is bound to the LIF receptor and activates the signal transducer and activator of transcription STAT-3. Phosphorilated STAT-3 translocates into the nucleus and regulates target genes transcription. Mouse ES cells growing without feeder cells begin to differentiate after several days of LIF withdrawal. On the other hand, human ES cells are not sensitive to LIF absence and the supplement to this factor to culture media does not prevent differentiation [48]. With the presence of LIF, bone morphogenetic protein BMP4 enhance the self-renewal of ES cells and activate Id (inhibitor of differentiation) genes. On the contrary, without LIF, BMP4 activates other signaling cascades that promote the differentiation of mouse ES cells. BMP4 also stimulates human ES cells to differentiate into trophoblast cell or mesodermal precursors [41, 49-51].

The activation of the WNT pathway leads to inhibition of glycogen-synthase kinase (GSK3) in undifferentiated mouse and human ES cells and blocks their differentiation [52-54]. Several groups demonstrated that the preserving of an undifferentiated state of human ES cells requires Activin and Nodal signaling interaction with FGF2 cascade [55, 56]. Our experiments for study expression of TGFβ superfamily factors and their receptors at the early stage of differentiation of human and mouse ES and EC do not reveal significant differences in expression profiles despite the diverse origin and species differences of studied cell lines [57]. We suppose that expression of Nodal, Activin, BMP and TGFβ factors in ES and EC cells reflects the situation in pre-gastrulating epiblast where spatial-temporal distribution of this factor drives the development of different areas of an embryo. However, the position information characteristic for the developing embryo is disturbed in ES and EC cells growing in vitro and spatial-temporal gradients of these signal factors are absent and therefore, every cell secrets whole set of ligands. The strict control of transcription and protein activity balance of TGFβ superfamily factors prevents differentiation more probably, than promote the self-renewal ES and EC cells. The unique combinatorial complex of signal pathways existing in ES cells provides the equal expectancies to initiate the differentiation of ectodermal, endodermal and mesodermal precursors. It is still unclear why nullipotent EC F9 cells that have similar to ES cells signaling pathways cannot initiate the spontaneous differentiation in vitro and in vivo. It is necessary to ascertain the disrupted components of regulation pathways that can direct EC cell differentiation and prevent their overgrowth.

SPONTANEOUS AND EXPERIMENTAL TERATOMAS AND TERATOCARCINOMAS

Germ cell tumors of the testis and the ovary have been studied extensively in humans and experimental animals. These spontaneous and experimentally induced tumors provide numerous data about the differentiation of tumor stem cells and the regulation of their growth. Teratomas and teratocarcinomas proved to be one of the best experimental models for elucidating the histogenesis of these tumors and the nature of their undifferentiated stem cells. The malignancy of teratocarcinoma stem cells is determined genetically but can be regulated epigenetically. Development of teratocarcinoma stem cells parallels the events in the normal embryo, suggesting that events in the tumor have their normal regulatory counterparts in the embryogenesis. Cumulative data indicate that neoplastic development of murine embryonic cells is just one of the possible ontogenic pathways these cells can take while proliferating in various developmental fields.

Spontaneous testicular and ovarian teratomas and teratocarcinamas were described in human, mouse and horses as rare tumors [6,58-60]. Stevens and Little demonstrated that teratomas arised in the testes of about 1% male of 129 strain mice [6]. Ovarian teratomas or benign ovarian cysts arisen from parthenogeneticaly activated oocytes begun development and then became disorganized embryonic cell structures [58]. Testicular germ cell tumors that were detected in young post-pubertal man, probably, arose from abnormal gonocytes in seminal tubules and progressed after birth. These cancers can either be benign or malignant. All of the well-known germinal tumors are divided into seminomas that consist of the cells resembling primordial germ cells and non-seminomas that contain a heterogeneous somatic cell population with undifferentiated teratocarcinoma cells. Recently, it was shown in the diagnostic study of different types of germ cell tumor that specific cancer-testicular antigen MAGE-4 is expressed only in classical seminoma cells while non-seminoma cells are negative for this antigen [61]. Hypothesis about the origin of germinal tumor from primordial germ cells was confirmed in the numerous experimental studies of teratomas that were induced by transplantation of genital ridge cells of mouse fetuses, between 11-13,5 days of development, into ectopic sites [22, 62,63]. Some of these experimental tumors were evidently highly malignant and reproduced the parental tumor phenotype in serial transplantation experiments. Later, the tumorigenic cell populations were expanded in vitro and permanent embryonal teratocarcinoma (EC) cell lines were established. Kleinsmith and Pierce demonstrated the stem-cell feature of EC cells in experiment with EC cell transplantation into the secondary host [64]. Inner cell mass and epiblast cells as well as ES and EG cells can initiate experimental teratomas after transplantation of them into different tissue sites of adult animals [65,66]. After human ES and EG cell lines were derived they were tested on the capacity to form experimental teratomas for the confirmation of their pluripotent state.

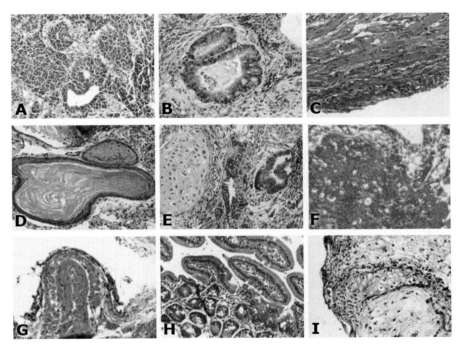

Figure 4. Differentiation of ES, EG and EC cells in experimental teratomas formed after transplantation into peritoneal cavities of immunocompromised hosts. Histological analysis revealed various types of differentiated cells in the tumors, including ectodermal, mesodermal and endodermal lineages: neural rosettes in mouse ES cell teratoma (A), ciliated epithelium of intestinal type in mouse ES cell teratoma (B), striated muscles in mouse (C) and human ES teratotoma (G), keratinized epithelium in mouse EG cell teratoma (D), hyaline cartilage in mouse EG cell teratoma (E) and human ES cell teratoma (I), intestinal crypts in human ES cell teratoma (H) and undifferentiated teratocarcinoma cell of mouse EC F9 line (F).

Teratomas test may also be helpful and informative to understand the developmental and tumorigenic potential of different precursor cells that originate from embryonic or adult stem cells differentiating in vitro. For example, developmental potential of undifferentiated mouse ES cells and embryoid bodies that have differentiated before in vitro during 4-5 days was compared in dynamic of the teratoma formation [67,68]. Approximately 3x105 cells in ES colonies or embryoid bodies growing on an acetate-cellulose membrane were implanted into peritoneal cavities of irradiated mice and then observed grafting cell differentiation within 2,3,4 and 6 week. Two weeks after the onset of each experimental series, cell aggregations resulting from proliferation and migration of the grafted cells appeared on the implanted membranes. By that time, the colonies of undifferentiated ESC had merged and acquired an asymmetric shape, while outgrowths of the embryoid bodies had increased in size. The cell aggregations contained no morphologically differentiated cell types. In addition to ESC, numerous fibroblasts-like cells of the recipient encapsulating the foreign body were found on the filters. These fibroblasts-like cells were also present on the membranes isolated from the abdominal cavity of the control animals. Note that small teratomas have been revealed in three out of five animals that received the implants of membranes with the embryoid bodies.

After three and six weeks, all experimental animals developed tumors in the region of contact between the membrane and loops of the small intestine, which were much larger than the tumors found after two weeks. No tumor growth was detected in other tissues.

Histological analysis revealed various types of differentiated cells in the tumors, including ectodermal (keratinized epithelium and neural ganglion cells, neural rosettes), mesodermal (hyaline cartilage and bone, striated and smooth muscles, adipocytes and connective tissue), and endodermal (secreted and ciliated epithelium of intestinal and respiratory types) lineages (Figure 4). Lacunar blood vessels (most likely originating from the recipient) and large hemorrhagic zones were found in the tumors.

Our experiments have revealed no significant differences in the types of differentiation of pluripotent cells in the ESC colonies and inner cells of the embryoid bodies, although the embryoid bodies attached to the substrate are a heterogeneous population including pluripotent, differentiated, and committed cells. On the other hand, the embryoid body cells have produced tumors much more rapidly, which agrees with the concept that they are an activated cell population.

To understand whether pluripotent cells remain in experimental teratomas we evaluated expression of pluripotent and germ line specific genes in ES cells and embryoid bodies prior to transplantation and in all types of experimental teratomas. Expression analysis showed that in all studied tumors cell populations exist, they expressed Oct4, Nanog, Stella, Fragilis, Dazl and Vasa/Mvh genes which are expressed by the initial transplanted cells [68, and unpublished data]. The same pattern of expression was revealed for mouse EG and EC cells and in teratomas formed by these cells into peritoneal cavities of Nude strain immuno-deficient mice (Figure 5).

Our results and that of other laboratories demonstrated that undifferentiated ES and EG cells and differentiating embryoid bodies have similar developmental potencies to differentiate into derivatives of three germ layers in teratomas that dramatically diverse from teratocarcinomas generating by EC F9 cell which contain only undifferentiated cells. It remains unclear whether these Oct4, Nanog, Stella, Dazl, Vasa positive cells in different types of experimental ES and EG teratomas have normal or cancer nature and why residual undifferentiated cells remained there so long together with well-differentiated structures. The first assumption, that undifferentiated cells in ES and EG teratomas are teratocarcinoma cells that resulted after transformation events during their differentiation in vivo. It was shown that human ES cells accumulate different mutations and epigenetic modifications during propagation in vitro and the number of aneuploid cells increases at the late passages especially when trypsin and collagenase are used for splitting cells [69-71]. Most likely, different genetic rearrangements may take place during experimental teratoma formation too.

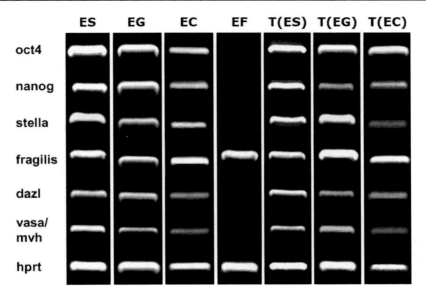

Figure 5. Expression of genes specific for pluripotent and germ line cells in mouse ES, EG and EC cells and in teratomas formed by these lines.

Another hypothesis, which explains the existence of residual undifferentiated cells in experimental teratomas, based on fundamental features of ES and EG cells. Comparative transcriptional profiling studies of ES, EG, EC cells and different embryonic and adult cells display the dissimilarity of ES cells from well-characterized cell types appearing during ontogenesis of this species. ES and EG cells have intermediate status between epiblast cells and primordial germ cells. This steady state provides them the same possibilities to proliferate actively (symmetric divisions) and to start differentiation of all the lineages with equal expectancy. During differentiation in teratomas ES and EG cells realize their developmental potentials and they give rise to the representative of all somatic lineages and early primordial germ cells. Precursors of germ cells stay immature like the most other histological structures presented in teratomas. This statement may be true for nullipotent teratocarcinomal cells that have only one cell destined to be abnormal intermediate progenitors of primordial germ cells. It will be interesting to model the experimental situations when teratomas would not contain the undifferentiated cell or these cells completely differentiate into different types of somatic cells. It is necessary to determine the critical cell number of grafted pluripotent and teratocarcinoma cells for growth and differentiation of experimental teratomas. What genetic mechanisms are involved in transformation of ES cells to EC cells? What are the ways to exterminate the cancer initiating cells? These questions need answers to understand the basic mechanisms underlying the early events of embryogenesis and for development of ES cell technologies for future therapeutic applications. Resent advances in stem cells research provide new insight in mechanisms of tissues development and function in embryo and adult individual and open new perspectives in understanding the cause of many pathologies including different cancers.

CONCLUSION

One of the most important lessons that came from the recent studies of stem cells biology postulates that the deregulation of signaling pathways that involved control of self-renewal and differentiation of stem cells and progenitors leads to tumorigenesis in tissues with high cell turnover [1,5]. Pluripotent cells that originate all cell types of organisms and some extraembryonic tissues theoretically can be transformed into wide variety of embryonic tumors. ES and EG cells are artificial counterparts of pluripotent cells of embryos and they retain their features. Obviously, genetic failures and epigenetic modifications in stem cells resulting in uncontrolled growth are true cases of tumorigenesis. Embryonic stem cells and different rapidly dividing multipotent cells deriving from pluripotent cells can became cancer initiating cells after long-term propagation in vitro and may be dangerous for therapeutic stem cells application.

On the other hand, embryonic stem cell lines may be used as a powerful experimental model and tool to develop new approaches in cancer research that directed towards the understanding of lineages of different embryonic and neonatal tumors. The combination of different genetic engineering technologies with transplantation assays provides new opportunities for cancer research focused on searching target genes involved in development of teratomas, teratocarcinomas or other embryonic malignancies. Utilizing of mutant ES cell lines may help us to discover many connections between normal stem cells and tumor initiating cells and to develop effective drugs target in cancer stem cells.

REFERENCES

[1]   Reya, T., Morrison, S.J., Clarke, M.F. and Weissman, I.L. (2001). Stem cells, cancer, and cancer stem cells. *Nature,* 414, 105-111.

[2]   Appelbaum, F.R., Rowe, J.M., Radich, J. and Dick, J.E. (2001*).* Acute myeloid leukemia. *Hematology Am Soc Hematol Educ Program.*, 62-86.

[3]   Dick, J.E. (2003). Breast cancer stem cells revealed. *PNAS,* 100, 3547-3549.

[4]   Clarke, M.F. and Becker, M.W. (2006). *Stem cells: The Real Culprits in Cancer?* Scientific American, July, 53-59.

[5]   Morrison, S.J. and Kimble, J. (2006). Asymmetric and symmetric stem-cell divisions in development and cancer. *Nature,* 441, 1068-1074.

[6]   Stevens, L.C. and Little, C.C. (1954). Spontaneous testicular teratomas in an inbred strain of mice. *Proc Natl Acad Sci U S A,* 40, 1080-1087.

[7]   D'Amour K.A. and Gage F.H. (2003). Genetic and functional differences between multipotent neural and pluripotent embryonic stem cells. *Proc. Natl. Acad. Sci.* USA., 100 (suppl 1), 11866-11872.

[8]   Ramalho-Santos, M., Yoon S., Matsuzaki Y., Mulligan R.C. and Melton D.A. (2002). «Stemness»: transcriptional profiling of embrionic and adult stem cells. *Science,* 298, 597-600

[9]   Tanaka, T.S., Kunath, T., Kimber, W.L., Jaradat, S.A., Stagg, C.A., Usuda, M., Yokota, T., Niwa, H., Rossant. J. and Ko, M.S. (2002). Gene expression profiling of embryo-derived stem cells reveals candidate genes associated with pluripotency and lineage

specificity. *Genome Res*, 12, 1921-1928

[10] Tanaka, T.S., Jaradat, S.A., Lim, M.K., Kargul, G.J., Wang, X., Grahovac, M.J., Pantano, S., Sano, Y., Piao, Y., Nagaraja, R., Doi, H., Wood, W.H. 3rd, Becker, K.G. and Ko. M.S (2000). Genome-wide expression profiling of mid-gestation placenta and embryo using a 15,000 mouse developmental cDNA microarray. *Proc. Natl. Acad. Sci. U S A.*, 97(16), 9127-9132.

[11] Palmieri, S.L., Peter, W., Hess, H. and Scholer, H.R. (1994). Oct-4 transcription factor is differentially expressed in the mouse embryo during establishment of the first two extraembryonic cell lineages involved in implantation. *Dev Biol.*, 166, 259-267.

[12] Evans, M.J.and Kaufman, M.H. (1981). Establishment in culture of pluripotential cells from mouse embryos. *Nature*, 292, 154-156.

[13] Martin, G.R. (1981). Isolation of pluripotent cell line from early mouse embryo cultured in medium conditioned by teratocarcinoma stem cells. *Proc. Natl. Acad. Sci.* USA., 78, 7634-7638.

[14] Rossant, J. (2001). Stem cells from mammalian blastocyst. *Stem Cells*, 19, 477-482.

[15] Thomson, J.A., Itskovitz-Eldor, J., Shapiro, S.S., Waknitz, M.A., Swiergiel, J.J, Marshall, V.S. and Jones J.M. (1998). Embryonic stem cell lines derived from human blastocysts. *Science*, 282(5391), 1145-1147.

[16] Matsui, Y., Zsebo, K., Hogan, B.L. (1992). Derivation of pluripotential embryonic stem cells from murine primordial germ cells in culture. *Cell*, 70, 841-847

[17] Resnick, J.L., Bixler, L.S., Cheng, L and Donovan, P.J. (1992). Long-term proliferation of mouse primordial germ cells in culture. *Nature*, 359, 550-551

[18] Bradley, A., Evans, M., Kaufman, M.H. and Robertson, E. (1984). Formation of germ-line chimaeras from embryo-derived teratocarcinoma cell lines. *Nature,* 309,255-256.

[19] Kanatsu-Shinohara, M., Inoue, K., Lee, J., Yoshimoto, M., Ogonuki, N., Miki, H., Baba, S., Kato, T., Kazuki, Y., Toyokuni, S., Toyoshima, M., Niwa, O., Oshimura, M., Heike, T., Nakahata, T., Ishino, F., Ogura, A. and Shinohara, T.(2004). Generation of pluripotent stem cells from neonatal mouse testis. *Cell*, 119, 1001-1012.

[20] Guan, K., Nayernia, K., Maier, L.S., Wagner, S., Dressel, R., Lee, J.H., Nolte, J., Wolf, F., Li, M., Engel, W. and Hasenfuss, G. (2006). Pluripotency of spermatogonial stem cells from adult mouse testis. *Nature*, 440, 1199-1203.

[21] Martin, G.R. and Evans, M.J. (1975). Differentiation of clonal lines of teratocarcinoma cells: formation of embryoid bodies in vitro. *Proc Natl Acad Sci U S A*, 72, 1441-1445.

[22] Andrews, P.W. (2002*).* From teratocarcinomas to embryonic stem cells. *Philos Trans R Soc Lond B Biol Sci.*, 357, 405-417.

[23] Mintz, B. and Illmensee, K. (1975). Normal genetically mosaic mice produced from malignant teratocarcinoma cells. *Proc Natl Acad Sci U S A.*, 72, 3585-3589.

[24] Illmensee, K. and Mintz, B. (1976). Totipotency and normal differentiation of single teratocarcinoma cells cloned by injection into blastocysts. *Proc Natl Acad Sci U S A*, 73, 549-553.

[25] Stewart, T.A. and Mintz, B. (1981). Successive generations of mice produced from an established culture line of euploid teratocarcinoma cells. *Proc Natl Acad Sci U S A*, 78, 6314-6318.

[26] Rossant, J. and McBurney, M.W (1982). The developmental potential of a euploid male teratocarcinoma cell line after blastocyst injection. *J Embryol Exp Morphol*, 70, 99-112.

[27] Przyborski, S.A. (2005). Differentiation of Human Embryonic Stem Cells After Transplantation in Immune-Deficient Mice. *Stem Cells*, 23, 1242-1250.

[28] Hochedlinger, K. and Jaenisch, R. (2006). Nuclear reprogramming and pluripotency. *Nature*, 441, 1061-1067

[29] Blelloch, R.H., Hochedlinger, K., Yamada, Y., Brennan, C., Kim, M., Mintz, B., Chin, L. and Jaenisch, R. (2004). Nuclear cloning of embryonal carcinoma cells. *Proc Natl Acad Sci U S A*, 101, 13985-13990.

[30] Hochedlinger, K., Blelloch, R., Brennan, C., Yamada, Y., Kim, M., Chin, L. and Jaenisch, R. (2004). Reprogramming of a melanoma genome by nuclear transplantation. *Genes Dev.*, 18, 1875-1885.

[31] Tada, M., Tada, T., Lefebvre, L., Barton, S.C. and Surani, M.A. (1997). Embryonic germ cells induce epigenetic reprogramming of somatic nucleus in hybrid cells. *EMBO J.*, 16, 6510-6520.

[32] Tada, M., Takahama, Y., Abe, K., Nakatsuji, N. and Tada, T. (2001). Nuclear reprogramming of somatic cells by in vitro hybridization with ES cells. *Curr Biol.*, 11, 1553-1558.

[33] Tada, M., Morizane, A., Kimura, H., Kawasaki, H., Ainscough, J.F., Sasai, Y., Nakatsuji, N. and Tada, T. (2003). Pluripotency of reprogrammed somatic genomes in embryonic stem hybrid cells. *Dev Dyn.*, 227, 504-510.

[34] Bortvin, A., Eggan, K., Skaletsky, H., Akutsu, H., Berry, D.L., Yanagimachi, R., Page, D.C. and Jaenisch, R. (2003). Incomplete reactivation of Oct4-related genes in mouse embryos cloned from somatic nuclei. *Development*, 130, 1673-1680.

[35] Cowan, C.A, Atienza, J., Melton, D.A. and Eggan, K. Nuclear reprogramming of somatic cells after fusion with human embryonic stem cells. *Science*, 309, 1369-1373.

[36] Niwa, H., Miyazaki. J. and Smith, A.G. (2000). Quantitative expression of Oct-3/4 defines differentiation, dedifferentiation or self-renewal of ES cells. *Nat Genet.*, 24, 372-376.

[37] Boiani, M. and Schöler, H.R. (2005). Regulatory networks in embryo-derived pluripotent stem cells. *Nat. Rev. Mol. Cell Biol.*, 6, 872-884.

[38] Chambers, I., Colby, D., Robertson, M., Nichols, J., Lee, S., Tweedie, S. and Smith, A. (2003). Functional expression cloning of Nanog, a pluripotency sustaining factor in embryonic stem cells. Cell, 113, 643-655.

[39] Mitsui, K., Tokuzawa, Y., Itoh, H., Segawa, K., Murakami, M., Takahashi, K., Maruyama, M., Maeda, M. and Yamanaka, S. (2003). The homeoprotein Nanog is required for maintenance of pluripotency in mouse epiblast and ES cells. *Cell*, 113, 631-642.

[40] Hart, A.H., Hartley, L., Ibrahim, M. and Robb, L. (2004). Identification, cloning and expression analysis of the pluripotency promoting Nanog genes in mouse and human. *Dev Dyn.*, 230, 187-198.

[41] Chambers, I. and Smith, A. (2004). Self-renewal of teratocarcinoma and embryonic stem cells. *Oncogene*, 23, 7150-7160.

[42] Boyer, L.A., Plath, K., Zeitlinger, J., Brambrink, T., Medeiros, L.A., Lee, T.I., Levine, S.S., Wernig, M., Tajonar, A., Ray, M.K., Bell, G.W., Otte, A.P., Vidal, M., Gifford, D.K., Young, R.A. and Jaenisch, R. (2006). Polycomb complexes repress developmental regulators in murine embryonic stem cells. *Nature*, 441, 349-353.

[43] Lee, T.I., Jenner, R.G., Boyer, L.A., Guenthe, M.G., Levine, S.S., Kumar, R.M., Chevalier, B., Johnstone, S.E., Cole, M.F., Isono, K., Koseki, H., Fuchikami, T., Abe, K., Murray, H.L., Zucker, J.P., Yuan, B., Bell, G.W., Herbolsheimer, E., Hannett, N.M., Sun, K., Odom, D.T., Otte, A.P., Volkert, T.L., Bartel, D.P., Melton, D.A., Gifford, D.K., Jaenisch, R. and Young, R.A. (2006). Control of developmental

regulators by Polycomb in human embryonic stem cells. *Cell*, 125, 301-313.

[44] Smith, A.G., Heath, J.K., Donaldson, D.D., Wong, G.G., Moreau, J., Stahl, M. and Rogers, D. (1988). Myeloid leukaemia inhibitory factor maintains the developmental potential of embryonic stem cells. *Nature,* 336, 684-687.

[45] Boeuf, H., Hauss, C., Graeve, F.D., Baran, N. and Kedinger, C. (1997). Leukemia inhibitory factor-dependent transcriptional activation in embryonic stem cells. *J Cell Biol.,* 138, 1207-1217.

[46] Niwa, H., Burdon, T., Chambers, I. and Smith, A. (1998). Self-renewal of pluripotent embryonic stem cells is mediated via activation of STAT3. *Genes Dev.,* 12, 2048-2060.

[47] Nichols, J., Davidson, D., Taga, T., Yoshida, K., Chambers, I. and Smith, A. (1996). Complementary tissue-specific expression of LIF and LIF-receptor mRNAs in early mouse embryogenesis. *Mech Dev.,* 57, 123-131.

[48] Daheron, L., Opitz, S.L., Zaehres, H., Lensch, W.M., Andrews, P.W., Itskovitz-Eldor, J. and Daley, G.Q. (2004). LIF/STAT3 signaling fails to maintain self-renewal of human embryonic stem cells. *Stem Cells,* 22, 770-778.

[49] Ying, Q.L., Nichols, J., Chambers, I. and Smith, A. (2003). BMP induction of Id proteins suppresses differentiation and sustains embryonic stem cell self-renewal in collaboration with STAT3. *Cell*, 115, 281-292.

[50] Gerami-Naini, B., Dovzhenko, O.V., Durning, M., Wegner, F.H., Thomson, J.A. and Golos, T.G. (2004). Trophoblast differentiation in embryoid bodies derived from human embryonic stem cells. *Endocrinology*, 145, 1517-1524.

[51] Schuldiner, M., Yanuka, O., Itskovitz-Eldor, J., Melton, D.A. and Benvenisty, N. (2000). Effects of eight growth factors on the differentiation of cells derived from human embryonic stem cells. *Proc Natl Acad Sci U S A,* 97, 11307-11312.

[52] Sato, N., Meijer, L., Skaltsounis, L., Greengard, P., Brivanlou, A.H. (2004). Maintenance of pluripotency in human and mouse embryonic stem cells through activation of Wnt signaling by a pharmacological GSK-3-specific inhibitor. *Nat Med.*, 10, 55-63.

[53] Paling, N.R., Wheadon, H., Bone, H.K. and Welham, M.J. (2004). Regulation of embryonic stem cell self-renewal by phosphoinositide 3-kinase-dependent signaling. *J Biol Chem.*, 279, 48063-48070.

[54] Hao, J., Li, T.G., Qi, X., Zhao, D.F. and Zhao, G.Q. (2006). WNT/beta-catenin pathway up-regulates Stat3 and converges on LIF to prevent differentiation of mouse embryonic stem cells. *Dev Biol.*, 290, 81-91.

[55] Beattie, G.M., Lopez, A.D., Bucay, N., Hinton, A., Firpo, M.T., King, C.C. and Hayek, A. (2005). Activin A maintains pluripotency of human embryonic stem cells in the absence of feeder layers. *Stem Cells*, 23, 489-495,

[56] Vallier, L., Alexander, M. and Pedersen, R.A. (2005). Activin/Nodal and FGF pathways cooperate to maintain pluripotency of human embryonic stem cells. *J Cell Sci.*, 118, 4495-4509.

[57] Krasnikova, N.Y. and Gordeeva, O.F. (2006). Nodal signaling in the regulation of pluripotent state ofhuman and mouse ES and EC cells. *FEBS*, 273(suppl 1), 126.

[58] Stevens, L.C. and Varnum, D.S. (1974). The development of teratomas from parthenogenetically activated ovarian mouse eggs. *Dev Biol.,* 37, 369-380.

[59] Lefebvre, R., Theoret, C., Dore, M., Girard, C., Laverty, S. and Vaillancourt, D. (2005). Ovarian teratoma and endometritis in a mare. *Can Vet J.,* 46, 1029-1033.

[60] Carver, B.S., Bianco, F.J. Jr., Shayegan, B., Vickers, A., Motzer, R.J., Bos, G.J. and Sheinfeld, J. (2006). Predicting teratoma in the retroperitoneum in men undergoing

post-chemotherapy retroperitoneal lymph node dissection. *J Urol., 176*, 100-103;

[61]   Aubry, F., Satie, A.P., Rioux-Leclercq, N., Rajpert-DeMeyts, E,, Spagnoli, G.C., Chomez, P., De Backer, O., Jegou, B. and Samson, M. (2001). MAGE-A4, a germ cell specific marker, is expressed differentially in testicular tumors. *Cancer*, 92, 2778-2785.

[62]   Stevens, L.C. (1964). Experimental production of testicular teratomas in mice. *Proc Natl Acad Sci U S A*, 52,654-561

[63]   Bendel-Stenzel, M., Anderson, R., Heasman, J. and Wylie, C. (1998). The origin and migration of primordial germ cells in the mouse. *Semin Cell Dev Biol.*, 9, 393-400.

[64]   Kleinsmith, L.J. and Pierce, G.B. Jr. (1964). Multipotentiality of single embryonal carcinoma cells. *Cancer Res.*, 24, 1544-1551

[65]   Solter, D., Skreb, N. and Damjanov, I. (1970). Extrauterine growth of mouse egg-cylinders results in malignant teratoma. *Nature*, 227,503-504.

[66]   Stevens, L.C. (1970). The development of transplantable teratocarcinomas from intratesticular grafts of pre- and postimplantation mouse embryos. *Dev Biol.*, 21, 364-382.

[67]   Gordeeva, O.F., Manuilova, E.S., Paiushina, O.V., Nikonova, T.M., Grivennikov, I.A. and Khrushchev, N.G. (2003*)*. Differentiation of pluripotent embryonic stem cells in peritoneal cavity of irradiated mice. *Izv Akad Nauk Ser Biol.*, 3, 371-374.

[68]   Gordeeva, O., Zinovieva, R., Smirnova, Y., Payushina, O., Nikonova, T. and Khrushchov, N. (2005). Differentiation of embryonic stem cells after transplantation into peritoneal cavity of irradiated mice and expression of specific germ cell genes in pluripotent cells. *Transplant Proc.*, 37, 295-298.

[69]   Rugg-Gunn, P.J., Ferguson-Smith, A.C. and Pedersen, R.A. (2005). Epigenetic status of human embryonic stem cells. *Nat Genet.*, 37, 585-587.

[70]   Mitalipova, M.M., Rao, R.R., Hoye,r D.M., Johnson, J.A., Meisner, L.F., Jones, K.L., Dalton, S., Stice, S.L. (2005). Preserving the genetic integrity of human embryonic stem cells. *Nat Biotechnol.*, 23, 19-20.

[71]   Maitra, A., Arking, D.E., Shivapurkar. N., Ikeda, M., Stastny, V., Kassauei, K., Sui, G., Cutler, J., Liu, Y., Brimble, S.N., Noaksson, K., Hyllner, J., Schulz, T.C, Zeng, X., Freed, W.J., Crook, J., Abraham, S., Colman, A., Sartipy, P., Matsu,i S., Carpenter, M., Gazdar, A.F., Rao, M., Chakravarti, A. (2005). Genomic alterations in cultured human embryonic stem cells. *Nat Genet.*, 37, 1099-1103.

In: Encyclopedia of Stem Cell Research (2 Volume Set)   ISBN: 978-1-61761-835-2
Editor: Alexander L. Greene   © 2012 Nova Science Publishers, Inc.

Chapter LIV

LEGAL ISSUES RELATED TO HUMAN EMBRYONIC STEM CELL RESEARCH[*]

Edward C. Liu

SUMMARY

Human embryonic stem cells are often described as "master cells," able to develop into any other type of cell in the human body. Research on embryonic stem cells has given rise to ethical debates, as the removal of an embryonic stem cell from an embryo typically involves the destruction of that embryo. In 2007, researchers in Japan and the United States published reports that they had successfully induced adult human somatic cells to exhibit characteristics similar to embryonic stem cells. Some have argued that these new induced pluripotent stem cells render embryonic stem cell research unnecessary, while others contend that continued embryonic stem cell research is still important.

Restrictions on the federal funding of research using stem cell lines were recently lifted by an executive order issued by President Obama. Pursuant to that order, the National Institutes of Health is directed to issue guidance on human stem cell research within 120 days. This change reversed an existing executive branch policy that limited federal funds to stem cell lines that were already in existence on August 9, 2001, and were derived (1) with the informed consent of the donors; (2) from excess embryos created solely for reproductive purposes; and (3) without any financial inducements to the donors.

In contrast, the federal funding of most methods of human embryonic stem cell procurement is still prohibited by federal legislation. No federal funds may be used for the derivation of stem cell lines from newly destroyed embryos; the creation of any human embryos for research purposes; or cloning of human embryos for any purposes. Recipients of

---

[*] This is an edited, reformatted and augmented version of a Congressional Research Service publication, Report RS21044, dated March 9, 2009.

federal funds may also be prohibited from discriminating against individuals who are opposed to stem cell research.

Several bills have been introduced in the 111th Congress that would direct the Secretary of Health and Human Services to conduct and support stem cell research. Some of these bills would appear to sanction continued federal funding of human embryonic stem cell research, while others would not.

BACKGROUND INFORMATION ON HUMAN EMBRYONIC STEM CELLS

Human embryonic stem cells are often described as "master cells," able to develop into any other type of cell in the human body.[1] Potential sources for human embryonic stem cells include embryos created via *in vitro* fertilization for either research or reproduction; five to nine week old embryos or fetuses obtained through elective abortion; and embryos created through cloning or somatic cell nuclear transfer. Stem cells which are derived from adult tissues, such as umbilical cord blood or bone marrow, are distinct from embryonic stem cells and do not naturally exhibit the same developmental characteristics or behaviors.

In 1998, researchers at the University of Wisconsin isolated cells from a human embryo early in the developmental cycle and developed the first human embryonic stem cell lines.[2] Controversy surrounds the removal of stem cells from human embryos and fetuses because most techniques require the destruction of the embryo during the removal process. However, human embryonic stem cells are regarded as possibly having more therapeutic or research potential than stem cells derived from adult tissue. Whereas embryonic stem cells are often classified as either totipotent[3] or pluripotent,[4] stem cells found in adult sources may only have the capacity to differentiate into a few types of cells.[5]

Recent discoveries may lessen the demand for embryonic stem cells. In 2007, researchers in Japan and the United States published reports that they had successfully induced human somatic cells to exhibit pluripotent characteristics.[6] This advancement notwithstanding, many stem cell researchers continue to argue that embryonic stem cell procurement is necessary in order to provide, among other things, the "gold standard" against which other means of pluripotent stem cell procurement are measured.[7]

Research utilizing human embryonic stem cell lines has focused on the potential that these cells can offer to advance the treatment or mitigation of diseases and conditions and to generate replacement tissues for disfunctioning cells or organs.[8] Examples of research efforts include spinal cord injury, multiple sclerosis, Parkinson's disease, Alzheimer's disease, and diabetes. Researchers also hope to use specialized cells to replace dysfunctional cells in the brain, spinal cord, pancreas, and other organs.[9] In January of 2009, the Food and Drug Administration approved a clinical trial to evaluate a therapy for spinal cord injuries that was developed using embryonic stem cell lines.[10]

FEDERAL FUNDING OF EMBRYONIC STEM CELL RESEARCH

Historically, there have been two sequential phases of research involving human embryonic stem cells: (1) research in which stem cells are produced from human embryonic tissue; and (2) research in which embryonic stem cells are used to study human development or illness. As the state of scientific knowledge and expertise has advanced, the federal government has taken various positions regarding the propriety of federally funding research at each stage. Currently, the use of federal funds for embryonic stem cell procurement is prohibited. In contrast, the guidelines governing the use of federal funds to support research using embryonic stem cell lines already in existence are currently being drafted by the National Institutes of Health (NIH).

Restrictions on Federal Funding of Research Using Embryos

While federal law has regulated federal funding of fetal research since 1974,[11] federal funding of embryonic research has only been restricted since 1994, when President Clinton, through an executive directive, prohibited federal funding of such research.[12] Subsequently, in 1996, Congress enacted a legislative ban in the funding measure of the NIH and has continued to pass a similar ban annually since that time.[13]

The congressional ban, often referred to as the Dickey Amendment,[14] prohibits federally appropriated funds from being used for either the creation of human embryos for research purposes or for research in which a human embryo or embryos are destroyed, discarded, or knowingly subjected to risk of injury or death.[15] The ban defined "human embryo or embryos" to include any organism, not protected as a human subject under 45 C.F.R. § 46 (Human Subject Protection regulations) that is derived by fertilization, parthenogenesis, cloning, or any other means from one or more human gametes.[16] As the collection of embryonic stem cells often entails the destruction of or harm to an embryo, the Dickey Amendment effectively forecloses federal funding of embryonic stem cell procurement.[17]

Despite the absence of federal funding, embryonic research has continued with other sources of funding. In 1998, after the inclusion of the Dickey Amendment, landmark developments were recognized by scientists at the University of Wisconsin when researchers were able to isolate stem cells from human embryos and coax them to grow into specialized cells.[18] This development led some to question whether federal funds could be used in subsequent research involving these cell lines.

Research on Embryonic Stem Cell Lines under the Dickey Amendment

In January of 1999, the General Counsel of Health and Human Services (HHS) concluded that the Dickey Amendment's prohibitions against the use of HHS appropriated funds for human embryo research would not apply to research using stem cells "because such cells are not a human embryo within the statutory definition."[19] HHS concluded that NIH could fund research that uses stem cells derived from the embryo by private funds. However, because of the language in the Dickey Amendment, NIH could not fund research that derived the stem cells from embryos.

Some Members of Congress strongly opposed HHS's interpretation and believed that the legislative ban covered and prohibited funding such research. In response to this opposition, HHS Secretary Shalala stated in a letter that the definition of embryo used in the HHS legal opinion relied on the definition of embryo in the statute and that the ban applied only to research in which human embryos are discarded or destroyed, but not to research preceding or following "on such projects."[20] Secretary Shalala also noted that "there is nothing in the legislative history to suggest that the provision was intended to prohibit funding for research in which embryos—organisms—are not involved."[21]

NIH published draft guidelines for funding of stem cell research in the Federal Register in December of 1999 and final guidelines were issued in August of 2000.[22] Based upon HHS's interpretation, the guidelines stated that funds could not be used to extract or derive stem cells from an embryo, thereby destroying it. However, studies utilizing pluripotent stem cell lines derived from human embryos could be conducted using NIH funds provided that the cells were derived (1) without federal funds, (2) from human embryos that were created for the purposes of fertility treatment, and (3) were in excess of the clinical need of the individuals seeking such treatment. NIH initiated the applications process, but that process was overtaken by events and a new administration's policy was set forth.

Recent Executive Branch Policies

When President George W. Bush took office in January of 2001, he announced his intent to conduct a review of the stem cell research issue and ordered HHS to review the NIH guidelines issued by the previous administration. During this transition period, NIH suspended its review of applications from researchers seeking federal funds to perform embryonic stem cell research. Subsequently, on August 9, 2001, President Bush announced that federal funds would be available to human embryonic stem cell research on a restricted basis. The new policy would provide federal funds to be used for research only on existing stem cell lines that were already in existence as of the date of the announcement.[23] In identifying the stem cell lines as being eligible for federal funding, President Bush said these embryos, from which the existing stem cell lines were created, had been destroyed previously and could not develop as human beings.

Under the policy announced on August 9, 2001, federal agencies, primarily NIH, would be permitted to fund embryonic stem cell research if certain eligibility criteria were met. Federal funds could only be used for research on existing stem cell lines that were derived (1) with the informed consent of the donors, (2) from excess embryos created solely for reproductive purposes, and (3) without any financial inducements to the donors.[24]

On March 9, 2009, President Obama issued an executive order revoking the restrictions on human embryonic stem cell funding established under the Bush administration. President Obama's executive order also directed the Director of NIH to review existing NIH guidance and other widely recognized guidelines on human stem cell research, including provisions establishing appropriate safeguards, and issue new NIH guidance on such research that is consistent with this order.[25]

Such guidelines must be issued within 120 days of the date of the executive order.

Recent Congressional Activity

Congressional interest in stem cell research continued steadily since President Bush's policy announcement in 2001. Despite the introduction of various bills to both promote and limit federal funding of stem cell research, there exists no legislative enactment defining what types of postprocurement embryonic stem cell research are eligible to receive federal funding.

During the 109th Congress, at least seven bills involving stem cell research were introduced, two of which were enacted.[26] A third measure, H.R. 810, the Stem Cell Research Enhancement Act of 2005, was passed by Congress, but vetoed by President Bush on July 19, 2006.[27] H.R. 810 would have amended the Public Health Service Act (PHSA) to direct the Secretary of HHS to conduct and support research that utilizes human embryonic stem cells without regard to the date on which the stem cells were derived from a human embryo. To be eligible for use in research conducted or supported by the Secretary, the stem cells would have been required to meet certain conditions. For example, only stem cells derived from human embryos that were donated from in vitro fertilization clinics, were created for the purposes of fertility treatment, and were in excess of the clinical need of the individuals seeking such treatment would have been eligible for use.[28] A vote to override the veto was unsuccessful.[29]

Finally, S. 2754, the Alternative Pluripotent Stem Cell Therapies Enhancement Act, would have amended the PHSA to direct the Secretary of HHS to conduct and support basic and applied research to develop techniques for the isolation, derivation, production, or testing of stem cells that are not derived from a human embryo. S. 2754 indicated that the research contemplated by the measure would not have affected any policy, guideline, or regulation regarding embryonic stem cell research or human cloning by somatic cell nuclear transfer. S. 2754 was passed by the Senate on July 18, 2006 by a vote 100-0. The House did not vote on the measure.

In the 110th Congress, at least 10 bills involving stem cell research were introduced.[30] H.R. 3, the Stem Cell Research Enhancement Act of 2007, a measure that was identical in language to the Stem Cell Research Enhancement Act of 2005, was passed by the House on January 11, 2007, by a vote of 253-174. A companion measure, S. 5, was passed by the Senate on April 11, 2007, by a vote of 63-34. S. 5 included the language of H.R. 3, as well as the language of the Alternative Pluripotent Stem Cell Therapies Enhancement Act from the 109th Congress. On June 7, 2007, the House passed S. 5 by a vote of 247-176, but it was ultimately vetoed by President Bush.[31]

In the 111th Congress, H.R. 872, the Stem Cell Research Improvement Act of 2009, contains language that is largely similar to the earlier Stem Cell Research Enhancement Acts of 2005 and 2007, and would amend the PHSA to direct the Secretary of HHS to conduct and support research involving embryonic stem cell lines that met the same criteria enumerated in the prior bills. This bill would additionally require guidelines governing such research to be issued by the Director of NIH within 90 days of enactment, and periodically reviewed every three years. H.R. 873, the Stem Cell Research Enhancement Act of 2009, would also amend the PHSA to direct the Secretary of HHS to conduct and support the same type of embryonic stem cell research. This bill would also require guidelines to be issued within 60 days of enactment, but would not require further periodic review of those guidelines. S. 487, also entitled the Stem Cell Research Enhancement Act of 2009, is identical to S. 5 in the 110th Congress.

Other bills introduced during the 111th Congress are aimed at supporting some types of stem cell research, but appear to exclude most embryonic stem cell research. H.R. 877, the Patients First Act of 2009 would direct the Secretary of HHS to conduct and support research on pluripotent stem cells, but appears to exclude research upon stem cell lines that were derived from embryonic sources. S. 99, the Ethical Stem Cell Research Tax Credit Act of 2009, would provide businesses a credit equal to 30% of "qualified stem cell research expenses."[32] Qualified stem cell research expenses do not appear to include embryonic stem cell procurement activities, insofar as those activities would subject a human embryo to destruction, discarding, or risk of injury. Research activities using embryonic stem cell lines that were derived in a manner which subject a human embryo to destruction, discarding, or risk of injury would not appear to be eligible for the tax credit proposed by this bill.

CONSCIENCE PROTECTIONS

Federal law protects individuals from being required to perform or assist in the performance of federally funded research that is morally or religiously objectionable to them.[33] This protection, which would likely encompass objections to research on embryonic stem cell lines, is only triggered in instances where the objectionable research is federally funded.[34] Therefore it is unlikely to arise in the context of embryonic stem cell procurement, as federal funds may not be used for those purposes.

Facilities that receive biomedical or behavioral research grants are additionally prohibited from discriminating among any employment or staff privileges based upon an individual's opinions of, or prior refusals to participate in, health services or research activities that are contrary to his religious beliefs or moral convictions.[35] This would appear to prevent recipients of NIH grants from discriminating against individuals that are opposed to stem cell research.

In December of 2008, the Bush administration issued final regulations reiterating these protections and additionally requiring recipients of federal funds to certify, in writing, that they will refrain from these prohibited actions.[36] The Obama administration has indicated that it intends to rescind these regulations.[37]

End Notes

[1] In contrast, differentiated somatic cells, which perform the "day to day" functions of the body, are not thought to give rise to other types of cells absent human intervention. *See, e.g., infra* footnote 6 and accompanying text.

[2] Nat'l Inst. of Health, U.S. Dep't of Health & Hum. Services, *Stem Cells: Scientific Progress and Future Research Directions* 4 (2001), *available at* http://stemcells.nih.gov/ info/scireport/2001report.htm.

[3] The earliest embryonic stem cells are called totipotent cells as they can develop into an entire organism, producing both the embryo and tissues required to support it in the uterus. PRESIDENT'S COUNCIL ON BIOETHICS, *Alternative Sources of Human Pluripotent Stem Cells*, at 5 n.* (2005), *available at* http://www.bioethics.gov.

[4] Pluripotent stem cells can develop into almost any type of cell in the body, but these stem cells cannot form the supporting tissues necessary for gestation, as seen with totipotent cells. *Id.*

[5] For example, hematopoietic stem cells found in adult bone marrow and umbilical cord blood only appear to naturally give rise to various types of blood cells. PRESIDENT'S COUNCIL ON BIOETHICS, *Monitoring Stem Cell Research*, at 3 (2004), *available at* http://www.bioethics.gov.

[6] James A. Thomson et al., *Induced Pluripotent Stem Cell Lines Derived from Human Somatic Cells*, 318 SCIENCE 1917 (2007); Shinya Yamanaka et al., *Induction of Pluripotent Stem Cells from Adult Human Fibroblasts by Defined Factors*, 131(5) CELL 861 (2007).

[7] Robert Lee Holtz, *Stem-Cell Researchers Claim Embryo Labs Are Still a Necessity*, THE WALL ST. J., Jan. 4, 2008, at B1.

[8] For additional information on stem cell research, see CRS Report RL33540, *Stem Cell Research: Federal Research Funding and Oversight*, by Judith A. Johnson and Erin D. Williams.

[9] *Id.* at 4-6.

[10] Andrew Pollack, *Milestone in Research in Stem Cells*, NEW YORK TIMES, Jan. 23, 2009, at 1.

[11] National Research Service Award Act of 1974, P.L. 93-348, § 213, 88 Stat. 342 (1974).

[12] Statement on Federal Funding of Research on Human Embryos, 30 Weekly Comp. Pres. Doc. 2459 (December 2, 1994).

[13] Balanced Budget Downpayment Act, 1996, P.L. 104-99, § 128, 110 Stat. 26, 34 (1996).

[14] The amendment is so named for its principal sponsor, Rep. Jay Dickey.

[15] This term was defined as risk greater than that allowed for research on fetuses in utero under 45 C.F.R. § 46.208(a)(2) and 42 U.S.C. § 289g(b).

[16] The rider language has not changed significantly over the years and is currently found in Title V of the Labor, HHS, and Education appropriations acts. P.L. 110-161, § 509 (2007).

[17] *But see* CRS Report RL33554, *Stem Cell Research: Ethical Issues*, by Erin D. Williams and Judith A. Johnson, at 14-15 (discussing potential methods of creating embryonic stem cell lines without destroying human embryos).

[18] James A. Thomson et al., *Embryonic Stem Cell Lines Derived from Human Blastocysts*, 282 SCIENCE 1145 (1998).

[19] Letter from HHS Gen. Counsel Harriet Rabb to Harold Varmus, Director, NIH, January 15, 1999. General Counsel Rabb determined that the statutory ban on human embryonic research defined an embryo as an "organism" that, when implanted in the uterus, is capable of becoming a human being. The opinion stated that pluripotent stem cells are not, and cannot, develop into an organism, as defined in the statute.

[20] Letter from Secretary Shalala to Rep. Jay Dickey, February 23, 1999.

[21] *Id.*

[22] 64 Fed. Reg. 67,576 (Dec. 2, 1999); 65 Fed. Reg. 51,976 (Aug. 25, 2000).

[23] President's Address to the Nation on Stem Cell Research From Crawford, Texas, 37 Weekly Comp. Pres. Doc. 1149 (August 9, 2001).

[24] *Id.* The policy also required the creation of the President's Council on Bioethics to study stem cells and embryonic research as well as other issues.

[25] Exec. Order No. _____, § 3, Mar. 9, 2009, *available at* http://www.whitehouse.gov/ the_press_office/Removing-Barriers-to-Responsible-Scientific-Research-Involving-Human-Stem-Cells/.

[26] H.R. 2520, 109th Cong., Stem Cell Therapeutic and Research Act of 2005 (providing for the collection and maintenance of human cord blood stem cells) (enacted as P.L. 109-129). S. 3504, 109th Cong., Fetus Farming Prohibition Act of 2006 (making it unlawful to either solicit or knowingly acquire, receive, or accept a donation of human fetal tissue knowing that a human pregnancy was deliberately initiated to provide such tissue or obtained from a human embryo or fetus that was gestated in the uterus of a nonhuman animal) (enacted as P.L. 109-242).

[27] A companion bill, S. 471, was introduced by Sen. Arlen Specter on February 28, 2005.

[28] The President argued that the bill would compel taxpayers "to fund the deliberate destruction of human embryos," and that "crossing this line would ... needlessly encourage a conflict between science and ethics that can only do damage to both and harm our Nation as a whole." 152 Cong. Rec. H5435 (daily ed. July 19, 2006) (Stem Cell Research Enhancement Act of 2005—Veto Message From the President of the United States (H. Doc. No. 109-127)).

[29] *See* 152 Cong. Rec. H5450 (daily ed. July 19, 2006) (the vote was 235-193).

[30] For additional discussion of stem cell research legislation in the 110th Congress, see CRS Report RL33540, *Stem Cell Research: Federal Research Funding and Oversight*, by Judith A. Johnson and Erin D. Williams, supra footnote 8 at 25-29.

[31] Message   to   the   Senate   of   the   United   States   (June   20,   2007),   *available   at* http://www.whitehouse.gov/news/releases/2007/06/print/20070620-5.html. The President observed, "S. 5, like the bill I vetoed last year, would overturn today's carefully balanced policy on stem cell research. Compelling American taxpayers to support the deliberate destruction of human embryos would be a grave mistake."

[32] This bill is similar to S. 2863 in the 110th Congress.

[33] 42 U.S.C. § 300a-7(d).

[34] *Id.*

[35] 42 U.S.C. § 300a-7(c)(2).

[36] 45 C.F.R. §§ 88.4(d), 88.5. *See* 73 Fed. Reg. 78,071-101.

[37] *See* Rob Stein, *Health Workers' Conscience Rule Set to Be Voided*, WASHINGTON POST, Feb. 28, 2009, at A1.

In: Encyclopedia of Stem Cell Research (2 Volume Set)   ISBN: 978-1-61761-835-2
Editor: Alexander L. Greene   © 2012 Nova Science Publishers, Inc.

Chapter LV

STEM CELL RESEARCH: ETHICAL ISSUES[*]

Erin D. Williams and Judith A. Johnson

SUMMARY

The central question before Congress in the debate over human stem cell research is how to treat human embryonic stem cell research (ESR), which may lead to lifesaving treatments, but which requires the destruction of embryos. Current federal law and policy address this question primarily through restrictions on federal funding for ESR. The Dickey amendment prohibits the use of Department of Health Human Services (HHS) funds for the creation of human embryos for research purposes or research in which a human embryo or embryos are destroyed, discarded, or knowingly subjected to certain risks of injury or death. The Dickey amendment thus prohibits the use of HHS funds to establish ES lines (line establishment involves embryo destruction), but not to conduct research using established lines. President Obama established current federal ESR policy with a March 9, 2009, executive order: *Removing Barriers to Responsible Scientific Research Involving Human Stem Cells* (Obama policy). The Obama policy authorizes HHS's National Institutes of Health (NIH) to support and conduct responsible, scientifically worthy human stem cell research, including ESR, to the extent permitted by law. It also requires NIH to issue a guidance consistent with the order. The Obama policy reversed one established by President George W. Bush, which had been the first to allow federal ESR funding, but only for a limited number of ES lines.

Congress has several sets of policy options, each one prompting a set of ethical dilemmas. The first set of options involves permitting or expanding federal ESR funding, as proposed in H.R. 872, H.R. 873, and S. 487. One such option is to take no action, allowing the Obama policy to persist. This option would permit federal funding for ESR with a range of lines, and would allow the executive branch to change the ESR policy in the future. Another such option is to enact a law permitting ESR. Even if consistent with the Obama policy, this course would limit

---

[*] This is an edited, reformatted and augmented version of a Congressional Research Service publication, Report RL33554, dated March 18, 2009.

the opportunity for the executive branch to change the policy in the future. A final such option involves expanding ESR by eliminating the Dickey amendment, thus allowing the use of federal funds for the establishment of ES lines, and/or for the creation of embryos for ESR. Some supporters this set of options assert that unused frozen embryos that are created for in vitro fertilization (IVF) could be used for federally regulated research instead of being destroyed. Other supporters seek federally regulated and funded research on embryos created specifically for research purposes, which might help to facilitate more targeted research. Critics seek to protect embryos and/or egg donors, and assert that federal funds should not be used for such purposes.

Congress's second set of options involves funding additional research that may eventually generate embryonic stem cells without destroying embryos, as proposed in H.R. 877. Supporters assert that this facilitates research without ethical dilemmas. Critics characterize it as unnecessary, costly, and a diversion from developing treatments. Congress's third set of options involves discouraging ESR via tax measures, or limiting or eliminating it by restricting research funding, banning certain cloning techniques, or giving embryos the Constitutional right to life. Examples include H.R. 110, H.R. 227, H.R. 881, H.R. 1050, H.R. 1654, S. 99, and S. 346. Supporters claim their approaches respect human dignity; critics claim they harm people already living.

It details the ethical arguments that surround ESR. The broadest is the balance of embryo destruction and relief of human suffering. More subtle issues focus on the relative importance of the viability of embryos, the purpose of embryo creation, new versus existing cell lines, the consent of donors, the ethics of egg procurement, the effectiveness of alternatives, the possibility of generating embryonic stem cells without destroying human embryos, and the use of federal funding.

INTRODUCTION

Human stem cell research is controversial not because of its goals, but rather because of the means of obtaining some of the cells. Research involving most types of human stem cells, such as those derived from adult tissues and umbilical cord blood, has been uncontroversial, except when its effectiveness as an alternative to embryonic stem cells is debated. The crux of the debate centers around embryonic stem cells, which enable research that may facilitate the development of medical treatments and cures, but which require the destruction of an embryo to derive.[1] In addition, because cloning is one method of producing embryos for research, the ethical issues surrounding cloning are also relevant.

Current Policy

Federal regulation of human embryonic stem cell research (ESR) primarily consists of one law and one policy: the Dickey amendment and the Obama policy, respectively.[2] Both address the use of federal funding to support ESR. Neither restricts or regulates ESR conducted solely with private, local and/or state government funding, or with funding from other non-federal sources. The Dickey Amendment, the Obama policy, and also the previous policy, which had been established by the George W. Bush Administration, are discussed below.

The Dickey Amendment

Since FY1996, the Dickey amendment, a provision added to each year's Labor-Health and Human Services-Education appropriations legislation, has prohibited the use of Department of Health and Human Services (HHS) funds for the creation of human embryos for research purposes or research in which a human embryo or embryos are destroyed, discarded, or knowingly subjected to risk of injury or death greater than that allowed for research on fetuses in utero under 45 CFR 46.204(b). This policy effectively precludes the use of federal funding to derive stem cells from embryos, which typically are produced via in vitro fertilization (IVF). However, the extracted embryonic stem cells can be used to generate embryonic stem cell lines that may continue to divide for many months to years. According to a legal opinion issued by the HHS General Council in 1999, by contrast to funding restrictions that Dickey places on the derivation of stem cells from embryos, federal funding for research performed with embryonic stem cells themselves (which does not itself involve embryos or the extraction of stem cells from embryos) is not proscribed by the Dickey amendment.[3] It is funding for research with these embryonic stem cell lines that is the subject of the Obama policy and of much of the current legislation before Congress.

The Obama Policy

The Obama policy took effect on March 9, 2009, in the form of an executive order.[4] In the executive order, President Barack Obama authorized the HHS Secretary, including the National Institutes of Health (NIH), to support and conduct responsible, scientifically worthy human stem cell research, including human embryonic stem cell research, to the extent permitted by law. The executive order also directed the NIH to review existing NIH guidance and other widely recognized guidelines on human stem cell research, including provisions establishing appropriate safeguards, and issue new NIH guidance on such research that is consistent with the executive order within 120 days (by early July 2009). On the same day that the executive order was issued, President Obama issued a memorandum on scientific integrity directing the head of the White House Office of Science and Technology Policy "to develop a strategy for restoring scientific integrity to government decision making."[5]

Historical Note: The Bush Policy

Prior to the Obama policy, ESR had been regulated by the policy that President George W. Bush had established in August 2001 (Bush policy). The Bush policy had, for the first time, allowed federal money to be used to support ESR. It had also restricted that funding to research using ES lines created (1) with appropriate informed consent of the donors, (2) using embryos created for reproductive purposes, and (3) before the date of the policy. This date restriction was the most controversial component of the Bush policy. President Bush had later issued a companion policy in the form of *Executive Order: Expanding Approved Stem Cell Lines in Ethically Responsible Ways* (E.O. 13435), which had directed the NIH to fund research on sources of pluripotent stem cells that did not involve the destruction of embryos.[6]

President Bush had issued E.O. 13435 on June 20, 2007, which was the same day that he vetoed a bill to expand federal funding for ESR (S. 5, 110th).

The Obama policy reversed the Bush policy, and also revoked E.O. 13435. The Obama policy thus allowed for the possibility of federal funding for ESR using many more stem cell lines than were previously eligible. While the Obama policy did not mandate funding for alternatives to ESR, it specifically authorized support for non-embryonic as well as embryonic stem cell research.

Legislation

Since ESR emerged bringing hope for medical cures and fears about ethical implications, a number of bills have been introduced that touch upon the subject. Enactment of any of these bills, even if consistent with the current executive policy, would limit or eliminate the opportunity for the executive branch to set the ESR policy in the future.

One set of bills would enact into law the authority to expend federal funds on ESR. Some of these bills were introduced prior to the Obama policy, and include restrictions greater than of those Obama policy. For example, some bills require that embryos used in federally funded ESR have been created for reproductive purposes, and/or that there have been no financial inducements made to embryo donors. However, none of these bills contains the August 2001 date restriction that had been imposed by the Bush policy. Examples of these bills in the 111th Congress include H.R. 872, H.R. 873, and S. 487.

A second set of bills would create incentives for activities that avoid ESR. Some of these bills would require federal support or tax benefits for research or activities that avoid damaging embryos. Others would create additional oversight for the conduct of ESR. Still others would create a bank of non-embryonic stem cells from amniotic fluid and placentas. Examples of these bills in the 111th Congress include H.R. 877, S. 99, and H.R. 1654.

A third set of bills would further restrict or prohibit ESR. Some would accomplish this through legislation placing the language of the Dickey amendment in statute, and/or extending it by prohibiting federal funding using stem cells derived in violation of the other restrictions. Others would allow funding only in very specific circumstances, such as when using techniques with non-living embryos created for reproductive purposes. Still others would amend other law (such as that governing the right to life, organ transplantation,[7] cloning, or the creation of animal-human hybrids) to prohibit ESR or restrict some aspect its conduct. Examples of such bills in the 111th Congress include H.R. 110, H.R. 227, H.R. 881, H.R. 1050, and S. 346.

Along with the policy options articulated in the above bills, Congress has additional options thathave been discussed in various forums. One of these is eliminating the Dickey amendment, thus allowing the use of federal funds for the establishment of ES lines, and/or for the creation of embryos for ESR. Another is to take no action, thus allowing the Obama policy to persist. This option would permit federal funding for ESR with a range of lines, and would allow the executive branch some latitude to change the ESR policy in the future.

Proponents and Opponents

In the ES debate, the Obama Administration, George W. Bush Administration (Bush Administration), a group of Representatives, a group of Senators, and a group of Nobel Laureates have each presented their respective positions on ESR. In addition, various other organizations, individuals, and councils have issued opinions and reports on the topic. Some groups, such as the National Academies,[8] the Coalition for the Advancement of Medical Research (CAMR),[9] former First Lady Nancy Reagan,[10] former Presidents Gerald Ford, Jimmy Carter, and Bill Clinton,[11] and the Union of Orthodox Jewish Congregations of America (UOJCA),[12] favor federal support ESR that is generally keeping with the Obama policy. Other groups, such as the Christian Legal Society,[13] Focus on the Family,[14] and the Christian Coalition[15] favor restrictions on ESR, and had supported the Bush policy. Still others, such as the National Right to Life Committee[16] and the United States Conference of Catholic Bishops,[17] oppose all ESR.

Two presidential bioethics advisory panels have considered the issues involved in ESR. The President's Council on Bioethics (President's Council)[18] published one report directly on the topic, *Monitoring Stem Cell Research*,[19] in which it sought to characterize the issues. While the Council made no recommendations there, in two other reports it has recommended that "Congress should ... [p]rohibit the use of human embryos in research beyond a designated stage in their development (between 10 and 14 days after fertilization),"[20] and unanimously recommended "a ban on cloning-to-produce-children," with a 10-member majority also favoring "a four-year moratorium on cloning-for-biomedical-research," and a seven-member minority favoring "regulation of the use of cloned embryos for biomedical research."[21] More recently, the President's Council published Alternative Sources of Human Pluripotent Stem Cells, a white paper exploring the ethics of four proposals to attempt to generate human embryonic stem cells "without creating, destroying, or harming human embryos."[22] A predecessor to the President's Council, the National Bioethics Advisory Commission (NBAC),[23] recommended federal funding for stem cell research using "embryos remaining after infertility treatments," but not for the "derivation or use of embryos ... made for research purposes."[24]

DISCUSSION OF ETHICAL ISSUES

Detailed review of the assorted reports and statements reveals that while positions on ESR may be broadly categorized as *for* or *against*, there is an array of finer distinctions present. These finer distinctions, in turn, reveal the variation in ethical and moral as well as factual beliefs. The following discussion breaks down the arguments about ESR according to these finer distinctions, demonstrating both the complexity of the issues and the points of resonance among the groups.

Embryo Destruction and Relief of Human Suffering

Most positions on ESR rest at least in part on the relative moral weight accorded to embryos and that accorded to the prospect of saving, prolonging, or improving others' lives. For some, the inquiry begins and ends with this question. For instance, one opponent of the research, the American Life League, posits that "human life begins at conception/fertilization and that there is never an acceptable reason for intentionally taking an innocent human life."[25] Similarly, the United States Conference of Catholic Bishops states that the research is immoral because it "relies on the destruction of some defenseless human beings for the possible benefit to others."[26]

Some groups explore the moral standing of human embryos, and also consider the "duty to relieve the pain and suffering of others."[27] Others take the position that embryos do not have the same moral status as persons. They acknowledge that embryos are genetically human, but hold that they do not have the same moral relevance because they lack specific capacities, including consciousness, reasoning, and sentience.[28] They also argue that viewing embryos as persons would "rule out all fertility treatments that involve the creation and discarding of excess embryos," and further assert that we do not have the same "moral or religious" response to the natural loss of embryos (through miscarriage) that we do to the death of infants.[29] Some have also rooted their arguments in religious texts, which inform them that an "isolated fertilized egg does not enjoy the full status of person-hood and its attendant protections."[30] They conclude that performing research to benefit persons justifies the destruction of embryos. Acceptance of the notion that the destruction of embryos can be justified in some circumstances forms the basis of pro-ESR opinions—including those of the Bush and Obama Administrations—and is usually modified with some combination of the distinctions and limitations that follow.

Viability of Embryos

Some proponents of ESR base their support on the question of whether an embryo is viable. The relevance of the viability distinction rests on the premise that it is morally preferable for embryos that will not grow or develop beyond a certain stage and/or those that would otherwise be discarded to be used for the purpose of alleviating human suffering.

The Obama policy does not reference the viability of embryos, but allows for the possibility that NIH guidance will do so. By contrast, the Bush policy had directly referenced viability, requiring, among other things, use of stem cells derived from only excess (non-viable) embryos for federally funded research. One report of the President's Council explores the moral significance of viability that is based upon "human choices" rather than an embryo's "own intrinsic nature," but draws no conclusions.[31] A second report broaches the subject of viability, recommending that Congress ban both the transfer of a human embryo to a woman's uterus for any purpose other than to produce a live-born child, and also research conducted on embryos more than 10 to 14 days after fertilization.[32] The NBAC report touches on the moral status of embryos in utero and those in vitro,[33] though NBAC does not specify whether viability was a key rationale for its recommendations. A group of Representatives,[34] a group of Senators,[35] and CAMR imply but do not state a distinction based on viability by expressly calling for the use of "excess" embryos developed for IVF, and making no mention of those in utero.[36] UOJCA makes a similar argument in its letter. By contrast, the National Academies and the group of Nobel Laureates more broadly support research on embryos, making no mention of viability.

Purpose of Embryo Creation

A separate distinction that often leads to the same conclusions as viability is the purpose for which embryos are created. This distinction draws an ethical line based upon the intent of the people creating embryos. In the view of some, it is permissible to create an embryo for reproductive purposes (such as IVF), but impermissible to create one with the intention of destroying it for research. Others worry that moral lines will erode quickly—from using only "spare" embryos left over in fertility clinics to creating human embryos solely for research to creating (or trying to create) cloned embryos solely for research.[37]

As is the case regarding embryo viability, the Obama policy does not reference the purpose of embryo creation, but allows for the possibility that NIH guidance will do so. Most groups at least note the potential ethical significance of reproductive versus research motives for creating embryos. The Bush policy had drawn a motive distinction by including a requirement that federally funded research be conducted only on embryonic stem cell lines derived from embryos created solely for reproductive purposes. NBAC draws the same distinction by recommending that federal funding be used for embryos remaining after infertility treatment but not for research involving the derivation or use of stem cells from embryos made for research purposes or from cloned embryos produced by SCNT.[38] UOJCA argue similarly that they "believe it is entirely appropriate to utilize for this research existing embryos, such as those created for IVF purposes that would otherwise be discarded but for this research. We think it another matter to create embryos ab initio for the sole purpose of conducting this form of research."[39]

The President's Council recommends that Congress ban attempts at conception by any means other than the union of egg and sperm (essentially banning cloning via SCNT) but does not specify whether embryos might be created in vitro specifically for research purposes.[40] Two Council members expressed a dissenting opinion in a medical journal article, arguing that SCNT "resembles a tissue culture" and that the products of SCNT should be available for research.[41] A group of Representatives, a group of Senators, and CAMR imply but do not state that embryos should not be created for research purposes. They overtly call for the use of "excess" embryos developed for IVF and make no mention of embryos created expressly for research.[42] By contrast, the National Academies supports the creation of embryos for research purposes, including via cloning (SCNT), to "ensure that stem cell-based therapies can be broadly applied for many conditions and people [by] overcoming the problem of tissue rejection."[43] Mrs. Nancy Reagan, her supporters, and the group of Nobel Laureates also take this position.

New and Existing Cell Lines

A further distinction has been drawn based upon the timing of the creation of embryonic stem cell lines. Here, the premise is that it is unacceptable to induce the destruction of embryos for the creation of new lines. However, in cases in which embryos have already been destroyed and the lines already exist, it is morally preferable to use those lines for research to improve the human condition.

The Obama policy makes no distinction based on the timing of when ES lines were created. By contrast, the timing of ES-line creation was one central concept in the Bush policy, which had limited the use of federal funding to research on lines derived on or before the date of the policy. Supporters of a distinction based on timing favor this distinction as a compromise because allows research on some embryonic stem cell lines and deters the future destruction of embryos for research. The President's Council writes that a policy based on timing mixes "prudence" with "principle, in the hope that the two might reinforce (rather than undermine) each other."[44] The Council notes that a timing-based policy is supported by what it titled a *moralist's* notion of when one may benefit from prior bad acts (referring to embryo destruction): it prevents the government from complying in the commission of or encouraging the act in the future, and it reaffirms the principle that the act was wrong.[45] The same report also contains alternative analyses that characterize the act of drawing a distinction between new and existing cell lines as "arbitrary," "unsustainable," and "inconsistent."[46] The Council itself takes no position in the report on this or any other issue.

Opponents of any distinction based on timing come from both sides of the issue. They view the distinction between new and existing stem cell lines with reproach. One side, which includes the National Right to Life Committee and the United States Conference of Catholic Bishops, objects because the distinction validates destruction of embryos, and rewards those who did so first with a monopoly. The other side, which includes the National Academies, a group of Representatives, a group of Senators, Nancy Reagan and her supporters, Gerald Ford, CAMR, and the group of Nobel Laureates, objects because the distinction limits the number of embryonic stem cell lines available for research, particularly since the number of authorized lines are dwindling[47] and are "contaminated with mouse feeder cells."[48] Likewise, though NBAC recognized the distinction between destroying embryos and using ones previously destroyed (e.g., "derivation of [embryonic stem] cells involves destroying the embryos, whereas abortion precedes the donation of fetal tissue and death precedes the donation of whole organs for transplantation"),[49] it still recommended future development of embryonic stem cell lines. UOJCA also recognizes a distinction between new and existing lines: "research on embryonic stem cells must be conducted under careful guidelines [that] ... relate to where the embryonic stem cells to be researched upon are taken from."[50]

Consent of Donors

There is consensus throughout a wide array of viewpoints about ESR that embryos should only be obtained for research with the consent of their biological donors. This consent requirement necessitates that embryos be taken only with donors' knowledge, understanding, and uncoerced agreement, which may, in fact, be complicated by conflicting studies regarding the long-term health effects of egg donation.[51] The donor consent requirement is consistent with the rules governing human beings' participation in research, and with individuals' general legal authority to make decisions regarding embryos they procreate. A potential drawback of the requirement is that it may restrict the number of embryos available for research purposes.

While the Obama policy does not explicitly require the consent of the donors, it does require that NIH support ESR conducted responsibly, which may include informed consent requirements.[52] The Bush policy had contained a donor consent requirement that had limited approved stem cell lines to those derived with the informed consent of the donors, and obtained without any financial inducements to the donors. Despite the policy, a 2008 report raised questions about whether one quarter of the lines eligible for federal funding actually met policy's the informed consent requirements.[53]

Like the Bush policy, the NBAC, the President's Council, and the UOJCA also favor donor consent requirements. The National Academies notes the importance of informed consent in its discussion of stem cell research oversight requirements.[54] A group of Representatives and a group of Senators mention and imply their support for donor consent requirements.[55]

Egg Procurement

Egg procurement from women has raised a number of issues, most notably, those of informed consent and payment. The topic of informed consent in egg procurement came to the public's attention in November 2005 with allegations that some human eggs used in South Korean scientist Dr. Hwang's laboratory had been obtained under coercive conditions. Informed consent can be undermined when a coercive situation prevents a free choice from being made, or when insufficient information is provided to the person making a decision. The situation alleged in Dr. Hwang's laboratory raises the issue of coercion both because subordinate women in the laboratory allegedly donated eggs, and because some women were allegedly paid for their eggs. A 2002 study conducted by a University of Pennsylvania student raised the issue of insufficient information, finding that a number of programs seeking donor eggs for reproductive purposes downplayed the risks involved in egg retrieval.[56] The wide consensus regarding the need for informed consent necessarily implies similar consensus on the need for an information-rich, coercion-free method of obtaining eggs, however there is some disagreement on the specifics of whether payment for eggs necessarily constitutes coercion.

Paying women for their eggs, which has been debated in the context of seeking donor eggs both for reproductive purposes (for example, to enable women who do not produce their own eggs to become pregnant), and for research purposes, is not unheard of in the United States. According to a 2000 study by the American Society of Reproductive Medicine (ASRM), some IVF programs reportedly offered as much as $5,000 for one egg retrieval cycle, though $2,500 appeared to be a more common amount.[57] Offers of much higher amounts ($50,000-$100,000) have been reported elsewhere.[58] Dr. Huang's laboratory reportedly made payments of $1,400 to each woman who donated eggs.[59] Payments are not illegal in the Unites States, nor were they illegal in South Korea at the time Dr. Huang's laboratory allegedly made them. The questions are, is payment for egg donation ever acceptable, and if so, what amount is appropriate?

Several arguments have been put forth in favor of payment for egg donation, many focused on donation for reproductive purposes.[60] First, some have argued that payment creates incentives to increase the number of egg donors, thus facilitating research and benefitting infertile couples. Second, some reason that payment for eggs gives women parity with sperm donors, who may be compensated for donating gametes at a lower rate given that they require a much less involved procedure. In addition, some argue that participants should be offered an amount commensurate with the time, inconvenience, discomfort, and risks of the procedure, as is the general practice in biomedical research.[61] Third, some allege that fairness dictates that women who donate eggs ought to be able to benefit from their action. Fourth, some claim that pressures created by financial incentives may be no greater than those experienced by women asked to make altruistic egg donations for relatives or friends, and may thus not rise to the level of coercion. These are the types of arguments that led ASRM to recommend in 2000 that sums of up to $5,000 may be appropriate for typical egg donation, while sums of up to $10,000 may possibly be justified if there are particular difficulties a woman must endure to make her donation.

Several arguments have also been put forth against payment for egg donation. First, some voiced fears that payment might lead to the exploitation of women, particularly poor women, and the commodification of reproductive tissues.[62] Second, some have argued that payment for eggs for research purposes might undermine public confidence in endeavors such as human ESR.[63] Arguments such as these have prompted both the National Academies and the President's Council to recommend that women not be paid for donating their eggs for research purposes. It also led the President's Council to note that in theory, there is the possibility that eggs could be procured from ovaries harvested from cadavers, which might at least alleviate concerns related to coercion.

It is worth noting that a woman may choose to undergo egg retrieval for her own reproductive purposes, which would effectively take the process of egg procurement out of the research arena and avoids the question of payment entirely. (For example, this could be an option for a woman seeking IVF because her fallopian tubes are blocked). While not making specific recommendations about payment for research-related egg donation, several groups' recommendations that only embryos left over from IVF procedures be used for stem cell research (noted above in the *Purpose of Embryo Creation* section) effectively takes the process of egg procurement from women out of the research arena. As is the case regarding other issues, the Obama policy does not reference the topic of egg donation, but allows for the possibility that NIH guidance will do so. The Bush policy had kept the consent process for egg retrieval separate from donation by funding research only on lines derived from embryos originally created for fertility treatments.

Effectiveness of Alternatives

One factual distinction that has been used to support competing ethical viewpoints is the efficacy of alternatives to ESR. The promise of stem cell therapies derived from adult tissue and umbilical cord blood have buttressed opposition to ESR. A report that stem cells similar to embryonic stem cells can be found in amniotic fluid may do the same, although the lead scientist conducting research on the amniotic cells and others have stated that amniotic cells will not make embryonic stem cells irrelevant.[64] Perhaps more promising, scientists claim to have generated pluripotent stem cells from adult cells, though technical and safety concerns regarding the cells' therapeutic use remain unresolved.[65] Alternatives such as those proposed for consideration by the President's Council are discussed in the next section. Some opponents of the current method of obtaining embryonic stem cells argue that therapies and cures can be developed without the morally undesirable destruction of embryos. The Obama policy neither requires not precludes research into ESR alternatives on its face, but does require that research be responsible and scientifically worthy. By contrast, E.O. 6/20 had affirmatively directed the pursuit of alternative methods of deriving embryonic stem cells, implying both a belief in the promise and necessity of such actions.

Not all scientists agree that adult stem cells or pluripotent stem cells derived from adult tissue hold as much potential as embryonic stem cells. Notably, during a congressional subcommittee hearing, when the NIH Director, Dr. Elias Zerhouni, was asked if other avenues of research should be pursued instead, he stated that "the presentations about adult stem cells holding as much or more potential than embryonic stem cells, in my view, do not hold scientific water. I think they are overstated."[66] Concerns have been raised that pluripotent stem cells derived from adult tissue may not be as versatile as embryonic stem cells, and may induce tumors.[67] Most supporters of ESR believe that it is the quickest and, perhaps in some cases, the only path that will yield results. Supporters also stress that embryonic and other stem cell research should be conducted collaboratively, so that they can inform one another. On a related note, some have pointed out that benefits from one alternative to ESR, umbilical cord blood banking, may only be available to families who can afford to pay private companies' storage fees.

Findings regarding the effectiveness of alternatives to ESR are mixed. The President's Council notes that there is a "debate about the relative merits of embryonic stem cells and adult stem cells."[68] Focus on the Family cites promising non-embryonic stem cell research: "adult stem cells may be as 'flexible' as embryonic ones and equally capable of converting into various cell types for healing the body."[69] By contrast, the National Academies finds that the "best available scientific and medical evidence indicates that research on both embryonic and adult human stem cells will be needed."[70] NBAC finds in its deliberations that "the claim that there are alternatives to using stem cells derived from embryos is not, at the present time, supported scientifically."[71] CAMR supports both embryonic and adult stem cell research, and adds that "many scientists believe and studies show that embryonic stem cells will likely be more effective in curing diseases because they can grow and differentiate into any of the body's cells and tissues and thus into different organs."[72] Mrs. Nancy Reagan and her supporters favor expedient approaches including ESR.[73]

Several laws have supported the development of stem cells from sources other than embryos. For each of fiscal years 2004 through 2006, Congress allocated money in the HHS appropriations for the establishment and continuation of a National Cord Blood Stem Cell Bank within the Health Resources and Services Administration. In 2005, Congress enacted

P.L. 109-129 for the collection and maintenance of human cord blood stem cells for the treatment of patients and for research.

Generating Embryonic Stem Cells without Destroying Human Embryos

One possible alternative to ESR as it has typically been conducted, the ability to generate embryonic stem cells without destroying human embryos, was explored by the President's Council in its 2005 white paper,[74] described in the introductory section of this report. The white paper discusses four potential methods of obtaining embryonic stem cells without having to destroy embryos. Those methods, the scientific and practical merits of which remain far from settled, are (1) extracting cells from organismically dead embryos; (2) non-harmful biopsy of living embryos; (3) bioengineering embryo-like artifacts; and (4) dedifferentiating somatic cells.[75]

In the white paper, the President's Council examined the ethical acceptability of each method. The first two seek to avoid the destruction of embryos either by developing standards for declaring an embryo "dead" when its cells have stopped dividing or by removing a cell from an embryo without destroying the embryo itself. The other two methods would avoid having to use an embryo altogether, by attempting to obtain embryonic stem cells through the destruction of something that is not an embryo.

The Council concluded that the use of organismically dead embryos raises a number of ethical questions that have yet to be answered. They include whether it is possible to be certain that an embryo is really dead, whether the proposal would put embryos at additional risk, and whether IVF practitioners would be encouraged to create extra embryos. A September 2006 report that a team based in Serbia and England had derived stem cells from "dead" embryos prompted precisely these types of questions, as well some regarding whether the stem cells might carry some defect that had made the embryos non-viable.[76]

Regarding the use of non-harmful biopsy, the Council found that it would be ethically unacceptable to test in humans because risks should not be imposed on living embryos destined to become children for the sake of getting stem cells for research. This same response was prompted by an August 2006 report in the journal *Nature* that a California company had used the nonharmful biopsy method to derive stem cells.[77] In addition, the technique was criticized on one side for effectively "creating a twin and then killing that twin,"[78] and on the other for being an inefficient method for deriving stem cell lines.[79] In November 2006, *Nature* issued an addendum to the August article to clarify that, while the company's lead scientist maintained that his method could be used to derive stem cells without destroying embryos, in fact, he had destroyed all of the embryos during his own experiments.[80]

The Council also concluded that bioengineering embryo-like artifacts raises many serious ethical concerns, including whether the artifact would really be a very defective embryo, the ethics of egg procurement, concerns about the use of genetic engineering itself, and the possibility of its use creating a "slippery slope." Finally, the Council found the proposal to dedifferentiate somatic cells to be ethically acceptable if and when it became scientifically practical, provided that de facto embryos were not created.

Although some Council members expressed their support for efforts to identify means of obtaining human embryonic stem cells for biomedical research that do not involve killing or harming human embryos, not all of the members agreed. Some expressed concern that all four methods would "use financial resources that would be better devoted to proposals that are likely to be more productive." One member wrote that he did not support publishing the white paper "with the implied endorsement that special efforts be made in the scientific areas described. While some of the suggestions could be explored in a scientific setting, most are high-risk options that only have an outside chance of success and raise their own complex set of ethical questions."

As is generally the case regarding alternatives to ESR, on its face the Obama policy neither requires not precludes funding research to obtain ES without destroying embryos, but does require that research be responsible and scientifically worthy. By contrast, E.O. 6/20 had specifically directed the HHS Secretary to consider the techniques outlined by the President's Council, and to fund attempts to generate sources of pluripotent stem cell therapies that were not derived from human embryos.

Use of Federal Funding

Some division over the support for and opposition to ESR focuses on the question of whether the use of federal funding is appropriate. Those who oppose federal funding argue that the government should not be associated with embryo destruction.[81] They point out that embryo destruction violates the "deeply held moral beliefs of some citizens," and suggest that "funding alternative research is morally preferable."[82] Proponents of federal funding argue that it is immoral to discourage life-saving research by withholding federal funding. They point out that consensus support is not required for many federal spending policies, as it "does not violate democratic principles or infringe on the rights of dissent of those in the minority."[83] They argue that the efforts of both federally supported and privately supported researchers are necessary to keep the United States at the forefront of what they believe is a very important, cutting edge area of science. Furthermore, supporters believe that the oversight that comes with federal dollars will result in better and more ethically controlled research in the field. Requirements attached to federal funding are one traditional mechanism that Congress has used to regulate scientific research that might otherwise be conducted without federal oversight.[84]

Groups' positions on federal funding tend to mirror their positions on stem cell research generally. The Obama policy authorizes federal funding for ESR, and requires funded research be responsible and scientifically worthy. The Bush policy had also authorized federal funding, but not in a way designed to effect how stem cell lines were established.[85] The President's Council does not take a position on the issue, but notes the pros and cons and stresses that there is a "difference between *prohibiting* embryo research and *refraining from funding* it."[86] Focus on the Family opposes ESR, including federal funding for it.[87] NBAC finds the arguments in favor of federal funding more persuasive than those against it.[88] The National Academies, a group of Representatives, a group of Senators, Mrs. Nancy Reagan and her supporters, CAMR, the Nobel Laureates, and the UOJCA favor federal funding for ESR.[89]

End Notes

[1] For an overview of various religious perspectives on embryonic stem cell research, see LeRoy Walters, "Human Embryonic Stem Cell Research: An Intercultural Perspective," *Kennedy Institute of Ethics Journal*, vol. 14, no. 1, March 2004, p. 3.

[2] For further information, see CRS Report RL33540, *Stem Cell Research: Federal Research Funding and Oversight*, by Judith A. Johnson and Erin D. Williams.

[3] For further information about the Dickey amendment and the HHS General Council's opinion, see CRS Report RL33540, *Stem Cell Research: Federal Research Funding and Oversight*, by Judith A. Johnson and Erin D. Williams.

[4] "Removing Barriers to Responsible Scientific Research Involving Human Stem Cells," March 9, 2009, at http://www.whitehouse.gov/the_press_office/Removing-Barriers-to-Responsible-Scientific-Research-Involving-Human-Stem-Cells/.

[5] The White House, Office of the Press Secretary, Remarks of President Barack Obama-As Prepared for Delivery, Signing of Stem Cell Executive Order and Scientific Integrity Presidential Memorandum, March 9, 2009, at http://www.whitehouse.gov/the_press_office/Remarks-of-the-President-As-Prepared-for-Delivery-Signing-of-Stem-Cell-Executive-Order-and-Scientific-Integrity-Presidential-Memorandum/.

[6] George W. Bush, Executive Order: Expanding Approved Stem Cell Lines in Ethically Responsible Ways, June 20, 2007, at http://www.whitehouse.gov/news/releases/2007/06/20070620-6.html.

[7] For further information about 42 U.S.C. 274e and valuable consideration, see CRS Report RL33902, *Living Organ Donation and Valuable Consideration*, by Erin D. Williams, Bernice Reyes-Akinbileje, and Kathleen S. Swendiman.

[8] The National Academies brings together "committees of experts in all areas of scientific and technological endeavor" as "advisors to the Nation." For statements on ESR and cloning, see National Research Council, Institute of Medicine, National Academies, *Stem Cells and the Future of Regenerative Medicine* (Washington: National Academies, 2001); and Committee on Science, Engineering and Public Policy and Global Affairs Division, et al., *Scientific and Medical Aspects of Human Reproductive Cloning* (Washington, National Academy Press, 2002) at http://www.nationalacademies.org/about/#org.

[9] CAMR was formed in 2001 to ensure that the voices of patients, scientists, and physicians were heard in the debate over stem cell research and the future of regenerative medicine http://www.camradvocacy.org/about_us.aspx; visited January 18, 2007. For a statement on ESR, see Coalition for the Advancement of Medical Research, "The Promise of Embryonic Stem Cells, http://www.camradvocacy.org/resources/The_Promise_of_Embryonic_Stem_Cells. htm, visited Jan 18, 2007.

[10] "Nancy Reagan plea on stem cells," *BBC News*, May 10, 2004, at http://news.bbc.co.uk/2/hi/americas/3700015.stm, visited January 18, 2007; Letter from Nancy Reagan to Senator Orrin Hatch, May 1, 2006, at http://www.camradvocacy.org/resources/ Nancy_Reagan.pdf, visited January 18, 2007.

[11] Ibid.

[12] Letter from Harvey Blitz, President, UOJCA et al., to President George W. Bush, July 26, 2001, at http://www.ou.org/public/statements/2001/nate34.htm, visited July 14, 2005. (Hereafter cited as UOJCA letter.)

[13] The Christian Legal Society is a "national grassroots network of lawyers and law students, committed to ... advocating biblical conflict reconciliation, public justice, religious freedom and the sanctity of human life." At http://www.clsnet.org/clsPages/vision.php, visited July 15, 2005.

[14] *Focus on the Family* was founded in 1977 by Dr. James Dobson to promote the teachings of Jesus Christ. See http://www.family.org.

[15] The Christian Coalition is "the largest and most active conservative grassroots political organization in America," at http://www.cc.org.

[16] The National Right to Life Committee was founded in 1973 to "restore legal protection to innocent human life," at http://www.nrlc.org/Missionstatement.htm.

[17] The United States Conference of Catholic Bishops "is an assembly of the hierarchy of the United States and the U.S. Virgin Islands who jointly exercise certain pastoral functions on behalf of the Christian faithful of the United States," at http://www.usccb.org/whoweare.shtml.

[18] The *President's Council* was created by President Bush in November 2001 to "advise the President on bioethical issues that may emerge as a consequence of advances in biomedical science and technology." George W. Bush, "Creation of The President's Council on Bioethics," Executive Order 13237, November 28, 2001.

[19] The President's Council on Bioethics, *Monitoring Stem Cell Research*, January 2004.

[20] The President's Council on Bioethics, *Reproduction and Responsibility*, March 2004, p. xlviii.

[21] The President's Council on Bioethics, Human Cloning and Human Dignity, July 2002, pp. xxxv-xxxviii). Note: At the June 20, 2002, meeting, 9 of 17 Council members voted to support cloning for medical research purposes, without a moratorium, provided a regulatory mechanism was established. Because one member of the Council had not attended the meetings and was not voting, the vote seemed to be 9 to 8 in favor of research cloning. However, draft versions of the Council report sent to Council members on June 28, 2002, indicated that 2 of the group of 9 members had changed their votes in favor of a moratorium. Both made it clear that they have no ethical problem with cloning for biomedical research, but felt that a moratorium would provide time for additional discussion. The changed vote took many Council members by surprise, and some on the Council believe that the moratorium option, as opposed to a ban, was thrown in at the last minute and did not receive adequate discussion. In addition, some on the Council believe that the widely reported final vote of 10 to 7 in favor of a moratorium does not accurately reflect the fact "that the majority of the council has no problem with the ethics of biomedical cloning." (Transcripts of the Council meetings and papers developed by staff for discussion during Council meetings can be found at http://www.bioethics.gov; S. S. Hall, "President's Bioethics Council Delivers," *Science*, vol. 297, July 19, 2002, pp. 322-324.) "Wise Words from Across the Pond?," *BioNews*, no. 252, March 29, 2004.

[22] The President's Council on Bioethics, *Alternative Sources of Human Pluripotent Stem Cells* (May 2005), at http://www.bioethics.gov/reports/white_paper/index.html, visited July 14, 2005.

[23] In 1995, President Clinton created the National Bioethics Advisory Commission by Executive Order, to advise him on bioethical issues. The Order expired in 2001. "Former Bioethics Commissions," *President's Commission on Bioethics* website, at http://www.bioethics.gov/reports/past_commissions/index.html, visited June 30, 2004.

[24] National Bioethics Advisory Commission, *Ethical Issues in Human Stem Cell Research*, vol. 1, September 1999, pp. 70-71.

[25] American Life League, *The Bush Stem Cell Decision*, 2001, athttp://www.all.org/article. php?id=10746&search=2001,visited January 18, 2007.

[26] Office of Communications, United States Conference of Catholic Bishops, *Catholic Bishops Criticize Bush Policy on Embryo Research* (August 9, 2001), at http://www.usccb.org/comm/ archives/2001/01-142.shtml.

[27] The President's Council on Bioethics, *Monitoring Stem Cell Research*, January 2004, pp. 58, 62.

[28] Presentation by B. Steinbock, Department of Philosophy, SUNY, Albany, NY, NIH Human Embryo Research Panel Meeting, February 3, 1994.

[29] Michael Sandel, "Embryo Ethics—The Moral Logic of Stem-Cell Research," *New England Journal of Medicine*, vol. 351, no. 3, July 15, 2004, p. 208.

[30] UOJCA letter.

[31] The President's Council on Bioethics, *Monitoring Stem Cell Research*, January 2004, p. 87.

[32] The President's Council on Bioethics, *Reproduction and Responsibility*, March 2004.

[33] National Bioethics Advisory Commission, *Ethical Issues in Human Stem Cell Research*, vol. 1, September 1999, p. 50.

[34] Letter from 206 Members of the House of Representatives to President George W. Bush, April 28, 2004, at http://www.house.gov/degette/news/releases/040428.pdf. (Hereafter cited as Letter from 206 Members of the House of Representatives.)

[35] Letter from 58 Senators to President George W. Bush, June 7, 2004, at http://feinstein.senate.gov/04Releases/rstemcell-ltr.pdf. (Hereafter cited as Letter from 58 Senators.)

[36] International Society for Stem Cell Research, "Alternative Methods of Producing Stem Cells: No Substitute for Embryonic Stem Cell Research," *Press Release*, (August 2, 2005), at http://www.isscr.org/press_releases/camr_alternatives.htm, visited April 10, 2007.

[37] See, e.g., Eric Cohen and Robert George, "Stem Cells Without Moral Corruption: Congress Can Give Research a Boost Without Supporting the Misuse of Human Embryos," *Washington Post*, July 6, 2006, p. A21.

[38] National Bioethics Advisory Commission, *Ethical Issues in Human Stem Cell Research*, vol. 1, September 1999, pp. 70-72. In SCNT the nucleus of an egg is removed and replaced by the nucleus from a mature body cell, such as a skin cell obtained from a patient. In 1996, scientists in Scotland used the SCNT procedure to produce Dolly the sheep, the first mammalian clone.

[39] UOJCA letter.

[40] The President's Council on Bioethics, *Reproduction and Responsibility*, March 2004, p. xlviii.

[41] Paul McHugh, "Zygote and 'Clonote'—The Ethical Use of Embryonic Stem Cells," *New England Journal of Medicine*, vol. 351, no. 3, July 15, 2004, p. 210.

[42] Letter from 206 Members of the House of Representatives; Letter from 58 Senators.

[43] National Research Council, Institute of Medicine, National Academies, *Stem Cells and the Future of Regenerative Medicine* (Washington: National Academies, 2001), p. 58.

[44] The President's Council on Bioethics, *Monitoring Stem Cell Research*, January 2004, pp. 33-34.

[45] Ibid.

[46] The President's Council on Bioethics, *Monitoring Stem Cell Research*, January 2004, pp. 63-67.

[47] Bridget M. Kuehn, "Genetic Flaws Found in Aging Stem Cell Lines," *Journal of the American Medical Association*, vol. 294, no. 15 (October 2005), p. 1883.

[48] Letter from 206 Members of the House of Representatives; Letter from 58 Senators.

[49] National Bioethics Advisory Commission, *Ethical Issues in Human Stem Cell Research*, vol. 1, September 1999, p. 49.

[50] UOJCA letter.

[51] Kathy Hudson, "International Society for Stem Cell Research Draft Guidelines," *Genetics & Public Policy Center ENews,* Issue 10 (July 2006), available online at http://www.dnapolicy. org/news.enews.article.nocategory.php? action=detail&newsletter_id=13&article_id=31.

[52] The HHS regulations that generally require informed consent for research involving human subjects research do not generally apply to gametes, embryos, or other tissue, once donated or discarded. (See 45 C.F.R. § 46, subparts A & B.)

[53] See the "Consent of Donors" section of this report for more information.

[54] National Research Council, Institute of Medicine, National Academies, *Stem Cells and the Future of Regenerative Medicine* (Washington: National Academies, 2001), p. 53.

[55] Letter from 206 Members of the House of Representatives; Letter from 58 Senators.

[56] "Egg Donation Ethics Study Wins Award," *Research at Penn*, (March 7, 2005), at http://www.upenn. edu/researchatpenn/article.php?113&soc, visited December 5, 2005.

[57] American Society of Reproductive Medicine, "Financial Incentives in Recruitment of Oocyte Donors," *Fertility and Sterility*, vol. 74, no. 2 (August 2000), p. 216.

[58] See e.g., "Egg Donation Ethics Study Wins Award," *Research at Penn*, (March 7, 2005), at http://www.upenn. edu/researchatpenn/article.php?113&soc, visited December 5, 2005.

[59] James Brooke, "Korean Leaves Cloning Center in Ethics Furor," Professional Ethics website (November 25, 2005), at http://ethics.tamucc.edu/article.pl?sid=05/11/26/1524206&mode=t hread visited December 12, 2005.

[60] Unless otherwise noted, these arguments can be found, among other places, at American Society of Reproductive Medicine, "Financial incentives in recruitment of oocyte donors," *Fertility and Sterility*, vol. 74, no. 2 (August 2000), p. 218; and Claudia Kalb, "Ethics, Eggs and Embryos," *MSNBC.com, Newsweek website*, at http://www.msnbc.msn.com/id/8185339/site/newsweek/, visited December 12, 2005.

[61] Kathy Hudson, "International Society for Stem Cell Research Draft Guidelines," *Genetics & Public Policy Center ENews,* Issue 10 (July 2006), available online at http://www.dnapolicy. org/news.enews.article.nocategory.php?action=detail&newsletter_id=13&article_id=31.

[62] See e.g., President's Council on Bioethics, *White Paper: Alternative Sources of Pluripotent Stem Cells* (May 2005), pp. 40-41 at http://www.bioethics.gov/reports/white_paper/index.html, visited December 12, 2005.

[63] National Academies, *Guidelines for Human Embryonic Stem Cell Research*, (Washington, DC: National Academies Press, p. 87, at http://books.nap.edu/books/0309096537/html/87.html, visited, December 12, 2005.

[64] Rick Weiss, "Scientists See Potential In Amniotic Stem Cells," *Washington Post*, January 8, 2007, p. A1, at http://www.washingtonpost.com/wp-dyn/content/article/2007/01/07/AR2007010 700674. html, visited January 8, 2007.

[65] Junying Yu et al., "Induced Pluripotent Stem Cell Lines Derived from Human Somatic Cells," *Science*, vol. 318, no. 5858 (21 December 2007; originally published in *Science Express* on 20 November 2007).

[66] Dr. Elias Zerhouni's answer to a question during the "Fiscal 2008 budget for the National Institutes of Health," *Hearing of the U.S. Senate Appropriations Subcommittee on Labor, Health and Human Services, Education, and Related Agencies* (March 19, 2007).

[67] "The News: Scientists for the first time have generated human stem cells from adult cells," *Bioethics Responder from the Hastings Center*, (20 November 2007).

[68] The President's Council on Bioethics, *Monitoring Stem Cell Research*, January 2004, p. 10.

[69] Carrie Gordon Earll, "Talking Points on Stem Cell Research," *Focus on the Family*, September 17, 2003 at http://www.family.org/cforum/fosi/bioethics/faqs/a0027980.cfm.

[70] National Research Council, Institute of Medicine, National Academies, *Stem Cells and the Future of Regenerative Medicine* (Washington: National Academies, 2001), p. 56.

[71] National Bioethics Advisory Commission, *Ethical Issues in Human Stem Cell Research*, vol. 1, September 1999, p. 53.

[72] Coalition for the Advancement of Medical Research, "The Promise of Embryonic Stem Cells," at http://www.camradvocacy.org/resources/The_Promise_of_Embryonic_Stem_Cells.htm, visited January 18, 2007.

[73] Nancy Reagan plea on stem cells," *BBC News*, May 10, 2004, at http://news.bbc.co.uk/2/hi/ americas/3700015. stm, visited January 18, 2007; Letter from Nancy Reagan to Senator Orrin Hatch, May 1, 2006, at http://www.camradvocacy.org/resources/Nancy_Reagan.pdf, visited January 18, 2007.

[74] The President's Council on Bioethics, *White Paper: Alternative Sources of Human Pluripotent Stem Cells*, May 2005, online at http://www.bioethics.gov/reports/white_paper/index.html.

[75] For more information, see CRS Report RL33540, *Stem Cell Research: Federal Research Funding and Oversight*, by Judith A. Johnson and Erin D. Williams.

[76] See, e.g., Rick Weiss "Researchers Report Growing Stem Cells From Dead Embryos," *Washington Post*, September 23, 2006, p. A03, available online at http://www.washingtonpost.com/wp-dyn/content/article/2006/09/22/AR2006092201377.html.

[77] See e.g., Nicholas Wade, "Stem Cell News Could Intensify Political Debate," *New York Times*, August 24, 2006, available online at http://www.nytimes.com/2006/08/24/science/ 24stem.html?ex=1164862800&en =1d51ef92cddc3e82&ei=5070.

[78] Ibid.

[79] See e.g., Josephine Quintavalle, "The Lanza Protocol: Damned With Very Faint Praise," *BioNews*, vol. 373, (August 22-28, 2006), available online at http://www.bionews.org.uk/commentary. lasso?storyid=3157.

[80] Robert Laza et al., "Human Embryonic Stem Cell Lines Derived from Single Blastomeres," *Nature*, vol. 444, p. 481 (November 23, 2006), available online at http://www.nature.com/nature/journal/v444/n7118/full/nature05366.html.

[81] National Bioethics Advisory Commission, *Ethical Issues in Human Stem Cell Research*, vol. 1, September 1999, p. 57.

[82] Ibid.

[83] Ibid.

[84] For further information about Congressional regulation of research involving human subjects, see CRS Report RL32909, *Federal Protection for Human Research Subjects: An Analysis of the Common Rule and Its Interactions with FDA Regulations and the HIPAA Privacy Rule*, by Erin D. Williams.

[85] Because the Bush policy only allowed funding for work with previously established ES lines, researchers who had created stem cell lines before the policy took effect could not have been influenced by its ethical constraints regarding the derivation of stem cells from embryos, as their work preceded the policy. Similarly, researchers who created stem cell lines after the policy took effect would not have been motivated to follow the Bush policy's ethical guidelines regarding the creation of stem cell lines, because the results of their work would have remained ineligible for federal funding regardless of their methodology. By contrast, E.O. 6/20 may have affected the future derivation of embryonic stem cells to the extent that it encouraged that such activities take place without creating embryos for research or harming, endangering, or destroying them.

[86] The President's Council on Bioethics, *Monitoring Stem Cell Research*, January 2004, p. 37.

[87] *Stem Cell Research: Our Position (Stem Cells)*, Focus on The Family, 2009,http://www.focusonthe family.com/socialissues/sanctity_of_life/stem_cell_research/our_position.aspx. The group had previously expressed general support for President Bush and his ESR policy, but was "disappointed by his decision to allow federal funding of research on the existing stem cell lines." Carrie Gordon Earll, "Talking Points on Stem Cell Research," *Focus on the Family*, September 17, 2003 at http://www.family.org/cforum/fosi/bioethics/faqs/a0027980.cfm.

[88] National Bioethics Advisory Commission, *Ethical Issues in Human Stem Cell Research*, vol. 1, September 1999, p. 70.

[89] See, e.g., National Research Council, Institute of Medicine, National Academies, *Stem Cells and the Future of Regenerative Medicine* (Washington: National Academies, 2001), p. 49.

In: Encyclopedia of Stem Cell Research (2 Volume Set)   ISBN: 978-1-61761-835-2
Editor: Alexander L. Greene   © 2012 Nova Science Publishers, Inc.

Chapter LVI

STEM CELL RESEARCH: FEDERAL RESEARCH FUNDING AND OVERSIGHT*

Judith A. Johnson and Erin D. Williams

SUMMARY

Embryonic stem cells have the ability to develop into virtually any cell in the body, and may have the potential to treat injuries as well as illnesses, such as diabetes and Parkinson's disease. In January 2009, the Food and Drug Administration approved a request from Geron, a California biotechnology company, to begin a clinical trial involving safety tests of embryonic stem cells in patients with recent spinal cord injuries.

Currently, most human embryonic stem cell lines used in research are derived from embryos produced via in vitro fertilization (IVF). Because the process of removing these cells destroys the embryo, some individuals believe the derivation of stem cells from human embryos is ethically unacceptable. In November 2007, research groups in Japan and the United States announced the development of embryonic stem cell-like cells, called induced pluripotent stem (iPS) cells, via the introduction of four genes into human skin cells. Those concerned about the ethical implications of deriving stem cells from human embryos argue that researchers should use iPS cells or adult stem cells (from bone marrow or umbilical cord blood). However, many scientists believe research should focus on all types of stem cells.

On March 9, 2009, President Barack Obama signed an executive order that reversed the nearly eight-year old Bush Administration restriction on federal funding for human embryonic stem cell research. In August 2001, President George W. Bush had announced that for the first time, federal funds would be used to support research on human embryonic stem cells, but funding would be limited to "existing stem cell lines." NIH established a registry of 78 human embryonic stem cell lines eligible for use in federally funded research, but only 21

---

* This is an edited, reformatted and augmented version of a Congressional Research Service publication, Report RL33554, dated March 13, 2009.

cell lines were available due to technical reasons and other limitations. Over time scientists became increasingly concerned about the quality and longevity of these 21 stem cell lines. These scientists believe that research advancement requires access to new human embryonic stem cell lines.

H.R. 873 (DeGette), the Stem Cell Research Enhancement Act of 2009, was introduced on February 4, 2009. The text of H.R. 873 is identical to legislation introduced in the 110th Congress, H.R. 3 (DeGette), and the 109th Congress, H.R. 810 (Castle). The bill would allow federal support of research that utilizes human embryonic stem cells regardless of the date on which the stem cells were derived from a human embryo. Stem cell lines must meet ethical guidelines established by the NIH, which would be issued within 60 days of enactment. H.R. 872 (DeGette), the Stem Cell Research Improvement Act of 2009, was also introduced on February 4, 2009. It is similar to H.R. 873 in that it adds the same Section 498D, "Human Embryonic Stem Cell Research," to the PHS Act, but it also adds another Section 498E, "Guidelines on Research Involving Human Stem Cells," which would require the Director of NIH to issue guidelines on research involving human embryonic stem cell within 90 days of enactment; updates of the guidelines would be required every three years. S. 487 (Harkin), introduced on February 26, 2009, is the same as H.R. 873, except it has an additional section supporting research on alternative human pluripotent stem cells. It is identical to a bill introduced in the 110th Congress, S. 5 (Reid).

During the 110th Congress, the Senate passed legislation (S. 5) in April 2007 that would have allowed federal support of research that utilizes human embryonic stem cells regardless of the date on which the stem cells were derived from a human embryo. The bill would have also provided support for research on alternatives, such as iPS cells. The House passed the bill in June 2007, and President Bush vetoed it on June 20, 2007. (The 109th Congress passed a similar bill, which also was vetoed by President Bush, the first veto of his presidency; an attempt to override the veto in the House failed.) On the related issue of human cloning, in June 2007 the House failed to pass a bill (H.R. 2560) that would have imposed penalties on anyone who cloned a human embryo and implanted it in a uterus.

INTRODUCTION

On March 9, 2009, President Barack Obama signed an executive order reversing the nearly eightyear old Bush Administration restriction on federal funding for human embryonic stem cell research.[1] President George W. Bush had announced on August 9, 2001, that for the first time federal funds would be used to support research on human embryonic stem cells. However, the Bush decision limited funding to research on stem cell lines that had been created prior to the date of the policy announcement.

The Obama executive order directs the National Institutes of Health (NIH) to issue new guidelines for the conduct of human embryonic stem cell research within 120 days of the date of the executive order. The Obama decision will allow scientists to use federal funds for research utilizing the hundreds of human embryonic stem cell lines that have been created since the Bush 2001 policy. NIH anticipates using some of the $10 billion in funds provided by the stimulus package (American Recovery and Reinvestment Act of 2009, P.L. 111-5) for research on human embryonic stem cells under the new guidelines.[2] President Obama also issued a memorandum on scientific integrity directing the head of the White House Office of Science and Technology Policy "to develop a strategy for restoring scientific integrity to government decision making."[3]

In order to codify the Obama stem cell policy and prevent future administrations from reversing it, Members of the 111th Congress have introduced legislation (H.R. 872, H.R. 873, S. 487) and stated their intention to quickly pass a stem cell bill.[4] Similar legislation was twice vetoed by President George W. Bush during the 109th and 110th Congress. However, scientists still will not be able to use federal funds for the derivation of new human embryonic stem cell lines or for research involving somatic cell nuclear transfer (SCNT) using human eggs unless Congress removes the existing Dickey Amendment from appropriations legislation.

Research involving human embryonic stem cells is of concern for some individuals because the stem cells are located inside the embryo, and the process of removing the cells destroys the embryo.[5] Many religious and socially conservative individuals believe the destruction of embryos for the purpose of harvesting embryonic stem cells is morally and ethically unacceptable. They argue that researchers should use other alternatives, such as iPS cells or adult stem cells (both discussed below), instead of embryonic stem cells.

Federal funding for the support human embryonic stem cell research was limited under the Bush 2001 policy. NIH identified 78 human embryonic stem cell lines that would be eligible for use in federally funded research, but most were found to be either unavailable or unsuitable for research. Only 21 cell lines were available under the Bush policy. Over time, scientists became increasingly concerned about the quality and longevity of these 21 stem cell lines. Many believe research advancement requires the use of new human embryonic stem cell lines.

The former Director of NIH, Elias Zerhouni, stated in a hearing on March 19, 2007, before the Senate Labor, Health and Human Services (HHS), Education, and Related Agencies Appropriations Subcommittee that "It's not possible for me to see how we can continue the momentum of science and research with the stem cell lines we have at NIH that can be funded."[6] When asked if other avenues of research should be pursued instead, Dr. Zerhouni stated that "the presentations about adult stem cells holding as much or more potential than embryonic stem cells, in my view, do not hold scientific water. I think they are overstated."[7] He noted that competitors in Europe, China, and India are investing heavily in human embryonic stem cell research. "I think it is important for us not to fight with one hand tied behind our back here. I think it's time to move forward on this area. It's time for policy makers to find common ground, to make sure that NIH does not lose its historical leadership.... To sideline NIH on such an issue of importance in my view is shortsighted."[8] On May 8, 2008, Dr. Zerhouni made similar statements about the need for additional embryonic stem cell lines and the value of pursuing all avenues of stem cells research at a hearing before the House Energy and Commerce Subcommittee on Health.[9]

Several states, such as California, Connecticut, Illinois, Maryland, and New Jersey, responded to the Bush stem cell policy limitations by moving forward with their own initiatives to encourage or provide funding for stem cell research, and many others have considered similar action. Proponents of these state stem cell research initiatives want to remain competitive, as well as prevent the relocation of scientists and biotechnology firms to other states or overseas. However, without the central direction and coordinated research approach that the federal government can provide, many are concerned that the states' actions will result in duplication of research efforts among the states, a possible lack of oversight for ethical concerns, and ultimately a loss of U.S. preeminence in this important area of basic research. States may be reconsidering their funding of stem cell research given the change in federal policy that occurred under the Obama Administration.

The 110th Congress addressed the topic of stem cell research early in the first session. H.R. 3 (DeGette) was introduced on January 5, 2007, with 211 cosponsors, and passed the House on January 11, 2007.[10] The bill would have allowed federal support of research that utilizes human embryonic stem cells regardless of the date on which the stem cells were derived from a human embryo, and thus would have negated the August 2001 Bush stem cell policy limitation. The Senate passed S. 5 (Reid) on April 11, the House passed S. 5 on June 7, and President Bush vetoed the bill on June 20, 2007. S. 5 was the same as H.R. 3 except it has an additional section supporting research on alternative human pluripotent stem cells.[11]

BASIC RESEARCH AND POTENTIAL APPLICATIONS

Most cells within an animal or human being are committed to fulfilling a single function within the body. In contrast, stem cells are a unique and important set of cells that are not specialized. Stem cells retain the ability to become some or all of the more than 200 different cell types in the body, and thereby play a critical role in repairing organs and body tissues throughout life. Although the term stem cells is often used in reference to these repair cells within an adult organism, a more fundamental variety of stem cells is found in the early-stage embryo. Embryonic stem cells may have a greater ability to become different types of body cells than adult stem cells.

Embryonic Stem Cells from IVF Embryos or Fetal Tissue

Embryonic stem cells were first isolated from mouse embryos in 1981 and from primate embryos in 1995. Animal embryos were the only source for research on embryonic stem cells until November 1998, when two groups of U.S. scientists announced the successful isolation of human embryonic stem cells. One group, at the University of Wisconsin, derived stem cells from fiveday-old embryos produced via *in vitro* fertilization (IVF).[12] The work is controversial because the stem cells are located within the embryo and the process of removing them destroys the embryo. Many individuals who are opposed to abortion are also opposed to research involving embryos. The second group, at Johns Hopkins University, derived stem cells with very similar properties from five- to nine-week-old embryos or from fetuses obtained through elective abortion.[13] Both groups reported the human embryos or fetuses were donated for research following a process of informing one or more parents and obtaining their consent. The cells removed from embryos or fetuses were manipulated in the laboratory to create embryonic stem cell lines that may continue to divide for many months to years. The vast majority of research on human embryonic stem cells, both in the United States and overseas, utilizes cell lines derived via the University of Wisconsin method.

Induced Pluripotent Stem (iPS) Cells

In November 2007, two research groups, one at Kyoto University in Japan and the second at the University of Wisconsin, Madison, announced the development of embryonic stem cell-like cells, called induced pluripotent stem (iPS) cells, through the introduction of four genes into human skin cells.[14] Until this breakthrough, the characteristics displayed by the iPS cells were thought to occur only in cells found within the embryo. The research teams accomplished the reprogramming of the adult skin cells by using a retrovirus to transport the four genes into the skin cells. The teams each used a different set of four genes; the Kyoto group has subsequently achieved reprogramming using three genes.[15] The work on human iPS cells is based on earlier studies by the Kyoto group in mouse embryos that identified the genes active in early embryos and then used combinations of these genes to try and reprogram adult mouse cells. The successful mouse reprogramming study, using four mouse genes, was announced in June 2006. The analogous four human genes were used by the Kyoto group on the human skin cells.

Although development of iPS cells may one day lessen the need to study stem cells derived from the human embryo, scientists insist that work on human embryonic stem cells must continue for several reasons.[16] For example, it is unclear whether iPS cells share all the characteristics of embryonic stem cells, and therefore multiple comparisons between the two types of cells will be necessary. In addition, because scientists have used potentially cancer-causing retroviruses to transfer the reprogramming genes, these iPS cells would not desirable for therapeutic uses in patients. Therefore, alternative mechanisms to accomplish reprogramming would need to be developed. Scientists are in the process of investigating the use of other safer viruses to transfer the genes. Some groups are exploring chemical methods of achieving the same results by switching on genes in the adult cell rather than transferring in additional gene copies with a virus.

Embryonic Stem Cells Obtained via SCNT (Cloning)

Another potential source of embryonic stem cells is somatic cell nuclear transfer (SCNT), also referred to as cloning.[17] For certain applications, stem cells derived using SCNT may offer the best hope for understanding and treating disease. In SCNT the nucleus of an egg is removed and replaced by the nucleus from a mature body cell, such as a skin cell obtained from a patient. In 1996, scientists in Scotland used the SCNT procedure to produce Dolly the sheep, the first mammalian clone.[18] When SCNT is used to create another individual, such as Dolly, the process is called reproductive cloning. In contrast, scientists interested in using SCNT to create cloned stem cells would allow the cell created via SCNT to develop for a few days, and then the stem cells would be removed for research. Stem cells created via SCNT would be genetically identical to the patient, and thus would avoid any tissue rejection problems that could occur if the cells were transplanted into the patient. Creating stem cells using SCNT for research purposes is sometimes referred to as therapeutic cloning.

Although various scientific groups have reported success in using SCNT to create cloned embryos (which are then used to produce stem cell lines or live births) of a variety of different mammals (sheep, rabbits, cows), attempts at creating primate embryos via SCNT had been unsuccessful. However, in June 2007, researchers at the Oregon National Primate Research Center at Oregon Health and Science University announced the successful derivation of stem cells from a rhesus monkey embryo created via SCNT.[19] Results of the Oregon group were confirmed in November 2007.[20]

The unsubstantiated announcement by Clonaid in December 2002 of the birth of a cloned child have contributed to the controversy over research on human embryos.[21] More recently, charges of ethical and scientific misconduct have clouded the reputation of scientists involved in deriving stem cells from human embryos created via SCNT. In February 2004, scientists at the Seoul National University (SNU) in South Korea announced the first isolation of stem cells from a cloned human embryo and in May 2005 announced advances in the efficiency of creating cloned human embryos and in isolating human stem cells. Concerns about the SNU work arose in November 2005 when a U.S. co-author of the 2005 paper accused Hwang Woo Suk, the lead SNU researcher, of ethical misconduct.[22] In December 2005, a Korean co-author of the May 2005 paper stated that the research was fabricated and the paper should be retracted; Hwang agreed to the retraction. On January 10, 2006, SNU stated that results of the 2004 paper were also a deliberate fabrication.[23] Despite these difficulties, scientists in a number of labs are continuing to work on deriving patient-matched stem cells from cloned human embryos.[24]

Stem Cells from Adult Tissue or Umbilical Cord Blood

Stem cells obtained from adult organisms are also the focus of research. In April 2007, researchers in Brazil published a preliminary report on attempts to treat 15 newly diagnosed type 1 diabetes patients with high-dose immunosuppressive chemotherapy followed by transplantation of the patient's own stem cells.[25] Although this experiment was first proposed by U.S. scientists, the risks associated with the procedure were judged to be to high (5% mortality) for a treatable disease that affects children.[26] Type 1 diabetes is thought to be an autoimmune disease in which the patient's immune system attacks the insulin-producing cells in the pancreas. Scientists are not certain about the exact mechanism of how the treatment works. One hypothesis is that the chemotherapy suppresses the patient's immune system and stops the destruction of the remaining insulin-producing cells in the patient's body, which is why early diagnosis is crucial in this approach. The patient's stem cells are then transfused back into the body, hopefully becoming part of an immune system that will not continue to attack the patient's insulin-producing cells.

A January 2007 report found that cells similar to embryonic stem cells can be found in amniotic fluid. However, the lead author of the report, as well as others in the field, caution that these cells are not a replacement for embryonic stem cells.[27] There have been a number of other publications on the abilities and characteristics of adult stem cells from a variety of different sources, such as bone marrow and the umbilical cord following birth. Bone marrow transplantation, a type of adult stem cell therapy, has been used for 50 years to treat patients for a variety of blood-related conditions.[28] Several private companies (such as MorphoGen, NeuralStem, Osiris Therapeutics, StemSource, ViaCell) are working on additional therapeutic uses of adult stem cells.

In 1999, David A. Prentice of the Family Research Council and other biomedical researchers founded Do No Harm: The Coalition of Americans for Research Ethics, a group that opposes stem cell research on the grounds that it is unethical because it destroys embryos and is unnecessary due to the success of adult stem cell therapy. Do No Harm has compiled a list of 73 diseases that it claims can be treated using adult stem cells.[29] In a July 2006 letter to *Science,* Smith et al. accuse Prentice of misleading the public and deceiving patients with the list because only nine of the adult stem cell treatments have been "fully tested in all required phases of clinical trials and approved by the U.S. Food and Drug Administration."[30] Prentice responded in a January 2007 letter that "Our list of [then] 72 applications, compiled from peer-reviewed articles, documents observable and measurable benefit to patients, a necessary step toward formal FDA approval and what is expected of new, cutting-edge medical applications."[31] Prentice also accused Smith et al. of "cruelly deceiving patients and the public" by promoting the "falsehood that embryonic stem cell cures are imminent." In a June 2007 exchange, Smith et al. continue to emphasize that the majority of treatments on the list haven't met FDA standards.[32] Prentice defended the list by pointing to tangible benefits to some patients.[33] Both sides again accused the other of misleading laypeople and deceiving patients.

Opponents of stem cell research advocate that adult instead of embryonic stem cell research should be pursued because they believe the derivation of stem cells from either IVF embryos or aborted fetuses is ethically unacceptable. Others believe that adult stem cells should not be the sole target of research because of important scientific and technical limitations. Adult stem cells may not be as long lived or capable of as many cell divisions as embryonic stem cells. Also, adult stem cells may not be as versatile in developing into various types of tissue as embryonic stem cells, and the location and rarity of the cells in the body might rule out safe and easy access. For these reasons, many scientists argue that both adult and embryonic stem cells should be the subject of research, allowing for a comparison of their various capabilities. Reports issued by the NIH and the Institute of Medicine (IoM) state that both embryonic and adult stem cell research should be pursued.[34]

In FY2004, the Consolidated Appropriations Act, 2004 (P.L. 108-199) provided $10 million to establish a National Cord Blood Stem Cell Bank within the Health Resources and Services Administration (HRSA). HRSA was directed to use $1 million to contract with the IoM to conduct a study that would recommend an optimal structure for the program. The study, *Cord Blood: Establishing a National Hematopoietic Stem Cell Bank Program*, was released in April 2005. The blood cell forming stem cells found in cord blood can be used as an alternative to bone marrow transplantation in the treatment of leukemia, lymphoma, certain types of anemia, and inherited disorders of immunity and metabolism. The IOM report provides the logistical process for establishing a national cord blood banking system, establishes uniform standards for cord blood collection and storage, and provides recommendations on ethical and legal issues associated with cord blood collection, storage and use.

On December 20, 2005, the President signed the Stem Cell Therapeutic and Research Act of 2005 (P.L. 109-129). The act provides for the collection and maintenance of human cord blood stem cells for the treatment of patients and for research. It stipulates that amounts appropriated in FY2004 or FY2005 for this purpose shall remain available until the end of FY2007, and authorizes $60 million over FY2007-FY2010. The act also reauthorizes the national bone marrow registry with $186 million over FY2006-FY2010. In addition, it creates a database to enable health care workers to search for cord blood and bone marrow matches and links all these functions under a new name, the C.W. Bill Young Cell Transplantation program.

Potential Applications of Stem Cell Research

Stem cells provide the opportunity to study the growth and differentiation of individual cells into tissues. Understanding these processes could provide insights into the causes of birth defects, genetic abnormalities, and other disease states. If normal development were better understood, it might be possible to prevent or correct some of these conditions. Stem cells could be used to produce large amounts of one cell type to test new drugs for effectiveness and chemicals for toxicity. The damaging side effects of medical treatments might be repaired with stem cell treatment. For example, cancer chemotherapy destroys immune cells in patients, decreasing their ability to fight off a broad range of diseases; correcting this adverse effect would be a major advance. Stem cells might be transplanted into the body to treat disease (e.g., diabetes, Parkinson's disease) or injury (e.g., spinal cord).

In January 2009, the Food and Drug Administration approved a request from Geron, a California biotechnology company, to begin a Phase I clinical trial involving safety tests of embryonic stem cells in 8 to 10 patients with recent spinal cord injuries.[35] In this first human subject trial using embryonic stem cells, the injected cells are intended to "help repair the insulation, known as myelin, around nerve cells, restoring the ability of some nerve cells to carry signals. There is also hope that growth factors produced by the injected cells will spur damaged nerve cells to regenerate."[36] Some scientists have expressed concern over the possibility that the transplanted cells may form a type of tumor called a teratoma, but extensive studies in rodents were performed to assure FDA that the stem cells did not causes tumors in animals.[37]

Before stem cells can be applied to human medical problems, substantial advances in basic cell biology and clinical technique are required. In addition, very challenging regulatory decisions will be required on any individually created tissue-based therapies resulting from stem cell research. Such decisions would likely be made by the Center for Biologics Evaluation and Research (CBER) of the Food and Drug Administration (FDA). The potential benefits mentioned above would be likely only after many more years of research. Technical hurdles include developing the ability to control the differentiation of stem cells into a desired cell type (like a heart or nerve cell) and to ensure that uncontrolled development, such as cancer, does not occur. Some experiments may involve the creation of a chimera, an organism that contains two or more genetically distinct cell types, from the same species or different species.[38] If stem cells are to be used for transplantation, the problem of immune rejection must also be overcome. Some scientists think that the creation of many more embryonic stem cell lines will eventually account for all the various immunological types needed for use in tissue transplantation therapy. Others envision the eventual development of a "universal donor" type of stem cell tissue, analogous to a universal blood donor.

However, if the method used to create iPS cells or if the SCNT technique was employed (using a cell nucleus from the patient), the stem cells created via these methods would be genetically identical to the patient, would presumably be recognized by the patient's immune system, and thus might avoid any tissue rejection problems that could occur in other stem cell therapeutic approaches. Because of this, scientists believe that these techniques may provide the best hope of eventually treating patients using stem cells for tissue transplantation.

REGULATION OF RESEARCH

A Brief History of Federal Policy on Human Embryo Research

Federal funding of *any* type of research involving human embryos, starting with *in vitro* fertilization (IVF) then later the creation of stem cell lines from embryos, had been blocked by various policy decisions dating back 30 years.

Ethics Advisory Board

Following the birth of the first IVF baby, Louise Brown, in July 1978, the federal Ethics Advisory Board (EAB) was tasked with considering the scientific, ethical, legal, and social issues surrounding human IVF.[39] The EAB released its report on May 4, 1979, which found that IVF research was acceptable from an ethical standpoint and could be supported with federal funds. The EAB's recommendations were never adopted by HHS, the EAB was dissolved in 1980, and no other EAB was ever chartered. Because federal regulations that govern human subject research (45 C.F.R. Part 46) stipulated that, at the time, federally supported research involving human IVF must be reviewed by an EAB, a so-called "de facto moratorium" on human IVF research resulted. Other types of embryo research ensuing from the development and use of IVF, such as cloning and stem cells, were therefore also blocked. The de facto moratorium was lifted with the enactment of the National Institutes of Health (NIH) Revitalization Act of 1993 (P.L. 103-43, Section 121(c)), which nullified the regulatory provision (45 C.F.R. § 46.204(d)) requiring EAB review of IVF proposals.

NIH Human Embryo Research Panel

In response, the NIH established the Human Embryo Research Panel to assess the moral and ethical issues raised by this research and to develop recommendations for NIH review and conduct of human embryo research. The NIH Panel released a report providing guidelines and recommendations on human embryo research in September 1994. The panel identified areas of human embryo research it considered to be unacceptable, or to warrant additional review. It determined that certain types of cloning[40] without transfer to the uterus warranted additional review before the panel could recommend whether the research should be federally funded. However, the panel concluded that federal funding for such cloning techniques followed by transfer to the uterus should be unacceptable into the foreseeable future. The NIH Panel recommended that some areas of human embryo research should be considered for federal funding, including SCNT, stem cells and, under certain limited conditions, *embryos created solely for the purpose of research.*[41] The panel's report was unanimously accepted by the NIH Advisory Committee to the Director (ACD) on December 2, 1994.

After the ACD meeting on December 2, 1994, President Clinton directed NIH *not* to allocate resources to support the *"creation of human embryos for research purposes."* The President's directive did not apply to research involving so-called "spare" embryos, those that sometimes remain from clinical IVF procedures performed to assist infertile couples to become parents. Nor did it apply to human parthenotes, eggs that begin development through artificial activation, not through fertilization. Following the Clinton December 2, 1994, directive to NIH, the agency proceeded with plans to develop guidelines to support research using spare embryos. NIH plans to develop guidelines on embryo research were halted on January 26, 1996, with the enactment of P.L. 104-99, which contained a rider that affected FY1996 funding for NIH. The rider, often referred to as the Dickey Amendment, prohibited HHS from using appropriated funds for the creation of human embryos for research purposes or for research in which human embryos are destroyed.

The Dickey Amendment

Prior to an August 2001 Bush Administration decision (see below), no federal funds had been used to support research on stem cells derived from either human embryos or fetal tissue.[42] The work at the University of Wisconsin and Johns Hopkins University was supported by private funding from the Geron Corporation. Private funding for experiments involving embryos was required because Congress attached a rider to legislation that affected FY1996 NIH funding. The rider, an amendment originally introduced by Representative Jay Dickey, prohibited HHS from using appropriated funds for the creation of human embryos for research purposes or for research in which human embryos are destroyed. The Dickey Amendment language has been added to each of the Labor, HHS, and Education appropriations acts for FY1997 through FY2008.[43] Funding for FY2009 is provided in the Omnibus Appropriations Act, 2009, P.L. 111-8 The Dickey Amendment is found in Section 509 of Division F—Departments of Labor, Health and Human Services, and Education, and Related Agencies Appropriations Act, 2009, of P.L. 111-8. It states that:

(a) None of the funds made available in this Act may be used for—
   the creation of a human embryo or embryos for research purposes; orresearch in which a human embryo or embryos are destroyed, discarded, or knowingly subjected to risk of injury or death greater than that allowed for research on fetuses in utero under 45 CFR 46.204(b) and Section 498(b) of the Public Health Service Act (42 U.S.C. 289g(b)).
   For purposes of this section, the term 'human embryo or embryos' includes any organism, not protected as a human subject under 45 CFR 46 [the Human

Subject Protection regulations] as of the date of enactment of this Act, that is derived by fertilization, parthenogenesis, cloning, or any other means from one or more human gametes [sperm or egg] or human diploid cells [cells that have two sets of chromosomes, such as somatic cells].

Clinton Administration Stem Cell Policy

Following the November 1998 announcement on the derivation of human embryonic stem cells by scientists at the University of Wisconsin and Johns Hopkins University, NIH requested a legal opinion from HHS on whether federal funds could be used to support research on human stem cells derived from embryos. The January 15, 1999, response from HHS General Counsel Harriet Rabb found that the Dickey Amendment would not apply to research using human stem cells "because such cells are not a human embryo within the statutory definition." The finding was based, in part, on the determination by HHS that the statutory ban on human embryo research defines an embryo as an *organism* that when implanted in the uterus is capable of becoming a human being. Human stem cells, HHS said, are not and cannot develop into an organism; they lack the capacity to become organisms even if they are transferred to a uterus. As a result, HHS maintained that NIH could support research that uses stem cells derived through private funds, but could not support research that itself, with federal funds, derives stem cells from embryos because of the federal ban in the Dickey Amendment.

Shortly after the opinion by the HHS General Counsel was released, NIH disclosed that the agency planned to fund research on stem cells derived from human embryos once appropriate guidelines were developed and an oversight committee established. NIH Director Harold Varmus appointed a working group that began drafting guidelines in April 1999. Draft guidelines were published in the *Federal Register* on December 2, 1999. About 50,000 comments were received during the public comment period, which ended February 22, 2000. On August 25, 2000, NIH published in the *Federal Register* final guidelines on the support of human embryonic stem cell research. The guidelines stated that studies utilizing "stem cells derived from human embryos may be conducted using NIH funds only if the cells were derived (without federal funds) from human embryos that were created for the purposes of fertility treatment and were in excess of the clinical need of the individuals seeking such treatment." Under the guidelines, NIH would not fund research directly involving the derivation of human stem cells from embryos; this was prohibited by the Dickey Amendment.

Other areas of research ineligible for NIH funding under the guidelines include (1) research in which human stem cells are utilized to create or contribute to a human embryo; (2) research in which human stem cells are combined with an animal embryo; (3) research in which human stem cells are used for reproductive cloning of a human; (4) research in which human stem cells are *derived* using somatic cell nuclear transfer (i.e., the transfer of a human somatic cell nucleus into a human or animal egg); (5) research *utilizing* human stem cells that were derived using somatic cell nuclear transfer; and (6) research utilizing stem cells that were derived from human embryos created for research purposes, rather than for infertility treatment.

NIH began accepting grant applications for research projects utilizing human stem cells immediately following publication of the guidelines; the deadline for submitting a grant application was March 15, 2001. All such applications were to be reviewed by the NIH Human Pluripotent Stem Cell Review Group (HPSCRG), which was established to ensure compliance with the guidelines. James Kushner, director of the University of Utah General Clinical Research Center, served briefly as chair of the HPSCRG. Applications would also have undergone the normal NIH peer-review process.[44] The first meeting of the HPSCRG was scheduled for April 25, 2001. The HPSCRG was to conduct an ethical review of human pluripotent stem cell lines to determine whether the research groups involved had followed the NIH guidelines in deriving the cell lines. However, in mid April 2001, HHS postponed the meeting until a review of the Clinton Administration's policy decisions on stem cell research was completed by the new administration following the election of George W. Bush.[45] According to media sources, the 12 HPSCRG members, whose names were not made public, represented a wide range of scientific, ethical and theological expertise and opinion, as well as at least one "mainstream Catholic."[46]

The Bush Administration conducted a legal review of the policy decisions made during the Clinton Administration regarding federal support of stem cell research, as well as a scientific review, prepared by NIH, of the status of the research and its applications. The scientific review was released on July 18, 2001, at a hearing on stem cell research held by the Senate Appropriations Subcommittee on Labor, Health and Human Services and Education.[47] The NIH report did not make any recommendations, but argued that both embryonic and adult stem cell research should be pursued.

George W. Bush Administration Stem Cell Policy

On August 9, 2001, President George W. Bush announced that for the first time federal funds would be used to support research on human embryonic stem cells, but funding would be limited to "existing stem cell lines where the life and death decision has already been made."[48] President Bush stated that the decision "allows us to explore the promise and potential of stem cell research without crossing a fundamental moral line, by providing taxpayer funding that would sanction or encourage further destruction of human embryos that have at least the potential for life." The President also stated that the federal government would continue to support research involving stem cells from other sources, such as umbilical cord blood, placentas, and adult and animal tissues, "which do not involve the same moral dilemma."

Under the Bush policy, federal funds may only be used for research on existing stem cell lines that were derived (1) with the informed consent of the donors, (2) from excess embryos created solely for reproductive purposes, and (3) without any financial inducements to the donors.[49] NIH was tasked with examining the derivation of all existing stem cell lines and creating a registry of those lines that satisfy the Bush Administration criteria. According to the White House, this will ensure that federal funds are used to support only stem cell research that is scientifically sound, legal, and ethical. Federal funds will not be used for (1) the derivation or use of stem cell lines derived from newly destroyed embryos, (2) the creation of any human embryos for research purposes, or (3) the cloning of human embryos for any purpose.

Impact of Bush Policy on Research

Over time, a growing number of scientists, disease advocates and others became concerned that federally supported research on human embryonic stem cells was limited to the number of cell lines that met the criteria of the August 9, 2001, Bush policy. Under the policy, only 21 cell lines were available for research with federal dollars. Because these pre-August 2001 cell lines were developed in the early days of human stem cell research using older 1990s techniques, the cell lines not only have the problems of xenotransplantion (described in the section below on FDA regulation), but they are harder to work with, are not as well characterized, and are genetically unstable compared to newer stem cell lines. In reaction to the limitations imposed by the Bush policy, several U.S. research groups decided to develop additional human embryonic stem cell lines using private funding or funds provided by state governments. In order to perform this work, the research groups were required to build new separate laboratories so that the group's federally funded research was conducted separately from research on the new stem cell lines.

A worldwide survey of laboratories conducted by the Boston Globe found that as of May 23, 2004, 128 human embryonic stem cell lines had been created since August 9, 2001; all were ineligible for use in federally funded research under the Bush policy on stem cell research.[50] Another survey of the number of human embryonic stem cell lines released in June 2006 found that as of January 1, 2006, 414 human embryonic stem cell lines had been created in at least 20 countries.[51]

Congressional Response to the Bush Policy

In response to concerns over access to human embryonic stem cell lines, in April 2004, a group of over 200 Members of the House of Representatives sent a letter to President George W. Bush requesting that the Administration revise the stem cell policy and utilize the embryos that are created in excess of need during the treatment of infertile couples.[52] The letter pointed out that an estimated 400,000 frozen IVF embryos[53] "will likely be destroyed if not donated, with informed consent of the couple, for research." According to the letter,

> scientists are reporting that it is increasingly difficult to attract new scientists to this area of research because of concerns that funding restrictions will keep this research from being successful. ... We have already seen researchers move to countries like the United Kingdom, which have more supportive policies. In addition, leadership in this area of research has shifted to the United Kingdom, which sees this scientific area as the cornerstone of its biotech industry.

Under the direction of the White House, then NIH Director Elias A. Zerhouni sent a letter in response to the House Members that restated the Bush Administration position against using federal funds for research involving the destruction of human embryos.[54] The letter from Dr. Zerhouni did contain the following sentence, which some observers believed in 2004 indicated a potential future policy shift: "And although it is fair to say that from a purely scientific perspective more cell lines may well speed some areas of human embryonic stem cell research, the president's position is still predicated on his belief that taxpayer funds should not 'sanction or encourage further destruction of human embryos that have at least the potential for life."[55] At the time, White House spokesperson Claire Buchan stated that the sentence did not indicate the president's position had changed. Supporters of stem cell research point out that the letter concedes that science could benefit from additional stem cell lines and that the president's position now rests solely on ethical arguments.

A letter signed by 58 Senators urging President Bush to expand the federal policy concerning embryonic stem cell research was sent on June 4, 2004.[56] The letter stated that "despite the fact that U.S. scientists were the first to derive human embryonic stem cells, leadership in this area of research is shifting to other countries such as the United Kingdom, Singapore, South Korea an dAustralia."[57]

On July 14, 2004, former HHS Secretary Tommy Thompson announced in a letter to then Speaker of the House Dennis Hastert that NIH would establish Centers of Excellence in Translational Stem Cell Research and a National Embryonic Stem Cell Bank.[58] The centers investigate how stem cells can be used to treat a variety of diseases and the bank collects in one location many of the stem cell lines that are eligible for federal research funding. In the letter to Speaker Hastert, Secretary Thompson stated that "before anyone can successfully argue the stem cell policy should be broadened, we must first exhaust the potential of the stem cell lines made available with the policy."[59] In reaction to the announcement, the President of the Coalition for the Advancement of Medical Research stated that "creating a bank to house stem cell lines created before August 2001 does nothing to increase the wholly inadequate supply of stem cell lines for research."[60] On October 3, 2005, NIH announced that it had awarded $16.1 million over four years to the WiCell Research Institute in Wisconsin to fund the National Stem Cell Bank.[61]

NIH also awarded $9.6 million over four years to fund two new Centers of Excellence in Translational Human Stem Cell Research, one at the University of California, Davis and the other at Northwestern University.

During the first session of the 109th Congress, the House passed H.R. 810 (Castle), the Stem Cell Research Enhancement Act of 2005, in May 2005. In July 2006, the Senate passed H.R. 810 and President George W. Bush immediately vetoed it, the first veto of his presidency. An attempt in the House to override the veto was unsuccessful.

During the 110th Congress, H.R. 3 (DeGette), the Stem Cell Research Enhancement Act of 2007, was introduced on January 5, 2007, with 211 cosponsors, and passed the House by a vote of 253 to 174 on January 11, 2007.[62] The Senate passed a companion bill, S. 5 (Reid), on April 11. 2007, by a vote of 63 to 34. The House passed S. 5 on June 7. 2007, by a vote of 247 to 176. President George W. Bush vetoed the bill on June 20, 2007, and signed Executive Order 13435, which directed the Secretary of HHS to "conduct and support research on the isolation, derivation, production and testing of stem cells that are capable of producing all or almost all of the cell types of the developing body and may result in improved understanding of or treatments for diseases and other adverse health conditions, but are derived without creating a human embryo for research purposes or destroying, discarding, or subjecting to harm a human embryo or fetus."[63] S. 5 was the same as H.R. 3, except it had an additional section supporting research on alternative human pluripotent stem cells.

Obama Administration Stem Cell Policy

On March 9, 2009, President Barack Obama signed an executive order revoking the Bush Presidential statement of August 9, 2001, as well as Executive Order 13435 signed by President Bush on June 20, 2007.[64] The Obama decision directs NIH to issue new guidelines for the conduct of human embryonic stem cell research within 120 days of the date of the executive order. NIH anticipates using some of the $10 billion in funds provided by the stimulus package (American Recovery and Reinvestment Act of 2009, P.L. 111-5) for research on human embryonic stem cells under the new guidelines.[65] The Obama decision will allow scientists to use federal funds for research utilizing the hundreds of human embryonic stem cell lines that have been created since the Bush 2001 policy. The International Society for Stem Cell Research estimates there are more than 800 such cell lines cited in the scientific literature, "but it is unclear how many to these lines would be eligible under the NIH guidelines."[66] The policy will also eliminate the need to separate federally funded research from research conducted with private funds on cell lines that were previously ineligible for federal funding under the Bush policy; this often required building new but duplicative laboratories under the Bush policy using funds that could have been spent on actual research.

On the same day, President Obama issued a memorandum on scientific integrity directing the head of the White House Office of Science and Technology Policy "to develop a strategy for restoring scientific integrity to government decision making."[67]

Stem Cell Research Regulation by Federal Agencies and other Entities

The Common Rule (45 CFR 46, Subpart A) is a set of regulations that govern most federally funded research conducted on human beings. Its three basic requirements are aimed at protecting research subjects: the informed consent of research subjects, a review of proposed research by an Institutional Review Board (IRB), and institutional assurances of compliance with the regulations. However, ex vivo embryos (those not in a uterus) are not considered "human subjects" for these purposes, but federally funded research on human embryos is regulated by the Dickey Amendment as described above. Stem cells and stem cell lines are also not considered "human subjects," nor are they governed by the Dickey Amendment.

Because of the lack of federal regulation of stem cell research, the National Academies developed voluntary guidelines for deriving, handling and using human embryonic stem cells.[68] Two HHS agencies, FDA and NIH, regulate some aspects of stem cell research, even if research on stem cell lines is not classified as "human subjects" research. FDA, the agency that ensures the safety and efficacy of food, drugs, medical devices and cosmetics, regulates stem cell research aimed at the development of any "product" subject to its approval. NIH, the medical and behavioral research agency within HHS, regulates stem cell research that it funds in compliance with President Bush's 2001 policy. NIH has created a Human Embryonic Stem Cell Registry that lists the human embryonic stem cell lines that meet the eligibility criteria as outlined in the Bush Administration stem cell policy.

National Academies Guidelines

In July 2004 the National Academies established the committee on Guidelines for Human Embryonic Stem Cell Research to develop voluntary guidelines for deriving, handling and using human embryonic stem cells due to the current lack of federal regulation of such research. The stated position of the National Academies is that there should be a global ban on human reproductive cloning and therefore the guidelines will focus only on therapeutic and research uses of human embryonic stem cells and somatic cell nuclear transfer.

The committee released its "Guidelines for Human Embryonic Stem Cell Research" on April 26, 2005. The document provides guidance on informed consent of donors and states that there should be no financial incentives in the solicitation or donation of embryos, sperm, eggs, or somatic cells for research purposes. The guidelines recommend that each institution conducting human embryonic stem cell research establish an oversight committee, including experts in the relevant areas of science, ethics, and law, as well as members of the public, to review all proposed experiments. The guidelines recommend that a national panel be established to oversee the issue in general on a continuing basis.

The Human Embryonic Stem Cell Research Advisory Committee met for the first time in July 2006 and held a number of meetings to gather information about the need to revise the guidelines. In February 2007, a revised version of the guidelines was published with minor changes affecting Sections 1 (Introduction) and Section 2 (Establishment of an Institutional Embryonic Stem Cell Research Oversight Committee).[69] The guidelines were updated again in September 2008 to reflect the advances with iPS cells by including a new section entirely devoted to this new area of research.[70]

International Society for Stem Cell Research Guidelines

In February 2007, the International Society for Stem Cell Research (ISSCR) released its "Guidelines for the Conduct of Human Embryonic Stem Cell Research."[71] The ISSCR guidelines were developed by a committee of scientists, ethicists, and legal experts from 14 countries in order to "facilitate international collaboration by encouraging investigators and institutions to adhere to a uniform set of practices."[72] In drafting the guidelines, the ISSCR committee used as a model the National Academies guidelines, the regulations of the California Institute for Regenerative Medicine, and "governmental regulations already in place in other countries, particularly that of the Human Fertilisation and Embryology Authority of the United Kingdom."[73]

In order to ensure the responsible development of safe and effective stem cell therapies for patients, the ISSCR released in December 2008 a second guidance document, "Guidelines for the Clinical Translation of Stem Cells." In addition, due to concerns over unproven stem cell therapies being marketed directly to patients, the ISSCR also developed a handbook to be used by patients and their doctors in evaluating a stem cell therapy.[74] In the press release for the guidelines they noted "[t]oo often rogue clinics around the world exploit patients' hopes by offering unproven stem cell therapies, typically for large sums of money and without credible scientific rationale, oversight or patient protections."[75] According to ISSCR, this concern was substantiated by a study conducted by the University of Alberta, Canada, which analyzed the claims of 19 internet sites offering "stem cell therapies," the vast majority of which "over promise results and gravely underestimate the potential risks of their offered treatments."[76]

FDA Regulation

All of the human embryonic stem cell lines listed on the NIH Human Embryonic Stem Cell Registry (see **Table 2**) have been grown on beds of mouse "feeder" cells. The mouse cells secrete a substance that prevents the human embryonic stem cells from differentiating into more mature cell types (nerve or muscle cells). Infectious agents, such as viruses, within the mouse feeder cells could transfer into the human cells. If the human cells were transplanted into a patient, these infected human cells may cause disease in the patient which could be transmitted to close contacts of the patient and eventually to the general population. Public health officials and regulatory agencies such as the FDA are specifically concerned about retroviruses, which may remain hidden in the DNA only to cause disease many years later, as well as any unrecognized agents which may be present in the mouse cells.

The FDA defines "xenotransplantation" as "any procedure that involves the transplantation, implantation, or infusion into a human recipient of either (a) live cells, tissues, or organs from a nonhuman source, or (b) human body fluids, cells, tissues or organs that have had ex vivo contact with live nonhuman animal cells, tissues or organs."[77] Under FDA guidelines, transplantation therapy involving Bush approved stem cell lines, which all have been exposed to mouse feeder cells, would constitute xenotransplantation. Xenotransplantation products are subject to regulation by the FDA under Section 351 of the Public Health Service Act (42 USC 262) and the Federal Food, Drug and Cosmetic Act (21 USC 321 et seq.). FDA has developed guidance documents and the U.S. Public Health Service has developed guidelines on infectious disease issues associated with xenotransplantation.[78]

During a Senate hearing on stem cell research held by the Health, Education, Labor and Pensions Committee on September 5, 2001, the HHS Secretary stated that the FDA was overseeing 17 investigational protocols involving xenotransplantation in other areas of clinical research that involve patients. Therefore, he said, the xenotransplantation-related public health concerns over the human embryonic stem cell lines may not necessarily preclude the development of treatments for patients. While the problems presented by xenotransplantation for clinical research are neither unique to stem cell research nor insurmountable, many scientists believe it will be preferable to use sterile cell lines when attempting to treat patients via stem cell transplantation, and scientists have been successful in developing human embryonic stem cells that can be maintained without the use of mouse feeder cells.[79]

NIH Research Funding and Stem Cell Registry under the Bush Policy

The August 9, 2001, Bush Administration policy statement on stem cell research and the NIH Stem Cell Registry effectively replaced the NIH stem cell guidelines that were developed under the Clinton Administration and never fully implemented. Grant proposals for embryonic stem cell research underwent only the normal peer-review process without the added review of the HPSCRG as had been specified under the Clinton NIH stem cell guidelines. In February 2002, NIH announced the approval of the first expenditures for research on human embryonic stem cells. Funding for stem cell research by NIH is shown in Table 1. The NIH website provides additional information about stem cell activities and funding opportunities.[80]

Table 1. National Institutes of Health Funding ($ in millions)

Stem Cell Research	FY04	FY05	FY06	FY07	FY08
Human Embryonic	24	40	38	74	88
Non-Human Embryonic	89	97	110	120	150
Human Non-Embryonic	203	199	206	226	297
Non-Human Non-Embryonic	236	273	289	400	497
Human Cord Blood/Placenta	16	15	16	38	38
Non-Human Cord Blood/Placenta	3	3	4	9	9
Total, Stem Cell Research	**553**	**609**	**643**	**968**	**938**

Source: NIH website, January 15, 2009, http://report.nih.gov/rcdc/categories/ PFSummaryTable.aspx.

The NIH Human Embryonic Stem Cell Registry lists stem cell lines that were eligible for use in federally funded research under the Bush policy.[81] As shown in **Table 2**, the NIH registry originally listed universities and companies that had derived a total of 78 human embryonic stem cell lines which were eligible for use in federally funded research under the August 2001 Bush Administration policy. However, many of these stem cell lines were found to be either unavailable or unsuitable for research. As of May 4, 2007, the NIH registry listed a total of 21 stem cell lines available from six sources.

State Laws that Restrict Stem Cell Research[82]

Many states restrict research on aborted fetuses or embryos, but research is often permitted with consent of the parent or parents. Almost half of the states also restrict the sale of fetuses or embryos. Louisiana is the only state that specifically prohibits research on in vitro fertilized (IVF) embryos. Illinois and Michigan also prohibit research on live embryos. Arkansas, Indiana, Michigan, North Dakota and South Dakota prohibit research on cloned embryos. Virginia may also ban research on cloned embryos, but the statute may leave room for interpretation because human being is not defined. (There may be disagreement about whether human being includes blastocysts, embryos or fetuses.) California, Connecticut, Illinois, Iowa, Massachusetts, New Jersey, New York, and Rhode Island have laws that prohibit cloning for the purpose of initiating a pregnancy, but allow cloning for research.

Several states limit the use of state funds for cloning or stem cell research. Missouri forbids the use of state funds for reproductive cloning but not for cloning for the purpose of stem cell research, and Maryland's statutes prohibit state-funded stem cell researchers from engaging in reproductive cloning. Arizona law prohibits the use of public monies for reproductive or therapeutic cloning. Nebraska statutes limit the use of state funds for embryonic stem cell research. Restrictions only apply to state healthcare cash funds provided by tobacco settlement dollars. State funding available under Illinois Executive Order 6 (2005) may not be used for reproductive cloning or for research on fetuses from induced abortions.

**Table 2. NIH List of Human Embryonic Stem Cell Lines Eligible for
Use in Federal Research**

Namea	Number of stem cell lines	
	Eligible	Available
BresaGen, Inc., Athens, GA	4	3
Cell & Gene Therapy Institute (Pochon CHA University), Seoul, Korea	2	
Cellartis AB, Goteborg, Sweden	3	2
CyThera, Inc., San Diego, CA	9	0
ES Cell International, Melbourne, Australia	6	6
Geron Corporation, Menlo Park, CA	7	
Goteborg University, Goteborg, Sweden	16	
Karolinska Institute, Stockholm, Sweden	6	0
Maria Biotech Co. Ltd.—Maria Infertility Hospital Medical Institute, Seoul, Korea	3	
MizMedi Hospital—Seoul National University, Seoul, Korea	1	0
National Center for Biological Sciences/Tata Institute of Fundamental Research,		
Bangalore, India	3	
Reliance Life Sciences, Mumbai, India	7	
Technion University, Haifa, Israel	4	3
University of California, San Francisco, CA	2	2
Wisconsin Alumni Research Foundation, Madison, WI	5	5
Total	**78**	**21**

Source: NIH website, February 3, 2009,
   http://stemcells.nih.gov/research/registry/eligibilityCriteria.asp.
   a. Six table entries do not have stem cell lines available for shipment to U.S. researchers because of a variety of scientific, regulatory and legal reasons. The zeros entered in the "Available" column indicate that "the cells failed to expand into undifferentiated cell cultures."

Despite restrictive federal and state policies, several states (California, Connecticut, Illinois, Indiana, Maryland, Massachusetts, New Jersey, New York, Ohio, Washington, Wisconsin, Virginia) are encouraging or providing funding for stem cell research (adult, embryonic, and in some cases SCNT as well), as they seek to remain competitive and prevent the relocation of scientists and biotechnology firms to other states or overseas.

LEGISLATION IN THE 111ᵀᴴ CONGRESS

H.R. 873 (DeGette), the Stem Cell Research Enhancement Act of 2009, was introduced on February 4, 2009. The text of H.R. 873 is identical to legislation introduced in the 110ᵗʰ

Congress, H.R. 3 (DeGette), and the 109th Congress, H.R. 810 (Castle). The bill would allow federal support for research that utilizes human embryonic stem cells regardless of the date on which the stem cells were derived from a human embryo, and thus if passed would negate the August 2001 Bush stem cell policy limitation. It would amend the Public Health Service (PHS) Act by adding a new Section 498D, "Human Embryonic Stem Cell Research." The new section would direct the Secretary of HHS to conduct and support research that utilizes human embryonic stem cells regardless of the date on which the stem cells were derived from a human embryo. Stem cell lines must meet ethical guidelines established by the NIH. In order to be eligible for federal research, stem cell lines must have be derived from embryos that were originally created for fertility treatment purposes and were in excess of clinical need. In addition, only embryos that the individuals seeking fertility treatments had determined would not be implanted in a woman, and would be discarded, would be eligible for stem cell derivation. Written consent would be required for embryo donation. The Secretary, in consultation with the Director of NIH, would promulgate guidelines 60 days after enactment. No federal funds would be used to conduct research on unapproved stem cell lines. The Secretary would annually report to Congress about stem cell research.

H.R. 872 (DeGette), the Stem Cell Research Improvement Act of 2009, was also introduced on February 4, 2009. It is similar to H.R. 873 in that it adds the same Section 498D, "Human Embryonic Stem Cell Research," to the PHS Act, but it also adds another Section 498E, "Guidelines on Research Involving Human Stem Cells," which would require the Director of NIH to issue guidelines on research involving human embryonic stem cell within 90 days of enactment; updates of the guidelines would be required every three years.

S. 487 (Harkin), the Stem Cell Research Enhancement Act of 2009, was introduced on February 26, 2009. S. 487 is the same as H.R. 873, except it has an additional section supporting research on alternative human pluripotent stem cells.[83] This section would amend the Public Health Service Act by adding a new Section 498E, "Alternative Human Pluripotent Stem Cell Research." The new section would require the Secretary of HHS to develop techniques for the isolation, derivation, production, and testing of stem cells that are capable of producing all or almost all of the cell types of a developing body, and may result in improved understanding of treatments for diseases, but that are not derived from a human embryo. The Secretary, after consulting with the Director of NIH, would be required to (1) provide guidance concerning the next steps for additional research, (2) prioritize research that holds the greatest potential for near-term clinical benefit, and (3) take into account techniques outlined by the President's Council on Bioethics and any other appropriate techniques and research. The Secretary would be required to prepare and submit to the appropriate committees of Congress an annual report describing the activities and research conducted. S. 487 would authorize such sums as may be necessary for FY2010 through FY2012. The bill is identical to a bill in the 110th Congress, S. 5 (Reid), which passed the Senate and House and was vetoed by President Bush in June 2007.

End Notes

[1] "Removing Barriers to Responsible Scientific Research Involving Human Stem Cells," March 9, 2009, at [http://www.whitehouse.gov/the_press_office/Removing-Barriers-to-Responsible-Scientific-Research-Involving- Human-Stem-Cells/].

[2] "Obama Signs Executive Order Reversing Bush's Embryonic Stem Cell Research Policy," *Health Care Daily Report*, March 10, 2009.

[3] The White House, Office of the Press Secretary, Remarks of President Barack Obama-As Prepared for Delivery, Signing of Stem Cell Executive Order and Scientific Integrity Presidential Memorandum, March 9, 2009, at [http://www.whitehouse.gov/the_press_office/Remarks-of-the-President-As-Prepared-for-Delivery-Signing-of-Stem-Cell-Executive-Order-and-Scientific-Integrity-Presidential-Memorandum/].

[4] Alex Wayne, "With Obama Reversal of Stem Cell Policy, Democrats Look to Expand Funding," *CQ Today*, March 9, 2009.

[5] For further information, see CRS Report RL33554, *Stem Cell Research: Ethical Issues*, by Erin D. Williams and Judith A. Johnson.

[6] Drew Armstrong, "NIH Chief's Opinion on Stem Cell Research Goes Afield of White House Policy," *CQ Today*, March 19, 2007.

[7] Ibid.

[8] John Reichard, "Zerhouni Makes Strong Case Against Bush Policy on Stem Cells, NIH Funding," *CQ Today*, March 19, 2005.

[9] An archived audio webcast of the May 8, 2008, hearing can be found athttp://energycommerce.house.gov/ cmte_mtgs/110-he-hrg.050808.StemCell.shtml.

[10] During the first session of the 109th Congress, the House passed identical legislation, H.R. 810 (Castle), in May 2005. In July 2006, the Senate passed H.R. 810 and President Bush immediately vetoed it, the first veto of his presidency. An attempt in the House to override the veto was unsuccessful.

[11] A pluripotent cell has the ability to differentiate into all of the various cell types that make up the body, but not the "extra-embryonic" tissues such as the components of the placenta.

[12] The IVF embryos were originally created for the treatment of infertility. Excess embryos are often frozen for future use. A couple may elect to discard their excess embryos, donate the embryos for research, or allow another couple to adopt an embryo. The Society for Assisted Reproductive Technology and RAND conducted a survey of more than 430 infertility clinics to determine the number of frozen embryos in the United States; 340 clinics responded to the survey. Nearly 400,000 embryos have been frozen and stored since the late 1970s. The vast majority of embryos are being held to help couples have children at a later date. Patients have designated 2.8%, or about 11,000 embryos, for research. Scientists estimate these 11,000 could form up to 275 stem cell lines, perhaps much less http://www.rand.org/pubs/research_briefs/ RB9038/index1.html.

[13] Scientists and physicians use the term "embryo" for the first eight weeks after fertilization, and "fetus" for the ninth week through birth. In contrast, the Department of Health and Human Services (HHS) regulations define "fetus" as "the product of conception from the time of implantation" (45 C.F.R. § 46.203).

[14] Gretchen Vogel and Constance Holden, "Field Leaps Forward with New Stem Cell Advances," *Science*, v. 318, November 23, 2007, pp. 1224-1225.

[15] Dennis Normile, "Shinya Yamanaka: Modest Researcher, Results to Brag About," *Science*, v. 319, February 1, 2008, p. 562.

[16] Constance Holden and Gretchen Vogel, "A Seismic Shift for Stem Cell Research," *Science*, v. 319, February 1, 2008, pp. 560-563.

[17] A somatic cell is a body cell. In contrast, a germ cell is an egg or sperm cell.

[18] Dolly was euthanized in February 2003 after developing a lung infection. Some claim her death at six years was related to being a clone, but her ailment may also have occurred because she was raised indoors (for security reasons) rather than as a pastured sheep, which often live to 12 years of age. G. Kolata, "First Mammal Clone Dies," *New York Times*, February 15, 2003, p. A4.

[19] Elizabeth Finkel, "Researchers Derive Stem Cells From Monkeys," *ScienceNOW Daily News*, June 19, 2007.

[20] Vogel and Holden, "Field Leaps Forward with New Stem Cell Advances," p. 1224.

[21] For further information, see CRS Report RL31358, *Human Cloning*, by Judith A. Johnson and Erin D. Williams.

[22] Gretchen Vogel, "Collaborators Split over Ethics Allegations" *Science*, November 18, 2005, p. 1100.

[23] Nicholas Wade and Choe Sang-Hun, "Researcher Faked Evidence of Human Cloning, Koreans Report," *The New York Times*, January 10, 2006, p. A1.

[24] Dennis Normile, Gretchen Vogel, and Constance Holden, "Cloning Researcher Says Work is Flawed but Claims Results Stand," *Science*, December 23, 2005, p. 1886-1887; Carl T. Hall, "UCSF Resumes Human Embryo Stem Cell Work," *The San Francisco Chronicle*, May 6, 2006, p. A.1.

[25] Julio C. Voltarelli, et al., "Autologous Nonmyeloablative Hematopoietic Stem Cell Transplantation in Newly Diagnosed Type 1 Diabetes Mellitus," *Journal of the American Medical Association*, April 11, 2007, v. 297, p. 1568-1576.

[26] Comments made by NIH Director Elias Zerhouni during a May 8, 2008 hearing before the House Energy and Commerce Subcommittee on Health, audio webcast available at http://energycommerce.house.gov/cmte_mtgs/110-he-hrg.050808.StemCell.shtml.

[27] Rick Weiss, "Scientists See Potential in Amniotic Stem Cells; They Are Highly Versatile And Readily Available," *The Washington Post*, January 8, 2007, p. A1, A5.

[28] Frederick R. Appelbaum, "Hematopoietic-Cell Transplantation at 50," *The New England Journal of Medicine*, v. 357, October 11, 2007, pp. 1472-1475.

[29] http://www.stemcellresearch.org/facts/treatments.htm.

[30] Shane Smith, William Neaves and Steven Teitelbaum, "Adult Stem Cell Treatments for Diseases?" *Science*, v. 313, July 28, 2006, p. 439; as well as online in *Sciencexpress*, July 13, 2006, p. 1 http://www.sciencexpress.org.

[31] David A. Prentice and Gene Tarne, "Treating Diseases with Adult Stem Cells," *Science*, v. 315, January 19, 2007, p. 328.

[32] Shane Smith, William Neaves and Steven Teitelbaum, "Adult Versus Embryonic Stem Cells: Treatments," *Science*, v. 316, June 8, 2007, p. 1422.

[33] David A. Prentice and Gene Tarne, "Adult Versus Embryonic Stem Cells: Treatments—Response," *Science*, v. 316, June 8, 2007, p. 1422-1423.

[34] National Institutes of Health, Department of Health and Human Services, *Stem Cells: Scientific Progress and Future Research Directions*, June 2001, available at http://stemcells.nih.gov/info/scireport/. Institute of Medicine, *Stem Cells and the Future of Regenerative Medicine*, 2002, available at http://www.nas.edu.

[35] Andrew Pollack, "FDA approves a stem cell trial," *New York Times*, January 23, 2009.

[36] Ibid.

[37] Jennifer Couzin, "Celebration and concern over U.S. trial of embryonic stem cells," *Science*, vol. 323 (January 30, 2009), p. 568.

[38] Chimeras have been created by scientists in a variety of different ways and have been the subject of research studies for many years. Human chimeras occur naturally when two eggs become fertilized and, instead of developing into twins, they fuse in the uterus creating a single embryo with two distinct sets of genes. For one example, see Constance Holden, "Chimera on a Bike?" *Science*, June 24, 2005, p. 1864.

[39] The EAB was created in 1978 by the Department of Health Education and Welfare (HEW), the forerunner of the Department of Health and Human Services (HHS). The EAB was formed at the recommendation of the National Commission for the Protection of Human Subjects of Biomedical and Behavioral Research. The National Commission operated from 1974 to 1978 and issued 10 reports, many of which formed the basis of federal regulations for research involving human subjects (45 C.F.R. Part 46).

[40] These were *blastomere separation*, where a two- to eight-cell embryo is treated causing the cells (blastomeres) to separate, and *blastocyst division*, in which an embryo at the more advanced blastocyst stage is split into two.

[41] National Institutes of Health, *Report of the Human Embryo Research Panel*, Sept. 27, 1994.

[42] However, federal funds have been provided for research on both human and animal adult stem cells and animal embryonic stem cells.

[43] The rider language has not changed significantly from year to year (however there was a technical correction in P.L. 109-149). The original rider can be found in Section 128 of P.L. 104-99; it affected NIH funding for FY1996 contained in P.L. 104-91. For subsequent fiscal years, the rider is found in Title V, General Provisions, of the Labor, HHS and Education appropriations acts in the following public laws: FY1997, P.L. 104-208; FY1998, P.L. 105-78; FY1999, P.L. 105-277; FY2000, P.L. 106-113; FY2001, P.L. 106-554; FY2002, P.L. 107-116; FY2003, P.L. 108-7; FY2004, P.L. 108-199; FY2005, P.L. 108-447; FY2006, P.L. 109-149; FY2007, P.L. 110-5; FY2008, P.L. 110-161.

[44] According to media sources, as of April 2001 only three grant applications had been submitted to NIH, and one was subsequently withdrawn. (*Washington FAX*, April 19, 2001.) Presumably, scientists were reluctant to invest the time and effort into preparing the necessary paperwork for the NIH grant application process when the prospects of receiving federal funding were uncertain under the new Bush Administration. (P. Recer, "Stem Cell Studies Said Hurt by Doubt," *AP Online*, May 2, 2001.) In a related development, one of the leading U.S. researchers on stem cells, Roger Pederson of the University of California, San Francisco, decided to move his laboratory to the United Kingdom for "the possibility of carrying out my research with human embryonic stem cells with public support." (Aaron Zitner, "Uncertainty Is Thwarting Stem Cell Researchers," *Los Angeles Times*, July 16, 2001, pp. A1, A8.) Human embryonic stem cell research was approved overwhelmingly by the House of Commons in December 2000 and the House of Lords in January 2001.

[45] Rick Weiss, "Bush Administration Order Halts Stem Cell Meeting; NIH Planned Session to Review Fund Requests," *Washington Post*, April 21, 2001, p. A2.

[46] Ibid.

[47] National Institutes of Health, Department of Health and Human Services. *Stem Cells: Scientific Progress and Future Research Directions*, June 2001. The NIH scientific report can be found at http://stemcells.nih.gov/info/scireport/.

[48] The August 9, 2001, *Remarks by the President on Stem Cell Research* can be found http://georgewbush whitehouse.archives.gov/news/releases/2001/08/20010809-2.html

[49] The White House, *Fact Sheet on Embryonic Stem Cell Research*, August 9, 2001, found at http://georgewbushwhitehouse.archives.gov/news/releases/2001/08/20010809-1.html

[50] Gareth Cook, "94 New Cell Lines Created Abroad since Bush Decision," *Boston Globe*, May 23, 2004, p. A14.

[51] Anke Guhr, et al., "Current State of Human Embryonic Stem Cell Research: An Overview of Cell Lines and Their Use in Experimental Work," *Stem Cells 2006*, v. 24, p. 2187-2191, found at http://www.StemCells.com.

[52] See http://www.house.gov/degette/news/releases/040428.pdf.

[53] A survey conducted in 2002 and published in 2003 by the Society for Assisted Reproductive Technology and RAND determined that nearly 400,000 frozen embryos are stored in the United States, but most are currently targeted for patient use. See David I. Hoffman et al., "Cryopreserved Embryos in the United States and Their Availability for Research," *Fertility and Sterility*, vol. 79, May 2003, pp. 1063-1069.

[54] Rick Weiss, "Bush's Stem Cell Policy Reiterated, but Some See Shift," *The Washington Post*, May 16, 2004, p. A18.

[55] Letter from Elias A. Zerhouni, Director, National Institutes of Health, to The Honorable Diana DeGette and The Honorable Michael Castle, May 14, 2004.

[56] See http://feinstein.senate.gov/04Releases/r-stemcell-ltr.pdf.

[57] Ibid.

[58] Andrew J. Hawkins, "NIH Stem Cell Bank, Centers of Excellence Will Fast-Track Translational Research, Says Thompson," *Washington FAX*, July 15, 2004.

[59] Ibid.

[60] Ibid.

[61] NIH Press Office, "NIH Awards a National Stem Cell Bank and New Centers of Excellence in Translational Human Stem Cell Research," October 3, 2005, http://www.nih.gov/news/pr/ oct2005/od-03.htm. The website for WiCell and the National Stem Cell Bank can be found at http://www.wicell.org/.

[62] During the first session of the 109th Congress, the House passed identical legislation, H.R. 810 (Castle), in May 2005. In July 2006, the Senate passed H.R. 810 and President Bush immediately vetoed it, the first veto of his presidency. An attempt in the House to override the veto was unsuccessful.

[63] The White House, Office of the Press Secretary, "Executive Order: Expanding Approved Stem Cell Lines in Ethically Responsible Ways," June 20, 2007, found at http://georgewbushwhitehouse.archives.gov/news/releases/2007/06/20070620-6.html

[64] "Removing Barriers to Responsible Scientific Research Involving Human Stem Cells," March 9, 2009, at [http://www.whitehouse.gov/the_press_office/Removing-Barriers-to-Responsible-Scientific-Research-Involving- Human-Stem-Cells/].

[65] "Obama Signs Executive Order Reversing Bush's Embryonic Stem Cell Research Policy," *Health Care Daily Report*, March 10, 2009.

[66] Ibid.

[67] The White House, Office of the Press Secretary, Remarks of President Barack Obama-As Prepared for Delivery, Signing of Stem Cell Executive Order and Scientific Integrity Presidential Memorandum, March 9, 2009, at [http://www.whitehouse.gov/the_press_office/Remarks-of-the-President-As-Prepared-for-Delivery-Signing-of-Stem-Cell-Executive-Order-and-Scientific-Integrity-Presidential-Memorandum/].

[68] The National Academies bring together committees of experts in all areas of science and technology to address critical national issues and give advice on a pro bono basis to the federal government and the public. The National Academies is comprised of four organizations: the National Academy of Sciences (NAS), established by Abraham Lincoln in 1863; the National Academy of Engineering, established by NAS in 1964; the Institute of Medicine, established by NAS in 1970; and, the National Research Council, established in 1916 by NAS at the request of President Wilson.

[69] The 2007 Amendment to the 2005 Guidelines for Human Embryonic Stem Cell Research can be found at http://www.nap.edu/catalog/11278.html.

[70] The original 2005 Guidelines as well as the 2007 amended version and the 2008 amended version can be found at http://www.nap.edu/catalog.php?record_id=12553.

[71] The ISSCR Guidelines can be found at http://www.isscr.org/guidelines/index.htm.

[72] George Q. Daley, Lars Ahrlund-Richter, and Jonathan M. Auerbach, et al., "The ISSCR Guidelines for Human Embryonic Stem Cell Research," *Science*, vol. 315 (February 2, 2007), pp. 603-604.

[73] Ibid.

[74] The ISSCR Guidelines and the Patient Handbook are at http://www.isscr.org/clinical_trans/index.cfm.

[75] International Society for Stem Cell Research, "The ISSCR Releases New Guidelines to Shape Future of Stem Cell Therapy," press release, December 3, 2008, http://www.isscr.org/ press_releases/clinicalguidelines.html.

[76] Ibid.

[77] Xenotransplantation Action Plan: FDA approach to the regulation of xenotransplantation. Available at http://www.fda.gov/cber/xap/xap.htm.

[78] These documents are available at http://www.fda.gov/cber/xap/xap.htm.

[79] National Institutes of Health, Department of Health and Human Services, *Stem Cells: Scientific Progress and Future Research Directions*, June 2001, pp. 95-96; Susanne Rust, "UW Grows Animal-Free Stem Cell Lines," *The Milwaukee Journal Sentinel*, January 2, 2006, p. A1.

[80] See http://stemcells.nih.gov/research/funding/.

[81] Information about the NIH Human Embryonic Stem Cell Registry iavailable at http://stemcells.nih.gov/research/registry/index.asp.

[82] The information in this section was obtained from "State Embryonic and Fetal Research Laws," updated January 2008 on the National Council of State Legislatures website, at http://www.ncsl.org/programs/health/genetics/embfet.htm, visited February 3, 2009.

[83] A pluripotent cell has the ability to differentiate into all of the various cell types that make up the body, but not the "extra-embryonic" tissues such as the components of the placenta.

In: Encyclopedia of Stem Cell Research (2 Volume Set)   ISBN: 978-1-61761-835-2
Editor: Alexander L. Greene   © 2012 Nova Science Publishers, Inc.

Chapter LVII

TESTIMONY TO BE PRESENTED TO THE HOUSE COMMITTEE ON ENERGY AND COMMERCE'S SUBCOMMITTEE ON HEALTH

Joseph R. Bertino[*]

Good Morning, Mr. Chairman, Members of the Committee. Thank you for inviting me to present my testimony today.

"Stem Cells" are defined as cells capable of self-renewal as well as differentiation. The investigators funded by the New Jersey State Commission on Science are exploring every type of stem cell for the purpose of understanding function, regulation, and potential therapeutic benefit. These studies range from very basic studies to studies that will soon be translated into the clinic.

The promise of stem cell research is compelling and far-reaching. No other line of scientific inquiry offers better hope for curing intractable medical conditions. Indeed, therapies based on stem cells are a paradigm shift in the modern medical revolution. The potential to treat currently incurable conditions is both real and achievable in our lifetimes.

As a society, we have an obligation to pursue scientific discoveries that offer a clear potential to help those living with devastating illnesses. At the same, we recognize the legitimate moral, social and religious concerns raised by new technologies.

To address such concerns, nationally respected science associations, federal agencies and the State of New Jersey have set forth policies and procedures that ensure stem cell research meets the highest scientific and ethical standards. The Stem Cell Institute of New Jersey is committed to conducting responsible research that complies fully with these stringent requirements.

---

[*] These remarks were delivered as testimony given on May 8, 2008. Joseph R. Bertino, presented to the House Committee on Energy and Commerce's Subcommittee on Health.

HISTORY OF STEM CELL RESEARCH IN NEW JERSEY

On May 12, 2004, the Stem Cell Institute of New Jersey was created by a memorandum of understanding between Rutgers, the State University of New Jersey and UMDNJ-Robert Wood Johnson Medical School.

The State committed $8.5 million in state funds to support work at the Stem Cell Institute in financial year 2006, including $5.5 million in capital funds to Robert Wood Johnson Medical School and Rutgers University to support laboratory renovation and GMP facilities to support stem cell research, as well as two clinical trials using umbilical cord-derived stem cells.

In December 2005, NJ became the first state to finance research using human embryonic stem cells. The Commission on Science and Technology awarded a total of $5 million to 17 research teams.

On October 19, 2006, the finance committee of the General Assembly passed a $250 million bill to support stem cell research facilities in New Brunswick, Camden, and Newark.

In October 2006, monthly meetings of investigators interested in stem cell research were initiated at Rutgers and Robert Wood Johnson Medical School. Over fifty investigators from academic and pharmaceutical companies have been meeting to report their work in stem cell research, to discuss progress in the field and to plan collaborative experiments.

In 2007, New Jersey awarded 17 grants, totaling $10 million to stem cell researchers, including two grants to fund core laboratories for embryonic stem cell research.

Despite polls that showed that the majority of New Jerseyans were in favor of supporting embryonic stem cell research, a referendum was defeated in November 2007 that would have provided $450 million dollars, for ten years in support of stem cell research. Major reasons for the defeat of the referendum were the off-year election, with fewer than 30% of voters coming to the polls, and the concern that this would add to the public's tax burden, as well as put New Jersey even further in the red.

Governor Corzine continues to be a strong supporter of stem cell research and the building of the joint Rutgers/UMDNJ-RWJMS Stem Cell Institute in New Brunswick. Key members of the NJ legislature also continue to strongly support stem cell research.

In June 2008, an additional 10 million dollars will be made available for investigators in New Jersey from the State for stem cell research via a peer-reviewed grant program.

Examples of studies in progress are as follows below

Two types of stem cells are found in the bone marrow: hematopoetic stem cells, that form blood cells, and mesenchymal stem cells, capable of differentiating or forming bone, cartilage, nerve cells, fat cells, etc. Hematopoeitic stem cells are now used at the RWJUH and throughout the world to treat patients with cancer following chemotherapy. Mesenchymal stem cells from bone marrow or cord blood are being tested for their ability to prevent graft vs. host disease, after marrow transplantation. Other uses for mesenchymal stem cells under study by NJ investigators include targeting tumors with mesenchymal stem cells carrying toxins, and use in regenerative medicine (spinal cord injury, heart injury and brain disorders (Parkinson's, Alzheimer's)).

Researchers at both Rutgers and UMDNJ have special expertise and interest in neural stem cells that may have important implications for brain disorders as well as serve as models to promote drug discovery.

Cord blood, placenta and amniotic fluid are also a rich source of stem cells. Clinical trials are in progress in collaboration with investigators in China, using a subset of these cells to treat spinal cord injury (Dr. Wise Young). The characterization of stem cells from placenta is under study by RJWMS investigators in collaboration with Celgene, a NJ-based biotech company.

Work on human embryonic stem cells has been hampered by Federal guidelines that limit studies to 20 cell lines that have been around for several years. The two core laboratories at Rutgers and RWJMS, established with NJ State funding, have allowed investigators to expand research activities using newly established embryonic cell lines.

Importantly, the completion of a GMP facility at the Cancer Institute/Stem Cell Institute will allow stem cells to be produced in quantities necessary for clinical studies.

The funding provided by the State of New Jersey has provided key support for both the research outlined above and additional research programs focused on a variety of important disease conditions including multiple sclerosis, Parkinson's disease, Alzheimer's disease and diabetes. A key part of our efforts has been the establishment of stem cell banking of umbilical cord blood and other stem cells. New Jersey's stem cell banks are leaders in this field.

I would be happy to answer the committee's questions. Thank you.

In: Encyclopedia of Stem Cell Research (2 Volume Set)   ISBN: 978-1-61761-835-2
Editor: Alexander L. Greene   © 2012 Nova Science Publishers, Inc.

Chapter LVIII

TESTIMONY TO HOUSE COMMITTEE ON ENERGY AND COMMERCE, SUBCOMMITTEE ON HEALTH "STEM CELL SCIENCE: THE FOUNDATION FOR FUTURE CURES"[*]

Thank you for the invitation to speak today on the subject of stem cell science. My name is George Daley and I am an Associate Professor of Biological Chemistry, Medicine, and Pediatrics at Children's Hospital Boston and Harvard Medical School, a core faculty member of the Harvard Stem Cell Institute, an investigator of the Howard Hughes Medical Institute, and the current President of the International Society for Stem Cell Research (ISSCR), the major professional organization of stem cell scientists worldwide. My laboratory studies blood development, blood cancer, and experimental transplant therapies for diseases like sickle cell anemia, immune deficiency and leukemia. In my clinical duties at Children's Hospital, I care for patients with these devastating blood diseases, and see first hand the need for better treatments. Stem cell research offers hope.

Let me recount the stories of two patients I cared for recently at Children's Hospital that illustrate the shortcomings of current therapies. One was a young African-American boy with sickle cell anemia, suddenly struck down by what we call a pain crisis. When I saw him in the emergency room, he was writhing on the gurney, and whimpering in pain. Despite powerful, high doses of intravenous morphine, I was unable to give that child adequate relief from his pain and suffering for several days. A second case was an infant who suffered repeated infections and had spent half his young life in the hospital hooked up to intravenous antibiotics. His disease was immune-deficiency, and unfortunately he had no sibling donors for a potentially curative adult stem cell transplant. Stem cell research is laying the foundation for improved treatments for these kids, and countless other children and adults with debilitating, life-threatening diseases.

---

[*] These remarks were delivered as testimony given on May, 8, 2008. George Q. Daley, Associate Professor of Biological Chemistry, Medicine, and Pediatrics at Children's Hospital Boston and Harvard Medical School, presented to the House Committee on Energy and Commerce's Subcommittee on Health "Stem Cell Science: The Foundation for Future Cures".

All stem cells—whether from embryonic, fetal, neonatal, or adult sources—hold great promise. The crowning scientific achievement of the twentieth century was the sequencing of the human genome, and the dominant mission of twenty-first century science is to discover how that blueprint drives the formation of tissues and organs, and how tissues are sustained, repaired, and rejuvenated over time. Stem cell research goes to the core of human biology and medicine.

Much excitement in stem cell research has focused on a property of embryonic cells called pluripotency—the capacity to generate all of the tissues in an organism. Recently, several laboratories, including my own, reported that a small set of genes linked to pluripotency in embryonic stem (ES) cells can be inserted into human skin cells to induce pluripotency—to endow skin cells with this same remarkable capacity to become a seed for all tissues in the body. By using gene-based reprogramming to make these so-called induced pluripotent stem cells (called "iPS cells"), scientists can now produce customized, patient-specific stem cells in the Petri dish. In a matter of weeks, we can take cells from a patient's forearm and transform them into pluripotent stem cells that we believe closely approximate embryonic stem cells. This is a major breakthrough in medical research, empowering scientists to create cellular models of human disease. It may also mean that one day we will treat patients with rejuvenated and repaired versions of their own tissues.

Realizing this promise will take time. A key concern is that the viruses used to carry the reprogramming genes into human skin cells can cause cancer. Moreover, the genes and pathways the viruses stimulate are themselves associated with cancer, raising the concern that even if viruses can be eliminated from the process, the reprogrammed cells might remain predisposed to cancer. For these reasons, iPS cells may never be suitable for use in patients. I sincerely hope that iPS cells are the long-sought-after customized patient-specific stem cell, but much more research must be done.

Even with iPS cells in hand, my laboratory will continue to study embryonic stem cells. First, we need to directly compare the capacity of these two types of stem cells to generate specific tissues. Some very preliminary data has suggested that iPS cells may be less potent than embryonic stem cells in making blood, while others are noting a deficiency in making heart muscle cells. It will take years for scientists to understand the similarities and differences between these two valuable classes of pluripotent stem cells. Even with iPS cells in hand, my laboratory will continue to investigate somatic cell nuclear transfer as a means of generating pluripotent stem cells. Reprogramming by nuclear transfer is faster and may entail very different mechanisms than gene-based reprogramming. Learning why may lead to better methods for making iPS cells.

The iPS breakthrough is being heralded by opponents of embryonic stem cell research as a solution to the long-smoldering debate over the necessity of embryonic stem cell research. We have heard the arguments for many years, first made when multi-potential adult progenitor cells (MAPCs) were reported in 2002, and later when stem cells were isolated from Fat and Amniotic fluid: we are told that alternatives are available that preclude the need for embryonic stem cell research. Congress has been wise to not yield to such arguments. Indeed, it was embryonic stem cell research that led directly to the breakthrough in iPS cells, and my own laboratory was poised to generate iPS cells in large part because of our experience and expertise in deriving and culturing human embryonic stem cells. Today, it would again be a mistake to place limits on the tools available to biomedical scientists to pursue the next medical breakthroughs. The right course for biomedical science and ultimately the right decision for patients and our health care system, is to expand the scope of federal funding for all forms of stem cell research, including the many lines of embryonic stem cells created after the President's artificial deadline of August 9th, 2001.

Yesterday, in my address to the Congressional Biomedical Research Caucus, I was asked the question: "Do we still need research on embryonic stem cells?" to which I replied a resounding "Yes." Embryonic stem cells remain the gold standard today and will remain so for the foreseeable future. If we are to maximize the pace of scientific discovery and accelerate development of new treatments for disease, we must continue to vigorously pursue all forms of stem cell research, using ES cells derived from embryos, pluripotent stem cells generated by nuclear transfer and gene-based reprogramming, and adult stem cells. Passage of the bill HR-810 originally proposed by members Castle and Degette remains a worthy goal.

In: Encyclopedia of Stem Cell Research (2 Volume Set)   ISBN: 978-1-61761-835-2
Editor: Alexander L. Greene   © 2012 Nova Science Publishers, Inc.

Chapter LIX

TESTIMONY OF JOHN K. FRASER[*]

John K. Fraser

Good morning, my name is John Fraser, and I am Principal Scientist at Cytori Therapeutics Inc, a publically-traded stem cell company in San Diego, California. Cytori is at the forefront of brining adult stem cells to patients, as we are currently selling a stem cell-based product in Europe, are conducting three separate clinical trials, and have a technology, which has been used in over 200 patient procedures.

From my graduate studies in New Zealand, through to a postdoctoral and then faculty appointment at UCLA, and now at Cytori, my entire research career has been centered on adult stem cells.

The topic of today's meeting is consideration of stem cells as the future of medicine. Indeed, stem cells will be an important part of the clinical armamentarium going forward. But this is nothing new; hematopoietic stem cells have been used in medicine for at least 50 years. In pioneering work started in the late 1950's E. Donnall Thomas performed bone marrow transplant studies that ultimately led to the award of the Nobel Prize for Medicine in 1990 (1-3). Many consider 1961 as the birth date of the stem cell field as that was the year that James E Till and Ernest A McCulloch published research (4) that led to the description of the first stem cell (5), the hematopoietic stem cell; which is still widely considered to be the model for all adult stem cells (6).

Hematopoietic stem cells make bone marrow transplantation possible. This is because they have the ability to regenerate the entire blood system of the recipient for the rest of that person's life. Simply put, hematopoietic stem cells are the regenerative engine of the blood system.

In my opinion, this is a key point of distinction between adult stem cells and embryonic stem cells. Embryonic stem cells are capable of immense proliferation and essentially universal plasticity. This is because they are, first and foremost, developmental cells; they are derived from a cell mass from which the entire organism develops.

---

[*] These remarks were delivered as testimony given by John K. Fraser, Principal Scientist, Cytori Therapeutics Inc.

By contrast, adult stem cells are, first and foremost, regenerative cells, responsible for maintaining and healing organs and tissues in the face of daily wear and tear, injury, and disease. They are, by their nature, repair cells; they activate in response to a need and shut off once healing is completed. One way to look at this is to view embryonic stem cells as responsible for generating all the tissues of an organism, while adult stem cells are responsible for maintaining and healing them.

The natural role of adult stem cells in repair and regeneration makes them ideally suited for clinical use. This has been proven in tens of thousands of bone marrow transplant patients in the last 40 years. This paradigm is now increasingly being repeated as other adult cell types associated with repair and regeneration are being applied in different diseases.

For example, Cytori has initiated several clinical studies using cells obtained from the patient's own fat tissue, which is recognized as one of the richest and most accessible sources for adult stem cells. The goal of these studies is to bring forth new treatments for the millions of patients suffering from heart disease as well as to help reconstruction breast defects in women who have undergone partial mastectomy. We also intend to start studies in intervertebral disc repair and potentially several other clinical applications, which look promising.

Other researchers have published case reports and clinical studies using fat tissue-derived stem cells in treating certain types of wound (7-9), in treating complications associated with bone marrow transplantation (10-14), and in bone defects (15). Published preclinical studies have indicated potential in treating renal damage associated with chemotherapy (16), preserving dopaminergic neurons in a Parkinson's disease model (17), treating liver damage (18), ischemic (19) and hemorrhagic (20) stroke, and in tissues as disparate as the cornea (21), the lung (22,23), and the vocal fold (24).

Published clinical studies with other types of adult stem cell have shown improvement in cardiac function (25-27), in an inherited brittle bone disease (28-30), in liver disease (31-33), and peripheral vascular disease (34) to name but a few.

However, there are still many unanswered questions and clearly additional science is needed. In certain settings, the mechanisms through which adult stem cells provide benefit are not well understood. It is also not yet clear which adult stem cell sources provide greatest clinical efficacy in which diseases. These are important questions that companies such as Cytori have neither the resources nor oftentimes the incentive to address.

For example, certain potentially beneficial cell populations fall outside of patent protections limiting the incentive of companies to invest resources in proving a technology that may then be applied without their participation. Without federal support much of this promise could be left to wither on the vine.

Cytori believes that ultimately science and the marketplace will determine which technologies will succeed. We have looked at the field of regenerative medicine, performed our own basic science, pre-clinical and now clinical research and we are very optimistic regarding the ability of our approach to harness the natural role of adult stem and regenerative cells to provide clinically and cost-effective treatments for a range of human diseases in the near future. We urge your continuing support of adult stem cell research.

Thank you.

REFERENCES

[1] Hamblin, T.J. E. & Donnall Thomas, M.D. (1991*). Nobel laureate 1990. Leuk Res 15*, 71.

[2] Thomas, E. D., Lochte, H. L., Jr., Lu,W. C., & Ferrebee,J. W. (1957). Intravenous infusion of bone marrow in patients receiving radiation and chemotherapy. *N Engl J Med 257,* 491-496.

[3] Thomas, E. D., Lochte, H. L., Jr., & Ferrebee,J. W. (1959). Irradiation of the entire body and marrow transplantation: some observations and comments. *Blood 14,* 1-23.

[4] Till, J. E. & McCulloch, E. A. (1961). A direct measurement of the radiation sensitivity of normal mouse bone marrow cells. *Radiat Res 14,* 213-222.

[5] Becker, A. J., McCulloch, E., & Till,J. (1963). Cytological demonstration of the clonal nature of spleen colonies derived from transplanted mouse marrow cells. *Nature 197,* 452-454

[6] Bryder, D., Rossi, D. J., & Weissman, I. L. (2006). Hematopoietic stem cells: the paradigmatic tissue-specific stem cell. *Am J Pathol 169*, 338-346.

[7] Garcia-Olmo, D., Garcia-Arranz, M., Garcia, L. G., Cuellar, E. S., Blanco, I. F., Prianes, L. A., Montes, J. A., Pinto, F. L., Marcos, D. H., & Garcia-Sancho, L. (2003). Autologous stem cell transplantation for treatment of rectovaginal fistula in perianal Crohn's disease: a new cell-based therapy. *Int J Colorectal Dis 18*, 451-454.

[8] Garcia-Olmo, D., Garcia-Arranz, M., Herreros, D., Pascual, I., Peiro, C., & Rodriguez-Montes, J. A. (2005). A phase I clinical trial of the treatment of Crohn's fistula by adipose mesenchymal stem cell transplantation. *Dis Colon Rectum 48*, 1416-1423.

[9] Alvarez, P. D., Garcia-Arranz, M., Georgiev-Hristov, T., & Garcia-Olmo, D. (2008). A new bronchoscopic treatment of tracheomediastinal fistula using autologous adipose-derived stem cells. *Thorax 63,* 374-376.

[10] Fang, B., Song, Y., Liao, L., Zhang, Y., & Zhao, R. C. (2007). Favorable response to human adipose tissuederived mesenchymal stem cells in steroid-refractory acute graft-versus-host disease. *Transplant Proc 39*, 3358-3362.

[11] Fang, B., Song, Y., Lin, Q., Zhang, Y., Cao, Y., Zhao, R. C., & Ma, Y. (2007). Human adipose tissue-derived mesenchymal stromal cells as salvage therapy for treatment of severe refractory acute graft-vs.-host disease in two children. *Pediatr Transplant 11,* 814-817.

[12] Fang, B., Song, Y., Zhao, R. C., Han, Q., & Cao, Y. (2007). Treatment of resistant pure red cell aplasia after major abo-incompatible bone marrow transplantation with human adipose tissue-derived mesenchymal stem cells. *Am J Hematol 82,* 772-773.

[13] Fang, B., Song, Y. P., Liao, L. M., Han, Q., & Zhao, R. C. (2006). Treatment of severe therapy-resistant acute graft-versus-host disease with human adipose tissue-derived mesenchymal stem cells. *Bone Marrow Transplant 38,* 389-390.

[14] Fang, B., Song, Y., Zhao, R. C., Han, Q., & Lin, Q. (2007). Using human adipose tissue-derived mesenchymal stem cells as salvage therapy for hepatic graft-versus-host disease resembling acute hepatitis. *Transplant Proc 39*, 1710-1713.

[15] Lendeckel, S., Jodicke, A., Christophis, P., Heidinger, K., Wolff, J., Fraser, J. K., Hedrick, M. H., Berthold, L., & Howaldt, H. P. (2004). Autologous stem cells

(adipose) and fibrin glue used to treat widespread traumatic calvarial defects: case report. *J Craniomaxillofac. Surg 32,* 370-373.

[16] Bi, B., Schmitt, R., Israilova, M., Nishio, H., & Cantley, L. G. (2007). Stromal cells protect against acute tubular injury via an endocrine effect. *J Am Soc Nephrol 18,* 2486-2496.

[17] McCoy, M. K., Martinez, T. N., Ruhn, K. A., Wrage, P. C., Keefer, E. W., Botterman, B. R., Tansey, K. E., & Tansey, M. G. (2007). Autologous transplants of Adipose-Derived Adult Stromal (ADAS) cells afford dopaminergic neuroprotection in a model of Parkinson's disease. *Exp Neurol.*

[18] Banas,A., Tokuhara,T., Teratani,T., Quinn,G., Yamamoto,Y., & Ochiya,T. Adipose tissue-derived mesenchymal stem cells as a source of human hepatocytes. *Hepatology 45,* (in press) (2007).

[19] Kang, S. K., Lee, D. H., Bae, Y. C., Kim, H. K., Baik, S. Y., & Jung, J. S. (2003). Improvement of neurological deficits by intracerebral transplantation of human adipose tissue-derived stromal cells after cerebral ischemia in rats. *Exp Neurol. 183,* 355-366.

[20] Kim, J. M., Lee, S. T., Chu, K., Jung, K. H., Song, E. C., Kim, S. J., Sinn, D. I., Kim, J. H., Park, D. K., Kang, K. M., Hyung, H. N., Park, H. K., Won, C. H., Kim, K. H., Kim, M., Kun, L. S., & Roh, J. K. (2007). Systemic transplantation of human adipose stem cells attenuated cerebral inflammation and degeneration in a hemorrhagic stroke model. *Brain Res 1183C,* 43-50.

[21] Arnalich-Montiel, F., Pastor, S., Blazquez-Martinez, A., Fernandez-Delgado, J., Nistal, M., Alio, J. L., & De Miguel, M. P. (2007). Adipose-Derived Stem Cells are a Source for Cell Therapy of The Corneal Stroma. *Stem Cells.*

[22] Shigemura, N., Okumura, M., Mizuno, S., Imanishi, Y., Nakamura, T., & Sawa, Y. (2006). Autologous transplantation of adipose tissue-derived stromal cells ameliorates pulmonary emphysema. *Am J Transplant 6,* 2592-2600.

[23] Shigemura, N., Okumura, M., Mizuno, S., Imanishi, Y., Matsuyama, A., Shiono, H., Nakamura, T., & Sawa, Y. (2006). Lung tissue engineering technique with adipose stromal cells improves surgical outcome for pulmonary emphysema. *Am J Respir. Crit Care Med 174,* 1199-1205.

[24] Lee, B. J., Wang, S. G., Lee, J. C., Jung, J. S., Bae, Y. C., Jeong, H. J., Kim, H. W., & Lorenz, R. R. (2006). The prevention of vocal fold scarring using autologous adipose tissue-derived stromal cells. *Cells Tissues Organs 184,* 198-204.

[25] Schachinger, V., Assmus, B., Britten, M. B., Honold, J., Lehmann, R., Teupe, C., Abolmaali, N. D., Vogl, T. J., Hofmann, W. K., Martin, H., Dimmeler, S., & Zeiher, A. M. (2004). Transplantation of progenitor cells and regeneration enhancement in acute myocardial infarction: final one-year results of the TOPCARE-AMI Trial. *J Am Coll Cardiol 44,* 1690-1699.

[26] Dimmeler, S., Burchfield, J., & Zeiher, A. M. (2008). Cell-based therapy of myocardial infarction. *Arterioscler Thromb Vasc Biol 28,* 208-216.

[27] Schachinger, V., Erbs, S., Elsasser, A., Haberbosch, W., Hambrecht, R., Holschermann, H., Yu, J., Corti, R., Mathey, D. G., Hamm, C. W., Suselbeck, T., Werner, N., Haase, J., Neuzner, J., Germing, A., Mark, B., Assmus, B., Tonn, T., Dimmeler, S., & Zeiher, A. M. (2006). Improved clinical outcome after intracoronary

administration of bone-marrow-derived progenitor cells in acute myocardial infarction: final 1-year results of the REPAIR-AMI trial. *Eur Heart J 27,* 2775-2783.

[28] Horwitz, E. M., Gordon, P. L., Koo, W. K., Marx, J. C., Neel, M. D., McNall, R. Y., Muul, L., & Hofmann, T. (2002). Isolated allogeneic bone marrow-derived mesenchymal cells engraft and stimulate growth in children with osteogenesis imperfecta: Implications for cell therapy of bone. *Proc Natl Acad Sci U S A 99,* 8932-8937.

[29] Horwitz, E. M. (2001). Marrow mesenchymal cell transplantation for genetic disorders of bone. *Cytotherapy. 3,* 399-401.

[30] Horwitz, E. M., Prockop, D. J., Fitzpatrick, L. A., Koo, W. W., Gordon, P. L., Neel, M., Sussman, M., Orchard, P., Marx, J. C., Pyeritz, R. E., & Brenner, M. K. (1999). Transplantability and therapeutic effects of bone marrow-derived mesenchymal cells in children with osteogenesis imperfecta. *Nat Med 5,* 309-13.

[31] Sakaida, I. (2008). Autologous bone marrow cell infusion therapy for liver cirrhosis. *J Gastroenterol Hepatol.*

[32] Sakaida, I. (2006). Clinical application of bone marrow cell transplantation for liver diseases. *J Gastroenterol 41,* 93-94.

[33] Sakaida, I., Terai, S., & Okita, K. (2005). Use of bone marrow cells for the development of cellular therapy in liver diseases. *Hepatol Res 31,* 195-196.

[34] Kajiguchi, M., Kondo, T., Izawa, H., Kobayashi, M., Yamamoto, K., Shintani, S., Numaguchi, Y., Naoe, T., Takamatsu, J., Komori, K., & Murohara, T. (2007). Safety and efficacy of autologous progenitor cell transplantation for therapeutic angiogenesis in patients with critical limb ischemia. *Circ J 71,* 196-201.

NIH Research Contract and Grant Funding Received by Dr Fraser

1R44HL076045 "Adipose Derived Cell Therapy for Myocardial Infarction" awarded by the National Heart, Lung, and Blood Institute of the National Institutes of Health. January 2004 to July 2006: Total $950,000

1R43HL088871-01 "Adipose Tissue-Derived Cells for Vascular Cell Therapy" awarded by the National Heart, Lung, and Blood Institute of the National Institutes of Health. September 2007 to August 2008: Total $250,000

1N01HB067142 "Collection and Storage Centers for Clinical Research on Umbilical Cord Blood Stem and Progenitor Cell Transplantation". September 1996 – September 2001: Total ~$11 million.

In: Encyclopedia of Stem Cell Research (2 Volume Set)   ISBN: 978-1-61761-835-2
Editor: Alexander L. Greene   © 2012 Nova Science Publishers, Inc.

Chapter LX

TESTIMONY ON STEM CELL SCIENCE: THE FOUNDATION FOR FUTURE CURES BEFORE THE U.S. HOUSE OF REPRESENTATIVES SUBCOMMITTEE ON HEALTH OF THE COMMITTEE ON ENERGY AND COMMERCE[*]

John Gearhart and C. Michael Armstron

Mr. Chairman and Members of the Subcommittee, I am John Gearhart, a stem cell biologist at Johns Hopkins Medicine. I am pleased to appear before you to discuss the foundation for future cures through stem cell science.

It is rare that a field of scientific research can have both an enormous potential impact of human health and quality of life and be a fount of new basic research discovery. What crystallized the scientific and medical communities' interest in stem cell research was the derivation of human embryonic stem cell lines. These cell lines are unique in that they are capable of forming all the different cell types (>220) that are present in the body (a property that is referred to as pluripotentiality) and they can produce more cells like themselves indefinitely (self-renew). This development, first reported ten years ago, has been among the most heralded as well as contentious issues of the modern scientific era. Heralded, as now we had in the laboratory a source of cells from which we could grow any and all cells of the human body for much needed replacement therapies and contentious, because embryos are destroyed to derive the cells. No wonder that stem cell research has impacted many areas of our society – science, medicine, religion, ethics, policy and economics. Seldom has a week gone by without some new revelation about stem cells reaching the front pages of the press or

---

[*] These remarks were delivered as testimony given on May 8, 2008. John Gearhart for "Stem Cell Science: The Foundation for Future Cures," before the United States House of Representatives Subcommottee on Health of the Committee on Energy and Commerce.

the top news stories of the day and what this means for our society, invariably hyped. It is recognized that stem cell research has the potential to revolutionize the practice of medicine and to improve the quality of life and in some cases, the length of life for many people suffering from devastating illnesses and injuries. Also, it is believed by many that there will be no realm of medicine that will not be impacted by stem cell research.

Research over the past ten years is setting the foundation for the use of embryonic stem cells and the knowledge derived from this research for developing and designing therapies, therapies that will be safe as well as effective. To envision what lies ahead for the use of these cells in human therapies, it is informative to mention the progress that has been made over the past decade while keeping in mind that the progress made by US investigators has been compromised by current policy on federal funding. In the very first Congressional hearing on these stem cells (December 2, 1998, Before the Senate Appropriations Committee, Subcommittee on Labor, Health and Human Services, Education and Related Agencies) and one in which I had participated, Harold Varmus, MD, then the Director of the National Institutes of Health (now the President of the Memorial Sloan-Kettering Cancer Center) outlined the potential uses of these cells in biomedicine and it is appropriate to use his list in evaluating what has transpired in laboratories since then.

(Varmus) At the most fundamental level, pluripotent stem cells could help us to understand the complex events that occur during human development. A primary goal of this work would be the most basic kind of research --the identification of the factors involved in the cellular decision-making process that determines cell specialization. We know that turning genes on and off is central to this process, but we do not know much about these "decision-making" genes or what turns them on or off. Some of our most serious diseases, like cancer, are due to abnormal cell differentiation and growth. A deeper understanding of normal cell processes will allow us to further delineate the fundamental errors that cause these deadly illnesses.

There is no question that we have learned a great deal about these stem cells and the molecular mechanisms underlying the bases of pluripotentiality and of cell differentiation, that is, the conversion of these cells into one of the types of specialized cells of the body. This is what we call basic science, a prerequisite first step in understanding cellular processes. We have utilized studies of other organisms to first give us insight into these mechanisms and then confirmed these mechanisms or variations on these mechanisms in the human cells. Much of our progress has been informed by such studies and as has been pointed out recently by Bruce Alberts, Ph.D., there are no shortcuts to medical progress: *But, as has been repeatedly demonstrated, the shortest path to medical breakthroughs may not come from a direct attack against a specific disease. Critical medical insights frequently arise from attempts to understand fundamental mechanisms in organisms that are much easier to study than humans; in particular, from studies of bacteria, yeasts, insects, plants, and worms. For this reason, an overemphasis on "translational" biomedical research (which focuses on a particular disease) would be counterproductive, even for those who care only about disease prevention and cures. (Bruce Alberts, Shortcuts to Medical Progress? Science Vol 319, 28 March 2008).* Embryonic stem cells provide another link in the biomedical investigation and discovery chain that leads to human application.

So, we now know a handful of the critical genes and of the regulation of the expression of these genes that enable cells to be pluripotential. This knowledge was at the basis of the most recent and exciting development in our field in which skin cells were converted to cells that had properties of embryonic stem cells by the addition of just a few genes to the cells. The skin cells had these genes but they were not being expressed. Adding exogenous version genes that were expressed caused these cells to be reprogrammed, eventually expressing their own, endogenous genes. The embryonic stem cell-like cells are called induced pluripotent stem (iPS) cells. This is a major paradigm shift in stem cell biology and I will comment more on this later but it was through the study of embryonic stem cells that this advance was made.

There have now been hundreds of research reports on studies of in which embryonic stem cells are differentiating to specialized cells. We are learning the mechanisms involved in the earliest decisions made by cells to become neurons or gut cells or muscle cells, etc. It has been know for decades that cell-cell interactions in the embryo determine the fates of cells during development as summarized by the Noble laureate Hans Spemann (1943): *We are standing and walking with parts of our body which we could have used for thinking if they had been developed in another position in the embryo.* With these embryonic stem cells in culture, we are learning how different factors influence cell fate decisions. By experimentally manipulating these factors we can then direct cell differentiation to a desired cell type through the use of growth factors, attempting to mimic the environment of the embryo.

Personally, I have been interested in human embryology and development for decades and have felt strongly as Samuel Taylor Coleridge (1934) stated so beautifully: *The history of man for the nine months preceding his birth would probably be far more interesting and contain events of far greater moment, than all the three-score and ten years that follow.* These stem cells have provided a unique resource to learn about the biologic mechanisms underlying our development, both normal and abnormal, so that we may eventually understand the basis of birth defects and perhaps guide us in correcting these malformations, etc. We have learned much about the mechanisms of cell decision making in the early embryo, such as within the conceptus, becoming embryonic or extra-embryonic, and within the germ layers of the embryo, what determines cell fate. In our own current work with embryonic stem cells, we have recently discovered ~40 new genes that are critical to the formation of the heart and great vessels. There are many other examples for the use of these important cells in studying human development.

Recent findings have discovered and solidified the understanding that many of the same cellular mechanisms found in the development of a tissue or organ play critical roles when rebuilding or regenerating that tissue. Investigators have gone on to show that manipulation of these developmental factors, the understanding for which has been often discovered, expanded and/or validated in embryonic stem cells, can greatly influence regenerative capacity, even recovering the capacity to regenerate in animals that did not possess it. It is of the outmost importance that studies continue in order to discover these and utilize this knowledge in designing therapies for the many maladies affecting us. As all of you have observed, we humans don't regenerated body parts like some of our lower relatives in the animal kingdom. Imagine the possibility of harnessing the capacity of zebrafish, for example, who using the same families of genes that we use in the development of our heart can regrow a large part of their heart when amputated. We must determine the reasons why humans fail to display this capacity in most organs, emboldened by the knowledge that our livers can regenerate, in order to combat many common debilitating diseases such as heart attacks and strokes.

(Varmus) Human pluripotent stem cell research could also dramatically change the way we develop drugs and test them for safety and efficacy. Rather than evaluating safety and efficacy of a candidate drug in an animal model of a human disease, these drugs could be tested against a human cell line that had been developed to mimic the disease processes. This would not replace whole animal and human testing, but it would streamline the road to discovery. Only the most effective and safest candidate would be likely to graduate to whole animal and then human testing.

There have now been many examples of use of what are called high throughput screens for testing the effect of various chemicals, molecules and drugs on the stem cells and their specialized derivatives. The use of this approach for studies with 'diseased' cells is just beginning as embryonic stem cells have been derived from embryos diagnosed with mutations that can lead to disease later in life.

(Varmus) Perhaps the most far-reaching potential application of human pluripotent stem cells is the generation of cells and tissue that could be used for transplantation, so-called cell therapies. Many diseases and disorders result from disruption of cellular function or destruction of tissues of the body. Today, donated organs and tissues are often used to replace the function of ailing or destroyed tissue. Unfortunately, the number of people suffering from these disorders far outstrips the number of organs available for transplantation. Pluripotent stem cells stimulated to develop into specialized cells offer the possibility of a renewable source of replacement cells and tissue to treat a myriad of diseases, conditions and disabilities including Parkinson's and Alzheimer's disease, spinal cord injury, stroke, burns, heart disease, diabetes, osteoarthritis and rheumatoid arthritis. There is almost no realm of medicine that might not be touched by this innovation

There are now many reports on the use of embryonic stem cell sources of cells for grafting into animals with various injuries or that serve as models for a variety of human diseases. The results have been highly variable (as it has been using stem cells from any source, adult or embryonic) but in many cases, they are encouraging. Our laboratory has been working with cell-based therapies for the heart. Currently there are no adult stem cells that have been identified to date that have shown robust cardiac muscle formation in vivo (in the heart), or for that matter, in vitro (in the dish). We and other laboratories have identified a stem cell that gives rise to most of the cells within the heart and these cells, when grafted to infarcted rodent hearts robustly undergo cardiac muscle formation, integrate into the heart and restore function.

There are three further important points that I want to make in considering the future of providing cures or ameliorating diseases and injuries through stem cell science.

- Time frame for developing safe and effective therapies.
- Where disease is involved, we must determine the underlying pathogenesis of the disease and stop it. I have talked only about having a source of cells (or the knowledge of how to control cell fates) in establishing a foundation for future therapies. What is as important, is the understanding of the pathogenesis of

devastating diseases for we must stop this process for grafted cells will surely succumb to the same fate.

- How do the iPS cells factor into the future?

Quite simply I believe that they are important part of the future. They require further vetting as true embryonic stem cells. At the moment, we can only measure what can measure with embryonic stem cells and induced pluripotent stem cells. More must be learned about each. They represent a powerful example of our goal to instruct our cells to do what we want; but this is just the beginning. Is this a farewell to embryonic stem cells in research? Not at all, for they represent the gold standard. For my studies focused on human embryology, I will continue to use embryonic cells but, like many of my colleagues, I will vigorously pursue the direct reprogramming of adult cells.

SUMMARY

Mr. Chairman, I am grateful to you for providing a forum to discuss this promising arena of science and medicine. Learning to instruct our cells to get them to do what we want is the ultimate control of our own cells and the basis of future medicine. Based on current research results with stem cells, the future is, as Yogi Berra has said, not what it used to be. We look to stem cells not only to provide cells for replacements in therapies, but also to provide us with the knowledge of how cells work and to use this information to instruct patients' cells to effect repair and regeneration of damaged or diseased tissues. We must recognize that the development therapies that are safe and effective is going to take time and resources and that circumspection is not a retreat from promise. I would be pleased to answer any questions you might have.

In: Encyclopedia of Stem Cell Research (2 Volume Set)   ISBN: 978-1-61761-835-2
Editor: Alexander L. Greene   © 2012 Nova Science Publishers, Inc.

Chapter LXI

WRITTEN TESTIMONY OF WEYMAN JOHNSON, INDIVIDUAL LIVING WITH MULTIPLE SCLEROSIS, CHAIRMAN OF THE BOARD, NATIONAL MULTIPLE SCLEROSIS SOCIETY, ENERGY AND COMMERCE COMMITTEE SUBCOMMITTEE ON HEALTH U.S. HOUSE OF REPRESENTATIVES[*]

- Summary of my personal and family experiences with a chronic, disabling disease.
- Speak to a patient perspective on my own diagnosis with multiple sclerosis.
- Speak to the position of a national voluntary health organization, as chairman of the board of the National Multiple Sclerosis Society.
- Speak to the need for continued research and the hope it brings for people living with chronic diseases and conditions nationwide.
- Support the need for the Committee and Congress to remain committed to legislation like the Stem Cell Research Enhancement Act.
- Embryonic stem cell research holds an incredibly unique promise for people living with chronic diseases and conditions, and the progress made to date on embryonic stem cell lines should not be abandoned.

Thank you Chairman Pallone and Ranking Member Deal. Thank you members of the Committee. I am honored to be invited to speak here today among many distinguished panelists and to represent patients who live with chronic disease.

Many diseases could benefit from expanded embryonic stem cell research. But today I will focus on one—multiple sclerosis. Not because it is more important than others, but because I know multiple sclerosis.

---

[*] These written remarks were delivered as testimony given on May 8, 2008. Weyman Johnson, Individual living with Multiple Sclerosis, Chairman of the Board, National Multiple Sclerosis Society to the Energy and Commerce Committee, Subcommittee on Health, United States House of Representatives, "Stem Cell Science."

I remember multiple sclerosis and how it entered my life as a child, in 1964, just barely 13 years old. My father received a diagnosis of MS suddenly. He died in 2001. His sister, my aunt Allene, also had MS. Research into this disease, into genetics was just starting to evolve in the 1960s.

There were good doctors then, but they did not recognize a genetic connection. They said MS in my family was a mere coincidence. Because of research, we now know that is not true.

My own sister, who's only a few years older than I, lives with MS. She uses a power wheelchair, her hands don't work well anymore, she can no longer teach the way she did, or play the piano the way she did. A few years after she was diagnosed, so was I. We hate this disease, its impact on our family, and the threat it poses to our future generations.

We are making progress into the genetic factors involved in multiple sclerosis. However there are still more questions than answers. The research must continue.

I remember being told that MS is a disease that doesn't affect my friends in the African American community. This is only for white people from Minnesota. With good science, we have found that's not true. The research must continue.

We also used to hear that this disease does not happen to children. But that is not true either. We now know there are thousands of children in the United States, thousands of children throughout the world, who live with this disease. The research must continue.

Before 1993, there were no treatments at all for multiple sclerosis. Now we have six. But there is a wide spectrum among people living with MS. Most of the therapies will only work for those of us on the lucky end of the spectrum like me. But for people like my sister, on the more unlucky end, there's still not much out there that provides effective treatment. So the research must continue.

Every hour, someone new is diagnosed with MS. It's an unpredictable, often disabling disease of the central nervous system. The progress, severity, and specific symptoms of MS in any one person still cannot be predicted. The cause is unknown, and there is no cure. But embryonic stem cell research holds an incredibly unique promise to repair nerve cells, to slow the progression of MS, to help find a cure.

One area that holds great promise, but is often misunderstood, is Somatic Cell Nuclear Transfer. We have seen some exciting breakthroughs. But as with all science, this research takes time. We are still exploring this avenue for medical research. I have hope that SCNT will succeed because of its promise to repair nerve cells, creating new tissues, and more. I know that researchers are focused on the idea of creating cells and tissues for transplantation and research. They are trying to understand how different genes are turned on and off. They are not focused on cloning. I know that as we explore somatic cell nuclear transfer research more, we will see greater potential for developing individualized cell and tissue therapies. That holds great promise for people living with MS like me, whose body's own defense system is attacking the myelin surrounding and protecting our central nervous system.

I am but one person living with a chronic disease. But I am also fortunate to serve as chairman of the board of the National Multiple Sclerosis Society. We believe that all promising avenues of research that could lead to new ways to prevent, repair, slow the progression, or cure MS *must* be explored, with adherence to the strictest ethical and procedural guidelines. The National Multiple Sclerosis Society believes that all promising avenues of research that could lead to the cure or prevention of multiple sclerosis or relieve its symptoms must be explored. The Society supports the Stem Cell Research Enhancement Act to expand the number of approved stem cell lines that are available for federally funded research. The Society supports the conduct of scientifically meritorious medical research, including research using human cells, in accordance with federal, state, and local laws and with adherence to the strictest ethical and procedural guidelines.

Research on all types of stem cells is critical because we have no way of knowing which type of stem cell will be of the most value in MS research. Stem cells — adult or embryonic — could have the potential to be used to protect and rebuild tissues that are damaged by MS, and to deliver molecules that foster repair or protect vulnerable tissues from further injury.

So I ask you to expand the federal policy on embryonic stem cell research and ensure that research continues ... for the more than 400,000 other Americans who live with MS and 100 million Americans with other diseases and conditions. Research on all types of stem cells is critical because we have no way of knowing at this point which type of stem cell will be of the most value ... for multiple sclerosis, for Parkinson's, for Alzheimer's, for cancer, for heart disease, for spinal cord and brain injuries, for many other conditions.

Just like with genetics and race and age, there is so much left to learn about how to treat and cure MS ... about how to treat and cure other diseases. Expanding our embryonic stem cell research is just one avenue. But it is an avenue of research that must continue. Federal barriers must be lifted.

You might see that I am not the only person living with MS on Capitol Hill today. *Hundreds* of MS activists are visiting with their legislators on the Hill right now, talking about the need to advance medical research.

Embryonic stem cell research remains one of the most promising avenues of research to cure diseases and end suffering. I am not a scientist, but I am an observer of science. And I know that science is a matter that requires some patience. That's why we must expand the important work done to date with embryonic stem cell lines. The research must continue. So we can improve the lives of people with chronic diseases and conditions. So we can improve the lives of families for generations to come. For my grandchildren and for yours.

We need your commitment to not give up on legislation like the Stem Cell Research Enhancement Act. We don't have the luxury of time. Like many others who live with a chronic disease, I know ... maybe not today, maybe not next week, but I pray soon ... with patience and continued research ... that there will be no more disease. Thank you for helping us move closer, and thank you for your time.

NATIONAL MULTIPLE SCLEROSIS SOCIETY POLICY POSITION EMBRYONIC STEM CELL LINES AVAILABLE FOR FEDERALLY FUNDED RESEARCH

Position

The National Multiple Sclerosis Society believes that all promising avenues of research that could lead to the cure or prevention of multiple sclerosis or relieve its symptoms must be explored. The Society supports the Stem Cell Research Enhancement Act (H.R. 3 and S. 5) to expand the number of approved stem cell lines that are available for federally funded research.

The Society supports the conduct of scientifically meritorious medical research, including research using human cells, in accordance with federal, state, and local laws and with adherence to the strictest ethical and procedural guidelines. Research on all types of stem cells is critical because we have no way of knowing which type of stem cell will be of the most value in MS research. Stem cells — adult or embryonic — could have the potential to be used to protect and rebuild tissues that are damaged by MS, and to deliver molecules that foster repair or protect vulnerable tissues from further injury.

Request

We urge Congress to support the Stem Cell Research Enhancement Act of 2007 (H.R. 3 and S. 5) at all levels of the legislative process. This legislation would increase the number of approved embryonic stem cell lines that can be used in federally funded research by allowing new lines to be generated from embryos that have been donated for research purposes by people using the services of in vitro fertilization clinics, while establishing important ethical protections.

Supporting Rationale

There is broad agreement that the policy limiting the number of stem cell lines available for federally funded research is flawed.

An insufficient supply of stem cell lines currently exists, as only 22 of the 70 approved lines are available to researchers. In addition, all of the available lines are contaminated by nutrients from mouse feeder cells. Many in the scientific community believe that these stem cell lines are unsuitable for research and hinder U.S. scientists' ability to capitalize on the potential breakthroughs from embryonic stem cell research.

At the same time, it has become increasingly clear that stem cell research holds tremendous promise for MS and many other diseases and disorders. Research suggests that stem cells might have many uses: for delivery of growth factors and drugs, for tissue culture systems for drug and gene discovery, for understanding and modeling MS, and for repairing or protecting brain tissue.

However, our scientific advisors have told us that we still don't know which type of stem cells will be most valuable for MS research, and thus we must support policies that promote the conduct of research using all types of stem cells.

In: Encyclopedia of Stem Cell Research (2 Volume Set) ISBN: 978-1-61761-835-2
Editor: Alexander L. Greene © 2012 Nova Science Publishers, Inc.

Chapter LXII

Testimony for "Stem Cell Science: The Foundation for Future Cures" before the Subcommittee on Health of the Committee on Energy and Commerce[*]

Amit N Patel

Chairman and members of the Committee, thank you for inviting me to testify before you. My name is Amit Patel. Please note that the testimony I am giving today is my own opinion and not necessarily that of the institution where I am currently employed. I am a translational scientist for cardiovascular diseases where my research is focused on working with regenerative therapies taking the science from the lab bench to the patients. I am also a cardiovascular surgeon who on daily basis sees patients who have exhausted all medical and surgical options available who may benefit from the science of stem cell research.

My goal today is to give both a scientific and real life perspective of the impact that cardiovascular disease has in the United States and potential use of stem cell therapies.

CARDIOVASCULAR DISEASE

Heart disease is the leading cause of death in the United States. Nearly 930,000 Americans die of cardiovascular diseases each year, which amounts to one death every 33 seconds. About 70 million Americans have some form of cardiovascular disease, which is responsible for more than 6 million hospitalizations each year. There are over a one million patients with heart attacks every year, along with six million patients with chronic angina

---

[*] These remarks were delivered as testimony by Amit N Patel, Director, Cardiovascular Cell Therapies, McGowan Institute of Regenerative Medicine, for "Stem Cell Science: The Foundation for Future Cures" before the Subcommittee on Health of the Committee on Energy and Commerce.

(chest pain), and five millions patients with heart failure. In 2005, the cost of heart disease and stroke in the United States exceeded $394 billion: $242 billion for health care expenditures and $152 billion for lost productivity from death and disability. Patients with end-stage cardiovascular disease have over $30 billion dollars in health care expenditures per year. Also, up to 20% of patients over the age 70 have limb ischemia.

Problem

The patients with end stage cardiovascular disease have at least one of two major problems:

- Heart failure, where there is inadequate pumping function of heart due to decreased blood supply or lack of sufficient muscle.
- Critical limb ischemia, where there is inadequate blood supply to the leg.

Current Treatment Options

Heart failure management involves optimal treatment with oral and/or intravenous medications along with surgical therapies. As patients continue to deteriorate the use of artificial hearts and heart transplantation remain the gold standard for end-stage therapy. There are many problems with the surgical options such as infection, stroke, rejection, and the overall costs associated with treatment. However, even with all these options there are limited organs for transplant and fifty percent of endstage heart failure patients die within five years.

Critical limb ischemia management involves oral medical therapy followed by surgical revascularization by bypass grafts. If the graft fails and further reoperative therapy is not possible, then amputation of the leg is performed. This problem is more severe in patients who also have diabetes.

The Role of Stem Cells

Based on the current science, human stem cells have been shown both in a lab dish and in the pre-human work to make new blood vessels and in rare cases new heart muscle.

CURRENT CLINICAL THERAPIES

Human stem cell therapies for cardiovascular disease have been performed under legitimate clinical trials since early 2000. The first group of patients had cells from thigh muscle (skeletal myoblasts) injected into their heart at the time of coronary bypass surgery hoping to grow new heart muscle in Europe. The early data demonstrated some issues with the therapy but larger trials were performed which also did not show significant improvement in heart function. This was truly an example of too rapid translation which could have destroyed the field. However, when these cells where used in a heart failure population and delivered via a catheter in U.S., the results where positive and have led to a large scale clinical trial. Also, using bone marrow cell therapy for the same patient population, both surgically and catheter based delivery has been performed in over one thousand patients in registered trials demonstrating no safety issues. This is the most important issue when performing translational therapies even though all the mechanisms of action have not been defined. As patient safety has been established, the next goal is to identify the patient population which may benefit the most from this therapy, which in the lab dish and pre-human work has shown to grow blood vessels and may improve cardiac muscle function. In these early clinical trials there has been modest improvement in heart function but there has been a significant decrease in adverse events, readmission for heart failure and new heart attacks in the randomized controlled studies. It is true that improvement in overall pumping has not been as large as most people had anticipated but that is most likely related to baseline function of the patient being enrolled in the studies. The analysis of the more severely impaired patients has shown a very dramatic increase which could not be attributed to medical therapy alone. The problem is, that most of these trials have been conducted in Europe or South America.

Similarly, the use of bone marrow stem cells for critical limb ischemia has also been studied since 2000. Most of the early clinical work was performed in Japan, with later translation to Europe and then most recently to the U.S. There has been a decrease in the rate of amputations which has been significant enough that the German government has approved certain centers of expertise which perform the therapy on patients as standard of care and obtain reimbursement from the equivalent of CMS.

Phase III	Country	# Patients	Funding	Results
Acute Myocardial Infarction	Germany	200, 800 pending	Government/ Private/ Corporate	Safe, Mild improvement in heart function and decease mid term adverse events
Acute Myocardial Infarction	Brazil	300	Government	Ongoing
Heart Failure	Brazil	300	Government	Ongoing
Limb Ischemia	Germany	90	Government	Ongoing
Phase II/III				
Heart Failure-myoblasts	USA	390	Corporate	Ongoing
CABG + cells	Germany	100	Government	Pending
Phase II				
Chronic Angina	USA	120	Corporate	Completed awaiting results

Both of these examples are of the first generation of cardiovascular cell therapy. There are many other multi- and pluri-potent stem cells which also have potential for clinical use in cardiovascular disease but the safety still needs to be established before large scale clinical trials are performed such as adipose (fat), amniotic, menstrual, umbilical cord, cardiac stem cells, fetal, and embryonic. Some of these cells are in phase I safety trials both here in the U.S. and Europe. I have attached a table below which shows some of the larger cardiovascular studies in the U.S. and the rest of the world based on the international registry clinicaltrials.gov.

Problems in Clinical Use

There are a number of clinical issues related to translation into reliable therapy. I have listed them below but also have attached a supplement which goes into further detail for each question: 1. What is the best source of stem cells? 2. Is a variety or combination of cells required for different types of heart disease? 3. What are the doses of cells required in humans compared to animals? 4. Are therapeutic doses available? 5. If so, what will be necessary to acquire them? 6. What is the best delivery method for the cells into the heart? 7. When is the best time after myocardial injury to deliver the cells? 8. Are the cells going to stay in the heart and, if not, where do they go and will they cause any harm? 9. How do we follow applied cells over time? 10. Will a tissue engineered scaffold be required to enhance effect? 11. Is it worth the risk to the patient?

Roles of the National Institutes of Health & Food and Drug Administration

The NIH has done a great job in terms of supporting cardiovascular cell based therapies by developing Cell Therapy Network, Heart Failure Network, and the Cardiac Surgery Network. They will all play a significant role in answering the above questions and advancing clinical cardiac cell therapy and the science that is needed to make it a reliable, safe and reproducible therapy.

The FDA has also been very helpful in approving clinical trials with adult based cell therapies. However, the use of both outside basic and clinical scientists in the field early in the development and approval of the trials may expedite approval but more importantly help in ensuring safety to the patients, which is most important.

SUMMARY

Cardiovascular cell therapies using the first generation adult stem cell have great potential to help our patients today. The science needs to continue to improve and help support the safety and efficacy of the therapies. Continued development of other multipotent stem cells along with tissue engineering to make new large blood vessels, heart valves, and the entire heart are the future of cardiac cell therapy. However, significant improvement in the amount of funding is required to keep pace with other countries but most importantly help our patients here in the U.S. I am a realist that these early therapies are a treatment for cardiovascular disease and not a cure. They are experimental but without our current work, the future cures that everyone hopes for and needs will be very difficult if not impossible to achieve.

In: Encyclopedia of Stem Cell Research (2 Volume Set)   ISBN: 978-1-61761-835-2
Editor: Alexander L. Greene   © 2012 Nova Science Publishers, Inc.

Chapter LXIII

ADULT STEM CELL RECIPIENT FOR THE HEART[*]

Douglas T. Rice

My name is Douglas T. Rice. I am 62 years old, have Congestive Heart Disease, and Diabetes. I could be one of over 750,000 people that die in the United States yearly, BUT I am not dead. Not because I shouldn't be, but because there is a resolution to this problem. I am not a miracle, a phenomenon, but a living person that by the grace of God was saved from a disease that kills approximately 2,000 people daily. However, I had to travel to Bangkok, Thailand and go in debt to do something that should be readily available in the United States. I used my own Adult Stem Cells, and a simple angioplasty procedure to have my life given back to me. Your own Adult Stem Cells have so much more to give than we give them credit for; a lot of other diseases are being treated successfully by just using the Adult Stem Cells.

My story is simple. In 1992 I had my first Heart Attack and was also diagnosed with Diabetes. That same year my mother died of Congestive Heart Failure and Diabetes, just like what I have. Also, just last year my sister died of what I have. I have had numerous Heart Attacks and Diabetes episodes as well as having to be jump-started at least three times. I have had a TMR (Trans Myocardial Revascularization), a procedure that uses a laser to drill holes in the Left Ventricle to get better blood flow--this did not help. In 1998, I was given only two years to live unless I received a Heart Transplant. Because of my Diabetes, I did not qualify for it. We tried different things that helped and then in November of 2005, I could not walk but a few feet, had to sleep sitting up, and was just worn out. My Ejection Fraction (the amount of blood my heart pumps out each beat) was around 11% (average is 50%+) and my Cardiologist, Dr. Donald Canaday, said at best I had 4 months without a mechanical heart pump to survive. It was battery operated and I decided I did not want to be battery powered.

That night my best friend, Sheba Rice, went on the Internet looking for new heart treatments. She found TheraVitae, a company in Bangkok, Thailand, that had been having

---

[*] This website information has been edited, reformatted and augmented from www.douglastrice.org adult stem cell recipient, presented by Douglas T. Rice, Adult Stem Cell Recipient for the heart, dated May 8, 2008.

success using the Adult Stem Cells. We contacted them, went to Bangkok in January of 2006, and other than drawing blood, shipping it to Israel, and then having the Adult Stem Cells shipped back and implanted in me via a simple angioplasty procedure, it was simple. The hardest part was the 20-hour flight there. When I returned to Spokane, within a month my Ejection Fraction was tested. It was 28% and going up. I felt better than I had felt in years. I was motivated to tell the world and that is when I found out that over 750,000 Americans die every year from Heart Disease.

These 750,000 heart patients that will die do not make the mainstream press, no newspaper articles of any significance, and certainly most politicians in Washington, D.C. don't even like to discuss it. Sadly, it is a fact, if a family dies in a car wreck, children are gunned down in a school, or a disgruntled person shoots or maims his or her co-workers, it is BIG NEWS.

BUT, 750,000 people die at a rate of over 2,000 a day and no one takes the time to talk for them. Not all are old, some very young and with families and friends to care about. Most people just don't realize that they die although almost everyone knows someone that has died or will die from this disease.

The Federal Government has spent millions of dollars on Embryonic Stem Cells, but not one person has been treated and the animals tested often get tumors.

By some estimates over 400,000 people with various cancers and other diseases have been successfully treated and most are alive to talk about the Adult Stem Cell treatment using their own stem cells or ones from cord blood stem cells.

The honest experts say maybe in 10 or 20 years embryonic stem cells might have potential to treat someone, but not now, and there is something that works "NOW," the Adult Stem Cells!! What does it take to make people realize that a bird in the hand is worth two in the bush, especially when it comes to people's lives?

If you ask most people about stem cells, they only know about Embryonic, because that is all they hear about. Education, Education, Education and the Facts regarding Adult Stem Cells are the only way to succeed in moving this issue to the forefront for funding and actual treatments "NOW."

I get many calls on a daily basis because I have been treated with my Adult Stem Cells, and the most frequent question is, "Why did you have to go toThailand?" Answer: Because there were no adult stem cell clinical trials in the US that I could participate in, and FDA has been slow to approve treatments that are being conducted overseas in countries like Thailand and Germany. My insurance did not cover the cost of this treatment (though I heard that in Germany insurance covers stem cell treatments for heart disease). I also know that much of the stem cell debate in recent years has led to drastically increased funding for embryonic stem cell research despite the fact they have not treated patients for any disease. More money needs to be spent in the United States to prevent a brain drain here for treatments, and siphoning off federal funding for embryonic stem cell research has not helped patients like me. Patients are being increasingly treated with adult stem cells, but we need drastically more federal funding for adult stem cell treatments. These cells aren't patentable, so private investment is far behind. The government should spend more on clinical trials so Americans like me can have the same chance at a treatment that I had.

Listen, I am but one man, a very lucky man to have had my best friend, Sheba Rice, find the solution on the Internet while looking for new technology for heart disease. Without her efforts, I would be in an urn on the fireplace. But, she cared and wanted me alive for whatever reason. We all need to do the same for someone we know or people that need the help. We that care need to educate everyone we meet. Not because I say it, because of the 750,000 people that will die this year!

I would get down on my knees and beg if I thought that I alone could do it. I can't. I doubt if I make a difference, but you can. You Congressmen, your Doctors, News Media and friends can make a difference. I will do whatever I can do to move this forward, but I need your help! Ask me for anything that will help and I will do my best. I am asking everyone that reads this to do their best. One day you may be where I have been, or your mother, father, brother or sister as well as relatives and friends. This is so serious I can't imagine everyone not getting involved.

Feel free to contact me if I can be of help. dtrice@douglastrice.org

Sincerely,

Douglas T. Rice

Links for information: www.vescell.com

In: Encyclopedia of Stem Cell Research (2 Volume Set)   ISBN: 978-1-61761-835-2
Editor: Alexander L. Greene   © 2012 Nova Science Publishers, Inc.

Chapter LXIV

TESTIMONY BEFORE THE SUBCOMMITTEE ON HEALTH COMMITTEE ON ENERGY AND COMMERCE UNITED STATES HOUSE OF REPRESENTATIVES STEM CELL SCIENCE: THE FOUNDATION OF FUTURE CURES.

Elais A. Zerhouni[*]

Good morning, Mr. Chairman, Ranking Member Deal and Members of the Subcommittee. I am Elias Zerhouni, the Director of the National Institutes of Health (NIH), an agency of the U.S. Department of Health and Human Services (HHS), and I am pleased to appear before you today to testify about the science of stem cell research. I look forward to discussing ongoing federal support of both embryonic and non-embryonic stem cell research and scientific progress, including the recently published findings on induced pluripotent stem cells and other updates provided during the NIH Symposium on Cell-Based Therapies, which we hosted just two days ago.

Stem cell research has the potential to lead to therapies for injuries and illnesses that could not even have been imagined when I first began studying medicine. As this new field of discovery advances, nothing we have learned has dissuaded us from the belief that these cells, representing the building blocks of life itself, offer the possibility of becoming a renewable source of replacement cells and tissues to treat such common diseases and disorders as Parkinson's disease, spinal cord injury, stroke, burns, heart disease, diabetes, osteoarthritis, and rheumatoid arthritis.

A great deal of progress has already occurred. When I first became the Director of NIH, scientists were still struggling with learning how to grow embryonic stem cell lines. Since then, experiments have occurred in animals where embryonic stem cells actually replaced damaged cells and tissues. But we have a very long way to go.

---

[*] These remarks were delivered as testimony given on May 8, 2008. Elias A. Zerhouni, Director, National Institutes of Health, United States Department of Health and Human Services, before the Subcommittee on Health Committee on Energy and Commerce United States House of Representatives.

THE NEED FOR RESEARCH TO EXPLORE THE POTENTIAL OF HUMAN STEM CELLS

Stem cells can multiply without changing – that is, self-renew – or can differentiate to produce specialized cell types. This ability to renew and eventually replace damaged cells and tissues fuels the excitement of stem cell researchers across the world. But all stem cells do not come from the same source; they have different characteristics and are difficult to harness and grow. Stem cells have been derived from both embryonic and non-embryonic tissues, and these cell types have different properties. Both pluripotent and nonpluripotent types show potential for developing treatments for human diseases and injuries, and there are many ways in which they might be used in basic and clinical research. We are still early in the learning process. This is an exciting but new field of discovery, and additional research is needed to realize the potential of stem cells and their uses. Before we reach the promised land of stem cell therapies, scientists must learn to reliably manipulate the cells so that they possess the necessary characteristics for successful differentiation, transplantation, and engraftment.

To be useful for transplant purposes, differentiated stem cells must:

- Proliferate extensively and generate sufficient quantities of specialized cells;
- Differentiate into the desired cell type(s);
- Survive in the recipient after transplant;
- Integrate into the surrounding tissue after transplant;
- Function appropriately for extended periods of time; and
- Avoid harming the recipient.

As this field of research advances, stem cells will yield still unknown information about the complex events that occur during the initial stages of human development. At present, a primary goal of this research is to identify the molecular mechanisms that allow undifferentiated stem cells to differentiate into one of the several hundred different cell types that make up the human body. Scientists have learned that turning genes on and off is central to this process. But we do not yet fully understand the signals that turn specific genes on and off to influence the differentiation of the stem cell into a specialized cell with a specific function, such as a nerve cell. This knowledge will not only offer the opportunity to learn how to control stem cells from both embryonic and non-embryonic sources, but also provide better understanding of the causes of a number of serious diseases, including those that affect infants and children, which in turn could lead to new and more effective intervention strategies and treatments.

Human stem cells are also being used to speed the development of new drugs. Initially testing thousands of potential drugs on cells in cell culture is typically far more efficient and informative than testing drugs in live animals. *In vitro* systems are useful in predicting *in vivo* responses and provide the benefits of requiring fewer animals, requiring less test material, and enabling higher throughput. New medications can be tested for safety on the specific types of human cells that are affected in disease by deriving these cells from human stem cell lines. Other kinds of cell lines are similarly used in this way. Cancer cell lines, for example, are used to screen potential anti-tumor drugs. The availability of useful stem cell lines would allow drug testing in a wider range of cell types. Potentially, stem cell research will result in a more efficient, effective, safer and faster way of developing drug treatments for a vast array of illnesses, but not until we produce the fundamental discoveries that will pave the way for the widespread use of stem cells in this manner.

ADVANCES IN STEM CELL RESEARCH

Over the past year, scientists have made remarkable discoveries about the potential of stem cells. For example, NIH-funded scientists have developed a method to coax human embryonic stem cells (hESCs) into becoming cells that resemble lung epithelial cells. The scientists engineered a virus (modified to eliminate its disease-transmitting function) to infect cells with two genes simultaneously, one that drives them into becoming a specialized type of lung cell and another that enables them to resist being killed by a drug (neomycin). Only those cells that express the two genes survived when the scientists treated the culture dish with neomycin. In this way, they were able to generate a pure population of lung-like cells, with no contaminating cells. The surviving cells had the appearance and shape of lung-lining cells called alveolar type 2 cells, which help maximize air exchange, remove fluid from the lungs, serve as a pool of repair cells, and fight airborne diseases. (*Proceedings of the National Academy of Sciences of the USA* 104(11):4449–4454, laboratory of R.A. Wetsel. 2007 March.)

In another experiment, NIH-funded investigators developed a new technique to generate large numbers of pure cardiomyocytes (heart muscle cells) from hESCs. They also formulated a "prosurvival" cocktail (PSC) of factors designed to overcome several known causes of transplanted cell death. The scientists then induced heart attacks in rats and injected the rat hearts with either hESC-derived human cardiomyocytes plus PSC (treatment group) or one of several control preparations. Four weeks later, the scientists identified human cardiomyocytes being supported by rat blood vessels in the treated rat hearts. The treated rat hearts also demonstrated an improved ability to pump blood. The control animals presented no improvement in heart function. This work demonstrates that hESC-derived cardiomyocytes can survive and improve function in damaged rat hearts. Scientists now hope to learn how the human cells improved the rat hearts, and eventually to test this method to treat human heart disease. (*Nature Biotechnology* 25(9):1015–1024, laboratory of CE Murry. 2007 Sept.)

In a significant advance, Japanese scientists and a team of NIH-supported scientists reported that they each succeeded at reprogramming adult human skin cells to behave like hESCs. The Japanese team forced adult skin cells to express the proteins *Oct3/4*, *Sox2*, *Klf4*, and c-Myc, while the NIH-supported team forced adult skin cells to express *OCT4*, *SOX2*, *NANOG*, and *LIN28*. The genes were all chosen for their known importance in maintaining the so-called "stemness" properties of stem cells. In both reports, the adult skin cells are thus reprogrammed into human induced pluripotent stem (iPS) cells that demonstrate important characteristics of pluripotency. The techniques reported by these research teams will enable scientists to generate patient-specific and disease-specific human stem cell lines for laboratory study, and to test potential drugs on human cells in culture. However, these human iPS cells are not yet suitable for use in transplantation medicine. The current techniques use viruses that could generate tumors or other undesirable mutations in cells derived from iPS cells.

Scientists are now working to accomplish reprogramming in adult human cells without using potentially dangerous viruses. (*Cell* 131:861–72, laboratory of S. Yamanaka, 2007 Nov 30; *Science* 318:1917–1920, laboratory of J. Thomson, 2007 Dec 21

Researchers from Japan were the first to successfully generate germ cells (the cells that give rise to sperm or eggs) from mouse iPS cells, and their results were verified and extended by another independent laboratory (Rudolf Jaenisch) in the United States. Recent publications from the same Japanese scientists, a team of NIH-supported scientists from University of Wisconsin-Madison, and the Harvard Stem Cell Institute report that they have each succeeded at reprogramming adult human skin cells to become human iPS cells.

There is no doubt that this finding is a remarkable scientific achievement, providing non-embryonic sources of pluripotent cells. Human ESCs and iPS cells are excellent tools to study differentiation, reversal of differentiation, and re-differentiation. In addition, both types of pluripotent cells may be useful for studying the cell biologic changes that accompany human disease. However, from a purely scientific view, it is essential to pursue all types of stem cell research simultaneously, including hESC research, since we cannot predict which type of stem cell will lead to the best possible therapeutic application.

In addition, reprogramming adult human cells would not have been possible without years of prior research studying the properties of hESCs. Two fundamental factors critical to the development of human iPS cells are based upon the knowledge gained from studying hESCs: knowledge of "stemness" genes whose expression or repression is essential to maintain pluripotency; and hESC culture conditions. NIH is proud of the role it has played in supporting this work since 2001 and advancing non-embryonic sources of pluripotent cells.

Scientists must now focus on understanding the mechanism by which retroviral transduction and consequent expression of "stemness" genes induce pluripotency in somatic cells. The consequences of using retroviral vectors to induce pluripotentiality for normal cell functions are unclear, and because the retroviral vectors integrate into the genome of the somatic cell, it can cause the cell to function abnormally. Scientists are now looking for safer methods to reprogram adult cells to a pluripotent state that do not disrupt the genome.

NIH STEM CELL SYMPOSIUM ON CELL-BASED THERAPIES

Two days ago, on May 6, the NIH hosted a symposium entitled "Challenges and Promise of Cell-Based Therapies." Notable stem cell researcher Dr. Stuart Orkin opened the symposium by explaining how 25 years of active research using blood stem cells has led to their successful use in the treatment of blood cancers and other blood disorders. He described the critical characteristics of blood-forming stem cells that have enabled their use in therapies, and how this knowledge will help scientists understand ways to use these and other types of stem cells for treating human diseases. Prominent scientists then discussed how they are developing stem cells as therapies for diseases of the nervous system, heart, muscle and bone, and metabolic disorders. The scientists shared their research results, the technical hurdles they must overcome, and what they ultimately hope to achieve with stem cells. Dr. George Daley of the Harvard Stem Cell Institute gave the final presentation on patient-specific pluripotent stem cells, also known as induced pluripotent stem cells.

FEDERAL FUNDING OF STEM CELL RESEARCH

NIH has acted quickly and aggressively to provide support for this research in accordance with the President's 2001 stem cell policy. Since 2001, NIH has invested approximately $3.7 billion on all types of stem cell research. Within this total, NIH has funded: more than $174 million in research studying human embryonic stem cells; more than $1.3 billion on research using human non-embryonic stem cells; more than $628 million on nonhuman embryonic stem cells; and more than $1.5 billion on nonhuman non-embryonic stem cells.

Additionally, in FY 2009, it is projected that NIH will spend approximately $41 million on human embryonic stem cell research and about $203 million on human non-embryonic stem cell research, while also investing approximately $105 million on nonhuman embryonic stem cell research and nearly $306 million on nonhuman non-embryonic stem cell research.

In addition, NIH is conducting activities under the President's July 2007 directive in Executive Order 13435, which directs HHS and NIH to ensure that the human pluripotent stem cell lines on research that it conducts or supports are derived without creating a human embryo for research purposes or destroying, discarding, or subjecting to harm a human embryo or fetus. The order expands the NIH Embryonic Stem Cell registry to include all types of ethically produced human pluripotent stem cells, and renames the registry as the Human Pluripotent Stem Cell Registry. The order invites scientists to work with the NIH, so we can add new ethically derived stem cell lines to the list of those eligible for federal funding.

Further, NIH has encouraged stem cell research through the establishment of an NIH Stem Cell Task Force, a Stem Cell Information Web Site, an Embryonic Stem Cell Characterization Unit, training courses in the culturing of human embryonic stem cells, support for multidisciplinary teams of stem cell investigators, and a National Stem Cell Bank and Centers of Excellence in Translational Human Stem Cell Research, as well as through extensive investigator initiated research. NIH determined that obtaining access to hESC lines listed on the Human Pluripotent Stem Cell Registry and the lack of trained scientists with the ability to culture hESCs were obstacles to moving this field of research forward. To remove these potential barriers, the National Stem Cell Bank and the providers on the Human Pluripotent Stem Cell Registry together have currently made over 1400 shipments of the hESC cell lines that are eligible for federal funding, as posted on the Human Pluripotent Stem Cell Registry web site. In addition, the NIH-supported hESC training courses have taught several hundred scientists the techniques necessary to culture these cells. We plan to continue to aggressively fund this exciting area of science.

Thank you for the opportunity to present these exciting developments to you. I will be happy to try to answer any questions.

CHAPTER SOURCES

Expert Commentary A, B, Short Communication B, C, D, Chapters VI, XII, XIX - XXIV have been previously published in *Stem Cell Applications in Diseases*, edited by Mikkel L. Sorensen, published by Nova Science Publishers, Inc.

Expert Commentary C, D, Chapters XXVII, XXXVI – ILII have been previously published in *Hematopoietic Stem Cell Transplantation Research Advances*, edited by Karl B. Neumann, published by Nova Science Publishers, Inc.

Short Communication A, Chapters I – V, VII – XI, XIII – XVIII have been previously published in *Progress in Stem Cell Applications*, edited by Allen V. Faraday and Jonathon T. Dyer, published by Nova Science Publishers, Inc.

Chapters XXV, XXVI, XXVIII – XXXV have been previously published in *Stem Cell Transplantation, Tissue Engineering and Cancer Applications*, edited by Bernard N. Kennedy, published by Nova Science Publishers, Inc.

Chapters ILIII – LIII have been previously published in *Pluripotent Stem Cells*, edited by Derek W. Rosales and Quentin N. Mullen, published by Nova Science Publishers, Inc.

Chapters LIV – LXIV have been previously published in *Stem Cell Research and Science: Background and Issues*, edited by Brendan E. Aylesworth, published by Nova Science Publishers, Inc.

INDEX

C

D

E

F

G

H

I

J

K

L

M

N

O

Q

S

U

V